The American Psychiatric Publishing

Textbook of Geriatric Psychiatry

THIRD EDITION

The American Psychiatric Publishing

Textbook of
Geriatric Psychiatry

THIRD EDITION

Edited by

Dan G. Blazer, M.D., Ph.D.

David C. Steffens, M.D., M.H.S.

Ewald W. Busse, M.D.

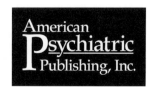

Washington, DC
London, England

Copyright © 2004 American Psychiatric Publishing, Inc.
ALL RIGHTS RESERVED

Manufactured in the United States of America on acid-free paper
08 07 06 05 04   5 4 3 2 1
Third Edition

Typeset in Adobe's Revival and Caecilia

American Psychiatric Publishing, Inc.
1000 Wilson Boulevard
Arlington, VA 22209-3901
www.appi.org

Library of Congress Cataloging-in-Publication Data
The American Psychiatric Publishing textbook of geriatric psychiatry / edited by Dan G.
 Blazer, David C. Steffens, Ewald W. Busse.—3rd ed.
     p. cm.
   Previous ed. has title: American Psychiatric Press textbook of geriatric psychiatry.
   Includes bibliographical references and index.
   ISBN 1-58562-065-3 (alk. paper)
   1. Geriatric psychiatry. I. Title: Textbook of geriatric psychiatry. II. Blazer, Dan G.
 (Dan German), 1944– III. Steffens, David C., 1962– IV. Busse, Ewald W., 1917– V.
 American Psychiatric Press textbook of geriatric psychiatry

 RC451.4.A5A518 2004
 618.97′689–dc22
                                                                                      2003060887

British Library Cataloguing in Publication Data
A CIP record is available from the British Library.

Contents

PART I

The Basic Science of Geriatric Psychiatry

PART II

The Diagnostic Interview in Late Life

PART III

Psychiatric Disorders in Late Life

PART IV

Treatment of Psychiatric Disorders in Late Life

PART V

Special Topics

Contributors

Marc E. Agronin, M.D.
Director of Mental Health Services, Miami Jewish Home
& Hospital for the Aged; Assistant Professor of Psychiatry,
University of Miami School of Medicine, Miami, Florida

Ann K. Aspnes
Clinical psychology graduate student, Department of
Psychology, Duke University, Durham, North Carolina

Deborah K. Attix, Ph.D.
Assistant Clinical Professor of Medical Psychology,
Department of Psychiatry and Behavioral Sciences and
Department of Medicine (Division of Neurology), Duke
University Medical Center, Durham, North Carolina

John L. Beyer, M.D.
Assistant Clinical Professor of Psychiatry, Duke University
Medical Center, Durham, North Carolina

Garth Bissette, Ph.D.
Professor, Department of Psychiatry and Human Behavior,
The University of Mississippi Medical Center,
Jackson, Mississippi

Dan G. Blazer, M.D., Ph.D.
J.P. Gibbons Professor of Psychiatry, Department of
Psychiatry and Behavioral Sciences, Duke University
Medical Center, Durham, North Carolina

Elise J. Bolda, M.S.P.H., Ph.D.
Consultant, Long Term Care Resources Program, Duke
University Medical Center, Durham, North Carolina;
National Program Director, Community Partnerships for
Older Adults, a Robert Wood Johnson Program and
Associate Professor, Edmund S. Muskie School of Public
Service, University of Southern Maine, Portland, Maine

Lauren T. Bonner, M.D.
Private practice of psychiatry, Glendale, Arizona

Ewald W. Busse, M.D.
J.P. Gibbons Professor of Psychiatry Emeritus, Associate
Provost and Dean of Medical Education Emeritus, Duke
University Medical Center, Durham, North Carolina

Christopher E. Byrum, M.D., Ph.D.
Staff Psychiatrist, Psychiatric Associates of the Carolinas,
Gastonia, North Carolina

Harvey Jay Cohen, M.D.
Professor, Department of Medicine; Director, Center for
the Study of Aging and Human Development; Chief, Division of Geriatrics, Duke University Medical Center, and
Director, Geriatric Research, Education and Clinical Center, Veterans Administration Medical Center, Durham,
North Carolina

Peggye Dilworth-Anderson, Ph.D.
Professor, Health Policy and Administration, School of
Public Health, The University of North Carolina at Chapel
Hill and UNC Institute on Aging, Chapel Hill,
North Carolina

Christian R. Dolder, Pharm.D., B.C.P.S.
Assistant Clinical Professor, Wingate School of Pharmacy,
Wingate, North Carolina

P. Murali Doraiswamy, M.D.
Associate Professor, Department of Psychiatry and Behavioral Sciences, Duke University, Durham, North Carolina

Jack D. Edinger, Ph.D.
Senior Psychologist, Veterans Affairs Medical Center;
Clinical Professor, Department of Psychiatry and Behavioral Sciences, Duke University Medical Center, Durham,
North Carolina

Richard B. Ferrell, M.D.
Associate Professor of Psychiatry, Department of Psychiatry, Dartmouth Medical School, Lebanon, New Hampshire

Dolores Gallagher-Thompson, Ph.D., A.B.P.P.
Professor of Research, Department of Psychiatry and
Behavioral Sciences, Stanford University School of
Medicine, Palo Alto, California; Director, Older Adult and
Family Center, Veterans Affairs Palo Alto Health Care
System, Menlo Park, California

Linda K. George, Ph.D.
Professor, Division of Social and Community Psychiatry,
Department of Psychiatry and Behavioral Sciences and
Professor, Department of Sociology, Duke University
Medical Center, Durham, North Carolina

Lisa P. Gwyther, M.S.W.
Associate Clinical Professor, Department of Psychiatry and
Behavioral Sciences, Duke University Medical Center,
Durham, North Carolina

Judith C. Hays, R.N., Ph.D.
Associate Research Professor, Department of Psychiatry and Behavioral Sciences, Center for the Study of Aging and Human Development, Duke University Medical Center, Durham, North Carolina

Christine M. Hulette, M.D.
Associate Professor, Department of Pathology, Duke University Medical Center, Durham, North Carolina

Celia F. Hybels, Ph.D.
Assistant Research Professor, Department of Psychiatry and Behavioral Sciences, Center for the Study of Aging and Human Development, Duke University Medical Center, Durham, North Carolina

Dilip V. Jeste, M.D.
Estelle and Edgar Levi Chair in Aging, Professor of Psychiatry and Neurosciences, University of California, San Diego; Chief, Division of Geriatric Psychiatry, VA San Diego Healthcare System, San Diego, California

Robert M. Kaiser, M.D.
Associate Professor of Clinical Internal Medicine, Division of Geriatrics, University of South Carolina School of Medicine; Attending Physician, Geriatrics and Extended Care and Medical Director, Home-Based Primary Care Program, Dorn Veterans Affairs Medical Center, Columbia, South Carolina

Ira R. Katz, M.D., Ph.D.
Professor of Psychiatry, Department of Psychiatry, University of Pennsylvania, Philadelphia Veterans Administration Medical Center, Philadelphia, Pennsylvania

Joel L. Kaye, Ph.D.
Consulting Psychologist, New York, New York

Harold G. Koenig, M.D., M.H.Sc.
Associate Professor of Psychiatry and Associate Professor of Medicine, Duke University Medical Center, Durham, North Carolina

Andrew D. Krystal, M.D., M.S.
Director, Sleep Research Laboratory; Associate Professor, Department of Psychiatry and Behavioral Sciences, Duke University Medical Center, Durham, North Carolina

J. Pierre Loebel, M.D.
Clinical Professor of Psychiatry and Behavioral Sciences, University of Washington, Seattle, Washington

Thomas R. Lynch, Ph.D.
Assistant Professor, Department of Psychiatry and Psychology, Duke University, Durham, North Carolina

David J. Madden, Ph.D.
Professor of Medical Psychology, Department of Psychiatry and Behavioral Sciences, Duke University Medical Center, Durham, North Carolina

George L. Maddox, Ph.D.
Professor Emeritus, Department of Sociology, and Program Director, Long Term Care Resources Program, Duke University Medical Center, Durham, North Carolina

Scott D. Moore, M.D., Ph.D.
Associate Professor, Department of Psychiatry and Behavioral Medicine, Duke University Medical Center, Durham, North Carolina

Benoit H. Mulsant, M.D.
Associate Professor of Psychiatry and Associate Director, Geriatric Psychiatry Fellowship, University of Pittsburgh School of Medicine, Western Psychiatric Institute and Clinic, Pittsburgh, Pennsylvania

Thomas E. Oxman, M.D.
Professor of Psychiatry and Director of Geriatric Psychiatry, Department of Psychiatry, Dartmouth Medical School, Lebanon, New Hampshire

Elaine R. Peskind, M.D.
Assistant Professor of Psychiatry and Behavioral Sciences, University of Washington School of Medicine, Seattle, Washington

Brenda L. Plassman, Ph.D.
Associate Research Professor, Department of Psychiatry and Behavioral Sciences, Duke University Medical Center, Durham, North Carolina

Bruce G. Pollock, M.D., Ph.D.
Professor of Psychiatry, Pharmacology, and Pharmaceutical Sciences and Chief, Academic Division of Geriatrics and Neuropsychiatry, University of Pittsburgh School of Medicine, Western Psychiatric Institute and Clinic, Pittsburgh, Pennsylvania

Leonard W. Poon, Ph.D.
Professor of Psychology; Chair, Faculty of Gerontology; Director, Gerontology Center, University of Georgia, Athens, Georgia

Murray A. Raskind, M.D.
Professor of Psychiatry and Behavioral Sciences, University of Washington School of Medicine, Seattle, Washington

William E. Reichman, M.D.
Professor of Psychiatry and Senior Associate Dean for Clinical Affairs, University of Medicine and Dentistry of New Jersey–Robert Wood Johnson Medical School, New Brunswick, New Jersey

Contributors

Burton Scott, Ph.D., M.D.
Assistant Clinical Professor, Division of Neurology, Department of Medicine, Duke Movement Disorders Clinic, Duke University Medical Center, Durham, North Carolina

Joseph M. Sharpe, M.D.
Private practice of psychiatry, Nashville, Tennessee

Ilene C. Siegler, Ph.D., M.P.H.
Professor of Medical Psychology, Department of Psychiatry and Behavioral Sciences, Duke University Medical Center, Durham, North Carolina; Professor of Psychology, Social and Health Sciences, Duke University; Adjunct Professor of Epidemiology, University of North Carolina School of Public Health, Chapel Hill, North Carolina

David C. Steffens, M.D., M.H.S.
Associate Professor, Department of Psychiatry and Behavioral Sciences, Duke University Medical Center, Durham, North Carolina

Joel E. Streim, M.D.
Associate Professor of Psychiatry, Department of Psychiatry, University of Pennsylvania, Philadelphia Veterans Administration Medical Center, Philadelphia, Pennsylvania

Robert J. Sullivan Jr., M.D., M.P.H.
Associate Professor, Department of Community and Family Medicine and Department of Medicine, Duke University Medical Center, Durham, North Carolina

Paulette C.Y. Tang, Ph.D.
Postdoctoral Fellow, Department of Psychiatry and Behavioral Sciences, Stanford University School of Medicine, Stanford, California

Warren D. Taylor, M.D.
Assistant Professor, Department of Psychiatry and Behavioral Sciences, Duke University, Durham, North Carolina

Larry W. Thompson, Ph.D.
Co-Director, Older Adult Center, Department of Veterans Affairs Medical Center; Professor of Medicine (Research), Division of Endocrinology, Gerontology, and Metabolism, Stanford University School of Medicine, Palo Alto, California

Richard D. Weiner, M.D., Ph.D.
Professor, Department of Psychiatry and Behavioral Sciences, Duke University Medical School; Chief, Mental Health Service Line, Department of Veterans Affairs Medical Center, Durham, North Carolina

Kathleen A. Welsh-Bohmer, Ph.D.
Professor of Medical Psychology, Department of Psychiatry and Behavioral Sciences; Associate Director, Joseph and Kathleen Bryan Alzheimer's Disease Research Center—Division of Neurology, Department of Medicine, Duke University Medical Center, Durham, North Carolina

Julie Loebach Wetherell, Ph.D.
Assistant Professor of Psychiatry, University of California, San Diego; Staff Psychologist, VA San Diego Healthcare System, San Diego, California

William K. Wohlgemuth, Ph.D.
Assistant Clinical Professor, Department of Psychiatry and Behavioral Sciences, Duke University Medical Center, Durham, North Carolina

Preface

The first edition of this textbook, titled *Geriatric Psychiatry*, was published in 1989. In 1996, the second edition was published with the title *The American Psychiatric Press Textbook of Geriatric Psychiatry*. The decision to publish a third edition rested on an appreciation of the enormous expansion of scientific knowledge about aging and the diseases of late life, as well as on advances in biological psychiatry and neuropsychiatry that have greatly altered the practice of geriatric psychiatry. *The American Psychiatric Publishing Textbook of Geriatric Psychiatry*, Third Edition, is designed to provide both the scholar and the clinician with the current state of scientific understanding as well as the practical skills and knowledge base required for dealing with mental disorders in late life. Consequently, this volume covers not only the wide range of important mental diseases of late life but also the so-called normal age changes that result in biological, social, and behavioral changes in older adults.

As in previous editions, the chapters are presented in a sequential and integrated fashion, which we have found enhances the accessibility and usefulness of the information presented. The contributors include both basic and clinical scholars who have a clear ability to make complex material understandable to our readers. We maintained an eclectic orientation regarding theory and practice in geriatric psychiatry. Although most contributors are psychiatrists, we also called on colleagues from relevant biomedical and behavioral disciplines, especially for chapters covering the basic sciences, because of their expertise and ability to incorporate such knowledge into a comprehensive approach to patient care.

We targeted this text to psychiatrists and other health professionals who have an interest in and a commitment to older adults. This book is of particular value to candidates seeking certification in geriatrics from the American Board of Psychiatry and Neurology, the American Board of Internal Medicine, and the American Board of Family Practice. All of these examinations place considerable emphasis on geriatric psychiatry and the behavioral aspects of aging.

We wish to express our deepest appreciation for the assistance of our staff assistant, Jill Gabel, for her long hours typing, editing, and organizing the manuscripts.

The Basic Science of Geriatric Psychiatry

The Myth, History, and Science of Aging

Ewald W. Busse, M.D.

Dan G. Blazer, M.D., Ph.D.

For thousands of years, scholars, physicians, theologians, philosophers, and others have written on the subjects of life, aging, and death. Some of their observations and conclusions are casual, a few are frivolous, and some are based on careful study and considered judgment. Some of the older writings are interesting because they provide information about social values, the influence of political and economic factors, the level of scientific knowledge, and, in particular, the interpretation of the significance and application of existing knowledge.

The Prolongation of Youth and Life: A Retrospective

Attempts to prolong youth or to restore sexual vigor and physical vitality have been made for many centuries and still occur today. Many such attempts at rejuvenation carry a distinct risk. Greek mythology actually teaches that the risk is greater than the gain. The goddess Aurora (also called Eos) with great effort persuaded Zeus to grant her husband Tithonus immortality. Regrettably, she neglected to mention that she also wanted him to remain eternally young. As the years passed, Tithonus became more and more disabled, praying frequently for death. Eternal life did not equate with eternal youth.

The belief that in remote parts of the world there are people who enjoy remarkably long lives appears in the mythology of many cultures. The Greek legend of the Hyperboreans held that there was a group of people who lived beyond the north wind in a region of perpetual sunshine. These fortunate people were free from all natural

ills. Writing in the first century, Pliny (23–79 A.D.) noted that the Hyperboreans were extremely happy and "aloof from toil and conflict" and that they lived to an extreme old age until, "sated with life and luxury, they leaped into the sea" (Gruman 1966, p. 22). This idea of people living in remote parts of the world who enjoy a long life persists in the mythology of the centenarians that occurs periodically in news media and scientific literature (see section "The Centenarians" later in this chapter).

The Fountain of Youth

In America, the myth of the fountain of youth is well known because it was instrumental in Ponce de Leon's discovery of what is now the state of Florida. The fountain of youth legend is traced by scholars to several possible origins. In ancient Greek and Roman writings, there are two interesting references to fountains with properties that conferred a prolonged life span. Hera, the wife of Zeus, bathed each year in a spring that renewed her maidenhood. In another classical reference, Herodotus (c 484–425 B.C.) recounted a search for a spring and pool whose constant use made people live longer.

Roger Bacon promoted his belief that the life span of his day, which usually was not more than 45–50 years, could be tripled. His reasoning was in part based on the long life spans of Methuselah and Noah: if life spans had once been that long and then had shortened, some reversal must be possible. Bacon became a Franciscan monk in order to pursue a moral and physically clean life. He did recommend the rejuvenating breath of a young virgin, but as a monk he cautioned against any accompanying licentiousness. Bacon reasoned that if disease were contagious, why not vitality (Gruman 1966).

The Myth of Cell Immortality

Alexis Carrel (1873–1944) was born and educated in France. Carrel was a skillful and creative surgeon who encountered frustrations in his career. He left for America in May 1904. At the University of Chicago and later at the Rockefeller Institute, he devoted his work to vascular and cardiac surgery and wound healing. This interest in wound healing led him to an interest in growing tissues outside the body. For his surgical contributions, he won the 1912 Nobel prize for physiology and medicine. He rapidly developed his studies in tissue culture, and on the basis of some of his own apparent successes, he became convinced that some human cells grown in culture were immortal. This claim of possible cell immortality was reported by Carrel and Ebeling beginning in 1912. Despite numerous objections to his work, Carrel was very persuasive, and his belief was widely accepted. In January 1912, Carrel established a series of chick heart fibroblast cultures, one of which was destined to become the "immortal" cell strain.

Subsequently, it was shown that Carrel and Ebeling had made an error in their methodology that resulted in improper conclusions. The Carrel-Ebeling cell culture was fed an extract taken from chick embryos. This extract actually contained a very few but significant number of new viable cells; hence, the introduction of new cells permitted the culture to survive. It was found that if the extract was carefully prepared, removing all new cells, the cell colony would die. Although other experiments have suggested that animal and human cells have the capacity to be immortal, all such immortal cell colonies are abnormal in one way or another. At present, it appears that the only human cells that may be immortal are transformed or abnormal mixoploid cells such as the HeLa cells, which were originally taken from cancerous cervical tissue and grown in culture by George O. Gey in 1950 (Gey 1955).

Before 1961, the accepted dogma was that cell and tissue cultures were potentially immortal. The death of a cell line was usually attributed to failure to use proper laboratory methods. Hayflick and Moorhead (1961) first described the finite replicative capacity of cultured normal human fibroblasts and interpreted the phenomenon to be aging at the cellular level. They reported that even when normal human embryonic cells were grown under the most favorable conditions, death was inevitable after about 50 population doublings. Thus, the death of the cell line was an inherent property of the cells themselves.

In 1965, Hayflick reported that culture fibroblasts derived from older human donors divided fewer times than did those derived from embryos. Since then, several investigators have replicated the work of Hayflick, finding that the number of population doublings of cultured human cells is inversely proportional to donor age. It was subsequently shown that freezing viable normal human cells at subzero temperatures does not alter the memory in the cells for the number of doublings that had previously occurred. These cells had been held for more than 24 years in a frozen state and, when thawed, replicated only the amount of times they would have had they never been frozen.

Zhores Medvedev, a Russian scientist, made many contributions to the study of biological aging, including the redundant theory of aging (i.e., the amount of deoxyribonucleic acid [DNA] reserve within the genome that can be called on to maintain vital function plays an important role in determining life span) (Busse 1983). Medvedev recounts how, between 1937 and 1964, Lysenko used a false doctrine and fabricated scientific data to achieve fame and power. Of particular interest to the geriatric psychiatrist is Medvedev's account of a technique of rejuvenation advocated by a disciple of Lysenko's, a woman named O.B. Lepeshinskaya. Around 1949, Lepeshinskaya began to advocate the use of soda baths to prolong life and restore vigor, a practice warmly supported by Lysenko. This approach quickly moved to the drinking of soda water and finally to the introduction of soda into the body by enema. Apparently the latter two techniques were used as alternatives for those who were unable to take frequent soda baths. Lepeshinskaya also claimed that she could make living matter from nonliving material. This account is a vivid example of how vulnerable geriatrics is to the practice of pseudoscience.

The Centenarians

Reports of life spans exceeding 100 years have involved three wide-ranging pockets of people. One group, the Viejos, live in Vilcabamba, a small mountain village in Ecuador. The other two pockets are in widely separated regions of Asia—the Hunzukuts of the Karakoram region in Kashmir and the Abkhazians of the Republic of Georgia in the former Soviet Union. Over the past decade, a number of individuals have visited the two groups in Ecuador and Georgia. In February 1978, the National Institute on Aging brought together several scientists who had visited Vilcabamba. After three visits to Vilcabamba, they concluded that the oldest person in the community was 96 years old. Similar visits to the Soviet Caucasus and reevaluations found that the reports of longevity had been grossly exaggerated (Palmore 1984).

In recent years, however, centenarians are becoming more prevalent, not because the life span is extended but rather because more persons are pushing the limits of the life span. In addition, centenarians are found to be more heterogeneous. In 1990, approximately 28,000 centenarians lived in the United States (Velkoff 2000). They were more likely to be women, to have lower educational levels than younger cohorts, and to be widowed; one-half were living in nursing homes. Diversity from a racial and ethnic perspective will increase among them, and biological diversity is apparent now as well (Hazzard 2001). For example, the ε2 allele of apolipoprotein E (APOE) (either homozygous or heterozygous) is found more frequently but not exclusively in centenarians compared with younger persons. The ε2 allele appears to be associated with lower cholesterol levels in persons at these advanced ages.

Attitudes Toward Aging

Marcus Tullius Cicero, the Roman orator and statesman of the first century (106–43 B.C.), incorporated into his elegant speeches and writings the philosophical views and social values of his time (Gruman 1966). Cicero, at age 62, produced an essay on senescence ("de Senectute"; 44 B.C.) in which he suggested that old age was not welcomed equally by different human races. The status the elderly held within a society apparently made a difference. The Spartans capitalized on the experience of older men, and the gerotes, a council of 28 men past 60 years old, controlled the city-state (Thewlis 1924). Cicero argued that successful aging was obtainable if one developed an appropriate attitude and dealt effectively with the four major complaints associated with aging. It is interesting that these same four complaints exist today.

The first complaint was that society excluded the aged from important work of the world. Cicero replied by saying that courageous elders can find a way to make themselves useful in various advisory, intellectual, and administrative functions. The second charge was that aging undermines physical strength and reduces the individual's value. Cicero answered that bodily decline counts for little compared with the cultivation of mind and character. The third complaint was that aging prevents or reduces the enjoyment of sensual pleasures, particularly sexual enjoyment. Cicero replied that such a loss has some merit because it allows the aged to concentrate on the promotion of reason and virtue.

The fourth, and final, charge was that old age brings with it increasing anxiety about death. In response to this charge, Cicero followed Plato by saying that death could be considered a blessing, freeing individuals and their immortal souls from their bodily prison on this very imperfect earth. Cicero concluded by saying that the wise individual is one who submits to the dictates of nature and passes through the vicissitudes of life with a tranquil mind. He implied that the prolongation of life seemed undesirable, particularly if, in old age, one had to go back to being "a crying child in the cradle."

Gerontocomia, perhaps the first practical manual on the problems of old age, was published in Latin by Gabriele Zerbi in 1482. Zeman (1967) reported finding this fascinating volume and said that Zerbi's work had not previously been quoted by any medical or lay writer since its original publication. Zerbi dealt with the care of the aged in a rest home, especially selected with regard to climate, exposure, equipment, and staff. He described all of his ideas regarding longevity and maintaining health, advocating exercise, bathing, massage, rest, and diet. He referred to medications that are useful to old people and discussed their ingredients and dosages. One of Zerbi's most fascinating recommendations was the continuing use of human milk for the aged. Recognizing that death and old age are inevitable, Zerbi stated, "It is impossible therefore to prevent the wasting away of old age, but it is possible to combat and resist it considerably" (Lind 1988, p. 26).

Sir William Osler, a superb observer, an excellent teacher, and a scholar, was knowledgeable about medicine, literature, and the humanities (Belkin and Neelon 1992). At age 56, he delivered the farewell address to the Johns Hopkins faculty (Berk 1989). In that address, he expressed the belief that with advancing age, professors often lose their usefulness. Osler held the position that productivity in life occurs before age 40. This farewell speech resulted in negative reaction both by his colleagues and by the public press. An effort was made to explain it away by characterizing it as an attempt in humor. However, in answer to this storm, Osler said the following:

> The criticisms have not shaken my convictions that the telling work of the world has been done and is done by men under forty years of age. The exceptions which have been given only illustrate the rule. It would also be to the general good if men at sixty were retired from active work. We should miss the energies of some young-old men, but on the whole be of greater service to the sexagenarii themselves. (Belkin and Neelon 1992, p. 863)

Osler died in 1919 at age 70. In contrast to his observations, until approximately a year before his death, he is said to have remained an active teacher, researcher, and statesman.

Many writers seem to have difficulty finding the advantages of aging. Somerset Maugham was being honored by the Garrick Club as part of his eightieth birthday celebration. He spoke the customary salutations, paused for a moment and said, "There are many…virtues in…growing old." He paused, he swallowed, he wet his lips, he looked about. The pause stretched out; he looked dumbstruck. The pause became too long—far too long. He looked down, studying the tabletop. A terrible tremor of nervousness went through the room. Was he ill? Would he ever be able to get on with it? Finally he looked up and said, "I'm just…trying…to think what they are!" (Kanin 1966).

Palmore (1979), in contrast, documented what he believed to be some major advantages of aging. These include the fact that the aged are the most law abiding of all age groups, except for young children. The aged are much better citizens and are interested and active in public issues and political affairs. They make an enormous contribution to society by maintaining voluntary participation in community organizations, churches, and recreational groups. Although many are not gainfully employed, they are quite capable of participating in performance tasks. Older workers are stable and dependable and have less absenteeism. Although older persons are equally exposed to crimes of certain types, they are much less likely to be the victims of crime in general than are people in other age groups.

Although some of the apparent advantages of aged individuals are under constant pressure, it is obvious that Social Security and other pension systems have improved their economic status, as have lower taxes and other economic benefits such as reduced rates in many hotels, motels, and recreational facilities. Medicare, in spite of its limitations, provides health insurance for many older people who would otherwise not be covered. Undoubtedly there are other advantages. The disadvantages, as is true in all medical publications, appear repeatedly throughout this book.

A Definition of Aging

Aging, in living organisms, usually refers to a series of time-dependent anatomical and physiological changes that reduce physiological reserve and functional capacity, although occasionally the term refers to the positive processes of maturation or acquiring a desirable quality (Ahmed and Tollefsbol 2001). Biological aging is not necessarily confined to the latter years of life; some declines begin with conception. In general, the term does designate those physical changes that develop in adulthood,

result in a decline in efficiency of function, reduce homeostasis, and terminate in death.

The multiple processes of decline that are associated with growing old can be separated into primary and secondary aging (Busse 1987). *Primary aging* is held to be intrinsic to the organism, and the decremental factors are determined by inherent or hereditary influences. The rate of aging as a functional decline varies widely between individuals. Furthermore, there are extreme aging variations in systems, organs, and cells. *Secondary aging* refers to the appearance of defects and disabilities that are caused by hostile factors in the environment, including trauma and acquired disease.

This operational separation of primary and secondary aging processes has limitations because both inherent (hereditary) and acquired decremental age changes are often of multiple etiologies. Inherent defects that make the organism vulnerable may not appear unless and until the organism is exposed to hostile precipitating events. Definitions of aging that have been offered, including those for primary and secondary aging, are not consistently accepted and applied. The aging of living organisms is a universal phenomenon, but the rate of aging can vary between individuals and groups. In humans, aging differences are in part genetically determined but also are substantially influenced by nutrition, lifestyle, and environment (Busse 1987). Some scientists define primary aging as first cause and secondary aging as the pathological processes that ensue from the first cause.

Many age changes are relatively benign and allow a person to continue to function, meet personal needs, and maintain a place in society. Age changes are recognized as a decline in efficiency or performance but in the extreme are often labeled a disease. Examples of age changes that can become sufficiently severe to be a disease include a decline in kidney function (creatinine clearance), reduced respiratory performance (forced expiratory volume), an increase in systolic blood pressure (isolated systolic hypertension), and an impaired response to oral glucose tolerance tests (type 2 diabetes mellitus) (Tobin 1984).

The chronological age of a person is often estimated by changes in appearance and the person's ability to perform tasks associated with activities of daily living and working. As humans age, the skin often becomes wrinkled, dry, and seborrheic, and actinic keratosis appears. Hair becomes gray and thinner; baldness increases. Teeth decay and are lost. In addition, height tends to decrease, as does weight. Chest depth and abdominal depth both increase. The ears lengthen and the nose broadens. Fat cells invade muscle, and muscle strength decreases. Posture and height are affected by musculoskeletal changes. Bone densities, influenced by gender and race, decrease with age; in women especially, the trabecular bones of the hip, wrist, and vertebrae are particularly affected.

The metabolic dimensions that are affected by age include drug absorption, distribution, destruction, excretion; the kinetics of drug binding; and alterations in biological rhythms. Drugs are therefore metabolized in elderly people differently from the way they are metabolized in younger adults.

Another important age change is the loss of irreplaceable cells, most noticeably in the skeletal muscle tissue, heart, and brain (although recent studies suggest that cells that were originally thought not to have the capability to reproduce, such as neurons, may under certain circumstances reproduce). Striated musculature diminishes by about one-half by approximately age 80 years. As these muscle cells disappear, they are replaced by fat cells and fibrous connective tissue. Hence, the body achieves increased storage capacities for certain drugs that are stored in fat cells. The loss of brain cells alters important aspects of body metabolism and affects circadian rhythms. The decrease in heart cells results in alterations in certain cardiac functions. Cellular and supportive tissue changes cause pulmonary changes.

In the brain, neurons shrink and are lost, and alterations occur in neuronal synapses and networks. The loss of nerve cells, particularly those in vulnerable areas of the hypothalamus, may contribute to placing the elderly at risk for certain physiological changes and associated mental and emotional aberrations. Aging results in a decline of neurotransmitters such as dopamine, norepinephrine, serotonin, tyrosine hydroxylase, and cholinesterase. The activity of monoamine oxidase increases with age.

Biological Theories of Aging

There are many theories and processes of aging. A satisfactory, unified theory of aging does not exist. In part, this is due to variability in the "aging" of various organs and tissues. Similar age changes have been identified in one or two of the body components, but rarely are the same changes seen in all simultaneously. Some theories of aging lack adequate scientific proof. For example, at present, there is substantial—although not conclusively definitive—evidence that intrinsic cellular or molecular aging changes underlie many of the neuronal or endocrine changes associated with the brain.

In 1993, the National Institute on Aging published a booklet, "In Search of the Secrets of Aging" (National Institute on Aging 1993a, 1993b). It divides the major theories of aging into two categories: program theories and error theories. Program theories hold that aging is the result of sequential switching on and off of certain genes. Defects develop during this switching on and off, and these defects are manifested by senescence. Those who subscribe to error theories maintain that aging is the result of wear and tear processes; these theorists hold that in many mechanisms, important parts wear out and cannot be replaced or repaired. Included among the error theories is the "somatic mutation theory," whose proponents maintain that, with increasing age, genetic mutations occur and accumulate, causing cells to deteriorate and malfunction.

In a review of biological theories of aging, Hart and Turturro (1985) categorized theories into cellular, organ, and population based; integrative approaches; and meta-aging. The cellular-based theories are those that emphasize the importance of the inherent limited potential proliferation of cells. These theories are consistent with the fact that animals have decreased cellularity in several organs as aging advances. Consequently, aging stem cells have a progressively limited ability to repopulate differentiated daughter cells. The capacity for limited proliferation is linked to some experiments that have shown that the limited proliferation of cells is the result of stochastic changes.

Other experiments have been concerned with the somatic-mutation theory of aging and the closely associated "error theory." Finally, cellular aging may be attributed to accumulated effects of damage from the expression of "cell death genes" important to development. This is linked with the observation that during embryogenesis the number of cells retained for further development is reduced by some genetic mechanism. Because cell numbers are reduced in late life, it would be important to understand the underlying mechanism that is needed by the organism early in life but that may be detrimental late in life. In a similar manner, the Hart and Turturro review identifies those theories of aging that are related to mechanisms of cell death. The final category of aging theories mentioned by Hart and Turturro is meta-aging. This encompasses what the authors refer to as "the theory of the theory of aging." The complexity of such a discussion is obvious, and the development of a unified theory of aging will be extremely difficult because such a theory of biosenescence would have to take into consideration all of the processes an individual undergoes as well as the sequence of environmental interactions that occur within the individual over a lifetime.

The Watch-Spring Theory

One early biological explanation of aging rested on the assumption that a living organism contained a fixed store of energy not unlike that contained within a coiled watch spring. When the spring of the watch was unwound, life ended. This is a type of exhaustion theory. Another simple theory relates to the accumulation of deleterious material. This particular theory is given some support by the observation that pigments such as lipofuscin accumulate in some cells throughout life. Although these two simple theories may make some contribution to the aging process, there is little evidence that they have any substantial role.

The "Master Clock"

The hypothalamus is said to be the location of the "master clock." Age changes within the hypothalamus play a particularly important role in losses of homeostatic mechanisms in the body. Cell loss, an event that is common in late life, occurs within clusters of cells in the hypothalamus. The disappearance of a few critical cells in the hypothalamus may have far-reaching consequences. The remaining aging cells may become less efficient. These changes in the hypothalamus undoubtedly cause important changes within the pituitary that affect other glands and organs within the body. As a consequence, the aging body undergoes many endocrine changes. Alterations within the hypothalamus also affect numerous connections within the brain and play a major role in age changes associated with chemical messengers of the brain. Nevertheless, there is debate as to where this timing mechanism might lie or how it might control aging from molecule to organ (Miller 1999).

Stochastic Theories

Processes of aging that are associated with random changes such as cell loss or mutation are often termed *stochastic* processes. Stochastic implies "a process or a series of events for which the estimate of the probability of certain outcomes approaches the true possibility as the number of events increases" (Busse 1977, p. 16). The atomic scientist Leo Szilard advanced a stochastic theory based on what he termed "a hit." A hit was not solely the result of radiation, but rather could be considered any event that would alter a chromosome. In addition, Szilard believed that every animal carries a load of what he termed "faults." A fault is a congenital absence or impairment of one of the genes essential to cell function. A cell is capable of operating as long as one of the pair of genes

continues to function; however, when both members of a pair of essential genes are incapable of functioning, the cell declines and dies. Therefore, a cell will cease to function effectively if one of the pair carries the fault and the other is the victim of a hit or if both of the pair are the victims of hits.

Deliberate Biological Programming

The theory of deliberate biological programming has received considerable attention. This theory holds that within a normal cell are stored the memory and the capability of determining the life of a cell. This theory is consistent with the research and conclusions of Hayflick (1965). The memory and capacity to terminate life are found in all normal human diploid cells. In mixoploid or cancer cells, this memory or capacity apparently is destroyed, and the cells can duplicate indefinitely.

Cristafalo (1972) reported that the number of doublings is the same for both male and female cells. (Female cells are easily identified by the presence of a Barr body, the second sex chromosome.) This observation suggests that the difference in life expectancy between human males and females cannot be attributed to intracellular differences (Weiss 1974).

The Telomere Theory

A variant of the deliberate biological programming theory and also of the genetic theories is the telomere theory. DNA damage is the centerpiece of many theories of aging. Recently, telomere shortening has been described to be associated with DNA damage (Ahmed and Tollefsbol 2001). Located at the ends of eukaryotic chromosomes, telomeres are specialized DNA sequences that maintain the length of chromosomes. When they are lost, DNA damage results. Telomere shortening and cellular senescence have been well established in the laboratory. In addition, many human cancer cells (which replicate without control) show high telomerase activity (telomerase is the enzyme that stimulates telomere activity). In other words, telomerase activity is essential for cellular immortalization, and its absence may constitute a fundamental basis for cellular aging.

The Free Radical Theory

A free radical is a chemical molecule or compound that has an odd number of electrons (an unpaired electron) and is highly reactive, in contrast to most chemical compounds, which have an even number of electrons and are stable. Often considered molecular fragments, free radicals are highly reactive and destructive, but they are produced by normal metabolic processes and are ubiquitous in living substances. They can also be produced by ionizing radiation, ozone, and chemical toxins such as insecticides. The oxygen free radical, superoxide, is an important agent of oxygen toxicity and the aging process. Scavengers of oxygen free radicals exist within cells. Enzymatic defenses involve superoxide dismutase, catalases, and perioxidases. Oxygen free radicals have been linked to DNA damage, the cross-linkage of collagen, and the accumulation of age pigments and cancers (Busse 1983). Nutrient antioxidants include vitamins C and E and beta-carotene (National Institute on Aging 1993a).

Immune System

The immune system performs both surveillance and protective tasks. It is a complex, widespread bodily function that is essential for the preservation of life (Suskind 1980). The destruction of the immune system is well known to people because it is identified with acquired immunodeficiency syndrome (AIDS) (Laurence 1985). Traditionally the immune system has been considered to have two major components. One is the humoral immune response, characterized by the production of antibody molecules that specifically bind the introduced foreign substance. The second is the cellular immune response, by which cells are mobilized that can specifically react with and destroy the invader. Considerable evidence has accumulated that a decrease in the immune competence and alterations in the regulation of the immune system are associated with aging. With increasing age, surveillance is impaired, and the efficiency of the protective mechanism declines. Furthermore, there is a loss of control so that immune functions become so distorted that they are self-destructive. The impairment of the immune system results in an increased incidence of certain diseases in the aging population. Certain tumors in the aged appear to be related to the failure of the body to recognize and eliminate abnormal cells. Autoantibodies increase with the passage of time, and the presence of autoantibodies identifies subpopulations at risk for early death. The older body has an increased susceptibility to infection, and, in general, effective immunization cannot be induced in late life (Finkelstein 1984).

The Eversion (Cross-Linkage) Theory

The eversion, or cross-linkage, theory of aging is based on the observation that changes in collagen structure are associated with aging. Collagen is probably the most important protein in the human body. The two types of collagen are interstitial and basement membrane. With the passage of time, the ester bonds from within the collagen molecule switch to binding together individual collagen molecules. This aging chain alters the characteristics of connective tissue. Modification of proteins may, in addition, be caused by glycosylation. Glycated forms of human collagen do accumulate with age in tendon and skin (Miller 1999).

Genetics of Human Aging

Brown and Wisniewski (1983) stated that the genetic nature of the aging process is reflected by the wide range of maximal life spans that animal species may attain. Among mammals, the life span range is from 1 year in the smoky shrew to more than 114 years in humans. This wide variation in life spans emphasizes that the aging process is likely to have an underlying basis that is in part encoded in our genes. The genetic basis may involve two types of inherited species-specific differences. The first type relates to development of the organism. This mechanism governs program timings in developmental stages as well as rates of maturation. The second genetic determinant relates to self-maintenance. This mechanism influences the efficiency of enzymatic systems as well as protection and repair of internal and external insults to the machinery.

If the DNA process in itself is damaged or declines in efficiency, the functioning capacity of the organism is severely impaired. It is obvious that the numerous biological changes that take place over the life span are very complicated. It is likely that many interacting genes are involved. However, specific genetic defects have been identified that are particularly relevant to certain life-shortening conditions. It is possible that there are other genes that contribute to longer life; however, at this stage of our knowledge, only rarely have specific "longevity" genes been identified that are consistently associated with increased life expectancy. Examples are genes that overproduce superoxide dismutase and catalase; such genes are antioxidants and appear to increase life expectancy (National Institute on Aging 1993b).

Martin (1977) reviewed a long list of human genetic conditions to select out those in which physical and physiological changes usually were associated with senescence. He identified the 10 genetic disorders that had the highest number of senescent features and thus that were considered to be associated with the aging process: Down syndrome, Werner's syndrome, Cockayne's syndrome, progeria, ataxia-telangiectasia, Lawrence-Seip syndrome, cervical lipodysplasia, Klinefelter's syndrome, Turner's syndrome, and myotonic dystrophy.

The progerias are syndromes that are linked with premature aging. The presence of these disorders does, to a limited extent, provide an opportunity to study accelerated bodily changes that resemble those attributable to aging. Although all of these syndromes are quite rare, two have received particular attention: Hutchinson-Gilford syndrome (Hastings 1904; Hutchinson 1886) and Werner's syndrome.

The early-onset Hutchinson-Gilford syndrome is characterized by dwarfism, physical immaturity, and pseudosenility. Individuals with this syndrome have a peculiar form of hypermetabolism, and they generally die during their mid-teens of coronary heart disease. Hutchinson-Gilford syndrome affects both sexes and has been described in white, black, and Asian races. The affected individuals look like very old, wizened, small humans with distorted features. This is because their heads are large in comparison to the face, and the ears and nose are small. Scalp hair, eyebrows, and eyelashes are lost. Some of the features that are commonly associated with aging are not increased in Hutchinson-Gilford syndrome. These include tumors, cataracts, and osteoporosis. A biochemical defect found in patients with Hutchinson-Gilford syndrome or Werner's syndrome is decreased excretion of urinary hyaluronic acid.

The search for the mode of inheritance of Hutchinson-Gilford syndrome continues. The syndrome has been considered to be a rare autosomal recessive condition, but it has been argued that it is more likely a sporadic autosomal dominant mutation because of several observations, including 1) a lower frequency of consanguinity than might be expected, 2) the low frequency of recurrence in families, and 3) a possible parental age effect. The vast majority of cases occur with no siblings affected. For this reason, all of the progerias—and particularly Hutchinson-Gilford syndrome—may be sporadic dominant-type mutations.

Although the life span of fibroblasts of progeria is affected, reports on the life spans of individuals with these disorders have varied, making it unclear whether the life span reduction is modest or severe. Furthermore, the suspicion that a basic defect in protein synthesis fidelity is a basic defect in progeria lacks confirmation (Goldstein et al. 1985). Similarly, there is confusion regarding the existence or nonexistence of definitive immune abnormalities. As to DNA repair capability, although such a defect is not uncommon, it is not a consistent marker for progeria. One must conclude that the basic metabolic defect is, at this time, unknown.

Werner's syndrome is a later-onset type of progeria. Werner (1904) described, in his doctoral dissertation for graduation from the Ophthalmological Clinic in Kiel, an unusual disorder, under the title "Cataract in Connection With Scleroderma." Werner reported the condition in siblings, two brothers and two sisters, between ages 36 and 40 years. The parents, grandparents, and one sister were healthy. Because Werner's syndrome differs from normal aging in several respects, Martin (1985) classified this condition as a "segmental progeroid syndrome."

The appearance of an individual affected by Werner's syndrome is indeed striking because the initial impression is that the person is very old. As the disease develops, affected individuals look 20–30 years older than their actual years, and their life span is shortened. Because the disease usually appears before growth is completed, patients with this syndrome frequently have thin limbs and typically are of smaller stature and are less developed than would be expected. Their appearance is striking in that the face develops a tightly drawn, pinched expression. Pseudoexophthalmos, a beak nose, protuberant teeth, and a recessive chin are characteristic features. Cataracts develop early, and, in addition to hypogonadism, individuals are likely to have diabetes. Not infrequently, they develop cancer, which contributes to their shortened life expectancy. The connective tissue cells and fibroblasts of these patients have been studied. For instance, Hayflick (1977) mentioned that fibroblast cells derived from such individuals and cultured in vitro undergo significantly fewer doublings than do cell samples from age-matched control subjects. The WRN locus on chromosome 8 produces a base that encodes a special protein, a helicase. Loss of function of this protein via mutation, which appears in Werner's syndrome, can result in genomic instability and subsequently a hastening of the aging process (Turner and Martin 1999).

Finch (1990) suggests that approximately 35% of the factors that influence the life span are inherited. The remainder are chance events that occur during biological development and random environmental changes during the life span. Species and even populations can vary tremendously in regard to the duration of the developmental phase and the adult life span as well as phenotypic variations. He concluded that little evidence indicates that the life span is generally set by molecular or cellular mechanisms that are intrinsically time dependent.

Length of Life: The Sex Differential

In humans and in many other animal species, females outlive males. It is easy to assume that the differences between the two sexes are genetically determined by the presence or absence of the Y chromosome. It has been suggested that the greater constitutional weakness of males may be the result of their having only one X chromosome.

Before 1900, in those nations where data are available, it appears there were slightly more older men than older women. After the turn of the century, this situation gradually changed, and by 1940 the situation had reversed itself. Thereafter, the preponderance of older women increased rapidly. In 1985 in the population older than 65 years, the sex ratio was 147 women for every 100 men; this discrepancy is increasing.

Contrary to the reasonable expectation of the equal balance in males and females at birth, there are in the United States approximately 106–110 white males born for every 100 white females and approximately 104 black males born for every 100 black females. It has been reported, but not confirmed, that in black populations of several islands in the West Indies, there are fewer males than females at birth (American Association of Retired Persons 1987).

Numerous environmental factors have been investigated to determine their influence on sex ratio at birth. In England and Wales, it has been reported that upper socioeconomic groups are likely to have a higher ratio of males to females than do lower socioeconomic groups. During World War II, many European countries observed that the ratio of males to females was higher than during times of peace. It is possible that this was because the births were occurring in younger parents as opposed to older parents during peacetime.

At birth, the female in the more developed nations has a life expectancy of 8 or more years beyond that of the male. In 1978, France had the most extreme male/female differences for life expectancy at birth: 8.21 years. Canada was second with a difference of 7.59 years. In 1981, Japan had the best life expectancy at birth: 79.1 years for females and 73.8 years for males, a difference of 5.3 years. In Japan this male/female difference is increasing rather than decreasing—in 1970, there was a difference of 4.4 years, and in 1952, there was a difference of 3.4 years.

Waldron (1986) reviewed the literature as to causes of sex differences in mortality. She noted that in contemporary industrial societies, the single most important cause of higher mortality for males has been a greater incidence of cigarette smoking among men. Other sex differences in mortality are related to behaviors that contribute to the males' higher mortality. Such behaviors include heavier alcohol consumption and employment in hazardous occupations. In many nonindustrial societies, where, in many instances, the sex differences in mortal-ity are not as great as in the industrial societies, these factors play a less important role.

In nonindustrial societies, women are more vulnerable to infectious diseases. This may be related to less adequate nutrition and health care for women. Waldron described a wide variety of factors that influence sex differences in mortality. In contrast to men in undeveloped nations, men in the United States tend to have a higher death rate from infectious and parasitic diseases than do women; American men were more vulnerable in 1930 than in 1978. However, one must be cautious in interpreting this information because, as Waldron pointed out, sex differences do vary somewhat for different types of infections and parasitic diseases.

Death rates by accidents and other violent causes are much higher for men than for women. Motor vehicle accidents account for a significant percentage of these differences. Although Waldron did not mention it, the differences caused by motorcycle accidents involving young men is a factor that appears in other United States statistics. Men have a much higher death rate than do women from accidental drownings and fatal gun accidents. Suicide is also more prevalent among men, and the incidence increases with age. As noted above, the higher death rate among men may be related to behavioral factors such as heavier alcohol consumption and other types of risk-taking behavior; these behaviors may or may not have a biological component, and cultural influences also may have an effect.

Ischemic heart disease has been consistently higher for men than for women in almost all available international and historical data. However, the magnitude of sex differences for ischemic heart disease has varied considerably in different regions, historical periods, and ethnic groups. The relation between cigarette smoking and heart disease cannot be ignored. Of interest is the fact that women who smoke do not have the same risk as men. This is attributable to different smoking habits. Men not only smoke more cigarettes per day but also inhale more deeply. As to smoking, an often-overlooked consideration is that females "may often feel sick as a result of smoking their first cigarette" (Waldron 1986, p. 64), and this may be a deterrent to their developing a smoking habit. Coronary-prone behavior also plays a significant role. There is a greater prevalence of type A coronary-prone behavior among men than among women. Type A behavior is marked by impatience, competitive drive, and hostility (Busse and Walker 1986).

As to the influence of menopause, there is contradictory evidence regarding the risk of women before or after menopause. There continues to be a debate regarding early onset of menopause. Early onset of natural menopause has been reported to be higher among women who smoke, and this may account in part for the increased risk of myocardial infarction among women with early natural menopause (Waldron 1986).

Mortality due to malignancies is more frequent among males than among females over most of the life span. Because of the large variety of cancers, the patterns and causes of sex differences vary for many different types of malignant neoplasms. Furthermore, occupational exposures contribute to the higher cancer rate among men.

Behavioral factors cannot be ignored for either sex. Clearly, the complex interaction of cultural, anatomical, physiological, and behavioral characteristics must be taken into consideration when discussing sex differences in aging, longevity, and mortality.

Waldron (1987) discussed mortality of "older adults"—a category that includes all adults age 40 and older. Ordinarily, the years from 40 to 65 would be considered to constitute middle age, with old age beginning at 65. In this older age group, a reversal of certain trends is beginning to show—for example, the gradual decline of ischemic heart disease. Waldron added some additional statistical information about the causes of the sex differential in longevity. Of deaths from ischemic heart disease, 50% are attributable to smoking. Ischemic heart disease is the major cause of death linked to atherosclerosis, but atherosclerosis linked to cerebrovascular disease accounts for only 2% of the sex differential in total mortality (National Center for Health Statistics 1984). Waldron concluded that smoking's effects on hormones and on atherosclerosis are responsible for, at most, 25% of the sex differential and total mortality in the United States. She noted that other observations point to behavioral factors as more important causes of sex differences in mortality. Taking high-risk behaviors as a group, behavioral differences appear to be responsible for at least 50% of the sex differential in total mortality in the United States. A question that remains unanswered is, What are the important factors that influence this difference in behavioral risks?

A Note on Stem Cells and Aging

Stem cell research will have a significant effect on the biology of aging and perhaps on the prevention and treatment of the diseases common in late life. Various types of stem cells are associated with stages of embryonic development, including totipotential cells (which develop into a genetically identical organism), pluripotential cells (which can produce many but not all types of cells neces-

sary for fetal development), and multipotential cells (which can produce limited types of cells that have a specific function, such as blood stem cells, which can supplement existing blood cells). The cells capable of production of specialized cells that can potentially supplement cells that have been destroyed or that deteriorate with aging are of special interest.

For example, conditionally immortal neuroepithelial stem cell grafts appear to reverse age-associated memory impairments in rats (Hodges et al. 2000). Age-associated memory impairments in rats have been linked to degeneration of cholinergic neurons. The rats were divided based on prior performance in a water maze into two groups: impaired and unimpaired. One half of the impaired rats were grafted with a hippocampal stem cell line. In a subsequent water maze test, the engrafted rats were substantially superior to the control rats in this task (improving function to the level of unimpaired aged control rats). The results suggest that the cognitive decline was not simply retarded but actually reversed. The findings demonstrate the capacity of a migratory stem cell line to repair diffuse damage in the aged brain.

Psychological Theories of Aging

Birren and Renner (1977) expressed the opinion that there was no pressure on the field of psychology to formulate a unified theory of aging or to explain how behavior is organized over time. They did offer a definition of aging for the behavioral sciences that recognizes that there can be incremental functions as well as decremental changes that occur over the adult life span. "Aging refers to the regular changes that occur in mature, genetically representative organisms living under representative environmental conditions" (Birren and Renner 1977, p. 4). Later, Birren and Cunningham (1985) said, "The psychology of aging is concerned with differences in behavior, changes in behavior with age, and patterns of behavior shown by persons of different ages in different periods of time" (p. 18). They also noted that "much of contemporary psychology of aging is a collection of segments of knowledge" (p. 19). Furthermore, this statement implies that most theories of the psychology of aging are actually microtheories because they do not embrace large amounts of data derived from various domains of behavior.

Baltes and Willis (1977) reached a somewhat similar conclusion: "All existing theories of psychologic aging and development are of the prototheoretical kind and are incomplete" (p. 148). The psychological theories that have appeared are often the extension of personality and developmental theories into middle and late life. Personality theories usually consider the innate human needs and forces that motivate thought and behavior and a modification of these biologically based energies by the experience of living in a physical and social environment.

Baltes (1993) later extended and clarified his concept of the process of the aging mind. He emphasized that it is important to know the full range of human mental performance and potential. Baltes begins with two major aggregations of mental processes: fluid and crystallized intelligence (Hebb 1949). *Fluid intelligence* is described as the cognitive mechanics and *crystallized intelligence* as the cognitive pragmatics. The fluid mechanisms are considered the basic information processes and are referred to as the hardware. In contrast, the crystallized pragmatics are culturally based and acquired; this cognitive function is the software of the mind. Baltes is also interested in reaching a better understanding of wisdom, as it is often believed to be a characteristic of many elderly persons. Baltes holds that wisdom is the ability to deal with important and difficult matters that are associated with how people conduct their lives and the meaning of life. Wisdom reflects a superior knowledge and includes judgment and sound advice; it is one of the few attributes of late life that is frequently recognized by a large segment of the population. One characteristic of wisdom that directly leads to better adaptation to aging is selective optimization and compensation. The wise elder selects carefully where her or his effort should be placed, optimizes the chances of success, and compensates when success is not attainable according to previous expectations.

Schaie (1977–1978) advanced what he called a "stage theory of adult cognitive development" (p. 129). His tentative scheme involved four possible cognitive stages: 1) acquisitive (childhood, adolescence); 2) achieving (young adulthood); 3) responsible and executive (middle age); and 4) reintegrative (old age). Schaie postulated two overlapping cognitive patterns during middle life—a "responsible" component and "executive" abilities—neither of which can be judged by common psychometric testing. He suggested that during the life span, a transition occurs from "what should I know" through "how should I use what I know" to a "why should I know" phase of life. Schaie stated the belief that numerous new strategies and techniques will have to be developed to fully test a stage theory and that alterations in the theory will emerge.

Kalish and Knudtson (1976) recommended the extension of the concept (theory) of attachment, common in infant and child psychology, to a lifetime conceptual scheme for understanding the relationships and involvements of older people. They further stated their belief that the concept (theory) of disengagement is not functional and that it should be eliminated. Attachment is a relationship established and maintained by "social bonds" and is distinguished from social contact. Elderly people lose significant early objects of attachment. New attachments are often much weaker, frequently are not mutual, and therefore are vulnerable. Kalish and Knudtson argued that an appreciation and understanding of attachments will provide a better approach to explaining the psychological changes in elderly people. Relevant to the attachment concept is the finding by Lowenthal and Haven (1968) that, more than any other single factor, having a confidant appeared to discriminate between elderly persons who were institutionalized and those who could remain in the community.

There are obvious limitations in the psychological theories of aging; these are quite realistic in view of the complexity of the research. Furthermore, recognizing the complexity of psychological experimentation and theory is essential to an awareness of the considerable psychological investigations that have contributed to a better understanding of human aging.

Social Theories of Aging

Palmore (1981) proposed five categories of social theories: 1) disengagement, activity, and continuity theories; 2) age stratification; 3) minority group theory; 4) life events and stress theory; and 5) homogeneity versus heterogeneity. *Disengagement theory* states that aging invariably causes physical, psychological, and social disengagement (Cumming and Henry 1961). Physical disengagement is attributable to a decline in physical energy, a decline in strength, and the slowing of responses. Psychological disengagement refers to the withdrawal of concern from a rather diffuse interest in many people to a focus on those who are directly related to the individual. Some describe this as a shift of attention from the outer world to the inner world of one's own feelings and thoughts. Social disengagement means the reduction of all types of social interaction, including activities such as those related to family, friends, community actions, church participation, and so forth. This theory of disengagement originally held that it was actually good—both for the older person and for society— for the older person to disengage. It was proposed that disengaged older persons tend to be happier and healthier than those who remain active.

Shortly after the appearance of the disengagement theory, the *activity theory* was published (Havighurst 1963). This theory holds that activity positively affects health, happiness, and longevity and that remaining active is good for both the aging individual and society.

The *continuity approach* is something of a compromise position between the disengagement and activity theories (Neugarten 1964). Proponents of the continuity approach maintain that older people tend to behave according to a pattern that has been established before late life. At times the person may disengage and at other times remain active. It is also apparent that some elderly people will drop one type of activity only to replace it with something that is more suitable to their health status and environment.

Age stratification is really a model of life-span development but obviously includes late life as a part of the conceptualization. According to Palmore (1981), age stratification conceptualizes society as being composed of different age groups with different roles and different expectations. Each age group must move up through time while responding to changes in environment. Age stratification focuses on distinguishing between age, period, and cohort effects.

The *minority group theory* relates to differences such as those attributed to race and ethnic groups. According to this theory, the aged are a minority group and frequently experience the same kind of discrimination that society inflicts on other minority groups (Busse 1970). The *life events and stress theory* holds that those major events usually associated with advancing age are particularly important to health and well-being in late life. A study using this approach must distinguish events that may be welcomed or resisted from those that do not affect all people in a similar manner. Some people resist retirement, whereas others welcome it. Some are unhappy in retirement, and others see it as an opportunity to attain life satisfactions.

Some social theories are related to the age distribution of the population and economic influences. One of these theories holds that the status of the aged is high in static societies and tends to decline with the acceleration of social change (Ogburn and Nimkoff 1940). Another theory is that the status of the aged is inversely related to the proportion of the aged in the population. For the most part, the aged are highly valued in societies in which they are scarce, and their value and status decrease as they become more numerous. The modernization theory of Cowgill and Holmes (1972) suggests that elderly persons are more highly respected in agricultural societies than they are in urbanized societies and that the status of the aged is inversely proportional to the rate of social change. A more recent study suggests that in some societies in the process of modernization, the status of the aged population goes through phases. During a developmental phase toward modernization, family control of resources increases, but as modernization continues, the

status of elderly people is likely to decline (Gilleard and Gurkan 1987).

Homogeneity and heterogeneity are concerned with the issue of whether individuals become more like one another or increasingly different from one another as they age (Maddox and Douglass 1974). One interesting consideration is the possibility that those who survive into late life (i.e., those who are 85 years and older) have identifiable characteristics that are very similar, whereas these individuals may have been quite different from the other people in the same age group 10–15 years earlier. Another consideration concerns the differences between men and women. Do men and women become increasingly different or increasingly similar as they age?

References

Ahmed A, Tollefsbol T: Telomeres and telomerase: basic science implications for aging. J Am Geriatr Soc 49:1105–1109, 2001

American Association of Retired Persons: A Profile of Older Americans, 1986. Washington, DC, American Association of Retired Persons, 1987

Baltes PB: The aging mind: potential and limits. Gerontologist 33:580–594, 1993

Baltes PB, Willis SL: Toward psychological theories of aging and development, in Handbook of the Psychology of Aging. Edited by Birren JE, Schaie KW. New York, Van Nostrand Reinhold, 1977, pp 128–147

Belkin BM, Neelon FA: The art of observation: William Osler and the method of Zadig. Ann Intern Med 116:863–866, 1992

Berk SL: Sir William Osler, ageism, and "the fixed period": a secret revealed. J Am Geriatr Soc 37:263–266, 1989

Birren JE, Cunningham WR: Research on the psychology of aging: principles, concepts, and theory, in Handbook of the Psychology of Aging, 2nd Edition. Edited by Birren JE, Schaie KW. New York, Van Nostrand Reinhold, 1985, pp 5–45

Birren JE, Renner VJ: Research on the psychology of aging, in Handbook of the Psychology of Aging. Edited by Birren JE, Schaie KW. New York, Van Nostrand Reinhold, 1977, pp 3–34

Brown TW, Wisniewski HM: Genetics of human aging. Review of Biological Research in Aging 1:81–99, 1983

Busse EW: The aged: a deprived minority. North Carolina Journal of Mental Health 4:3–7, 1970

Busse EW: Theories of aging, in Behavior and Adaptation in Late Life, 2nd Edition. Edited by Busse EW, Pfeiffer E. Boston, MA, Little, Brown, 1977, pp 11–32

Busse EW: Biologic and psychosocial bases of behavioral changes in aging, in American Psychiatric Association Annual Review, Vol 2. Washington, DC, American Psychiatric Press, 1983, pp 96–106

Busse EW: Primary and secondary aging, in The Encyclopedia of Aging. Edited by Maddox GL, Roth G, Atchley R, et al. New York, Springer, 1987, pp 5–34

Busse EW, Walker JI: Heart and neuropsychiatric disorders, in The International Text of Cardiology. Edited by Cheng TO. New York, Pergamon, 1986, pp 976–987

Carrel A: On the permanent life of tissues outside of the organism. J Exp Med 15:516–528, 1912

Cowgill D, Holmes L (eds): Aging and Modernization. New York, Appleton-Century-Crofts, 1972

Cristafalo VS: Animal cell cultures as a model for the study of aging, in Advances in Gerontological Research. Edited by Strehler BL. New York, Academic Press, 1972, pp 68–72

Cumming E, Henry W: Growing Old. New York, Basic Books, 1961

Finch CE: Longevity, Senescence and the Genome. Chicago, IL, University of Chicago Press, 1990

Finkelstein MS: Defenses against infection in the elderly: the compromises of aging. Triangle 23:57–64, 1984

Gey GO: Some aspects of the constitution and behavior of normal and malignant cells maintained in continuous culture. Harvey Lectures 50:154–229, 1955

Gilleard CJ, Gurkan AA: Socioeconomic development and the status of elderly men in Turkey: a test of modernization theory. J Gerontol 42:353–357, 1987

Goldstein S, Wojtyk RI, Harley CB, et al: Protein synthetic fidelity in aging human fibroblasts, in Werner's Syndrome and Human Aging (Advances in Experimental Medicine and Biology, Vol 190). Edited by Salk D, Fujiwara Y, Martin GM. New York, Plenum, 1985, pp 495–508

Gruman GJ: A History of Ideas About the Prolongation of Life: The Evolution of Prolongevity Hypotheses to 1880. Philadelphia, PA, American Philosophical Society, 1966

Hart RW, Turturro A: Review of recent biological research theories of aging. Review of Biological Research in Aging 2:3–12, 1985

Hastings G: Progeria: a form of senilism. Practitioner 73:188–217, 1904

Havighurst R: Successful aging, in Processes of Aging. Edited by Williams R, Tibbitts C, Donahue W. New York, Atherton Press, 1963, pp 81–90

Hayflick L: The limited in vitro lifetime of human diploid cell strains. Exp Cell Res 37:614–616, 1965

Hayflick L: Cellular basis for biological aging, in Handbook of Biology of Aging. Edited by Finch CE, Hayflick L. New York, Van Nostrand Reinhold, 1977, pp 73–86

Hayflick L, Moorhead PS: The serial cultivation of human diploid cell strains. Exp Cell Res 25:585–621, 1961

Hazzard WR: What heterogeneity among centenarians can teach us about genetics, aging, and longevity. J Am Geriatr Soc 49:1568–1569, 2001

Hebb DO: The Organization of Behavior. New York, Wiley, 1949

Hodges H, Veizovic T, Bray N, et al: Conditionally immortal neuroepithelial stem cell grafts reverse age-associated memory impairments in rats. Neuroscience 101:945–955, 2000

Hutchinson J: Case of congenital absence of hair and mammary glands with atrophic condition of the skin and its appendages. Lancet 1:473–477, 1886

Kalish RA, Knudtson FW: Attachment versus disengagement: a life-span conceptualization. Human Development 19:171–181, 1976

Kanin G: Remembering Mr. Maugham. New York, Atheneum, 1966

Laurence J: The immune system in AIDS. Sci Am 252:84–93, 1985

Lind LR (trans): Gabriele Zerbi, Gerontocomia: On the Care of the Aged and Maximianus, Elegies on Old Age and Love, translated from the Latin. Philadelphia, PA, American Philosophical Society, 1988

Lowenthal MF, Haven C: Interaction and adaptation: intimacy as a critical variable, in Middle Age and Aging. Edited by Neugarten BL. Chicago, IL, University of Chicago Press, 1968, pp 390–400

Maddox GL, Douglass EB: Aging and individual differences. J Gerontol 29:555–563, 1974

Martin GM: Genetic syndromes in man with potential relevance to the pathobiology of aging: genetics of aging. Birth Defects 14:5–39, 1977

Martin GM: Genetics and aging: the Werner syndrome as a segmental progeroid syndrome, in Werner's Syndrome and Human Aging (Advances in Experimental Medicine and Biology, Vol 190). Edited by Salk D, Fujiwara Y, Martin GM. New York, Plenum, 1985, pp 161–170

Miller RA: The biology of aging and longevity, in Principles of Geriatric Medicine and Gerontology, 4th Edition. Edited by Hazzard WR, Blass JP, Ettinger WH, et al. New York, McGraw-Hill, 1999, pp 1–19

National Center for Health Statistics: Monthly Vital Statistics Report 33(9), 1984

National Institute on Aging: Biochemistry and aging, in In Search of the Secrets of Aging (NIH Publ No 93-2756). Washington, DC, National Institute on Aging, May 1993a. Also available at http://www.healthandage.net/html/min/nih/content/booklets/in_search_of_the_secrets/in_search_of_the_secrets.htm. Accessed October 20, 2003.

National Institute on Aging: The genetic connection, in In Search of the Secrets of Aging (NIH Publ No 93-2756). Washington, DC, National Institute on Aging, September 1993b. Also available at http://www.healthandage.net/html/min/nih/content/booklets/in_search_of_the_secrets/in_search_of_the_secrets.htm. Accessed October 20, 2003.

Neugarten B: Personality in Middle and Later Life. New York, Atherton Press, 1964

Ogburn WF, Nimkoff MF: Sociology. Boston, MA, Houghton Mifflin, 1940

Palmore E: Advantages of aging. Gerontologist 19:220–223, 1979

Palmore E: Social Patterns in Normal Aging: Findings From the Duke Longitudinal Study. Durham, NC, Duke University Press, 1981

Palmore EB: Longevity in Abkhasia: a reevaluation. Gerontologist 24:95–96, 1984

Paul R: Alchemy altercation at Texas A&M. Science 262:1367, 1993

Schaie KW: Toward a stage theory of adult cognitive development. Int J Aging Hum Dev 8:129–138, 1977–1978

Suskind GW: Immunological aspects of aging: an overview. Paper presented at the National Institute on Aging Conference on Biological Mechanisms of Aging, Washington, DC, 1980

Thewlis MW: The history of geriatrics, in The Care of the Aged. Edited by Thewlis MW. St. Louis, MO, CV Mosby, 1924

Tobin JD: Physiological indices of aging, in The Baltimore Longitudinal Study of Aging (NIH Publ No 84-2450). Edited by Shock NW. Rockville, MD, National Institutes of Health, 1984, pp 387–395

Turner MS, Martin GM: Genetics of human disease, longevity, and aging, in Principles of Geriatric Medicine and Gerontology, 4th Edition. Edited by Hazzard WR, Blass JP, Ettinger WH, et al. New York, McGraw-Hill, 1999, pp 21–44

Velkoff V: Centenarians in the United States, 1990 and beyond. Statistical Bulletin–Metropolitan Insurance Companies 81:2–9, 2000

Waldron I: What do we know about causes of sex differences in mortality: a review of the literature. Population Bulletin of the United Nations 18:59–76, 1986

Waldron I: Causes of the sex differential in longevity. J Am Geriatr Soc 35:365–366, 1987

Weiss AK: Biomedical gerontology: the Hayflick hypothesis. Gerontologist 14:491–493, 1974

Werner O: Uber Katarakt im Verbindung mit Sklerdermie. Doctoral dissertation, Ophthalmological Clinic, Kiel, Germany, 1904

Zeman FD: Some little-known classics of old-age medicine. JAMA 200:150–152, 1967

Demography and Epidemiology of Psychiatric Disorders in Late Life

Dan G. Blazer, M.D., Ph.D.

Celia F. Hybels, Ph.D.

Judith C. Hays, R.N., Ph.D.

The epidemiology of psychiatric disorders in late life is the study of the distribution of psychiatric disorders among the elderly and those factors that influence this distribution (MacMahon and Pugh 1970). Roberts (1977) suggested that epidemiology is not only the basic science of preventive and community medicine but also may serve as the basic science of clinical practice. In this chapter, the findings of demographers and epidemiologists are reviewed as they relate to the care of the psychiatrically impaired older adult.

Demography

Of the more than 275 million persons enumerated during the United States census of 2000, nearly 35 million, or 13% of the population, are age 65 years or older (Federal Interagency Forum on Aging Related Statistics 2000). The average age in the United States is now 36 years. Even more astounding, more than 4 million, or 1.6% of the United States population and 12.5% of the 65 and older age group, are age 85 years or older. These oldest old among us are projected to reach 20 million by the year 2050 and to make up 5% of the United States population at that time. The "old-old" are more likely to experience poverty, to have less education, and to receive far more federal transfer payments (Blazer 2000). More than 50% of the nursing home residents in the United

States are age 80 years or older, representing a cost of more than $30 million per year (Suzman 1995). At least half of these residents are placed in nursing homes because of psychiatric disorders, especially the behavior problems that result from Alzheimer's disease.

The size of the elderly population in the United States is expected to dramatically increase in the next decades, reaching 70 million by the year 2030 (Figure 2-1) (Federal Interagency Forum on Aging Related Statistics 2000). Most of these elders are women (58%) and white (84%). Women are expected to continue to survive longer than men, yet the racial/ethnic composition of the elderly will change dramatically over the next few decades. Currently, 8% of elders are non-Hispanic black, 2% are non-Hispanic Asian and Pacific Islander, and fewer than 1% are non-Hispanic American Indian/Alaska natives. Hispanic elders make up 6% of the 65 and older age group. By 2050, the percentage of white non-Hispanic elders will decline to 64%, and Hispanic persons will account for 16% (a growth of 11 million persons), with non-Hispanic blacks accounting for 12% (Federal Interagency Forum on Aging Related Statistics 2000).

In 1900, the life expectancy at birth in the United States was 49 years (Federal Interagency Forum on Aging Related Statistics 2000). In 1997, the life expectancy at birth was 79 years for women and 74 years for men. Persons who survive to age 65 can expect to live an average of nearly 18 more years. Life expectancy of persons who

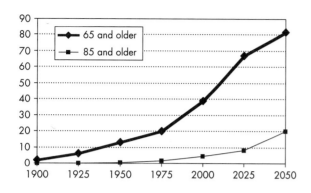

FIGURE 2–1. Population of older adults in the United States (in millions) from 1900 and projected to 2050.

survive to age 85 is 7 years for women and 6 years for men. The higher percentage of the elderly who are women and the increased life expectancy of women compared with men have been the subject of much discussion. Contributions to this difference in longevity may derive from both environmental and genetic factors. Cigarette smoking, more prevalent among men, has contributed to the difference. The more stressful and physically demanding occupations in which men engaged through much of the twentieth century may partially explain the difference as well. These potential mortality risks are dynamic across the sexes because more women are entering the workplace at all levels, and more women are smoking. Women may have a genetic advantage in life expectancy.

If the average retirement age remains the same and persons continue the trend to enter the workforce in their early 20s, the effect of an aging population on the economy of the United States—not to mention the need for health care—will be dramatic. This can be seen in the profound increase in the age-to-dependency ratio—that is, the ratio of persons in the workforce compared with children or retired people. Flexibility in retirement and other social and economic changes will help modify the effect of this "squaring" of the population pyramid. Nevertheless, this demographic revolution will affect every individual and every institution in our society (Pifer and Bronte 1986).

If an older person develops a psychiatric disorder, that disorder may become chronic, and the years of life that are associated with a decreased quality of life because of psychiatric morbidity are substantial. In addition, with increasing age, the great majority of older persons with psychiatric disorders experience a comorbid physical illness (Blazer 2000).

What can psychiatric epidemiological studies contribute to mental health services for older adults? Morris (1975) suggested the following uses of epidemiology:

- Identify cases (e.g., can the symptom pattern of depression in elderly persons be readily identified in community-dwelling and clinical [e.g., hospitalized] populations of older adults?).
- Reveal the distribution of psychiatric disorders in the population (e.g., what is the prevalence and/or incidence of dementia?).
- Trace historical trends of mental illness among elderly persons (e.g., has the incidence of suicide increased among this population over the past 10 years?).
- Determine the etiology of psychiatric disorders in late life (e.g., do social factors contribute more to the etiology of late-life psychiatric disorders than to such disorders in midlife, given lower potential for genetic contributions?).
- Examine the use of psychiatric and other mental health services by elderly persons (e.g., do psychiatrically impaired older adults in the community underutilize psychiatric services?).

Each of these functions of epidemiology is reviewed in this chapter.

Case Identification

Clinicians constantly face the task of distinguishing abnormality from normality. Although most epidemiologists and clinicians agree on the core symptoms of psychiatric disorders throughout the life cycle, the absolute distinction between a case and a noncase—that is, persons requiring psychiatric attention versus those who do not require such care—is not easily established. Many of the symptoms and signs of a psychiatric disorder in late life may be ubiquitous with the aging process, thus blurring the distinction between cases and noncases. Epidemiologists can assist the clinician in identifying meaningful clusters of symptoms and significant degrees of symptom severity. Case identification is also the foundation of descriptive epidemiology: "cases" are the numerator of the equation from which prevalence and incidence estimates are derived in community and clinical samples (the denominator).

What is a case? Copeland (1981) suggested that the question be turned by epidemiologists, with advantage, to "A case for what?" The choice of a construct for a case depends on the particular scientific or clinical inquiry of the investigator. If, to determine the value of a new short-acting sedative-hypnotic agent, the clinician wishes to identify a group of older adults with initial insomnia, the prevalence and severity of a target symptom—initial insomnia—define the case. The sleep difficulty may result from several different underlying disorders, but diagnosis would be irrelevant to the purpose of the study. For most clinicians, however, the goal of case identification is to identify subjects experiencing uniform underlying psychopathology, as is implicit in DSM-IV and DSM-IV-TR (American Psychiatric Association 1994, 2000).

According to D. Goodwin and Guze (1979), diagnosis is prognosis. Diagnostic categories that approximate true disease processes have several characteristics, including the following (Weissman and Klerman 1978):

1. A category should be distinguished on the basis of patterns of symptomatology (e.g., the clustering of symptoms in vascular depression) (Alexopoulos et al. 1997).
2. A category should predict the outcome of a disorder (e.g., Alzheimer's disease should predict a steady decline in cognitive functioning) (Shoghi-Jadid et al. 2002).
3. A category should reflect underlying biological reality, confirmed by family and genetic studies (e.g., Alzheimer's disease) (Roses 1994).
4. Laboratory studies should eventually validate a diagnostic category (e.g., the use of specific imaging studies to diagnose Alzheimer's disease) (Roses 1997).
5. The classification scheme should identify persons who may respond to a specific therapeutic intervention, such as a particular form of psychotherapy or a specific group of medications (Reynolds et al. 1999).

The goal of DSM-IV-TR is to provide categories that eventually will meet each of these characteristics. At present, however, these categories are defined by operational criteria (such as the symptom criteria for the diagnosis of major depression). One method of case identification is the use of diagnostic instruments. These instruments (usually standardized interviews) have been developed and used in community- and clinic-based epidemiological studies to identify persons with symptoms that meet these criteria. The Structured Clinical Interview for DSM-IV (SCID; First et al. 1997) and the Diagnostic Interview Schedule (DIS; Robins et al. 1981) are examples of the most frequently used interview schedules. For example, the DIS was used in the Epidemiologic Catchment Area (ECA) study, from which a 1-month national estimate of the prevalence of affective disorders in persons age 65 years and older was 2.5% (compared with 6.4% for persons age 25–44 years) (Regier et al. 1988).

A second approach to case identification is the use of self-administered symptom scales and personality inventories. Frequently used scales in epidemiological surveys include the Center for Epidemiologic Studies Depression Scale (CES-D; Radloff 1977) and the Geriatric Depression Scale (Yesavage et al. 1983), which screen for depressive symptoms, and the Short Portable Mental Status Questionnaire (Pfeiffer 1975) and the Mini-Mental State Exam (MMSE; Folstein et al. 1975), which screen for cognitive impairment. The advantage of these scales is that, unlike diagnostic interviews, they do not subjectively assign patients to a particular diagnostic category; a disadvantage is the lack of diagnostic specificity that can be achieved with their use. For example, the severity of depressive symptoms after the loss of a loved one may be similar to that associated with a major depressive episode with melancholia. A symptom checklist cannot be used to distinguish one from the other, although the diagnosis of, and intervention for, these two disorders would be very different. Blazer et al. (1991a) estimated the prevalence of clinically significant depression symptoms among community-dwelling elders in North Carolina to be 9%, although most of these individuals would not receive diagnoses of major depression.

Other authors define a case on the basis of severity of physical, psychological, and social impairment secondary to the symptoms. This approach to case identification is less popular among clinicians, who are more inclined to "treat a disease" than to "improve function." Improved function, in theory, should derive from remission of the disease. Nevertheless, function has special relevance in the care of older adults, especially the oldest old (Blazer 2000). When managing chronic psychiatric disorders, such as primary degenerative dementia of the Alzheimer's type, the improvement or maintenance of physical, psychological, and social functioning is a clinician's primary goal (Hazzard 1994). Family members are often more concerned with improved functioning than with alleviation of symptoms. Improved sleep and appetite and a decline in suicidal ideation in a depressed older adult may not translate into a perceived recovery from a depressive episode by the family. Rather, the family may focus on the quality of interpersonal interactions and social functioning.

Regardless of the approach taken to identify cases, most clinicians and clinical investigators want to achieve perfection in the separation of cases from noncases (e.g., case identification is critical for entry into a clinical trial). The epidemiological method depends, for the most part, on a clear distinction between cases and noncases (Kleinbaum et al. 1982), yet most older adults do not ideally fit the psychiatric diagnosis that they receive (Strauss et al. 1981). Regardless of the diagnostic system, unusual or borderline cases that cannot be clearly placed in a single category exist. This has led some investigators to consider the possibility of "fuzzy sets" as a means by which cases can be more realistically distinguished (Blazer et al. 1989). Not infrequently, older adults manifest more than one disease simultaneously—for example, major depression and primary degenerative dementia. In addition, the prescribed categories of DSM-IV-TR do not always match the symptoms that individuals in this population may be experiencing; generalized anxiety, for instance, is not easily disentangled from a major depressive episode in an agitated older adult.

Most natural clustering of older adults into categories is perceptually "fuzzy" (Rosch 1978), for natural processes rarely show necessary and sufficient criteria for sharp distinctions. Boundaries between closely related categories are ill defined. Some of the methods of case identification, such as the symptom checklist and standardized interview approaches that archive symptoms, are adaptive to the development of clusters of both symptoms and subjects with fuzzy boundaries. For example, depressed elderly persons are more likely to express cognitive dysfunction than are depressed middle-aged persons, yet cognitive dysfunction is part of the depressed syndrome across the life cycle (Blazer et al. 1988). Therefore, psychiatric syndromes—rather than discrete disorders—are more realistic as diagnostic entities in geriatric psychiatry. The most common of these syndromes are memory loss, confusion, depression, anxiety, suspiciousness and agitation, sleep disturbance, and hypochondriasis (Blazer 2000).

Regardless of the approach taken to case identification, a diagnosis must be reliable and valid for it to be a useful means of communicating clinical information. To pass the test of reliability, a diagnosis must be consistent and repeatable. Standardized or operational methods for identifying psychiatric symptoms and the availability of specific criteria for psychiatric diagnoses have greatly improved the reliability of case identification by psychiatrists and by lay interviewers in psychiatric epidemiological surveys. Reliability, however, does not ensure validity—that is, the test of whether a case identified by a particular method reflects underlying reality (meeting only one of the five criteria listed earlier in this discussion) (Blazer and Kaplan 2000).

Distribution of Psychiatric Disorders

The authors of descriptive studies of the epidemiology of psychiatric impairment in older adults have concentrated on either overall mental health functioning or the distribution of specific psychiatric disorders in the population. Reports from these studies usually begin as general observations of the relation of impairment or specific disorders to characteristics such as age, gender, race/ethnicity, and socioeconomic status. These trends provide the template for more in-depth studies of the hereditary, biological, and psychosocial contributors to the etiology of disorders and the effect of the distribution of the disorders on mental health care utilization. Frequencies of disorders within the population are usually presented in terms of prevalence—the proportion or percentage of persons within the population with a defined impairment or specific disorder at a particular time or within a particular period. Almost all such studies provide estimates based on community samples of larger populations. Smaller studies of the prevalence of impairment or specific disorders in institutional or clinical settings provide important data about service use.

Longitudinal epidemiological studies of older adults also can provide data on the incidence of impairment or psychiatric disorders; that is, the proportion of persons who develop the disorder during a specified period of observation. In addition, longitudinal studies provide data on outcomes associated with impairment or specific psychiatric disorders.

The National Institute of Mental Health (NIMH) established the ECA program in the United States to determine the prevalence of specific psychiatric disorders in both community and institutional populations (Regier et al. 1984). Data were collected in five communities, and the DIS was used to identify persons who met criteria for specific disorders. Although conducted more than two decades ago, the ECA study remains the landmark study in the United States for addressing the prevalence of psychiatric impairment in older adults. More than 18,000 persons were interviewed in the ECA study, including 5,702 persons who were age 65 years or older. All disorders, with the exception of cognitive impairment, were more prevalent in younger or middle-aged adults, compared with older adults. A total of 12.3% (13.6% of the women and 10.5% of the men) of those age 65 or older met criteria for one or more psychiatric disorders in the month before the interview. The two most prevalent disorders in this age group were an anxiety disorder (5.5%) and severe cognitive impairment (4.9%) (Regier et al. 1988).

Specific disorders will be addressed in detail in subsequent chapters, but Tables 2–1 through 2–5 provide a summary of the prevalence of psychiatric symptoms and specific disorders in both community and institutional samples based on studies conducted in the United States, Canada, Europe, and Australia over the last several decades.

The prevalence of cognitive impairment in selected community and institutional populations is presented in Table 2–1. As shown in Table 2–1, the prevalence of cognitive impairment reported from the ECA studies was 2.9% in those age 65–74, 6.8% in those age 75–84, and 15.8% in those age 85 or older (Regier et al. 1988). The overall prevalence of 4.9% (Regier et al. 1988) was within the range found in three of the sites of the Established Populations for Epidemiologic Studies of the Elderly (EPESE) conducted by the National Institute on Aging (Cornoni-Huntley et al. 1986). The prevalence of cognitive impairment among primary care patients and in institutional samples is higher than that obtained from community samples and, as shown in Table 2–1, can range from 15.7% in primary care patients to 59.4% in institutionalized Medicaid patients (Burns et al. 1988; Callahan et al. 1995; Teeter et al. 1976). The Canadian Study of Health and Aging reported a prevalence of 16.8% for a diagnosis they identified as "cognitive impairment, no dementia" in their sample of both community and institutionalized older adults (Graham et al. 1997).

It is important to note that these studies reporting the prevalence of cognitive impairment are measuring cognitive function by standardized screening tests such as the Short Portable Mental Status Questionnaire and the MMSE. Therefore, these studies are not reporting the prevalence of dementia or Alzheimer's disease or actual cerebral impairment. The prevalence of cognitive impairment can be affected by educational level of the population being studied, as well as by other sociocultural factors that may affect performance on cognitive tasks.

The prevalence of dementia and Alzheimer's disease in both community and institutional samples is shown in Table 2–2. Kay et al. (1970) reported that 6.2% of their community sample met the criteria for chronic brain syndromes. The prevalence of dementia reported from community studies is similar. In a study of 1,070 community-dwelling adults age 65 or older in Liverpool, England, the prevalence of probable dementia was 5.2% (Copeland et al. 1987), whereas in the Canadian Study of Health and Aging, the reported prevalence of dementia was 8.0% (Canadian Study of Health and Aging Working Group 1994). As expected, the prevalence of dementia in community-dwelling older adults is higher in older age groups. Heeren et al. (1991) reported that the prevalence of dementia in a sample of adults age 85 or older was 23%, with 11% classified as having moderate or severe dementia. The prevalence of dementia is also higher in institutional samples. In their sample of nursing home patients, Rovner et al. (1986) found that the prevalence of primary degenerative dementia was 56%, whereas the prevalence of multi-infarct dementia was 18% and the prevalence of Parkinson's dementia was 4%.

Several studies have provided data on the prevalence of Alzheimer's disease. Evans et al. (1989) reported that the prevalence of probable Alzheimer's disease was 10.3% in a sample of community-dwelling adults age 65 or older. The prevalence increased with age. Specifically, the prevalence was 3.0% in those age 65–74, 18.7% in those age 75–84, and 47.2% in those age 85 or older. Copeland et al. (1992) used different diagnostic criteria and found that the prevalence of Alzheimer's disease in their study in Liverpool was 3.3%. In the Canadian Study of Health and Aging, the prevalence of Alzheimer's disease was 5.1% (Canadian Study of Health and Aging Working Group 1994). That the prevalence of Alzheimer's disease is estimated to be higher than the prevalence of cognitive impairment may at first appear counterintuitive. Nevertheless, a careful diagnostic evaluation may establish Alzheimer's disease even when overall cognitive impairment is not severe.

The prevalence of psychiatric symptoms in community populations of older adults is presented in Table 2–3. The most frequently reported symptoms are problems with sleep and symptoms of anxiety. In the Iowa EPESE, more than 30% of the respondents reported awakening during the night and/or feeling sleepy during the day, and more than 14% reported having trouble falling asleep (Cornoni-Huntley et al. 1986). In a study of adults age 78 or older in Sweden, a total of 24.4% of the respondents reported feelings of anxiety (Forsell and Winblad 1998). Henderson et al. (1998) reported from Australia that the prevalence of psychotic symptoms among community-dwelling older adults was 5.7%, which is similar to the prevalence rate of persecutory ideation of 4% reported from North Carolina (Christenson and Blazer 1984). Blazer and Houpt (1979) reported that 14% of their sample of elders in North Carolina had symptoms of hypochondriasis. The prevalence of alcohol use is low in older adults, but the proportion of drinkers who drink in excess is greater than 19% (P.A. Saunders et al. 1989).

Numerous studies have reported a high prevalence of depressive symptoms among community-dwelling older adults. In the New Haven, Connecticut EPESE, the prevalence of depressive symptomatology as defined by the CES-D was 15.1% (Cornoni-Huntley et al. 1986). Copeland et al. (1999) found a similar prevalence in data from the European Concerted Action on Depression of Older People (EURODEP). Specifically, 12.3% of the sample age 65 or older were either cases or subcases of depression. Finally, Beekman et al. (1995) found that the prevalence of minor depression (depressive symptomatology not meeting criteria for major depression) was 12.9% in the Longitudinal Aging Study Amsterdam (LASA), a study of community-dwelling adults age 55–85. In addi-

TABLE 2–1. Prevalence of cognitive impairment in community and institutional populations of older adults

Study/site	Reference	Sample	N	Age (years)	Measurement	Prevalence
ECA	Regier et al. 1988	Five U.S. communities	5,702	65+	MMSE	4.9%
				65–74	MMSE	2.9%
				75–84	MMSE	6.8%
				85+	MMSE	15.8%
New Haven EPESE	Cornoni-Huntley et al. 1986	Community	2,811	65+	SPMSQ	5.3%
Iowa EPESE	Cornoni-Huntley et al. 1986	Community	3,673	65+	SPMSQ	1.3%
East Boston EPESE	Cornoni-Huntley et al. 1986	Community	3,812	65+	SPMSQ	6.0%
Minnesota	Teeter et al. 1976	Institutionalized Medicaid patients	74	Mean age = 81	SPMSQ	59.4%
U.S. national sample	Burns et al. 1988	Institution	526	Mean age = 79	Chart review and nurse interview	39.0%
Canadian Study of Health and Aging	Graham et al. 1997	Community and institution	2,914	65+	Modified MMSE and clinical assessment	16.8% cognitive impairment, no dementia
Indiana	Callahan et al. 1995	Primary care patients	3,594	60+	SPMSQ	15.7%
Germany	Busse et al. 2003	Community	1,045	75+	SIDAM	3.1% mild cognitive impairment 8.8% age-associated cognitive decline

Note. ECA = Epidemiologic Catchment Area; EPESE = Established Populations for Epidemiologic Studies of the Elderly; MMSE = Mini-Mental State Exam (Folstein et al. 1975); SIDAM = Structured Interview for Diagnosis of Dementia of Alzheimer Type, Multi-Infarct Dementia and Dementias of Other Aetiology According to ICD-10 and DSM-III-R (Zaudig et al 1991); SPMSQ = Short Portable Mental Status Questionnaire (Pfeiffer 1975).

TABLE 2–2. Prevalence of dementia and Alzheimer's disease in community and institutional populations of older adults

Study/site	Reference	Sample	N	Age (years)	Measurement	Prevalence
England	Kay et al. 1970	Community	758	65+	Psychiatric interviews	6.2% chronic brain syndromes
Netherlands	Heeren et al. 1991	Community	1,259	85+	Standardized interviews	23% dementia (11% with moderate or severe dementia)
Maryland	Rovner et al. 1986	Institution	50	Mean age = 83	Standardized interviews	56% primary degenerative dementia; 18% multi-infarct dementia; 4% Parkinson's dementia
East Boston EPESE	Evans et al. 1989	Community	467	65+	Standardized interviews and clinical evaluation	10.3% probable Alzheimer's disease
Liverpool	Copeland et al. 1987	Community	1,070	65+	GMS-AGECAT	5.2% probable dementia
Liverpool	Copeland et al. 1992	Community	1,070	65+	GMS-AGECAT	3.3% Alzheimer's disease
Canada	Canadian Study of Health and Aging Working Group 1994	Community and institution	10,263	65+	3MS and clinical examination	8.0% dementia 5.1% Alzheimer's disease
Germany	Riedel-Heller et al. 2001	Community and institution	1,692	75+	SIDAM	17.4% DSM-III-R dementia 12.4% ICD-10 dementia
London	Stevens et al. 2002	Community	1,085	65+	Short-CARE	9.86% dementia

Note. EPESE = Established Populations for Epidemiologic Studies of the Elderly; GMS-AGECAT = Geriatric Mental State (Copeland et al. 1976); 3MS = Modified Mini-Mental State (Teng and Chui 1987); Short-CARE = Short Comprehensive Assessment and Referral Evaluation (Gurland et al 1984); SIDAM = Structured Interview for Diagnosis of Dementia of Alzheimer Type, Multi-Infarct Dementia and Dementias of Other Aetiology According to ICD-10 and DSM-III-R (Zaudig et al 1991).

TABLE 2–3. Prevalence of psychiatric symptoms in community populations of older adults

Study/site	Reference	N	Age (years)	Measurement	Disorder/syndrome	Prevalence
New Haven EPESE	Cornoni-Huntley et al. 1986	2,811	65+	CES-D	Depressive symptoms	15.1%
Durham County, NC	Blazer and Houpt 1979	997	65+	Selected questions	Hypochondriasis	14%
Durham County, NC	Christenson and Blazer 1984	997	65+	MMPI	Persecutory ideation	4%
Australia	Henderson et al. 1998	1,377	70+	Structured psychiatric interviews	Psychotic symptoms	5.7%
Iowa EPESE	Cornoni-Huntley et al. 1986	3,673	65+	Selected questions	Trouble falling asleep Awakens during night Sleepy during day	14.1% 33.7% 30.7%
EURODEP	Copeland et al. 1999	13,808	65+	GMS-AGECAT	Cases and subcases of depression	12.3% Males 8.6% Females 14.1%
Liverpool	P.A. Saunders et al. 1989	1,070	65+	GMS-AGECAT	Among drinkers, proportion exceeding sensible limits	Males 19.5% Females 19.6%
Stockholm	Forsell and Winblad 1998	966	78+	Selected questions	Feelings of anxiety	24.4%
LASA	Beekman et al. 1995	3,056	55–85	CES-D	Minor depression	12.9%

Note. CES-D = Center for Epidemiologic Studies Depression Scale (Radloff 1977); EPESE = Established Populations for Epidemiologic Studies of the Elderly; EURODEP = European Concerted Action on Depression of Older People; GMS-AGECAT = Geriatric Mental State (Copeland et al. 1976); LASA = Longitudinal Aging Study Amsterdam; MMPI = Minnesota Multiphasic Personality Inventory (Hathaway and McKinley 1970).

tion, Beekman et al. (1999) recently reviewed studies of major depression and depressive symptoms among persons age 55 or older and found that the average prevalence of depressive syndromes deemed clinically relevant was 13.5%.

Across the entire life cycle, many psychiatric symptoms, especially hypochondriasis and sleep disorders, have their highest frequencies among elderly adults. A relatively high frequency of certain symptoms in elderly populations, however, does not necessarily signify an increased frequency of specific psychiatric disorders. The paradox of relatively high reports of depressive symptoms and relatively low reports of the prevalence of major depressive episodes illustrates this point (Blazer 1982). Diagnostic categories, such as those found in DSM-IV-TR, are clusters of symptoms and signs that derive their validity not from the overall weight of symptomatology but, rather, from regularities in the clustering of history, the persistence of symptoms over time, a predictable outcome, a common pathophysiology, and possibly common biochemical disturbances. As biological markers of psychiatric disorders are identified, laboratory diagnostic techniques will provide information that is complementary to the symptoms reported. As our knowledge progresses in the area of nomenclature, new categories of symptoms may be lumped together to define a particular syndrome. As Morris (1975) noted, each succeeding generation will split and lump groups of symptoms and signs to suit its own purposes, given the current biomedical and clinical understanding of disease entities.

Symptoms, the most objective clinical indicators of psychopathology, may reflect more than one diagnostic entity. On the other hand, symptoms may not be associated with any disorder of interest to the clinician. For example, decreased appetite can result from several sources. At a given time, grief reactions, more frequent in late life than at other stages of the life cycle, may be virtually indistinguishable from major depressive episodes if appetite alone is considered. Loss of appetite also accompanies major life adjustments such as a forced change of residence or a decline in economic resources. Most commonly, loss of appetite in late life is a result of poor physical health.

The prevalence of selected psychiatric disorders in community populations of older adults is shown in Table 2–4. The prevalence of psychiatric disorders is lower than the prevalence of related psychiatric symptoms. The most prevalent disorders, other than dementia disorders, are mood and anxiety disorders. Numerous studies of older adults have reported that the prevalence of major depression is approximately 1%–2%, with a higher prev-

alence in females (Beekman et al. 1995; Bland et al. 1988; Regier et al. 1988). Henderson et al. (1993) reported that the prevalence of ICD-10 (World Health Organization 1992) depressive episodes in persons age 70 or older was 3.3%. Kay et al. (1985) reported an increase in DSM depression with age, with a prevalence of 6.3% in those age 70–79 and 15.5% in those age 80 or older. Copeland et al. (1987) reported that the prevalence of depressive neurosis was 8.3% in their Liverpool sample, whereas the prevalence of depressive psychosis was 2.9%. The prevalence of generalized anxiety was lower, estimated from the ECA study to be 2.2% (Blazer et al. 1991b). The prevalence of any anxiety disorder in adults age 65 or older in the ECA study was 5.5%, with a higher prevalence in females (6.8%) compared with males (3.6%) (Regier et al. 1988). Among adults age 65 or older in Edmonton, Canada, the prevalence of phobic disorder was 3.0% (Bland et al. 1988), whereas the prevalence of phobic disorder in a community sample of adults in the same age group in London was 10.0% (Lindesay et al. 1989). The prevalence of alcohol abuse or dependence was low in this population, with an overall 1-month prevalence of 0.9% reported from the ECA study (Regier et al. 1988). Similarly, the 1-month prevalence of schizophrenia reported from the ECA study in adults age 65 or older was 0.1% (Regier et al. 1988).

Overall, psychiatric disorders are found at a lower prevalence among the elderly than at other stages of the life cycle. The virtual absence of alcohol abuse or dependence and schizophrenia in those age 65 or older in the ECA data may reflect selective mortality. On the other hand, it also may reflect the case-finding techniques used. For example, the investigators did not attempt to assess the homeless population. The community data do not include individuals in institutions, and many persons in late life with chronic schizophrenia may be institutionalized. In addition, early-onset schizophrenia may be associated with a "burned-out" symptom picture; this fact, coupled with poor reporting, may mean that an individual's clinical presentation does not meet the criteria for a diagnosis of schizophrenia.

Another question derives from these data: Do unique late-life symptom presentations render the Research Diagnostic Criteria (RDC; Spitzer et al. 1978) and DSM-IV-TR inadequate as systems of nomenclature? DSM-IV-TR provides age-specific categories for children but not for elderly persons. Clinicians who work with older adults, however, have often commented that depression may be masked in late life by symptoms of poor physical health or pseudodementia. Yet there is no compelling evidence for developing a new diagnostic classification specific to older adults. Although DSM-IV-TR may not identify all persons

TABLE 2–4. Prevalence of selected psychiatric disorders in community populations of older adults

Study/site	Reference	Sample	N	Age (years)	Measurement	Disorder	Prevalence
ECA	Regier et al. 1988	Five U.S. communities	5,702	65+	DIS	Major depression	Males 0.4% / Females 0.9%
						Dysthymia	Males 1.0% / Females 2.3%
						Alcohol abuse/dependence	Males 1.8% / Females 0.3%
						Schizophrenia	Males 0.1% / Females 0.1%
						Any anxiety disorder	Males 3.6% / Females 6.8%
ECA	Blazer et al. 1991b	Three U.S. communities	784	65+	DIS	Generalized anxiety	2.2%
LASA	Beekman et al. 1995	Netherlands	3,056	55–85	DIS	Major depression	2.0%
Edmonton	Bland et al. 1988	Canada	358	65+	DIS	Major depression	1.2%
						Phobic disorder	3.0%
						Panic disorder	0.3%
Liverpool	Copeland et al. 1987	England	1,070	65+	GMS-AGECAT	Depressive neurosis	8.3%
						Depressive psychosis	2.9%
Guy's/Age Concern Survey	Lindesay et al. 1989	London	890	65+	Structured interview	Phobic disorder	10.0%

Note. DIS = Diagnostic Interview Schedule (Robins et al. 1981); ECA = Epidemiologic Catchment Area; GMS-AGECAT = Geriatric Mental State (Copeland et al. 1976); LASA = Longitudinal Aging Study Amsterdam.

with significant psychiatric symptoms, those who do qualify for a DSM-IV-TR diagnosis are not unlike persons at other stages of the life cycle (Blazer 1980b; Blazer et al. 1987a). The deficiency inherent in DSM-IV-TR is that it poorly differentiates psychiatric symptoms from those that signify the presence of physical illness and impaired cognition—a situation that also may occur in younger individuals, although it is far more common as a diagnostic problem in late life than in midlife.

The prevalence of psychiatric disorders, especially major depression, in treatment facilities is presented in Table 2–5. Burns et al. (1988) found among nursing home patients with mental disorders, excluding organic brain syndrome, an average of 1.3 mental disorder diagnoses per person. As is evident, the prevalence of both minor and major depression is much higher than that found in community populations. The prevalence of major depression is estimated to be 6.0%–14.4% (Koenig et al. 1988; Lyness et al. 1999; Parmelee et al. 1989; Rovner et al. 1986; Teresi et al. 2001) and the prevalence of minor depression to be as high as 30.5% (Parmelee et al. 1989). Many depressed older adults may be selectively admitted to medical inpatient units or long-term care facilities (because older adults are less likely to use specialty psychiatric care). The lower prevalence of these disorders in the community, therefore, should not lull clinicians into believing that psychiatric problems are of little consequence for older adults.

Fewer data regarding the incidence of psychiatric disorders in late life are available because most disorders begin earlier in adulthood. In a study of 875 nondepressed older adults, the 3-year incidence of depression was 4.1% (Forsell and Winblad 1999). Henderson et al. (1997) reported that the 3- to 6-year incidence of depression in a sample of community-dwelling elders age 70 or older was 2.5%. The incidence of schizophrenia among older adults is estimated to be 3.0 per 100,000 persons per year for new cases (Copeland et al. 1998). Finally, the incidence of dementia increases with age. Bachman et al. (1993) reported from the Framingham data that the 5-year incidence of dementia was 7.0 per 1,000 in those age 65–69 and 118.0 per 1,000 at ages 85–89. A similar increase with age in the 1-year incidence of Alzheimer's disease was reported from the East Boston EPESE: 0.6% in those age 65–69 and 8.4% in those age 85 or older (Hebert et al. 1995).

Historical Studies

Psychiatrists typically follow up patients for relatively short periods during the course of their illnesses. In addition, they usually interact with each patient within a relatively brief window of historical time. Epidemiological studies add a historical perspective to current cross-sectional findings in population and clinical surveys. Some diseases, such as tuberculosis, are known to wax and wane; new diseases, such as acquired immunodeficiency syndrome (AIDS) dementia, may emerge; and old diseases, such as smallpox, are eradicated or disappear naturally (Morris 1975). Historical studies in psychiatric epidemiology are rare, especially of the elderly. Unlike changes observed with infectious diseases, however, temporal changes that occur with most behaviors that are of psychiatric interest must be determined over years rather than months; exceptions are the clustering of psychiatric emergencies after the Christmas season and the increase in suicide during the spring season of each year (Hilliard et al. 1981; Lester 1979). Constructs of case identification have changed over the years, and so it is rare to find a study in which similar methods of case identification were applied at two points distant enough in time to establish historical trends. Longitudinal studies are also fraught with methodological problems, especially problems with follow-up.

The study of changes in suicide frequency among older adults during the twentieth century illustrates the value of longitudinal studies, despite the methodological problems associated with these designs. Suicide rates have been positively correlated with age. The highest suicide rates are consistently evident among persons older than 65 (McIntosh et al. 1994; Moscicki 1997). As is shown in Figure 2–2, the correlation is largely explained by the elevated rates of suicide among white men older than 70 years. Rates among white men age 70 and older have fallen since 1940, from a high of 60–65 per 100,000 in 1940 (Bureau of the Census 1973) to a low of 39 per 100,000 in 2000 (data from WISQARS injury mortality report database, see Centers for Disease Control and Prevention 2003).

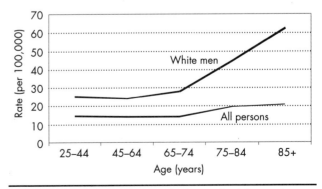

FIGURE 2–2. Suicide rates in the United States by age in 1998.

TABLE 2–5. Prevalence of selected psychiatric disorders among older adults in selected treatment facilities

Study/site	Reference	N	Age (years)	Measurement	Disorder	Prevalence
Intermediate-care facility	Rovner et al. 1986	50	Mean age = 83	Standardized interviews	Major depression	6.0%
Long-term care facility	Parmelee et al. 1989	708	Mean age = 84	DSM-III-R checklist	Major depression	12.4%
				GDS	Minor depression	30.5%
Acute-care facility	Koenig et al. 1988	171	65+	Screening and modified DIS	Major depression	11.5%
					Minor depression	23.0%
Primary care facility	Lyness et al. 1999	224	60+	SCID	Major depression	6.5%
				Ham-D	Minor depression	5.2%
Long-term care facility	Teresi et al. 2001	319	Mean age = 85	Structured psychiatric interviews	Major depression	14.4%

Note. DIS = Diagnostic Interview Schedule (Robins et al. 1981); GDS = Geriatric Depression Scale (Yesavage et al. 1983); Ham-D = Hamilton Rating Scale for Depression (Williams 1988); SCID = Structured Clinical Interview for DSM-III-R (Spitzer et al. 1992).

The century-long trend for suicide rates increasing with age has flattened. Why has this happened? The suicide rate at any point in time is determined by at least three factors: age, generational or cohort effects, and unique stressors for a particular age group at a particular point in time (i.e., period effects). Both age and generational effects were shown to be predictors of suicide in the United States since 1900 in a study by G. E. Murphy and Wetzel (1980). The generational effect was illustrated in a study by Haas and Hendin (1983). Age groups were studied at four points in time from 1908 to 1970. Cohorts in the 15- to 24-year-old age group showed significantly different suicide rates. The 15- to 24-year-olds in 1908 showed a suicide rate of 13.5 per 100,000; in contrast, the rate of the same age group in 1923 showed a rate of 6.3 per 100,000. The 1908 cohort continued to show higher rates of suicide than the 1923 cohort at every age through life, although both cohorts showed increases in suicide rates with age.

In 2000, the suicide rate was 12.6 per 100,000 for those age 65–74, 17.7 per 100,000 for those age 75–84, and 19.4 per 100,000 for those age 85 or older (Centers for Disease Control and Prevention 2002). For all cohorts combined, annual national suicide rates have stabilized at about 10–13 per 100,000 since 1941 (McIntosh et al. 1994).

In a study of suicides in England and Wales, E. Murphy and colleagues (1986) were able to show a marked period effect. In a cohort analysis of recorded suicides from 1921 to 1980, a decline in suicide rates of successively older cohorts was identified. (This finding contrasts with figures in the United States.) Murphy postulated the effect of period events—specifically, World War II and the detoxification of domestic gas. The last hypothesis is especially intriguing. Before the early 1960s, domestic gas in England and Wales contained large amounts of carbon monoxide. One of the more popular means of suicide, particularly among middle-aged and elderly individuals, was putting one's head in a gas oven. As domestic gas was converted to a methane-based product in the 1960s, the rate of gas poisoning in the more elderly groups decreased dramatically. This decrease was not offset by increasing rates of suicide by other means, suggesting that withdrawal of a method of suicide could result in a net saving of life.

It is clear from these historical studies that many factors contribute to changing rates in at least one indicator of psychiatric disorder—that is, suicide. Concomitant changes in other factors are less well understood but may be especially relevant to the study of psychiatric disorders in elderly persons. Klerman et al. (1985) suggested that the relatively low prevalence of depression in the 1980s among late-life cohorts might have been the result of a cohort effect. Current cohorts of older adults appear remarkably protected against severe or clinically diagnosed depressive disorders. Younger cohorts, in contrast, have had higher rates of major depression throughout the life cycle. Because there is no reason to expect the rates for younger cohorts to decrease as they enter late life—that is, there is no evidence of a period effect—the prevalence of major depression in late life may increase in future years.

Age, period, and cohort effects on suicide rates also have been anticipated for future decades. Aging is assumed to be a risk factor for suicide, as in the past. Period effects could work for or against increased age effects. Proliferation of how-to manuals for suicide and dramatic erosion of economic conditions could elevate risk; enhanced pain management and palliative care services, improvement in economic conditions, and advances in treatment of depression and Alzheimer's disease could decrease risk (McIntosh et al. 1994). The sheer size of the baby-boom cohort may presage extremely high absolute frequency and rates of suicide in the decades ahead, although earlier elevated rates in this cohort may mean that surviving members are more suicide resistant (Manton et al. 1987; McIntosh et al. 1994). If the baby-boom cohort depletes economic resources, there is some concern for elevated suicide rates among subsequent cohorts (the baby busters, followed by the baby boomlet or echo cohort). A historical perspective enables public health workers to anticipate future needs and plan preventive services targeted to subgroups of the population at potentially high risk.

An additional historical consideration in the study of psychiatric disorders is the study of incidence and duration of these disorders. Cumulative incidence, the probability of developing a disorder over a specified time (usually 1 year), is less important to the health care provider at a given point in time but is very relevant to planning for services in the future. The duration of a psychiatric disorder in late life, such as senile dementia, interacts with both incidence and prevalence. For example, the incidence of primary degenerative dementia or senile dementia of the Alzheimer's type appears to have been relatively unchanged over the past 15–20 years (although accurate studies are still lacking). Nevertheless, patients with dementia currently receive better health care and appear to follow the general trend of the aging population—an increased life expectancy. Therefore, in addition to a higher number of cases because there are more older adults at risk, the prevalence of the disorder over time is increasing, leading to a greater burden of dementia within the community (Gruenberg 1978).

Etiological Studies

One of the more important tasks in epidemiology is to identify factors that can either predispose individuals to developing psychiatric disorders or precipitate such disorders (Blazer and Jordan 1985). Other factors can be identified that are associated with the prevalence of a disorder, but the antecedent/consequent relationship has not been established. For practical purposes in this discussion, we identify all of these as "risk factors." These factors generally fall into several categories, including genetic or biological factors, environmental or chemical factors, and social factors. Examples of each are provided below. In addition, the presence of a comorbid physical or mental condition or disorder often leads to the development of psychiatric symptoms or another disorder.

The contribution of epidemiology to uncovering hereditary trends in mental disorders is best illustrated by the work in senile dementia. Heston et al. (1981) studied the relatives of 125 probands who had dementia of the Alzheimer's type (as identified at autopsy). The risk of dementia in first-degree relatives varied with the age of the person at the onset of dementia. Those persons who were first-degree relatives of someone with Alzheimer's disease were more likely to develop the disease earlier in life, suggesting that the inherited form of Alzheimer's disease is associated with an accelerated onset. Barclay et al. (1986) reported that a family history for dementia was positive in 35.9% of the patients with Alzheimer's disease, compared with 5.6% of the individuals who were cognitively intact.

Folstein and Breitner (1981) suggested that a subtype of Alzheimer's disease may be transmitted as an autosomal dominant trait with complete penetrance (Chase et al. 1983). In their original investigation, Folstein and Breitner found that the presence of aphasia and apraxia distinguished patients with a primary degenerative dementia who had a family history of the disease from those who did not have such a history. In a study of 39 cases of Alzheimer's disease, patients with relatives who had the disease were less often able to complete a sentence on the MMSE than were those who did not have afflicted relatives ($P<0.05$). Among those individuals who were unable to write a sentence, the investigators found a fourfold increased risk of dementia compared with the general population. In a follow-up study, Folstein and colleagues (1985) found that among 54 nursing home patients diagnosed with Alzheimer's disease, 40 were considered aphasic and agraphic and 14 were not. The first-degree relatives of the aphasic and agraphic patients with primary degenerative disorder had a 44% risk

of senile dementia by age 90, approaching the 50% rate for a genetic disorder that is autosomal dominant with complete penetrance.

Other biological risk factors have been identified. Research in Alzheimer's disease and dementia has focused on the ε4 allele of the *APOE* gene (Evans et al. 1997; A.M. Saunders et al. 1993). That is, the ε4 allele is a susceptibility gene in that some (but not all) persons with the allele develop dementia. Some studies have also found a relation between the *APOE3* and *APOE4* alleles and the onset of late-life depression (Krishnan et al. 1996), whereas other studies did not find a link between genotype and change in the number of depressive symptoms (Mauricio et al. 2000).

Investigators have suggested an association between early-onset Alzheimer's disease and Down syndrome, suggesting a common biological or genetic mechanism. Heyman et al. (1983) studied 68 patients with Alzheimer's disease who had experienced clinical onset before age 70. Secondary cases of dementia were found in 17 (25%) of the families, affecting 22 of the probands' siblings and parents. An increased frequency of Down syndrome was observed among relatives of the probands, a rate of 3.6 per 1,000, compared with the expected rate of 1.3 per 1,000. Heston et al. (1981) not only found an excess of Down syndrome in the families of patients with Alzheimer's disease but also identified an increased frequency of lymphoma and immune system disorder diatheses among family members, suggesting that immune system disorders and an increased risk for Alzheimer's disease are associated.

Physical agents in the environment may lead to cognitive problems and other psychiatric symptoms. Two illustrative studies show the effect of such agents on the brain. J.S. Goodwin et al. (1983) studied 260 noninstitutionalized men and women between ages 60 and 94. On clinical examination, these individuals were not found to have serious illness or to be clinically malnourished or vitamin deficient. Dietary intake for these subjects was calculated: the nutrients measured included protein, vitamin C, vitamin B_{12}, folic acid, riboflavin, thiamine, niacin, and pyridoxine. Blood samples were obtained to determine the blood levels of these specific nutrients. The investigators discovered a significant relation between scores on memory tests and blood levels of vitamin C and folic acid in these generally well-functioning older adults. Henderson et al. (1992) found a relation between Alzheimer's disease and starvation/malnutrition in a case-control study. These results suggest that variables, such as nutrient levels, may provide an opportunity for intervention in the relation between cognitive functioning and primary (innate) and secondary (environmentally induced) changes with aging. Gerontologists have long sought such intervening variables that may allow clinical intervention to prevent or mitigate deficits that were previously ascribed to primary aging.

Parker et al. (1983) investigated the relation between alcohol use and cognitive functioning. In the study, 1,937 employed men and women who were asked about their alcohol consumption during the previous month. In addition, vocabulary skills and abstraction abilities were examined. Results from the study suggested a linear relation between the amount of alcohol consumption during the previous month and cognitive impairment. The relation held both for the men and for the women whose drinking patterns resembled the men's. This model suggests that cognitive performance may be decreased by alcohol consumption before the postintoxication period, and because this relationship is linear, even moderate alcohol intake may lead to impairment in cognitive functioning. The implications of these findings for the elderly are evident.

Environmental agents such as bodily injury also can be factors. Studies of the association between prior head trauma and the development of Alzheimer's disease have been inconclusive. Mortimer et al. (1991) pooled data from 11 retrospective studies and concluded that head trauma increased the risk of Alzheimer's disease (relative risk = 1.82). In a prospective study of 6,645 patients age 55 or older, however, mild head trauma was not a risk factor for dementia or Alzheimer's disease (Mehta et al. 1999). Other chemical agents such as medication have the potential to affect the brain. Estrogen has been shown in some studies to have a protective effect against dementia (Kawas et al. 1997), yet other studies have found that estrogen was not protective against cognitive decline (Fillenbaum et al. 2001). Some research has found a protective effect of nonsteroidal anti-inflammatory drug use in Alzheimer's disease (Anthony et al. 2000).

By far the most frequently investigated environmental factors associated with psychiatric disorders are social factors. Many investigators believe that the changing roles and circumstances of older adults can cause stress and therefore contribute to the onset of psychiatric disorders and cognitive difficulties in older adults. In a study of 986 community-dwelling older adults, Blazer (1980a) found the crude estimate of relative risk for mental health impairment to be 2.14, given a life event score of 150 or greater on the Schedule of Recent Events (Holmes and Rahe 1967). A relative risk of 1.73 ($P < 0.01$) was estimated when a binary regression procedure was used, controlling for physical health, economic status, social support, and age. In a study of individuals age 55 or older, Murrell et al. (1983) found that social factors, including widowhood, divorce, separation, and decreased income, were related to depressive symptomatology in the community.

In the LASA study, major depression was associated with being unmarried; having functional limitation, perceived loneliness, internal locus of control, and poorer self-perceived health; and not receiving instrumental social support (Beekman et al. 1995). In the Duke ECA study, the recent experience of negative life events and poor social support were associated with major depression (Blazer et al. 1987b). Cognitive impairment has been shown to be associated with poorer self-rated health (Christensen et al. 1994). Impairment or dissatisfaction with the social network has been reported to be associated with anxiety symptoms in late life (Forsell and Winblad 1998). Patterson et al. (1997) found that older patients with schizophrenia had more impairments in social functioning compared with control subjects.

Nevertheless, the study of social factors in relation to psychiatric disorders must not be viewed simplistically. The mitigating effect of social support, the perception of a stressful life event (as well as the actual occurrence of the event), the expectancy of an event, and the perceived importance of an event all may contribute to the effect of environmental stress on the older adult. Blazer (2002) suggested several possible hypotheses by which social factors, specifically social stressors and social support, may influence the onset of depressive disorders in late life:

- Demographic factors, such as age, gender, and race, may contribute to the onset of depression. For example, prejudice related to age, such as loss of social roles, may contribute to depression onset.
- Early experiences, especially childhood traumas and impoverishment, may increase the risk for the onset of depression, regardless of age. For example, childhood deprivation may determine in part adult social relationships, which may indirectly contribute to late-life depression.
- Recent social stressors may precipitate a depressive disorder in older adults or aggravate the outcome of a disorder.
- An impaired social network, such as the absence of a spouse, few family members, and few friends, increases the risk for depression in late life.
- A decline in social interaction, perception of social support, and tangible (or instrumental) support leads to depression in late life.
- Poor social integration may lead directly to the onset and persistence of late-life depression. The absence of strong religious affiliations and an unstable environ-

ment may contribute to the onset and outcome of depression.

• The causal relation between social stressors and late-life depression may be buffered by both the social network and social support.

Finally, issues of comorbidity between psychiatric symptoms and disorders and physical health are important in late life. Psychiatric symptoms and physical and mental conditions may themselves lead to the development of other psychiatric symptoms and impairment. Depression has been shown to be a risk factor for declines in physical functioning (Penninx et al. 1998), and declines in physical functioning have been shown to be a risk factor for depression (Kennedy et al. 1990). Studies also have shown that disability in daily life is associated with hallucinations and delusions in late life (Ostling and Skoog 2002). In cross-sectional studies, cognitive impairment has been associated with depressive symptoms (Yaffe et al. 1999). In addition, some studies have shown depression to be a risk factor for decline in cognitive function (Devanand et al. 1996). Finally, a history of depression or anxiety has been shown to be a risk factor for depression or anxiety symptoms in late life (Forsell 2000).

From these examples, it is clear that both psychiatric disorders and symptoms in late life can have multiple causes and that these factors may interact with one another to produce adverse outcomes.

Health Service Utilization

Epidemiological studies provide a disturbing profile of the use of mental health services by elderly persons. Although older adults are less likely than those in any other age group to use community-based psychiatric services, they are more likely to use psychotropic medication. In a study of three of the ECA communities (New Haven, Connecticut; Baltimore, Maryland; and St. Louis, Missouri), Shapiro et al. (1984) found that 6%–7% of older adults had made a visit to a health care provider for mental health reasons during the previous 6 months. Those in the group age 65 or older infrequently received care from mental health specialists, even if they were identified in the community as having a DSM-III (American Psychiatric Association 1980) psychiatric disorder or severe cognitive impairment. German et al. (1985) analyzed the data from Baltimore in greater detail. Of those persons younger than 65, 8.7% had made a visit to a specialty or primary care provider for mental health care during the

6 months prior to the interview. For those age 64–74, the rate was 4.2%; of those age 75 or older, only 1.4% received such care. In the 75 or older age group, not one person among the 292 individuals interviewed saw a specialty mental health care provider. The investigators concluded that the likeliest source of care for older individuals with emotional or psychiatric problems is their primary care provider, within the context of a visit for physical medical problems.

In contrast, the use of psychotropic drugs is high among older adults. Hanlon et al. (1992) found that only 12.5% of community-dwelling persons older than 65 years during 1986 were taking central nervous system drugs, and psychotropic medications were the second most frequently used therapeutic class of medication. Blazer et al. (2000a) recently reported that the use of antidepressants in community-dwelling older adults increased from 1986 to 1996. Blazer et al. (2000b) also noted a simultaneous increase in the use of antianxiety, sedative, and hypnotic medications in this population.

Even though a high proportion of older adults uses psychotropic medications, their disorders, such as depression, remain untreated. Unutzer et al. (2000) found in a study of health maintenance organization enrollees that 4%–7% of the older adults received treatment for depression, but most individuals with probable depression did not receive treatment. Similarly, Steffens et al. (2000) recently found in the Cache County Study that only 35.7% of the older adults with major depression were taking an antidepressant. A total of 27.4% of those with major depression were taking a sedative-hypnotic.

The value of community surveys does not end with a description of patterns of health services use, however. Such investigations are especially useful for determining the need for service for noninstitutionalized and institutionalized elderly persons. By sampling elderly community-dwelling populations, researchers can collect data on the proportion of older adults with impairment, need for services, and perceived needs or demands for services and the current use of services. This information can be used by government and private agencies to chart effective assessment, treatment, and prevention programs. This development is especially relevant to the care of older adults because they tend to be isolated, their psychiatric impairment may be masked, and they are less active advocates for their mental health needs than are younger persons. In summary, community studies of older adults have shown that the prevalence of psychiatric disorders and psychiatric symptoms in older adults is significant, which has implications for all types of health service utilization.

References

Alexopoulos GS, Meyers BS, Young RC, et al: 'Vascular depression' hypothesis. Arch Gen Psychiatry 54:915–922, 1997

American Psychiatric Association: Diagnostic and Statistical Manual of Mental Disorders, 3rd Edition. Washington, DC, American Psychiatric Association, 1980

American Psychiatric Association: Diagnostic and Statistical Manual of Mental Disorders, 3rd Edition, Revised. Washington, DC, American Psychiatric Association, 1987

American Psychiatric Association: Diagnostic and Statistical Manual of Mental Disorders, 4th Edition. Washington, DC, American Psychiatric Association, 1994

American Psychiatric Association: Diagnostic and Statistical Manual of Mental Disorders, 4th Edition, Text Revision. Washington, DC, American Psychiatric Association, 2000

Anthony JC, Breitner JC, Zandi PP, et al: Reduced prevalence of AD in users of NSAIDs and H2 receptor antagonists: the Cache County Study. Neurology 54:2066–2071, 2000

Bachman DL, Wolf PA, Linn RT, et al: Incidence of dementia and probable Alzheimer's disease in a general population: the Framingham Study. Neurology 43:515–519, 1993

Barclay LL, Kheyfets S, Zemcov A, et al: Risk factors in Alzheimer's disease, in Alzheimer's Disease and Parkinson's Disease: Strategies for Research and Development. Edited by Fisher A, Hanin I, Lachman C. New York, Plenum, 1986, pp 141–146

Beekman ATF, Deeg DJH, van Tilberg T, et al: Major and minor depression in later life: a study of prevalence and risk factors. J Affect Disord 36:65–75, 1995

Beekman ATF, Copeland JRM, Prince MJ: Review of community prevalence of depression in late life. Br J Psychiatry 174:307–311, 1999

Bland RC, Newman SC, Orn H: Prevalence of psychiatric disorders in the elderly in Edmonton. Acta Psychiatr Scand Suppl 338:57–63, 1988

Blazer DG: Life events, mental health functioning and the use of health care services by the elderly. Am J Public Health 70:1174–1179, 1980a

Blazer DG: The diagnosis of depression in the elderly. J Am Geriatr Soc 28:52–58, 1980b

Blazer DG: The epidemiology of late life depression. J Am Geriatr Soc 30:587–592, 1982

Blazer DG: Psychiatry and the oldest old. Am J Psychiatry 157:1915–1924, 2000

Blazer DG: Depression in Late Life, 3rd Edition. New York, Springer, 2002

Blazer DG, Houpt JL: Perception of poor health in the healthy older adult. J Am Geriatr Soc 27:330–334, 1979

Blazer DG, Jordan K: Epidemiology of psychiatric disorders and cognitive problems in the elderly, in Psychiatry, Vol 3. Edited by Michels R, Cavenar JO. Philadelphia, PA, JB Lippincott, 1985, pp 1–12

Blazer D, Kaplan B: Controversies in community-based psychiatric epidemiology. Arch Gen Psychiatry 57:227–228, 2000

Blazer D, Bachar JR, Hughes DC: Major depression with melancholia: a comparison of middle-aged and elderly adults. J Am Geriatr Soc 35:927–932, 1987a

Blazer D, Hughes DC, George LK: The epidemiology of depression in an elderly community population. Gerontologist 27:281–287, 1987b

Blazer D, Swartz M, Woodbury M, et al: Depressive symptoms and depressive diagnoses in a community population. Arch Gen Psychiatry 45:1078–1084, 1988

Blazer D, Woodbury M, Hughes D, et al: A statistical analysis of the classification of depression in a mixed community and clinical sample. J Affect Disord 16:11–20, 1989

Blazer D, Burchett B, Service C, et al: The association of age and depression among the elderly: an epidemiologic exploration. J Gerontol A Biol Sci Med Sci 46:M210–215, 1991a

Blazer D, Hughes D, George L: Generalized anxiety disorder, in Psychiatric Disorders in America: The Epidemiologic Catchment Area Study. Edited by Robins L, Regier D. New York, Free Press, 1991b, pp 180–203

Blazer DG, Hybels CF, Simonsick E, et al: Marked differences in antidepressant use by race in an elderly community sample: 1986–1996. Am J Psychiatry 157:1089–1094, 2000a

Blazer DG, Hybels CF, Simonsick E, et al: Sedative, hypnotic and anti-anxiety medication use in an aging cohort over ten years: a racial comparison. J Am Geriatr Soc 48:1073–1079, 2000b

Bureau of the Census: Vital Statistics Special Reports, Vol 15, No 21. Washington, DC, U.S. Census Bureau, 1973, pp 217–243

Burns BJ, Larson DB, Goldstrom ID, et al: Mental disorder among nursing home patients: preliminary findings from the National Nursing Home Survey Pretest. Int J Geriatr Psychiatry 3:27–35, 1988

Busse A, Bischkopf J, Riedel-Heller SG, et al: Mild cognitive impairment: prevalence and incidence according to different diagnostic criteria. Results of the Leipzig Longitudinal Study of the Aged (LEILA /5+). Br J Psychiatry 182:449–454, 2003

Callahan CM, Hendrie HC, Tierney WM: Documentation and evaluation of cognitive impairment in elderly primary care patients. Ann Intern Med 122:422–429, 1995

Canadian Study of Health and Aging Working Group: Canadian Study of Health and Aging: study methods and prevalence of dementia. CMAJ 150:899–912, 1994

Centers for Disease Control and Prevention, National Center for Health Statistics: Death rates for suicide, 1950–2000, in Health, United States, 2002. Centers for Disease Control and Prevention, National Center for Health Statistics. Available at: http://infoplease.com/ipa/A0779940.html. Accessed August 18, 2003.

Centers for Disease Control and Prevention, National Center for Health Statistics: WISQARS injury mortality report, suicide injury deaths and rates per 100,000 white, non-Hispanic males, ages 70–85+, ICD-10 codes: X60–X84, Y87.0. Available at http://webapp.cdc.gov/sasweb/ncipc/mortrate10.html. Accessed September 23, 2003.

Chase GA, Folstein MF, Breitner JCS, et al: The use of life tables and survival analyses in testing genetic hypotheses with an application to Alzheimer's disease. Am J Epidemiol 7:590–597, 1983

Christensen H, Jorm AF, Henderson AS, et al: The relationship between health and cognitive functioning in a sample of elderly people in the community. Age Ageing 23:204–212, 1994

Christenson R, Blazer D: Epidemiology of persecutory ideation in an elderly population in the community. Am J Psychiatry 141:1088–1091, 1984

Copeland J: What is a "case"? A case for what?, in What Is a Case: The Problem of Definition in Psychiatric Community Surveys. Edited by Wing J, Bebbington P, Robins L. London, Grant McIntyre, 1981, pp 9–11

Copeland JRM, Kelleher MJ, Kellett JM, et al: A semi-structured clinical interview for the assessment of diagnosis and mental state in the elderly. Psychol Med 6:439–449, 1976

Copeland JRM, Dewey ME, Wood N, et al: Range of mental illness among the elderly in the community: prevalence in Liverpool using the GMS-AGECAT package. Br J Psychiatry 150:815–823, 1987

Copeland JRM, Davidson IA, Dewey ME, et al: Alzheimer's disease, other dementias, depression, and pseudodementia: prevalence, incidence, and three-year outcome in Liverpool. Br J Psychiatry 161:230–239, 1992

Copeland JRM, Dewey ME, Scott A, et al: Schizophrenia and delusional disorder in older age: community prevalence, incidence, comorbidity, and outcome. Schizophr Bull 24:153–161, 1998

Copeland JRM, Beekman ATF, Dewey ME, et al: Depression in Europe: geographic distribution among older people. Br J Psychiatry 174:312–321, 1999

Cornoni-Huntley J, Brock D, Ostfeld A, et al: Established Populations for Epidemiologic Studies of the Elderly: Resource Data Book. Bethesda, MD, National Institute on Aging, 1986

Devanand DP, Sano M, Tang M-X, et al: Depressed mood and the incidence of Alzheimer's disease in the elderly living in the community. Arch Gen Psychiatry 53:175–182, 1996

Evans DA, Funkenstein HH, Albert MS, et al: Prevalence of Alzheimer's disease in a community population of older persons: higher than previously reported. JAMA 262:2551–2556, 1989

Evans DA, Beckett LA, Field T: Apolipoprotein E e4 and incidence of Alzheimer's disease in a community population of older persons. JAMA 277:822–824, 1997

Federal Interagency Forum on Aging Related Statistics: Older Americans 2000: Key Indicators of Well-Being. Washington, DC, Federal Interagency Forum on Aging Related Statistics, 2000

Fillenbaum GG, Hanlon JT, Landerman LR, et al: Impact of estrogen use on decline in cognitive function in a representative sample of older community-resident women. Am J Epidemiol 153:137–144, 2001

First MB, Spitzer RL, Gibbon M, et al: Structured Clinical Interview for DSM-IV Axis I Disorders, Research Version. Washington, DC, American Psychiatric Association, 1997

Folstein MF, Breitner JCS: Language disorder predicts familial Alzheimer's disease. Johns Hopkins Medical Journal 149:145–147, 1981

Folstein MF, Folstein SE, McHugh P: Mini-Mental State: a practical method for grading the cognitive state of patients for clinicians. J Psychiatr Res 12:189–198, 1975

Folstein MF, Anthony JC, Parhad I, et al: The meaning of cognitive impairment in the elderly. J Am Geriatr Soc 33:228–235, 1985

Forsell Y: Predictors for depression, anxiety and psychotic symptoms in a very elderly population: data from a 3-year follow-up study. Soc Psychiatry Psychiatr Epidemiol 35:259–263, 2000

Forsell Y, Winblad B: Feelings of anxiety and associated variables in a very elderly population. Int J Geriatr Psychiatry 13:454–458, 1998

Forsell Y, Winblad B: Incidence of major depression in a very elderly population. Int J Geriatr Psychiatry 14:368–372, 1999

German PS, Shapiro S, Skinner EA: Mental health of the elderly: use of health and mental health services. J Am Geriatr Soc 33:246–252, 1985

Goodwin D, Guze S: Psychiatric Diagnosis. New York, Oxford University Press, 1979

Goodwin JS, Goodwin JM, Garry PJ: Association between nutritional status and cognitive functioning in a healthy elderly population. JAMA 249:2917–2921, 1983

Graham JE, Rockwood K, Beattie BL, et al: Prevalence and severity of cognitive impairment with and without dementia in an elderly population. Lancet 349:1793–1796, 1997

Gruenberg EM: Epidemiology of senile dementia, in Neurological Epidemiology. Edited by Schoenberg BS. New York, Raven, 1978, pp 437–457

Gurland B, Golden RR, Teresi JA, et al: The SHORT-CARE: an efficient instrument for the assessment of depression, dementia and disability. J Gerontol 39:166–169, 1984

Haas AP, Hendin H: Suicide among older people: projections for the future. Suicide Life Threat Behav 13:147–154, 1983

Hanlon JT, Fillenbaum GG, Burchett B, et al: Drug-use patterns among Black and nonblack community-dwelling elderly. Ann Pharmacother 26:679–685, 1992

Hathaway SR, McKinley JC: Minnesota Multiphasic Personality Inventory, Revised Edition. Minneapolis, University of Minnesota, 1970

Hazzard W: Introduction: the practice of geriatric medicine, in Principles of Geriatric Medicine and Gerontology. Edited by Hazzard W, Bierman E, Blass J, et al. New York, McGraw-Hill, 1994, pp xxiii–xxiv

Hebert LE, Scherr PA, Beckett LA, et al: Age-specific incidence of Alzheimer's disease in a community population. JAMA 273:1354–1359, 1995

Heeren TJ, Lagaay AM, Hijmans W, et al: Prevalence of dementia in the 'oldest old' of a Dutch community. J Am Geriatr Soc 39:755–759, 1991

Henderson AS, Jorm AF, Korten AE, et al: Environmental risk factors for Alzheimer's disease: the relationship to age of onset and to familial or sporadic types. Psychol Med 22:429–436, 1992

Henderson AS, Jorm AF, MacKinnon A, et al: The prevalence of depressive disorders and the distribution of depressive symptoms in later life: a survey using Draft ICD-10 and DSM-III-R. Psychol Med 23:719–729, 1993

Henderson AS, Korten AE, Jacomb PA, et al: The course of depression in the elderly: a longitudinal community-based study in Australia. Psychol Med 27:119–129, 1997

Henderson AS, Korten AE, Levings C, et al: Psychotic symptoms in the elderly: a prospective study in a population sample. Int J Geriatr Psychiatry 13:484–492, 1998

Heston LL, Mastri AR, Anderson E, et al: Dementia of the Alzheimer's type: clinical genetics, natural history, and associated conditions. Arch Gen Psychiatry 38:1085–1090, 1981

Heyman A, Wilkinson WE, Hurwitz BJ, et al: Alzheimer's disease: genetic aspects and associated disorders. Ann Neurol 14:507–515, 1983

Hilliard JR, Holland JM, Ramm D: Christmas and psychopathology: data from a psychiatric emergency room population. Arch Gen Psychiatry 38:377–381, 1981

Holmes TH, Rahe RH: The Social Readjustment Rating Scale. J Psychosom Res 11:213–218, 1967

Kawas C, Resnick S, Morrison A, et al: A prospective study of estrogen replacement therapy and the risk of developing Alzheimer's disease: the Baltimore Longitudinal Study of Aging. Neurology 48:1517–1521, 1997

Kay DWK, Bergmann K, Foster EM, et al: Mental illness and hospital usage in the elderly: a random sample followed up. Compr Psychiatry 11:26–35, 1970

Kay DWK, Henderson AS, Scott R, et al: Dementia and depression among the elderly living in the Hobart community: the effect of the diagnostic criteria on the prevalence rates. Psychol Med 15:771–788, 1985

Kennedy GJ, Kelman HR, Thomas C: The emergence of depressive symptoms in late life: the importance of declining health and increasing disability. J Community Health 15:93–103, 1990

Kleinbaum DG, Kupper LL, Morgenstern H: Epidemiologic Research. New York, Van Nostrand Reinhold, 1982, pp 320–376

Klerman GL, Lavori PW, Rice J, et al: Birth-cohort trends in rates of major depression among relatives of patients with affective disorder. Arch Gen Psychiatry 42:689–694, 1985

Koenig HG, Meador KG, Cohen HJ, et al: Depression in elderly hospitalized patients with medical illness. Arch Intern Med 148:1929–1936, 1988

Krishnan KRR, Tupler LA, Ritchie JC, et al: Apolipoprotein E-e4 frequency in geriatric depression. Biol Psychiatry 40:69–71, 1996

Lester D: Temporal variation in suicide and homicide. Am J Epidemiol 109:517–520, 1979

Lindesay J, Briggs K, Murphy E: The Guy's/Age Concern Survey: prevalence rates of cognitive impairment, depression and anxiety in an urban elderly community. Br J Psychiatry 155:317–329, 1989

Lyness JM, King DA, Cox C, et al: The importance of subsyndromal depression in older primary care patients: prevalence and associated functional disability. J Am Geriatr Soc 47:647–652, 1999

MacMahon B, Pugh TF: Epidemiology: Principles and Methods. Boston, MA, Little, Brown, 1970

Manton KG, Blazer DG, Woodbury MA: Suicide in middle age and later life: sex- and race-specific life table and cohort analyses. J Gerontol 42:219–227, 1987

Mauricio M, O'Hara R, Yesavage JA, et al: A longitudinal study of apolipoprotein-E genotype and depressive symptoms in community-dwelling older adults. Am J Geriatr Psychiatry 8:196–200, 2000

McIntosh JL, Santos JF, Hubbard RW, et al: Elder Suicide: Research, Theory, and Treatment. Washington, DC, American Psychological Association, 1994

Mehta KM, Ott A, Kalmijn S, et al: Head trauma and risk of dementia and Alzheimer's disease: the Rotterdam Study. Neurology 53:1959–1962, 1999

Morris JN: Uses of Epidemiology, 3rd Edition. London, Churchill Livingstone, 1975

Mortimer JA, van Duijn CM, Chandra V, et al: Head trauma as a risk factor for Alzheimer's disease: a collaborative re-analysis of case-control studies. EURODEM Risk Factors Research Group. Int J Epidemiol 20 (suppl 2):S28–35, 1991

Moscicki EK: Identification of suicide risk factors using epidemiologic studies. Psychiatr Clin North Am 20:499–517, 1997

Murphy E, Lindesay J, Grundy E: Sixty years of suicide in England and Wales. Arch Gen Psychiatry 43:969–977, 1986

Murphy GE, Wetzel RD: Suicide risk by birth cohort in the United States, 1949–1974. Arch Gen Psychiatry 37:519–523, 1980

Murrell SA, Himmelfarb S, Wright K: Prevalence of depression and its correlates in older adults. Am J Epidemiol 117:173–185, 1983

Ostling S, Skoog I: Psychotic symptoms and paranoid ideation in a nondemented population-based sample of the very old. Arch Gen Psychiatry 59:53–59, 2002

Parker DA, Parker ES, Brody JA, et al: Alcohol use and cognitive loss among employed men and women. Am J Public Health 73:521–526, 1983

Parmelee PA, Katz IR, Lawton MP: Depression among institutionalized aged: assessment and prevalence estimation. J Gerontol A Biol Sci Med Sci 44:M22–M29, 1989

Patterson TL, Semple SJ, Shaw WS, et al: Self-reported social functioning among older patients with schizophrenia. Schizophr Res 27:199–210, 1997

Penninx BWJH, Guralnik JA, Ferrucci L, et al: Depressive symptoms and physical decline in community-dwelling older persons. JAMA 279:1720–1726, 1998

Pfeiffer E: A Short Portable Mental Status Questionnaire for the assessment of organic brain deficit in elderly patients. J Am Geriatr Soc 23:433–441, 1975

Pifer A, Bronte D: Introduction: Squaring the pyramid. Daedalus 115:1–12, 1986

Radloff LS: The CES-D scale: a self-report depression scale for research in the general population. Applied Psychological Measurement 1:385–401, 1977

Regier DA, Myers JK, Kramer M, et al: The NIMH Epidemiologic Catchment Area Program: historical context, major objectives and study population characteristics. Arch Gen Psychiatry 41:934–994, 1984

Regier DA, Boyd JH, Burke JD, et al: One-month prevalence of mental disorders in the United States. Arch Gen Psychiatry 45:977–986, 1988

Reynolds C, Frank E, Perel J, et al: Nortriptyline and interpersonal psychotherapy as maintenance therapies for recurrent major depression: a randomized controlled trial in patients older than 59 years. JAMA 281:39–45, 1999

Riedel-Heller SG, Busse A, Aurich C, et al: Prevalence of dementia according to DSM-III-R and ICD-10: results of the Leipzig Longitudinal Study of the Aged (LEILA 75+) Part 1. Br J Psychiatry 179:250–254, 2001

Roberts CJ: Epidemiology for Clinicians. London, Pitman Medical, 1977

Robins LN, Helzer JE, Croughan J, et al: National Institute of Mental Health Diagnostic Interview Schedule: its history, characteristics, and validity. Arch Gen Psychiatry 38:381–389, 1981

Rosch E: Principles of categorization, in Cognition and Categorization. Edited by Rosch E, Lloyd B. Hillsdale, NJ, Lawrence Erlbaum, 1978, pp 3–27

Roses AD: Apolipoprotein E affects the rate of Alzheimer's disease expression: beta-amyloid burden is a secondary consequence dependent on APOE genotype and duration of disease. J Neuropathol Exp Neurol 53:429–437, 1994

Roses AD: Genetic testing for Alzheimer disease: practical and ethical issues. Arch Neurol 54:1226–1229, 1997

Rovner BW, Kafonek S, Filipp L, et al: Prevalence of mental illness in a community nursing home. Am J Psychiatry 143:1446–1449, 1986

Saunders PA, Copeland JRM, Dewey ME, et al: Alcohol use and abuse in the elderly: findings from the Liverpool Longitudinal Study of Continuing Health in the Community. Int J Geriatr Psychiatry 4:103–108, 1989

Saunders AM, Schmader K, Breitner J: Apolipoprotein E epsilon 4 allele distributions in late-onset Alzheimer's disease and in other amyloid forming disease. Lancet 342:710–711, 1993

Shapiro S, Skinner EA, Kessler LG, et al: Utilization of health and mental health services. Arch Gen Psychiatry 41:971–982, 1984

Shoghi-Jadid K, Small G, Agdeppa E, et al: Localization of neurofibrillary tangles and beta-amyloid plaques in the brains of living patients with Alzheimer's disease. Am J Geriatr Psychiatry 10:24–35, 2002

Spitzer RL, Endicott J, Robins E: Research Diagnostic Criteria: rationale and reliability. Arch Gen Psychiatry 35:773–782, 1978

Spitzer R, Williams J, Gibbon M, et al: The Structured Clinical Interview for DSM-III-R (SCID), I: history, rationale, and description. Arch Gen Psychiatry 49:624–629, 1992

Steffens DC, Skoog I, Norton M, et al: Prevalence of depression and its treatment in an elderly population: the Cache County Study. Arch Gen Psychiatry 57:601–607, 2000

Stevens T, Livingston G, Kitchen G, et al: Islington study of dementia subtypes in the community. Br J Psychiatry 180:270–276, 2002

Strauss J, Gabriel K, Kokes R: Do psychiatric patients fit their diagnoses? Patterns of symptomatology as described with a biplot. J Nerv Ment Dis 167:105–113, 1981

Suzman R: Oldest old, in Encyclopedia of Aging. Edited by Maddox G. New York, Springer, 1995, pp 712–715

Teeter RB, Garetz FK, Miller WR, et al: Psychiatric disturbances of aged patients in skilled nursing homes. Am J Psychiatry 133:1430–1434, 1976

Teng EL, Chui HC: The Modified Mini-Mental State (3MS) Examination. J Clin Psychiatry 48:314–318, 1987

Teresi J, Abrams R, Holmes D, et al: Prevalence of depression and depression recognition in nursing homes. Soc Psychiatry Psychiatr Epidemiol 36:613–620, 2001

Unutzer J, Simon G, Belin T, et al: Care for depression in HMO patients aged 65 or older. J Am Geriatr Soc 48:871–878, 2000

Weissman M, Klerman G: Epidemiology of mental disorders. Arch Gen Psychiatry 25:705–715, 1978

Williams JBW: A structured interview guide for the Hamilton Depression Rating Scale. Arch Gen Psychiatry 45:742–747, 1988

World Health Organization: International Statistical Classification of Diseases and Related Health Problems, 10th Revision. Geneva, World Health Organization, 1992

Yaffe K, Blackwell T, Gore R, et al: Depressive symptoms and cognitive decline in nondemented elderly women. Arch Gen Psychiatry 56:425–430, 1999

Yesavage JA, Brink TL, Rose TL, et al: Development and validation of a geriatric depression screening scale. J Psychiatr Res 17:37–49, 1983

Zaudig M, Mittelhammer J, Hiller W, et al: SIDAM—a structured interview for the diagnosis of dementia of the Alzheimer type, multi-infarct dementia and dementias of other aetiology according to ICD-10 and DSM-III-R. Psychol Med 21:225–236, 1991

Physiological and Clinical Considerations of Geriatric Patient Care

Robert M. Kaiser, M.D.

Harvey Jay Cohen, M.D.

Grow old along with me!
The best is yet to be…

—*Robert Browning*

Will you still need me,
will you still feed me
When I'm sixty-four?

—*John Lennon and
Paul McCartney*

The burgeoning of the geriatric population is an unquestioned demographic fact in the early twenty-first century. People older than 65 years constitute one of the fastest growing segments of the United States population (Bureau of the Census 1996; Fried 2000). The conquest of childhood infectious disease, improvements in sanitation, and better nutrition all have contributed to increased survival (McKeown 1979), and medical innovation also has had a beneficial effect on morbidity and mortality (Hunick et al. 1997). People are living longer, and the numbers of elderly grow with each passing year. The average life span has lengthened significantly (Fried 2000; W. J. Hall 1997; Valliant and Mukamal 2001). Careful and sophisticated longitudinal studies of elderly populations in the United States, such as the Established Populations for the Epidemiological Studies of the El-

derly (Cornoni-Huntley et al. 1986) and the Baltimore Longitudinal Study of Aging (Shock 1984), have addressed how and why people are living to the eighth decade and beyond. Basic science has yielded fundamental anatomical, physiological, and genetic information about the aging process. A more complete picture of what aging entails has emerged.

How does aging occur? According to Armbrecht (2001), that perplexing question has been answered (to date incompletely) by two main theories: 1) a "programmed" theory of aging, in which genetics dictates how fast one ages and how long one lives; and 2) a "wear and tear" theory, in which continued injury overwhelms the organism's capacity to repair it. Of the several programmed theories, the cellular senescence theory is one of the best known. The number of times a cell can divide is fixed; this was noted by Hayflick when he cultivated human diploid fibroblasts in vitro. This theory is not without flaws. It fails to explain why nondividing cells such as brain cells age. The free radical theory is an excellent example of one widely endorsed wear and tear theory of aging. Free radicals, the products of oxidative metabolism, accumulate in cells and cause considerable damage over time; this cumulative damage affects the function of cells, tissues, and organs. This theory also has inconsistencies it cannot explain; the weakening in antioxidant defenses over time, which theoretically leads to more free radical damage, has not been definitively shown. The free radical theory does, however, provide a reasonable explanation for the age-related deterioration in physiological function (Armbrecht 2001).

The hallmarks of physiological change in the elderly are twofold: impaired homeostasis (also called *homeostenosis*) and increased vulnerability because of decreased reserve capacity (Armbrecht 2001; Taffet 1999). The ability of the organism to maintain a steady state—homeostasis—lessens with time. Consider two straightforward, representative examples: 1) in the elderly, the baroreceptor reflex, which triggers vasoconstriction in order to maintain normal blood pressure, is less robust, and the elderly are less able to respond quickly to intravascular volume depletion; and 2) when faced with repelling an invading microorganism, an older patient is less able to mount a strong immune response, therefore making it more difficult to fight infection effectively. Both of these situations clearly show how altered physiology leads the elderly patient to be more susceptible to harm. Thus, in the first situation above, an older person might become light-headed and possibly fall to the floor; in the second situation, the inability to repel a virulent streptococcus might lead to a severe upper respiratory infection or perhaps even a life-threatening pneumonia.

"Grow old along with me! The best is yet to be," proclaims Robert Browning optimistically in his famous poem. One might endorse Browning's belief that human relationships become deeper and richer with time, but the inevitability of physiological decline is also a reality that all human beings must face as they age. Lennon and McCartney's rather endearing song, which has a young man wondering what life will be like in the seventh decade, underscores that widespread apprehension about approaching infirmity. As time passes, none of us can expect—like an aspiring Olympic athlete—to run faster, throw farther, and leap higher. Age brings with it expected decrements in function. In this chapter, we detail the various physiological changes that occur with "normal aging"—in other words, those progressive changes that take place over time but not as a result of disease. We discuss

- Physiological changes in the major organ systems
- Geriatric syndromes
- Special implications for prescribing medications in the elderly because of age-related physiological changes
- Fundamental principles of geriatric assessment that follow from those expected physiological changes

Central Nervous System

The central nervous system undergoes several anatomical changes with age. In the brain, significant neuronal loss occurs in the locus coeruleus and the substantia nigra, and Purkinje's cells decrease in the cerebellum. Other areas of the brain also lose neurons, including the entorhinal cortex, hypothalamus, pons, medulla, and nucleus basalis of Meynert. Aging neurons nevertheless maintain the ability to make new synapses; and although the number of synapses may decrease, the size of the synapses may increase. The protein and myelin content of the brain decreases, and the brain becomes smaller and lighter. Both increases and decreases in the production of neurotransmitters in the brain occur with age, but the effect on brain function is unclear. Cholinergic transmission decreases but not uniformly. Dopamine levels decline, particularly in the striatum, and dopaminergic transmission is affected. Levels of norepinephrine rise with age, whereas serotonin decreases. Levels of glutamate receptors decline, but any connection to impaired glutamatergic transmission is unknown. Structural changes in cytoskeletal proteins occur, although the level of proteins is constant. The deposition of the amyloid in neurons damages them and may hasten cell death (Mattson 1999; Oskvig 1999; Taffet 1999; Whalley 2001).

Cognition and Aging

Various studies have documented a decline in cognitive function with age. Such decline may occur in several areas, including intelligence, ability to maintain attention, language, memory, learning, visuospatial function, and psychomotor function. These deficits do not occur uniformly across all areas nor do they occur in every person. Crystallized intelligence, an indication of accumulated knowledge or experience, does not change with age, but fluid intelligence, or novel problem-solving ability, begins to decline in the middle of the sixth decade and accelerates thereafter. Practical intelligence, which tracks procedural skills, may be stable or even improve with age. Aging adults may lose their ability to sustain attention over long periods. The capacity to recognize words does not change, but elderly adults are less able to name items. Short-term, or working, memory is unaffected, but there may be problems in accessing data from long-term memory. The time needed for the elderly to learn new information increases. Visuospatial tasks are more difficult, and both motor speed and response times decline with aging. Some evidence suggests that executive function, or the ability to conceive, organize, and carry out a plan or activity, may remain intact in the elderly (Ashman et al. 1999; Oskvig 1999).

Vision and Hearing

The elderly develop significant changes in the eye, which have important effects on vision. The weakening of the ciliary muscle, combined with the loss of elasticity in the lens, results in presbyopia; it then becomes difficult for an individual to focus on near objects, and bifocals may be needed. It is also difficult for the elderly to adapt to light because of rigidity of the pupil and increasing opacity of the lens. The elderly also show a decline in their ability to view objects at rest (static acuity) and in motion (dynamic acuity). Photooxidation leads to yellowing of the lens. As the lens changes with age, the increased scattering of light produces glare, which may be bothersome to elderly patients. With age, the lens opacifies, and a cataract can form; the lens becomes less transparent as a result of protein aggregations. Elderly patients are also at risk for age-related macular degeneration, which causes loss of central vision when drusen (yellowish-white deposits) accumulate in the retina (Kalina 1999; Taffett 1999).

Along with changes in vision, the elderly can expect alterations in the ear, which may lead to hearing loss in both high and low frequencies. In the middle ear, thickening of the tympanic membrane and degenerative changes in the ossicles occur, but these changes have an insignificant effect on function. In the inner ear, cochlear neurons are lost, and there are changes in the organ of Corti, basilar membrane, stria vascularis, and spiral ligament that also affect hearing. The degeneration of the organ of Corti is associated with high-frequency sensorineural hearing loss, whereas atrophy of the stria vascularis may cause hearing loss across all frequencies. The stiffening of the basilar membrane and atrophy of the spiral ligament both can result in loss of speech discrimination (Reed et al. 1999; Taffett 1999).

Cardiovascular System

The heart and blood vessels in the aging patient undergo significant anatomical alterations. These structural changes lead to changes in function. In addition, age-associated changes occur in the autonomic nervous system, and the response of the cardiovascular system to it, which have important physiological effects. The ability of the heart to beat faster and pump efficiently and the ease with which blood vessels dilate or constrict are markedly affected. Both cardiac output and cardiac reserve decrease (Lakatta 1999; Oskvig 1999; Taffet 1999).

With age, human blood vessels stiffen. Anatomically, the intimal layer of large arteries has a higher content of collagen, and the internal elastic lamina becomes frayed; the medial layer also undergoes significant changes with age, with disorientation, fragmentation, and degeneration of elastin fibers, followed by deposition of collagen, calcification, and cystic degeneration. The vessels are thicker and less distensible. The physiological results are a greater pulse wave velocity, early reflected pulse waves, and higher systolic blood pressures in older individuals. Higher pressures can increase the load on the heart and lead to left ventricular enlargement (Lakatta 1999; Oskvig 1999).

Higher aortic impedance caused by early reflected pulse waves requires longer myocardial contraction to maintain left ventricular function at rest. With prolonged contraction comes a reduction in the early ventricular filling rate and resultant diastolic dysfunction in some, but not all, older patients. To compensate for this reduction, the left atrium enlarges. The enlarged left atrium facilitates filling of the ventricle and raises left ventricular end-diastolic volume and stroke volume, thereby maintaining systolic heart function (Lakatta 1999).

The function of the heart during exercise, including the force and rate of contraction, is mediated by the sympathetic nervous system. Age-related changes in that system affect the adaptability of the heart and blood vessels to stress. In general, sympathetic nervous activity rises in the elderly patient, as evidenced by higher circulating levels of norepinephrine. Norepinephrine fills cardiac and vascular surface cell receptors, making them less sensitive. The β-adrenergic response of the heart during exercise is attenuated; a lower maximum heart rate and decreased force of contraction are the result. Similarly, large arteries do not respond as well to β-adrenergic stimulation. Their ability to dilate is reduced (Lakatta 1999; Seals and Esler 2000).

The older heart dilates during exercise to increase end-diastolic volume and maintain stroke volume, but cardiac output nonetheless declines with age. Because the heart stiffens, it empties less completely. This is the result of several factors, including increased afterload, decreased contractility of the heart, and the reduced inotropic effect of β-adrenergic stimulation to the heart. The decline in cardiac output also adversely affects oxygen use in the elderly adult. The decline in cardiac function with age may explain 50% of the reduction in maximum oxygen consumption that occurs (Lakatta 1999).

Respiratory System

Notable changes in the chest wall develop with age (Oskvig 1999; Taffett 1999). The thoracic cage becomes rounder, and the cartilaginous conducting airways enlarge, resulting in an increase in dead space. Neither of these changes is thought to have a significant effect on respiratory function. However, a more rigid chest wall does negatively affect the mechanical process of breathing. In the older individual, more work is required to expand the chest wall. Declining respiratory muscle strength, particularly in the intercostal muscles, and decreased endurance also affect the ability to breathe normally.

Changes in the lung itself and in the control of breathing negatively affect the respiratory system (Oskvig 1999; Taffet 1999). A loss of elastic tissue in the lung occurs, and the alveolar ducts and respiratory bronchioles enlarge. This enlargement leads to a loss of alveolar surface area; less tissue is available for gas exchange, and partial pressure of oxygen (PO_2) decreases at a rate of 0.5% per year. Higher closing volumes make full expansion of the airways more difficult, especially in the dependent areas of the lung. The loss of surface area combined with decreased expansion results in ventilation-perfusion mismatch and decreased oxygenation. The control of breathing is also altered in elderly patients. Low oxygen tension and high carbon dioxide levels fail to provide the same physiological stimulus to breathe. Furthermore, when the elderly are short of breath, the age-associated decrease in slow and forced vital capacity impairs their ability to respond as vigorously.

The elderly lung is less able to guard itself against infection (Taffet 1999). The mucociliary tree lining the respiratory tract lacks the same speed in rapidly ridding the lung of invading particles and microorganisms. With age, the ability to generate a sufficiently strong cough declines. The development of higher closing volumes further complicates defense against infection by making it harder to expel secretions from the lower areas of the lungs.

Some studies suggest that exercise training can slow the respiratory decline that occurs with aging. The age-related decrease in maximum oxygen consumption as well as the decreased responsiveness to low oxygen tension or high carbon dioxide levels can all improve with exercise. Although exercise is helpful, it cannot prevent the ultimate decline in pulmonary function (R.S. Schwartz and Buchner 1999).

Gastrointestinal System

As human beings age, numerous anatomical changes take place throughout the gastrointestinal tract, some of which are functionally significant (K.E. Hall and Wiley 1999; Majumdar et al. 1997; Taffet 1999). For the most part, the production of saliva is adequately maintained. Receding gums make the teeth more susceptible to den-

tal caries and subsequent tooth loss. The mastication of food may be incomplete. There are fewer myenteric ganglion cells, which affects the coordination of swallowing and may predispose some elderly patients to aspiration. The strength of esophageal contractions is diminished, but food nonetheless traverses the length of the esophagus uneventfully. The production of acid and pepsin by the stomach is mostly preserved. Both the stomach and the small intestine do not as easily dilate as a bolus of food enters, and transit through the large bowel may be slower. The small bowel less effectively absorbs vitamins and minerals (such as vitamin D, calcium, and iron) and sugars (such as xylose and lactose).

The liver, gallbladder, and pancreas continue to function well in the elderly patient (K.E. Hall and Wiley 1999; Majumdar et al. 1997; Taffet 1999). The liver loses hepatocytes and becomes smaller. Those cells remaining are less able to regenerate. In general, the liver's ability to manufacture binding proteins and metabolize drugs is stable, although considerable variability can be found between individuals. The liver makes fewer vitamin K–dependent factors. Liver transaminases and alkaline phosphatase remain unchanged. Few significant anatomical changes occur in the gallbladder, and its function remains intact. In the aging pancreas, there is parenchymal fibrosis, acinar atrophy, and fatty infiltration but no resulting impairment in the synthesis of pancreatic enzymes and bicarbonate. The role of the pancreas in digestive function is therefore unaffected.

Endocrine System

Prolactin

Levels of prolactin in aging women have been reported to increase, decrease, or remain the same, whereas those in men are slightly increased. None of these changes are believed to have an effect on normal function (Gruenewald and Matsumoto 1999).

Antidiuretic Hormone

Aging causes significant changes in antidiuretic hormone (ADH), and the body's response to it, which alter the older patient's ability to excrete free water—resulting in hyponatremia—or to prevent volume losses—resulting in dehydration. Basal ADH levels are normal to increased in the elderly; because renal free water clearance decreases with age, hyponatremia can more easily occur. However, when volume loss takes place, with subsequent hypotension, less ADH is released in older persons. In this particular clinical situation, other age-related changes are also at work to produce dehydration: 1) the kidney is less responsive to ADH, which impairs its effort to make more concentrated urine; and 2) aldosterone activity decreases, and natriuretic hormone activity increases, both of which inhibit renal conservation of sodium and restoration of normal volume. The impaired thirst mechanism in elderly people further exacerbates this scenario by preventing them from drinking adequate amounts of fluid to correct free water losses, thereby contributing further to dehydration (Gruenewald and Matsumoto 1999; Oskvig 1999; Perry 1999).

Corticotropin and Cortisol

Basal corticotropin levels are normal in the elderly. Neither the corticotropin pulse frequency nor its circadian rhythm of secretion is altered. Stimulation of the hypothalamic-pituitary-adrenal (HPA) axis by exogenous corticotropin produces the expected cortisol response, but the cortisol secretion rate actually declines. Cortisol levels remain the same because of a decrease in the cortisol metabolic clearance rate. When subjected to stress, the HPA axis produces higher peak cortisol levels, which then dissipate more slowly; this occurs because the negative feedback of cortisol on the HPA axis is less effective (Gruenewald and Matsumoto 1999).

Adrenal Androgens

Both dehydroepiandrosterone (DHEA) and dehydroepiandrosterone sulfate (DHEA-S) decrease significantly in the elderly. DHEA production peaks at age 20 and then declines (Fried and Walston 1999; Gruenewald and Matsumoto 1999).

Adrenal Medulla and Sympathetic Nervous System

In the elderly, secretion of norepinephrine increases and clearance decreases; plasma levels therefore increase. Epinephrine secretion and clearance both increase with age, so the level of epinephrine does not change. The level of sympathetic nervous system activity is increased in older persons, but both α-adrenergic and β-adrenergic receptors are less sensitive to stimulation (Gruenewald and Matsumoto 1999; Oskvig 1999; Seals and Esler 2000).

Renin, Angiotensin, and Aldosterone

An age-related decrease in plasma renin activity leads to reduced aldosterone secretion; aldosterone levels are thus reduced significantly. The rise in natriuretic hormone secretion in the elderly also serves to decrease aldosterone levels; higher levels of natriuretic hormone suppress renin secretion, plasma renin activity, and angiotensin II, further lowering aldosterone secretion. In addition, natriuretic hormone itself can inhibit aldosterone secretion. The ability of corticotropin to stimulate aldosterone secretion is unchanged in the aging adult. The overall decrease in aldosterone adversely affects sodium retention in the kidney and predisposes the elderly to dehydration, as discussed earlier in this chapter. Another consequence of lower aldosterone levels is an increased likelihood of hyperkalemia (Gruenewald and Matsumoto 1999).

Growth Hormone

Growth hormone levels peak at puberty and then decrease by 14% per decade. Both a decrease in growth hormone releasing hormone secretion and an increase in somatostatin are responsible for the decline in growth hormone. Insulin-like growth factor (IGF-1), which is produced by the liver and mediates the actions of growth hormone in the body, also diminishes gradually, at a rate of 7%–13% per decade. The decline in growth hormone with age may result in a decrease in both lean body mass and bone mass (Gruenewald and Matsumoto 1999; Perry 1999).

PTH, Vitamin D, and Calcium Regulation

The elderly generally consume insufficient calcium in the diet; in addition, calcium is less efficiently absorbed in the small intestine. Vitamin D is essential to that absorption, and levels of vitamin D, 25-hydroxy (25,D) and vitamin D, 1,25-dihydroxy (1,25D) both decrease as a result of several factors, including 1) decreased sunlight exposure and less efficient photoconversion in the skin of 2-dehydrocholesterol to vitamin D_3; 2) insufficient dietary intake of vitamin D; 3) intestinal malabsorption of, or resistance to, vitamin D; 4) decreased 1-α-hydroxylase activity in the kidney; and 5) the use of medications that cause the liver to break down vitamin D.

The decline in both serum calcium and 1,25D levels triggers a compensatory increase in parathyroid hormone (PTH). PTH then 1) stimulates osteoclasts to resorb bone; and 2) acts on the renal distal tubule to promote calcium reabsorption, thereby increasing serum calcium levels. PTH levels are higher in the elderly because of increased secretion and decreased renal clearance. This is thought to represent a form of secondary, rather than primary, hyperparathyroidism and can have a deleterious effect on bone mass in older patients (Baylink et al. 1999; Perry 1999).

Testosterone

As men age, the number of Leydig's cells in the testis declines, and testosterone secretion gradually decreases. Two other factors influence the age-related decline in testosterone: 1) a loss of the circadian variation in testosterone levels, and (2) an increase in sex-hormone binding globulin levels, which limits the amount of free testosterone available. The action of the hypothalamus and pituitary on the testis also may be affected by aging. The pituitary in some older men may be less responsive to gonadotropin-releasing hormone, with lower follicle-stimulating hormone and luteinizing hormone levels as a result. The overall decline in testosterone causes a decrease in both the number of Sertoli's cells and daily sperm production; the sperm produced may have defects in motility as well as chromosomal abnormalities. The volume of the seminiferous tubules and the testis itself also decreases. Both libido and fertility may decline. The effect of declining testosterone levels on sexual function is thought to be less important than chronic medical or psychiatric illness, vascular disease, neuropathy, or medications. Declining testosterone may indeed adversely affect bone mass as well as muscle mass and strength in older men. The changes in testosterone secretion are common but not universal, and some men have normal serum testosterone levels as they age (Gruenewald and Matsumoto 1999; Perry 1999).

Estrogen

Estrogen declines precipitously with menopause. Both fibrosis and involution of the ovary, as well as atrophy of the uterus and vagina, take place. The number of ovarian follicles declines, and a corresponding decrease in the secretion of both estrogen and androgens occurs; after menopause, the ratio of estrogens to androgens decreases. Menopause is also marked by an alteration in gonadotropin-releasing hormone secretion and high follicle-stimulating hormone levels, although luteinizing hormone levels remain the same. The loss of estrogen affects bone mass and places women at risk for osteoporosis. Women also lose the beneficial effects of estrogen on lipids, with rising low-density lipoprotein levels, and are at higher risk for cardiovascular disease. The lack of estrogen causes atrophy of the vaginal endothelium, the endothelium thins, less lubrication occurs with intercourse, and dyspareunia can result (Gruenewald and Matsumoto 1999; Perry 1999; Taffet 1999).

Thyroid

Although there are age-related changes in the thyroid gland, these changes have no corresponding effect on thyroid function. The aging thyroid is more fibrotic and nodular in composition; there have been conflicting reports about whether its size increases, decreases, or remains unchanged. The renal and thyroidal iodide clearance rate declines in older persons. Thyrotropin has been reported to be higher, lower, or normal in elderly patients. A study of older men documented decreased responsiveness to thyrotropin-releasing hormone stimulation, with decreased thyrotropin production, but other studies have reported no change or an increase in response to thyrotropin-releasing hormone. Although the thyroid continues to make sufficient amounts of thyroxine (T_4), it fails to metabolize T_4 as well. The synthesis of T_4 actually declines, but its level is unchanged. Peripheral deiodination of T_4 to triiodothyronine (T_3) also decreases, and the level of T_3 declines by 10%–20% in the elderly. Reverse T_3 levels do not change. Thyroxine-binding globulin levels remain normal with age (Hassani and Hershman 1999; Perry 1999).

Insulin

Elderly patients have a tendency toward hyperglycemia. Circulating insulin levels may rise but are less efficiently utilized. Although insulin secretion by the pancreatic beta cells is preserved with age, insulin clearance declines, and insulin levels increase. Peripheral uptake of insulin is affected by insulin resistance in peripheral tissues; some of these tissues, particularly adipocytes, have fewer receptors, thereby decreasing their sensitivity to insulin. Elderly patients have decreased muscle mass and a higher percentage of fat and therefore an increased number of adipocytes. These notable changes in insulin secretion and tissue sensitivity in the periphery may lead to observed increases in fasting glucose in the elderly. In addition, another factor leads to higher glucose levels. IGF-1, which acts at insulin receptors to promote glucose uptake, is less abundant in the elderly (Halter 1999; Perry 1999; Taffet 1999).

Musculoskeletal System

In general, the elderly person is less muscular and weaker. A decline in skeletal muscle mass, or sarcopenia, occurs. In the fourth decade, both muscle mass and strength begin to decrease. There are smaller numbers of type II fast-twitch fibers and fewer motor units and synapses; slow muscle fibers predominate. The motor units may enlarge. There are fewer and smaller ventral spinal motor neurons in the cervical and lumbar regions. Age, however, does not affect conduction velocity. Biochemical changes also occur, with decreased activity of glycolytic enzymes, including triosephosphate dehydrogenase, lactate dehydrogenase, glycerolphosphate dehydrogenase, and citrate synthase. Exercise may modify age-associated changes in muscle mass and strength. Sarcopenia places the elderly at risk for significant physical disability and a decline in their ability to perform activities of daily living and may ultimately undermine their ability to live independently (Loeser and Delbono 1999; Taffet 1999).

The elderly also develop demonstrable changes in cartilage, tendons, and ligaments. Cartilage becomes less cellular with age. Alterations in the structure of proteoglycans affect the ability of these molecules to bind water and maintain the hydration of cartilage. Cartilage weakens as the number of proteoglycan monomers decreases and the protein links between the monomers are broken. An increase in collagen cross-linking and in the diameter of collagen fibrils occurs, which makes collagen stiffer; this stiffness results in the compression of proteoglycans, which further interferes with water retention. The overall effect of age-related changes in cartilage is to decrease both its tensile strength and its stiffness, adversely affecting its response to mechanical stress (Loeser and Delbono 1999; Taffet 1999).

Older tendons and ligaments also may be stiffer because of an increase in cross-linking of type I collagen; their water content is also decreased. This alteration may make them less able to withstand mechanical stress and more susceptible to fatigue. Biomechanical studies confirm the weakening of tendons and ligaments with age. These changes may decrease the range of motion of joints in the elderly and make them more prone to tendonitis, ligament tears, and ligament ruptures (Loeser and Delbono 1999; Taffet 1999).

Age-related changes in the structure of both cortical and trabecular bone occur. Cortical bone becomes thinner and more porous; trabecular bone also thins, and whole trabeculae are lost. Bones are therefore weaker. With age, the number of osteoblasts and osteocytes may decrease. Osteoclasts continue to function normally. Mechanical strain, an important stimulus to bone formation, has less of an effect in the elderly, and less bone is made. The elderly are at increased risk for bone loss. Without estrogen replacement, women can lose significant bone mass after menopause. Elderly men with testosterone deficiency also may develop osteoporosis. Other factors that contribute to bone loss in both men and women include low peak bone density, poor calcium intake, secondary hyperparathyroidism (as discussed earlier), and insufficient exercise (Baylink et al. 1999).

Hematological and Immune Systems

The aging adult does not lose the ability to produce normal numbers of red blood cells, white blood cells, and platelets—despite a decrease in the bone marrow mass—but when challenged to produce more red blood cells by the occurrence of blood loss or by the presence of hypoxic conditions, the bone marrow is less able to respond quickly. Red blood cells and white blood cells retain normal function. The red blood cell's capacity to carry oxygen is essentially unchanged. The white blood cell continues to engulf and kill bacteria, but the respiratory burst activity of polymorphonuclear neutrophils decreases with age. Platelets, however, may be more sensitive to substances that trigger them to form blood clots. Although the prothrombin time and partial thromboplastin time are unchanged, fibrinogen increases, and Factor VII, Factor VIII, and D-dimer are all elevated (Chatta and Lipschitz 1999; Taffet 1999).

When confronted with a new infection, the elderly are less able to mount an adequate cell-mediated response. With age, the thymus decreases in size, the number of naïve T lymphocytes is diminished, and the individual's capacity to respond is adversely affected. Although the number of memory T lymphocytes increases with age, these are less easily activated. Age appears to have little, or at most a small, effect on the function of natural killer cells. The humoral, or antibody, response in the elderly is also impaired. The elderly respond less vigorously to the first presentation of an antigen as well as to the reintroduction of antigen. These decreased primary and secondary responses may explain why the elderly respond less well to vaccination (Miller 1999; Taffet 1999).

The body's primary defenses against infection are also affected by age. The thinner skin of the elderly is more vulnerable to injury; when the integrity of this barrier is compromised, surface bacteria may enter, resulting in cellulitis or a potentially serious bacteremia. The mucous membranes of the genitourinary and respiratory tracts of the elderly may become more easily colonized with gram-negative organisms, thereby serving as a potential source of infection. The decreased concentration, acidity, and amount of urea in the urine itself deprive it of an intrinsic defense against possible bacterial infection. Microorganisms also may find their way into the body by other means; those elderly patients with swallowing dysfunction may subsequently aspirate bacteria from the oral cavity, or those unable to produce an adequate cough will leave infectious material in the airways (Taffet 1999).

Renal System

Aging brings with it a progressive decrease in the size of the kidney from fatty infiltration, fibrosis, and the drop-out of cortical nephrons. The rate of decline of nephrons is 0.5%–1% per year; by age 60, 30%–50% of functioning glomeruli have been eliminated. Cortical nephrons become diffusely sclerotic. Glomeruli outside the cortex have fewer capillary loops and epithelial cells but more mesangial cells. Other areas of the kidney also may be affected; interstitial fibrosis may adversely affect the renal pyramids. These losses do not automatically lead to a failure of the kidney to keep fluids and electrolytes in balance, but decreased reserve capacity does predispose the kidney to possible dysfunction or failure. Creatinine clearance, a widely accepted measure of kidney function, declines 7.5%–10% per decade (Oskvig 1999; Taffet 1999).

These anatomical changes have important physiological consequences, including the decreased ability of the kidney to acidify urine or to excrete an acid or a water load. The response of the renin-angiotensin-aldosterone system is less supple, renin activity declines, and less renin is produced in the face of decreased intravascular volume or a depletion of salt. The kidney is able to maintain its output of erythropoietin, but the hydroxylation of vitamin D declines. Levels of atrial natriuretic peptide rise. The kidney less reliably metabolizes hormones such as glucagon, calcitonin, and parathyroid hormone; drug metabolism is also significantly affected (Oskvig 1999; Taffet 1999) and is discussed below in "Effects of Aging on Pharmacokinetics and Pharmacodynamics."

Considerations in Geriatric Prescribing

Effects of Aging on Pharmacokinetics and Pharmacodynamics

The effect of aging on pharmacokinetics (absorption, volume of distribution, clearance rate, and elimination half-life) and pharmacodynamics (the effect of a drug at a given dose) is crucial to understanding how drugs should be prescribed in the elderly patient (Leipzig 1999; J.B. Schwartz 1999).

Absorption

Age has no significant effect on absorption; although acid secretion, gastrointestinal perfusion, and membrane transport all may decrease and thereby *lower* absorption, gastrointestinal transit time is prolonged and *increases* absorption, and thus no net change occurs.

Volume of Distribution

The volume of distribution is significantly affected by the changes in body mass and total body water that occur with aging; older patients, with decreased lean body mass and total body water, have a smaller volume of distribution. This is particularly relevant when choosing proper doses for drugs such as antibiotics or lithium, which are primarily distributed in water. Protein binding also can affect the volume of distribution; it is generally unaffected by age. In frail elderly patients, there may be significant decreases in albumin levels, which affect the binding of potentially harmful drugs such as warfarin, which must be vigilantly titrated.

Clearance Rate

With age, renal mass and renal blood flow are decreased, resulting in a decline in glomerular filtration rate and creatinine clearance. This decrease in clearance can alter the rate at which drugs are excreted, and dosages must be appropriately adjusted. Certain drugs, such as nonsteroidal anti-inflammatory drugs and angiotensin-converting enzyme inhibitors, also may alter renal blood flow and thereby depress kidney function. Hepatic drug clearance is decreased by an age-related decline in hepatic blood flow; oxidative metabolism in the cytochrome P450 system is slower, thereby affecting elimination, but conjugation is not. Underlying hepatic disease and drug interactions also may significantly affect the metabolism of drugs by the liver.

Elimination Half-Life

The elimination half-life—the time required for the drug concentration to decrease by half—of certain drugs increases in the elderly and may be affected by the relation between volume of distribution or clearance; this may require adjustment of the drug dosing interval. For example, aspirin, certain antibiotics (such as vancomycin), digoxin, and the calcium-channel blockers (diltiazem, felodipine, and nifedipine) all have higher elimination half-lives, and the dosages must be adjusted downward.

Pharmacodynamic Effects

One also must consider the pharmacodynamic effects of drugs in the elderly. Frequently, the elderly are more sensitive to medications, and drugs often must be given in lower doses. For example, the response to anticholinergic drugs in particular is increased; elderly patients develop side effects more frequently than in younger patients, including constipation, urinary retention, and delirium. Other notable examples of drugs with enhanced pharmacodynamic effects in the elderly include diazepam, morphine, and theophylline.

Chronic Disease in the Elderly

Some chronic diseases are more prevalent in the elderly, and these predominantly occur as a result of "usual aging." The cumulative effect of environment and heredity on the individual over time makes these diseases more common, and they account for significant morbidity and mortality. Among the most formidable and omnipresent are cardiovascular disease, cerebrovascular disease, and cancer. Hypercholesterolemia and hypertension are frequently diagnosed. With age, weight and the incidence of obesity increase; patients are at higher risk for the development of type 2 diabetes mellitus. Age also brings an increased occurrence of joint problems, particularly osteoarthritis, which can result in chronic pain and the need for joint replacement. The elderly can develop cataracts and macular degeneration and therefore impaired vision; hearing loss in the elderly, caused by either previous exposure to noise or age-related anatomical changes in the ear, is also prevalent. Postmenopausal women and some hypogonadal elderly men are prone to develop osteoporosis. Benign prostatic hypertrophy, often with resultant urinary frequency and nocturia, becomes more of a clinical problem as men age. Polymyalgia rheumatica and temporal arteritis are collagen vascular diseases that occur often in elderly patients. The increasing prevalence of multisystem disease in the older patient can impose a substantial burden on the individual; in the face of already diminished physiological reserves, such an individual is considerably more vulnerable to declining health (Fried 2000).

Geriatric Syndromes

In addition, several common syndromes—known generally as *geriatric syndromes*—are found more frequently in older patients. Geriatric syndromes include falls, a multifactorial phenomenon that increases with age. Both elderly men and elderly women also often develop chronic difficulty with control of urination, or urinary incontinence. The elderly can be predisposed to delirium, a waxing and waning disorder of inattention; many elderly patients develop dementia, which doubles in the population every 5 years after age 65. The tendency of the elderly to use multiple drugs—or polypharmacy—is also a well-known geriatric syndrome. Frailty is a complex geriatric syndrome in which the health of the elderly individual declines after cumulative loss of physiological reserve, with sarcopenia, osteopenia, weight loss, and progressive functional deterioration. Four of the most characteristic geriatric syndromes—dementia, falls, urinary incontinence, and polypharmacy—are discussed in the following subsections; frailty is discussed later in conjunction with geriatric assessment.

Dementia

Dementia is a prevalent condition in the elderly but not a result of normal aging (Morris 1999). It is defined as the development of significant deficits in two or more areas of cognition—an impairment of memory and at least one other area such as abstract thinking, judgment, language, or visuospatial ability—that are severe enough to affect day-to-day functioning of the individual (Nyenhuis and Gorelick 1998). With the inevitable decline in intellectual functioning and the ability to perform activities of daily living that occurs, dementia poses particular challenges for the clinician as well as special burdens for caregivers.

Two-thirds of all dementia is caused by Alzheimer's disease. Vascular dementia accounts for 15%–25% of disease. Lewy body dementia constitutes 10%. The natural history and symptomatology of dementia vary according to its etiology (Marin et al. 2002).

- In Alzheimer's disease, symptoms begin gradually and steadily progress. Early on, a loss of short-term memory occurs; difficulty learning also may be evident. With progression, long-term memory is affected as well as orientation, judgment, word finding, performance of motor tasks, and visuospatial function. In late disease, patients lose their ability to perform their activities of daily living; they may become increasingly depressed or agitated. They may develop motor or gait problems and urinary and fecal incontinence (Marin et al. 2002).
- Vascular dementia occurs in patients with underlying cerebrovascular disease. Its clinical course is more abrupt in onset and less linear than Alzheimer's disease; the progressive nature of vascular dementia has not been precisely defined. In some cases of vascular dementia, there may be some overlap with Alzheimer's disease (Nyenhuis and Gorelick 1998).

- Lewy body dementia is distinguished by its unique set of presenting symptoms. Patients not only present with cognitive deficits but also may report visual hallucinations. The neurological examination may identify rigidity, bradykinesia, and postural changes (Gomez-Tortosa et al. 1998).

The accurate diagnosis of dementia requires a comprehensive assessment by the clinician, including a detailed history; thorough physical, neurological, and mental status examinations; and a depression screen. Because the patient may have significant deficits, the history needs to be gathered from the patient along with someone who is extremely familiar with the history of the patient's illness, medications, and social history. The evaluating clinician should order laboratory studies to rule out vitamin B_{12} deficiency, syphilis, and hypothyroidism and examine the patient for evidence of anemia, electrolyte abnormalities, renal failure, and liver dysfunction. This laboratory evaluation enables the clinician to detect reversible causes of dementia and uncover evidence of metabolic abnormalities that might point to a diagnosis of delirium rather than dementia (Marin et al. 2002).

Above all, the proper treatment of dementia involves the building of a proper support system for the patient. Pharmacological treatment of Alzheimer's disease may be appropriate in some cases. Acetylcholinesterase inhibitors, including donepezil, galanthamine, and rivastigmine, have shown some effectiveness in clinical trials of patients with mild to moderate disease, with documented improvements in the Alzheimer's Disease Assessment Scale Cognitive Subscale score (Frisoni 2001; Sramek et al. 2001). Patients with Alzheimer's disease are at risk for the development of depressive symptoms as well as major depression, and clinicians can provide effective medical treatment for this. Because agitation is also a prevalent symptom, particularly in patients with late disease, this symptom also may require treatment; atypical antipsychotic agents such as risperidone may be helpful in this context (Defilippi and Crismon 2000; Tune 2001).

Falls

Falls are a common phenomenon in older patients; every year, half of all nursing home residents and one-third of all community-dwelling elderly have a fall. These falls produce notable morbidity: 2% cause hip fractures, 5% cause other fractures, and 10% cause head injuries or other significant injuries. Half of the persons who fall experience minor injuries. In the aftermath of falls, disability may result. Those who fall frequently are at risk for a decline in their instrumental activities of daily living and their activities of daily living (assessment of such functions is discussed later in this chapter in "Fundamentals of Geriatric Assessment"). A decline in these functions can ultimately undermine independence and also might result in hospitalization (Alexander 1999; Fried 2000; King and Tinetti 1995; Rubenstein et al. 1994).

Falls are generally multifactorial and are caused by 1) intrinsic factors, 2) situational factors, 3) extrinsic factors, and 4) medications (Alexander 1999; King and Tinetti 1995). *Intrinsic factors* are disease-specific deficits in an individual patient that might contribute to falling; these factors include neurological problems (central, neuromuscular, vestibular, visual, and proprioceptive) as well as systemic illness. *Situational factors* relate to the particular activity that is taking place. *Extrinsic factors* relate to the demands and hazards of a particular environment. *Medications* may adversely affect mental status, cognition, balance, circulation, and neuromuscular function and predispose patients to falls.

The proper evaluation of a fall requires a) taking a detailed history and review of systems and b) performing a thorough physical examination and neurological examination as well (Alexander 1999). The fall may indeed be a nonspecific presentation of a serious medical illness such as cardiac ischemia, infection, intravascular volume depletion, or hypothyroidism, and these should be initially considered. The clinician should ask about any symptoms and situational or extrinsic factors that might have led to the fall and determine exactly how the fall occurred. A medication list should be compiled. The physical examination should rule out any cardiac abnormalities; the neurological examination must carefully assess the patient for any deficits in vision, strength, sensation, joint mobility, balance, cerebellar function, gait, or proprioception.

The prevention of falls focuses on altering both intrinsic and extrinsic factors (Alexander 1999; Gillespie et al. 2000; King and Tinetti 1995). With regard to intrinsic factors, one can 1) prescribe medication appropriately, 2) optimally treat disease, 3) improve balance and gait through physical therapy, and 4) improve conditioning and strength through exercise. With regard to extrinsic factors, one can 1) improve the environment by reducing or eliminating hazards, 2) monitor patients more carefully by increasing staff supervision and using motion detection, 3) eliminate restraints and the risk of injury they pose, 4) encourage patients to wear hip protectors, and 5) install protective flooring. Preventing falls ultimately requires multiple steps to produce successful results.

Urinary Incontinence

Urinary incontinence is a prevalent condition in the elderly that causes significant morbidity and affects quality of life (DuBeau 1999; Tannenbaum et al. 2001). Half of all nursing home residents and up to one-third of persons older than 65 residing in the community carry the diagnosis. It is a condition with multiple causes, including age-related changes, genitourinary tract abnormalities, and coexisting illnesses.

Urinary incontinence can be classified into two main categories: 1) transient incontinence and 2) established incontinence. Transient incontinence is reversible and can be easily treated; for example, transient incontinence could be a consequence of an acute urinary tract infection, inadequately controlled diabetes mellitus, or recent prescription of a diuretic and will resolve with the correction of those conditions. Established incontinence is further subdivided into the following three subcategories:

1. *Urge incontinence:* This form of incontinence has the highest prevalence in older patients. Urge incontinence results from detrusor overactivity, sometimes with simultaneous impaired contractility. Detrusor overactivity is more common with aging but can also occur for other reasons, including neurological dysfunction (such as stroke) or irritation of the bladder (secondary to cancer, urolithiasis, or infection); it can also occur in elderly patients without other illnesses. Patients usually complain of a sudden urge to urinate. They also classically have urinary frequency and nocturia. They experience varying amounts of leakage.
2. *Stress incontinence:* Stress incontinence occurs when increased abdominal pressure, triggered by cough or sneezing, results in urinary leakage. It happens commonly in women with weak pelvic muscles, although it also may occur as a consequence of failed anti-incontinence surgery or vaginal mucosal atrophy in women or prostatectomy in men. It is a frequent form of incontinence among elderly women, ranking second.
3. *Overflow incontinence:* Detrusor underactivity and bladder outlet obstruction can both produce overflow incontinence. Detrusor underactivity can be caused by fibrosis of the detrusor muscle, peripheral neuropathy, disc herniation, or spinal stenosis. Detrusor underactivity is an infrequent cause of urinary incontinence in the elderly. Urethral strictures, benign prostatic hypertrophy, and prostate cancer can cause bladder outlet obstruction in elderly men; this form of incontinence is the second most prevalent in this population. Bladder outlet obstruction in women occurs much less frequently; the etiology is either the presence of a large cystocele or a history of anti-incontinence surgery.

In general, the treatment of incontinence in the elderly begins with behavioral interventions and is followed by medical treatment. Surgery is considered the last option and is only appropriate for stress incontinence or outlet obstruction. Because urinary incontinence in the elderly is invariably the result of more than one cause, clinicians must appreciate that a single intervention may not be effective. Medications must be reviewed to determine whether they are contributing to incontinence. Patients must be cautioned against intake of fluids such as alcohol, coffee, tea, and soft drinks, which stimulate urination. Fluid restriction at bedtime may be appropriate to decrease nocturia.

Several specific interventions can be undertaken to treat the three forms of established incontinence.

1. Urge incontinence is best treated by frequent voluntary voiding and bladder retraining. Patients are placed on a voiding schedule that corresponds to their usual minimal interval of urination. They are taught how to voluntarily inhibit the urge to void. The goal of therapy is to increase gradually the interval between urination. For patients with cognitive impairment, bladder retraining is not appropriate; instead, timed voiding, scheduled voiding, or prompted voiding is instituted to decrease episodes of incontinence. For those who fail behavioral methods, medications such as oxybutynin, tolterodine, or imipramine may be helpful, but patients should be monitored carefully for anticholinergic side effects.
2. Stress incontinence is also amenable to nonmedical therapy. The mainstay of this approach is to strengthen the pelvic muscles that support the urethra by performing repeated isometric exercises, thereby preventing urinary leakage. The patient should be referred to a physical therapist to initiate an exercise program. In some cases, medical treatment also may be helpful. In women, oral or topical estrogen sometimes has been beneficial. Proponalamine also can be a useful adjunct, although this is not an option in patients with hypertension. For women who fail physical therapy and medical treatment, surgery remains another option.
3. Overflow incontinence in men is most often the result of outlet obstruction due to benign prostatic hypertrophy, which can be treated by both medical and surgical modalities. α-Blockers have been proven most effective for benign prostatic hypertrophy in clinical trials,

although finasteride may be used as a second-line treatment. Transurethral resection of the prostate and prostatectomy are available options for those who fail medical therapy. In women, previous vaginal or urethral surgery may be the cause of overflow incontinence; this is surgically correctable by lysis of adhesions or unilateral suture removal. For cases of overflow incontinence caused by detrusor underactivity, appropriate interventions include avoidance of constipation as well as careful management of medications to exclude those that adversely affect detrusor function. Intermittent catheterization is most often recommended for treatment of detrusor underactivity.

Incontinence can ultimately have harmful medical consequences, including pressure ulcers, cellulitis, falls, and fractures. It can interfere with sleep. It can also result in sexual dysfunction and depression. The proper treatment of incontinence is therefore important and can yield significant benefits.

Polypharmacy

Polypharmacy, defined as the simultaneous use of multiple medications or the prescribing of more medications than is clinically appropriate, is a common problem in the elderly (Hanlon et al. 2001; Leipzig 1999; Stewart 2001). Their use of drugs is attributable to several factors. Chronic illness is more common in older patients, and they experience more symptoms. They are also more frequent consumers of medical care. Drug use is also influenced by individual physician prescribing practices and by drug advertising. According to studies conducted in outpatients, elderly patients typically use 3.1–7.9 prescription and nonprescription drugs simultaneously. Polypharmacy carries with it certain consequences, including adverse drug reactions, drug interactions, and patient noncompliance; polypharmacy also increases the incidence of geriatric syndromes such as urinary incontinence, falls, cognitive impairment, and delirium.

Clinicians should take several steps to ensure that medicines are prescribed appropriately. They should take a careful, comprehensive medication history, including allergies and adverse drug reactions. Current use of alcohol, tobacco, and recreational drugs should be documented. Medicines should be prescribed only if they have a known benefit, and if so, they should be given at the lowest effective dose. Instructions about medication use should be communicated clearly to patients. Patients taking medication should be carefully monitored for therapeutic effectiveness and for side effects (Leipzig 1999). Two randomized controlled trials have reported a reduction of inappropriate prescribing and polypharmacy when clinical pharmacists were asked to review drug regimens, consult with physicians, and meet with patients (Hanlon et al. 2001).

Geriatric Assessment

The presentation of acute illness in the elderly may not be typical of that in younger adults, and diagnosis in the geriatric patient therefore poses special challenges. For example, the geriatric patient may experience a change in mental status that suggests an acute neurological event but is instead due to pneumonia, urinary tract infection, myocardial infarction, or an adverse reaction to medication. The symptoms of the older patient are very often nonspecific. The astute clinician must consider this carefully when constructing a differential diagnosis. Something as straightforward as functional decline might signal a more serious medical problem. The physiological changes that occur in the elderly also may alter markedly how patients present. Older persons may not always develop fever and leukocytosis in response to infection, and one must recognize other clues. The decline in functional reserve in many organ systems may predispose the elderly to harm even when a precipitating event seems minor. An elderly person with an impaired thirst mechanism may not replenish water losses quickly enough on a hot summer day, and dehydration could then happen very suddenly. The challenges of deciphering symptoms and preventing harm are heightened by the difficulty of gathering information from elderly patients; those who are capable of giving a good history may be reluctant to report that anything is wrong; they may be depressed, fearful of a new diagnosis, convinced that their problem is nothing but "old age," or skeptical that any doctor or medical system can help them. In some cases, medical illness can exacerbate psychiatric illness—making the depressed patient more disengaged or the schizophrenic patient become more agitated—and clinicians must be willing to consider diagnoses beyond mere worsening of an ongoing psychiatric condition and other possibilities.

Frailty

The sum effect of physiological decline in the older patient, combined with the cumulative and simultaneous burden of chronic disease, may result in the geriatric syndrome known as *frailty* (Cohen 2000; Hamerman 1999). Frailty has been defined by Fried and Walston (1999) as "a state of age-related physiologic vulnerability resulting from impaired homeostatic mechanisms and a reduced capacity of the organism to withstand stress" (p. 1389). Older patients have less pulmonary, cardiac, and renal reserve. They are less able to mount an effective immune response. Older patients also have higher sympathetic nervous tone, which may increase cortisol production and further impair the immune system. In these patients, cortisol also may have catabolic effects on bone and muscle and result in insulin resistance; older patients also may have higher levels of circulating cytokines—such as interleukin-6 (IL-6), IL-1B, and tumor necrosis factor-α—which also may have deleterious catabolic effects on muscle. Changes in neuroendocrine function—the decline in sex steroids, growth hormone, and DHEA—can have corresponding negative effects on the size and strength of muscle and, in the case of estrogen and testosterone, on bone mass. The frail older individual is characteristically weak as a result of declining muscle and bone mass; a tendency toward a sedentary state may lead to deconditioning, further weakness, and fatigue. Poor oral intake may lead to weight loss and nutritional compromise, adding even more to the tendency to tire easily. Progressive weakness may adversely affect balance and the ability to ambulate. Ultimately, the frail older patient loses the capacity to function independently and may require skilled assistance in a facility outside the home. Frailty also carries with it a higher risk of medical illness and mortality (Fried and Walston 1999).

Fundamentals of Geriatric Assessment

The effective evaluation and treatment of the geriatric patient—from the fully functioning community-dwelling older adult to the frail older adult in decline—require a global approach, which includes, but reaches beyond, a consideration of the patient's medical problems.

Reuben (1999) defined *geriatric assessment* as a comprehensive patient evaluation, conducted by an individual clinician or an interdisciplinary team, which considers the effect of key medical, social, psychological, and environmental factors on health and pays careful attention to function. During the medical assessment, the clinician performs a complete history and physical examination. He or she reviews the medication list for appropriateness and evidence of polypharmacy; checks for deficits in vision, hearing, ambulation, and balance; and screens for common geriatric problems such as falling, incontinence, and malnutrition. Vision is tested with Snellen's eye chart. Hearing is screened with the "whispering voice test" or a hand-held audiometer. The patient is weighed, the height is measured, and the body mass index is calculated. In addition to the standard neurological examina-

tion, the patient's mobility and balance can be determined by a "get up and go" test; the patient is asked to stand, walk 10 feet, turn around, return, and be seated. The task is timed; a time greater than 20 seconds suggests that more extensive evaluation is needed.

Cognitive assessment is performed with the Folstein Mini-Mental State Exam. The Geriatric Depression Scale is used to screen for depression. Fundamental day-to-day functioning is determined by documenting activities of daily living—bathing, dressing, toileting, feeding, transferring—and instrumental activities of daily living—driving, shopping, cooking, housekeeping, using the telephone, and managing finances. The clinician also must gather other important information about function: 1) the extent, strength, and reliability of the patient's social support system (this is most often the patient's family); 2) the patient's economic resources; and 3) the safety of the patient's home and its proximity to medical care and other essential services. The patient's spiritual preferences and needs are also assessed. After the assessment is completed, recommendations are developed and a care plan is implemented.

Although the results across clinical trials have not been consistent, the effectiveness of comprehensive geriatric assessment and management has been validated in a few studies. Increased diagnostic accuracy has been noted. Patients have shown significant improvements in functional status. Affect and cognition have improved. The use of health care services, as measured by nursing home days, hospital services, and medical costs, has been reduced. The use of medications has improved, with fewer drugs being prescribed (Hanlon et al. 2001; Reuben 1999; Stuck et al. 1993). A recent multi-institutional randomized controlled trial of geriatric evaluation and management units clearly showed a positive effect on functional status and quality of life for inpatients and on mental health and quality of life for outpatients, with overall costs equivalent to those for usual care (Cohen et al. 2002). As suggested by the evidence, comprehensive geriatric assessment and management therefore serves as a useful tool in both the diagnosis and the care of older patients. The geriatrician therefore may serve as a valuable and essential resource in the evaluation and treatment of this population.

References

Alexander NB: Falls and gait disturbances, in Geriatrics Review Syllabus: A Core Curriculum in Geriatric Medicine. Edited by Cobbs E, Duthie EH, Murphy JB. Dubuque, IA, Kendall/Hunt, 1999, pp 145–149

Armbrecht HJ: The biology of aging. J Lab Clin Med 138:220–225, 2001

Ashman TA, Miohs RC, Harver PD: Cognition and aging, in Principles of Geriatric Medicine and Gerontology. Edited by Hazzard WR, Blass JP, Ettinger WH, et al. New York, McGraw-Hill, 1999, pp 1219–1228

Baylink DJ, Jennings JC, Mohan S: Calcium and bone homeostasis and changes with aging, in Principles of Geriatric Medicine and Gerontology. Edited by Hazzard WR, Blass JP, Ettinger WH, et al. New York, McGraw-Hill, 1999, pp 1041–1057

Bureau of the Census, US Department of Commerce: Current Population Reports: 65+ in the United States (Special Studies Series P-23, No 190). Washington, DC, US Government Printing Office, 1996

Chatta GS, Lipschitz DA: Aging of the hematopoietic system, in Principles of Geriatric Medicine and Gerontology. Edited by Hazzard WR, Blass JP, Ettinger WH, et al. New York, McGraw-Hill, 1999, pp 889–897

Cohen HJ: In search of underlying mechanisms of frailty. J Gerontol A Biol Sci Med Sci 55(12):M706–M708, 2000

Cohen HJ, Feussner JR, Weinberger M, et al: A controlled trial of inpatient and outpatient geriatric evaluation and management. N Engl J Med 346:905–912, 2002

Cornoni-Huntley J, Brock DB, Ostfield A, et al (eds): Established Populations for the Epidemiologic Study of the Elderly: Resource Data Book. Bethesda, MD, National Institutes of Health, 1986

Defilippi JL, Crismon ML: Antipsychotic agents in patients with dementia. Pharmacotherapy 20:23–33, 2000

DuBeau CW: Urinary incontinence, in Geriatrics Review Syllabus: A Core Curriculum in Geriatric Medicine. Edited by Cobbs E, Duthie EH, Murphy JB. Dubuque, IA, Kendall/Hunt, 1999, pp 115–123

Fried LP: Epidemiology of aging. Epidemiol Rev 22:95–106, 2000

Fried LP, Walston J: Frailty and failure to thrive, in Principles of Geriatric Medicine and Gerontology. Edited by Hazzard WR, Blass JP, Ettinger WH, et al. New York, McGraw-Hill, 1999, pp 1387–1402

Frisoni GB: Treatment of Alzheimer's disease with acetylcholinesterase inhibitors: bridging the gap between evidence and practice. J Neurol 248:551–557, 2001

Gillespie LD, Gillespie WJ, Cumming R, et al: Interventions for preventing falls in the elderly. Cochrane Database Syst Rev 2:CD000340, 2000

Gomez-Tortosa E, Ingraham AO, Irizarry MC, et al: Dementia with Lewy bodies. J Am Geriatr Soc 46:1449–1458, 1998

Gruenewald DA, Matsumoto AM: Aging of the endocrine system, in Principles of Geriatric Medicine and Gerontology. Edited by Hazzard WR, Blass JP, Ettinger WH, et al. New York, McGraw-Hill, 1999, pp 949–966

Hall KE, Wiley JW: Age-associated changes in gastrointestinal function, in Principles of Geriatric Medicine and Gerontology. Edited by Hazzard WR, Blass JP, Ettinger WH, et al. New York, McGraw-Hill, 1999, pp 835–842

Hall WJ: Update in geriatrics. Ann Intern Med 127:557–564, 1997

Halter JB: Diabetes mellitus, in Principles of Geriatric Medicine and Gerontology. Edited by Hazzard WR, Blass JP, Ettinger WH, et al. New York, McGraw-Hill, 1999, pp 991–1012

Hamerman D: Toward an understanding of frailty. Ann Intern Med 130:945–950, 1999

Hanlon JT, Schmader KE, Ruby CM, et al: Suboptimal prescribing in older inpatients and outpatients. J Am Geriatr Soc 49:200–209, 2001

Hassani S, Hershman JM: Thyroid diseases, in Principles of Geriatric Medicine and Gerontology. Edited by Hazzard WR, Blass JP, Ettinger WH, et al. New York, McGraw-Hill, 1999, pp 949–966

Hunick MG, Goldman L, Tosteson AN, et al: The recent decline in mortality from coronary heart disease. JAMA 277:535–542, 1997

Kalina R: Aging and visual function, in Principles of Geriatric Medicine and Gerontology. Edited by Hazzard WR, Blass JP, Ettinger WH, et al. New York, McGraw-Hill, 1999, pp 603–615

King MB, Tinetti ME: Falls in community-dwelling older persons. J Am Geriatr Soc 43:1146–1154, 1995

Lakatta EG: Cardiovascular aging research: the next horizons. J Am Geriatr Soc 47:613–625, 1999

Leipzig RM: Pharmacology and appropriate prescribing, in Geriatrics Review Syllabus: A Core Curriculum in Geriatric Medicine. Edited by Cobbs E, Duthie EH, Murphy JB. Dubuque, IA, Kendall/Hunt, 1999, pp 30–35

Loeser RF, Delbono O: Aging and the musculoskeletal system, in Principles of Geriatric Medicine and Gerontology. Edited by Hazzard WR, Blass JP, Ettinger WH, et al. New York, McGraw-Hill, 1999, pp 1097–1112

Majumdar AP, Jaszewski R, Dubick MA: Effect of aging on gastrointestinal tract and the pancreas. Proc Soc Exp Biol Med 215:134–144, 1997

Marin DB, Sewell MC, Schlecter A: Alzheimer's disease: accurate and early diagnosis in the primary care setting. Geriatrics 57:36–40, 2002

Mattson MP: Cellular and neurochemical aspects of the aging human brain, in Principles of Geriatric Medicine and Gerontology. Edited by Hazzard WR, Blass JP, Ettinger WH, et al. New York, McGraw-Hill, 1999, pp 1193–1208

McKeown T: The role of medicine: dream, mirage, or nemesis. Princeton, NJ, Princeton University Press, 1979

Miller RA: The biology of aging and longevity, in Principles of Geriatric Medicine and Gerontology. Edited by Hazzard WR, Blass JP, Ettinger WH, et al. New York, McGraw-Hill, 1999, pp 3–19

Morris JC: Is Alzheimer's disease inevitable with age? Lessons from clinicopathologic studies of healthy aging and very mild Alzheimer's disease. J Clin Invest 104:1171–1173, 1999

Nyenhuis DL, Gorelick PB: Vascular dementia: a contemporary review of epidemiology, diagnosis, prevention and treatment. J Am Geriatr Soc 46:1437–1448, 1998

Oskvig RM: Special problems in the elderly: perioperative cardiopulmonary evaluation and management. Chest 155 (suppl):158S–164S, 1999

Perry HM: The endocrinology of aging. Clin Chem 45:1369–1376, 1999

Reed RS, Duckert LG, Carey JP: Auditory and vestibular dysfunction, in Principles of Geriatric Medicine and Gerontology. Edited by Hazzard WR, Blass JP, Ettinger WH, et al. New York, McGraw-Hill, 1999, pp 617–631

Reuben DB: Principles of geriatric assessment, in Principles of Geriatric Medicine and Gerontology. Edited by Hazzard WR, Blass JP, Ettinger WH, et al. New York, McGraw-Hill, 1999, pp 467–482

Rubenstein LZ, Josephson KR, Robbins AS: Falls in the nursing home. Ann Intern Med 121:442–451, 1994

Schwartz JB: Clinical pharmacology, in Principles of Geriatric Medicine and Gerontology. Edited by Hazzard WR, Blass JP, Ettinger WH, et al. New York, McGraw-Hill, 1999, pp 303–332

Schwartz RS, Buchner DM: Exercise in the elderly: physiological and functional effects, in Principles of Geriatric Medicine and Gerontology. Edited by Hazzard WR, Blass JP, Ettinger WH, et al. New York, McGraw-Hill, 1999, pp 143–158

Seals DR, Esler MD: Human ageing and the sympathoadrenal system. J Physiol (Lond) 528:407–417, 2000

Shock NW: Normal Human Aging: The Baltimore Longitudinal Study of Aging. Washington, DC, National Institute on Aging, U.S. Government Printing Office, 1984

Sramek JJ, Alexander BD, Cutler NR: Acetylcholinesterase inhibitors for the treatment of Alzheimer's disease. Annals of Long Term Care 9(10):15–22, 2001

Stewart RB: Drug use in the elderly, in Therapeutics in the Elderly, 3rd Edition. Edited by Delafuente JC, Stewart RB. Cincinnati, OH, Harvey Whitney, 2001, pp 235–256

Stuck AE, Siu AL, Wieland GD, et al: Comprehensive geriatric assessment: a meta-analysis of controlled trials. Lancet 342:1032–1036, 1993

Taffet GE: Age-related physiologic changes, in Geriatrics Review Syllabus: A Core Curriculum in Geriatric Medicine. Edited by Cobbs E, Duthie EH, Murphy JB. Dubuque, IA, Kendall/Hunt, 1999, pp 10–23

Tannenbaum C, Perrin L, DuBeau CE, et al: Diagnosis and management of urinary incontinence in the older patient. Arch Phys Med Rehabil 82:134–138, 2001

Tune LE: Risperidone for the treatment of behavioral and psychological symptoms of dementia. J Clin Psychiatry 62 (suppl 21):29–32, 2001

Vaillant GE, Mukamal K: Successful aging. Am J Psychiatry 158:839–847, 2001

Whalley LJ: The Aging Brain. New York, Columbia University Press, 2001

Neuroanatomy, Neurophysiology, and Neuropathology of Aging

Christopher E. Byrum, M.D., Ph.D.

Scott D. Moore, M.D., Ph.D.

Christine M. Hulette, M.D.

Neuroanatomy and the Aging Brain

Much has been revealed about the human brain in the past few decades. In vivo visualization of the human brain is much more accessible to psychiatrists and other clinicians with the emergence of high-resolution magnetic resonance imaging (MRI). Functional neuroimaging has broken the great barrier separating human from animal neuroscience research. Positron emission tomography (PET) and single photon emission computed tomography (SPECT) have begun to reduce the blindness that has kept neuropsychiatry in the realm of too much speculation. These radioligand tomographic techniques have had limited resolution, but functional MRI (fMRI) has great promise because of greatly improved resolution and availability.

As images of the brain become readily available to the clinician, a working knowledge of neuroanatomy becomes very useful. Unfortunately, neuroanatomy tends to be overwhelming, indigestible, and frustrating. The difficulties inherent in human neuroanatomy research, along with the enormous gaps in understanding that remain, have meant that a treatise on the anatomy of the human brain lacks the simplicity and elegance that come with a real grasp of the subject. What is left is a flood of information that leaves one numb and confused. Given that the understanding of the brain is still quite limited, especially regarding the qualities and functionality

unique to the human brain, many clinicians lack a clear understanding of the basic framework of brain anatomy and function. Few clinicians have the time to read neuroanatomy textbooks cover to cover. As a result, a working knowledge of neuroanatomy tends to be patchy and vague.

This discussion is intended to be a brief and concise review of neuroanatomy—almost a contradiction in terms. To enhance the basic understanding of how the brain may work, it is helpful to step back and look at a simplified, more essential picture. This review will err on the side of being too simple, perhaps glossing over controversy, but also will avoid misrepresenting speculation as fact. The intent is to allow the reader to obtain a picture of the whole brain, a simple functional framework, which will allow the clinician and other readers to have a better idea of where to dig more deeply for more comprehensive information. Several excellent neuroanatomy texts are noted in the references, some exhaustive, some more readable.

A review of the terminology used by radiologists and neuroanatomists may be helpful. Literature describing the animal central nervous system (CNS) includes terms such as *dorsal* and *ventral*, which do not really fit when applied to the human neuraxis. The dorsal and ventral horns of the spinal cord are not dorsal and ventral in the human spinal cord but anterior and posterior. However, especially in the spinal cord, the animal nomenclature is retained. This is also true to some degree in the human brain stem, although the terms *rostral* (or cranial) and *caudal* are preferred, meaning toward the forebrain and toward the spinal cord, respectively. In the human forebrain, the terms *rostral* and *caudal* are less useful. Preferred are the terms *anterior* and *posterior*, referring to the front and back of the brain (i.e., toward the frontal pole and the occipital pole, respectively). The terms *superior* and *inferior* mean toward the top of the brain (the vertex) and toward the bottom of the brain (i.e., toward the base of the skull). The term *neuraxis* refers to the entire CNS, excluding cranial nerves and spinal nerves, and *extra-axial* refers to anything outside the CNS, including the skull and vertebral column and the dural and vascular spaces, as well as the nerves traversing the spaces.

Several concepts can facilitate gaining a basic but sophisticated understanding of brain function. First, for those of us raised on cellular physiology, is the obvious but important fact that *the brain is not the liver.* In the brain, precise anatomical connections are virtually everything. That drugs can act on a particular cell type belies the fact that neuronal *systems* in the brain mediate experience and behavior. Neurons with a particular type of receptor may respond to a drug, but it is the anatomical connections of that neuron that determine what parts of the brain have their activity altered. The targets of the given neuron may be distant in the brain, may be myriad, and may respond in a variety of ways to the given neuronal impulse. A certain type of drug may influence several (or more) neuronal types simultaneously and may interact with a given cell type to produce quite different changes in neuronal activity in different target areas in the brain. For this reason, pharmacological treatments are determined empirically. Thus, the basic concept is this: in the brain, anatomy and function are inseparable, and so any discussion of any part of the brain will be in terms of its known or suspected function.

Second, our current understanding of the roles played by identified brain structures may need to be reexamined. Neuroscience research is not just adding to our understanding of brain function. Sometimes what we already knew was not quite right. For example, the basal ganglia have traditionally been associated with motor functions. These structures are now known to have extensive limbic system connections and participate in cognitive and emotional functioning and in fact can play a role in mood disorders.

The third and probably most important concept in neuroanatomy today is that of *distributed systems*. It has become abundantly clear that cortical and subcortical structures are so extensively interconnected that it is not possible to assign a behavior or an emotional or cognitive experience to a discrete area of the brain. Individual neurons in the human brain can receive thousands of afferent connections, and each neuron may in turn directly influence many other neurons simultaneously, some nearby and some in relatively remote areas of the CNS. Some functional systems in the brain are relatively well defined, other systems are becoming clearer, and others lie undiscovered. As research progresses, behaviors and experiences are now being seen to arise from one or more distributed systems in the brain, with components that may lie in far-flung parts of the brain, including the brain stem. This is not to say that every locus in the distributed system performs some homogeneous or interchangeable function. A particular part of the system may contribute some unique or relatively unique aspect to the overall brain function. Moreover, a given brain structure may participate in several or more systems, perhaps contributing its unique processing to a multitude of behaviors and experiences. An example of a distributed system is the limbic system (Parent 1996).

Brain Stem

Although the initial impression may be that the brain stem has little to do with issues of mood or cognition relevant to geriatric psychiatry, this is definitely not the case. The brain stem is of course of central importance in neurological dysfunction because of its control of vegetative functions and because the brain stem either mediates or gives passage to the great majority of sensory and motor impulses. The geriatric patient is at greater risk for neurological events. The brain stem can be a locus of important and serious drug side effects, and these frequently need to be differentiated from acute cerebrovascular events. Moreover, because of decreased reserves and other factors, the geriatric patient is much more sensitive to these medication side effects. In addition, the neuronal perikarya of the monoamine systems are in the brain stem, and these systems can affect virtually any part of the brain and can affect the brain in a global way. Thus, a brief description of the brain stem from a functional standpoint is important and will make a neuroanatomical survey more complete.

The brain stem, or *rhombencephalon,* is composed of several subdivisions (from caudal to rostral): the medulla, the pons, and the midbrain, plus the cerebellum, which has large and direct connections with all three. From an anatomical and functional (and even embryological) perspective, the brain stem is the cranial extension of the spinal cord and shares the basic anatomical organization. The brain stem contains elements of both motor and sensory systems, including systems intrinsic to the brain stem (the cranial nerves) as well as prominent ascending and descending *fibers of passage,* which pass through the brain stem to or from the spinal cord without synapsing in the brain stem.

Although from a gross anatomical perspective, the pons is most notable for the corticocerebellar connections making up the middle cerebellar peduncle, it otherwise is fairly similar to the medulla, and for our purposes, we consider them as a unit. The medulla and pons contain the subcortical aspects of the sensory systems for all the cranial nerves (CNs) except CNs I (olfaction) and II (vision). The massive somatosensory system of the head and neck is mediated by the sensory division of the trigeminal nerve (CN V). The cochlear (and some secondary auditory structures) and the vestibular nuclei of the eighth cranial nerve, now known as the vestibulocochlear nerve, mediate the sense of hearing and the special sense related to the vestibular system. The sense of taste (gustation) is mediated by the solitary nucleus in the medulla, with input from CNs VII, IX, and X. Sensory input from the viscera is considered a special sense and is mediated by the sensory division of the vagus nerve (CN X). The somatosensory, auditory, and gustatory senses send fiber bundles ascending toward the thalamus, joining the sensory pathways ascending from the spinal cord. The auditory system has special characteristics, projecting first to the tectum of the midbrain and then to the thalamus.

The medulla and pons contain the motor nuclei and related pathways mediating control of skeletal muscle of the head and neck. They are also involved in the parasympathetic control of visceral organs, pupillary responses, and exocrine function. The facial motor nucleus (CN VII) controls all the muscles of facial expression. The motor division of the trigeminal nerve (CN V) controls the muscles of mastication. The nucleus of the spinal accessory nerve (CN XI) controls the large muscles responsible for rotating and tilting the head. This nucleus has important connections with the tectum of the midbrain, constituting special systems mediating head and neck reflexes such as orienting and tracking in response to auditory or visual stimuli.

The tongue is controlled by the hypoglossal nerve (CN XII). The muscles of the larynx and pharynx are controlled by the nucleus ambiguus, with its motor fibers split between the glossopharyngeal (CN IX) and vagus (CN X) nerves. Other motor fibers of the vagus nerve, part of the parasympathetic arm of the autonomic nervous system (ANS), originate in the dorsal motor nucleus of the vagus nerve and modulate the intrinsic activity of the cardiac muscle and the smooth muscle of the viscera.

The extraocular muscles of the eyes are controlled by the nuclei of CNs III and IV (midbrain) and VI (pontomedullary), which are tightly interconnected with one another and with the vestibular nuclei. Another small nucleus in the midbrain, the Edinger-Westphal nucleus, contributes to parasympathetic control of the iris and pupillary reflexes.

The brain stem also contains the cerebellar system, best known for controlling balance, posture, coordination, and gait. The system is extensive and includes precerebellar nuclei (including the inferior olivary nucleus and several reticular formation nuclei) and their connection to the cerebellum through the inferior cerebellar peduncle. The corticocerebellar pathway includes the massive corticopontine tract, the pontine gray nuclei, and their connection to the cerebellum through the middle cerebellar peduncle. The output of cerebellar cortical activity is mediated by the deep cerebellar nuclei, which project via the superior cerebellar peduncle mainly to the motor nuclei of the thalamus. The vestibular part of the cerebellum also projects to the spinal cord via the red nucleus and the rubrospinal tract, *directly* facilitating balance and posture.

Prominent fiber bundles course through all three subdivisions of the brain stem, including the large *corticospinal tract*, composed mainly of descending cortical motor neuron axons. At the level of the medulla, the corticospinal tract is relatively superficial, forming bulges on the anterior surface known as the pyramids, giving the more common name *pyramidal tract*. Rostrally, at the level of the pons, the corticospinal tract is broken up into many fascicles by the pontine gray nuclei. At the most rostral level of the brain stem—the midbrain—the corticospinal tract is again united into single bundles bilaterally, now completely superficial and known as the *cerebral peduncles*. Among the many descending motor neuron axons of the corticospinal tract, some terminate in the brain stem (*corticobulbar* fibers) to influence the cranial nerve motor nuclei. A large proportion of the descending corticospinal axons are *corticopontine* fibers, which synapse in the pontine gray nuclei (thus, *corticospinal tract* is a misnomer), giving rise to axons that innervate the cerebellum through the middle cerebellar peduncle. The remaining fibers course through the brain stem to the spinal cord. Similarly, ascending sensory neuron axons from the spinal cord and cranial nerve sensory nuclei form several large bundles as they pass through the brain stem toward the thalamus.

The sensory and motor nuclei of the cranial nerves and the ascending and descending fiber bundles are embedded in a loose matrix of many short neurons, collectively called the *reticular formation*. The reticular formation extends throughout the brain stem from the medulla into the diencephalon. In addition to other roles, these neurons constitute the *reticular activating system*, which plays a critical role in regulating the sleep-wake cycle and level of arousal or *vigilance*. The reticular formation plays several other roles, including that of a slower sensory pathway from the spinal cord and brain stem to the thalamus. The sensory information transmitted along this pathway serves less to provide specific information about stimulus features, instead functioning to change the level of arousal in relation to stimuli.

The reticular formation also contains centers for control of the primary functions, including respiration and cardiac and vascular control of blood pressure. This is mediated through the ANS, via direct connections from reticular formation cells to sympathetic preganglionic cells in the spinal cord and through the parasympathetic influence of the vagus nerve (CN X).

The midbrain differs somewhat from the medulla-pons, although the reticular formation continues to be prominent (called the *tegmentum* in the midbrain). The ascending fiber tracts remain embedded in the reticular formation, but the corticospinal/pontine/bulbar tract is superficial to the tegmentum as the cerebral peduncles. The posterior aspect of the midbrain (covered by the cerebellum at lower levels) forms four bumps known as the *superior* and *inferior colliculi* and collectively known as the *tectum*. The superior and inferior colliculi receive direct visual and auditory input, respectively, and mediate head and neck reflexes (via the tectospinal tract) and other functions not involving the cerebral sensory cortex. The core of the midbrain is composed of a dense area of neurons surrounding the cerebral aqueduct and is known as the *periaqueductal gray*, an area significantly involved in pain control.

Finally, the brain stem gives rise to the monoamine systems, which are of great relevance to psychiatry. All three subdivisions of the brain stem contain the neuronal cell bodies of the monoamine systems—small groups of cells that together innervate virtually the entire CNS. The monoamines include norepinephrine (a catecholamine), comprising several groups, the largest and most compact of which is the *locus coeruleus* (LC). This nucleus is highly significant for several reasons, most notably because it innervates virtually the entire forebrain, giving it the potential to profoundly influence the cerebrum. Moreover, the LC is considered critical in mood disorders, anxiety, and certain types of drug withdrawal. A second catecholamine, dopamine, arises from the midbrain in a large, compact group known as the *substantia nigra* and from a smaller, diffuse group lying in the anterior tegmental area known as the *ventral tegmental area*. Dopamine deficiencies and excesses figure prominently in certain neurological and psychiatric diseases.

Another monoamine, serotonin, is an indoleamine rather than a catecholamine. Some small groups of serotoninergic neurons lie throughout the brain stem along the midline anterior to the ventricular system. These collectively are known as the *raphe nuclei*, and individually these groups each innervate certain areas of the CNS from spinal cord to cerebellum to forebrain. The largest and most rostral of the raphe nuclei is called the *dorsal raphe nucleus*, and like the LC, it innervates virtually the entire cerebrum, giving the dorsal raphe nucleus the capacity to influence the brain in a global way. Serotonin has been implicated in major psychiatric illness, especially mood disorders, and has been found to influence numerous behaviors and experiences.

Prosencephalon

The *prosencephalon*, or forebrain, contains all the parts of the "higher brain" that makes us human but more importantly contains all of the higher control of the critical physiological machinery that keeps us alive. The forebrain, which is synonymous with cerebrum, has two main parts: the *diencephalon* and the *telencephalon*.

Diencephalon

The diencephalon forms the core of the forebrain, both anatomically and functionally. Some neuroanatomists include the diencephalon as part of the brain stem, which is based mainly on the continuity of the reticular formation from the midbrain tegmentum into the hypothalamus and thalamus. No discrete border exists between the posterior hypothalamus and the reticular formation of the midbrain. This reticular formation also continues rostrally from the midbrain into the thalamus, forming the intralaminar nuclei. This is a less obvious continuation than seen in the hypothalamus but in fact is a very clear continuity from a functional standpoint. The intralaminar nuclei, especially the centromedian nuclei, form a critical part of the reticular activating system, essentially governing the level of activation of the forebrain, from deep sleep to waking to a state of hypervigilance.

Conversely, however, the hypothalamus and thalamus are integral parts of the cerebral systems and participate fully in cortical functioning on multiple levels. In contrast to the anatomical landmarks, from a functional standpoint the boundary between the diencephalon and telencephalon is arbitrary. Thus, the term *cerebrum* is synonymous with prosencephalon, which represents the diencephalon and telencephalon as an anatomical and functional unit.

The diencephalon is mainly composed of the hypothalamus and thalamus but generally is considered to include several smaller structures. These include the subthalamus, functionally part of the basal ganglia, and the epithalamus, which lumps together the habenula (part of the limbic system) and the pineal body or gland, which secretes the hormone melatonin into the cerebrospinal fluid in relation to circadian rhythms. Finally, the pituitary gland hangs off the bottom of the hypothalamus, forming the endocrine effector interface between the hypothalamus and the body.

Hypothalamus. The hypothalamus is a relatively small, heterogeneous structure at the base of the cerebrum. It is roughly divisible into medial and lateral halves, which are extensively interconnected. The medial portion is characterized by discrete nuclei embedded in a loose matrix of small neurons. The pituitary gland hangs by a stalk, the infundibulum, from the medial hypothalamus. The lateral half of the hypothalamus more closely resembles the reticular formation of the brain stem, with which it is continuous. The lateral hypothalamus is dominated by a large fiber bundle known as the *median forebrain bundle*, running longitudinally from brain stem to basal forebrain.

The median forebrain bundle contains many short axons interconnecting nuclei in the midbrain, hypothalamus, and basal forebrain. However, the median forebrain bundle also contains many important fibers of passage—most notably, the monoamine projections from noradrenergic and serotoninergic cell groups in the brain stem that innervate virtually the entire forebrain. The fornix, another prominent fiber bundle that serves to delineate lateral from medial hypothalamus, interconnects the hippocampus with the mamillary nuclei of the hypothalamus and several other structures important in the formation, storage, and retrieval of memories.

The hypothalamus plays multiple roles, reflecting its diverse anatomical makeup. Most notably, the hypothalamus serves to coordinate endocrine, autonomic, and somatic motor responses to a broad array of physiological and psychological information to maintain physiological homeostasis. Among the factors regulated by the hypothalamus are body temperature, heart rate, blood pressure, blood osmolarity, metabolism, digestion, and water and food intake. The hypothalamus regulates sexual and reproductive functioning and growth. The hypothalamus also plays roles in the body's responses to stress, including control of adrenal cortical secretion of cortisol, which is part of the body's mechanism for coping with stress. These functions are mediated by a distributed system of interconnected hypothalamic nuclei.

The hypothalamus controls the endocrine system through the pituitary gland, to which it is directly connected by a system of small (portal) capillaries (anterior pituitary or adenohypophysis), or by a direct neuronal connection (posterior pituitary or neurohypophysis). Nuclei of the medial half of the hypothalamus produce many peptide hormones and hormone releasing factors. The hypothalamus also has receptors for the hormones it controls, as well as thermoreceptors and osmoreceptors. Control of the ANS occurs through projections from the lateral hypothalamus to the preganglionic sympathetic and parasympathetic neurons in the brain stem and spinal cord. Some functional division can be appreciated, with the anterior hypothalamus manifesting mainly parasympathetic aspects of the ANS and the posterior hypothalamus manifesting mainly the sympathetic autonomic responses.

The hypothalamus has widespread and often reciprocal connections with the brain stem, limbic structures, and prefrontal cortex. In addition to its well-defined role in maintaining physiological homeostasis, the hypothalamus participates in emotional expression and motivation through its broad interconnections with limbic structures, especially the amygdala. The hypothalamus integrates cortical and subcortical aspects of emotional states and coordinates concomitant physiological manifestations.

Thalamus. The thalamus is located superior to the hypothalamus, enclosing the upper part of the third ventricle. It is bounded laterally by the white matter of the internal capsule, which is comprised in part of thalamocortical and corticothalamic fibers. The thalamus is divided into lateral, medial, and anterior groups by white matter laminae.

The thalamus plays a critical role in the functioning of the cerebral cortex. No information enters the cortical mantle without going through the thalamus, with the notable exception of the olfactory system, the most primitive of the sensory systems.

The thalamus contains two different types of subnuclei. One type is called the *specific (or relay)* type. Each nucleus of the specific type receives a specific type of input that is projected to a discrete area of cerebral cortex. However, it is now known that these nuclei do not function as simple relays between afferent input and efferent projection to its area of neocortex. Each of these nuclei receives reciprocal afferent input from the area of cortex it is projecting to, allowing the thalamic nucleus to modulate its own output. In fact, it is now apparent that a considerable amount of processing takes place at the level of the thalamus.

Each *lateral thalamic nucleus* receives either unimodal (only one sensory type) sensory input or specially processed information related to control of movement and projects to and receives input from a specific region of sensory, motor, or association cortex. The ventral tier of the lateral nuclear group of the thalamus contains nuclei for each of the senses except olfaction, which is the only sensory modality that bypasses the thalamus on its way to the cerebral cortex. Each of these thalamic nuclei then sends its sensory-specific information to the appropriate primary sensory cortex for that modality. The lateral group also receives information related to movement from the cerebellum and basal ganglia, relaying information to the primary motor cortex.

The *dorsal tier* of the lateral thalamic nuclear group contains the pulvinar, the largest of the thalamic nuclei. The pulvinar processes sensory information, but the information is polymodal (i.e., representing the integration of two or more sensory modalities). The pulvinar receives input from the superior colliculus, parietal-temporal-occipital association cortex, and primary visual cortex and, in turn, projects back to the parietal-temporal-occipital association cortex. Its diverse connections suggest that the pulvinar is performing a high-level integration of sensory information (see discussion of multimodal association cortex in the "Association Cortex" section later in this chapter).

Other specific-type nuclei in the thalamus receive input from limbic structures and project to limbic association cortex. The anterior nuclear group receives input from the hippocampus by way of the mamillary nuclei and the mamillothalamic tract and projects to the limbic association cortex of the cingulate gyrus. Similarly, the dorsomedial nucleus of the medial thalamic group receives afferent input from the amygdaloid complex and temporal neocortex, projecting in turn to the limbic association cortex of the prefrontal lobe.

In contrast to the specific nuclei, the other type of thalamic nuclei is known as the *diffuse projection* type. These include the intralaminar nuclei, which have precisely organized connections with the striatum and also project diffusely to several cortical areas in the frontal lobe, influencing the sensitivity of cortical neurons. The reticular thalamic nucleus is a second type of diffuse projection nucleus, which forms a shell around the lateral aspect of the thalamus on each side so that corticothalamic and thalamocortical fibers are contacted as they pass through it. The reticular nucleus does not project to the cerebral cortex and instead has an inhibitory influence on the activity of the specific-type nuclei. The activity of the reticular nucleus is closely correlated with electroencephalogram (EEG) activity during sleep and wakefulness and is associated with the control of attention to sensory stimuli.

Telencephalon

The telencephalon is about 40% white matter by volume—huge bundles of myelinated axons that provide vital connectivity within the cerebral hemispheres and which connect the cerebral cortex with subcortical structures and the rest of the CNS. In addition to the thin layer of gray matter of the cerebral cortex, the forebrain contains several subcortical gray matter structures. The basal ganglia lie deep in the cerebrum, forming a sort of outer core surrounding the diencephalon. A loose group of nuclei and diffuse cell groups collectively called the *basal forebrain* lies anterior to the diencephalon. Unlike the basal ganglia, this gray matter is superficial but does not form anything resembling a layered cortical structure. The amygdalohippocampal complex forms the ventromedial surface of the temporal lobes, overlapping with the olfactory brain (rhinencephalon) that comprises the anterior region of the temporal lobes. The phylogenetically old hippocampal formation and the olfactory structures are in fact cortical in structure but differ from the rest of the cerebral cortex in structure and are designated *allocortex* (discussed later in this chapter in the "Classification and Parcellation of Cerebral Cortex" section). The amygdaloid complex is a heterogeneous collection of subnuclei that has been called *corticoid* (i.e., showing only a suggestion of the neuronal layering characteristic of cortex).

At the level of the midbrain, ascending and descending tracts of myelinated axons coalesce to form the large white matter fiber bundles called the *cerebral peduncles* (discussed earlier in this chapter in the "Brain Stem" section). Rostral to the midbrain, at the most inferior levels of the cerebrum, the cerebral peduncles spread to form a capsule around the diencephalon and are given the name *internal capsule*. At this level, a large amount of two-way traffic leading into and out of the thalamus mixes with the fibers of the corticospinal tract, forming a thick sheet of white matter, which separates the gray matter of the thalamus from the gray matter of the globus pallidus and also splits the caudate nucleus from the putamen. Superior to the level of the basal ganglia, the internal capsule splays out anteriorly, laterally, and posteriorly to form the *corona radiata*. These fibers are joined by the medial and laterally oriented fibers of the corpus callosum to form a dense core of white matter in the superior part of the cerebrum known as the *centrum semiovale*. This collection of myelinated axons includes corticothalamic and thalamocortical fibers, commissural fibers from the corpus callosum (interhemispheric association fibers), descending projections from motor cortex to multiple levels of the CNS, and long intrahemispheric association fibers interconnecting areas of cortex. Finally, just below the thin layer of gray matter making up the cerebral cortex are short association fibers interconnecting neurons in one gyrus with those in the next gyrus.

Basal ganglia. Deep in the cerebrum are several nuclei constituting the basal ganglia, although a sometimes confusing multitude of names are given to these structures in various combinations. The superior portion of the basal ganglia is known as the *dorsal striatum*, which includes the caudate nucleus and the putamen, which are very similar in structure and essentially split into the two nuclei by fibers of the internal capsule. The striped appearance of the small white matter bundles of the internal capsule and the gray matter bridges still joining the two nuclei in places gave rise to their original, collective name of *striatum* (or rarely *neostriatum*). Ventromedial to the putamen are the inner and outer segments of the globus pallidus, making up the third major element of the dorsal striatum. This structure is sometimes just called the *pallidum* (or rarely the *paleostriatum*), so named because the greater content of whitish myelinated axons gives this structure a pale appearance in fresh sections. The putamen and globus pallidus are nestled snugly together, giving the appearance of a lens shape with the convex surface oriented laterally and narrowing to somewhat of a point ventromedially, pointing toward the base of the diencephalon. The term *lenticular nucleus* is given to the putamen–globus pallidus combination; this term has usefulness as a gross anatomical term but little usefulness from a functional standpoint.

The inferior division of the basal ganglia, known as the *ventral striatum*, has a structure that parallels that of the dorsal striatum but differs significantly in connectivity and function. The ventral striatum is usually considered to include the nucleus accumbens and the olfactory tubercle; the nucleus accumbens represents the fused inferior extent of the caudate and putamen. Similarly, the ventral pallidum is the inferior extent of the globus pallidus, so no clear separation exists between dorsal and ventral striatopallidum from a gross anatomical standpoint, although the differences in connectivity clearly justify the nomenclature.

The basal ganglia consist of input nuclei and output nuclei. The input nuclei, comprising the caudate, putamen, and ventral striatum, receive afferent input from virtually all areas of cortex. Cortical input to the striatum has a distinctly regional pattern. The putamen is innervated by sensorimotor cortex, whereas the caudate nucleus preferentially receives input from association areas of frontal, temporal, parietal, and cingulate cortex. Furthermore, afferent input from limbic and paralimbic cortex, hippocampus, and amygdala primarily terminates in the ventral striatum. Based on this corticostriatal innervation pattern, the striatum is divided into sensorimotor, associative, and limbic territories. This regional organization is maintained throughout the basal ganglia as parallel,

segregated pathways from input to output. In addition to the massive cortical innervation, the striatum receives prominent afferent input from the thalamus, originating primarily in the intralaminar nuclei. Both striatal divisions are innervated by dopaminergic cell groups in the midbrain; the dorsal striatum receives input from the substantia nigra (considered part of the basal ganglia), and the ventral division receives input from the more diffuse *ventral tegmental area*. In addition, like most of the forebrain, both divisions receive serotoninergic input from the dorsal raphe nucleus and noradrenergic input from the LC.

The striatal nuclei project exclusively to the globus pallidus, which is the main output nucleus of the basal ganglia, and to the substantia nigra. The effects exerted by the dorsal striatopallidum on other parts of the nervous system are mediated primarily by efferent fibers from the internal segments of the globus pallidus and from the substantia nigra to the thalamus (the ventral tier and centromedian nuclei). The ventral striatopallidum similarly projects to the thalamus, to the limbic-related dorsomedial nucleus. However, in contrast to the globus pallidus, which has connections exclusively to other elements of the basal ganglia and the thalamus, the ventral pallidum also has direct reciprocal connections with limbic structures, especially the amygdala.

The basal ganglia are thus intercalated in a loop of neuronal connections from the cerebral cortex and back to the cerebral cortex via the thalamus (corticostriatal-thalamocortical loops). Although the basal ganglia receive afferent input from almost all parts of the cortex, a high degree of topographic organization is maintained throughout the basal ganglia, from input to output. It is now believed that the basal ganglia process different kinds of information in parallel rather than being primarily concerned with integration of information from large parts of the cortex. Thus, every cortical area has a separate functional pathway through the striatum that lies adjacent to and interdigitates with that of functionally related cortical areas. In other words, the striatum is processing information of different kinds simultaneously, although it remains segregated.

There are thought to be five or more lines or circuits through the basal ganglia in which the flow of information remains segregated. Presumably, the basal ganglia are performing some particular type of processing common to all the pathways. Because of the parallel processing and the segregation, the output of each functional pathway will be dissimilar, reflecting the unique and varying type of input to each pathway. Within each pathway, convergence on a local scale is evident, reflecting the considerable processing that is occurring during the transit through the basal ganglia system.

The nature of the processing that occurs in the basal ganglia system is unclear; thus, the function of the basal ganglia system, within each pathway and as a whole, remains speculative. It is believed, at least for the systems involving sensorimotor cortex, that the basal ganglia system is involved in the planning and production of movement. In contrast to the putamen, which mainly receives input from sensorimotor cortex and projects back to sensorimotor cortex via the thalamus, the caudate nucleus receives highly processed information from association areas and acts primarily on prefrontal cortex. Several corticostriatal-thalamocortical loops involving the caudate nucleus and prefrontal cortex have been proposed, which may involve primarily cognitive tasks. A similar corticostriatal-thalamocortical loop exists between limbic cortex of orbitofrontal and temporal lobes and the cingulate gyrus through the ventral striatopallidum to the dorsomedial thalamus and back to the same cortex. The connections of the ventral striatopallidum with limbic structures suggest involvement in motivation and emotion. The specific role played by the various loops of the basal ganglia system may be analogous to the motor role played by part of the dorsal aspect of the system, acting to suppress or select potentially competing cognitive or limbic mechanisms.

As a final note, diseases affecting the basal ganglia have long been known to affect motor functioning, resulting in disturbances of movement and of resting muscle tone. Before modern tract-tracing technologies, it was believed there was a second, *extrapyramidal* pathway from motor cortex to the brain stem and spinal cord. This has been proven incorrect, so the term *extrapyramidal* is inappropriate and misleading. However, the term *extrapyramidal* is fairly entrenched in psychiatric literature in relation to medication side effects and may continue to persist as an occasionally confusing relic.

Basal forebrain. The basal forebrain is one of several subcortical gray matter areas in the telencephalon. Unlike the basal ganglia or the amygdalohippocampal complex, the basal forebrain does not have a real structure. Rather, it is largely a collection of diffuse cholinergic cell groups and several nuclei of apparently unrelated function. The basal forebrain region lies anterior to the diencephalon and inferomedial to the basal ganglia. The basal forebrain's three functional entities are

1. The ventral striatopallidum or ventral striatum, which was discussed with the basal ganglia.
2. The *extended amygdala*, which primarily comprises the bed nucleus of the stria terminalis. The stria terminalis is one of two main efferent pathways from the amygdala, and the extended amygdala thus represents a rostral extension of the medial amygdala, with which it shares neurotransmitter properties.
3. A system of large cholinergic neurons in a thin disk close to the basal surface of each hemisphere, which is the most diffuse component of the basal forebrain. The most lateral collection of these magnocellular cholinergic neurons is known as the *basal nucleus* (or the basal nucleus of Meynert), an area of great notoriety. The basal nucleus, which receives an extensive and diverse afferent input, provides cholinergic innervation to virtually the entire neocortex, in a manner analogous to the monoamine systems originating in the LC and raphe system. The loss of acetylcholine in the cerebral cortex in certain degenerative dementias has been traced to degeneration of this small group of neurons. The other magnocellular cholinergic neurons are found in the septal nuclei, the most medial and least diffuse grouping of these neurons. The septal nuclei are part of the limbic system and, with some adjacent neurons, provide cholinergic innervation of the hippocampal formation.

Classification and Parcellation of Cerebral Cortex

In the adult human brain, the cerebral cortex has about 1,500–2,200 cm^2 of surface area, with a thickness that varies from 1.5 to 4.5 mm. Only about one-fourth of the cortex is visible, and the rest is buried in sulci and fissures.

Cerebral cortex can be classified in several different ways: 1) by the sizes and shapes and arrangements of neuronal perikarya, or *cytoarchitectonics*; 2) by the pattern of layering of cortical neurons; or 3) by connectivity. One fundamental classification of cerebral cortex looks at the layering of small and large neurons and neuronal axons in different areas of cortex. Most (≥95%) of the cerebral cortex consists of six layers and is known as *neocortex*, *isocortex*, or *homotypic cortex*. Phylogenetically older parts of cerebral cortex contain fewer layers and are known as *allocortex* or *heterotypic cortex*. Allocortex often contains only three layers and includes areas related to olfaction and the hippocampal formation. Notably, whereas neocortex develops in parallel with the thalamus and receives most of its subcortical afferents from the thalamus, allocortex receives afferents from other subcortical nuclei.

A second classification scheme was developed by Brodmann based on cytoarchitectonics. Brodmann identified 47 different areas of neocortex, which can be approximately classified into three functional categories. Some of the more readily recognizable areas are noted here for those interested. One category is termed *agranular cortex* and is characteristic of motor cortex (Brodmann's areas 4 and 6). This type of cortex is characterized by a poorly developed inner granular layer and prominent pyramidal cell layers. The large pyramidal cells provide long axons to project long distances to the brain stem or spinal cord. A second cytoarchitectonic category is termed *granular cortex* or *koniocortex*, characterized by a prominent inner granular layer and a paucity of large projection neurons. The inner granular layer, so named for the many small neurons concentrated there, is specialized to receive afferent axons and is best developed in sensory cortex, which receives dense thalamocortical input. Granular cortex includes somatosensory cortex (Brodmann's areas 1–3), auditory cortex (areas 41 and 42), gustatory cortex (area 43), and visual cortex (areas 17–19). The large remaining areas of cortex are designated association cortex, with variable cytoarchitectonics reflecting both input and output functions.

The third classification scheme is based on connectivity. All areas of cortex receive thalamic input, which in a real sense determines the identity of each cortical area. Cerebral cortex can thus be divided into sensory, motor, and association areas. Some areas of association cortex are identified as limbic cortex, based on their connections with subcortical limbic structures.

Afferent and Efferent Connections of Cerebral Cortex

Afferent input to the cerebral cortex is of several types: thalamocortical, corticocortical, and the diffuse modulatory neurotransmitter systems. As described earlier, two types of thalamic input reach the cerebral cortex. The first arises from specific thalamic nuclei, which contribute topographically organized projections to all parts of the neocortex. These are generally reciprocated and are not simple relays (i.e., some degree of processing takes place at the level of the thalamus). The second arises from the diffuse projection thalamic nuclei, which contribute diffusely organized connections and represent primarily the projections of the intralaminar thalamic nuclei. These nuclei exert general effects on the excitability of cortical neurons. Corticocortical connections include association fibers and commissural fibers. Association fibers interconnect areas of cortex within the hemispheres, are generally reciprocal, and are a vital part of the distributed neuronal systems mediating many brain activities. Commissural fibers generally interconnect corresponding areas in the two hemispheres, virtually all crossing in the corpus callosum.

In addition to the diffuse thalamic innervation, most of the forebrain, including the entire cerebral cortex, is diffusely innervated by two monoamine neurotransmitter systems that originate in the brain stem. The LC in the pons provides noradrenergic innervation, and the dorsal raphe nucleus in the midbrain provides serotoninergic innervation of the forebrain. In both cases, a relatively small number of neurons innervate vast areas of cortex, as well as subcortical structures, by widely ramifying axonal collaterals. Thus, the modulatory actions mediated by these systems would act in a global way, perhaps affecting the whole of distributed systems simultaneously. A third monoamine system in the ventral tegmental area of the midbrain that uses dopamine affects more restricted areas of cortex, primarily frontal and temporal neocortex. A fourth neurotransmitter system that uses acetylcholine arises in the basal nucleus in the basal forebrain and diffusely innervates the cerebral neocortex. By virtue of their extremely widespread distribution, these systems can affect the brain in comprehensive ways. Each of these systems is now known to have profound implications for geriatric psychiatry.

Efferent connections of cerebral cortex include the corticocortical connections described above, in addition to the subcortical targets of cortical projection neurons. These targets include the thalamus, in part reciprocating corticothalamic projections, and the striatum, which receives projections from all areas of cortex except primary auditory and visual cortex. The remaining subcortical projections of cerebral cortical neurons are corticopontine (innervating the cerebellum via the pontine gray nuclei and the middle cerebellar peduncle), corticobulbar (innervating various brain stem nuclei), and corticospinal (projecting primarily to spinal motor neurons).

Organization of Sensorimotor Systems

Sensory cortex is organized such that thalamic projections for each sensory modality innervate a single area of neocortex, designated *primary sensory cortex*. Olfactory cortex is exceptional because it is allocortical and because the thalamus is bypassed, but the organization is similar. Adjacent to the primary sensory cortex for each modality are one or two areas of secondary sensory cortex, which receive sensory input from the primary sensory cortex after initial processing. In the case of *visual cortex*, the area surrounding the calcarine sulcus near the posterior (occipital) pole of the brain (Brodmann's area 17), known as *striate cortex* or *calcarine cortex*, receives direct thalamic input from the lateral geniculate nucleus (ventral tier of the lateral thalamus). Striate cortex sends its output to secondary and then to tertiary visual cortex (areas 18 and

19), which lie adjacent to primary visual cortex. There are extensive, reciprocal connections between these three areas of visual cortex. Different aspects of visual processing take place in different areas, with the development of progressively more complex analysis. For example, recognition of stimuli in the visual system goes from simple spots of light or color in primary visual cortex to detection of shapes, direction, and speed of movement in secondary and tertiary visual cortex. Thus, the overall movement of information from primary to secondary to tertiary visual cortex shows a progressively higher level of processing at each step, but the information being analyzed remains unimodal and still lacks meaningful context.

Somatosensory (somesthetic) cortex has some unique features because of its relationship with motor cortex. Somesthetic cortex and motor cortex can be seen as a unitary system, not only because of their proximity but also because they are extensively interconnected at each level. Activation of muscles can even occur with electrical stimulation of somesthetic cortex, albeit at higher stimulus intensities than direct stimulation of motor cortex. Primary somesthetic cortex (S-1) is located in the postcentral gyrus and its medial extension (Brodmann's areas 1–3). Thalamic input comes from the lateral and medial ventral posterior thalamic nuclei (VPL and VPM). An additional unique feature is that the secondary somesthetic area (S-2) also receives direct input from VPL and VPM and from S-1 bilaterally. Both S-1 and S-2 project to multimodal sensory association cortex in the posterior parietal lobe (areas 5 and 7). However, both somesthetic areas also project directly to primary motor cortex, and, moreover, both make a significant contribution to the corticospinal tract, allowing direct control of sensory signal transmission from caudal levels of the CNS.

Primary *motor cortex* (M-1), located in the precentral gyrus (Brodmann's area 4), is the locus of voluntary movement control and is the main source of corticospinal tract axons. M-1 receives afferent input from primary and secondary somesthetic areas. Thalamic input to M-1 comes from the ventral anterior and ventral lateral thalamic nuclei, which provide critical input from the two subcortical adjunctive motor control systems: the basal ganglia and the cerebellum, respectively. Brodmann's area 6 contains "supramotor" areas: the premotor area and the supplementary motor area. Both of these adjunctive motor areas receive afferent input from prefrontal cortex and project primarily to M-1 and are important for precise movements of the hands (especially rhythmic movements). The supplementary motor area is important for organizing and planning fairly complex movements and for mediating an appropriate motor response to sensory

stimuli. The premotor area is important for control of visually guided movements. Just anterior to the premotor area is the frontal eye field, the center for voluntary eye movements.

Primary *auditory cortex* (A-1) is located in a part of the superior temporal gyrus of the posterior temporal lobe known as *Heschl's gyrus* (Brodmann's areas 41 and 42) and receives thalamic input from the medial geniculate body (ventral tier of lateral thalamus). The rest of the superior temporal gyrus represents secondary auditory cortex (A-2), necessary for the interpretation of auditory information. Damage to A-2 can result in *acoustic agnosia*, the inability to recognize tones in particular patterns, such as laughter or the sounds of various animals, in the absence of impaired hearing.

Gustatory cortex is found in Brodmann's area 43, part of insular cortex buried in the lateral sulcus (also known as the *sylvian fissure*). This primary sensory cortex is less well defined than other sensory cortices and is not discussed further.

The oldest part of the human cerebral cortex is the *rhinencephalon*, or *olfactory brain*. This includes the olfactory structures, the anterior olfactory nucleus, the corticomedial and anterior parts of the amygdaloid complex, and the piriform lobe in the anteromedial temporal lobe. Part of the piriform lobe is *allocortex* and represents the primary sensory cortex of the olfactory system. The other subdivision of the piriform lobe is entorhinal cortex, which is *neocortex* (Brodmann's area 28) and represents secondary olfactory cortex. This area, located on the parahippocampal gyrus, forms the *uncus*, a gross anatomical landmark that can have critical clinical significance in cases of traumatic brain injury. Notably, olfactory cortex receives input directly from olfactory structures, making the olfactory system unique among the sensory systems in that the thalamus does not intervene between sensory neurons and sensory cortex.

Association Cortex

Sensorimotor cortex occupies a relatively small proportion of cerebral cortex, leaving a large amount of neocortex designated *association cortex*. Association cortex is found in parietal, temporal, and frontal lobes. Sensory and association cortices form a functional hierarchy, with primary sensory cortex forming the most basic level (Table 4–1). What has been traditionally described as secondary and tertiary sensory cortex for each sensory modality is *unimodal sensory association cortex*. This level of association cortex is responsible for integrating the most basic elements of sensory information that have been identified by the primary sensory cortex. For example,

TABLE 4–1. Distribution of major cortical types

Cortical type	Specific type	Lobe	Location in lobe
Primary sensorimotor cortex	Motor	Frontal	Precentral gyrus
	Somesthetic	Parietal	Postcentral gyrus
	Visual	Occipital	Calcarine fissure
	Auditory	Temporal	Heschl's gyrus
	Olfactory	Temporal	Piriform cortex (anteromedial temporal lobe)
	Gustatory	Parietal	Insular cortex
Unimodal sensory association cortex	Somesthetic	Parietal	Anterior inferior parietal lobe at the lateral sulcus (sylvian fissure)
	Visual	Occipital	Gyri surrounding calcarine fissure
	Auditory	Temporal	Superior temporal gyrus
	Olfactory	Temporal	Entorhinal cortex (parahippocampal gyrus)
Multimodal sensory association cortex	Somesthetic-visual	Parietal, occipital	Parietal-occipital junction
	Auditory-visual	Temporal	Middle and inferior temporal gyri
Nonsensory association cortex	Premotor	Frontal	Anterior to precentral gyrus
	Limbic	Temporal, parietal, frontal	Cingulate gyrus, parahippocampal gyrus, temporal pole, orbitofrontal cortex
Integrative association cortex	Posterior: final sensory integration	Parietal, temporal, occipital	Junction of parietal, temporal, occipital lobes
	Anterior: higher cortical functions	Frontal	Dorsolateral prefrontal cortex; this is the bulk of the outer surface (the convexity)

visual association cortex could integrate information such as the shape and color of an object and the direction and velocity of its movement.

Within primary sensory cortex and unimodal sensory association cortex, sensory information is processed sequentially. Each of the sensory modalities is operating in parallel. Subsequently, sensory information from the unimodal sensory association cortices converges in *multimodal sensory association cortex*. This level of association cortex takes highly processed unimodal sensory information from several sensory modalities and begins the process of weaving a comprehensive sensory experience. Multimodal sensory association cortex is found at the junction of parietal, temporal, and occipital lobes, near the visual, auditory, and somesthetic cortices.

Multimodal sensory association cortex in the posterior parietal area is responsible for the integration of visual and somesthetic information, essential for defining spatial relationships (visuospatial localization). This area is important for movement and motor control, specifically for the execution of more complex movements. Lesions of parietal association areas can result in a variety of neurological deficits, including apraxias (inability to perform certain learned complex movements in the absence of paralysis, sensory loss, or ataxia). Other deficits include agnosias (impairment of the ability to recognize or compre-

hend the meaning of various sensory stimuli), neglect (the inability to recognize or interact with part of one's personal or extrapersonal space), and problems with visually guided movements.

Multimodal sensory association cortex in the temporal area (the middle and inferior temporal gyri) is responsible for the integration of visual and auditory information, essential for language. This area is important for object identification, with discrete lesions resulting in area-specific agnosias, such as the inability to recognize faces (prosopagnosia) or the inability to recognize movements (akinetopsia). The inferior temporal gyrus is dominated by input of processed visual information from extrastriate visual areas and is of importance for the interpretation and categorization of complex visual stimuli. As noted earlier in this chapter, the superior temporal gyrus comprises primary and unimodal auditory association cortex.

Motor and premotor cortex represent the effector end of the brain, acting on the progressive integration of sensory, emotional, motivational, and physiological information from other association areas. The premotor areas are in themselves integrative, receiving stimuli from integrative association cortex as well as directly from unimodal somesthetic cortex. The influence of bias introduced by noradrenergic, serotoninergic, cholinergic, and possibly dopaminergic innervation is integrated with excitatory input from the thalamus, which represents the influence of the cerebellum and basal ganglia.

Limbic Structures

A "limbic system" was originally proposed as the neuroanatomical substrate of emotion. It was conceived as a discrete, closed system of cortical and subcortical structures and addressed the mechanism by which the cerebral cortex influences the hypothalamus and vice versa. As sophisticated tract-tracing techniques have clarified the extensive interconnections between limbic and nonlimbic structures and the existence of distributed systems throughout the CNS, the limbic system is now accepted as an open system thoroughly integrated with structures at all levels of the CNS (Parent 1996).

The subcortical limbic structures include the amygdaloid complex, septal nuclei, ventral striatum, mamillary nuclei, hypothalamus, and several smaller structures, in addition to several thalamic nuclei. Cortical regions considered limbic include the neocortical parahippocampal gyrus, cingulate gyrus, orbitofrontal cortex, allocortical olfactory (piriform) cortex, and hippocampus. Several limbic structures, including the amygdaloid complex, hippocampal formation, and cingulate gyrus, have extensive and often reciprocal connections with broad areas of neocortex, including virtually all areas of multimodal sensory association cortex and integrative association cortex (discussed in the following section).

From a functional perspective, the limbic system may form the gateway for neocortical cognitive influences on hypothalamic mechanisms associated with motivation and emotion, and vice versa. The limbic system directly influences neuroendocrine, autonomic, and behavioral mechanisms associated with the diencephalon. Functions such as fight or flight, homeostasis, self-maintenance, feeding, and sexuality are thought to be linked to limbic structures. It is, however, involved in more complex behaviors, including the elaboration and expression of emotions, as well as learning and memory. For example, the amygdala is the CNS locus that attaches emotional significance to extensively processed sensory stimuli. Additionally, the hippocampal formation–mamillary body–fornix system is crucial in the formation of new memories.

Integrative Association Cortex

Following integration of sensory modalities, information progresses to *integrative association cortex*. Two areas come under this heading, differing somewhat in emphasis. Note that these two areas are extensively interconnected, so they should be considered as two aspects of a distributed system. The smaller of the two areas—the *posterior integrative association cortical area*—is found where three lobes converge: parietal, occipital, and temporal. This area can be considered the locus of final multimodal sensory integration. Along with adjacent multimodal sensory association areas, it is in this area that object identification and other meaningful features of the sensory experience are appreciated. This suggests an area where a completely integrated perceptual world might be accessed and an area where dysfunction, as in degenerative dementias, could leave a person essentially lost in the world.

The *anterior integrative association cortical area* is found in the broad convexity of the frontal lobes, usually designated *dorsolateral prefrontal cortex*. This area manifests extensive connections with occipital, parietal, and temporal lobes, especially the posterior integrative association cortical area, and the cingulate gyrus. Afferent input from the dorsomedial thalamic nucleus provides input from the amygdala and other limbic structures. It also has reciprocal connections with premotor and supplementary motor areas, the caudate nucleus, and the hypothalamus.

Frontal association cortex thus receives information from all sensory modalities, from all other cortical association areas, from subcortical structures such as the basal ganglia and limbic system, and from the hypothalamus, the master of the body's physiology and ANS. Limbic input, both cortical and subcortical, introduces the influence of emotion, attention, and motivation to the integrated and interpreted sensory information.

Frontal association cortex is considered the locus of executive functioning, insight, judgment, planning, abstract thought, and the ability to anticipate consequences of actions. This area uniquely does not fully mature until late adolescence, so some of these are capabilities of adult humans. Other abilities conferred by frontal association cortex include the ability to form and retain inner conceptions of objects, with dysfunction resulting in increased distractibility. Lesions restricted to the frontal lobes can produce disturbances of mood, including depression or mania, as well as marked personality changes and impairment of judgment. Schizophrenic patients show "hypofrontality" in measurements of regional blood flow, especially in tasks that require (and usually result in) increased blood flow to the frontal lobes.

Hemispheric Lateralization of Function

Lateralization of speech is the most extreme example of lateralization of function (or *hemispheric dominance*). Speech centers are located in the dominant hemisphere (usually the left) in at least 90% of people. The anterior speech area (Broca's area) is located in prefrontal association cortex, just anterior to the most inferior part of the motor strip, corresponding approximately to Brodmann's area 44. Broca identified this region as an essential component of the motor mechanisms governing articulated speech. Lesions of Broca's area result in *motor aphasia* or nonfluent aphasia, but the most descriptive term is *expressive aphasia*. It should be noted that the muscle systems necessary for generating speech are intact. These names emphasize that understanding of language is usually preserved, but the ability to produce more than a few words is markedly impaired. The impairment of speech production is often accompanied by *agraphia*, the inability to generate written communication. Thus, the inability to express oneself through language characterizes this form of aphasia.

The posterior speech area (Wernicke's area) is located in the superior part of the temporal lobe, corresponding approximately to Brodmann's area 22. Lesions of Wernicke's area result in *sensory aphasia* or fluent aphasia, but again, the most descriptive term is *receptive aphasia*. Receptive aphasia is characterized by impairment of the appreciation of the meaning of both spoken and written words. Speech can appear normal in terms of flow, but the content of the communication is notable for a paucity of meaning and the use of incorrect words. Other forms of aphasia have been noted to result from lesions interrupting the fiber bundle interconnecting the anterior and posterior speech areas.

Although we have just stated that speech centers are located in the dominant hemisphere in most people, this is an oversimplification. In fact, the verbal aspect of speech occupies the dominant hemisphere in most people. The nondominant hemisphere has corresponding speech centers that govern *nonverbal* aspects of speech, or *prosody*. Lesions can result in impairment of the ability to imbue speech with the intonation and melody that lend emotional meaning to speech (anterior area) or in impairment of the ability to appreciate or understand the prosody of other people's speech (posterior area).

Electrophysiological Studies in the Psychiatric Evaluation of the Elderly Patient

Electroencephalogram

The EEG is the oldest functional imaging technique in continued use by psychiatry and neurology. Although lack-

ing the spatial resolution of newer imaging techniques, it retains an exceptionally high degree of temporal resolution, as EEG recordings reflect brain activity essentially on the same time scale as the activity of cortical neurons. The EEG has traditionally been used to assist diagnosis of epilepsy, delirium, and gross neuropathology. Although no qualitatively specific EEG markers exist for psychopathology, the EEG is exquisitely sensitive to a variety of neuropathological conditions. In addition, the introduction of quantitative EEG analysis has greatly expanded the usefulness of the technique in the evaluation of dementia and delirium. Quantitative EEG has been an important research tool, showing promise for enhancing our understanding of the neurophysiology and neuropathology underlying these conditions (Cook and Leuchter 1996; Holschneider and Leuchter 1999; Knott et al. 2001). The APA Task Force on Quantitative Electrophysiological Assessment (1991) has suggested that the technique has particular clinical utility for detection of slow-wave abnormalities.

The surface and scalp EEG measures the integrated electrical activity of neuronal processes in the superficial layers of the cortex. The specific neuronal events constituting the EEG signal likely result from summated postsynaptic potentials rather than the relatively short-duration action potentials (Creutzfeldt et al. 1966). Although activity in only the most superficial layers of cortex is thought to produce the EEG signal, the influence of deeper brain structures on the activity of these cortical neurons is reflected in the frequency spectra and synchrony of the EEG (Holschneider and Leuchter 1999). In particular, synchronous pacemaker activity is thought to be generated by thalamocortical networks, whereas desynchronization (which reflects increased arousal) may be mediated by monoaminergic inputs from brain stem and basal forebrain. Normally, the resistive and capacitive characteristics of the scalp and skull significantly attenuate the electrical signal. Thus, pathologies that may reduce electrical resistance (skull fractures) or increase resistance (subdural hematomas) may result in localized alterations in the amplitude of the EEG (Pfurtscheller and Cooper 1975). On occasion, the EEG may provide the initial clue to the presence of these conditions.

The EEG is typically recorded with the patient awake and at rest in a comfortable position. Specific studies also may use sleep deprivation or hyperventilation to increase sensitivity for detection of abnormal electrical activity. Electrodes are placed on the scalp in an array, or *montage*, of 10–20 leads, although special studies may warrant the addition of nasopharyngeal or ethmoid electrodes. Visual inspection by a qualified electroencephalographer remains the best method for distinguishing paroxysmal activity, epileptiform activity, and asymmetries from artifacts. Subsequently, portions of the signal may be digitized and the various frequency spectra of background activity quantified with a computer. The spectra of EEG frequencies are conventionally divided into bands defined as delta (<4 Hz), theta (4–8 Hz), alpha (8-13 Hz), and beta (>13 Hz). These frequency bands can be characterized on the basis of *absolute power* (the magnitude of the signal amplitude of a specific frequency band, measured in microvolts squared) and *relative power* (the percent contribution of a specific frequency band to the total power), in addition to measures of ratios of particular frequencies ("spectral ratios"). Alterations in the frequency spectrum associated with neuropathology may be global (often seen in metabolic, toxic, or anoxic encephalopathy) or localized (seen in focal lesions such as tumors or strokes). Other useful quantitative EEG measures are *coherence*, which indicates the functional coupling of distinct brain regions based on common time-locked frequency elements, and *cordance*, which normalizes power across electrode sites and combines absolute and relative power into a single measure (Holschneider and Leuchter 1999). Cordance, in particular, appears to best correlate with measures of cerebral perfusion (Leuchter et al. 1999).

EEG Changes With Normal Aging

The EEG of a healthy awake adult is dominated by frequencies in the alpha range. This pattern shows little change with normal aging (Duffy et al. 1984). A small decline in the mean alpha frequency may be seen beginning in the fifth decade, but a significant drop suggests underlying neuropathology. When comparing healthy subjects across the entire span of the adult years, a small increase in beta frequency activity often correlates with age (Holschneider and Leuchter 1995). Small increases in theta activity are frequently seen in healthy aged subjects but also may be associated with the subclinical onset of cerebrovascular disease; however, normal aging is generally not associated with significant increases in delta activity (Holschneider and Leuchter 1999).

EEG Changes With Dementia

The most characteristic EEG findings associated with dementia are an increase in low-frequency (delta and theta) activity, along with a decrease in high-frequency beta activity and slowing of the dominant alpha frequencies. These separate findings are not necessarily statistically associated within populations of subjects with dementia, suggesting that they may reflect independent underlying processes (Claus et al. 2000; Leuchter et al. 1993a). Abnormal findings with conventional EEGs are most evident in the later stages of dementia but may be common even in the early stages (Leuchter et al. 1993b). The probability of early detection of these abnormalities is increased by combining several complementary quantitative EEG measures (Leuchter et al. 1993a). Thus, the change in the low-frequency band is best able to distinguish subjects with dementia from control subjects, although inclusion of additional parameters has cumulative diagnostic significance. Several studies have also shown decreased coherence in dementia, which may reflect the loss of long corticocortical connections (Knott et al. 2000; Leuchter et al. 1992). By combining measures of spectral ratios and coherence variables, quantitative EEG has accurately discriminated between subjects with Alzheimer's dementia, subjects with vascular dementia, and control subjects without dementia (Leuchter et al. 1987).

The cognitive dysfunction seen in Alzheimer's dementia is associated with loss of central cholinergic systems. Following treatment of dementia with the acetylcholinesterase inhibitor physostigmine (Gustafson 1993), tetrahydroaminoacridine (Minthon et al. 1993; Perryman and Fitten 1991), or rivastigmine (Adler and Brassen 2001), the quantitative EEG shows a decrease in slow-frequency power and an increase in high-frequency power. Thus, the quantitative EEG may parallel response to agents that enhance cognitive function in subjects with dementia (although this effect may not necessarily be specific to cholinergic agents).

EEG Changes With Delirium

Delirium refers to an acute confusional state, characterized by clouding of consciousness and impaired attentional capacity. The causes of delirium are numerous, with the most common being drug toxicity and metabolic imbalances. The EEG is a standard tool in the evaluation of delirium because EEG slowing is an almost universal finding in delirium. The quantitative EEG may be more sensitive than the conventional EEG to changes in slow-wave power during the course of delirium (Leuchter and Jacobson 1991). The quantitative EEG signal correlates with the severity and duration of the delirium (Koponen et al. 1989), whereas the normalization of the signal parallels and occasionally precedes the course of recovery (Leuchter and Jacobson 1991). The degree of slowing reflects the severity of the delirium even in the context of preexisting dementia and therefore may be of particular use in detecting delirium as a complication of dementia (Jacobson et al. 1993).

EEG Changes With Depression

The standard awake EEG is expected to have normal findings in otherwise healthy depressed subjects (Heyman et al. 1991). Thus, in the context of cognitive dysfunction suggestive of dementia, a normal EEG result may be useful in identifying depression-related pseudodementia (Brenner et al. 1989). However, several studies of subjects with pseudodementia or depression still documented more EEG abnormalities than in nondepressed control subjects (Brenner et al. 1986, 1989; Visser et al. 1985). In depressed elderly subjects, abnormal EEG findings are associated with an increased risk for subsequent cognitive dysfunction and may be indicative of underlying cerebrovascular disease. The EEG recorded during sleep (polysomnographic recording) often shows depression-related phenomena such as reduced slow-wave sleep and decreased REM latency (see Chapter 20, "Sleep and Circadian Rhythm Disorders," in this volume).

Epilepsy in the Elderly

The incidence of seizures in the elderly is quite high and may account for up to one-quarter of new epilepsy cases (Sander et al. 1990). Approximately half of these seizures are related to either strokes or tumors, whereas up to a quarter have unknown causes; as many as 80% become recurrent (Luhdorf et al. 1986b). Alzheimer's dementia is also a risk factor for refractory seizures in the elderly (Mendez et al. 1994). The EEG is commonly used to confirm epileptiform activity and to assist in classification of the seizure disorder. However, a high percentage of persons with seizures may have normal EEG findings, depending on the type of seizure and the interval between the seizure activity and the recording (Luhdorf et al. 1986a). In addition, the presence of interictal epileptiform activity (spike-and-wave complexes) alone does not establish a diagnosis of epilepsy. Various other clinical conditions can predispose to paroxysmal electrical activity unrelated to seizures. For example, elderly patients with syncopal episodes show an almost 50% incidence of epileptiform events (Hughes and Zialcita 2000). Increased diagnostic reliability may be facilitated by simultaneous EEG and videotape monitoring to assess motor and behavioral disturbance with concomitant EEG activity (Bridgers and Ebersole 1985). Ultimately, the diagnosis of epilepsy and the decision to treat with anticonvulsant medication should rely primarily on the clinical presentation.

Evoked Potentials

Evoked potentials refer to EEG signals recorded in response to a specific sensory stimulus. However, the amplitude of background EEG activity is typically 10–100 times that of single evoked responses. Averaging the stimulus-locked signal over multiple trials causes the background activity to average out to zero, allowing accurate measure of the amplitude and latency of the evoked response. Evoked potentials are frequently used to assess neuroanatomical pathways underlying the response to visual, auditory, or somatosensory stimuli. Most studies focus on particular components of the evoked potential waveform, designated according to the eliciting conditions or the electrophysiological signature (e.g., the P300, or P3, wave, seen as a positive-going wave 300 ms after the trigger stimulus). The P3 wave is elicited in response to infrequent target stimuli to which the subject must attend; these stimuli are typically intermixed with multiple irrelevant stimuli. As such, the P3 wave is thought to reflect neural processes underlying attention and immediate memory (Polich and Kok 1995). The P3 wave has been shown to increase in latency with age in neurologically normal subjects (Goodin et al. 1978a), with little age-related change in other components of the evoked waveform (Polich 1997). The P3 latency is increased further in most patients with dementia (Goodin et al. 1978b; Polich 1991). The P3 latency is related to the severity of the dementia, although less so with mild dementia (Polich et al. 1986). Although studies of the P3 latency have not been able to distinguish between subtypes of cortical dementias (Polich et al. 1986), other studies have suggested that evoked potentials may distinguish between cortical (e.g., Alzheimer's) and subcortical (Parkinson's or Huntington's disease) dementias (Goodin and Aminoff 1986, 1987).

Use of evoked potentials in the evaluation of dementias remains primarily a research tool, although studies to date suggest that, like quantitative EEG, evoked potentials may serve to elucidate aspects of the underlying neuropathologies of dementias (Polich 1991).

Magnetoencephalography (MEG)

Magnetoencephalography (MEG) is the technique of recording magnetic fields generated by neural activity, which according to the "right-hand rule," occur at right angles to the direction of current flow across the neuronal membranes. Thus, the MEG signal is related to the EEG but has the advantage of more accurately detecting current sources from deep brain structures (Reeve et al. 1989). For example, MEG recordings have localized the neural generators of the P300 in the frontal and posterior parietal cortices and have shown age-related decreases in the magnetic signal from these areas that parallel the

P300 (Anderer et al. 1998). Recent MEG studies have reported delayed preconscious auditory processing in patients with mild to moderate Alzheimer's dementia (Pekkonen et al. 1999). However, MEG remains primarily a research tool largely because of cost and the technical constraints of the recording.

Neuroanatomical and Neuropathological Processes of Aging

The facility of cognition is that function of the human brain that uniquely sets us apart from lower animals. Unfortunately, this unique ability is subject to degeneration as a consequence of aging. Much more extensive degeneration with significant loss of cognitive function occurs during the evolution of Alzheimer's disease and other neurodegenerative disorders that uniquely afflict the aging population.

We focus on the neuroanatomical and neuropathological processes that occur during normal aging. Subsequently, we address abnormal aging, discussing each of the major neurodegenerative disorders that affect the human brain and cause dementia.

Neuroanatomy

The average adult male human brain weighs 1,400 g (Sunderman and Boerner 1949). The organ is composed of neurons and supporting structures. The supporting structures are astrocytes, oligodendroglia, and ependyma, collectively known as *glia, blood vessels,* and *myelin.* Myelin is a complex lipoprotein that serves to protect axonal processes and to facilitate neurotransmission.

It has been estimated that the adult human brain contains some 20 billion neurons. Each neuron is an individual unit that can be thought of as a microprocessor. Individual neurons are functionally integrated into networks of allied nerve cells. Networks of neurons are assembled within subcortical structures that are known as *nuclei* (Vogel 1996). Networks of neurons in the neocortex, the outer layer of the cerebrum, are also organized into functional units so that some parts of the neocortex are devoted to cognitive function, whereas other parts command motor skills and the major senses, including vision, hearing, and smell.

The neuron develops during embryonic intrauterine life. Both neurons and glia originate from the germinal zone in the subpial and subependymal regions. During intrauterine development, neurons undergo mitotic divi-

sion and then migrate to the cerebral cortex. They are assisted in their migration by glial filaments that stretch from the subependymal germinal zone to the cortex (Marín-Padilla 1995). Once the neurons have reached their permanent location, the neurons differentiate and develop synaptic connections. Development of synaptic connections continues to progress rapidly after birth (Vogel 1996). The neuron is no longer capable of division after birth, but synaptic connections are continuously remodeled. This is the neuroanatomical basis of memory and learning. Loss of some of these synaptic connections is the neuroanatomical cause of normal age-related memory impairment. Pathological loss of these synaptic connections is the basis of dementia.

Each neuron is surrounded by a three-layer plasma membrane that is regionally specialized to form axons, dendrites, and synapses. As with all cells in the body, the plasma membrane of neurons controls the movement of metabolites between the neuron and its environment. Selected areas serve as synaptic sites. Synaptic transmission transfers messages from one neuron to other neurons and to end organs (Vogel 1996).

The neuronal nucleus is located in the cell body. It varies in size from 5 to 100 mm. The area around the nucleus, or perikaryon, contains ribosomes that synthesize the proteins that are necessary to maintain metabolism and synaptic transmission. Ribosomes may reside free within the cytoplasm, or they may be attached to the endoplasmic reticulum. The endoplasmic reticulum, being largely composed of proteins, is acidic in nature, and it appears as a blue granular Nissl substance on histological preparations (Vogel 1996).

Neurons are metabolically very active cells and thus require numerous mitochondria. Most of the neuronal mitochondria are contained in the perikaryon. Additionally, numerous proteins are turned over frequently in neuronal cell bodies as a function of their role in synaptic transmission. Some of these proteins are not metabolized entirely, and these nonmetabolized proteins are stored in structures known as *lysosomes.* Histologically, collections of these lysosomes are known as *lipofusion granules.* Increased numbers of lipofusion granules are evidence of normal metabolic wear and tear. As a consequence, they accumulate with age.

Microtubules, neurofilaments, and microfilaments are additional specialized structures within neurons. Microtubules measure 20–30 μm, neurofilaments 10 μm, and microfilaments 5 μm in length. Microtubules are long, unbranched cylinders composed almost entirely of the protein tubulin (Vogel 1996). Many neurodegenerative processes cause abnormal cross-linking of microtubules. This results in the formation of neurofibrillary tangles.

The synapse is a specialized structure that permits the flow of information from one neuron to another neuron or to the end organ. The synapse is analogous to an electronic circuit so that the flow of information is from sensory to motor neurons, for example, but never the reverse. The synapse consists of the approximation of two membranes physically separated by approximately 20 µm. The contact between an axon and a cell body is termed an *axosomatic synapse*. Contact between an axon and a dendrite is termed an *axodendritic synapse*. The synaptic connection between two axons is known as an *axoaxonic synapse*, and the synapse between two dendrites is known as a *dendrodendritic synapse*. When an electrical impulse is transmitted from the nerve cell body through the axon or dendrite to the synapse, the neuron releases a substance known as a *neurotransmitter*. Each neuron releases only one neurotransmitter (Vogel 1996). Groups of neurons that are collected into nuclei generally release the same neurotransmitter. For example, the neurons in the nucleus basalis of Meynert release the neurotransmitter acetylcholine. Suppression or enhancement of neurotransmission is the pharmacological basis of most neuroactive compounds.

Normal Aging

We all recognize that as we age, our fund of knowledge and experience increases, but regrettably, we may not always recollect this information with the same speed as we did when we were younger. When the process of remembering is slightly slowed, but still intact, this is recognized as normal aging. However, this normal slowing may progress in some individuals to mild cognitive impairment. In a further subgroup of unfortunate individuals, this mild cognitive impairment and memory loss may follow an inexorable downhill decline into dementia. Subsequent sections cover the changes observed in pathological aging. In this section, we discuss the neuropathological changes that are seen in persons who have aged normally.

Normal aging is sometimes associated with absolutely no neuropathological changes. Approximately 30%–50% of normally aged individuals show no evidence of cortical atrophy, no evidence of cell loss, no evidence of senile neuritic plaques, and no evidence of neurofibrillary tangles. However, in most elderly individuals, some pathological changes are evident (Hulette et al. 1998). Both senile neuritic plaques and neurofibrillary tangles can be observed in normally aged individuals. Nevertheless, the frequency and distribution of these pathological changes in the elderly without dementia are generally much less extensive than that observed in individuals at the same age who have dementia.

Senile plaques first begin to appear in the cortex, where they are observed as round smudges on silver impregnation studies. Plaques at this stage begin to become immunoreactive for β-amyloid, but there is no histological distortion of the surrounding neuropil. These are known as *diffuse plaques*. Diffuse plaques may occur quite early in individuals who are environmentally and genetically at risk for the development of Alzheimer's disease (Crain et al. 1995). Diffuse plaques are common in normally aged individuals and are considered to have no pathological significance. As the plaque matures, neurites that are filled with β-amyloid and other abnormally cross-linked proteins begin to accumulate around a central amyloid core. These plaques are now called *mature neuritic plaques*. A few mature neuritic plaques are common in normally aged individuals. Even frequent mature plaques may be seen. The distribution and frequency of mature neuritic plaques do not consistently correlate with cognitive function.

In contrast to this lack of correlation between neuritic plaques and cognition, neurofibrillary tangle frequency and distribution do predict cognitive status. Persons with neurofibrillary change limited to the entorhinal cortex and the inferior temporal lobe generally have functioned normally in their communities. Prior to death, they were able to live independently, to engage in conversation, and to be involved in all of the normal activities of daily living. However, when these persons are subjected to rigorous neuropsychological tests, they may show some slight slowing, especially on tests of frontal lobe function. Their ability to create trails is somewhat slowed compared with their counterparts who have absolutely no neuropathological changes. They also show some minor deficits in word list recall (Hulette et al. 1998; Welsh-Bohmer et al. 2001). When the neurofibrillary change has become more extensive, spreading to the neocortex, cognitive impairment develops (Mitchell et al. 2002). Further studies of normal aging may yield additional cognitive tests, which are sensitive indicators of early decline. There is hope that in the future, individuals who begin to show cognitive decline may be subjects for cognitive or pharmacological intervention.

Alzheimer's Disease

Alzheimer's disease is, by definition, associated with cognitive impairment before death. Pathologically, Alzheimer's disease frequently can be diagnosed by gross inspection of the brain. Generally, moderate to severe diffuse corti-

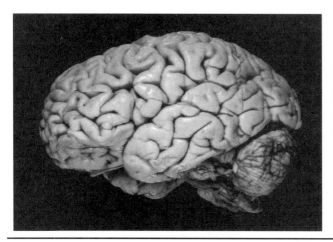
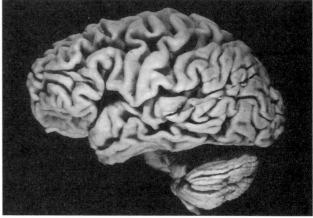

FIGURE 4–1. Normal brain—lateral view (left). Alzheimer's disease brain—lateral view (right).

In the Alzheimer's brain, notice moderate diffuse cortical atrophy. The gyri are narrowed and the sulci are widened.

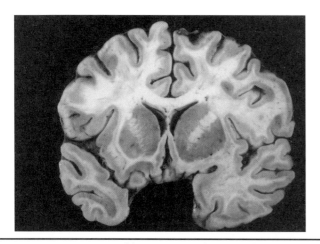
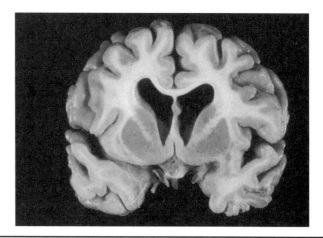

FIGURE 4–2. Normal brain—coronal section through the basal ganglia (left). Alzheimer's disease brain—coronal section through the basal ganglia (right).

In the normal brain, the lateral ventricles are small and there is no atrophy. In the Alzheimer's brain, the lateral ventricles are enlarged and dilated from neuronal loss and atrophy of the cortex.

cal atrophy is present. The gyri are narrowed, and the sulci are widened. This cortical atrophy may be readily apparent in imaging studies that may have been performed years prior to death (Figures 4–1A, 4–1B).

The atrophy associated with Alzheimer's disease results in a 200- to 500-g weight loss. The brain of an Alzheimer's patient generally weighs less than 1,200 g and may be as small as 800 g. The atrophy is bilaterally symmetrical and affects all lobes of the brain, with sometimes more severe involvement of the frontal and temporal lobes. The cerebellum is generally uninvolved. The meninges are grossly normal. The cranial nerves usually are normal, and the large cerebral vessels in cases of uncomplicated Alzheimer's disease are not affected by atherosclerosis. When the brain is sectioned, moderate to severe ventricular dilation is grossly evident (Figures 4–2A, 4–2B). In uncomplicated Alzheimer's disease, subcorti-

cal structures are grossly normal (Esiri et al. 1997).

When sections of the brain are stained and examined under the microscope, several characteristic features may be identified. The senile or neuritic plaque is one of the most-studied pathological hallmarks of Alzheimer's disease. The senile plaque is a discrete globular structure ranging from 50 to 200 μm in diameter. The plaque consists of a dense amyloid core surrounded by swollen axonal and dendritic processes that contain abnormally cross-linked microtubule proteins, extracellular amyloid deposits, reactive astrocytes, and microglial cells. Immunohistochemical studies of senile plaques indicate that they are largely composed of β-amyloid protein. This fibrillar β-amyloid protein has a β-pleated sheet structure that induces polarization of the planar dye Congo red. These polarized dye molecules result in apple green birefringence when viewed under polarized light. Senile neu-

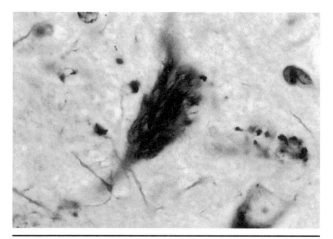

FIGURE 4–4. Alzheimer's disease brain—hippocampus, neurofibrillary tangle.

Note the fibrillary nature of this intraneuronal inclusion. The tangle is shaped like the neuron and fills the cell body. Tangle formation is due to cross-linking of abnormally phosphorylated microtubule-associated protein. These abnormal cross-linked proteins then form paired helical filaments. The paired helical filaments interfere with normal neuronal transport and synaptic transmission. (King's silver impregnation stain; original magnification ×1,000.)

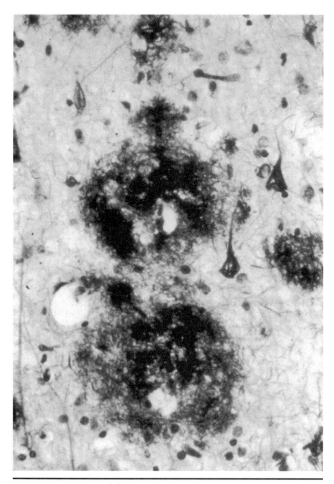

FIGURE 4–3. Alzheimer's disease brain.

The neocortex is filled with senile neuritic plaques and neurofibrillary tangles. (King's silver impregnation stain; original magnification ×400.)

ritic plaques are also sometimes termed *amyloid plaques* to denote this characteristic feature.

Studies of the molecular composition of plaques have shown that the senile plaque also contains multiple proteins that are involved in the inflammatory cascade (Hulette and Walford 1987; McGeer et al. 1999). Reactive microglial cells, which are the resident immunocompetent cells of the CNS, are prominent. The presence of inflammatory mediators and immunocompetent cells in the vicinity of senile plaques has led some investigators to believe that the immune system plays a significant role in senile plaque formation (McGeer et al. 1999). Indeed, there are ever-increasing reports of use of nonsteroidal anti-inflammatory agents to slow progression and even prevent or delay the onset of Alzheimer's disease.

The neurofibrillary tangle is the second characteristic microscopic feature observed in Alzheimer's disease brain tissue. In contrast to the senile neuritic plaques, which are unique to Alzheimer's disease, neurofibrillary tangles occur in a wide variety of neurodegenerative disorders, such as frontotemporal dementia, postencephalitic parkinsonism,

dementia pugilistica, amyotrophic lateral sclerosis–parkinsonism-dementia complex of Guam, subacute sclerosing panencephalitis, and Niemann-Pick disease (Hulette et al. 1991). Neurofibrillary tangles are neuronal inclusions composed of the abnormally cross-linked microtubule-associated protein known as tau. Their configuration is determined by the intrinsic shape of the neurons they affect so that tangles occurring in the hippocampal formation have a pyramidal or flame shape, and tangles occurring in subcortical structures may have a globoid shape (Figures 4–3 and 4–4).

Neurofibrillary tangles develop slowly. Early in the process of neurofibrillary degeneration, tangles may be difficult to discern. However, as disease progresses and normal proteins become increasingly cross-linked, intraneuronal tangles may be observed in routinely stained sections when examined by the skilled observer. As the degenerative progress continues, affected neurons die, but the abnormally cross-linked proteins are left behind. When this occurs, eosinophilic "ghost" tangles are readily observed, especially in the entorhinal cortex and hippocampus. Tangles are better demonstrated with silver impregnation studies and immunohistochemistry to visualize the proteins implicated in tangle formation. The major component of neurofibrillary tangles is the microtubule-associated protein tau, which plays a role in microtubule assembly and stabilization (Lantos and Cairns 2000). There are six normal isoforms of tau in the adult human brain. All of these isoforms are hyperphosphorylated in Alzheimer's disease. Antibodies to specific phosphorylation-dependent epitopes may be used to show pathological cross-linking because the antigenic properties of these abnormal proteins differ from those of their normal counterparts. Because tau or microtubule-associated protein forms the backbone of the neuron and its processes, cross-linking of the protein causes pathology not only within the neuronal cell body but also within its processes or "neurites." Abnormally cross-linked proteins within neurites are seen on histological sections as dystrophic neurites or neuropil threads.

Electron microscopy shows that neurofibrillary tangles are composed of dense bundles of long filaments. These filaments occupy most of the neuron's cytoplasm. Each filament has a diameter of 10–20 μm, with crossover points at 80 μm resulting in a double helix. These anatomical structures have been termed *paired helical filaments*. These paired helical filaments displace normal cellular organelles and distort the nucleus.

Large population studies of young and old adults without Alzheimer's disease and elderly persons with dementia have found that neurofibrillary change follows a stereotypical progression (Braak and Braak 1991). Neurofibrillary tangles first begin to appear in the entorhinal cortex and the hippocampus. The first appearance of neurofibrillary tangles is called Braak Stage I and II. At these stages, persons, even elderly persons, with neurofibrillary change restricted to the entorhinal cortex, hippocampus, and inferior temporal lobe structures generally do not have significant cognitive impairment. At the next stage, Braak Stage III or IV, tangles become more widespread, involving the inferior temporal lobe diffusely and parts of the neocortex. The individual may or may not develop significant cognitive impairment. However, when cognitive difficulties are present at this stage of neurofibrillary degeneration, they are frequently associated with other neuropathological processes known to cause dementia. Cognitive impairment at this stage of neurofibrillary tangle formation may actually be caused by the concurrence of several disorders, such as Alzheimer's disease plus cerebrovascular disease, Alzheimer's disease plus dementia with Lewy bodies, or Alzheimer's disease plus cardiovascular compromise. If neurofibrillary change progresses unimpeded to involve the cortex globally, including the occipital lobe and the primary visual cortex, Braak Stage V or VI is reached. Individuals at this stage always have dementia, and the dementia is due to Alzheimer's disease.

Other pathology seen in Alzheimer's disease includes granulovacuolar degeneration, which was first described in 1911. The granulovacuoles are abnormal cytoplasmic inclusions of 3.5-μm diameter surrounded by a clear halo. These granulovacuoles are considered to be age related and contain actin proteins (Figure 4–5). Granulovacuoles

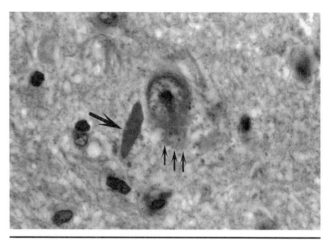

FIGURE 4–5. Alzheimer's disease brain—hippocampus. This neuron has undergone granulovacuolar degeneration (**small arrows**). Granulovacuolar degenerations are seen almost exclusively in the hippocampal formation. The frequency of granulovacuolar degeneration increases as neurofibrillary change increases elsewhere in the neocortex. Also seen here is a Hirano body (**large arrow**). Hirano bodies are eosinophilic extracellular aggregates of actin protein. Hirano bodies are usually closely associated with granulovacuolar degeneration. (Hematoxylin-eosin stain; original magnification ×1,000.)

occur within large pyramidal neurons of the hippocampal formation and amygdala. The frequency of neurons with granulovacuolar degeneration correlates with the frequency and distribution of neurofibrillary change and thus Braak stage (unpublished observations, November 2002).

Extracellular eosinophilic rods composed of actin filaments are known as *Hirano bodies*. They are seen as bright pink structures on hematoxylin-eosin-stained sections. They have a diameter of approximately 25 μm and are approximately 30 μm in length. Hirano bodies are most commonly seen surrounding pyramidal neurons in the hippocampal formation. The frequency of Hirano bodies increases with age and with the severity of neurofibrillary change.

Neuronal loss and gliosis are perhaps the essential pathological features of Alzheimer's disease. The neuronal loss accompanies the accumulation of senile plaques and neurofibrillary tangles that are seen pathologically in Alzheimer's disease. Neuronal loss results naturally in loss of synapses and abnormalities of neuronal processes (Einstein et al. 1998). This neuronal and synapse loss is nearly always accompanied by increased numbers and enlargement of astrocytes. This astrogliosis is readily observed on routine histological sections or by immunohistochemical preparations with an antibody to glial fibrillary acidic protein. In addition to astrogliosis, microgliosis occurs as a result of increased numbers of microglial cells, especially in the region of senile plaque formation. These microglia are the resident immunocompetent cells of the CNS. They are normally engaged in antigen presentation and phagocytosis. These cells are thought to represent the nidus for many of the inflammatory mediators that are associated with senile plaques (Hulette and Walford 1987).

Vascular abnormalities are common in Alzheimer's disease brain tissue. Many, but not all, cases of end-stage Alzheimer's disease are associated with extracellular deposits of vascular amyloid (Schmechel et al. 1993). This vascular amyloid is the same as the β-amyloid protein that is present in senile plaques. The severity of vascular amyloid deposition depends on many factors. Interestingly, we have determined that one of these factors is apolipoprotein E (apoE). Apolipoprotein E is a lipid transport molecule that occurs in three allelic forms: APOE2, APOE3, and APOE4. APOE4 is a major genetic risk factor for the development of Alzheimer's disease in late life (Corder et al. 1993; Roses et al. 1995, 1996; Saunders et al. 1993, 1996).

Individuals who have inherited one copy of the APOE4 allele have increased risk of vascular amyloid deposition, and individuals with two copies of the APOE4 gene invariably have very severe vascular amyloid deposition. In a recent study comparing the neuropathological changes of APOE3/APOE3- and APOE4/APOE4-related Alzheimer's disease, it was discovered that APOE4/APOE4 patients with severe vascular amyloid deposition also had markedly reduced smooth muscle actin in their cerebral vessels (Hulette et al. 1999a). It would thus appear that vascular amyloid replaces smooth muscle actin in the blood vessels of persons with APOE4/APOE4-related Alzheimer's disease. Interestingly, apoE knockout mice have a leaky blood-brain barrier (Fullerton et al. 2001). This presents the intriguing possibility that vascular pathology may be an inciting event in APOE4-related Alzheimer's disease.

Abnormalities in the white matter are also common in Alzheimer's disease. Whether these abnormalities are a cause or a consequence of the basic neuropathological process is a matter of intense debate. Nevertheless, people with severe Alzheimer's-type pathology have myelin loss in the white matter and perivascular retraction of the neuropil. Frequently, increased numbers of macrophages are present in the perivascular space. Sometimes areas of microinfarction develop.

Considerable effort has been expended to standardize the clinical and neuropathological assessment of patients with dementia (McKhann et al. 1984). Criteria based on neuritic plaque frequency and cognitive status, as well as criteria based on neurofibrillary tangle distribution and frequency, have been proposed (Braak and Braak 1991; Mirra et al. 1991). Recently, the National Institute on Aging (NIA) in cooperation with the Reagan Institute pro-

posed diagnostic guidelines that require the identification of both frequent senile neuritic plaques and frequent neurofibrillary tangles for a definitive diagnosis of Alzheimer's disease (Hyman and Trojanowski 1997). These criteria, known as NIA-Reagan criteria, have gained wide acceptance in research centers.

Dementia With Lewy Bodies

Dementia with Lewy bodies is the second most common neurodegenerative disorder manifesting as dementia (Ince et al. 2000). Dementia with Lewy bodies can best be thought of as combined Alzheimer's disease and Parkinson's disease. Clinical and pathological features of both disorders are present. Patients may present to medical attention first complaining of a movement disorder, or they may present with a primary complaint of dementia. Patients who present with dementia often show subtle signs of extrapyramidal dysfunction when subjected to careful neurological examination. This form of dementia is frequently associated with psychotic features such as delusions, hallucinations, and bizarre behaviors (Hulette et al. 1995). Like Alzheimer's disease, dementia with Lewy bodies may be familial (Ishikawa et al. 1997; Rosenberg et al. 2000; Trembath et al. 2003). Genetic studies indicate a potential locus for dementia with Lewy bodies on chromosome 12 (Scott et al. 2000).

Generally, the weight of the brain of the patient with dementia with Lewy bodies is greater than the weight of the brain of the patient with Alzheimer's disease and may closely approximate normal. Cortical atrophy occurs, but this atrophy is generally much less profound than that seen in Alzheimer's disease in its pure form. On sectioning of the brain, mild ventricular dilation is seen. The hippocampus is generally not grossly atrophic. Sectioning of the midbrain reveals pallor of the substantia nigra as seen in Figure 4–6.

When the substantia nigra is examined microscopically, neuronal loss and gliosis with pigment incontinence are detected. Lewy bodies are readily identified (Figure 4–7). Oddly enough, the frequency of Lewy bodies in the substantia nigra of patients with dementia with Lewy bodies may be greater than in patients dying of idiopathic Parkinson's disease. Even in patients with dementia, Lewy bodies may be confined to the brain stem. However, Lewy body pathology frequently has spread to involve the limbic system and the neocortex. The pathology of this disease forms a broad spectrum ranging from the occasional case with Lewy bodies confined to the midbrain to the more commonly observed cases with Lewy body formation in the limbic system and the cortex. Alzheimer's-type pathology, which frequently, but

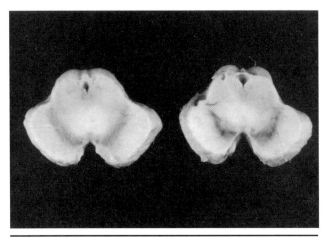

FIGURE 4–6. Dementia with Lewy bodies brain—section through the midbrain (left). Normal brain—section through the midbrain (right).

Note the loss of the black neuromelanin pigment in the substantia nigra of the patient with dementia with Lewy bodies. This degeneration of the substantia nigra may cause extrapyramidal symptoms such as tremor, rigidity, and bradykinesia.

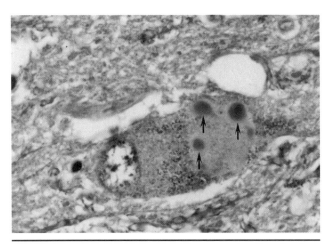

FIGURE 4–7. Dementia with Lewy bodies brain—pigmented neuron of the substantia nigra with several Lewy bodies (arrows).

Lewy bodies are intraneuronal cytoplasmic inclusions with a clear halo. (Hematoxylin-eosin stain; original magnification ×1,000.)

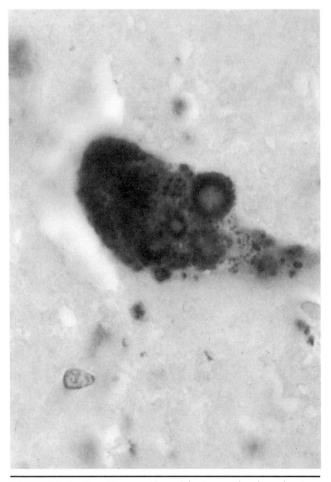

FIGURE 4–8. Dementia with Lewy bodies brain—pigmented neuron of the substantia nigra with numerous Lewy bodies.

Many more Lewy bodies are apparent with this α-synuclein immunostain than are seen in the routine preparation (Figure 4–7). (α-Synuclein immunostain; original magnification ×1,000.)

not always, complicates the pathological picture, is generally mild in nature. Diffuse and neuritic plaques may be frequent, but neurofibrillary change is generally less intense than in "pure" Alzheimer's disease. Braak stage neurofibrillary change of IV or less is very common in dementia with Lewy bodies (Rosenberg et al. 2001).

Although neurofibrillary tangles are less frequent in dementia with Lewy bodies than in Alzheimer's disease, new immunohistochemical studies have reported that Lewy bodies are more frequent than previously suspected. α-Synuclein is a protein that has been found to be mutated in rare families with early-onset familial Parkin-

son's disease. Spillantini and colleagues (1997) reported that this protein is expressed in Lewy bodies. Immunohistochemistry for α-synuclein has emerged as a sensitive and specific diagnostic tool for the evaluation of dementia with Lewy bodies (Hamilton 2000) (Figure 4–8).

Consensus guidelines have been proposed for the clinical and pathological evaluation of dementia with Lewy bodies (McKeith et al. 1996). These guidelines have begun to gain wide acceptance.

- *Brain stem category* implies that Lewy body pathology is confined to the substantia nigra, LC, and other brain stem nuclei such as the dorsal motor nucleus of the vagus nerve.
- *Limbic category* is defined as disease involving the brain stem and also limbic system structures including the amygdala, entorhinal cortex, insula, and cingulate gyrus.

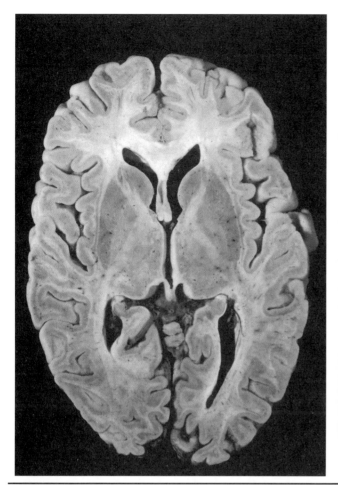 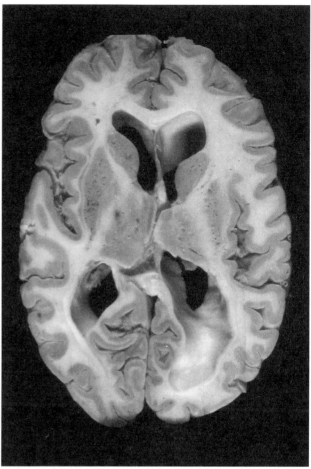

FIGURE 4–9. Normal brain—horizontal section through the basal ganglia (left). Vascular dementia, Binswanger's subcortical arteriosclerotic encephalopathy—horizontal section through the basal ganglia at the same level (right).
In the vascular dementia brain, the ventricles are dilated and the white matter is pitted and granular.

• *Neocortical category* includes cases in which Lewy body formation occurs throughout the neocortex, as well as in the midbrain and limbic system (McKeith et al. 1996).

Vascular Dementia

Cerebrovascular disease is associated with a high risk of cognitive impairment and dementia (Brun 2000). Because vascular causes of cognitive impairment are common and potentially reversible, this entity has received increasing attention in recent years. The risk factors for vascular dementia are identical to those for coronary atherosclerosis. These include arterial hypertension, atrial fibrillation, myocardial infarction, diabetes, systemic atherosclerosis, lipid abnormalities, and smoking.

Both small- and large-vessel disease may result in cognitive impairment (Meyer et al. 2000; Pasquier et al. 1999). Large-artery disease, particularly involving the anterior and posterior cerebral circulation, is likely to be associated with dementia. The pathological process may take the form of complete occlusion of the anterior or posterior cerebral artery with the evolution of complete infarcts. However, hypoperfusion syndromes due to severe nonocclusive cerebrovascular atherosclerosis are increasingly being recognized as a cause of dementia.

Small-vessel infarction or ischemia, especially when it occurs in a strategic location, such as the dorsal medial nucleus of the thalamus or the hippocampal formation, also may be associated with cognitive impairment (Hulette et al. 1997). Lacunes and infarcts in the subcortical structures, especially the basal ganglia and thalamus, also may cause or contribute to dementia (Zekry et al. 2002) (Figures 4–9A, 4–9B). Lacunes are seen pathologically as small defects in basal ganglia or cortex. Gliosis of the surrounding neuropil is seen, and the central infarcted tissue is gradually replaced by macrophages (Montine and Hulette 1997) (Figure 4–10).

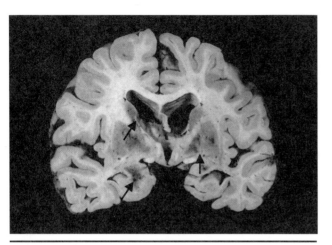

FIGURE 4–10. Vascular dementia with multiple lacunar infarcts (arrows)—coronal section of brain.

Multiple lacunar infarcts are seen in the basal ganglia. These may cause strokes. Because the individual lesions may occur at different times, there is a stepwise progression of dementia.

Alternatively, chronic hypertension and atherosclerosis may cause widespread profound white matter ischemic injury without frank infarction. This is recognized pathologically as Binswanger's subcortical arteriosclerotic encephalopathy. In addition to atherosclerosis in the cerebral vasculature, coronary atherosclerosis and cardiovascular injury may result in hypoperfusion injury and contribute to the dementing process (Hulette et al. 2002).

A rare inherited form of vascular dementia is cerebral autosomal dominant arteriopathy with subcortical infarcts and leukoencephalopathy. These patients have strokes at an early age and subsequently may develop dementia. Characteristically, a vasculopathy without amyloid or atherosclerosis affects the arterioles of the white matter (Gray et al. 1994; Zhang et al. 1994). The genetic defect has been mapped to chromosome 19 (Tournier-Lasserve et al. 1993).

Frontotemporal Dementia

The frontotemporal dementias include classic Pick's disease as well as a group of disorders that have distinctive clinical, psychiatric, and pathological features (Hodges 2000). Pick's disease was first described in 1907. Asymmetrical atrophy of the frontal and temporal lobes occurs with sparing of the parietal and occipital lobes (Figures 4–11 and 4–12). Histologically, the involved cortex undergoes profound cell loss, which is much greater than that usually seen in Alzheimer's disease. In addition, characteristic Pick's bodies are found within the neurons of the involved areas of cortex. Pick's bodies are globular intraneuronal inclusions that are best visualized with silver

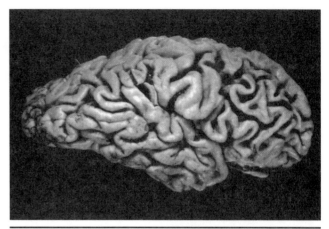

FIGURE 4–11. Pick's disease—lateral view of the brain.
Very severe atrophy ("knife blade") is most pronounced in the frontal and temporal lobes.

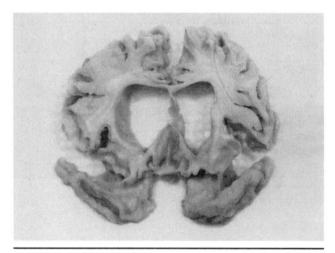

FIGURE 4–12. Pick's disease—coronal section through the basal ganglia.
This disease causes profound atrophy of the cortex. The ventricles are widely dilated. The caudate nucleus is flattened.

impregnation techniques (Figures 4–13 and 4–14). On immunohistochemical studies, they stain positively for tau epitopes.

In recent years, some distinct frontotemporal dementia variants that lack Pick's bodies have been described (Hulette and Crain 1992), prompting the use of several different nomenclatures to describe these disorders. Because we do not want to increase confusion, the reader is simply referred to appropriate references (Foster et al. 1997; Hulette et al. 1999b; Yamaoka et al. 1996).

A recent consensus conference has recommended the following simplified diagnostic terms (Trojanowski and Dickson 2001):

- *Pick's disease* is defined as frontotemporal dementia and lobar atrophy with Pick's bodies.

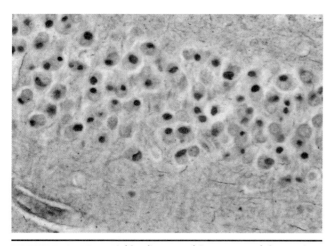

FIGURE 4–13. Pick's disease—hippocampal formation, fascia dentata.

Pick's bodies, which are round, densely homogeneous argyrophilic inclusions, fill the cytoplasm of virtually every neuron. Pick's bodies, like neurofibrillary tangles, contain abnormally cross-linked proteins. (Glees silver stain; original magnification ×400.)

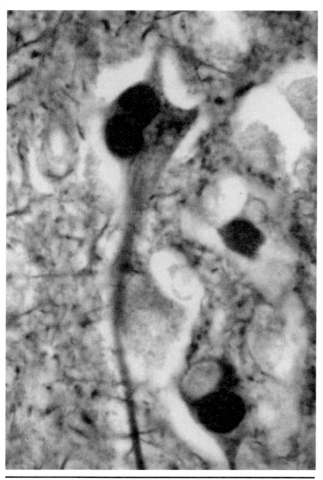

FIGURE 4–14. Pick's disease—hippocampal formation, Ammon's horn.

Pick's bodies are seen here within pyramidal neurons. (Glees silver stain; original magnification ×1,000.)

- *Frontotemporal dementia with parkinsonism linked to chromosome 17* has variable histopathology but is always associated with mutations in the *TAU* gene on chromosome 17.
- *Corticobasal degeneration* is a frontotemporal dementia distinguished by asymmetrical tau deposits, both tangles and characteristic tau plaques, in the basal ganglia and cortex, without genetic abnormalities in the *TAU* gene.
- *Progressive supranuclear palsy* may present clinically as dementia or as an extrapyramidal movement disorder with paresis of upward gaze. Pathologically, this frontotemporal dementia is characterized by bilaterally symmetrical tangles in the basal ganglia.
- *Neurofibrillary tangle dementia* shows extensive neurofibrillary change without plaques and without known *TAU* mutations.
- *Dementia lacking distinctive histopathology* is diagnosed if the brain has frontotemporal cell loss without plaques, tangles, or ubiquitin-positive inclusions.
- *Frontotemporal dementia with motor neuron disease inclusions* includes patients with dementia who may have experienced paresis due to motor neuron disease during life. Pathologically, frontotemporal cell loss with ubiquitin-positive, tau-negative inclusions in the hippocampal formation are seen (Figure 4–15).

Summary

The brain is a complex organ, which, when functioning optimally, is a source of wonder. However, as we age, normal wear and tear result in some loss of cognition. This loss is manifested pathologically by the formation of a few plaques and tangles. At some point, synapse loss and the pathology of plaques and tangles reach a critical threshold and dementia ensues. Plaques and tangles, and therefore Alzheimer's disease, are the most common pathological substrate of dementia. Second most common in incidence is dementia with Lewy bodies, which may be considered the convergence of Alzheimer's disease and Parkinson's disease. Third most common in frequency are vascular dementias, and the fourth most common cause of dementia is frontotemporal dementia.

Genetic studies are beginning to unravel some of the genetic risk factors and autosomal dominant genes associated with the development of dementia and cognitive impairment. In the future, cognitive and therapeutic interventions will be aimed at persons who are genetically and behaviorally at risk for the insidious development of dementia.

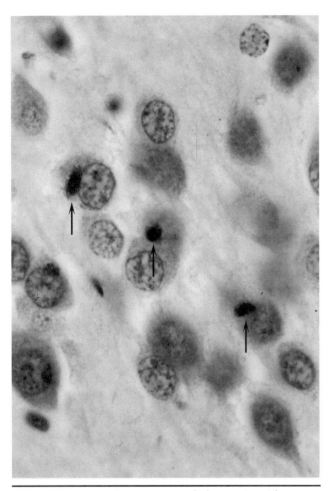

FIGURE 4–15. Frontotemporal dementia with motor neuron disease inclusions—hippocampal formation, fascia dentata.

Frontotemporal dementia with motor neuron disease inclusions (**arrows**) are small granular cytoplasmic inclusions that are best observed in the small neurons of the fascia dentata of the hippocampus. These inclusions cannot be seen on routine histological preparations. They stain positively only for ubiquitin. They lack tau, β-amyloid, α-synuclein, and other proteins that are present in the other major neurodegenerative disorders. (Ubiquitin immunostain; original magnification ×1,000.)

References

Adler G, Brassen S: Short-term rivastigmine treatment reduces EEG slow-wave power in Alzheimer patients. Neuropsychobiology 43:273–276, 2001

Anderer P, Pascual-Marqui RD, Semlitsch HV, et al: Electrical sources of P300 event-related brain potentials revealed by low resolution electromagnetic tomography, 1: effects of normal aging. Neuropsychobiology 37:20–27, 1998

APA Task Force on Quantitative Electrophysiological Assessment: Quantitative electroencephalography: a report on the present state of computerized EEG techniques. Am J Psychiatry 148:961–964, 1991

Braak H, Braak E: Neuropathological staging of Alzheimer-related changes. Acta Neuropathol 82:239–259, 1991

Brenner RP, Ulrich RF, Spiker DG, et al: Computerized EEG spectral analysis in elderly normal, demented and depressed subjects. Electroencephalogr Clin Neurophysiol 64:483–492, 1986

Brenner RP, Reynolds CF, Ulrich RF: EEG findings in depressive pseudodementia and dementia with secondary depression. Electroencephalogr Clin Neurophysiol 72:298–304, 1989

Bridgers SL, Ebersole JS: The clinical utility of ambulatory cassette EEG. Neurology 35:166–173, 1985

Brun A: Vascular dementia: pathological findings, in Dementia, 2nd Edition. Edited by O'Brien J, Ames D, Burns A. New York, Oxford University Press, 2000, pp 655–666

Claus JJ, Ongerboer De Visser BW, Bour LJ, et al: Determinants of quantitative spectral electroencephalography in early Alzheimer's disease: cognitive function, regional cerebral blood flow, and computed tomography. Dement Geriatr Cogn Disord 11:81–89, 2000

Cook IA, Leuchter AF: Synaptic dysfunction in Alzheimer's disease: clinical assessment using quantitative EEG. Behav Brain Res 78:15–23, 1996

Corder EH, Saunders AM, Strittmatter WJ, et al: Gene dose of apolipoprotein E type 4 allele and the risk of Alzheimer's disease in late onset families. Science 261:921–923, 1993

Crain BJ, Croom DW II, Hulette CM, et al: Argyrophilic plaques in children. Acta Neuropathol (Berl) 89:42–49, 1995

Creutzfeldt OD, Watanabe S, Lux HD: Relations between EEG phenomena and potentials of single cortical cells, II: spontaneous and convulsoid activity. Electroencephalogr Clin Neurophysiol 20:19–37, 1966

Duffy FH, Albert MS, McAnulty G: Age-related differences in brain electrical activity in healthy subjects. Ann Neurol 16:430–438, 1984

Einstein G, Hulette C, Schmechel DE, et al: Intraneuronal ApoE in human visual cortex reflects the staging of Alzheimer's disease pathology. J Neuropathol Exp Neurol 57:1190–1201, 1998

Esiri MM, Hyman BT, Beyreuther K, et al: Aging and dementia, in Greenfield's Neuropathology, 6th Edition. Edited by Graham DI, Lantos PL. New York, Oxford University Press, 1997, pp 153–234

Foster NL, Wilhelmsen K, Sima AAF, et al: Frontotemporal dementia and parkinsonism linked to chromosome 17: a consensus conference. Ann Neurol 41:706–715, 1997

Fullerton SM, Shirman GA, Strittmatter WJ, et al: Impairment of the blood-nerve and blood-brain barriers in apolipoprotein E knockout mice. Exp Neurol 169:13–22, 2001

Goodin DS, Aminoff MJ: Electrophysiological differences between subtypes of dementia. Brain 109 (Pt 6):1103–1113, 1986

Goodin DS, Aminoff MJ: Electrophysiological differences between demented and nondemented patients with Parkinson's disease. Ann Neurol 21:90–94, 1987

Goodin D, Squires KC, Starr A: Age-related variations in evoked potentials to auditory stimuli in normal human subjects. Electroencephalogr Clin Neurophysiol 44:447–458, 1978a

Goodin D, Squires KC, Starr A: Long latency event-related components of the auditory evoked potential in dementia. Brain 101:635–648, 1978b

Gray F, Rober F, Labrecque R, et al: Autosomal dominant arteriopathic leuko-encephalopathy and Alzheimer's disease. Neuropathol Appl Neurobiol 20:22–30, 1994

Gustafson L: Physostigmine and tetrahydroaminoacridine treatment of Alzheimer's disease. Acta Neurol Scand Suppl 149:39–41, 1993

Hamilton RL: Lewy bodies in Alzheimer's disease: a neuropathological review of 145 cases using alpha-synuclein immunohistochemistry. Brain Pathol 10:378–384, 2000

Heyman RA, Brenner RP, Reynolds CF, et al: Age at initial onset of depression and waking EEG variables in the elderly. Biol Psychiatry 29:994–1000, 1991

Hodges J: Pick's disease: its relationship to progressive aphasia, semantic dementia and frontotemporal dementia, in Dementia, 2nd Edition. Edited by O'Brien J, Ames D, Burns A. New York, Oxford University Press, 2000, pp 747–758

Holschneider DP, Leuchter AF: Beta activity in aging and dementia. Brain Topogr 8:169–180, 1995

Holschneider DP, Leuchter AF: Clinical neurophysiology using electroencephalography in geriatric psychiatry: neurobiologic implications and clinical utility. J Geriatr Psychiatry Neurol 12:150–164, 1999

Hughes JR, Zialcita ML: EEG in the elderly: seizures vs syncope. Clin Electroencephalogr 31:131–137, 2000

Hulette CM, Crain BJ: Lobar atrophy without Pick bodies. Clin Neuropathol 11:151–156, 1992

Hulette CM, Walford RL: Immunological aspects of Alzheimer's disease. Alzheimer Dis Assoc Disord 1:72–82, 1987

Hulette CM, Earl NL, Anthony DC, et al: Adult onset Niemann-Pick disease type C: a case presenting with dementia. Clin Neuropathol 11:293–297, 1991

Hulette CM, Mirra S, Heyman A, et al: A prospective clinical-neuropathological study of Parkinson's features in Alzheimer's disease: the CERAD experience, part IX. Neurology 45:1991–1995, 1995

Hulette CM, Mirra SS, Heyman A, et al: Clinical-neuropathologic findings in multi-infarct dementia: a report of six autopsied cases. Neurology 48:668–672, 1997

Hulette CM, Welsh-Bohmer K, MacIntyre L, et al: Neuropathological changes in normal aging. J Neuropathol Exp Neurol 57:1168–1174, 1998

Hulette CM, Ervin J, Saunders AM, et al: Vascular pathology in ApoE 3,3 and ApoE 4,4 dementia, in 1st International Congress on Vascular Dementia. Edited by Korczyn AD. Bologna, Italy, Monduzzi Editore, 1999a, pp 45–49

Hulette CM, Pericak-Vance MA, Spillantini MG, et al: Neuropathologic features of frontotemporal dementia and parkinsonism linked to chromosome 17q12–22 (FTDP-17): Duke family 1684. J Neuropathol Exp Neurol 58:859–866, 1999b

Hulette CM, Huang H, Pan Y-P, et al: Cardiovascular disease in demented and non-demented elderly (abstract). J Neuropathol Exp Neurol 61:443, 2002

Hyman BT, Trojanowski JQ: Consensus recommendations for the postmortem diagnosis of Alzheimer disease from the National Institute on Aging and the Reagan Institute Working Group on diagnostic criteria for the neuropathological assessment of Alzheimer disease. J Neuropathol Exp Neurol 56:1095–1097, 1997

Ince P, Perry R, Perry E: Pathology of dementia with Lewy bodies, in Dementia, 2nd Edition. Edited by O'Brien J, Ames D, Burns A. New York, Oxford University Press, 2000, pp 699–718

Ishikawa A, Takahashi H, Tanaka H, et al: Clinical features of familial diffuse Lewy body disease. Eur Neurol 38:34–38, 1997

Jacobson SA, Leuchter AF, Walter DO, et al: Serial quantitative EEG among elderly subjects with delirium. Biol Psychiatry 34:135–140, 1993

Knott V, Mohr E, Mahoney C, et al: Electroencephalographic coherence in Alzheimer's disease: comparisons with a control group and population norms. J Geriatr Psychiatry Neurol 13:1–8, 2000

Knott V, Mohr E, Mahoney C, et al: Quantitative electroencephalography in Alzheimer's disease: comparison with a control group, population norms and mental status. J Psychiatry Neurosci 26:106–116, 2001

Koponen H, Partanen J, Paakkonen A, et al: EEG spectral analysis in delirium. J Neurol Neurosurg Psychiatry 52:980–985, 1989

Lantos P, Cairns N. The neuropathology of Alzheimer's disease, in Dementia, 2nd Edition. Edited by O'Brien J, Ames D, Burns A. New York, Oxford University Press, 2000, pp 443–460

Leuchter AF, Jacobson SA: Quantitative measurement of brain electrical activity in delirium. Int Psychogeriatr 3:231–247, 1991

Leuchter AF, Spar JE, Walter DO, et al: Electroencephalographic spectra and coherence in the diagnosis of Alzheimer's-type and multi-infarct dementia. Arch Gen Psychiatry 44:993–998, 1987

Leuchter AF, Newton TF, Cook IA, et al: Changes in brain functional connectivity in Alzheimer-type and multi-infarct dementia Brain 115:1543–1561, 1992

Leuchter AF, Cook IA, Newton TF, et al: Regional differences in brain electrical activity in dementia: use of spectral power and spectral ratio measures. Electroencephalogr Clin Neurophysiol 87:385–393, 1993a

Leuchter AF, Daly KA, Rosenberg-Thompson S, et al: Prevalence and significance of electroencephalographic abnormalities in patients with suspected organic mental syndromes. J Am Geriatr Soc 41:605–611, 1993b

Leuchter AF, Uijtdehaage SG, Cook IA, et al: Relationship between brain electrical activity and cortical perfusion in normal subjects. Psychiatry Res 90:125–140, 1999

Luhdorf K, Jensen LK, Plesner AM: Epilepsy in the elderly: incidence, social function, and disability. Epilepsia 27:135–141, 1986a

Luhdorf K, Jensen LK, Plesner AM: Etiology of seizures in the elderly. Epilepsia 27:458–463, 1986b

Marín-Padilla M: Prenatal development of fibrous (white matter), protoplasmic (gray matter), and layer I astrocytes in the human cerebral cortex: a Golgi study. J Comp Neurol 357:554–572, 1995

McGeer PL, McGeer EG, Yasojima K: Alzheimer disease and neuroinflammation. J Neural Transm Suppl 59:53–57, 1999

McKeith IG, Galasko D, Kosaka K, et al: Consensus guidelines for the clinical and pathologic diagnosis of dementia with Lewy bodies (DLB): report of the Consortium on DLB international workshop. Neurology 47:1113–1124, 1996

McKhann G, Drachman D, Folstein M, et al: Clinical diagnosis of Alzheimer's disease: report of the NINCDS-ADRDA Work Group under the auspices of Department of Health and Human Services Task Force on Alzheimer's Disease. Neurology 34:939–944, 1984

Mendez MF, Catanzaro P, Doss RC, et al: Seizures in Alzheimer's disease: clinicopathologic study. J Geriatr Psychiatry Neurol 7:230–233, 1994

Meyer JS, Rauch G, Rauch RA, et al: Risk factors for cerebral hypoperfusion, mild cognitive impairment, and dementia. Neurobiol Aging 21:161–169, 2000

Minthon L, Gustafson L, Dalfelt G, et al: Oral tetrahydroaminoacridine treatment of Alzheimer's disease evaluated clinically and by regional cerebral blood flow and EEG. Dementia 4:32–42, 1993

Mirra SS, Crain BJ, Vogel FS, et al: The Consortium to Establish a Registry for Alzheimer's Disease (CERAD), part II: standardization of the neuropathologic assessment of Alzheimer's disease. Neurology 41:479–486, 1991

Mitchell TW, Mufson EJ, Schneider JA, et al: Parahippocampal tau pathology in healthy aging, mild cognitive impairment and early Alzheimer's disease. Ann Neurol 51:182–189, 2002

Montine TJ, Hulette CM: Pathology of ischemic cerebrovascular disease, in Neurosurgery, 2nd Edition. Edited by Wilkins RH, Rengachary SS. New York, McGraw-Hill, 1997, pp 2045–2052

Parent P: Carpenter's Human Neuroanatomy, 9th Edition. Philadelphia, PA, Williams & Wilkins, 1996

Pasquier F, Henon H, Leys D: Risk factors and mechanisms of post-stroke dementia. Rev Neurol (Paris) 155:749–753, 1999

Pekkonen E, Jaaskelainen IP, Hietanen J, et al: Impaired preconscious auditory processing and cognitive functions in Alzheimer's disease. Clin Neurophysiol 1942–1947, 1999

Perryman KM, Fitten LJ: Quantitative EEG during a double-blind trial of THS and lecithin in patients with Alzheimer's disease. J Geriatr Psychiatry Neurol 4:127–133, 1991

Pfurtscheller G, Cooper R: Frequency dependence of the transmission of the EEG from cortex to scalp. Electroencephalogr Clin Neurophysiol 38:93–96, 1975

Polich J: P300 in the evaluation of aging and dementia. Electroencephalogr Clin Neurophysiol Suppl 42:304–323, 1991

Polich J: EEG and ERP assessment of normal aging. Electroencephalogr Clin Neurophysiol 104:244–256, 1997

Polich J, Kok A: Cognitive and biological determinants of P300: an integrative review. Biol Psychol 41:103–146, 1995

Polich J, Ehlers CL, Otis S, et al: P300 latency reflects the degree of cognitive decline in dementing illness. Electroencephalogr Clin Neurophysiol 63:138–144, 1986

Reeve A, Rose DF, Weinberger DR: Magnetoencephalography: applications in psychiatry. Arch Gen Psychiatry 46:573–576, 1989

Rosenberg CK, Pericak-Vance MA, Hulette CM, et al: Lewy body (LB) and Alzheimer pathology in a family with the amyloid precursor protein APP717 gene mutation. Acta Neuropathol 100:145–152, 2000

Rosenberg CK, Roses AD, Hulette CM, et al: Dementia with Lewy bodies and Alzheimer disease. Acta Neuropathol 102:621–626, 2001

Roses AD, Hulette C, Strittmatter WJ, et al: Influence of the susceptibility genes apolipoprotein E-4 and apolipoprotein E-2 on the rate of disease expressivity of late-onset Alzheimer's disease. Azneimittel-Forschung/Drug Research 45:413–417, 1995

Roses AD, Hulette CM, Strittmatter WJ, et al: Apolipoprotein E and Alzheimer disease. International Academy for Biomedical and Drug Research 11:187–197, 1996

Sander JW, Hart YM, Johnson AL, et al: National General Practice Study of Epilepsy: newly diagnosed epileptic seizures in a general population. Lancet 336:1267–1271, 1990

Saunders AM, Hulette CM, Roses AD, et al: Association of apolipoprotein E allele ε4 with late onset familial and sporadic Alzheimer's disease. Neurology 43:1467–1472, 1993

Saunders AM, Hulette CM, Roses AD, et al: Specificity, sensitivity and predictive value of apolipoprotein E genotyping in a consecutive autopsy series of sporadic Alzheimer disease patients. Lancet 348:90–93, 1996

Schmechel DE, Hulette CM, Roses AD, et al: Increased amyloid β-peptide deposition as a consequence of apolipoprotein E genotype in late-onset Alzheimer's disease. Proc Natl Acad Sci U S A 90:9649–9653, 1993

Scott WK, Hulette CM, Pericak-Vance MA, et al: Fine mapping of the chromosome 12 late-onset Alzheimer disease locus: potential genetic and phenotypic heterogeneity. Am J Hum Genet 66:922–932, 2000

Spillantini MG, Schmidt ML, Lee V M-Y, et al: Alpha-synuclein in Lewy bodies. Nature 388:839–840, 1997

Sunderman FW, Boerner F: Normal Values in Clinical Medicine. Philadelphia, PA, WB Saunders, 1949, pp 641–642

Tournier-Lasserve E, Joutel A, Melki J: Cerebral autosomal dominant arteriopathy with subcortical infarcts and leucencephalopathy. Nat Genet 3:256–259, 1993

Trembath Y, Rosenberg C, Ervin JF, et al: Lewy body pathology is a frequent co-pathology in familial Alzheimer Disease. Acta Neuropathol (Berl) 105:484–488, 2003

Trojanowski JQ, Dickson D: Update on the neuropathological diagnosis of frontotemporal dementias. J Neuropathol Exp Neurol 60:1123–1126, 2001

Visser SL, Van Tilburg W, Hooijer C, et al: Visual evoked potentials (VEPs) in senile dementia (Alzheimer type) and in non-organic behavioural disorders in the elderly: comparison with EEG parameters. Electroencephalogr Clin Neurophysiol 60:115–121, 1985

Vogel FS: Neuroanatomy and neuropathology of aging, in The American Psychiatric Press Textbook of Geriatric Psychiatry, 2nd Edition. Edited by Busse EW, Blazer DG. Washington, DC, American Psychiatric Press, 1996, pp 61–70

Welsh-Bohmer KA, Hulette C, Schmechel D, et al: Neuropsychological detection of preclinical Alzheimer's disease: results of a neuropathological series of "normal" controls, in Alzheimer's Disease: Advances in Etiology, Pathogenesis and Therapeutics: The Proceedings of the 7th International Conference on Alzheimer's Disease and Related Disorders. Edited by Iqbal K, Sisodia SS, Winblad B. London, Wiley, 2001, pp 111–122

Yamaoka LH, Hulette CM, Pericak-Vance MA, et al: Linkage of frontotemporal dementia to chromosome 17: clinical and neuropathological characterization of phenotype. Am J Hum Genet 59:1306–1312, 1996

Zekry D, Duyckaerts C, Moulias R, et al: Degenerative and vascular lesions of the brain have synergistic effects in dementia of the elderly. Acta Neuropathol (Berl) 103:481–487, 2002

Zhang WW, Ma KC, Andersen O, et al: The microvascular changes in cases of hereditary multi-infarct disease of the brain. Acta Neuropathol (Berl) 87:317–324, 1994

Chemical Messengers

Garth Bissette, Ph.D.

In the time since the first version of this chapter appeared in the second edition of this textbook, the techniques of molecular biology have elucidated the sequence of several neurotransmitter-related proteins that had previously been unknown, the role of growth factors in neuronal repair and survival has been amplified, and the further development of imaging techniques has allowed assessment of some neuronal mechanisms that are altered with aging in living patients. Because the amount of literature in the domain of aging and brain neurotransmitter function has increased beyond the space this review can command, this revised chapter includes a discussion of some of the developments mentioned above and briefly mentions some of the most recent research findings regarding the various neurotransmitters covered in the previous version. The aim is to present a selected, rather than comprehensive, review of the current state of this research front with recent reports that may themselves provide a more thorough treatment of a particular subfield.

The concept of biochemical substances controlling the communication between nerve cells (or neurons) can be traced to the latter part of the nineteenth century when the famous argument between the classical anatomists Ramón y Cajal and Camillo Golgi was finally resolved in Cajal's favor. Cajal and Sherrington had described very small gaps between the processes of adjacent nerve cells, which they termed *synapses* after the Greek word meaning "to touch." Based on his technique of silver staining, Golgi had held that the nerve cells actually connected into a neural network. We now know that Golgi could claim partial victory in that such networks have been shown to exist in certain invertebrates; however, the vast majority of species that have been examined do, in fact, have synaptic clefts between neurons that are in communication with each other.

These areas are composed of specialized membrane thickenings across which biochemicals are released from the presynaptic neuron into the intracellular space. These substances then diffuse across this gap to their corresponding receptor sites on adjacent postsynaptic neurons or glial cells or to presynaptic autoreceptors. These receptors are also specialized areas of the cell membrane where proteins that span the receptive cell's membrane are able to recognize and bind their specific biochemical molecules (or *ligands*). The usual result of this binding is a conformational change in the receptor protein that can open a channel through the membrane that is selective for a particular ionic element, such as calcium, potassium, or sodium. Alternatively, the binding of the ligand to the receptor can initiate a cascade of changes on molecules that are associated with the receptor, so-called second-messenger species such as adenosine or guanosine triphosphate (ATP or GTP) or inosine 3'-triphosphate (IP3) and diacylglycerol (DAG). These, in turn, alter other membrane and intracellular proteins by a series of biochemical reactions, often involving the addition or deletion of a phosphate group on the target molecule. It is now well established that many different receptors may bind the same type of neurotransmitter molecule with very different postsynaptic effects. These events usually have one of two ultimate effects on the receiving neuron: a decrease in its firing rate, termed *inhibition*, or an increase in firing activity, termed *excitation*. The actual biomolecules that are released across the synapse and bind to a receptor that then produces a discrete physiological change are termed *chemical neurotransmitters*, and they come in a wide assortment of classes and molecular individuality within these classes (see Figure 5–1).

Signal transduction has exploded as a field within neurobiology and cellular physiology, and many more steps in the transduction cascades that are initiated by receptor activation have now been described and investigated (Nestler and Duman 1994). Much of this work has occurred with in vitro techniques that use cultured cells

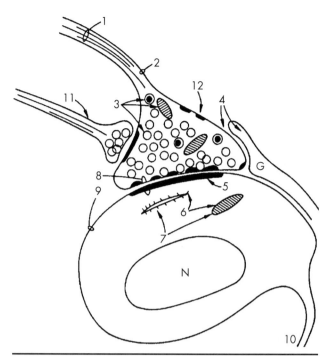

FIGURE 5–1. Twelve steps in the synaptic transmission process in an idealized synaptic connection.

1: Transport down the axon. 2: Electrically excitable membrane of the axon. 3: The organelles and enzymes present in the nerve terminal for synthesizing, storing, and releasing the transmitter, as well as for the process of active reuptake. 4: Enzymes present in the extracellular space and within the glia for catabolizing excess transmitter release from nerve terminals. 5: The postsynaptic receptor that triggers the response of the postsynaptic cell to the transmitter. 6: The organelles within the postsynaptic cells that respond to the receptor trigger. 7: Interaction between genetic expression of the postsynaptic nerve cell and its influences on the cytoplasmic organelles that respond to transmitter action. 8: The possible "plastic" steps modifiable by events at the specialized synaptic contact zone. 9: The electrical portion of the nerve cell membrane that, in response to the various transmitters, is able to integrate the postsynaptic potentials and produce an action potential. 10: Continuation of the information transmission by which the postsynaptic cell sends an action potential down its axon. 11: Release of transmitter, subjected to modification by a presynaptic (axoaxonic) synapse; in some cases an analogous control can be achieved between dendritic elements. 12: Release of the transmitter from a nerve terminal or secreting dendritic site may be further subject to modulation through autoreceptors that respond to the transmitter that the same secreting structure has released.

G = glia; N = nucleus.

Source. Reprinted from Cooper JR, Bloom FE, Roth RH (eds.): *The Biochemical Basis of Neuropharmacology.* New York, Oxford University Press, 1996, pp. 46–47. Used with permission.

of various lineages and cell types. Advances in molecular techniques have now allowed specific mutations to be expressed on both cellular and whole animal preparations as well as allowing targeted removal (knockout) of a specific gene and its protein product. This has further accelerated our knowledge of the actions of various proteins in the regulation and maintenance of neuronal signaling mecha-

nisms. Some of these tools have now been applied to the investigation of aging-induced behavioral and physiological deficits that may be mediated by chemical neurotransmitters in the brain.

With the advent of molecular techniques, not only could the amounts and locations of messenger RNA (mRNA) encoding neurotransmitter-related proteins be assessed, but also the regulatory sequences and different molecular subtypes of various gene products could be investigated. These techniques also have allowed discovery of heretofore unknown proteins related to proteins with similar sequence homology but often with subtly different functions. Many neurotransmitter receptors contain discrete protein subunits, and these techniques have allowed the characterization of a plethora of new subunits, which in various combinations often result in receptors with different binding affinities and ligand recognition sites.

Measurement of amounts of mRNA for neuropeptides, the enzymes that produce the classical neurotransmitters, their reuptake proteins, and receptors have now joined measures of neurotransmitter concentration and receptor binding in the descriptions of alterations in neurophysiological mechanisms due to disease or aging. However, interpretation of these data is complicated by parameters such as neuronal location and distribution, metabolic half-life and cellular compartmentalization, receptor affinity, and the physiological availability and proportion of the active signaling product that is able to access the synapse. Because the average half-life of an mRNA molecule is around 30 minutes and the amount of expression of the mRNA into protein product is controlled by so many cellular regulatory factors, knowledge of mRNA concentration in the absence of information on the amount of product is not very useful in determining whether synaptic availability of the protein or its product has changed. Similar problems occur with knowledge of only the chemical neurotransmitter's concentration. Because storage of transmitters in synaptic vesicles does not equate with amounts of released neurotransmitter, knowledge of synthetic capacity, releasability, and degradation rates is required to estimate "turnover" or amount of released versus manufactured neurotransmitter. Thus, if relative concentrations of a neurotransmitter are reported to be different during disease or aging, one must not automatically assume that increased or decreased rates of signaling are present until evidence for increased relative release, degradation, and appropriate receptor responses is known. This caveat is not always observed by those reporting or attempting to interpret the results of neurobiological experiments.

These molecular techniques are largely limited to in

vivo and in vitro investigation with cells or laboratory animals, but advances in electronics have allowed development of technology to allow noninvasive and repeatable methods for indirect assessment of anatomical and biochemical parameters in living subjects. This technology has shown great utility in human clinical and basic research and promises wondrous revelations of brain regions and neurochemistry associated with behavioral and cognitive processes that are unique to humans. Imaging techniques have evolved with increasing acceleration over the past decade, with initial limitations on anatomical resolutions being steadily improved and with the advent of imaging techniques to quantify endogenous concentrations of certain cellular components and the distribution of specific receptor populations. Thus, the anatomical resolution of computed tomography (CT) was improved with magnetic resonance imaging (MRI), which has been further improved to functional MRI, which uses metabolic contrasting agents in the visualization of task-activated anatomical structures within the working brain. Magnetic resonance spectroscopy (MRS) now allows quantitative measurement of nine endogenous compounds with millimolar concentrations in brain, whereas positron-emission tomography (PET) allows visualization and quantitation of levels of radioactive receptor ligands that can access the brain. These techniques hold the promise of evaluating individual subjects over their lifetime and into senescence (Sullivan et al. 2002), with the benefit of understanding a particular individual's neurobiological responses to increasing age.

The first substance identified as a chemical neurotransmitter was acetylcholine (ACh) in the 1920s. Otto Loewi and Sir Henry Dale independently demonstrated that this substance was secreted from the endings of nerve cells of the peripheral nervous system when their fibers were stimulated and that it had predictable and reproducible effects on heart rate and blood pressure. The subsequent identification in the 1940s of epinephrine (EPI) and norepinephrine (NE) in the peripheral nervous system set the stage for work that would eventually allow development of techniques for staining specific components of the synthetic and degradative biochemical pathways in the central nervous system (CNS).

Between 1950 and 1970, these and related procedures led to the identification of what are now considered to be the "classical" CNS neurotransmitters: ACh; the so-called biogenic amines, which include the catecholamines NE, EPI, and dopamine (DA); and the indoleamine serotonin (5-hydroxytryptamine; 5-HT). This work also led to the recognition that the amino acid γ-aminobutyric acid (GABA) was an inhibitory neurotransmitter. These classical neurotransmitters are de-

rived from amino acid precursors by sequential biochemical steps that are under the control of specific enzymes. The presence of these enzymes indicates that the neuron is capable of producing the particular neurotransmitter under investigation, and their presence, when coupled with selective staining procedures, allows mapping of the location of the nerve cells that are producing the neurotransmitter. This technique allowed the first practical application of this developing knowledge to the treatment of a neurodegenerative disease. The identification of the DA cells of the substantia nigra as the primary target of the degenerative process in Parkinson's disease led to an effective therapy that is still used today, although the cause of the neuronal degeneration and a cure have not yet been discovered. This success reinforced the interest in discovering neurochemical pathologies in other neurodegenerative diseases, such as Alzheimer's disease and Huntington's chorea, as well as offering hope for effective therapies in mental illness based on rational drug design.

Since the 1970s, a plethora of newly discovered transmitter substances have been reported. The discovery of the excitatory amino acids glutamate and aspartate, as well as the identification of other inhibitory amino acids (including glycine, serine, and several others), greatly expanded the list in this class of neurotransmitter substances. The nucleotides adenosine and guanosine have now been shown to be neurotransmitters as well as components of the genetic code and, when phosphorylated, second messengers. Chains of from 3 to more than 40 amino acids, termed *neuropeptides*, have been shown to act as messenger molecules and represent a new class of neurotransmitters whose final tally may include more than 200 distinct species. Only recently, the neuronal production and neurotransmitter status of the diffusible gases nitric oxide (NO) and carbon monoxide (CO) have been recognized.

To qualify as a neurotransmitter, most of the criteria discussed below must be met, although in many cases, technical problems or insufficient resources for the appropriate research have prevented the accumulation of sufficient evidence for all of the criteria to be met. First, the substance must be found within neurons in a subcellular compartment (usually synaptic vesicles) that allows its release into the synaptic cleft. Second, the biochemical machinery necessary to produce the substance must be localized within the same neuron. Third, the substance must be released from the neuron by physiological mechanisms. Fourth, synthetic forms of the molecule must evoke the same response as does the endogenous candidate when applied directly to the receptive neurons. Fifth, specific receptors linked to a physiological response must be present on the cells in communication with the neuron containing the neurotransmitter candidate. Sixth, mechanisms must be present to end the effect of the secreted putative neurotransmitter. (These mechanisms usually involve degradation of the neurotransmitter in the synaptic cleft by specific degradative enzymes or reuptake by the presynaptic neuron.) Seventh, and finally, it must be possible to block the action of the neurotransmitter substance by pharmacological agents that prevent binding to or activation of the receptor for the neurotransmitter.

In the review that follows, I focus on the neurotransmitters that have fulfilled all or almost all of these criteria. To allow adequate discussion of these neurotransmitters in the allotted space, however, it is necessary to omit from consideration many other interesting substances that have thus far been shown to meet only one or more of these criteria but that may eventually achieve the status of true neurotransmitters. For a more comprehensive review of the various neurotransmitters and their associated biochemistry, I encourage readers to refer to the excellent seventh edition of *The Biochemical Basis of Neuropharmacology* (Cooper et al. 2002).

Acetylcholine

ACh was the first biochemical recognized as a neurotransmitter substance. It produces initiation of skeletal muscle contraction and mediates parasympathetic effects and preganglionic autonomic neurotransmission in the peripheral nervous system. It is a simple molecule, constructed by joining an acetyl group from the donor molecule, acetylcoenzyme A (acetyl-CoA), with a molecule of choline derived from a variety of metabolic sources. The enzyme that couples these two molecules into one molecule of ACh is termed *choline acetyltransferase* (CAT), and its presence in neurons indicates that the neuron uses ACh as a neurotransmitter. The rate of ACh synthesis is directly coupled to the firing rate of the cholinergic neuron. However, it is not the rate of CAT activity that controls the amount of ACh synthesis when demand increases. Rather, it is the rate at which choline can be transported across the neuronal cell membrane from its extraneuronal pool that mediates availability of choline to CAT for synthesis. This transport process is performed by the high-affinity choline transporter that resides in the cell membrane of cholinergic neurons. The high-affinity characterization is to distinguish this mechanism from the alternative low-affinity choline transport mechanism that virtually all cells have to maintain membrane integrity through synthesis of choline-containing

phospholipids. The gene for the high-affinity transporter molecule has now been cloned from human (Apparsundaram et al. 2000; Okuda et al. 2000), rat (Misawa et al. 2001), and mouse (Apparsundaram et al. 2001) DNA, but it requires energy from neuronal metabolism to function, and this activity quickly degrades at death.

Research with laboratory animals has found that at death, the concentration of choline in brain tissue increases severalfold. This is thought to be due to the rapid hydrolysis of ACh by its degradative enzyme, acetylcholinesterase (AChE). One molecule of AChE can hydrolyze 5,000 molecules of ACh per second, and blockade of AChE is the mechanism of action of many insecticides and of nerve gases developed for use in war. This enzyme is found on the surface of cell membranes and in soluble form in the extracellular fluid but is not confined to cholinergic cells. Because it is present in large quantities in tissues such as the electric organ of freshwater electric eels, it was purified to homogeneity earlier than any other enzyme related to chemical neurotransmission in the brain; this allowed immunohistochemical mapping of its distribution in the brain relatively early in the history of this research. Imaging techniques now allow mapping of AChE in vivo (Kuhl et al. 1999). More recent work with the specific cholinergic marker CAT has confirmed that much of the previous AChE mapping evidence does truly delineate the major CNS cholinergic pathways. Many brain regions, such as the striatum, contain short interneurons that use ACh as a neurotransmitter; however, the long projection neurons that contain ACh are found in only a few discrete regions: the dorsal tegmental nuclei of the midbrain, where both descending projections to the brain stem and ascending projections to the limbic forebrain arise, and the magnocellular neurons of the septum and diagonal band/nucleus basalis region. The septal neurons give rise to cholinergic projections to the hippocampus, and the basal nucleus projects topographically to the entire cortex (Figure 5–2).

The cholinergic neurons in this latter region have been shown to be one of the major targets of degeneration in Alzheimer's disease; the dementia associated with Alzheimer's disease has been postulated to result from the decreased synaptic availability of ACh in these cortical projections from the nucleus basalis (Bierer et al. 1995). The nucleus basalis ACh neurons are often found to contain the neuropeptide galanin, and the galanin terminals that innervate the ACh neurons in this region become hypertrophied in persons with Alzheimer's disease (Mufson et al. 1993). In an attempt to achieve a therapeutic effect in these patients similar to that which has been successful in patients with Parkinson's disease, some investigators have tried using precursor enrichment

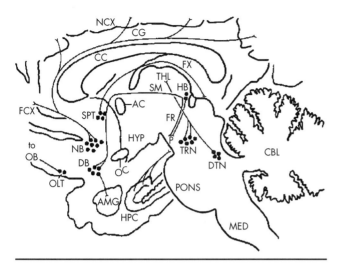

FIGURE 5–2. Cholinergic systems.

Parasagittal view of a schematized primate brain showing the distribution of cholinergic cell bodies **(solid circles)** and their projections. Note that although some of these systems also have been confirmed in the human brain, most of our current knowledge of cholinergic systems stems from studies in the rodent brain.

AC = anterior commissure; AMG = amygdala; CBL = cerebellum; CC = corpus callosum; CG = cingulate gyrus; DB = diagonal band; DTN = dorsal tegmental nucleus; FCX = frontal cortex; FR = fimbria; FX = fornix; HB = habenula; HPC = hippocampus; HYP = hypothalamus; MED = medulla; NB = nucleus basalis; NCX = neocortex; OB = olfactory bulb; OC = optic chiasm; OLT = olfactory tubercle; P = pineal; PONS = pons; SM = stria terminalis; SPT = septum; THL = thalamus; TRN = thalamic red nucleus.

Source. Reprinted from Watson SJ, Khachaturian H, Lewis ME, et al.: "Chemical Neuroanatomy as a Basis for Biological Psychiatry," in *American Handbook of Psychiatry.* Edited by Berger PA, Brodie HKH. New York, Basic Books, 1986, p. 17. Used with permission.

in the form of dietary choline. Disappointingly few practical benefits have been derived in terms of decreasing the dementia already present or in slowing its inexorable progress. Several drugs that block AChE are now approved by the U.S. Food and Drug Administration for use in treating Alzheimer's disease. Unfortunately, most patients taking these drugs do not experience gain of cognitive function or clearly demonstrable relief of other symptoms of dementia that would be expected of a truly effective therapy, and this equivocal success has led to proposed revisions in the definition of clinical efficacy for these drugs in Alzheimer's disease (Winblad et al. 2001). Imaging techniques now allow assessment of degree of cholinesterase inhibition by these drugs in living subjects (Kuhl et al. 2000).

Although few direct studies of the high-affinity transporter in humans have been attempted, a group of researchers at Duke University Medical School used a rapid autopsy protocol that enabled access to postmortem tissue within 2 hours of death, allowing measurement of the activity and amount of high-affinity choline uptake trans-

porter while it remained biochemically viable. The amount of high-affinity choline uptake transporter is regulated by its synthesis relative to its degradation, although its activity is believed to be regulated by the firing rate of the neuron that uses it. Large increases (400%) in the activity and the number of high-affinity choline uptake transporter sites were observed in cortical tissue from patients with Alzheimer's disease compared with control subjects without dementia and those with dementia from a cause other than Alzheimer's disease (Bissette et al. 1996; Slotkin et al. 1990, 1994). Thus, in individuals with Alzheimer's disease compared with control subjects, the mechanism for delivery of choline to the surviving cholinergic neurons appears to be upregulated, and the precursor replacement therapy should effectively raise intraneuronal choline levels. Imaging techniques directed at the vesicular subtype of the choline transporter recently have been developed and tested in Alzheimer's disease subjects but have not seen similar changes (Mulholland et al. 1998). Whether this large increase in high-affinity choline uptake activity is related to increased neuronal firing rates or represents a pathological increase remains unknown; however, it seems that attempts to increase the synthesis of ACh in patients with this disease are unlikely to succeed in the face of this already maximally accelerated uptake.

The flexibility of the choline moiety in the ACh molecule allows this neurotransmitter to interact at very different binding sites; this is represented physiologically by the presence of two general classes of receptors for ACh: nicotinic and muscarinic receptors. Named for the respective pharmacological agents that specifically stimulate these receptors, these two classes represent both ligand gated, ionic channel (nicotinic) type I receptors and second-messenger-linked membrane protein (muscarinic) type II receptors. Type I receptors usually have four or five membrane-spanning segments and mediate fast (millisecond) responses, whereas type II receptors have seven membrane-spanning domains and in most cases are linked to second messengers. The nicotinic receptors are present at the site of innervation of skeletal muscle, as well as in discrete regions of the CNS, including limbic areas thought to mediate emotion and reward. Muscarinic receptors are the predominant ACh receptors in the CNS and act either directly on ion channels for potassium, calcium, or chloride or through second messengers linked to the receptors by G proteins (phosphorylated guanine compounds used as an energy source). The effector systems activated by G proteins either can open or close channels or can stimulate or inhibit other components of the signal transduction cascade (such as adenylate or guanylate cyclase, phospholipases, and phosphodiesterases).

The tools of molecular biology have been used to identify four molecularly distinct forms of the nicotinic receptor and five forms of the muscarinic receptor. Previously, only a few of these receptor subtypes had been characterized pharmacologically, and thus the existence of different molecular phenotypes does not guarantee differences in ligand-binding affinity. It is a well-recognized neurobiological principle that, as endogenous ligand availability is altered over a long enough time, the corresponding receptor population usually will attempt to compensate for a reduced signal, often by increasing the number of receptors or, more rarely, by increasing the affinity for the ligand. Because some earlier postmortem reports and now imaging studies (Zubieta et al. 2001) have indicated that certain of these subtypes of muscarinic M_2 ACh receptor populations may be decreased in patients with Alzheimer's disease, efforts are now under way to develop specific agonists for muscarinic and nicotinic receptor subtypes that can be administered peripherally. Although such goals are laudable, the excitement generated by their potential achievement must be tempered with the realization that unless the cause of the degeneration can be identified and its progress halted, little more than temporary respite can be offered by such pharmacotherapies.

Specific alterations in various aspects of ACh neuronal systems in the aging brains of humans and laboratory animals have been recently reported. In a survey of several neurotransmitters in aged (30-month-old) rats compared with less-aged (20-month-old) or young (4-month-old) rats, Virgili et al. (2001) reported widespread deficits in cholinergic markers in the oldest group that were not seen in the intermediate-aged or younger groups. Old (22-month-old) Fischer 344 rats compared with young (6-month-old) and middle-aged (15-month-old) rats have been reported to have decreased numbers of several (M_1, M_2, M_3, M_5) muscarinic receptor subtypes depending on the specific region of the hippocampus examined (Tayebati et al. 2002), a finding that underscores the anatomical precision that must be used to investigate age-related changes. Neuroimaging studies of endogenous choline concentrations in various brain regions of otherwise normal, aging (40- to 61-year-old) subjects compared with younger (21- to 39-year-old) patients using MRS imaging (Angelie et al. 2001) have documented hippocampal and cortical decreases in percent choline in the older group. This technique is unable to distinguish between neurotransmitter-derived choline and choline in neuronal and glial membranes, and the choline hydrolyzed from ACh is much less than 1% of this signal. Others (Kadota et al. 2001) have reported a decrease in choline signal beginning in the middle of the third decade in both

gray and white matter with this imaging technique, but this was not confirmed in a similar study (Brooks et al. 2001).

The vesicular cholinergic transporter was assessed in 23 rhesus monkeys (age range = 10–37 years) by PET, and binding of the radioligand was reduced in the basal ganglia with increasing age (Voytko et al. 2001), but individual differences were large among these animals. In another PET study that used monkeys, muscarinic receptors in frontal and temporal cortex and in the striatum were reduced with age compared with younger animals (Kakiuchi et al. 2001). The response of the immediate-early gene, c-*fos*, to administration of the ACh release-enhancing agent linopirdine was found to be greater in aged (30-month-old) than in young (3-month-old) rats, and this effect on Fos was blocked by muscarinic receptor blockers (Dent et al. 2001). These studies indicate altered cholinergic regulation and stimulatory responses with increasing age rather than a generalized global decrease in cholinergic function. But others have argued that specific functional deficits in attention and executive processes are mediated by a gradual, age-related decrease in the integrity of cortical cholinergic systems (Sarter and Turchi 2002). This latter view is supported by reports of amounts of the vesicular cholinergic transporter, a presynaptic marker of cholinergic terminal boutons, in cortical layer 5 being reduced with age in rats (Turrini et al. 2001). Thus, both transport and release alterations in cholinergic circuits have been documented with increasing age, whereas the effects of age on muscarinic receptor populations call into question the specificity of the loss of M_2 muscarinic receptors in Alzheimer's disease.

These and earlier reports indicate that overall cholinergic function declines during normal aging and that ACh regulation is severely and adversely affected at all levels in brain regions affected in Alzheimer's disease. However, the assumption that all or most of the age-related changes in learning and memory are due to cholinergic deficiency should not be made without consideration of the many other neurotransmitter systems that are altered in aging (for review, see Decker and McGaugh 1991 and Palmer and DeKosky 1993).

γ-Aminobutyric Acid

The amino acids are part of the general metabolic pool, and this fact has hindered recognition of their role in synaptic transmission. It also poses problems in attempts to separate the metabolic components from the neurotransmitter component in assays using cellular homogenates. The amino acids are also components of larger neurotransmitter molecules, the neuropeptides and endocrine hormones, the cleavage of which also ultimately produces free amino acids. Several amino acids are now known to fulfill most of the criteria for neurotransmitter molecules, and they can be classified as producing predominantly excitatory or inhibitory effects on their postsynaptic target neurons.

The principal inhibitory neurotransmitter in mammalian brains is the amino acid GABA. Found almost exclusively in the CNS, GABA is produced through the decarboxylation of glutamic acid by the enzyme glutamic acid decarboxylase (GAD), which is the rate-limiting step in GABA formation. The GABA signal is terminated by transamination to yield glutamate and succinic semialdehyde. The enzyme responsible for this step is GABA transaminase, which is usually found in association with succinic semialdehyde dehydrogenase, the enzyme that metabolizes the by-product of GABA transamination. These degradative enzymes are found in many tissues, but GABA and GAD are almost exclusively confined to the CNS. A reuptake mechanism to retrieve synaptic GABA for reuse by the presynaptic neuron is mediated by the GABA transporter protein, which requires sodium for activity (Lam et al. 1993). Relatively high (micromolar) concentrations of GABA are found in certain areas of the brain, such as the hypothalamus and striatum. Neurons containing GAD are usually local circuit interneurons, but some projection neurons, such as the globus pallidus to substantia nigra projection, also use this inhibitory neurotransmitter (Figure 5–3).

Other neurotransmitters co-localized within certain GABAergic neurons are ACh, serotonin, DA, glycine, histamine, neuropeptide Y, vasoactive intestinal peptide, substance P, and somatostatin. The inhibitory effect of GABA is mediated by two distinct receptor subtypes: GABA-A and GABA-B. GABA-A receptors produce inhibition by hyperpolarization of the postsynaptic neuron through an increase in the permeability of chloride ion channels, whereas GABA-B receptors are linked to second messengers and act by decreasing calcium or increasing potassium ion channel conductance. Similar to the nicotinic ACh receptors, GABA-A receptors are composed of five subunits, whereas GABA-B receptors more closely resemble the muscarinic ACh receptor with its second-messenger linkage. The benzodiazepine anxiolytic drugs, the barbiturates, and ethanol all interact with the GABA-A receptor, and this interaction is the physiological basis for the pharmacological ability of these substances to potentiate each other's effects when they are administered concomitantly. Many anticonvulsant drugs act by stimulating GABA receptors, and blockade of GABA or glycine receptors initiates convulsions.

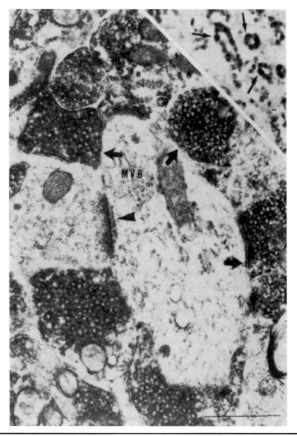

FIGURE 5–3. Terminals containing glutamic acid decarboxylase (GAD) in the substantia nigra from specimens incubated in anti-GAD serum.

Inset: Semithin (1 μm) section of the pars reticulata with obliquely and transversely sectioned dendrites that are encircled by punctate structures containing GAD-positive reaction product (**arrows**). Scale bar = 1 μm.

The accompanying electron micrograph shows an obliquely sectioned dendrite in the substantia nigra, surrounded by many axon terminals filled with GAD-positive reaction product that are equivalent to the puncta seen in the inset. Some of the terminals form symmetrical synapses (**arrows**), whereas the unstained terminal contains round synaptic vesicles and forms an asymmetrical synapse (**bold arrow head**) with this dendritic shaft, multivesicular body (MVB). Scale bar = 1 μm.

Source. Reprinted from Ribak CE, Vaughn JE, Saito K, et al.: "Immunocytochemical Localization of Glutamate Decarboxylase in Rat Substantia Nigra." *Brain Research* 116:288, 1977. Used with permission.

Age-related changes in GABA neuronal systems have been reported in laboratory animals and in human brain tissue. Recent work with aged (24-month-old), middle-aged (18-month-old), and young (3-month-old) rats reported no differences in the ability of a benzodiazepine drug to potentiate the ability of microiontophoretically applied GABA to inhibit the firing rate of cerebellar Purkinje's neurons (Bickford and Breiderick 2000), indicating no effect of aging on the ability of GABA to inhibit this cerebellar circuit. Unlike cerebellar GABA, hypothalamic GABA is reported to be decreased in older

(18-month-old) rats relative to young (3-month-old) rats, and this change is reversed if rats are fed a low-protein diet (Poddar et al. 2000) for a several-month period, indicating that the age-related change in hypothalamic GABA may indicate altered responses of appetitive circuits rather than a pathological development. Hippocampal efferents to the hypothalamus that produce GABA have been reported to have increased amounts of mRNA for GAD in their terminals found in the medial preoptic hypothalamus and posteromedial bed nucleus of the stria terminals in aged (30-month-old) F344 rats compared with middle-aged (15-month-old) and young (3-month-old) animals, which decreased with stress only in the older rats (Herman and Larson 2001). These studies add the hypothalamus to the other brain regions previously shown to be altered with age with respect to GABAergic neurons and indicate relative sparing of the cerebellar circuits using this inhibitory transmitter. The picture emerging from this research indicates that although it is clear that GABA systems are altered during the aging process, great care must be taken in extrapolating results from one or two brain regions or one species to other areas and species.

Dopamine

DA is one of three catecholamine neurotransmitters, the others being NE and EPI. The catecholamines share a similar molecular structure based on the amino acid tyrosine, with additions or deletions of certain biochemical side groups that distinguish one from the others. DA is formed by the decarboxylation of a previously hydroxylated tyrosine moiety under the control of the enzymes tyrosine hydroxylase and dopa decarboxylase. On release into the synapse, DA is recaptured by a specific DA transporter protein (for review, see Hitri et al. 1994) in the presynaptic membrane; unbound DA is metabolized by the enzymes monoamine oxidase (MAO) and catechol-O-methyltransferase (COMT) to the metabolic products homovanillic acid (HVA) and dihydroxyphenylacetic acid (DOPAC). In contrast to ACh synthesis, DA synthesis is rate limiting at the tyrosine hydroxylase step, and the activity of this enzyme is stimulus regulated. DA is heterogeneously distributed in the CNS, with most of the neurotransmitter found in projection neurons of the hypothalamus and midbrain. The DA neurons of the substantia nigra and the ventral tegmental areas of the midbrain project topographically to the striatum and limbic forebrain regions, where they appear to mediate voluntary movement and emotional aspects of pleasure and reward, respectively. DA-containing neurons have been ob-

served to include other neurotransmitters, such as the neuropeptides methionine enkephalin, cholecystokinin, and neurotensin (Figure 5–4).

DA receptors are pharmacologically divided into two classes, the D_1 and D_2 receptor subtypes; molecular techniques also have permitted identification of D_3, D_4, and D_5 forms of the D_1 and D_2 basic classes, as well as the existence of a long and a short form of the D_2 receptor. The D_1 receptor is predominantly postsynaptic and usually is found to stimulate adenylate cyclase activity and phosphoinositide turnover. The D_2 receptor is found at both postsynaptic sites and on the axons, dendrites, and soma of presynaptic, DA-producing neurons (autoreceptors). The D_2 receptor usually is found to inhibit adenylate cyclase activity, but it can also exert effects through inhibition of calcium channel passage and potassium conductance, as well as through phosphoinositide turnover changes. Autoreceptors can exert effects on DA release, synthesis, and storage through distinct mechanisms, allowing highly integrated regulation of DA synaptic availability. Drugs that alter DA synaptic availability either can exert effects directly at the receptor or can alter reuptake, synthesis, or degradation. The stimulant drugs cocaine, amphetamine, and methylphenidate inhibit reuptake of DA in the synaptic cleft by the DA transporter, whereas the classical antipsychotic drugs block D_2 receptors by binding to the DA recognition site. In patients with Parkinson's disease, the degeneration of the DA neurons of the substantia nigra produces tremor and bradykinesia, and these symptoms are temporarily reversed by precursor enrichment in the form of L-dopa administration. The remaining DA neurons increase their rate of DA synthesis to compensate for the reduced synaptic availability at the terminal sites of innervation, and increased amounts of precursor aid this process. However, as the remaining DA neurons degenerate, the synthetic acceleration of these neurons eventually fails to compensate for the reduced synaptic availability, and treatment becomes ineffective. In patients with schizophrenia, the blockade of DA D_2 receptors by antipsychotic drugs provides significant relief from the intrusive thoughts and auditory hallucinations that often accompany this disease. The long-term use of these drugs presents the risk of eventual development of tardive dyskinesia and its associated movement disorder. Thus, although these DA system-directed treatments are undeniably effective in treating certain symptoms in patients with these diseases, they do not cure the disease, they are associated with significant limitations, and the risk of side effects complicates their chronic use.

Research involving possible dopaminergic effects on age-related changes has focused on various parts of the brain, and initial evidence for striatal loss of DA has now

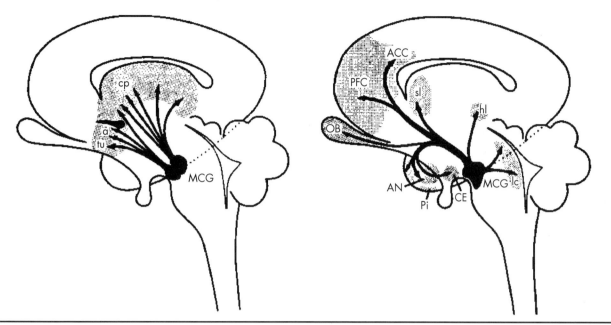

FIGURE 5–4. Dopamine neurons and their pathways in the human brain.

a = nucleus accumbens; ACC = anterior cingulate cortex; AN = amygdaloid nuclei; CE = entorhinal cortex; cp = nucleus caudatus–putamen; hl = lateral habenular nucleus; lc = locus coeruleus; MCG = mesencephalic dopamine cell groups; OB = olfactory bulb; PFC = prefrontal cortex; Pi = piriform cortex; sl = lateral septal nucleus; tu = olfactory tubercle.

Source. Reprinted from Lindvall O, Bjorklund A: "Neuroanatomical Localization of Dopamine in the Brain and Spinal Cord," in *Handbook of Schizophrenia, Vol. 2.* Edited by Henn FA, DeLisi LE. Amsterdam, the Netherlands, Elsevier, 1987, p. 63. Used with permission.

been extended to include several other regions. Reduced amounts of DA have been reported in the hippocampus, amygdala, and brain stem, with the DA metabolite DOPAC concomitantly decreased only in the hippocampus, of aged (24-month-old) rats relative to younger (3- and 12-month-old) rats (Miguez et al. 1999). Other studies (Lee et al. 2001) have reported decreased levels of DA and DOPAC but increased concentrations of HVA in the frontal cortex of aged (24-month-old) rats compared with younger (6- and 12-month-old) control groups. Functionally, alterations in the DA–to–DA metabolite ratio in frontal/parietal and occipital cortex and dorsal hippocampus of aged rats with severe impairments in spatial memory have been described, but other neurotransmitter systems (ACh and serotonin) also were altered in these memory-impaired, aged rats (Stemmelin et al. 2000).

In more recent efforts to characterize the apparent deficits in DA neurotransmission in aging, researchers have reported increased amounts of DA and DA metabolites from the auditory nerve innervation of the cochlea of aged male rats and interpreted these changes as a decreased functional release of DA in response to auditory stimuli (Vicente-Torres et al. 2001). The reduced plasticity of the striatal dopaminergic innervation to injury in aged rats was shown with 6-hydroxy-DA lesions. Striatal DA and DA neuronal activity were decreased in aged (18- or 23-month-old) rats relative to younger (4- or 12-month-old) animals before lesioning, and increased dopaminergic responses after lesioning in younger animals were not seen in the older groups (Ling et al. 2000). Other researchers (Gerhardt et al. 2002), who used nonhuman primates, measured DA in the substantia nigra with in vivo microdialysis and documented a decrease in the major DA metabolites HVA (44%) and DOPAC (79%) in aged (23- to 28-year-old) monkeys relative to younger (8- to 9-year-old and 14- to 17-year-old) groups. Postmortem tissue from these aged animals also showed decreased amounts of DA and metabolites in the putamen and decreased numbers and size of tyrosine hydroxylase–staining neurons and tyrosine hydroxylase fiber density in the substantia nigra relative to the younger groups. These age-related deficits may underlie the decreased locomotor ability of aged animals.

Many of the functions that decrease with aging, such as locomotion, motivation, memory, and learning, involve DA and DA receptors, and some researchers have postulated oxidative stress-mediated dopaminergic pathology as responsible for decreasing function with age (Luo and Roth 2000). The technology to visualize biochemical parameters in living patients, as realized by PET, has been used to show a loss of DA D_2 receptor binding of [^{11}C]raclopride in the frontal, temporal, and cingulate cortices that was significantly correlated with age-related decline in neuronal glucose metabolism in these regions (Volkow et al. 2000). Decreased numbers of D_2 receptors in the striatum with increasing age also have been correlated with decreasing cognitive function in another PET study (Backman et al. 2000). A recent imaging study (van Dyck et al. 2002), which used single photon emission computed tomography (SPECT) and measured the DA transporter in caudate and putamen of a series of patients from age 18 to 88 years, reported a symmetrically bilateral 45%–48% decrease in both regions in the oldest subjects relative to younger subjects, with an average decline of 6.6% per decade. The authors interpreted these data as indicating that the DA transporter declines slowly over the entire course of aging, not just at the end stages of life. Surprisingly, this effect of normal aging on the DA transporter is apparently not accelerated by Parkinson's disease–induced loss of DA neurons (Booij et al. 2001). Thus, strain and species differences are apparent in the research literature on DA and aging, although there is generally agreement as to striatal DA mechanism pathology in aging.

Serotonin

Serotonin is an indoleamine that is produced by enzymatic alteration of the amino acid tryptophan; it was named for its potent effects on the smooth muscle of blood vessels. Because only a small percentage of the total serotonin in the body is contained in the CNS, the neurotransmitter status of this molecule was not established until many years after its discovery. The rate-limiting step in the synthesis of serotonin is the hydroxylation of neuronally available tryptophan by tryptophan hydroxylase, which is subsequently decarboxylated by 5-hydroxytryptophan decarboxylase to yield the functional neurotransmitter molecule. MAO removes an amino group, and further oxidation yields the principal serotonin metabolite 5-hydroxyindoleacetic acid (5-HIAA).

Serotonin in the synaptic cleft can be recaptured by the presynaptic neuron via the specific serotonin transporter protein. This transporter protein, cloned relatively recently (Blakely and Berson 1991), is the target of a wide variety of drugs that are useful in reducing the symptoms of major depressive disorder, although this therapeutic result is achieved only after 2–3 weeks of treatment. A similar response also can be elicited, over the same time frame, by drugs that block the NE transporter.

Three classes of serotonin receptors in the CNS have been characterized pharmacologically: 5-HT$_1$, 5-HT$_2$, and 5-HT$_3$. Use of molecular techniques also has allowed identification of subtypes of some of these receptors. The category of 5-HT$_1$ receptors now includes 5-HT$_{1A}$, 5-HT$_{1B}$, 5-HT$_{1C}$, and 5-HT$_{1D}$ subtypes; the 5-HT$_2$ receptors include 5-HT$_{2A}$ and 5-HT$_{2B}$ subtypes (Teitler et al. 1994). At last count, 14 molecular subtypes of serotonin receptors had been identified (Oh et al. 2001). These subtypes all appear to be linked to second messengers via G proteins, yet the actual second messenger and the effect (stimulatory or inhibitory) of the receptor on these second messengers can be quite different for the various subtypes of serotonin receptors. The similarity in the shape of the serotonin molecule and the chemical shape of various psychoactive drugs has promulgated much research into the mechanisms of the effects of these compounds. The hallucinogenic drugs lysergic acid diethylamide (LSD), mescaline, and psilocin all have profound effects on the activity of serotonin-containing neuronal systems. Whether these effects are due to an agonist or antagonist effect at various serotonin receptor sites is an issue that has not yet been resolved; however, the current data indicate that a decrease in median raphe serotonin neuronal firing rates correlates with the effects of these drugs. The distribution of serotonin neurons in the CNS resembles that of the catecholamines, with the major concentrations of neuronal cell bodies in the midbrain dorsal raphe nucleus and smaller cell groups in the median raphe of the brain stem. The projections from the dorsal raphe course through the median forebrain bundle in the lateral hypothalamus to innervate the entire cortex and limbic systems and may mediate certain emotional states (Figure 5–5).

Aging-related changes in serotonin neuronal systems have been reported in both human and laboratory animal subjects. Recent reports of alterations in serotonin circuits with advancing age include PET imaging studies of 5-HT$_{1A}$ receptor binding in living subjects that reported a 10% decrease in binding per decade for this serotonin receptor subtype, which was present in a variety of cortical and subcortical regions (Tauscher et al. 2001). Another PET imaging study found evidence for a 17% per decade loss of 5-HT$_{2A}$ receptors in a variety of brain regions from age 20 to middle age, with losses subsiding at later ages (Sheline et al. 2002). Others (Pirker et al. 2000) have reported decreased serotonin transporter number in the striatum (6.6% per decade) and a 3%–4% per decade decrease in other serotonin transporter–rich regions with increasing age when SPECT imaging techniques were used. Postmortem brain tissue studies of young (5- to 29-year-old) and older (62- to 84-year-old) subjects have reported that the major midbrain serotonin neuronal population of the median raphe does not show alterations in the amount of the synthetic enzyme

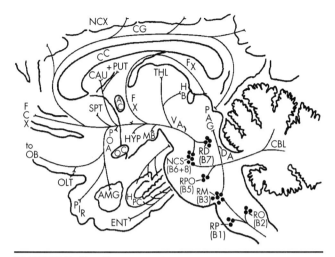

FIGURE 5–5. Serotonergic systems.

This schematic parasagittal view of a primate brain depicts the serotonin cell groups (**solid circles**) and their major projections. These groups were designated B_1 through B_9 by Dahlstrom and Fuxe (1964).

AC = anterior commissure; AMG = amygdala; CAU = caudate nucleus; CBL = cerebellum; CC = corpus callosum; CG = cingulate gyrus; DA = dorsal ascending pathway; ENT = entorhinal cortex; FCX = frontal cortex; FX = fornix; HB = habenula; HPC = hippocampus; HYP = hypothalamus; MB = mamillary bodies; NCS = nucleus centralis superior; NCX = neocortex; OB = olfactory bulb; OC = optic chiasm; OLT = olfactory tubercle; PAG = periaqueductal gray; PIR = piriform cortex; POA = preoptic anterior hypothalamus; PUT = putamen; RD = raphe dorsalis; RM = raphe magnus; RO = raphe obscurus; RP = raphe pallidus; RPO = raphe pontis; SPT = septum; THL = thalamus; VA = ventral ascending pathway.

Source. Reprinted from Nieuwenhuys R, Voogd J, van Huijzen C: *The Human Central Nervous System.* New York, Springer-Verlag, 1981, p. 230. Used with permission.

tryptophan hydroxylase with increasing age (Kloppel et al. 2001).

Researchers at Duke University Medical Center (Slotkin et al. 2000) reported different responses of serotonergic neurons in the cortex to the DA- and serotonin-toxic drug methylene dioxymethamphetamine (MDMA), with younger mice showing increased turnover and older mice having decreased serotonin turnover relative to similar degrees of serotonin damage. This article stated that even if basal conditions are similar across age groups, responses to injury and repair processes still may differ with age. In another study, Duncan et al. (2000) used three age groups of hamsters; the numbers of serotonin reuptake sites were increased, and $5\text{-}HT_{1B}$ receptors were decreased, in the suprachiasmatic nucleus of the hypothalamus of middle-aged and old hamsters versus young animals, leading the authors to suggest these changes may underlie the alterations in circadian rhythm seen in older subjects. Serotonin alterations with age have been documented in a variety of brain regions and

among various species but occur most often in terminal areas rather than in cell body regions.

Norepinephrine

The catecholamine NE was first shown to be a neurotransmitter in the peripheral nervous system and was later found to be a component of the CNS. The development of staining techniques for visualization of the catecholamines in tissue sections greatly facilitated research into NE's neurotransmitter role in both the CNS and the peripheral nervous system. As the neurotransmitter of postganglionic sympathetic peripheral nerves, NE's effects on a variety of organ systems are well known, although its role in the CNS is not as well delineated. Like DA, NE is synthesized by sequential modifications of a tyrosine amino acid substrate. DA is further hydroxylated by DA β-hydroxylase to yield NE after modifications of tyrosine induced by tyrosine hydroxylase and dopa decarboxylase. After release into the synapse, NE is metabolized by MAO and COMT to form the major degradative product 3-methoxy-4-hydroxyphenylglycol (MHPG). Similar to what happens with serotonin and DA, released NE is also recaptured by the presynaptic neuron via a NE transporter protein. This protein has now been cloned, and its sequence has been found to be highly homologous with that of the GABA transporter protein (Melikian et al. 1994) (see Figure 5–6).

Blockade of the NE transporter protein for 2–3 weeks by specific NE uptake inhibitor drugs results in amelioration of depressive symptoms in patients with major depressive disorder. However, because this therapeutic effect is also elicited by specific serotonin transporter inhibitors, it is probably mediated by some adaptive regulatory response to the sequelae of transporter inhibition rather than by the inhibition itself. The receptor subtypes that mediate the actions of NE at the postsynaptic site were originally divided into two classes (α and β adrenoreceptors) based on location and pharmacology, with further subdivision into α_1 and α_2 and β_1 and β_2. Use of molecular techniques has permitted expansion of this classification to seven specific subtypes to accommodate the very different effects on second-messenger systems mediated by these G protein–linked, seven-membrane domain receptors.

The NE neurons in the CNS reside predominantly in two distinct midbrain regions: the locus coeruleus and the dorsal tegmental nucleus. The locus coeruleus provides the major NE projection to the forebrain and the hypothalamus, where NE mediates a variety of behavior-

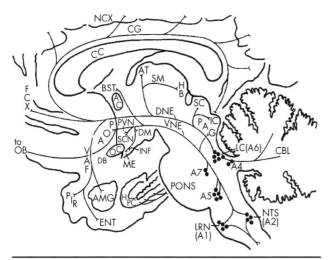

FIGURE 5–6. Noradrenergic systems.

This schematized parasagittal view of a primate brain shows the location of major norepinephrine-producing cell bodies **(solid circles)** and their major projections. These cell groups were designated A_1 through A_7 by Dahlstrom and Fuxe (1964).

AC = anterior commissure; AMG = amygdala; AT = anterior thalamus; BST = bed nucleus of the stria terminalis; CBL = cerebellum; CC = corpus callosum; CG = cingulate gyrus; DB = diagonal band; DM = dorsomedial hypothalamus; DNE = dorsal noradrenergic efferents; ENT = entorhinal cortex; FCX = frontal cortex; HB = habenula; HPC = hippocampus; IC = inferior colliculus; INF = infundibulum; LC = locus coeruleus; LRN = lateral reticular nucleus; ME = median eminence; NCX = neocortex; NTS = nucleus tractus solitarius; OB = olfactory bulb; OC = optic chiasm; PAG = periaqueductal gray; PIR = piriform cortex; POA = preoptic anterior hypothalamus; PONS = pons; PVN = paraventricular nucleus of the hypothalamus; SC = superior colliculus; SM = stria medullaris; SCN = suprachiasmatic nucleus; VAF = ventral ascending fibers; VNE = ventral noradrenergic efferents.

Source. Reprinted from Nieuwenhuys R, Voogd J, van Huijzen C: *The Human Central Nervous System.* New York, Springer-Verlag, 1981, p. 228. Used with permission.

al and endocrine effects associated with responses to physiological challenges; this region often shows degeneration of NE-containing neurons in patients with Alzheimer's disease. The neuropeptides galanin and neuropeptide Y have been identified within NE neurons, but the significance of this co-localization is not yet known. An intimate relation between the NE and the corticotropin-releasing factor (CRF) neuronal systems exists; CRF is released from nerve terminals in the locus coeruleus to elicit increases in NE neuronal firing rates in the locus coeruleus. Through NE projections to the hypothalamus, this noradrenergic activity in the locus coeruleus subsequently induces CRF mRNA production in the paraventricular nucleus of the hypothalamus, where CRF is available for transport to the median eminence and eventual release to the pituitary. Thus, the neurotransmitter that plays such an essential role in the sympathetic nervous

system's response to stress is apparently well placed to mediate the CNS responses to stressful stimuli in addition. Anxiolytic drugs, such as the benzodiazepines, reduce the firing rate of NE locus coeruleus neurons, a fact that further strengthens the hypothesis that this circuit mediates arousal states in mammals.

Although NE circuits are not as well known for alterations in aging as DA circuits are, some lines of evidence suggest alterations in NE brain systems with increasing age. In a study comparing aged (25-month-old) rats with younger (9-month-old) animals, the NE concentration in frontal cortex terminals arising from neurons in the locus coeruleus was not changed with increasing age despite decreased numbers of locus coeruleus neurons in the older rats (Ishida et al. 2001a). The authors interpreted their data as indicating increased dendritic branching in remaining locus coeruleus projections that would allow compensation for decreased numbers of locus coeruleus neurons while preserving regional synaptic availability. However, these researchers also quantified numbers of NE axonal varicosities in frontal cortex as being reduced in aged animals, which would require increased synthesis and release from remaining sites to maintain regional signaling strength (Ishida et al. 2001b). These findings indicate that NE systems do show age-related changes, but the distribution and complexity of these changes are not as great as those reported for some of the other classical neurotransmitters.

Glutamic Acid

Glutamic acid, or glutamate, is the prototypical excitatory amino acid neurotransmitter, although the evidence for its role in vertebrate neurotransmission has accumulated relatively slowly as a result of the many roles that glutamate plays in cellular metabolism. Because glutamate is both the precursor for GABA and a transmitter itself, its presence in nerve endings cannot indicate whether glutamic acid is being used as a transmitter, and the additional presence of the glutamate transporter protein (Kanner et al. 1993; Kawakami et al. 1994) does not disclose how a neuron is using glutamic acid. The additional problem of lack of regional specificity in neuronal excitation after application of the excitatory amino acids has been interpreted as being attributable to the fact that almost all neurons have receptors for the excitatory amino acids. The ability of these excitatory amino acid transmitters (including aspartate) to excite virtually all neurons to which they are applied has been exploited through the use of excitotoxic analogues of glutamic acid:

kainic acid, quisqualic acid, and ibotenic acid. These agents apparently stimulate the neurons to which they are applied until those neurons die of exhaustion, thus allowing the formation of a relatively discrete, localized lesion of cell bodies without an interruption of neighboring axons or adjacent terminals.

The best evidence for a neurotransmitter role of glutamic acid is derived from the various receptor subtypes that recognize this agent. Originally classified on the basis of whether the receptor would or would not bind the N-methyl-D-aspartate (NMDA) analogue, these glutamic acid receptors have now been divided into five distinct groups. The NMDA receptor recognizes aspartate as well as glutamic acid and contains at least four other functional subcomponents, making it similar to the benzodiazepine/GABA receptor complex. The NMDA receptor forms a membrane channel that is permeable to sodium and calcium ions when opened and that contains a modulatory site that recognizes glycine. The hallucinogenic drug phencyclidine (PCP, or "angel dust") and the investigative drug dizocilpine (MK801) bind to the NMDA receptor complex and prevent ion passage through the channel. The kainate glutamic acid receptor subtype (which preferentially binds kainic acid) and the quisqualate-preferring AMPA receptor subtype (which is named for its ability to specifically bind α-3-hydroxy-5-methyl-isoxazole-4-propionic acid, or AMPA) are both ligand-gated ion channels that pass sodium and potassium ions when open. The fourth glutamic acid receptor subtype is also an ion channel receptor and is named AP-4, after its specificity for the compound 1-2-amino-4-phosphonobutyrate. The fifth glutamic acid receptor subtype, the metabotropic, or ACPD, receptor (named for its specificity in binding trans-1-aminocyclopentane-1,3-dicarboxylic acid, or t-ACPD), is linked to the IP3/DAG second-messenger signal transduction pathway and thus represents a membrane receptor more like the muscarinic ACh receptor than the nicotinic (channel) receptor.

The neurons containing these various glutamic acid receptor subtypes are distributed among several brain regions and are particularly enriched in the hippocampus, where they form long projection neurons among the different hippocampal subfields. The pathological involvement of glutamic acid neurons in the devastating sequelae of cerebral infarction (stroke) and in epileptic foci, as well as in learning and memory disorders, and the potential for specific manipulation of the various receptor subtypes, makes this ubiquitous neurotransmitter system an attractive target for a wide variety of pharmacological agents.

Because glutamate is the predominant excitatory neurotransmitter in the CNS and its major receptor (NMDA)

is present in more than half of all brain synapses, theories of glutaminergic alterations during the aging process abound. However, evidence for altered glutaminergic function in aging rests on relatively few data. Some investigators have described altered glutamate transporter activity and decreased numbers of NMDA receptors as providing the mechanical basis for loss of function in the domains of cognition, locomotor activity, and emotion (Segovia et al. 2001). Others have argued that some of the changes in NMDA receptor populations in aging are the result of responses to alterations in other neurotransmitter systems that regulate these receptors. An example of this is the reported alteration of numbers of NMDAR2 receptors in hippocampus and cortex of aged (21- and 30-month-old) rats compared with younger (10-month-old) control rats and the protection of such hippocampal, but not cortical, receptors from age-induced loss by administration of insulin-like growth factor (Sonntag et al. 2000). In mice, cortical and hippocampal density of the zeta subunit of the NMDA receptor were reduced in aged (30-month-old) mice compared with young (3-month-old) control mice, leading to different responses to certain agonists and antagonists with age (Magnusson 2000).

Striatal metabotropic glutamate receptors in aged (24-month-old) rats have decreased ability to initiate second-messenger production or activate postsynaptic neurons and are less able to potentiate the effects of NMDA after administration of a glycine agonist than is seen in younger (3-month-old) rats (Pintor et al. 2000), confirming decreased function of these glutamate receptors in the aged striatum. Locomotor deficits in aged (30-month-old) rats relative to young (3-month-old) or middle-aged (20-month old) rats have been correlated with loss of NMDA receptors rather than DA receptor or neuron loss (Ossowska et al. 2001). Numbers of both NMDA and AMPA receptors have been reported to be decreased in the aging hippocampus of rats; NMDA receptors were decreased in the CA1 and CA3 regions and subiculum but were spared in the dentate hilus, whereas AMPA receptors were decreased in the latter but not the former regions (Wenk and Barnes 2000). Hypothalamic NMDA receptors on gonadotropin-releasing hormone neurons in female rats alter subunit mRNA content with age and become inhibitory rather than stimulatory with increasing age (Gore et al. 2000), which may underlie some of the reproductive endocrine changes seen in aging females. Alterations in NMDA subunit deficits also are partially reversed by diet restriction in aged (26-month-old) mice compared with young (3-month-old) or middle-aged (15-month-old) mice, further supporting the concept of altered subunit content of NMDA receptors contributing to the effects of age on NMDA receptor function (Magnusson 2001). Immunohistochemical studies of aged primate brain have documented age-related loss of NMDAR1 and GluR2 receptor subunits in both long and short projection neurons of the cerebral cortex, indicating decreased function in more than one type of subunit for glutamate receptors with age (Hof et al. 2002).

Imaging studies of young (19- to 31-year-old) compared with middle-aged (40- to 52-year-old) humans with MRS have documented decreased levels of glutamate and GABA in the dorsolateral prefrontal cortex (Grachev et al. 2001), which the authors interpreted as an adaptive or compensatory response to continued growth of neuronal processes rather than underlying functional deficits. Another MRS study found decreased levels of combined glutamate-glutamine signal in 18 subjects with clinical Alzheimer's disease compared with 12 control subjects without Alzheimer's disease (Antuono et al. 2001), and this measure may aid in an earlier diagnosis of probable Alzheimer's disease.

There is little doubt that glutamic acid systems are altered in normal aging and in persons with Alzheimer's disease (Francis et al. 1993), as these human and animal data indicate. What remains to be seen is whether these changes result from primary alterations in other neurotransmitter systems or occur independently and whether glutamic acid changes might contribute to the further loss of other neurotransmitters during the aging process.

Histamine

Because histamine is found in mast cells of the reticular activating system, and because it is difficult to separate the histamine component from the CNS tissue component, researchers experienced great difficulty in establishing the role of histamine in CNS neurotransmission. It is now confirmed that histamine is formed in specific neurons by decarboxylation from the amino acid histidine. Both dopa decarboxylase and a specific histidine decarboxylase can accomplish this step. Although histamine can be oxidized or methylated, the predominant inactivation step in the mammalian brain is methylation by histamine methyltransferase. Researchers used antibodies to histidine decarboxylase to map the distribution of histamine-containing neurons and identified two distinct cell groups. The major group is found in the mamillary body region of the posterior hypothalamus; the other group is found in the mesencephalic reticular formation. These

two regions send projections to the cortex and limbic system through fiber bundles in the lateral hypothalamus (median forebrain bundle).

Three forms of histamine receptors can be distinguished pharmacologically: H_1, H_2, and H_3. The H_1 receptor seems to mediate excitatory effects of histamine, whereas H_2 is inhibitory and linked to adenylate cyclase as a second messenger. The H_3 receptor may be an autoreceptor for histamine presynaptic neurons, and their activation inhibits histamine synthesis and release. There have been surprisingly few reports of age-associated changes in histamine neuronal systems in either humans or laboratory animals.

Neuroactive Peptides (Neuropeptides)

Neuropeptides are one of the most recently discovered classes of neurotransmitter substances. They were originally purified to obtain just a few milligrams from hundreds of thousands of sheep and pig hypothalami, the section of the brain in which several neuropeptides that function as regulators of pituitary hormones are found in relatively large concentrations (for a review of peptide biology, see Owens et al. 2000). Whereas the amino acid neurotransmitters such as GABA and glutamic acid are found in micromolar concentrations in enriched brain regions, and the biogenic amines (DA, NE, serotonin) and ACh are found in nanomolar concentrations in their neuronal terminal regions, the neuropeptides are found in picomolar and femtomolar concentrations per gram of brain tissue.

Ranging in size from 2 to more than 40 amino acids in length, these small proteins are constructed according to the same transcription/translation mechanism that provides the synthetic and degradative enzymes that are responsible for metabolism of the classical neurotransmitters. The DNA strand encoding the neuropeptide precursor, a larger protein termed a *prohormone*, is transcribed into mRNA sequences within the cell nucleus. The resulting prohormone mRNA sequence is translated into a protein at the ribosome and packaged into vesicles at the Golgi apparatus. The vesicles are transported to the nerve terminal presynaptic region; during this procedure, the active peptide is cleaved from the prohormone sequence at pairs of dibasic residues by specific cleavage enzymes. The active neuropeptide is then released into the synaptic cleft by vesicular fusion with the nerve terminal membrane and crosses the extracellular space in the synaptic cleft to bind to the appropriate receptors.

Because only a few of the amino acids in any peptide make up the recognition site at the receptor-binding site, it is possible for fragments of the active peptide to retain all or some of the activity of the intact active form. It is also possible for peptides with similar sequences, or with sequences that fit the active site of a particular receptor, to show cross-reactivity at a receptor. Similarly, the degradative peptidase enzymes that remove the active peptide from the synapse are designed to cleave the peptide bond at certain amino acids or at one end of the peptide chain and thus may degrade more than one neuropeptide substrate. In addition, several copies of the active peptide may be contained in the prohormone sequence, allowing quick amplification of the neuropeptide signal on demand.

The various neuropeptides known to reside in the CNS are grouped into families according to sequence similarities, receptor activity, and similarity of physiological effects. These include the tachykinins (substance P, kassinin, eledoisin, bradykinin), which mediate blood pressure responses; the endogenous opioids (endorphins, enkephalins, and dynorphin), which produce analgesia in neuronal systems associated with pain sensation; the posterior pituitary hormones vasopressin and oxytocin, which are involved in maintenance of water balance and milk production, respectively; the glucagon-related peptides (vasoactive intestinal peptide, peptide histidine leucine, and peptide histidine methionine); and the pancreatic polypeptide-related peptides (neuropeptide Y, peptide YY, avian pancreatic polypeptide, and human pancreatic polypeptide). Many of these related neuropeptides are derived from different regions of the same prohormone precursor protein.

Other interesting neuropeptides are apparently unrelated to larger families, as is the case for neurotensin and neuromedin N. These two neuropeptides are encoded in the same prohormone, and their respective coding sequences are separated by a single pair of dibasic amino acids. Neurotensin produces hypothermia, potentiates the effects of barbiturates, and induces analgesia after direct CNS delivery. This fascinating neuropeptide also blocks the effects of DA in various brain regions. Synthesis of neurotensin is induced by antipsychotic drug administration in laboratory animals. Because group mean neurotensin cerebrospinal fluid (CSF) concentrations are often decreased in schizophrenic patients relative to psychiatrically normal control subjects, the hypothesis that neurotensin may act as an endogenous neuroleptic or antipsychotic agent has been proposed. (For a comprehensive review of the neurobiology of neurotensin, see Bissette and Nemeroff 1994.) The current list of CNS neuropeptides approaches 100 distinct entities; three representative neuropeptides are discussed here: thyrotropin-releasing hormone (TRH), CRF, and somatostatin.

Thyrotropin-Releasing Hormone

The first hypothalamic releasing factor to be purified was TRH. The isolation of TRH was the result of an intense competition between two research teams, whose leaders eventually shared the Nobel Prize in medicine for this effort (for a review of TRH neurobiology, see Mason et al. 1994). The release of thyrotropin from the anterior pituitary is induced by the release of a TRH molecule from nerve terminals in the median eminence into the pituitary portal system; the TRH molecule eventually binds to a TRH receptor on thyrotrophs of the pituitary.

The TRH molecule is composed of three amino acids (glutamic acid–histidine–proline–amino [pGlu-His-Pro-NH_2]), which are joined between the amide terminus of one amino acid and the carboxyl terminus of the next amino acid in a (peptide) bond. The TRH molecule is further modified by a cyclized amino terminus (pGlu) and an amidated carboxyl terminus (NH_2) to protect it from degradation by the specific peptidase enzymes that degrade the neuropeptides into constituent amino acids. The TRH molecule is small enough to cross the blood-brain barrier after peripheral administration, which is not the case for larger neuropeptides and biomolecules, although the half-life of TRH in serum is only a couple of minutes.

The major metabolite of TRH is a cyclized His-Pro dipeptide that has biological activity of its own within the brain (Banks et al. 1993). The TRH receptor is membrane bound and is primarily associated with the IP3/DAG second-messenger signal transduction system; synthesis of TRH receptor mRNA is regulated by local concentrations of TRH. Two TRH receptors have now been cloned, and their discrete nervous system distributions have been mapped (O'Dowd et al. 2000). Neurons containing TRH are found in highest concentrations in the hypothalamus, but TRH is also found in neurons of the anterior preoptic hypothalamus and septal nuclei. TRH is found within serotonin neurons of the medullary raphe nuclei, and TRH nerve terminals impinge on the serotonin neurons of the dorsal raphe midbrain nuclei that project to the entire cortex. The ability of TRH to reverse the sedative effects of barbiturates and ethanol is thought to reside in the septal region, whereas TRH applied to thermosensitive neurons of the preoptic anterior hypothalamus increases the firing rate of cold-sensitive neurons and decreases the firing rate of warm-sensitive neurons. In laboratory animals, it has been found that TRH is released from the hypothalamus after exposure to cold, following hemorrhage, or in association with restraint.

Patients with major depressive disorder often have reduced activity (blunting) of TRH pituitary receptors, and an increased incidence of antithyroid antibodies has been identified in the blood of such patients; groups of depressed patients have shown increased mean TRH concentrations in CSF compared with psychiatrically healthy control subjects (Banki et al. 1988). These findings suggest that hypersecretion of TRH may be associated with depressive disorder (Bissette 1991b).

Human studies of TRH-stimulated release of thyrotropin in two groups of aged subjects (65–80 and 81–92 years) compared with younger control subjects (20–60 years) have reported decreased pituitary responses to TRH in the elderly, with further alterations in thyroid hormone levels indicating decreased activity of the hypothalamic-pituitary-thyroid (HPT) axis with increasing age (Monzani et al. 1996). Japanese researchers have investigated the effects of a compound, JTP-4819, that blocks the effects of one of the enzymes that destroys TRH after it is released from the presynaptic neuron and have reversed the age-induced decrease in amounts of TRH in the hippocampus and cerebral cortex in aged rats with a 21-day oral administration regimen (Shinoda et al. 1995). This compound also restores spatial memory and reverses the deficits in hippocampal choline uptake and cortical CAT levels in aged rats after 14 or 21 days of oral delivery (Toide et al. 1997) and may prove useful in cognitive disorders that occur with increasing age. Others (Cizza et al. 1995) have examined the HPT axis in aged (23-month-old) and young (3-month-old) F344 rats and reported decreased basal hypothalamic concentrations of TRH mRNA in the aged rats, and immobilization stress did not decrease these levels further in the aged rats as it did in the young group.

Thus, the endocrine activity of TRH systems appears to be affected by age, although there is little evidence for such changes in extraendocrine TRH systems.

Corticotropin-Releasing Factor

CRF was finally isolated and purified by Vale and colleagues (1981) in the early 1980s, after being intensively sought by various research teams for more than 20 years. The CRF molecule is 41 amino acids in length, and the sequence of CRF in rats and humans has been shown to be identical (for a review of CRF neurobiology, see De Souza and Nemeroff 1990). CRF-binding protein, a specific carrier protein present in blood and brain, somewhat sequesters bound CRF from the action of peptidases and prevents access to the CRF receptor in the bound configuration. The release of CRF from the median eminence,

where processes from cell bodies in the paraventricular nucleus of the hypothalamus terminate, into the pituitary portal system evokes the release of several related peptides derived from the prohormone precursor protein pro-opiomelanocortin (POMC), including β-endorphin and corticotropin. The CRF receptor active site is directed toward the carboxyl terminus of CRF; the receptor is linked to the adenyl cyclase second-messenger signal transduction system and stimulates the action of this enzyme when the receptor is activated. Outside the hypothalamus, CRF neurons project from the central nucleus of the amygdala to limbic and brain stem nuclei, and CRF is found in interneurons of the cortex and hippocampus. This distribution underscores CRF's putative role in mediating the higher CNS responses to stress and adumbrates a role for CRF in emotional responses to adverse stimuli (for reviews, see Bissette 1989, 1991a). The release of hypothalamic CRF is induced by a variety of stressful stimuli in laboratory animals (Chappell et al. 1986), and exogenous CRF administered directly into the CNS of laboratory animals has been shown to elicit fearful and anxious behaviors, behaviors that are blocked by regional application of specific CRF receptor antagonists (Bakshi et al. 2002). Traumatic sensitization of CRF endocrine circuits during early development has been hypothesized to contribute to vulnerability to mood and anxiety disorders in adults.

Patients with major depressive disorder often have a blunted corticotropin response after challenge with exogenous CRF; show early escape from the inhibition of corticotropin and cortisol secretion after administration of the synthetic glucocorticoid dexamethasone; have higher group mean concentrations of CRF in CSF than do non–psychiatrically ill control subjects (Banki et al. 1987; Nemeroff et al. 1984); and have reduced numbers of CRF receptors in the frontal cortex, as demonstrated by Nemeroff and co-workers (1988) on postmortem examination of brain tissue of depressed patients who committed suicide. These findings are consistent with the interpretation of a dysregulated hypersecretion of CRF in patients with mood disorders.

CRF in Alzheimer's Disease

Concentrations of CRF were reported to be decreased in frontal and temporal cortex of postmortem Alzheimer's disease brain relative to age-matched non–Alzheimer's disease control tissues in 1985 (Bissette et al. 1985). CRF concentrations in the Alzheimer's disease group were not altered in subcortical regions such as the nucleus basalis or hypothalamus in this patient population, although the caudate nucleus concentrations of CRF

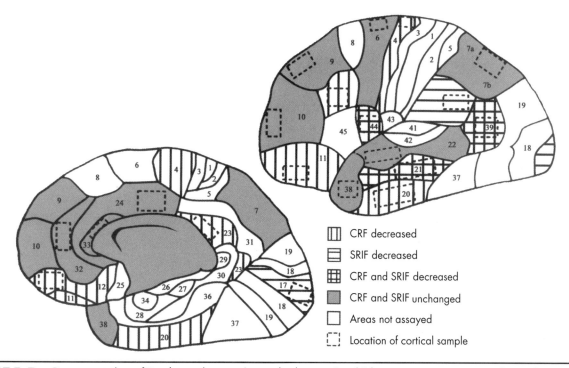

FIGURE 5–7.   Representation of Brodmann's areas in cerebral cortex in which postmortem concentrations of corticotropin-releasing factor (CRF) and somatostatin (somatotropin release-inhibiting factor, SRIF) are decreased in subjects with Alzheimer's disease relative to control subjects without Alzheimer's disease.

Regions are *shaded* to show decreased concentrations of CRF **(vertical lines)**, decreased concentrations of SRIF **(horizontal lines)**, or decreased concentrations of both neuropeptides **(both horizontal and vertical lines)** relative to control subjects. Gray areas had no changes in either peptide. *Dotted line rectangles* within the Brodmann's region indicate where sample was obtained within that region.

Source.   Adapted from Bissette G, Cook L, Smith W, et al.: "Regional Neuropeptide Pathology in Alzheimer's Disease: Corticotropin-Releasing Factor and Somatostatin." *Journal of Alzheimer's Disease* 1:91–105, 1998. Used with permission.

were decreased in the Alzheimer's disease group. Loss of cortical CRF in Alzheimer's disease was confirmed by De Souza and co-workers (1986), who also reported decreased CRF concentrations in occipital and parietal cortical regions of Alzheimer's disease subjects. These findings were extended to include increased numbers of CRF receptors that were roughly proportional to the decreased concentration of CRF and may have occurred in response to the reduced synaptic availability of CRF. The cortical distribution of CRF$_1$ receptors makes this subtype the most likely candidate for such upregulation. Immunohistochemical staining of Alzheimer's disease cortex has established that interneurons of the cortex containing CRF (Powers et al. 1987) degenerate, whereas regions such as the hypothalamus, cerebellum, or hippocampus maintain normal amounts of CRF immunoreactivity (Kelley and Kowall 1989). The normal amounts of CRF in the hypothalamus as assessed by immunohistochemistry have not supported findings of increased amounts of CRF mRNA in the postmortem paraventricular nucleus of the hypothalamus in Alzheimer's disease patients and even greater elevations in patients with a clinical history of major depression during life (Raadsheer et al. 1995). Our

laboratory has assessed different groups of subjects with Alzheimer's disease and found either a nonsignificant increase in CRF content of the postmortem hypothalamus (Bissette et al. 1985) or groups in which hypothalamic CRF and somatotropin release inhibiting factor were significantly decreased (Bissette et al. 1998) (Figure 5–7).

Increased hypothalamic CRF mRNA elevations in patients with Alzheimer's disease might be reflected in CSF concentrations of CRF if hypothalamic CRF contributes significantly to CSF concentrations. Increased concentrations of CRF in CSF from subjects with Alzheimer's disease have been reported (Martignoni et al. 1990), and increased levels of CRF in CSF from patients with dementia and depression have been described (Banki et al. 1992). However, CSF concentrations of CRF in clinical Alzheimer's disease also have been reported to be either unchanged (Banki et al. 1992; Edvinsson et al. 1993; Jolkkonen et al. 1990; Molchan et al. 1993; Nemeroff et al. 1984; Pomara et al. 1989) or decreased (Heilig et al. 1995; May et al. 1987; Mouradian et al. 1986; Suemaru et al. 1991, 1995). These differences may reflect individual variation and clinical diagnostic uncertainty.

Attempts to restore CRF levels in patients with Alzheimer's disease by releasing endogenous CRF from the CRF-binding protein have been successful in increasing postmortem CRF tissue levels to near concentrations seen in non–Alzheimer's disease control tissue (Behan et al. 1995) and confirmed that normal amounts of CRF-binding protein exist in Alzheimer's disease cortical tissue. Such a therapy may prove useful in light of recent data (Davis et al. 1999) indicating statistically significant CRF cortical deficits in postmortem tissue of confirmed Alzheimer's disease patients with a dementia severity score of 2 on the 5-point Clinical Dementia Rating Scale, whereas somatostatin and ACh deficits did not achieve significance until patients had reached a score of 4.

Thus, CRF deficits may precede those of the other neurotransmitters affected during the disease process and could become an important therapeutic target and diagnostic marker.

Hypothalamic-Pituitary-Adrenal Axis

Endocrine changes in aging are one of the most comprehensively researched aspects of this phenomenon, and alterations in just about every endocrine axis investigated to date have been reported with increasing age (for review, see Rehman and Masson 2001). Alterations in the numbers of neurons in hypothalamic nuclei with aging have been described (for review, see Hofman 1997 and Swaab 1995). Evidence for decreased resiliency to stress with increasing age in almost all levels of the hypothalamic-pituitary-adrenal (HPA) axis response is found in both laboratory animal studies and human studies (for a review of the human data, see Seeman and Robbins 1994; for a review of the animal data, see Sadow and Rubin 1992). Several advances recently have been made in understanding the physiology of the HPA axis and how it may evolve over the life span. The number of hypothalamic regulatory factors mediating age-related changes in the central control of this important endocrine system has grown exponentially in the past few years (for review, see Pedersen et al. 2001).

The original hypothalamic secretagogue, CRF, has now been joined by the urocortins (I, II, and III [Lewis et al. 2001]) and stresscopin and stresscopin-related peptide (Hsu and Hsueh 2001). All these new corticotropin-releasing agents are more active at the CRF_2 receptor than at the CRF_1 receptor subtype.

The overall activity of the HPA axis, as reflected in measures of CRF, CRF mRNA, and mRNA for the CRF_1 receptor, is increased both in basal tone and in response to novelty stress in aged (30-month-old) F344 rats compared with either young (3-month-old) or middle-aged (15-month-old) rats (Herman et al. 2001). Amounts of CRF mRNA in the paraventricular nucleus of the hypothalamus, amygdala, and bed nucleus of the stria terminalis were decreased in older (24-month-old) F344 rats compared with young (3-month-old) rats (Kasckow et al. 1999). Hypothalamic CRF mRNA deficits in older (18-month-old) male and female rats were partially reversed by treatment with dehydroepiandrosterone (DHEA), indicating preservation of androgen regulation mechanisms in aged animals (Givalois et al. 1997). Others (Pisarska et al. 2000) have reported differences in amygdala CRF and CRF binding protein mRNA levels of aged (24- and 12-month-old) rats compared with young (4-month-old) rats after restraint stress (1 hour/day for 14 days).

Vasopressin, which is synergistic with CRF in releasing corticotropin from the pituitary, also shows age-related changes in older (24-month-old) rats because blockade of vasopressin V_1 receptors prevented CRF-induced release of corticotropin in dexamethasone-pretreated old rats, and this did not occur in young (3-month-old) rats (Hatzinger et al. 2000). Basal vasopressin release from the hypothalamus was reported to be increased in aged Wistar rats relative to younger rats, with decreased vasopressin release to swim stress in the older group (Keck et al. 2000). Circadian alterations in type I glucocorticoid receptor (mineralocorticoid) regulation of corticosterone secretion also have been found to be increased in aged (average = 66.2 years) humans, with 8 days of spironolactone blockade of these receptors producing longer increases in corticosterone for the aged subjects compared with the young control subjects (Heuser et al. 2000). Thus, responses to stress change with increasing age and generally become less volatile but longer in duration.

Somatostatin

Somatostatin (somatotropin release-inhibiting factor) was isolated by Brazeau and colleagues (1973) soon after TRH was isolated. Somatostatin was originally described as consisting of 14 amino acid molecules with a disulfide bridge between the two cysteine residues in the naturally occurring form (for a review, see Rubinow et al. 1994). It was later shown that a larger, 28–amino acid form of somatotropin release-inhibiting factor was also produced when the somatotropin release-inhibiting factor prohormone was cleaved and that the distribution of these two forms of somatostatin (SRIF-14 and SRIF-28) was different in various brain regions. The larger version, SRIF-28, is the predominant form in the endocrine axes (where somatotropin release-inhibiting factor inhibits the release of growth hormone, thyrotropin, and corticotropin as part of a dual-control mechanism that regulates anterior pituitary hormone secretion) and in the gut (where somatotropin release-inhibiting factor inhibits the release of many digestive hormones). The smaller version, SRIF-14, although originally isolated from the hypothalamus, is the principal form of somatotropin release-inhibiting factor in the extrahypothalamic regions of the CNS. Somatotropin release-inhibiting factor functions as an inhibitory transmitter; in addition, it is often found to be localized in neurons containing the inhibitory amino acid GABA. Interneurons throughout the cerebral cortex contain somatotropin release-inhibiting factor, and scattered somatotropin release-inhibiting factor neurons are also seen in the amygdala, hippocampus, and limbic forebrain regions.

The receptors for somatotropin release-inhibiting factor are selective in their preference for either form of the somatotropin release-inhibiting factor molecule. Investigators have used molecular techniques to describe five somatotropin release-inhibiting factor receptor subtypes. Octreotide, a somatotropin release-inhibiting factor receptor agonist, is used to control secretion of gut hormones from tumors that produce excess hormone; however, no centrally acting somatotropin release-inhibiting factor receptor agonists or antagonists are approved for clinical use. Recent studies have shown that octreotide has similar effects on reducing growth hormone secretion in young (33- to 44-year-old) men compared with older (62- to 79-year-old) men (Mulligan et al. 1999), indicating preservation of pituitary responses to somatostatin in aging. Because somatotropin release-inhibiting factor is reduced in concentration in the CSF of patients with a wide variety of diseases that affect cognitive function (including Alzheimer's disease, Parkinson's disease with dementia, Huntington's chorea, multiple sclerosis, major depressive disorder, schizophrenia, and during states of delirium), a receptor agonist directed at CNS receptors for somatotropin release-inhibiting factor may be useful in reversing some symptoms of dementia (for review, see Bissette and Myers 1992). However, unlike the compensatory upregulation of CRF receptors, the decreased production of somatotropin release-inhibiting factor by cortical interneurons in patients with Alzheimer's disease is not accompanied by upregulation of somatotropin release-inhibiting factor receptor number or affinity.

Somatostatin and ACh changes in Alzheimer's disease apparently occur sometime after CRF loss (Davis et al. 1999), and they may interact. Studies comparing the effects of lesions of the cholinergic system with those directed at somatostatin reported similar loss of spatial memory performance or passive avoidance task acquisi-

tion in young animals, and endogenous levels of somatostatin were reported to be increased in the frontal cortex of aged (24-month-old) rats without such lesions (Matsuoka et al. 1995). Lesions of nucleus basalis cholinergic neurons with the neurotoxin 192-saporin were recently reported to decrease somatostatin neurons in cortex that are also decreased by normal aging in old (24-month-old) rats compared with middle-aged (12-month-old) and young rats (Zhang et al. 1998), although previous nucleus basalis lesion studies in rats reported increases rather than decreases in the numbers of somatostatin neurons (for review, see Bissette 1997). Others have reported that brain-derived neurotrophic factor (BDNF) increases the numbers of somatostatin neurons in the cortex and hippocampus of both young and aged rats (Croll et al. 1999). Both BDNF and somatostatin mRNA levels were decreased in the hippocampus and cortex of macaque monkeys older than 30 years compared with levels in 10- and 2-year-old macaque monkeys (Hayashi et al. 1997); these investigators attributed the somatostatin mRNA loss to the prior loss of BDNF. The amounts of pre-prosomatostatin mRNA in cortical neurons of aged (21-month-old) rats were reported to be decreased compared with middle-aged (7-month-old) and young (3-month-old) rats, whereas somatostatin receptor binding was relatively unchanged in another study (Nilsson et al. 1995). These findings are not without question because some researchers have not seen as much decrease in somatostatin neurons of the cortex in aged rats relative to other neuropeptides such as neuropeptide Y and vasoactive intestinal peptide (Cha et al. 1997). Thus, somatostatin levels may decrease with age, and this decrease may be partially reversible with application of growth factors such as BDNF.

Growth Factors

The role of trophic agents in nervous system development and maintenance has undergone great change in the past few years, with investigation of several known growth factors in processes leading to neuronal remodeling and repair. Nerve growth factor, BDNF, insulin-like growth factor-I, and epidermal growth factor are among these trophic agents and have been subjects of several recent reports concerned with changes in the aging brain. Aging macaque monkeys (26–32 years) were reported to have less BDNF immunoreactivity in all areas of the hippocampus, except CA-2, compared with adult (10–12 years) monkeys (Hayashi et al. 2001). Others (Yurek and Fletcher-Turner 2000) have reported a decreased response of striatal BDNF in old (33-month-old) F344/Brown-Norway rats compared with younger (4- to 5-month-old) animals after a 6-hydroxy-DA lesion, which supports the view that younger animals have better responses to neuronal injury than older animals. Restraint and cold-exposure stressors that increase nerve growth factor levels in the basal forebrain of young (3-month-old) rats apparently do not produce such changes in older (24-month-old) rats (Scaccianoce et al. 2000), which would indicate a lessened response to stress with age in this system.

Neuroactive Gases

NO (Schuman and Madison 1994) and CO (Verma et al. 1993) are gases that have now been shown to regulate neuronal firing rates by activation of second-messenger substances after diffusing into the reactive cell (Dawson and Snyder 1994). NO is formed by the action of NO synthetase on the amino acid arginine. Three isoforms of NO synthetase have been identified and cloned from neuronal tissues and appear related to the cytochrome P450 heme oxygenase enzymes involved in many metabolic reactions (Sessa 1994). On release after synthesis, NO diffuses across the synapse and activates soluble guanylate cyclase to produce cyclic guanosine monophosphate, which then activates various kinases. This diffusion of a gas rather than release of a neurotransmitter from synaptic vesicles conceivably allows a larger population of cells to be affected by the NO signal because specialized synapses are not required for signal detection. The presence of NO synthetase inhibitors blocks the effects of the glutaminergic excitatory receptor for NMDA, indicating the crucial role of NO in mediating the effects of this ubiquitous receptor population. Age-related alterations in NO signaling have been postulated as an important mechanism in endocrine changes during senescence (for review, see McCann 1997).

In Alzheimer's disease, NO has been hypothesized to contribute to oxidative damage that results at the cellular level during the neurodegenerative process (Calabrese et al. 2000). Interestingly, an endogenous NO synthetase inhibitor substance, asymmetrical dimethyl arginine, is decreased in the CSF of aged patients and further decreased in subjects with Alzheimer's disease (Abe et al. 2001), which would allow more NO synthetase activity with possible deleterious results from increased levels of NO. Increased levels of NO in several hypothalamic nuclei of aged male rats (Ferrini et al. 2001) and in the auditory brain stem of aged dwarf hamsters (Reuss et al. 2000) have been postulated to contribute to respective reproductive and hearing deficits in aging. Postmortem human brain studies have documented a decrease in cortical amounts of the soluble guanylyl cyclase receptor for NO that were significantly correlated with increasing age (Ibarra et al. 2001), which also could be a response to locally increased concentrations of NO.

Conclusion

Additional chemical messengers undoubtedly will be discovered in the future as the laborious and tedious biochemical methods of protein purification are replaced by the elegant techniques of molecular biology and as it becomes increasingly possible to ideally amplify a molecule and determine its structure. However, as discussed in this chapter, this is just the starting point for demonstrating neurotransmitter status. The successful wedding of the classical biochemical, physiological, and behavioral techniques to the exquisitely precise manipulations of molecular genetics promises to require ever-increasing complexity and interdependence among the various transmitter molecules and the neuronal systems that use them. Already drugs are being developed not on the basis of serendipitously discovered activity but according to a design intended to create a specific interaction with one or more receptor subtypes in the CNS. The results of using these rationally designed drugs to treat diseases with known pathological mechanisms will soon be known. However, the potential bonanza that drives the pharmaceutical industry in this area is the exciting possibilities inherent in being able to specifically affect the precise pathological target in diseases for which no effective treatment currently exists. It must be emphasized, however, that without funding for research to find the specific pathological targets and to sponsor the development of valid laboratory animal models to test nascent therapies, such a dream will remain unrealized for many more years. The increasing age of the United States population as the post–World War II demographic bulge approaches retirement amplifies the need for research into the neurochemical substrates of aging and the possible avenues for retarding or reversing deleterious changes.

References

Abe T, Tohgi H, Murata T, et al: Reduction in asymmetrical dimethylarginine, an endogenous nitric oxide synthase inhibitor, in the cerebrospinal fluid during aging and in patients with Alzheimer's disease. Neurosci Lett 312:177–179, 2001

Angelie E, Bonmartin A, Boudraa A, et al: Regional differences and metabolic changes in normal aging of the human brain: proton MR spectroscopic imaging study. AJNR Am J Neuroradiol 22:119–127, 2001

Antuono PG, Jones JL, Wang Y, et al: Decreased glutamate + glutamine in Alzheimer's disease detected in vivo with (1) H-MRS at 0.5 T. Neurology 56:737–742, 2001

Apparsundaram S, Ferguson SM, George AL, et al: Molecular cloning of a human, hemicholinium-3-sensitive choline transporter. Biochem Biophys Res Commun 276:862–867, 2000

Apparsundaram S, Ferguson SM, Blakely RD: Molecular cloning and characterization of a murine hemicholinium-3-sensitive choline transporter. Biochem Soc Trans 29:711–716, 2001

Backman L, Ginovart N, Dixon RA, et al: Age-related cognitive deficits mediated by changes in the striatal dopamine system. Am J Psychiatry 157:635–637, 2000

Bakshi VP, Smith-Roe S, Newman SM, et al: Reduction of stress-induced behavior by antagonism of corticotropin-releasing hormone 2 (CRH2) receptors in lateral septum or CRH1 receptors in amygdala. J Neurosci 22:2926–2935, 2002

Banki CM, Bissette G, Arato M, et al: Cerebrospinal fluid corticotropin-releasing factor–like immunoreactivity in depression and schizophrenia. Am J Psychiatry 144:873–877, 1987

Banki CM, Bissette G, Arato M, et al: Elevation of immunoreactive CSF TRH in depressed patients. Am J Psychiatry 145:1526–1531, 1988

Banki C, Karmacsi L, Bissette G, et al: Cerebrospinal neuropeptides in dementia. Biol Psychiatry 32:452–456, 1992

Banks WA, Kastin AJ, Akerstrom V, et al: Radioactively iodinated cyclo(His-Pro) crosses the blood-brain barrier and reverses ethanol-induced narcosis. Am J Physiol 164:723–729, 1993

Behan DP, Heinrichs SC, Troncoso JC, et al: Displacement of corticotropin-releasing factor from its binding protein as a possible treatment for Alzheimer's disease. Nature 378:284–287, 1995

Bickford PC, Breiderick L: Benzodiazepine modulation of GABAergic responses is intact in the cerebellum of aged F344 rats. Neurosci Lett 291:187–190, 2000

Bierer LM, Haroutunian V, Gabriel SM, et al: Neurochemical correlates of dementia severity in Alzheimer's disease: relative importance of the cholinergic deficits. J Neurochem 64:749–760, 1995

Bissette G: CNS CRF in stress: radioimmunoassay studies, in Corticotropin-Releasing Factor: Basic and Clinical Studies of a Neuropeptide. Edited by De Souza EB, Nemeroff CB. Boca Raton, FL, CRC Press, 1989, pp 21–28

Bissette G: Neuropeptides involved in stress and their distribution in the mammalian central nervous system, in Stress, Neuropeptides and Systemic Disease. Edited by Kaufman PG, McCubbin JA, Nemeroff CB. San Diego, CA, Academic Press, 1991a, pp 55–72

Bissette G: The role of thyrotropin-releasing hormone in depression. Biol Psychiatry 2:556–558, 1991b

Bissette G: Neuropeptides and Alzheimer's disease pathology. Ann N Y Acad Sci 814:17–29, 1997

Bissette G, Myers B: Mini review: somatostatin in Alzheimer's disease and depression. Life Sci 51:1389–1410, 1992

Bissette G, Nemeroff CB: The neurobiology of neurotensin, in Psychopharmacology: Fourth Generation of Progress. Edited by Bloom FE, Kupfer DJ. New York, Raven, 1994, pp 573–584

Bissette G, Reynolds GP, Kilts CD, et al: Corticotropin-releasing factor-like immunoreactivity in senile dementia of the Alzheimer type. JAMA 254:3067–3069, 1985

Bissette G, Seidler FJ, Nemeroff CB, et al: High affinity choline transporter status in Alzheimer's disease tissue from rapid autopsy. Ann N Y Acad Sci 777:197–204, 1996

Bissette G, Cook L, Smith W, et al: Regional neuropeptide pathology in Alzheimer's disease: corticotropin-releasing factor and somatostatin. Journal of Alzheimer's Disease 1:91–105, 1998

Blakely RD, Berson HE: Cloning and expression of a functional serotonin transporter from rat brain. Nature 354:66–70, 1991

Booij J, Bergsman P, Winogrodzka A, et al: Imaging of dopamine transporters with [123-I] FP-SPECT does not suggest a significant effect of age on the symptomatic threshold of disease in Parkinson's disease. Synapse 39:101–108, 2001

Brazeau P, Vale W, Burgus R, et al: Hypothalamic peptide that inhibits the secretion of immunoreactive pituitary growth hormone. Science 179:77–79, 1973

Brooks JC, Roberts N, Kemp GJ, et al: A proton magnetic resonance spectroscopy study of age-related changes in frontal lobe metabolite concentrations. Cereb Cortex 11:598–605, 2001

Calabrese V, Bates TE, Stella AM: NO synthase and NO-dependent signal pathways in brain aging and neurodegenerative disorders: the role of oxidant/antioxidant balance. Neurochem Res 25:1315–1341, 2000

Cha CI, Lee YI, Lee EY, et al: Age-related changes of VIP, NPY and somatostatin-immunoreactive neurons in the cerebral cortex of aged rats. Brain Res 753:235–244, 1997

Chappell PB, Smith MA, Kilts CD, et al: Alterations in corticotropin-releasing factor–like immunoreactivity in discrete rat brain regions after acute and chronic stress. J Neurosci 6:2908–2914, 1986

Cizza G, Brady LS, Pacak K, et al: Stress-induced inhibition of the hypothalamic-pituitary-thyroid axis is attenuated in the aged Fischer 344/N male rat. Neuroendocrinology 62:506–513, 1995

Cooper JR, Bloom FE, Roth RH (eds): The Biochemical Basis of Neuropharmacology, 8th Edition. New York, Oxford University Press, 2002

Croll SD, Chestnutt CR, Greene NA, et al: Peptide immunoreactivity in aged rat cortex and hippocampus as a function of memory and BDNF infusion. Pharmacol Biochem Behav 64:625–635, 1999

Dahlstrom A, Fuxe K: Evidence for the existence of mono-amine-containing neurons in the central nervous system. Acta Physiol Scand 62:1–55, 1964

Davis KL, Mohs RC, Marin DB, et al: Neuropeptide abnormalities in patients with early Alzheimer disease. Arch Gen Psychiatry 56:981–987, 1999

Dawson TM, Snyder SH: Gases as biological messengers: nitric oxide and carbon monoxide. J Neurosci 14:5147–5151, 1994

De Souza EB, Nemeroff CB: Corticotropin-Releasing Factor: Basic and Clinical Studies of a Neuropeptide. Boca Raton, FL, CRC Press, 1990

De Souza EB, Whitehouse PJ, Kuhar MJ, et al: Reciprocal changes in corticotropin-releasing factor (CRF)-like immu-noreactivity and CRF receptors in cerebral cortex of Alzheimer's disease. Nature 319:593–595, 1986

Decker MW, McGaugh JL: The role of interactions between the cholinergic system and other neuromodulatory systems in learning and memory. Synapse 7:151–168, 1991

Dent GW, Rule BL, Zhan Y, et al: The acetylcholine release en-hancer linopirdine induces Fos in neocortex of aged rats. Neurobiol Aging 22:485–494, 2001

Duncan MJ, Crafton CJ, Wheeler DL: Aging regulates 5-HT (1B) receptors and serotonin reuptake sites in the SCN. Brain Res 856:213–219, 2000

Edvinsson L, Minthon L, Ekman R, et al: Neuropeptides in cerebrospinal fluid of patients with Alzheimer's disease and dementia with frontotemporal lobe degeneration. De-mentia 4:167–171, 1993

Ferrini M, Wang C, Swerdloff RS, et al: Aging-related increased expression of inducible nitric oxide synthase and cytotox-icity markers in rat hypothalamic regions associated with male reproductive function. Neuroendocrinology 74:1–11, 2001

Francis PT, Webster M-T, Chessell IP, et al: Neurotransmitters and second messengers in aging and Alzheimer's disease. Ann N Y Acad Sci 695:19–26, 1993

Gerhardt GA, Cass WA, Yi A, et al: Changes in somatodendritic but not terminal dopamine regulation in aged rhesus mon-keys. J Neurochem 80:168–177, 2002

Givalois L, Li S, Pelletier G: Age-related decrease in the hy-pothalamic CRH mRNA expression is reduced by de-hydroepiandrosterone (DHEA) treatment in male and female rats. Brain Res Mol Brain Res 48:107–114, 1997

Gore AC, Yeung G, Morrison JH, et al: Neuroendocrine aging in the female rat: the changing relationship of hypothalamic gonadotropin-releasing hormone neurons and N-methyl-D-aspartate receptors. Endocrinology 141:4757–4767, 2000

Grachev ID, Swarnkar A, Szeverenyi NM, et al: Aging alters the multichemical networking profile of the human brain: an in vivo (1) H-MRS study of young versus middle-age sub-jects. J Neurochem 77:292–303, 2001

Hatzinger M, Wotjack CT, Naruo T, et al: Endogenous vaso-pressin contributes to hypothalamic-pituitary-adrenocortical alterations in aged rats. J Endocrinol 164:197–205, 2000

Hayashi M, Yamashita A, Shimizu K: Somatostatin and brain-derived neurotrophic factor mRNA expression in the pri-mate brain: decreased levels of mRNAs during aging. Brain Res 749:283–289, 1997

Hayashi M, Mistunaga F, Ohira K, et al: Changes in BDNF-immunoreactive structures in the hippocampal formation of the aged macaque monkey. Brain Res 918:191–196, 2001

Heilig M, Sjögren M, Blennow K, et al: Cerebrospinal fluid neu-ropeptides in Alzheimer's disease and vascular dementia. Biol Psychiatry 38:210–216, 1995

Herman JP, Larson BR: Differential regulation of forebrain glutamic acid decarboxylase mRNA expression by aging and stress. Brain Res 912:60–66, 2001

Herman JP, Larson BR, Speert DB, et al: Hypothalamo-pituitary-adrenocortical dysregulation in aging F344/Brown-Norway F1 hybrid rats. Neurobiol Aging 22:323–332, 2001

Heuser I, Deuschle M, Weber A, et al: The role of the mineralo-corticoid receptors in the circadian activity of the human hypothalamus-pituitary-adrenal system: effects of age. Neurobiol Aging 21:585–594, 2000

Hitri A, Hurd YL, Wyatt RJ, et al: Molecular, functional and bio-chemical characteristics of the dopamine transporter: regional differences and clinical relevance. Clin Neuropharmacol 17:1–22, 1994

Hof PR, Duan H, Page TL, et al: Age-related changes in GluR2 and NMDAR1 glutamate receptor subunit protein immu-noreactivity in corticocortically projecting neurons in macaque and patas monkeys. Brain Res 928:175–186, 2002

Hofman MA: Lifespan changes in the human hypothalamus. Exp Gerontol 32:559–575, 1997

Hsu SY, Hsueh AJ: Human stresscopin and stresscopin-related peptide are selective ligands for the type 2 corticotropin-releasing hormone receptor. Nat Med 7:605–611, 2001

Ibarra C, Nedvetsky PI, Gerlach M, et al: Regional and age-dependent expression of the nitric oxide receptor, soluble guanylyl cyclase, in the human brain. Brain Res 907:54–60, 2001

Ishida Y, Shirokawa T, Komatsu Y, et al: Changes in cortical nor-adrenergic axon terminals of locus coeruleus neurons in aged F344 rats. Neurosci Lett 307:197–199, 2001a

Ishida Y, Shirokawa T, Miyaishi O, et al: Age-dependent changes in noradrenergic innervations of the frontal cortex in F344 rats. Neurobiol Aging 22:283–286, 2001b

Jolkkonen J, Soikkeli R, Hartikainen P, et al: CSF neuropep-tides in Alzheimer's disease and Parkinson's disease. Anu-ario Psiquiatrico 1:251–257, 1990

Kadota T, Horinouchi T, Kuroda C: Development and aging of the cerebrum: assessment with proton MR spectroscopy. AJNR Am J Neuroradiol 22:128–135, 2001

Kakiuchi T, Ohba H, Nishiyama S, et al: Age-related changes in muscarinic cholinergic receptors in the living brain: a PET study using N-[11C]methyl-4-piperidyl benzilate combined with cerebral blood flow measurement in conscious monkeys. Brain Res 916:22–31, 2001

Kanner BI, Danbolt N, Pines G, et al: Structure and function of the sodium and potassium-coupled glutamate transporter from rat brain. Biochem Soc Trans 21:59–61, 1993

Kasckow JW, Regmi A, Mulchahey JJ, et al: Changes in brain corticotropin-releasing factor messenger RNA expression in aged Fischer 344 rats. Brain Res 822:228–230, 1999

Kawakami H, Tanaka K, Nakayama T, et al: Cloning and expression of a human glutamate transporter. Biochem Biophys Res Commun 199:171–176, 1994

Keck ME, Hatzinger M, Wotjak CT, et al: Ageing alters intrahypothalamic release patterns of vasopressin and oxytocin in rats. Eur J Neurosci 12:1487–1494, 2000

Kelley M, Kowall N: Corticotropin-releasing factor immunoreactive neurons persist throughout the brain in Alzheimers disease. Brain Res 501:392–396, 1989

Kloppel S, Kovacs GG, Boigtlander T, et al: Serotonergic nuclei of the raphe are not affected in human ageing. Neuroreport 12:669–671, 2001

Kuhl DE, Koeppe RA, Minoshima S, et al: In vivo mapping of cerebral acetylcholinesterase activity in aging and Alzheimer's disease. Neurology 52:691–699, 1999

Kuhl DE, Minoshima S, Frey KA, et al: Limited donepezil inhibition of acetylcholinesterase measured with positron emission tomography in living Alzheimer cerebral cortex. Ann Neurol 48:391–395, 2000

Lam DM, Fei J, Zhang XY, et al: Molecular cloning and structure of the human (GABATHG) GABA transporter gene. Brain Res Mol Brain Res 19:227–232, 1993

Lee JJ, Chang CK, Liu IM, et al: Changes in endogenous monoamines in aged rats. Clin Exp Pharmacol Physiol 28:285–289, 2001

Lewis K, Li C, Perrin MH, et al: Identification of urocortin III, an additional member of the corticotropin-releasing factor (CRF) family with high affinity for the CRF 2 receptor. Proc Natl Acad Sci U S A 98:7570–7575, 2001

Ling ZD, Collier TJ, Sortwell CE, et al: Striatal trophic activity is reduced in the aged rat brain. Brain Res 856:301–309, 2000

Luo Y, Roth GS: The roles of dopamine oxidative stress and dopamine receptor signalling in aging and age-related neurodegeneration. Antioxid Redox Signal 2:449–460, 2000

Magnusson KR: Declines in mRNA expression of different subunits may account for differential effects of aging on agonist and antagonist binding to the NMDA receptor. J Neurosci 20:1666–1674, 2000

Magnusson KR: Influence of diet restriction on NMDA receptor subunits and learning during aging. Neurobiol Aging 22:613–627, 2001

Martignoni E, Petraglia F, Costa A, et al: Dementia of the Alzheimer type and the hypothalamus-pituitary-adrenocortical axis: changes in cerebrospinal fluid corticotropin-releasing factor and plasma cortisol levels. Acta Neurol Scand 81:452–456, 1990

Mason GA, Garbutt JC, Prange AJ: Thyrotropin-releasing hormone: focus on basic neurobiology, in Psychopharmacology: Fourth Generation of Progress. Edited by Bloom FE, Kupfer DJ. New York, Raven, 1994, pp 493–504

Matsuoka N, Yamazaki M, Yamaguchi I: Changes in brain somatostatin in memory-deficient rats: comparison with cholinergic markers. Neuroscience 66:617–626, 1995

May C, Rapoport SI, Tomai TP, et al: Cerebrospinal fluid concentrations of corticotropin-releasing hormone (CRH) and corticotropin (ACTH) are reduced in Alzheimer's disease. Neurology 37:535–538, 1987

McCann SM: The nitric oxide hypothesis of brain aging. Exp Gerontol 32:431–440, 1997

Melikian HE, McDonald JK, Gu H, et al: Human norepinephrine transporter: biosynthetic studies using a site-directed polyclonal antibody. J Biol Chem 269:12290–12297, 1994

Miguez JM, Aldegunde M, Paz-Valinas L, et al: Selective changes in the contents of noradrenaline, dopamine and serotonin in rat brain areas during aging. J Neural Transm 106:1089–1098, 1999

Misawa H, Nakata K, Matsuura J, et al: Distribution of the high-affinity choline transporter in the central nervous system of the rat. Neuroscience 105:87–98, 2001

Molchan SE, Hill JL, Martinez RA, et al: CSF somatostatin in Alzheimer's disease and major depression: relationship to hypothalamic-pituitary-adrenal axis and clinical measures. Psychoneuroendocrinology 18:509–519, 1993

Monzani F, Del Guerra P, Caraccio N, et al: Age-related modifications in the regulation of the hypothalamic-pituitary-thyroid axis. Horm Res 46:107–112, 1996

Mouradian MM, Farah JM, Mohr E, et al: Spinal fluid CRF reduction in Alzheimer's disease. Neuropeptides 8:393–400, 1986

Mufson EJ, Cochran E, Benzing W, et al: Galaninergic innervation of the cholinergic vertical limb of the diagonal band (Ch2) and bed nucleus of the stria terminalis in aging, Alzheimer's disease and Down's syndrome. Dementia 4:237–250, 1993

Mulholland GK, Wieland DM, Kilbourn MR, et al: [18F]Fluoroethoxy-benzovesamicol, a PET radiotracer for the vesicular acetylcholine transporter and cholinergic synapses. Synapse 30:263–274, 1998

Mulligan T, Jaen-Vinuales JA, Godschalk M, et al: Synthetic somatostatin analog (octreotide) suppresses daytime growth hormone secretion equivalently in young and older men: preserved pituitary responsiveness to somatostatin's inhibition in aging. J Am Geriatr Soc 47:1422–1424, 1999

Nemeroff CB, Widerlov E, Bissette G, et al: Elevated concentrations of CSF corticotropin-releasing factor–like immunoreactivity in depressed patients. Science 226:1342–1344, 1984

Nemeroff CB, Owens MJ, Bissette G, et al: Reduced corticotropin-releasing factor (CRF) binding sites in the frontal cortex of suicides. Arch Gen Psychiatry 45:577–579, 1988

Nestler EJ, Duman RS: Intracellular messenger pathways as mediators of neural plasticity, in Psychopharmacology: Fourth Generation of Progress. Edited by Bloom FE, Kupfer DJ. New York, Raven, 1994, pp 695–704

Nilsson L, Winblad B, Bergstrom L: Diminution of preprosomatostatin-mRNA in cerebral cortex of the aged rat. Neurochem Int 27:481–487, 1995

O'Dowd BF, Lee DK, Huang W, et al: TRH-R2 exhibits similar binding and acute signaling but distinct regulation and anatomic distribution with TRH-1. Mol Endocrinol 14:183–193, 2000

Oh SJ, Ha HJ, Chi DY, et al: Serotonin receptor and transporter ligands—current status. Curr Med Chem 8:999–1034, 2001

Okuda T, Haga T, Kanai Y, et al: Identification and characterization of the high-affinity choline transporter. Nat Neurosci 3:120–125, 2000

Ossowska K, Wolfarth S, Schulze G, et al: Decline in motor functions in aging is related to the loss of NMDA receptors. Brain Res 907:71–83, 2001

Owens MJ, Nemeroff CB, Bissette G: Neuropeptides: biology, regulation and role in neuropsychiatric disorders, in The Comprehensive Textbook of Psychiatry, VII. Edited by Kaplan HI, Sadock BJ. Philadelphia, PA, Williams & Wilkins, 2000, pp 60–70

Palmer AM, DeKosky ST: Monoamine neurons in aging and Alzheimer's disease. J Neural Transm Gen Sect 91:135–159, 1993

Pedersen WA, Wan R, Mattson MP: Impact of aging on stress-responsive neuroendocrine systems. Mech Ageing Dev 122:963–983, 2001

Pintor A, Potenza RL, Domenici MR, et al: Age-related decline in the functional response of striatal group, I: mGlu receptors. Neuroreport 11:3033–3038, 2000

Pirker W, Asenbaum S, Hauk M, et al: Imaging serotonin and dopamine transporters with 123I-beta-CIT SPECT: binding kinetics and effects of normal aging. J Nucl Med 41:36–44, 2000

Pisarska M, Mulchahey JJ, Welge JA, et al: Age-related alterations in emotional behaviors and amygdalar corticotropin-releasing factors (CRF) and CRF-binding protein expression in aged Fischer 344 rats. Brain Res 877:184–190, 2000

Poddar MK, Bandyopadhyay BC, Chakrabarti L: Dietary protein alters age-induced change in hypothalamic GABA and immune response. Neuroscience 97:405–409, 2000

Pomara N, Singh RR, Deptula D, et al: CSF corticotropin-releasing factor (CRF) in Alzheimer's disease: its relationship to severity of dementia and monoamine metabolites. Biol Psychiatry 26:500–504, 1989

Powers RE, Walker LC, De Souza EB, et al: Immunohistochemical study of neurons containing corticotropin-releasing factor in Alzheimer's disease. Synapse 1:405–410, 1987

Raadsheer FC, van Heerikhuize JJ, Lucassen PJ, et al: Corticotropin-releasing hormone mRNA levels in the paraventricular nucleus of patients with Alzheimer's disease and depression. Am J Psychiatry 152:1372–1376, 1995

Rehman HU, Masson EA: Neuroendocrinology of ageing. Age Ageing 30:279–287, 2001

Reuss S, Schaeffer DF, Laages MH, et al: Evidence for increased nitric oxide production in the auditory brain stem of the aged dwarf hamster (Phodopus sungorus): an NADPH-diaphorase histochemical study. Mech Ageing Dev 112:125–134, 2000

Rubinow DR, Davis CL, Post RM: Somatostatin in the central nervous system, in Psychopharmacology: Fourth Generation of Progress. Edited by Bloom FE, Kupfer DJ. New York, Raven, 1994, pp 553–562

Sadow TF, Rubin RT: Effects of hypothalamic peptides on the aging brain (review). Psychoneuroendocrinology 17:293–314, 1992

Sarter M, Turchi J: Age- and dementia-associated impairments in divided attention: psychological constructs, animal models and underlying mechanisms. Dement Geriatr Cogn Disord 13:46–58, 2002

Scaccianoce S, Lombardo K, Angelucci L: Nerve growth factor brain concentration and stress: changes depend upon stressor and age. Int J Dev Neurosci 18:469–479, 2000

Schuman EM, Madison DV: Nitric oxide and synaptic function. Annu Rev Neurosci 17:153–160, 1994

Seeman TE, Robbins RJ: Aging and hypothalamic-pituitary-adrenal response to challenge in humans. Endocr Rev 15:233–260, 1994

Segovia G, Porras A, Del Arco A, et al: Glutaminergic neurotransmission in aging: a critical perspective. Mech Ageing Dev 122:1–29, 2001

Sessa WC: The nitric oxide synthetase family of proteins. J Vasc Res 31:131–139, 1994

Sheline YI, Mintun MA, Moerlein SM, et al: Greater loss of 5-HT(2A) receptors in midlife than in later life. Am J Psychiatry 159:430–435, 2002

Shinoda M, Okamiya K, Toide K: Effect of a novel prolyl endopeptidase inhibitor, JTP-4819, on thyrotropin-releasing hormone–like immunoreactivity in the cerebral cortex and hippocampus of aged rats. Jpn J Pharmacol 69:273–276, 1995

Slotkin TA, Seidler FJ, Crain BJ, et al: Regulatory changes in presynaptic cholinergic function assessed in rapid autopsy material from patients with Alzheimer's disease: implications for etiology and therapy. Proc Natl Acad Sci U S A 87:2452–2455, 1990

Slotkin TA, Nemeroff CB, Bissette G, et al: Overexpression of the high affinity choline transporter in cortical regions affected by Alzheimer's disease: evidence from rapid autopsy studies. J Clin Invest 94:696–702, 1994

Slotkin TA, Seidler FJ, Ali SF: Cellular determinates of reduced adaptability of the aging brain: neurotransmitter utilization and cell signaling responses after MDMA lesion. Brain Res 879:163–173, 2000

Sonntag WE, Bennett SA, Khan AS, et al: Age and insulin-like growth factor-1 modulate N-methyl-D-aspartate receptor subtype expression in rats. Brain Res Bull 51:331–338, 2000

Stemmelin J, Lazarus C, Cassel S, et al: Immunohistochemical and neurochemical correlates of learning deficits in aged rats. Neuroscience 96:275–289, 2000

Suemaru S, Hashimoto K, Ogasa T, et al: Cerebrospinal fluid and plasma corticotropin-releasing hormone in senile dementia. Life Sci 48:1871–1879, 1991

Suemaru S, Suemaru K, Kawai K, et al: Cerebrospinal fluid corticotropin-releasing hormone in neurodegenerative diseases: reduction in spinocerebellar degeneration. Life Sci 57:2231–2235, 1995

Sullivan EV, Pfefferbaum A, Adalsteinsson E, et al: Differential rates of regional brain change in callosal and ventricular size: a 4-year longitudinal MRI study of elderly men. Cereb Cortex 12:438–445, 2002

Swaab DF: Ageing of the human hypothalamus. Horm Res 43:8–11, 1995

Tauscher J, Verhoeff NP, Christensen BK, et al: Serotonin 5-HT1A receptor binding potential declines with age as measured by [11C]WAY-100635 and PET. Neuropsychopharmacology 24:522–530, 2001

Tayebati SK, Amenta F, El-Assouad D, et al: Muscarinic cholinergic receptor sub-types in the hippocampus of the aged rat. Mech Ageing Dev 123:521–528, 2002

Teitler M, Herrick-Davis K: Multiple serotonin receptor sub-types: molecular cloning and functional expression. Crit Rev Neurobiol 8:175–188, 1994

Toide K, Shinoda M, Fujiwara T, et al: Effect of a novel prolyl endopeptidase inhibitor, JTP-4819, on spatial memory and central cholinergic neurons in aged rats. Pharmacol Biochem Behav 56:427–434, 1997

Turrini P, Casu MA, Wong TP, et al: Cholinergic nerve terminals establish classical synapses in the rat cerebral cortex: synaptic pattern and age-related atrophy. Neuroscience 105:277–285, 2001

Vale W, Spiess J, Rivier C, et al: Characterization of a 41-residue ovine hypothalamic peptide that stimulates secretion of corticotropin and beta-endorphin. Science 213:1394–1399, 1981

van Dyck CH, Seibyl JP, Malison RT, et al: Age-related decline in dopamine transporters. Am J Geriatr Psychiatry 10:36–43, 2002

Verma A, Hirsch DJ, Glatt CE, et al: Carbon monoxide: a putative signalling molecule. Science 259:381–387, 1993

Vicente-Torres MA, Munoz E, Davila D, et al: Changes in the cochlear dopaminergic system of the aged rat. Brain Res 917:112–117, 2001

Virgili M, Monti B, Polazzi E, et al: Topography of neurochemical alterations in the CNS of aged rats. Int J Dev Neurosci 19:109–116, 2001

Volkow ND, Logan J, Fowler JS, et al: Association between age-related decline in brain dopamine activity and impairment in frontal and cingulate metabolism. Am J Psychiatry 157:75–80, 2000

Voytko ML, Mach RH, Gage HD, et al: Cholinergic activity of aged rhesus monkeys revealed by positron emission tomography. Synapse 39:95–100, 2001

Wenk GL, Barnes CA: Regional changes in the hippocampal density of AMPA and NMDA receptors across the lifespan of the rat. Brain Res. 885:1–5, 2000

Winblad B, Brodaty H, Gauthier S, et al: Pharmacotherapy of Alzheimer's disease: is there a need to redefine treatment success? Int J Geriatr Psychiatry 16:653–666, 2001

Yurek DM, Fletcher-Turner A: Lesion-induced increase of BDNF is greater in the striatum of young versus old animals. Exp Neurol 161:392–396, 2000

Zhang ZJ, Lappi DA, Wrenn CC, et al: Selective lesion of the cholinergic basal forebrain causes a loss of cortical neuropeptide Y and somatostatin neurons. Brain Res 800:198–206, 1998

Zubieta JK, Koeppe RA, Frey KA, et al: Assessment of muscarinic receptor concentrations in aging and Alzheimer disease with [1C]NMPB and PET. Synapse 39:275–287, 2001

CHAPTER 6

Genetics

Brenda L. Plassman, Ph.D.

David C. Steffens, M.D., M.H.S.

Genetics is a field of clinical science that has developed rapidly in recent years. Genetic mutations that cause specific diseases have been identified for many disorders, particularly those with early age at onset. However, it also has become evident that few diseases associated with aging have a single genetic etiology. In fact, it appears that most diseases in the elderly not only have multiple genetic and environmental etiologies, but these various causative factors also interact with one another to alter the risk of developing the disease.

Such diseases with multifactorial causes are called *complex*, and many of the disorders within the domain of geriatric psychiatry fall into this category. It is particularly difficult to localize genes for such diseases that have onset in late life because many individuals at risk for the disease will die before expressing the symptoms of the disease. One such disease, Alzheimer's disease (AD), has become a paradigm for studying complex diseases of the elderly. In this chapter, we provide a general overview of the current state of knowledge in the genetics of AD, some of the other tau-related dementias, Parkinson's disease (PD), and depression. Although this list does not entail all genetics-related psychiatric diseases of the elderly, the management of these conditions likely consumes most of a geriatric psychiatrist's time. The genetic principles of these conditions can likely be used as models for other psychiatric conditions in the elderly.

Alzheimer's Disease

Family and Twin Studies

As early as the 1920s, there were reports of a few families with many individuals with AD across more than one generation (for review, see Kennedy et al. 1994). These individuals typically had early-onset AD, which has arbitrarily been defined as onset of disease before age 65. Although these multigenerational kindreds with so-called familial AD probably represent no more than 2% of all AD cases, their existence was the impetus for further investigation of the genetic causes of AD.

Other early evidence suggesting that genes played a role in at least some cases of AD was based on studies examining family history of the disease in clinical and population-based samples. Most of these studies showed an increased risk of AD in first-degree relatives, regardless of whether the proband's age at onset was before or after 65. Generally, from 25% to 50% of the individuals with AD had a positive family history of the disease, as compared with 10%–15% or fewer of control subjects without dementia (Breitner 1991; van Duijn et al. 1991). This finding suggests that even in kindreds that do not appear to have familial AD, first-degree relatives of the individuals with AD may have as much as a fivefold increase in risk for developing the disease.

Most previous work focused on families at greater risk for developing AD. However, one family study (Silverman et al. 1999) took a different approach to this question by studying families that appeared to be at lower risk for acquiring AD. They showed that the first-degree relatives of individuals who reached age 90 and did not have dementia were less likely to have AD after age 60, as compared with the families of younger individuals without dementia. Based on these findings, it appears that genes may either increase or decrease the risk of AD.

When studying the role of genes in disease, family studies have advantages over studies of unrelated individuals (i.e., case-control studies, community studies). Twin studies can be even more informative on this issue when all of the culpable genes have not been identified. The twin design compares rates of disease concordance in monozygotic (identical) and dizygotic (fraternal) twin pairs. Members of monozygotic pairs share 100% of their genes, whereas dizygotic pairs share 50% of their genes on average. Thus, higher concordance in monozygotic pairs compared with dizygotic pairs implies a genetic etiology. *Heritability* is defined as the proportion of disease liability attributable to genes, and it can be estimated from these concordance rates. Simultaneously, one can also estimate the contribution of shared and unique environmental factors to disease risk (Plomin et al. 1990).

Generally, twin studies support a role for genes in the etiology of AD. Heritability estimates from three ongoing studies of AD in population-based twin registries range from 0.33 to 0.74 (Bergem et al. 1997; Breitner et al. 1995; Gatz et al. 1997). We suggest that the wide range of these estimates of heritability may reflect the differences in the age distribution of twins in the three registries. Others have shown that the risk of developing AD for a relative of a proband with AD increases with age at least until the mid-80s (Silverman et al. 1994). We speculate that the lowest heritability estimate (0.33), from our work on the National Academy of Sciences–National Research Council Registry of Aging Twin Veterans (Breitner et al. 1995), may underestimate the true heritability of AD because of the atypically young age (mean onset age = 67 years) of patients with AD in this sample. As the registry approaches the typical age at risk for AD of the late 70s, 80s, and even beyond, we anticipate that heritability in this twin sample will approximate that of the other two studies and that the consensus estimate of heritability will likely be between 0.5 and 0.65. Based on this estimate of heritability and the reports of identical twin pairs that remain discordant for AD as much as 20 years after the onset of the disease in the proband (Nee and Lippa 1999; B.L. Plassman, unpublished observation, August 2002), it appears that nongenetic factors also alter the risk for AD.

Alzheimer's Disease Genes

Autosomal Dominant Genes

Findings from family and twin studies have provided evidence of a genetic cause of AD in at least some cases, but they did not identify specific genes that may play a role in the disease. However, recent advances in molecular genetic techniques have now been used to identify mutations at three genetic loci that are associated primarily with early-onset AD. The first identified AD gene was the β-amyloid precursor protein (*APP*) gene located on chromosome 21 (Goate et al. 1991). Since the first report of a missense mutation (i.e., one amino acid is substituted for another) associated with AD on this gene, several other mutations pathogenic for AD have been identified (for review, see Alzheimer Research Forum 2003, APP mutations table; Van Broeckhoven 1995). Individuals with one of these *APP* mutations generally have onset of disease between ages 40 and 60; however, recently there has been some question of whether such mutations also may cause late-onset AD (i.e., onset at or later than age 65). Although the identification of *APP* as an AD gene has been key to advancing our understanding of the genetic causes of AD, all *APP* mutations combined appear to account for the disease in fewer than two dozen families worldwide (Van Broeckhoven 1995).

A second AD locus was found on chromosome 14 (Schellenberg et al. 1992; St. George-Hyslop et al. 1992) and is now called presenilin-1 (*PS1*) (Sherrington et al. 1995). More than 70 mutations in the *PS1* locus have now been reported in several hundred families throughout the world (Alzheimer Research Forum 2003, presenilin-1 mutations table; Selkoe 2001). Onset of symptoms for those with *PS1* mutations is often before age 50. Like the *APP* mutations, *PS1* mutations appear to act as autosomal dominant traits with nearly complete penetrance (Cruts et al. 1998). However, there has been at least one report of possible nonpenetrance of a *PS1* mutation in a healthy 68-year-old member of a pedigree with multiple affected members (Rossor et al. 1996). There has been conflicting information on the proportion of early-onset cases attributable to the *PS1* mutations. Some reports have suggested that *PS1* mutations may account for most early-onset familial AD cases (Campion et al. 1995, 1999; Hutton et al. 1996), but others have reported that a more realistic estimate is 20% or fewer of such cases (Cruts et al. 1998).

A third AD gene has been localized to chromosome 1 and termed presenilin-2 (*PS2*) (Levy-Lahad et al. 1995a, 1995b). These mutations appear to be rare; only a few families of different ethnicity have been identified with *PS2* mutations. In fact, in a population-based sample of early-onset AD cases, it was estimated that *PS2* mutations accounted for fewer than 1% of the cases (Cruts et al. 1998). Although the *PS2* mutations are autosomal dominant, they may not be fully penetrant. *PS2* mutations generally lead to onset of AD symptoms before age 65. Like *APP*, most *PS1* and *PS2* mutations are missense mutations.

It is estimated that AD mutations on chromosomes 21, 14, and 1 account for between 30% and 50% of the individuals with dominantly inherited AD, depending on the inclusion criteria and the source of the sample. For the remainder of this group, the genetic marker has yet to be identified (Finckh et al. 2000; Liddell et al. 2001; Rosenberg 2000). But it is important to note that these dominantly inherited genes are primarily associated with the relatively uncommon early-onset AD; thus, combined, the known mutations probably account for no more than 5% of all AD cases (Farrer 1997). Although identification of these mutations has led to major advances in understanding the etiology of this disease, the vast majority of AD cases are late onset. From a public health perspective, identifying genes associated with late-onset AD would have a greater effect.

Apolipoprotein E

Searching the genome for other AD genes, Pericak-Vance and colleagues (1991) reported linkage of disease to a locus on chromosome 19 in families with late-onset AD. The apolipoprotein E gene (APOE) was found to be located in the region of chromosome 19 implicated by the linkage study (Strittmatter et al. 1993). The ε4 allele at APOE was shown to be associated with both familial and sporadic AD cases (Brousseau et al. 1994; Mayeux et al. 1993; Rebeck et al. 1993; Saunders et al. 1993; Schmechel et al. 1993). Other studies reported that the risk of AD is elevated and the mean age at onset is reduced as the number of ε4 alleles increases from 0 to 2 (Corder et al. 1993).

A meta-analysis of data on more than 14,000 subjects from 40 research teams confirmed the basic findings noted above (Farrer et al. 1997). This study also reported that the risk associated with the APOE ε4 allele appears to vary by age, sex, and ethnicity. Findings from a recent population-based study that included many individuals age 90 and older have suggested that the ε4 allele influences when, but not if, a person gets AD (Miech et al. 2002). They found that APOE ε4 exerted only a modest effect on overall incidence of the disease.

Combined, these findings indicate that the association between AD and APOE ε4 is complex. It is generally estimated that APOE accounts for up to 50% of the genetic contribution to AD (Pericak-Vance and Haines 1995), thus supporting the idea that it plays a major role in the etiology of the disease. However, many individuals without an ε4 allele develop AD, and other individuals with an ε4 allele do not get the disease. Estimates are that for those who are disease-free at age 65, at most 50% of the ε4 homozygotes will develop AD within their lifetimes (Henderson et al. 1995; Seshadri et al. 1997). However, it is not clear why some individuals with the ε4 allele develop the disease but others do not.

Other Putative Genes

In aggregate, the AD genes identified to date account for at most 55% of the total genetic risk for the disease, suggesting that other genes have yet to be identified. The genomic screens of multiplex AD families by different research groups have shown promising results for linkage to regions on at least three chromosomes. The first region identified was on chromosome 12 (Pericak-Vance et al. 1997) in individuals without an APOE ε4 allele. Multiple research groups have now replicated this finding in regions near the initially implicated chromosome 12 locus, but the findings are somewhat discrepant regarding whether the association is strongest in individuals with or without an ε4 allele (Rogaeva et al. 1998; Wu et al. 1998).

Investigations of the region implicated on chromosome 12 have identified several candidate genes. Two of these genes have drawn particular interest both because of their biological function and because of the number of studies that have reported a positive association with AD. The first is the gene for the major apolipoprotein E receptor in the brain—the low-density lipoprotein receptor-related protein (LRP) that is selectively found in neurons and reactive astrocytes (Rebeck et al. 1995). LRP is biallelic, and the homozygous C genotype appears to be associated with increased risk of AD, earlier onset of AD, and significantly more neuritic plaques at postmortem, as compared with individuals with at least one T allele (Kang et al. 1997). Several groups have confirmed these initial results (Hollenbach et al. 1998; Lambert et al. 1998b; Lendon et al. 1997; Wavrant-De Vrièze et al. 1997), but others have not (Clatworthy et al. 1997; Fallin et al. 1997).

The second candidate locus of particular interest on chromosome 12 is the α_2-macroglobulin (A2M) gene (Pericak-Vance et al. 1997). At least three different A2M polymorphisms have been implicated so far (Blacker et al. 1998; Liao et al. 1998; Myllykangas et al. 1999). But as with LRP, other studies have not confirmed the association between A2M and AD in several large samples (Chen et al. 1999; Crawford et al. 1999; Dow et al. 1999; Rogaeva et al. 1999; Rudrasingham et al. 1999; Wang et al. 2001).

The inconsistent outcomes from the association studies on LRP and A2M imply that if these genes do alter AD risk, their effect may be limited to susceptible subgroups and that different polymorphisms may even be important in each of these subgroups. Discrepant findings on these two genes have prompted continued searches for influential genes on chromosome 12. Recently, another gene in the region of interest on chromosome 12 has been under investigation. In separate clinical and autopsy samples, the A allele of the 3'-untranslated region (3'UTR) biallelic polymorphism in the *LBP-1c/CP2/LSF* gene showed association with reduced risk of AD (Lambert et al. 2000; Taylor et al. 2001). Replication of these findings in other samples will determine this gene's role in AD.

A second locus of interest in the search for AD genes has been identified on chromosome 10. Recently, three groups that used different analytical approaches found strong evidence for a major late-onset AD susceptibility locus on chromosome 10 (Bertram et al. 2000; Ertekin-Taner et al. 2000; Myers et al. 2000). One group (Ertekin-Taner et al. 2000) used a novel approach to this issue; they used plasma Aβ-42 as a surrogate trait and performed linkage analysis on AD pedigrees based on the presence of high plasma Aβ levels in the patients with late-onset AD. With this novel approach, they reported linkage to a location near *D10S1225*, the region also identified by others (Myers et al. 2000).

In another genome screen, a third locus was identified on chromosome 9 (Pericak-Vance et al. 2000). A lod score of 4.31 was reported in an autopsy-confirmed sample of AD cases. Lod score reflects the strength of the linkage; a lod score of 3.0 or greater is the accepted threshold for evidence of linkage to a given locus. The value of 4.31 is the highest linkage reported to date in a genome screen for AD.

The linkage studies described above focused on loci that alter risk of AD. However, genes also may influence the age at onset of disease. Recent AD and PD linkage studies demonstrate this point. It has been estimated that the prevalence of AD doubles with every 5 years of age (Jorm et al. 1987). Thus, if the onset could be delayed a few years, many of those at risk for developing the disease would die from other causes before getting the disease. Some researchers have now used linkage techniques to identify putative age-at-onset genes for AD (Daw et al. 1999; Li et al. 2002) and PD (Li et al. 2002). Interestingly, a region on chromosome 10 showed linkage to age at onset in both AD and PD, suggesting a connection between these two neurodegenerative diseases (Li et al. 2002).

The pursuit of other AD genes has produced numerous reports of associations between specific genes and AD, but none of these has been consistently replicated. In fact, for many of these genes, there are more negative than positive findings (Emahazion et al. 2001). A partial list of the contending genes includes interleukin-1 (*IL1*) on chromosome 2 (Grimaldi et al. 2000; Nicoll et al. 2000); the K variant of butyrylcholinesterase (*BCHE-K*) on chromosome 3 (Brindle et al. 1998; Lehmann et al.

1997; Russ et al. 1998; Singleton et al. 1998; Wiebusch et al. 1999); the nonamyloid component precursor gene (*NACP*/α-synuclein) on chromosome 4 (Xia et al. 1996); the human leukocyte antigen (*HLA*) gene on chromosome 6 (Curran et al. 1997; Payami et al. 1997); tumor necrosis factor (*TNF*) gene on chromosome 6 (Collins et al. 2000); endothelial nitric oxide synthase gene (*NOS3*) on chromosome 7 (Dahiyat et al. 1999); the *FE65* gene on chromosome 11 (Hu et al. 1998); the dihydrolipoyl succinyltransferase (*DLST*) gene on chromosome 14 (Nakano et al. 1997; Sheu et al. 1999); α$_1$-antichymotrypsin (*ACT*), a gene on chromosome 14 (Egensperger et al. 1998; Ezquerra et al. 1998; Kamboh et al. 1995; Lamb et al. 1998; Muramatsu et al. 1996; Nacmias et al. 1998; Talbot et al. 1996; Thome et al. 1995; Yoshiiwa et al. 1997); bleomycin hydrolase (*BH*) on chromosome 17 (Montoya et al. 1998); the myeloperoxidase (*MPO*) gene on chromosome 17 (Crawford et al. 2001; Reynolds et al. 1999); phenylethanolamine *N*-methyltransferase (*PNMT*) on chromosome 17 (Mann et al. 2001); the dipeptidyl carboxypeptidase 1 (*DCP1*) gene on chromosome 17 (Mattila et al. 2000; Narain et al. 2000); the *APOE* promoter gene on chromosome 19 (Halimi et al. 2000; Lambert et al. 1998a); and the mitochondrial cytochrome c oxidase genes *CO1* and *CO* (Davis et al. 1997). To complicate the issue further, many of the genes listed above appear to interact in varying degrees with *APOE* or other genes to alter risk of AD (Wang et al. 1998).

In complex traits in which several genetic loci and/or environmental factors are believed to contribute to disease etiology, linkage studies might not be powerful enough to identify genetic factors of only moderate effect. However, association studies have their limitations, and there are several possible reasons for the contradictory results with the purported AD genes noted above. These reasons include 1) diverse disease etiologies in different ethnic populations; 2) lack of adjustment for multiple comparisons (type I statistical error, resulting from simultaneous screening of many different candidate loci); 3) linkage disequilibrium in some (or all) populations between the tested polymorphism and the functional polymorphism; and 4) inability to detect an effect because of limited statistical power or weak genetic effects (Cardon and Bell 2001; Katzman et al. 1998; Wu et al. 1998). Association studies are also more difficult to interpret when one does not know characteristics such as the mode of inheritance, age-dependent expression characteristics, interaction with other loci, misdiagnosis rate, and disease allele frequency. Finally, the inconsistent findings may reflect interactions with nongenetic factors.

Considering the lengthy list of purported loci, genes, and mutations associated with AD, one may wonder whether a common thread exists in the pathogenesis of AD. The pathogenic mechanisms of the *APP, PS1,* and *PS2* mutations are not completely understood, but each appears to be associated with increased production of the long form of Aβ (Aβ-42), relative to the production of the shorter forms (mostly Aβ-40) of Aβ (Hardy 1997). Aβ-42 seems to be a particularly pathogenic form of Aβ in AD. Both *LRP* and *A2M* are involved in the degradation of Aβ. It has been suggested that these links to Aβ may be the underlying common pathogenic event leading to AD for these genes (Kim and Tanzi 1997). One might predict that as other candidate genes are confirmed, they too may be linked to the known AD genes via such a common pathway.

Frontotemporal Dementia

Frontotemporal dementia (FTD) is characterized by a range of cognitive, behavioral, motor, and pathological findings. The variability in the presentation of the disorder has resulted in multiple names for the condition, including disinhibition-dementia-parkinsonism-amyotrophy complex, hereditary FTD, multiple system tauopathy dementia, and *pallidopontonigral dementia*. The various forms of the condition typically begin with insidious onset of behavior and personality changes, motor symptoms, and cognitive decline between ages 45 and 65 years (Neary 2000). It is difficult to estimate the prevalence of the condition because most studies have been based on specialty clinic samples. FTD has been the focus of genetic investigations in recent years because approximately 50% of those with FTD have a family history of the disorder (Neary 2000). Some of these cases that have motor involvement have now shown linkage to chromosome 17, and the preferred name for this particular condition has become FTD with parkinsonism linked to chromosome 17 (FTDP-17) (Foster et al. 1997). The search for the candidate gene for FTDP-17 has focused on *TAU* because biological evidence suggests that *TAU* may play a role in several neurodegenerative disorders, including FTDs, progressive supranuclear palsy, and corticobasal ganglionic degeneration (Lee et al. 2001; Poorkaj et al. 1998). To date, more than 20 *TAU* mutations have been identified (Alzheimer Research Forum 2001, tau mutation table; Lee et al. 2001), and there appear to be distinctive clinical and pathological features related to some of the different mutations. The complexity of the genetic influence on these conditions becomes even more apparent when one realizes that not only do some *TAU* gene mutations cause a similar phenotype in different family members or different families (Delisle et

al. 1999; Reed et al. 1998; Yasuda et al. 1999) but also examples of multiple phenotypes are found within and between families for the same genetic mutation (Bird et al. 1999; Mirra et al. 1999; Nasreddine et al. 1999; Spillantini et al. 1998). There is little information on the percentage of FTDP-17 cases accounted for by the known *TAU* mutations. However, it is noteworthy that *TAU* mutations were uncommon in at least one clinic sample of purportedly non-AD dementia patients who were thought to have FTDP-17 (Poorkaj et al. 2001). This finding suggests that, similar to AD, there may be additional FTDP-17 mutations and genes that are yet to be identified.

Parkinson's Disease

PD is a common progressive neurodegenerative disorder affecting 1%–2% of the population older than 65 years (de Rijk et al. 1997). It is characterized by a combination of motor symptoms, including akinesia, rest tremor, rigidity, and disturbance of postural reflexes. The age at onset for PD ranges from the 20s through late life. Much of PD is thought to be sporadic. In fact, the risk for first-degree family members of PD patients is increased only two- to threefold, and it is estimated that only about 5%–15% of families have more than one member with PD (Gasser 2001). In recent years, mutations in multiple genes have been identified that appear to cause PD via a mendelian mode of inheritance. But just as with AD, all of these mutations combined account for a relatively small number of affected families and are primarily associated with onset of PD before age 50 or 60 (for review, see Gasser 2001; Mouradian 2002). Consistent with this, results from a twin study of World War II male veterans suggested that genetics may be important in early-onset (before 50 years) PD but appeared negligible in those with onset after age 50 (Tanner et al. 1999).

To date, mutations on three genes associated with PD have been identified. They are α-synuclein on chromosome 4 (Kruger et al. 1998; Polymeropoulos et al. 1997), Parkin on chromosome 6 (Ishikawa and Tsuji 1996), and ubiquitin carboxy-terminal hydrolase L1 (*UCH-L1*) on chromosome 4 (Leroy et al. 1998). Linkage has been shown to four additional loci on chromosome 1 (Valente et al. 2001; van Duijn et al. 2001), chromosome 2 (Gasser et al. 1998), and chromosome 4 (Farrer et al. 1999); however, the culpable genes have not yet been identified. In addition, some studies have described an association between the triplet repeat expansions in the spinocerebellar ataxia *SCA3* and *SCA2* genes and clinical parkinsonism (Gwinn-Hardy et al. 2000, 2001). The mode of inheritance appears to differ among the loci and includes autosomal dominant transmission, autosomal recessive transmission, maternal transmission, and genetic anticipation (Mouradian 2002). Similar to other conditions discussed in this chapter, the genetic influence on phenotype appears to be complex. Not only does the phenotype sometimes vary within a family when the affected members have the same mutation, but also reports indicate that different loci sometimes cause virtually identical clinical syndromes. The pathology differs somewhat by loci, primarily regarding whether Lewy bodies are present. The genes identified to date appear to have a common mechanism, as all play a critical role in disrupting protein folding and degradation through the ubiquitin proteasome pathway, which then leads to cell death (Mouradian 2002).

The genetics of PD parallel the genetics of AD in several ways. Similar to AD, some evidence indicates that the age at onset of PD is inherited (Li et al. 2002; Zareparsi et al. 2002). In addition, there appear to be multiple susceptibility genes that may increase the risk of developing PD. However, as with AD, replication studies have not consistently confirmed any of the candidate genes under study (for review, see Gasser 2001).

Depression

Depression in the elderly represents a new field of inquiry for genetics researchers. Most of the published reports thus far used relatively small samples, often with fewer than 100 subjects. One challenge facing investigators is the heterogeneity of the condition, because depression at all ages is thought to have multifactorial etiologies. Thus, in designing genetic studies, one must strive to obtain a maximally homogeneous group. Without such homogeneity, it may be particularly difficult to find genetic influences. To this end, there have been attempts to subtype late-life major depression into categories, such as depression associated with cerebrovascular disease. Research criteria have been proposed for this "vascular depression" (Alexopoulos et al. 1997; Steffens and Krishnan 1998), but the sensitivity and specificity of the diagnosis have not been established.

Thus, one must keep heterogeneity in mind when examining the literature on the genetics of geriatric depression. Here, we briefly review the previous work that has focused on the following three areas: 1) association of specific genes and late-life depression, 2) association between different genetic alleles and response to treatment, and 3) association between genes and other biological markers in geriatric depression.

Several studies have examined the relation between *APOE* and late-life depression. Although some reports showed a positive relation between the *APOE* ε4 allele and late-life depression (Krishnan et al. 1996; Zubenko et al. 1996), many other studies have failed to find such a relation (Class et al. 1997; Schmand et al. 1998). Because the ε4 allele is associated with an increased risk for AD, one explanation for these inconsistent findings is the potential contamination of the depressed group with subjects who have dementia. Geriatric depression often is accompanied by cognitive impairment; indeed, the differential diagnosis of depression and dementia is a common challenge faced by geriatric psychiatrists. Inclusion in some studies of subjects with lower cognitive scores might explain the association between the ε4 allele and depression if such scores represent the early stages of dementia.

Genetic variation in the serotonin transporter gene, a key target for pharmacogenetic research, also has been examined in older depressed and nondepressed populations. We examined gender differences in the serotonin transporter-linked polymorphic region (*5HTTLPR*) among depressed patients and control subjects (Steffens et al. 2002). The prevailing genotype is two long alleles, with a long allele frequency of 0.629 in control subjects and 0.599 in depressed patients, and the most common variant is the short allele. In our study, we reported two significant findings. Twenty-three percent of the depressed men had two short alleles, compared with only 5% of the male control subjects. Among women, 67% of the depressed women with more than one episode had at least one short allele, compared with 41% of the single-episode female patients.

Therapeutic consequences of genetic mutations also have been examined. Study outcomes have included both altered drug metabolism and differential response to treatment. For example, genetic variability in cytochrome P450 2D6 activity has been hypothesized to affect plasma concentrations of a variety of antidepressants metabolized by the enzyme. One study found a significant association between mutations encoding decreased metabolism and plasma concentration of nortriptyline (Murphy et al. 2001).

The *5HTTLPR* gene also may affect response to antidepressant medications among elderly control subjects. In a group of elderly patients taking paroxetine and nortriptyline, on average, those with the long allele genotype showed a more rapid reduction in Hamilton Rating Scale for Depression score than did those with a short allele, despite equivalent paroxetine concentrations (Pollock et al. 2000). Onset of response to nortriptyline was not affected.

In keeping with the notion that the subtype "vascular depression" exists, investigators have examined the *APOE* genotype and occurrence of increased signal hyperintensities on magnetic resonance imaging that are thought to represent cerebrovascular disease. In a group weighted with elderly individuals carrying at least one *APOE* ε4 allele, those with depressive symptoms reported on the Geriatric Depression Scale had more white matter intensities on magnetic resonance imaging (Nebes et al. 2001). Our group reported an association between subcortical gray matter hyperintensities and presence of at least one *APOE* ε4 allele in elderly patients with major depression (Steffens et al. 2003).

Implications for Clinical Practice and Conclusion

How should the clinician use the information presented in this chapter? In recent years, patients and their families have frequently asked to what extent the patient's condition may be attributable to genes and the implications that this may have regarding risk of disease for their offspring. As more genetic advances are publicized, such queries will likely only increase. However, it is evident from the information provided here that these are not simple questions with clear-cut answers.

Several points need to be considered when advising patients on the role of genes in a specific disease. For all of the conditions discussed in this chapter, the identified genes account for only a subset of the individuals with the disease. Clearly, additional genes will be identified. Furthermore, except in a minority of cases, the disorders discussed in this chapter are not explained by single genes functioning in a mendelian inheritance pattern. For many illnesses of late life, "susceptibility genes" appear to account for most of the genetic risk for the disease. The effect of any one susceptibility gene may be influenced by the age, sex, and ethnicity of the individual at risk. Evidence also suggests that these genes may interact with other genes and nongenetic factors. Thus, although not everyone with a specific susceptibility gene or genotype will develop the disease, our current knowledge is too limited to predict which individuals at risk will get the disease.

Further complicating the picture in diseases of late life is that because of competing causes of death, individuals at risk may not express the disease symptoms during their lifetime. We use AD to illustrate this point. It has repeatedly been shown that the first-degree relatives of patients with AD have a 50% lifetime incidence rate of the disease. However, because of other causes of mortality, it is estimated that only about one-third of this theoretical familial predisposition to AD is realized in the usual life span (Breitner 1991; Breitner et al. 1988). This means that the actual predicted risk of developing AD in the first-degree relatives of probands with AD is likely between 15% and 19% compared with 5% in control subjects. Extrapolating from these findings, one could estimate that the risk to children of AD patients is one in five or one in six (Liddell et al. 2001).

The above information is useful when discussing widely confirmed gene-disease associations. But the deluge of information on novel candidate genes can be difficult to interpret for the clinician who has not had specialty training in this area. In response to this problem, the Centers for Disease Control and Prevention and the National Institutes of Health recently convened an expert panel to develop guidelines for reporting and evaluating epidemiological studies on gene-disease associations (Little et al. 2002). The guidelines include recommendations on assessing the validity of the genotyping, selection of subjects, confounding due to population stratification, and statistical issues. Others have suggested additional criteria that may be useful for the clinician in interpreting such results (Cardon and Bell 2001).

The final question the clinician faces is whether to use genetic testing for diagnostic purposes or to predict risk of developing disease in otherwise healthy individuals. As a result of the efforts of the expert panel noted above, guidelines for evaluating genetic tests have now been published (Burke et al. 2002). The recommendations include assessing 1) the accuracy of the specific genetic laboratory test, 2) the accuracy with which a test predicts a given clinical outcome, and 3) the likelihood that the test will lead to improved health outcome. The panel also stressed that the ethical, legal, and social implications of the test need to be considered, and some of these outcomes are not easily assessed.

Again, we use AD as the example; genetic testing does not appear to improve the accuracy of the AD diagnosis, except possibly in the small minority of individuals with early-onset disease with known AD mutations. Based on current treatment approaches, use of genetic testing in the diagnostic process would not modify the treatment. For the purpose of identifying individuals at risk, genetic testing likely predicts clinical outcome with good accuracy in the small subset of members of familial AD kindreds with known AD mutations. However, the predictive accuracy of other genes appears to have a large margin of error. Furthermore, no proven treatments currently exist to prevent or delay AD; thus, the test would not lead to improved health outcome.

Similar conclusions might be drawn for other dementias and for PD. As for mood disorders, it is difficult to predict when knowledge of genetic information will become useful in the management of such patients. Reliance on clinical history and mental status examination will likely continue to be paramount for diagnosis. However, advances in pharmacogenetics may come to guide the choice of psychotropic agent.

It is important to note that the value of genetic testing is not static or generalized to all diseases. The value will change with the identification of more genes and with improved or gene-specific treatments for each of these diseases. Moreover, genetics in geriatric psychiatry is a rapidly changing field. It is incumbent on the clinician to be able to interpret the published findings and to be able to assess the value of genetic testing for each disease.

References

Alexopoulos GS, Meyers BS, Young RC, et al: 'Vascular depression' hypothesis. Arch Gen Psychiatry 54:915–922, 1997

Alzheimer Research Forum: Tau mutation directory. Updated January 2001. Available at: http://www.alzforum.org/res/com/mut/tau/table1.asp. Accessed September 16, 2003.

Alzheimer Research Forum: APP mutations table. Updated March 2003. Available at: http://www.alzforum.org/res/com/mut/app/table1.asp. Accessed September 8, 2003.

Alzheimer Research Forum: The presenilin-1 mutations. Updated August 2003. Available at: http://www.alzforum.org/res/com/mut/pre/table1.asp. Accessed September 8, 2003.

Bergem ALM, Engedal K, Kringlen E: The role of heredity in late-onset Alzheimer disease and vascular dementia. Arch Gen Psychiatry 54:264–270, 1997

Bertram L, Blacker D, Mullin K, et al: Evidence for genetic linkage of Alzheimer's disease to chromosome 10q. Science 290:2302–2303, 2000

Bird TD, Nochlin D, Poorkaj P, et al: A clinical pathological comparison of three families with frontotemporal dementia and identical mutations in the tau gene (P301L). Brain 122:741–756, 1999

Blacker D, Wilcox MA, Laird NM, et al: Alpha-2 macroglobulin is genetically associated with Alzheimer disease. Nat Genet 19:357–360, 1998

Breitner JCS: Clinical genetics and genetic counseling in Alzheimer's disease. Ann Intern Med 115:601–606, 1991

Breitner JCS, Murphy EA, Silverman JM, et al: Age-dependent expression of familial risk in Alzheimer's disease. Am J Epidemiol 128:536–548, 1988

Breitner JCS, Welsh KA, Gau BA, et al: Alzheimer's disease in the National Academy of Sciences–National Research Council Registry of aging twin veterans, III: detection of cases, longitudinal results, and observations on twin concordance. Arch Neurol 52:763–771, 1995

Brindle N, Song Y, Rogaeva E, et al: Analysis of the butyrylcholinesterase gene and nearby chromosome 3 markers in Alzheimer disease. Hum Mol Genet 7:933–935, 1998

Brousseau T, Legrain S, Berr C, et al: Confirmation of the epsilon4 allele of the apolipoprotein E gene as a risk factor for late-onset Alzheimer's disease. Neurology 44:342–344, 1994

Burke W, Atkins D, Gwinn M, et al: Genetic test evaluation: information needs of clinicians, policy makers, and the public. Am J Epidemiol 156:311–318, 2002

Campion D, Flaman J-M, Brice A, et al: Mutations of the presenilin 1 gene families with early onset Alzheimer's disease. Hum Mol Genet 4:2373–2377, 1995

Campion D, Dumanchin C, Hannequin D, et al: Early onset autosomal dominant Alzheimer disease: prevalence, genetic heterogeneity, and mutation spectrum. Am J Hum Genet 65:664–670, 1999

Cardon LR, Bell JI: Association study designs for complex diseases. Nat Rev Genet 2:91–99, 2001

Chen L, Baum L, Ng HK, et al: Apolipoprotein E promoter and alpha2-macroglobulin polymorphisms are not genetically associated with Chinese late onset Alzheimer's disease. Neurosci Lett 269:173–177, 1999

Class CA, Unverzagt FW, Gao S, et al: The association between Apo E genotype and depressive symptoms in elderly African-American subjects. Am J Geriatr Psychiatry 5:339–343, 1997

Clatworthy AE, Gomez-Isla T, Rebeck W, et al: Lack of association of a polymorphism in the low-density lipoprotein receptor-related protein gene with Alzheimer disease. Arch Neurol 54:1289–1292, 1997

Collins JS, Perry RT, Watson JB, et al: Association of a haplotype for tumor necrosis factor in siblings with late-onset Alzheimer disease: the NIMH Alzheimer Disease Genetics Initiative. Am J Med Genet (Neuropsychiatric Genetics) 96:823–830, 2000

Corder EH, Saunders AM, Strittmatter WJ, et al: Gene dose of apolipoprotein E type 4 allele and the risk of Alzheimer's disease in late onset families. Science 261:921–923, 1993

Crawford F, Freeman M, Town T, et al: No genetic association between polymorphisms in the tau gene and Alzheimer's disease in clinic or population based samples. Neurosci Lett 266:193–196, 1999

Crawford FC, Freeman MJ, Schinka JA, et al: Association between Alzheimer's disease and a functional polymorphism in the myeloperoxidase gene. Exp Neurol 167:456–459, 2001

Cruts M, van Duijn CM, Backhovens H, et al: Estimation of the genetic contribution of presenilin-1 and -2 mutations in a population-based study of presenile Alzheimer disease. Hum Mol Genet 7:43–51, 1998

Curran M, Middleton D, Edwardson J, et al: HLADR antigens associated with major genetic risk for late-onset Alzheimer's disease. Neuroreport 8:1467–1469, 1997

Dahiyat M, Cumming A, Harrington C, et al: Association between Alzheimer's disease and the NOS3 gene. Ann Neurol 46:664–667, 1999

Davis RE, Miller S, Herrnstadt C, et al: Mutations in mitochondrial cytochrome c oxidase genes segregate with late-onset Alzheimer disease. Proc Natl Acad Sci U S A 94:4526–4531, 1997

Daw EW, Heath SC, Wijsman EM: Multipoint oligogenic analysis of age-at-onset data with applications to Alzheimer disease pedigrees. Am J Hum Genet 64:839–851, 1999

de Rijk MC, Breteler MMB, den Breeijen JH, et al: Dietary antioxidants and Parkinson disease. Arch Neurol 54:762–765, 1997

Delisle M-B, Murrell JR, Richardson R, et al: A mutation at codon 279 (N279K) in exon 10 of the tau gene causes a tauopathy with dementia and supranuclear palsy. Acta Neuropathol (Berl) 98:62–77, 1999

Dow DJ, Lindsey N, Cairns NJ, et al: α-2 macroglobulin polymorphism and Alzheimer disease risk in the UK. Nat Genet 22:16–17, 1999

Egensperger R, Herrmann H, Kosel S, et al: Association between ACT polymorphism, and Alzheimer's disease (letter). Neurology 50:575, 1998

Emahazion T, Feuk L, Jobs M, et al: SNP association studies in Alzheimer's disease highlight problems for complex disease analysis. Trends Genet 17:407–413, 2001

Ertekin-Taner N, Graff-Radford N, Younkin LH, et al: Linkage of plasma Abeta42 to a quantitative locus on chromosome 10 in late-onset Alzheimer's disease pedigrees. Science 290:2303–2304, 2000

Ezquerra M, Blesa R, Tolosa E, et al: Alpha-antichymotrypsin gene polymorphism and risk for Alzheimer's disease in the Spanish population. Neurosci Lett 240:107–109, 1998

Fallin D, Kundtz A, Town T, et al: No association between the low density lipoprotein receptor-related protein (LRP) gene and late-onset Alzheimer's disease in a community-based sample. Neurosci Lett 233:145–147, 1997

Farrer LA: Genetics and the dementia patient. Neurologist 3:13–30, 1997

Farrer LA, Cupples LA, Haines JL, et al: Effects of age, sex, and ethnicity on the association between apolipoprotein E genotype and Alzheimer disease. JAMA 278:1349–1355, 1997

Farrer M, Gwinn-Hardy K, Muenter M, et al: A chromosome 4p haplotype segregating with Parkinson's disease and postural tremor. Hum Mol Genet 8:81–85, 1999

Finckh U, Muller-Thomsen T, Mann U, et al: High prevalence of pathogenic mutations in patients with early onset dementia detected by sequence analyses of four different genes. Am J Hum Genet 66:110–117, 2000

Foster NL, Wilhelmsen K, Sima AAF, et al: Frontotemporal dementia and parkinsonism linked to chromosome 17: a consensus conference. Ann Neurol 41:706–715, 1997

Gasser T: Genetics of Parkinson's disease. J Neurol 248:833–840, 2001

Gasser T, Muller-Myhsok B, Wszolek ZK, et al: A susceptibility locus for Parkinson's disease maps to chromosome 2p13. Nat Genet 18:262–265, 1998

Gatz M, Pedersen NL, Berg S, et al: Heritability for Alzheimer's disease: the study of dementia in Swedish twins. J Gerontol 52A:M117–M125, 1997

Goate A, Chartier-Harlin MC, Mullan M, et al: Segregation of a missense mutation in the amyloid precursor protein gene with familial Alzheimer's disease. Nature 349:704–706, 1991

Grimaldi LME, Casadei VM, Ferri C, et al: Association of early onset Alzheimer's disease with an interleukin-1[alpha] gene polymorphism. Ann Neurol 47:361–365, 2000

Gwinn-Hardy K, Chen JY, Liu H-C, et al: Spinocerebellar ataxia type 2 with parkinsonism in ethnic Chinese. Neurology 55:800–805, 2000

Gwinn-Hardy K, Singleton A, O'Suilleabhain P, et al: Spinocerebellar ataxia type 3 phenotypically resembling Parkinson disease in a black family. Arch Neurol 58:296–299, 2001

Halimi G, Duplan L, Bideau C, et al: Association of APOE promoter but not A2M polymorphisms with risk of developing Alzheimer's disease. Neuroreport II:3599–3601, 2000

Hardy J: Amyloid, the presenilins and Alzheimer's disease. Trends Neurosci 20:154–159, 1997

Henderson AS, Easteal S, Jorm AF, et al: Apolipoprotein E allele ε4, dementia, and cognitive decline in a population sample. Lancet 346:1387–1390, 1995

Hollenbach E, Ackermann S, Hyman BT, et al: Confirmation of an association between a polymorphism in exon 3 of the low-density lipoprotein receptor-related protein gene and Alzheimer's disease. Neurology 50:1905–1907, 1998

Hu Q, Kukull WA, Bressler SL, et al: The human FE65 gene: genomic structure and an intronic biallelic polymorphism associated with sporadic dementia of the Alzheimer type. Hum Genet 103:295–303, 1998

Hutton M, Busfield F, Wragg M, et al: Complete analysis of the presenilin 1 gene in early onset Alzheimer's disease. Neuroreport 7:801–805, 1996

Ishikawa A, Tsuji S: Clinical analysis of 17 patients in 12 Japanese families with autosomal-recessive type juvenile parkinsonism. Neurology 47:160–166, 1996

Jorm AF, Korten AE, Henderson AS: The prevalence of dementia: a quantitative integration of the literature. Acta Psychiatr Scand 76:465–479, 1987

Kamboh M, Sanghera D, Ferrell R, et al: APOE*4-associated Alzheimer's disease risk is modified by alpha 1-antichymotrypsin polymorphism. Nat Genet 10:486–488, 1995

Kang DE, Saitoh T, Chen X, et al: Genetic association of the low-density lipoprotein receptor-related protein gene (LRP), an apolipoprotein E receptor, with late-onset Alzheimer's disease. Neurology 49:56–61, 1997

Katzman R, Kang D, Thomas R: Interaction of apolipoprotein E epsilon 4 with other genetic and non-genetic risk factors in late onset Alzheimer disease: problems facing the investigator. Neurochem Res 23:369–376, 1998

Kennedy AM, Brown J, Rossor M: The genetics of Alzheimer's disease. Baillieres Clin Neurol 3:217–240, 1994

Kim W, Tanzi RE: Presenilins and Alzheimer's disease. Curr Opin Neurobiol 7:683–688, 1997

Krishnan KR, Tupler LA, Ritchie JC, et al: Apolipoprotein E-e4 frequency in geriatric depression. Biol Psychiatry 40:69–71, 1996

Kruger R, Kuhn W, Muller T, et al: Ala30Pro mutation in the gene encoding alpha-synuclein in Parkinson's disease. Nat Genet 18:106–108, 1998

Lamb H, Christie J, Singleton AB, et al: Apolipoprotein E and alpha-1 antichymotrypsin polymorphism genotyping in Alzheimer's disease and in dementia with Lewy bodies: distinctions between diseases. Neurology 50:388–391, 1998

Lambert JC, Berr C, Pasquier F, et al: Pronounced impact of the Th1/E47cs mutation compared with -491 AT mutation on neural APOE gene expression and risk of developing Alzheimer's disease. Hum Mol Genet 7:1511–1516, 1998a

Lambert JC, Vrieze FW-D, Amouyel P, et al: Association at LRP gene locus with sporadic late-onset Alzheimer's disease. Lancet 351:1787–1788, 1998b

Lambert JC, Coumidi L, Vrieze FW, et al: The transcription factor LBP-1c/CP2/LSF gene on chromosome 12 is a genetic determinant of Alzheimer's disease. Hum Mol Genet 9:2275–2280, 2000

Lee VM-Y, Goedert M, Trojanowski JQ: Neurodegenerative tauopathies. Annu Rev Neurosci 24:1121–1159, 2001

Lehmann DJ, Johnston C, Smith AD: Synergy between the genes for butyrylcholinesterase K variant and apolipoprotein E4 in late onset confirmed Alzheimer disease. Hum Mol Genet 6:1933–1936, 1997

Lendon CL, Talbot CJ, Craddock NJ, et al: Genetic association studies between dementia of the Alzheimer's type and three receptors for apolipoprotein E in a Caucasian population. Neurosci Lett 222:187–190, 1997

Leroy E, Boyer R, Auburger G, et al: The ubiquitin pathway in Parkinson's disease. Nature 395:451–452, 1998

Levy-Lahad E, Wasco W, Poorkaj P, et al: Candidate gene for the chromosome 1 familial Alzheimer's disease locus. Science 269:973–977, 1995a

Levy-Lahad E, Wijsman EM, Nemens E, et al: A familial Alzheimer's disease locus on chromosome 1. Science 269:970–973, 1995b

Li Y, Scott WK, Hedges DJ, et al: Age at onset in two common neurodegenerative diseases is genetically controlled. Am J Hum Genet 70:985–993, 2002

Liao A, Nitsch RM, Greenberg SM, et al: Genetic association of an α2-macroglobulin (Val1000lle) polymorphism and Alzheimer's disease. Hum Mol Genet 7:1953–1956, 1998

Liddell MB, Lovestone S, Owen MJ: Genetic risk of Alzheimer's disease: advising relatives. Br J Psychiatry 178:7–11, 2001

Little J, Bradley L, Bray MS, et al: Reporting, appraising, and integrating data on genotype prevalence and gene-disease associations. Am J Epidemiol 156:300–310, 2002

Mann MB, Wu S, Rostamkhani M, et al: Phenylethanolamine n-methyltransferase (PNMT) gene and early onset Alzheimer disease. Am J Med Genet 105:312–316, 2001

Mattila KM, Rinne JO, Roytta M, et al: Dipeptidyl carboxypeptidase 1 (DCP1) and butyrylcholinesterase (BCHE) gene interactions with the apolipoprotein E ε4 allele as risk factors in Alzheimer's disease and in Parkinson's disease with coexisting Alzheimer pathology. J Med Genet 37:766–770, 2000

Mayeux R, Stern Y, Ottman R, et al: The apolipoprotein E4 allele in patients with Alzheimer's disease. Ann Neurol 34:752–754, 1993

Miech RA, Breitner JCS, Zandi PP, et al: Incidence of AD may decline in the early 90s for men, later for women: the Cache County Study. Neurology 58:209–217, 2002

Mirra SS, Murrell JR, Gearing M, et al: Tau pathology in a family with dementia and a P301L mutation in tau. J Neuropathol Exp Neurol 58:335–345, 1999

Montoya SE, Aston CE, DeKosky ST, et al: Bleomycin hydrolase is associated with risk of sporadic Alzheimer's disease. Nat Genet 18:211–212, 1998

Mouradian MM: Recent advances in the genetics and pathogenesis of Parkinson disease. Neurology 58:179–185, 2002

Muramatsu T, Matsushita S, Arai H, et al: Alpha 1-antichymotrypsin gene polymorphism and risk for Alzheimer's disease. J Neural Transm 103:1205–1210, 1996

Murphy GM Jr, Pollock BG, Kirshner MA, et al: CYP2D6 genotyping with oligonucleotide microarrays and nortriptyline concentrations in geriatric depression. Neuropsychopharmacology 25:737–743, 2001

Myers A, Holmans P, Marshall H, et al: Susceptibility locus for Alzheimer's disease on chromosome 10. Science 290:2304–2305, 2000

Myllykangas L, Polvikoski T, Sulkava R, et al: Genetic association of alpha$_2$-macroglobulin with Alzheimer's disease in a Finnish elderly population. Ann Neurol 46:382–390, 1999

Nacmias B, Marcon G, Tedde A, et al: Implication of α$_1$-antichymotrypsin polymorphism in familial Alzheimer's disease. Neurosci Lett 244:85–88, 1998

Nakano K, Ohta S, Nishimaki K, et al: Alzheimer's disease and DLST genotype. Lancet 350:1367–1368, 1997

Narain Y, Yip A, Murphy T, et al: The ACE gene and Alzheimer's disease susceptibility. J Med Genet 37:695–697, 2000

Nasreddine ZS, Loginov M, Clark LN, et al: From genotype to phenotype: a clinical pathological, and biochemical investigation of frontotemporal dementia and parkinsonism (FTDP-17) caused by the P301L tau mutation. Ann Neurol 45:704–715, 1999

Neary D: Frontotemporal dementia, in Dementia. Edited by O'Brien J, Ames D, Burns A. London, Arnold, 2000, pp 737–746

Nebes RD, Vora IJ, Meltzer CC, et al: Relationship of deep white matter hyperintensities and apolipoprotein E genotype to depressive symptoms in older adults without clinical depression. Am J Psychiatry 158:878–884, 2001

Nee LE, Lippa CF: Alzheimer's disease in 22 twin pairs—13-year follow-up: hormonal, infectious and traumatic factors. Dement Geriatr Cogn Disord 10:148–151, 1999

Nicoll JAR, Mrak RE, Graham DI, et al: Association of interleukin-1 gene polymorphisms with Alzheimer's disease. Ann Neurol 47:365–368, 2000

Payami H, Schellenberg GD, Zareparsi S, et al: Evidence for association of HLA-A2 allele with onset age of Alzheimer's disease. Neurology 49:512–518, 1997

Pericak-Vance MA, Haines JL: Genetic susceptibility to Alzheimer disease. Trends Genet 11:504–508, 1995

Pericak-Vance MA, Bebout JL, Gaskell PC, et al: Linkage studies in familial Alzheimer disease: evidence for chromosome 19 linkage. Am J Hum Genet 48:1034–1050, 1991

Pericak-Vance MA, Bass MP, Yamaoka LH, et al: Complete genomic screen in late-onset familial Alzheimer disease: evidence for a new locus on chromosome 12. JAMA 278:1237–1241, 1997

Pericak-Vance MA, Grubber J, Bailey LR, et al: Identification of novel genes in late-onset Alzheimer's disease. Exp Gerontol 35:1343–1352, 2000

Plomin R, DeFries JC, McClearn GE: Twin studies, in Behavioral Genetics—A Primer, Second Edition. New York, WH Freeman, 1990, pp 309–340

Pollock BG, Ferrell RE, Mulsant BH, et al: Allelic variation in the serotonin transporter promoter affects onset of paroxetine treatment response in late-life depression. Neuropsychopharmacology 23:587–590, 2000

Polymeropoulos MH, Lavedan C, Leroy E, et al: Mutation in the alpha-synuclein gene identified in families with Parkinson's disease. Science 276:2045–2047, 1997

Poorkaj P, Bird TD, Wijsman E, et al: Tau is a candidate gene for chromosome 17 frontotemporal dementia. Ann Neurol 43:815–825, 1998

Poorkaj P, Tsuang D, Wijsman E, et al: Tau as a susceptibility gene for amyotropic lateral sclerosis–parkinsonism dementia complex of Guam. Arch Neurol 58:1871–1878, 2001

Rebeck GW, Reiter JS, Strickland DK, et al: Apolipoprotein E in sporadic Alzheimer's disease: allelic variation and receptor interactions. Neuron 11:575–580, 1993

Rebeck GW, Harr SD, Strickland DK, et al: Multiple, diverse senile plaque-associated proteins are ligands of an apolipoprotein E receptor, α_2-macroglobulin receptor/low-density-lipoprotein receptor-related protein. Ann Neurol 37:211–217, 1995

Reed LA, Schmidt ML, Wszolek ZK, et al: The neuropathology of a chromosome 17-linked autosomal dominant parkinsonism and dementia ("pallido-ponto-nigral degeneration"). J Neuropathol Exp Neurol 57:588–601, 1998

Reynolds WF, Rhees J, Maciejewski D, et al: Myeloperoxidase polymorphism is associated with gender specific risk for Alzheimer's disease. Exp Neurol 155:31–41, 1999

Rogaeva E, Premkumar S, Song Y, et al: Evidence for an Alzheimer disease susceptibility locus on chromosome 12 and for further locus heterogeneity. JAMA 280:614–618, 1998

Rogaeva EA, Premkumar S, Grubber J, et al: An α-2-macroglobulin insertion-deletion polymorphism in Alzheimer disease. Nat Genet 22:19–21, 1999

Rosenberg R: The molecular and genetic basis of AD: the end of the beginning: the 2000 Wartenberg lecture. Neurology 54:2045–2054, 2000

Rossor MN, Fox NC, Beck J, et al: Incomplete penetrance of familial Alzheimer's disease in a pedigree with a novel presenilin-1 gene mutation (letter). Lancet 347:1560, 1996

Rudrasingham V, Wavrant-De Vrièze F, Lambert J-C, et al: α-2 macroglobulin gene and Alzheimer disease. Nat Genet 22:17–19, 1999

Russ C, Powell J, Loveston S, et al: K variant of butyrylcholinesterase and late-onset Alzheimer's disease. Lancet 351:881, 1998

Saunders AM, Strittmatter WJ, Schmechel D, et al: Association of apolipoprotein E allele E4 with late-onset familial and sporadic Alzheimer's disease. Neurology 43:1467–1472, 1993

Schellenberg GD, Bird TD, Wijsman EM, et al: Genetic linkage evidence for a familial Alzheimer's disease locus on chromosome 14. Science 258:668–671, 1992

Schmand B, Hooijer C, Jonker C, et al: Apolipoprotein E phenotype is not related to late-life depression in a population-based sample. Soc Psychiatry Psychiatr Epidemiol 33:21–26, 1998

Schmechel DE, Saunders AM, Strittmatter WJ, et al: Increased amyloid B-peptide deposition in cerebral cortex as a consequence of apolipoprotein E genotype in late-onset Alzheimer disease. Proc Natl Acad Sci U S A 90:9649–9653, 1993

Selkoe DJ: Alzheimer's disease: genes, proteins, and therapy. Physiol Rev 81:741–766, 2001

Seshadri S, Wolf PA, Beiser A, et al: Lifetime risk of dementia and Alzheimer's disease: the impact of mortality on risk estimates in the Framingham Study. Neurology 49:1498–1504, 1997

Sherrington R, Rogaev EI, Liang Y, et al: Cloning of a gene bearing missense mutations in early onset familial Alzheimer's disease. Nature 375:754–760, 1995

Sheu KFR, Brown AM, Haroutunian V, et al: Modulation by DLST of the genetic risk of Alzheimer's disease in a very elderly population. Ann Neurol 45:48–53, 1999

Silverman JM, Li G, Zaccario ML, et al: Patterns of risk in first-degree relatives of patients with Alzheimer's disease. Arch Gen Psychiatry 51:577–586, 1994

Silverman JM, Smith CJ, Marin DB, et al: Identifying families with likely genetic protective factors against Alzheimer disease. Am J Hum Genet 64:832–838, 1999

Singleton AB, Smith G, Gibson AM, et al: No association between the K variant of the butyrylcholinesterase gene and pathologically confirmed Alzheimer's disease. Hum Mol Genet 7:937–939, 1998

Spillantini MG, Crowther RA, Kamphorst W, et al: Tau pathology in two Dutch families with mutations in the microtubule-binding region of tau. Am J Pathol 153:1359–1363, 1998

St. George-Hyslop P, Haines J, Rogaev E, et al: Genetic evidence for a novel familial Alzheimer's disease locus on chromosome 14. Nat Genet 2:330–334, 1992

Steffens DC, Krishnan KR: Structural neuroimaging and mood disorders: recent findings, implications for classification, and future directions. Biol Psychiatry 43:705–712, 1998

Steffens DC, Svenson I, Marchuk DA, et al: Allelic differences in the serotonin transporter-linked polymorphic region in geriatric depression. Am J Geriatr Psychiatry 10:185–191, 2002

Steffens DC, Trost WT, Payne ME, et al: Apolipoprotein E genotype and subcortical vascular lesions in older depressed patients and control subjects. Biol Psychiatry 54:674–681, 2003

Strittmatter WJ, Saunders AM, Schmechel D, et al: Apolipoprotein E: high-avidity binding to B-amyloid and increased frequency of type 4 allele in late-onset familial Alzheimer disease. Proc Natl Acad Sci U S A 90:1977–1981, 1993

Talbot C, Houlden H, Craddock N, et al: Polymorphism in AACT gene may lower age of onset of Alzheimer's disease. Neuroreport 7:534–536, 1996

Tanner CM, Ottman R, Goldman SM, et al: Parkinson's disease in twins: an etiologic study. JAMA 281:341–346, 1999

Taylor AE, Yip A, Brayne C, et al: Genetic association of an LBP-1c/CP2/LSF gene polymorphism with late onset Alzheimer's disease. J Med Genet 38:232–233, 2001

Thome J, Baumer A, Kornhuber J, et al: Alpha-1-antichymotrypsin bi-allele polymorphism, apolipoprotein-E tri-allele polymorphism and genetic risk of Alzheimer's syndrome. J Neural Transm 10:207–212, 1995

Valente EM, Bentivoglio AR, Dixon PH, et al: Localization of a novel locus for autosomal recessive early onset parkinsonism, PARK6, on human chromosome 1p35-p36. Am J Hum Genet 68:895–900, 2001

Van Broeckhoven CL: Molecular genetics of Alzheimer disease: identification of genes and gene mutations. Eur Neurol 35:8–19, 1995

van Duijn CM, Clayton D, Chandra V, et al: Familial aggregation of Alzheimer's disease and related disorders: a collaborative re-analysis of case-control studies. Int J Epidemiol 20 (suppl 2):S13–S20, 1991

van Duijn CM, Dekker MC, Bonifati V, et al: Park7, a novel locus for autosomal recessive early onset parkinsonism, on chromosome 1p36. Am J Hum Genet 69:629–634, 2001

Wang X, DeKosky ST, Wisniewski S, et al: Genetic association of two chromosome 14 genes (presenilin 1 and α_1-antichymotrypsin) with Alzheimer's disease. Ann Neurol 44:387–390, 1998

Wang X, Luedecking EK, Minster RL, et al: Lack of association between α2-macroglobulin polymorphisms and Alzheimer's disease. Am J Hum Genet 108:105–108, 2001

Wavrant-De Vrièze F, Pérez-Tur J, Lambert JC, et al: Association between the low-density lipoprotein receptor-related protein (LRP) gene and Alzheimer's disease. Neurosci Lett 227:68–70, 1997

Wiebusch H, Poirier J, Sévigny P, et al: Further evidence for a synergistic association between APOE ε4 and BCHE-K in confirmed Alzheimer's disease. Hum Genet 104:158–163, 1999

Wu W, Holmans P, Wavrant-DeVrièze F, et al: Genetic studies on chromosome 12 in late-onset Alzheimer disease. JAMA 280:619–622, 1998

Xia Y, Rohan DeSilva HA, Rosi BL, et al: Genetic studies in Alzheimer's disease with an NACP/a-synuclein polymorphism. Ann Neurol 40:207–215, 1996

Yasuda M, Kawamata T, Komure O, et al: A mutation in the microtubule-associated protein tau in pallido-nigro-luysian degeneration. Neurology 53:864–868, 1999

Yoshiiwa A, Kamino K, Yamamoto H, et al: α_1-Antichymotrypsin as a risk modifier for late-onset Alzheimer's disease in Japanese apolipoprotein E ε4 allele carriers. Ann Neurol 42:115–117, 1997

Zareparsi S, Camicioli R, Sexton G, et al: Age at onset of Parkinson disease and apolipoprotein E genotypes. Am J Med Genet 107:156–161, 2002

Zubenko GS, Henderson R, Stiffler JS, et al: Association of the APOE epsilon 4 allele with clinical subtypes of late life depression. Biol Psychiatry 40:1008–1016, 1996

Psychological Aspects of Normal Aging

Ilene C. Siegler, Ph.D., M.P.H.

Leonard W. Poon, Ph.D.

David J. Madden, Ph.D.

Peggye Dilworth-Anderson, Ph.D.

In the years since this chapter was written for the second edition of the textbook, major changes in the aging field have been reflected in the psychology of normal aging as other disciplines, especially epidemiology, have become increasingly involved in studying psychological constructs as indexed by variables such as personality and cognition (see Zelinski et al. 1998) in population-based samples of normally aging persons (Fried 2000). This has made the distinction between normal aging and disease moot in many cases and a less useful indicator than it used to be (Siegler et al. 2003a). A revolution in neurosciences has had an effect on normative aging, age-related memory impairments, and pathologies such as stroke and Alzheimer's disease from both assessment and treatment viewpoints that again change our understanding of the psychological aspects of cognitive, personality, social, and intellectual functioning. The demographic revolution continues to expand the number of persons who survive, the number of generations that survive within a family, and the characteristics of the extreme aged themselves.

All of these factors have implications for social relationships in later life. Finally, there has been a new approach to attempting to understand and ameliorate the role of health disparities due to ethnic and minority status in the United States. These larger societal concerns have an effect on the psychology of normal aging because they make us aware of the full range of individual differences within cultural groups. As more data and more review chapters have accumulated, increasingly thoughtful chapters can now deal with the implications of the research.

In this chapter, we update five areas of research in the psychology of aging: 1) experimental and cognitive psychology; 2) neuroimaging and neuroscience; 3) personality and aging in the social context; 4) the role of age-related diseases, health, and behavior; and 5) extreme longevity and aging well. This chapter builds on previous reviews by Siegler (1980), Siegler and Poon (1989), Poon and Siegler (1991), and Siegler et al. (1996). These publications should be consulted for more

Work on this chapter was supported by a variety of grants to each of the coauthors: Dr. Siegler's work is supported by grants R01-HL55356 from the National Heart, Lung, and Blood Institute with additional support from the National Institute on Aging; P01-HL36587 from the National Heart, Lung, and Blood Institute; R01-AG12458 and R01-AG19605 from the National Institute on Aging; and P01 CA72099 from the National Cancer Institute; Dr. Poon's work is supported by grants P01-AG17553 from the National Institute on Aging and additional support from the AARP Andrus Foundation. Dr. Madden's work is supported by grants R01 AG11622 and R37 AG02163 from the National Institute on Aging. Dr. Dilworth-Anderson's work is supported by grant R01 AG12268 from the National Institute on Aging. We thank Susan Boos for her work on the coordination of this chapter.

detail on the work in psychology of aging published before 1995.

Experimental and Cognitive Psychology

The term *cognition* subsumes the range of human intellectual functioning, including perception, attention, memory, reasoning, decision making, problem solving, and formation of complex structures of knowledge. Investigations of age-related cognitive changes have used both cross-sectional and longitudinal research paradigms and have yielded a complex mosaic of results. Age-related decline can be measured in many cognitive tasks, but areas of preserved functioning are also observed.

When examining the literature comparing cognitive performances among age groups, one should keep in mind that the level of cognition can be affected by several individual, environmental, and task characteristics regardless of chronological age (Hultsch and Dixon 1990; Poon 1985). Depending on the task and the situation, some persons tend to excel in certain types of performance and not in others. For example, in some cognitive tasks, some adults with high intelligence and more education will show minimal decline in their performances with increasing age, whereas adults with lower intelligence and less education show significant decline (Bowles and Poon 1982; Poon and Fozard 1980). For those tasks, intelligence and education rather than chronological age are the important determinants of performance. In some cognitive tasks that are well practiced, the amount of age decline tends to be small or even nonexistent (Salthouse 1982). On the whole, however, there do appear to be age-related declines in several areas of cognitive performance, and these declines are largely independent of the amount of experience in related cognitive activities (Salthouse 1991). One influential distinction developed in the psychometric literature, applicable to the interpretation of many cognitive tasks, is the distinction between fluid and crystallized abilities (Cattell 1963; Horn 1982; Schaie 1990). *Fluid abilities*, involved with the novel manipulation of new information, tend to decline as a function of age, whereas *crystallized abilities*, related to the use of knowledge and previously learned skills, are more resistant to age-related decline. In current research, a related theoretical construct, that of the generalized slowing of information-processing speed, has been proposed to have a major role in age-related changes in cognitive performance (Madden 2001; Myerson et al. 1990; Salthouse 1991, 1996b).

Memory Functioning

Although all cognitive processes are intimately interrelated, age-related changes in memory functioning—in both normal and abnormal aging—have received by far the largest share of research effort (for reviews, see Balota et al. 2000; L.L. Light 1996; Zacks et al. 2000). The heightened emphasis on memory performance and aging may be the result of two factors. First, memory decline is a major concern articulated by community-dwelling elderly adults (Lowenthal et al. 1967). Second, memory dysfunction is a key behavioral benchmark in neuropsychopathology, such as dementia of the Alzheimer's type (Kaszniak et al. 1986).

Poon (1985) listed 20 reviews focusing on memory and normal aging that had been published since 1980 and noted the prevalence of the information-processing model in examining age-related differences in memory components, stages, and processes. The information-processing model postulates that information flows from input to output through a series of stages: registration, primary memory, secondary memory, and tertiary memory. *Registration* is sensory memory, a preattentive and highly unstable system. Primary (short-term) and secondary (long-term) memory (Waugh and Norman 1965) are responsible for the acquisition and retention of new information. *Primary memory* (or working memory) is conceptualized as a limited-capacity store in which information is still "in mind" as it is being used. If the information is not rehearsed instantaneously so that it can be stored in secondary memory, the information will be lost. *Secondary memory* is a repository of newly acquired information. *Tertiary memory* is the repository for well-learned and personal information.

This "linear" model is only one of several theoretical models of memory functioning. Others include the episodic and semantic memory model (Tulving 1972), the explicit and implicit memory model (Schacter 1987), the level-of-processing model (Craik and Lockhart 1972), and the parallel distributed model (McClelland et al. 1986). However, the information-processing model has been used extensively in the clinical domain, and the largest amount of data in the study of normal aging and in abnormal memory functioning has been gathered with this model (for a review, see Kaszniak et al. 1986). Findings on age-related differences in memory have been numerous, and only a brief review is attempted here.

A general theme of memory aging research is that age-related declines tend to increase as the environmental support provided by the task decreases (Craik and Jennings 1992). Memory tasks such as free recall (e.g., "Recall the 10 words presented earlier") provide little support for the retrieval processes required to perform the task. Recognition memory measures ("Is *chair* one of the words presented earlier?") provide more support. Age-related declines in memory performance are more evident in recall tasks, which involve self-directed retrieval, than in recognition tasks, although a decline is often observed in recognition as well. As noted earlier, an age-related decline is prominent in what have been termed *fluid abilities*, and this slowing in information-processing speed contributes to virtually all age differences in cognitive performance, including those in memory (Salthouse 1996a). Significant age-related slowing is evident in the initial registration of sensory input (Di Lollo et al. 1982) and in the retrieval of information from primary, secondary, and tertiary memory (Anders and Fozard 1973; Madden 1985). The capacity of primary memory (e.g., digit span) is relatively constant as a function of age, whereas a significant age-related decline occurs in the capacity of secondary memory. Consequently, aging appears to exert a profound effect on the acquisition and retrieval of new information in secondary memory. The age-related decline in memory performance, however, is most evident in tasks that are episodic, in the sense of referring to a particular study context or episode (e.g., a recently presented list of words or pictures). When the memory test is semantic, in the sense of referring to facts or knowledge that is relatively context-independent, age differences are typically either less pronounced or absent (Burke et al. 2000; Wingfield and Stine-Morrow 2000).

Attention

Age-related changes in attention are important to theories of cognitive aging, because the explanation of so many forms of cognitive performance—ranging from memory to skill acquisition—involves the concept of attention in some way. As with memory, the investigation of attentional processes has been an active area of cognitive aging research (for reviews, see Hartley 1992; Madden and Whiting, in press; McDowd and Shaw 2000). A fundamental distinction in this research is between selective attention and divided attention. In the former, the relevant and irrelevant sources of information are defined during task performance, allowing attention to be focused selectively on the relevant information. In the latter, multiple sources of information are relevant and must be attended simultaneously.

The general conclusion from research in this area is that age-related decline is more pronounced when attention must be divided or switched among several relevant stimulus inputs or tasks, as compared with conditions in which attention is focused on a single task or input. This decline appears in different forms in relation to task demands and the type of mental set (i.e., preparation) required for task performance. For example, older adults' performance is differentially impaired by the requirement to maintain two different types of task sets in working memory (Kray and Lindenberger 2000), to update the currently relevant task set (Mayr 2001), or to generate and execute two similar motor programs simultaneously (Hartley 2001). In contrast, several investigators have reported that older adults' selective attention performance (e.g., the use of advance information regarding the location or color of a target item) is virtually as efficient as that of younger adults (Hartley et al. 1990; Madden et al. 1999a; Plude and Hoyer 1986). This pattern of results has led to the view that older adults' ability to guide attention to task-relevant information is relatively preserved. Previous studies of age-related differences in selective attention, however, have nearly always used a mixture of different forms of attentional guidance (Wolfe 1998): top-down (endogenous, cognitively driven) and bottom-up (exogenous, stimulus driven) components. Some initial evidence indicates an age-related decline in top-down attentional guidance (Folk and Lincourt 1996). Thus, the differential degree of age-related change and constancy in attentional functioning remains an active area of investigation.

Understanding and Remembering Written Information

Understanding communication abilities is pertinent to our understanding of everyday cognition of older adults. Siegler (1980), Siegler and Poon (1989), Poon and Siegler (1991), and Siegler et al. (1996) provided reviews of these areas. These reviews showed the following:

- Earlier studies showed substantial age-related deficits in discourse, text, or prose processing among older adults.
- The next generations of research focused on the influence and contributions of the individual, the properties of the text to be processed, and the task demand on the observed processing performance. These studies found that these variables all can inhibit or facilitate performances of older adults.
- The level of education and verbal intelligence could account for some portion of the observed age effects on text recall performance.
- Older adults have been shown to have deficits in auditory processing in laboratory settings; however, older

adults do not seem to have disproportionate problems in processing everyday conversations or spoken input from television or radio. Peripheral hearing deficits may have an adverse effect on the understanding of conversations among adults with no central deficits.

- Tests of performance in everyday problem-solving tasks show that middle-aged adults can, in some situations, perform better than young adults, but performance decline remains evident for the older adults.
- Traditional laboratory-based problem-solving tasks seem to be predictive of everyday problem-solving performances for older adults.

For further updates on these areas, see Zacks et al. (2000) and Salthouse (2000).

Neuroimaging and Neuroscience

Neuropsychological research on aging is covered in Chapter 11, "Neuropsychological Assessment of Dementia," and age-related changes in brain morphology are summarized in Chapter 4, "Neuroanatomy, Neurophysiology, and Neuropathology of Aging." In this section, we briefly note some of the implications of neuroimaging and neuroscience research for understanding normal aging.

Research in neuropsychology has contributed to the understanding of normal aging through broad-based neurobehavioral studies of healthy elderly individuals and patients with cognitive syndromes (such as Alzheimer's disease) whose symptoms are often confused with normal aging processes. To separate normal age changes from disease effects, investigators often use longitudinal evaluation to confirm diagnostic placement (Flicker et al. 1993; Katzman et al. 1989), including, when possible, neuropathological verification (Hof et al. 1992; Morris et al. 1991). The interpretation of cognitive decline associated with Alzheimer's disease must be done with caution, however, because the variance in performance associated with Alzheimer's disease on a particular neuropsychological measure is likely shared with performance on other behavioral measures (Salthouse and Becker 1998). Researchers in this field also have taken advantage of the advances in neuroimaging to enhance diagnostic accuracy (Rapoport 1991). Excellent reviews of geriatric neuropsychology can be found in Albert and Moss (1988), Huppert (1994), Poon (1986), and Van Gorp and Mahler (1990).

Most studies involving examination of the cognitive changes associated with aging have focused on one functional domain in isolation—memory, intellect, or attention, for example. Studies focusing on multiple domains simultaneously, as is possible with broad-based neuropsychological designs, have provided some insight into how these different areas of information-processing functions interact and change with aging of the nervous system (Van Gorp and Mahler 1990). In one important early study (Benton et al. 1981), a large sample of normal older adults participated in a battery of neuropsychological tests. The results showed little evidence of generalized decline in cognitive function before age 80. Significant declines were seen in short-term visual memory, serial digit learning, and facial recognition. Subsequent studies have supported the findings that these particular functions (construction, speed of information processing, and nonverbal perceptual processing) are vulnerable to aging (Koss et al. 1991). Similarly, in studies that used the Wechsler Adult Intelligence Scales (WAIS, WAIS-R), selective decline in nonverbal performance and relative stability in verbal abilities were seen with advancing age (Botwinick 1977; Salthouse 1991).

Several interpretations have been proposed regarding the functional and anatomical significance of these findings. One interpretation is that age-associated degenerative changes are lateralized to the right hemisphere (Goldstein and Shelly 1981; Klisz 1978; Schaie and Schaie 1977). This hypothesis is based primarily on the observation that right hemisphere brain lesions often produce a discrepancy between verbal and nonverbal performance similar to that seen in aging individuals (Benton 1994; Lezak 1983). Neuroanatomical and neuroimaging studies of normal older adults, however, failed to show preferential deterioration of right hemisphere structures (Brody 1978; Coffey et al. 1992; Gur et al. 1987; Parashos and Coffey 1994; Welsh and Hoffman 1996). In addition, many investigators have pointed out that the nonverbal subtests of the WAIS/WAIS-R, used as evidence of right hemisphere function, are confounded by their reliance on speed of responding, thereby rendering them less than ideal for comparisons of right and left hemisphere integrity (Mittenberg et al. 1989). Thus, the more pronounced age-related decline on nonverbal psychometric tests may reflect the differential sensitivity of fluid versus crystallized abilities. An important component of this age-related decline in fluid ability is a slowing of elementary perceptual processing (Salthouse 1991). The results of at least two studies based on factor analysis of a broad-based neuropsychological assessment suggested that speed of information processing is a major determinant of age-related changes in performance (Koss et al. 1991; Van Gorp et al. 1990).

Although no specific hemispheric lateralization is predicted by the speed of processing model, the relevant fluid abilities (such as novel problem solving, attention, and perceptual-motor integration) all have been ascribed in the neuropsychological literature to frontal lobe function (Benton 1994; Lezak 1983). A current hypothesis, supported by converging lines of evidence from neuropsychology and cognitive psychology, is that normal aging leads to differentially greater declines in frontal lobe neocortex and interconnected subcortical brain structures (Raz 2000; Rubin 1999; West 1996). In line with this notion, neuropsychological changes reported in frontal lobe damage have been observed in normal aging (Huppert 1994; Van Gorp et al. 1990; Whelihan and Lesher 1985). In contrast, other cognitive changes—such as rapid forgetting—typically associated with Alzheimer's disease and mesial temporal lobe dysfunction (Welsh et al. 1991) are not typical of normal aging (Ivnik et al. 1991; Petersen et al. 1992; Welsh et al. 1994). However, again, caution in interpreting the psychometric data is warranted because age-related variance is shared across a wide range of neuropsychological tests (Salthouse et al. 1996).

More recently, a rapid development of research has applied neuroimaging techniques to investigate the changes in perceptual and cognitive functioning associated with aging. These techniques include measures of brain structure from computed tomography (CT) and magnetic resonance imaging (MRI), as well as functional measures of regional cerebral blood flow and other metabolic variables from positron emission tomography (PET) and functional MRI (fMRI). Reviews of this research are provided by Madden and Hoffman (1997), Grady (1998), Raz (2000), and Cabeza (2001). The neuroimaging research has provided some support for the frontal lobe hypothesis. Whereas generalized brain atrophy and decreases in resting cerebral blood flow with advanced age have been commonly noted (Raz 2000), some investigators report particularly pronounced reductions in frontal lobe blood flow (Gur et al. 1987) and volume (Coffey et al. 1992; Raz et al. 1997) in older adults. Demyelination of subcortical, periventricular brain structures is also common in aging and is associated with signs of frontal lobe deficits on neuropsychological examination (Boone et al. 1992; Coffey et al. 1992; Schmidt et al. 1993). Finally, histopathological studies show selective frontal lobe decline in the aging brain, with the most significant cell loss identified in the superior frontal, precentral, and superior temporal gyri (Creasey and Rapoport 1985; Haug et al. 1983).

Neuroimaging research also has focused on investigating the functional brain changes associated with aging in the absence of significant disease. Participants in this type of research are generally carefully screened, either through neuropsychological testing or through structural neuro-

imaging, and thus the changes that are observed are a conservative estimate of the age-related changes expected in the general population. This research is in its early stages, and methodology and interpretive issues are evolving rapidly. Much of the research has used a subtraction design in which the pattern of neural activation occurring during a specific cognitive task (e.g., read a list of words to be recalled later) is compared with a control condition (e.g., word reading without a memory requirement), so that specific cognitive processes can be isolated.

Age-related changes in frontal lobe functioning also have been implicated in this research. During memory retrieval tasks, in particular, it appears that younger adults show activation selectively in the prefrontal cortex of the right hemisphere, whereas older adults are more likely to activate left prefrontal cortex as well (Cabeza et al. 1997; Madden et al. 1999b). Thus, older adults' prefrontal activation during memory tasks may actually be more extensive than that of younger adults, perhaps as a result of compensatory processes. These latter processes would involve the recruitment of additional neural regions, outside of the task-relevant pathway, to support task performance. Age-related decline in activation also has been observed, particularly for functioning of occipitotemporal regions during perceptual processing (Grady et al. 1994; Madden et al. 1996). Interpretation of what appears to be an age-related decline in activation, however, is complicated by the fact that older adults may show higher levels of activation in the easier task conditions rather than lower activation in the more difficult conditions (Madden et al. 2002). In addition, the level of noise in the hemodynamic signal measured by PET and fMRI appears to be higher for older adults than for younger adults (D'Esposito et al. 1999; Huettel et al. 2001).

Applications

In addition to understanding the neurological correlates of age-related changes in cognition, neuroimaging has a ready-made application to further understand the efficacy of some cognitive intervention strategies. For example, studies comparing highly active and nonactive older adults showed that cognitive functions were also higher in adults who regularly engaged in exercise (e.g., Abourezk 1989; Dustman et al. 1990; Spirduso 1975; Spirduso and Clifford 1978). These findings are controversial in that some longitudinal exercise intervention studies with older adults showed that cognition can be improved with exercise (e.g., Dustman et al. 1984), but others showed no effects (e.g., Blumenthal and Madden 1988; Blumenthal et al. 1989). Several hypotheses on the exercise-cognition relation can be tested by the use of neuroimaging. For example, Kramer et al. (2002) postulated that because aging affects the frontal and prefrontal areas of the brain, improved aerobic fitness may activate these areas that may improve cognitive functioning. Similarly, Dustman and his colleagues (1984, 1990) noted that decreased cognitive functioning can be due to lower levels of blood flow and oxygenation to the brain, and improved aerobic fitness can overcome some of the cognitive deficits. These are fruitful research areas that can have direct benefits for older adults.

Aside from the basic science work in cognition, there has been increased interest in the everyday applications of cognitive processes for decision making, particularly in the area of risk perceptions that may guide medical and financial decision making, where poor decisions will have potentially serious consequences. Peters et al. (2000) reviewed the theoretical underpinnings of research in decision making. This is also important clinically because the older person may not be in the best position to make decisions about his or her own care and may require the input of concerned family members. Aldwin and Brustrom (1997) discussed the role of older couples, who adapt as a unit and are often involved in joint decision making. This increases in complexity when adult children are also involved.

Behavioral Medicine and Health and Behavior Relationships

Behavioral medicine seeks to understand the role that psychosocial factors play in medicine as well as the effect of specific physical illnesses on psychological functioning. Most physical disorders have behavioral aspects, which have been recently reviewed (see Smith et al. 2002). Age has a special role to play in understanding these relationships. Age may be a proxy for physical conditions in ways that make it difficult to interpret findings of age differences in psychological performance directly. Treating and controlling the medical condition in an older person often can make the age differences seem much less important (for reviews, see Manuck et al. 2000; Matthews 2000; Siegler et al. 2002, 2003a; R.B. Williams 2000a, 2000b). It is important to keep in mind that the burden of illness is not distributed evenly according to social class. House and co-workers (1992) have shown that 75-year-old persons of upper socioeconomic status (SES) have about 1.5 chronic conditions per person, the level that is reached in the lower SES ranges at about ages 42–43. Thus, the issue of individual differences in health status

is starting to be recognized in the psychology of aging (Siegler 1989, 1990). This recognition helped to form the basis of the health disparities work. The basis for these cultural differences is not well understood (Whitfield et al. 2002a, 2002b).

Health and Disease Interact With Intellectual and Cognitive Functioning

Research on intellectual functioning has one of the longest and most productive records in the psychology of aging. As noted previously, a consistent finding from this research is that crystallized abilities, or knowledge acquired in the course of the socialization process, tend to remain stable over the adult life span, whereas fluid abilities, or abilities involved in the solution of novel problems, tend to decline gradually from younger to older adulthood (Schaie 1990). Changes in cognitive functioning, especially those in the less expected crystallized domains, have been associated with earlier death (Bosworth and Siegler 2002). Disease and pathology exert profound effects on intellectual functioning. For example, in reviewing the role of age compared with particular health conditions in the Framingham population, Elias et al. (2000) compared the adjusted odds ratios (ORs) of performing at or below the twenty-fifth percentile on the Framingham neuropsychological test measurements, controlling for education, occupation, gender, alcohol consumption, history of cardiovascular disease, and antihypertensive treatment. They found that age itself was the strongest factor; getting 5 years older increased the odds to 1.61 of performing at or below the twenty-fifth percentile on a battery of neuropsychological tests, compared with having type II diabetes (OR = 1.21) or an increase in diastolic blood pressure of 10 mm Hg (OR = 1.30) (Siegler et al. 2002, 2003a, 2003b; Waldstein 2000). Zelinski et al. (1998) provided an excellent review of the literature on specific diseases on cognition and also reported on data from an ongoing national survey that had some measures of cognitive status and of health conditions; although these measures are not as good as those that can be assessed on direct examination, the data are quite remarkable for national survey data.

Modern work in neuropsychology and experimental psychology now routinely separates persons by age as well as by diagnosis and thus provides data on each component of functioning. This is an important advance in our study of cognitive aging. In studies of cognition and aging prior to the 1980s, participants' pathological status (e.g., dementia and depression) generally was not screened (other than general reported health). A consequence was that participants with early dementia might have been included in the "normal" samples of older adults; age-related differences might have been overestimated in these studies. Although only a limited number of studies have been done on the influence of pathology and functions on cognitive processes of the oldest old, some evidence cautions the generalization or projection of findings from data obtained from participants from 65–85 years (young-old) to 85 years and older (old-old) (Poon et al. 1992b). For example, prevalence of dementia of the Alzheimer's type is projected to double every 5 years after age 65, and 360,000 new cases will occur each year. This number will increase as the population ages (National Institute on Aging 2000). It is projected that all or most individuals who reach age 100 would have dementia. Centenarian studies from around the world (Poon 2001) have shown that about a quarter to a third of living centenarians may not have dementia and have maintained significant cognitive functions. If these studies are correct, then the trajectory of dementia over time may not be accurate for these long-lived individuals. Furthermore, cognition and functional capacities are closely related, with age, health, and diseases as potential contributing factors. These interactions are not clearly understood at present, but they should be important priority research areas.

Health and Self-Rated Health

Since Mossey and Shapiro (1982) found that self-ratings of health were predictive of 7-year survival among elderly adults, there has been an enhanced interest in the use of self-rated health (usually measured by asking respondents whether they would rate their health as excellent, very good, good, fair, or poor) as a measure of health status. Self-rated health is a specific component of health-related quality of life and also reflects psychological well-being (George and Clipp 1991; Hooker and Siegler 1992). To better interpret studies that use self-ratings of health, it is important to remember that 1) these findings will have an SES gradient related to timing and quality of medical care such that a more severe disease profile will tend to be seen earlier in the life cycle in the disadvantaged (Anderson and Armstead 1995; House et al. 1992); 2) the reports will be related to cognitive status because individuals need to remember what the diagnosis is to be able to report it; 3) the reports will be related to psychological symptoms because individuals are more

likely to seek medical care if symptomatic (Costa and McCrae 1985); and 4) the self-rated measures will be more highly correlated with psychosocial constructs that are also associated with the same underlying dimensions of personality (Siegler et al. 2003a).

Personality and Aging in the Social Context

Contrary to popular conceptions that personality changes dramatically throughout adulthood, several longitudinal studies have shown remarkable stability over long periods of the life span (Costa and McCrae 1989; Pederson and Reynolds 1998). Even cross-sectional studies that reflect differences between age groups failed to show striking change past age 30 (Costa et al. 1986). In contrast to adulthood and later years when changes in personality are subtle, substantial changes in personality occur at ages 18–30 (McCrae et al. 2000).

Recent findings from more than a dozen different countries indicate that these changes are not confined to North American samples. McCrae and colleagues (1999, 2000) found a consistency in the pattern of change during this age period. The American pattern of declines on the dimensions of neuroticism, extraversion, and openness to experience and increases in agreeableness and conscientiousness was consistently replicated in various cultures and nations, suggesting that these cross-sectional age differences were due to intrinsic maturational processes.

Despite its popularity and trendiness, the midlife period until recently has been relatively neglected. This situation has been dramatically rectified by two published reports on the University of North Carolina Alumni Heart Study (Siegler et al. 1992). More than 2,200 middle-aged University of North Carolina Alumni Heart Study participants were studied over a 6- to 9-year follow-up period. Rank-order or retest stability coefficients were uniformly high and large in magnitude for all personality traits. Also, mean levels showed only slight declines on the domains of neuroticism, extraversion, openness, and conscientiousness and no significant changes on the domain of agreeableness (Costa et al. 2000).

Analyses of life events showed that personality was largely resilient and uninfluenced by the sheer occurrence of positive or negative events. Costa et al. (2000) suggested that promising directions for future research concern events that influence or affect key aspects of self-concept or identity such as job loss or changes in marital status. The latter event led to the most significant changes, and the effects were different for men and women: "divorce seemed to be liberating for women and demoralizing for men" (Costa et al. 2000, p. 377). Another interesting finding from the University of North Carolina Alumni Heart Study data showed that people who felt that their personality had changed a good deal over a 6-year period had higher scores on the domains of neuroticism and openness to experience at baseline (Herbst et al. 2000). This finding is consistent with previous research in behavioral medicine showing that individuals with high neuroticism scores overreport or make many somatic complaints. These new data complement that picture by suggesting that perceived personality changes may be predicted from particularly emotional and imaginative individuals. Personality also can influence response to stressors. Patrick and Hayden (1999) examined the role of neuroticism in the prediction of coping and well-being for older mothers caring for adult children with chronic disabilities—either mental retardation or mental illness. They reported a complex structural model that indicated that neuroticism had both direct and indirect effects in terms of perceptions of the stressors and choice of coping mechanisms.

Personality Disorders

Advances in understanding personality from the aging literature have led to linkages to psychopathology, particularly personality disorders. The influence of the five-factor model in particular is spurring efforts to reconceptualize personality disorders as maladaptive variants of normal personality traits that are present in all individuals to varying degrees (Costa and Widiger 1994). Personality disorders were thought to age out and have little effect on older persons.

Recent clinical experience and study reflect the prevalence of personality disorders in older people; the roles they play in the onset, course, and treatment outcomes of other emotional, cognitive, and physical problems; and the lifelong continuity of these disorders (Costa et al. 1999; Rosowsky et al. 1999). An interesting area for future research might be to examine whether disordered personality patterns (i.e., personality disorders, especially borderline personality disorder) might mask or be mistaken for the disruption of Alzheimer's disease.

Does Alzheimer's Disease Cause Personality Change?

It has long been held that dementia affects characteristics, such as motivation, mood, and impulse control; however, assessment has been impaired by lack of a com-

prehensive model of personality to guide systematic study and difficulties in assessing personality among impaired patients.

An observer-rating form of the Revised NEO Personality Inventory (NEO-PI-R), a measure of the five-factor model, has been used to study some acute and chronic brain conditions or dementing diseases such as Alzheimer's disease and Parkinson's disease (Dawson et al. 2001; Siegler 2000). A series of studies by Siegler and colleagues (1991, 1994) that gathered information from caregivers and family members showed that patients with Alzheimer's disease undergo significant changes in personality—namely, they have diminished capacity for organization, punctuality, dependability, goal-setting, and planning. These results were clearly replicated in two other studies (Chatterjee et al. 1992; Welleford et al. 1995).

It is interesting to note that the neuroanatomical changes that accompany the progression of Alzheimer's disease profoundly affect planning and goal-directed behavior while leaving intact the quality of interpersonal orientation. As Costa and McCrae (2000) pointed out, studies of personality correlates of disease may offer insights into brain-behavior relationships, and a comparison of personality changes across many different disorders would be particularly informative.

Coping in Later Life

Lazarus (1998) examined age differences in coping by considering what older people must face in their lives. He writes from the perspective of his current age (76; see p. 112) and a long history of his own research in the area. He notes that compared with developmental changes in late life, the task is to "preserve endangered functions as much as possible in the face of increasing physical and mental losses" (p. 114). Basically, however, the process of coping with aging is a holding action designed to actualize personal values and goals that remain viable (p. 115).

Additionally, coping in later life is related to adaptive coping strategies such as spirituality, passive forbearance, positive appraisal, and reappraisal of negative situations (Chang et al. 1998; Diehl et al. 1996; Ellison 1995; Krause and Van Tran 1989; Levin 1994; Levin et al. 1995) that individuals have acquired throughout the life course. Researchers have found that older persons have higher levels of internal control and less emotional reactivity when faced with stress than do younger adults (Diehl et al. 1996; Lawton et al. 1992). Findings show that religious affiliation and involvement and strong spiritual beliefs serve to offset and buffer the negative effects of some life experiences such as health problems that are experienced in later life. In their study of the effects of religion on health status and life satisfaction, Levin et al. (1995) found that individuals who perceived themselves as religious had greater life satisfaction. In a study examining the health protective behaviors of black elderly women, Wilson-Ford (1992) found that more than 90% of the respondents in her study used relaxation, prayer, or the act of living by religious principles to protect their health. Idler (1987) found that the more religiosity a woman had, the less physically disabled or depressed she was likely to be.

The sociohistorical context of a group can shape coping strategies in later life, especially among groups that have been marginalized within this culture. For example, African Americans have had a long history of using spirituality and religious activity as coping strategies in the face of adversity and oppression (Billingsley 1992; Ellison 1995; Taylor and Chatters 1986). Other marginalized groups such as Native Americans and Hispanics also have used religion and spirituality as coping resources, which can be seen as a response to marginalization and oppression and the subsequent lack of access to other resources. Neighbors et al. (1983) reported that marginalized minority groups, unlike whites, used more religious coping when faced with problems, and they expressed greater satisfaction in using religion as a coping strategy.

Although the evidence is mixed regarding the effects of religiosity and spirituality on physical and emotional health outcomes, some research suggests that religious beliefs and practices are related to higher levels of well-being (Koenig et al. 1989) and lower levels of depression (Idler 1987; Miller 1998). It could be suggested from the available evidence that we have not adequately measured the positive effects of religiosity and spirituality on well-being in later life. Anecdotal information from minority elders illustrates that they have used spirituality throughout their adult lives as a major coping strategy, and they perceive great benefits, often intangible, from their strong sense of faith and their religious practices. Few studies, however, have examined the effects of these religious and spiritual experiences and practices on well-being in later life from a life course.

Social Interactions and Attributions

Research on the social nature of later life has reemerged with the publication of Carstensen's (1991) view of selectivity theory as a replacement for the disengagement/activity controversy of old. The term *selectivity* refers to the fact that social interactions are chosen for specific reasons and functions in later life. Rook (2000) reviewed the progression from disengagement to socioemotional selectivity and provided important theoretical perspectives that help to explain declines in participation that may be unrelated to well-being and the result of adaptive strategies on the part of the older person. Many social losses are far from voluntary and include widowhood, deaths of significant others, increasing disability, and forced relocations required to obtain needed supportive and medical care for many older persons. Rook suggests that research is needed on processes of substitution and compensation and suggests that the next generation of research should focus on the individual differences in strategies used.

There has been a developing interest in the role of social support as a moderating variable in the lives of middle-aged and older persons. Studies show a strong relation between the presence of social support and health, primarily in terms of survival (House et al. 1988). Berkman and colleagues (1993) reviewed the interactions between social support and both cardiovascular disease and mortality. They found that similar patterns of social support existed for men and women and noted equal consequences for lowered social support for both sexes. Several studies confirmed our expectation that a strong social support system is related positively to physical and mental health and to survival among middle-aged and older persons with heart disease (R. B. Williams et al. 1992). Data from a longitudinal study in Sweden indicated that social support also may protect against the development of dementia in older persons (Wang et al. 2002).

The benefits of a social support system in later life, however, may vary across different racial and ethnic groups. This variation often reflects the historical and social development of interpersonal relationships within groups, particularly in families. The long-standing history of racial discrimination against African Americans, issues of immigration and acculturation for Hispanics and Asians, and experiences of isolation and oppression for Native Americans in the United States can either hinder or foster social support systems in later life (Dilworth-Anderson and Burton 1999). For example, the history of discrimination against African Americans, in part, has fostered strong extended family support systems that have traditionally cared for all dependent persons within the family (Franklin 1997). At the same time, growing evidence suggests that the ability of African American families to maintain these support systems is being challenged by contemporary demographic and social changes (e.g., population aging, geographic mobility, and decreases in multigenerational households) (McDonald and Armstrong 2001; Roschelle 1997). Such changes in the social support systems of older persons may have a negative effect on their well-being because of their economic and social vulnerability and dependency.

Caregiving Issues in the Normal Psychology of Aging

Recognition of caregiving issues in patients with Alzheimer's disease has been long-standing (see E. Light et al. 1994, which was based on presentations given in 1990) because one could do so little for the patients. In cancer, now that there are increases in cancer survivorship and the need for palliative care (Foley and Gelband 2001), a caregiving literature is developing.

Variations in Caregiving

When examined within a cultural context, findings also show that the negative effects of caregiving can vary across racial and ethnic groups. Furthermore, findings show that depression and burden are higher among white caregivers than among African American caregivers, depression is similar between white caregivers and Hispanic caregivers, and burden is similar between Hispanic caregivers and African American caregivers. Researchers have suggested that these differences may be related to the appraisal of the caregiving situation across diverse groups. For example, African American caregivers tend to use more positive reappraisal than white caregivers when faced with the difficulty of caring for a dependent elder (Farran et al. 1997; Haley et al. 1996; Knight and McCallum 1998; Knight et al. 2000; Wood and Parham 1990). In particular, Haley et al. (1996) reported that African American caregivers appraised self-care, memory, and behavior problems of older care recipients as less stressful than did white caregivers. These researchers also found that caregivers' appraisals and other coping responses mediated the effects of race on well-being. Other evidence (Hinrichsen and Ramirez 1992) has shown that African American and white caregivers had similar use of appraisal when faced with stressful caregiving situations. Picot (1995) reported that African American caregivers who appraised greater caregiving rewards were most likely to be older and have lower levels of education.

Other researchers suggested that variations in caregiving may reflect the different norms and values across ethnic groups about reciprocity (giving back), filial obligation, and a sense of responsibility for providing care to older family members. Findings show that specific cultural values and norms in Hispanic (Clark and Huttlinger

1998; Cox and Monk 1993), Korean (Youn et al. 1999), Native American (Hennessy and John 1996; Strong 1984), Chinese (Ishii-Kuntz 1997), and African American families (Dilworth-Anderson et al. 1999) governed familial relationships and care provision for older family members. For example, Korean families have specific beliefs about familial roles, unlike those found among white families, wherein daughters-in-law are expected to serve as primary caregivers to their mothers- and fathers-in-law (Youn et al. 1999). Additional findings show that American Indians (Hennessy and John 1996) and African Americans (Nkongho and Archbold 1995; S. Williams and Dilworth-Anderson 2002) strongly value giving back to those who have provided for them in the past. Because of their influence on coping processes, cultural values, norms, and beliefs may indirectly affect well-being of elders and their caregivers.

Caregiving is a multigenerational problem, and the effects are not limited to caring for spouses and parents with Alzheimer's disease. Elderly persons may be caring for their adult children who have chronic mental illnesses or have survived into adulthood with mental retardation. The parents, who are still in the caregiving role, may be unable to maintain that role as their own marital or health status changes. Clinicians of both generations need to help families deal with these problems, which can be expected to increase in complexity with the aging of the family and increased community care of impaired adults. Lefley and Hatfield (1999) present an excellent summary of the issues from the point of view of family members of both adult generations and provide guidance to the clinicians who treat them. Dyck et al. (1999) studied middle-aged persons caring for relatives with schizophrenia and found that the stress levels were high and the effects equally serious. Seltzer et al. (1995) found that mothers of mentally ill adult children are worse off than are mothers of retarded adults. Greenberg et al. (1999) reported on differences in siblings of adults with disabling illnesses and found that siblings of mentally retarded adults are more likely to expect to provide care for them when the parents are unable to do so than are siblings of mentally impaired adults. As the population continues to age and care is shifted to the community, these issues will increase in complexity.

Interventions for Reducing the Stress on Caregivers

Regardless of the background of the caregivers (e.g., ethnicity or education) or the relationship between the caregiver and the care recipient (e.g., spouse, adult child, or sibling), caregiving to dependent older persons can be stressful. Research shows that caregiving can put the health of the caregiver at risk, especially among older spouse caregivers (Schulz and Beach 1999; Vitaliano et al. 1998, 2002). Telephone interventions have been found to be increasingly effective and are well suited to elderly persons for whom transportation to sites of care is often a problem, particularly so for those with caregiving responsibilities. Interventions to reduce the stress on the caregiver and to reduce the incidence of physical illness are needed. Interventions that are culturally sensitive and that reflect the norms, values, and customs of a people are also very useful and effective. These interventions typically integrate the language, food customs, and beliefs of a group.

Longevity and the Extreme Aged

In the study of the long-lived and longevity, a fundamental challenge is to understand *how* the oldest-old live longer and *what* specific biological, psychological, and sociological characteristics they possess that would allow them to survive longer (Lehr 1991; Poon et al. 1997). Another basic challenge is whether we could generalize the knowledge gained in our volumes of aging research on individuals of average life span (in their 70s) (e.g., the MacArthur Study, Rowe and Kahn 1998) to individuals who live 20–30 years longer. Studies of centenarians and the oldest-old remain a rarity within gerontological research (Vaupel et al. 1998), but interest in this area has increased steadily over the past 20 years (Lehr 1991; Poon et al. 1997). Completed studies conducted in the United States (e.g., Perls 1997; Poon et al. 1992a), Japan (e.g., Chan et al. 1997), Italy (e.g., Capurso et al. 1997), Hungary (Regius et al. 1994), France (Allard et al. 1994), Sweden (Samuelsson et al. 1997), Finland, and Denmark (Jeune and Kannisto 1997) have provided a foundation for further hypothesis testing. Centenarian studies have identified several characteristics associated with longevity. For example, food preferences (Fischer et al. 1995), marital status (Samuelsson et al. 1997), personal and coping strategies (Martin et al. 1992), levels of family support (Capurso et al. 1997), and education (Poon et al. 1992a; Ravaglia et al. 1997) all have been linked with successful late-life aging. However, the robustness of these findings awaits further research because of variations from different centenarian studies in sampling strategies, subject selection, and research methods. For example, the Georgia Centenarian Study examined community-dwelling and cognitively intact centenarians,

who are estimated to be about 20%–30% of the centenarian population. The findings await generalization to the other 70% of centenarians as well as research on predictors that could differentiate functional differences among centenarians.

Aging Well

For many individuals, old age is really just an extended phase of middle age, with only modest changes in mind and body. Furthermore, adaptation to these changes is well within the range of an individual's capability, and the use of certain behavioral strategies can help to maintain this optimistic pattern of successful aging (Rowe and Kahn 1998; Vaillant 2002). However, there is another side of the story—what might be called "the Grim Side of Gerontology." Cassel and co-workers (1992), in an article titled "The Price of Success," discussed the implications of the survival of frail elderly persons. A new movement is now concerned with care at the end of life. This palliative care movement seeks to provide comfort rather than cure at the end of life and recognizes that many survive frail. A psychology of aging of the frail elder has yet to emerge beyond those dealing with measures of functional health, most probably because the measurement problems are so daunting.

Changes in the 1990s indicate that cohorts who are becoming elderly are more elite because of better education and medical care earlier in their life cycle; also, elderly cohorts are living longer and spending more time in both active and impaired life expectancy. At the same time, variance resulting from differential treatment of ethnic and minority populations indicates that changes due to advanced education are not found in all groups that are currently aging. Thus, we may be reaching a new time in history when we need a psychology of normal aging for the frail and for the nonfrail elderly, with particular attention paid to the details of the life histories of the persons being studied and/or treated. As life expectancy increases, it becomes clear that very different subgroups exist among the elderly. Variations in health, rather than age, may be responsible for a large portion of observed age differences up to around age 85. These age/health interactions may be mediated by social class such that health disparities are apparent at younger ages for minority populations.

Age 85 and older, or what Paul Baltes (2002) would describe as the "Fourth Age," is no longer the province of "happy gerontology." Real declines in functioning and associated adaptive challenges are normative for most, but not all, who survive to be the extreme aged.

References

Abourezk T: The effects of regular aerobic exercise on short-term memory efficiency in the older adult, in Aging and Motor Behavior. Edited by Ostrow AC. Indianapolis, IN, Benchmark Press, 1989, pp 105–114

Albert MS, Moss M: Geriatric Neuropsychology. New York, Guilford, 1988

Aldwin CM, Brustrom J: Theories of coping with chronic stress: illustrations from the health psychology and aging literatures, in Coping With Chronic Stress. Edited by Gottlieb BH. New York, Plenum, 1997, pp 75–103

Allard M, Lèbre V, Robine J-M: Les 120 ans de Jeanne Calment, doyenne de l'humanité. Paris, Le Cherche Midi Editeur, 1994

Anders TR, Fozard JL: Effects of age upon retrieval from primary and secondary memory. Dev Psychol 9:411–415, 1973

Anderson NA, Armstead CA: Toward understanding the association of socioeconomic status and health: a new challenge for the bio-psychosocial approach. Psychosom Med 57:213–225, 1995

Balota DA, Dolan PO, Duchek JM: Memory changes in healthy older adults, in The Oxford Handbook of Memory. Edited by Tulving E, Craik FIM. Oxford, UK, Oxford University Press, 2000, pp 395–408

Baltes PB: Mastering the challenges of aging: towards a general theory of adaptive development. George Maddox Award Lecture, Duke University, Durham, NC, March 2002

Benton AL: Neuropsychological assessment. Annu Rev Psychol 45:1–23, 1994

Benton AL, Eslinger RJ, Damasio AR: Normative observations on neuropsychological test performances in old age. J Clin Neuropsychol 3:33–42, 1981

Berkman LF, Vaccarion V, Seeman T: Gender differences in cardiovascular morbidity and mortality: the contribution of social networks and social support. Ann Behav Med 15:112–117, 1993

Billingsley A: Climbing Jacob's Ladder: The Enduring Legacy of African American Families. New York, Simon & Schuster, 1992

Blumenthal JA, Madden DJ: Effects of aerobic training, age, and physical fitness on memory-search performance. Psychol Aging 3:280–285, 1988

Blumenthal JA, Emery CF, Madden DJ, et al: Cardiovascular and behavioral effects of aerobic exercise training in healthy older men and women. J Gerontol 44:147–157, 1989

Boone KB, Miller BL, Lesser IM, et al: Neuropsychological correlates of white-matter lesions in healthy elderly subjects: a threshold effect. Arch Neurol 49:549–554, 1992

Bosworth HB, Siegler IC: Terminal change in cognitive function: an updated review of longitudinal studies. Exp Aging Res 28:299–315, 2002

Botwinick J: Intellectual abilities, in The Handbook of the Psychology of Aging. Edited by Birren JE, Schaie KW. New York, Van Nostrand Reinhold, 1977, pp 580–605

Bowles NL, Poon LW: An analysis of the effect of aging on recognition memory. J Gerontol 37:212–219, 1982

Brody H: Cell counts in cerebral cortex and brainstem, in Alzheimer's Disease: Senile Dementia and Related Disorders. Edited by Katzman R, Terry RD, Bick KL. New York, Raven, 1978, pp 345–351

Burke DM, MacKay DG, James LE: Theoretical approaches to language and aging, in Models of Cognitive Aging. Edited by Perfect TJ, Maylor EA. Oxford, UK, Oxford University Press, 2000, pp 204–237

Cabeza R: Functional neuroimaging of cognitive aging, in Handbook of Functional Neuroimaging of Cognition. Edited by Cabeza R, Kingstone A. Cambridge, MA, MIT Press, 2001, pp 331–377

Cabeza R, Grady CL, Nyberg L, et al: Age-related differences in neural activity during memory encoding and retrieval: a positron emission tomography study. J Neurosci 17:391–400, 1997

Capurso A, Resta F, Damelio A, et al: Epidemiological and socioeconomic aspects of Italian centenarians. Arch Gerontol Geriatr 25:149–157, 1997

Carstensen LL: Selectivity theory: social activity in a life-span context, in Annual Review of Gerontology and Geriatrics, Vol 11. Edited by Schaie KW, Lawton MP. New York, Springer, 1991, pp 195–217

Cassel CK, Rudberg MA, Olshansky SJ: The price of success: health care in an aging society. Health Aff (Millwood) (Summer):87–99, 1992

Cattell RB: Theory of fluid and crystallized intelligence: a critical experiment. J Educ Psychol 45:1–22, 1963

Chan YC, Suzuki M, Yamamoto S: Nutritional status of centenarians assessed by activity and anthropometric, hematological and biochemical characteristics. J Nutr Sci Vitaminol (Tokyo) 43:73–81, 1997

Chang B, Noonan AE, Tennstedt SL: The role of religion/spirituality in coping with caregiving for disabled elders. Gerontologist 38:463–470, 1998

Chatterjee A, Strauss ME, Smyth KA, et al: Personality change in Alzheimer's disease. Arch Neurol 49:486–491, 1992

Clark M, Huttlinger K: Elder care among Mexican American families. Clin Nurs Res 7:64–81, 1998

Coffey CE, Wilkinson WE, Parashos IA, et al: Quantitative cerebral anatomy of the aging human brain: a cross-sectional study using magnetic resonance imaging. Neurology 42:527–536, 1992

Costa PT Jr, McCrae RR: Hypochondriasis, neuroticism, and aging: when are somatic complaints unfounded? Am Psychol 40:19–28, 1985

Costa PT Jr, McCrae RR: Personality, continuity and the changes of adult life, in The Adult Years: Continuity and Change. Edited by Storandt MK, VandenBos GR. Washington, DC, American Psychological Association, 1989, pp 41–78

Costa PT Jr, McCrae RR: Contemporary personality psychology, in Textbook of Geriatric Neuropsychiatry. Edited by Coffey CE, Cummings JL. Washington, DC, American Psychiatric Press, 2000, pp 453–462

Costa PT Jr, Widiger TA (eds): Personality Disorders and the Five-Factor Model of Personality. Washington, DC, American Psychological Association, 1994

Costa PT Jr, McCrae RR, Zonderman AB: Cross-sectional studies of personality in a national sample, II: stability in neuroticism, extraversion, and openness. Psychol Aging 1:144–149, 1986

Costa PT Jr, McCrae RR, Siegler IC: Continuity and change over the adult life cycle: personality and personality disorders, in Personality and Psychopathology. Edited by Cloninger CR. Washington, DC, American Psychiatric Press, 1999, pp 129–153

Costa PT Jr, Herbst JH, McCrae RR: Personality at midlife: stability, intrinsic maturation, and response to life events. Assessment 7:365–378, 2000

Cox C, Monk A: Hispanic culture and family care of Alzheimer's patients. Health Soc Work 18:92–100, 1993

Craik FIM, Jennings JM: Human memory, in The Handbook of Aging and Cognition. Edited by Craik FIM, Salthouse TA. Hillsdale, NJ, Lawrence Erlbaum, 1992, pp 51–110

Craik FIM, Lockhart RS: Levels of processing: a framework for memory research. Journal of Verbal Learning and Verbal Behavior 11:671–684, 1972

Creasey H, Rapoport SI: The aging human brain. Ann Neurol 17:2–10, 1985

Dawson DV, Welsh-Bohmer KA, Siegler IC: Informant rated personality change in Alzheimer's disease patients: replication, influence of premorbid profile, and covariate relationships. Research and Practice in Alzheimer's Disease 5:2–32, 2001

D'Esposito M, Zarahn E, Aguirre GK, et al: The effect of normal aging on the coupling of neural activity to the BOLD hemodynamic response. Neuroimage 10:6–14, 1999

Diehl M, Coyle N, Labouvie-Vief G: Age and sex differences in strategies of coping and defense across the life span. Psychol Aging 11:127–139, 1996

Di Lollo V, Arnett JL, Kruk RV: Age-related changes in rate of visual information processing. J Exp Psychol Hum Percept Perform 8:225–237, 1982

Dilworth-Anderson P, Burton L: Critical issues in understanding family support and older minorities, in Full Color Aging: Facts, Goals, and Recommendations for America's Diverse Elders. Edited by Miles T. Washington, DC, Gerontological Society of America, 1999, pp 93–105

Dilworth-Anderson P, Williams S, Cooper T: Family caregiving to elderly African Americans: caregiver types and structures. J Gerontol 54B:S237–S241, 1999

Dustman RE, Ruhling RO, Russell EM, et al: Aerobic exercise training and improved neuropsychological function of older individuals. Neurobiol Aging 5:35–42, 1984

Dustman RE, Emmerson RY, Ruhling RO, et al: Age and fitness effects on EEG, ERPs, visual sensitivity, and cognition. Neurobiol Aging 11:193–200, 1990

Dyck DG, Short R, Vitaliano PP: Predictors of burden and infectious illness in schizophrenia caregivers. Psychosom Med 61:411–419, 1999

Elias MF, Elias PK, Robbins MA, et al: Cardiovascular risk factors and cognitive functioning: an epidemiological perspective, in Neuropsychology of Cardiovascular Disease. Edited by Waldstein SR, Elias MF. Hillsdale, NJ, Lawrence Erlbaum, 2000, pp 83–104

Ellison CG: Race, religious involvement and depressive symptomatology in a southeastern U.S. community. Soc Sci Med 40:1561–1572, 1995

Farran CJ, Miller BH, Kaufman JE, et al: Race, finding meaning, and caregiver distress. Journal of Aging and Health 9:316–333, 1997

Fischer JG, Johnson MA, Poon LW, et al: Dairy product intake of the oldest old. J Am Diet Assoc 95:918–921, 1995

Flicker C, Ferris SH, Reisbert B: A two-year longitudinal study of cognitive function in normal aging and Alzheimer's disease. J Geriatr Psychiatry Neurol 6:84–96, 1993

Foley KM, Gelband (eds): Improving Palliative Care for Cancer. Washington, DC, National Academy Press, 2001

Folk CL, Lincourt AE: The effects of age on guided conjunction search. Exp Aging Res 22:99–118, 1996

Franklin D: Ensuring Inequality: The Structural Transformation of the African American Family. New York, Oxford University Press, 1997

Fried LP: Epidemiology of aging. Epidemiol Rev 22:95–106, 2000

George LK, Clipp EC: Subjective components of aging well. Generations 15:57–60, 1991

Goldstein G, Shelly CH: Does the right hemisphere age more rapidly than the left? J Clin Neuropsychol 3:65–78, 1981

Grady CL: Brain imaging and age-related changes in cognition. Exp Gerontol 33:661–673, 1998

Grady CL, Maisog JM, Horwitz B, et al: Age-related changes in cortical blood flow activation during visual processing of faces and location. J Neurosci 14:1450–1462, 1994

Greenberg JS, Seltzer MM, Orsmond GI, et al: Siblings of adults with mental illness or mental retardation: current involvement and expectation of future caregiving. Psychiatr Serv 50:1214–1219, 1999

Gur RC, Gur RE, Obrist WD, et al: Age and regional cerebral blood flow at rest and during cognitive activity. Arch Gen Psychiatry 44:617–621, 1987

Haley WE, Roth DL, Coleton MI, et al: Appraisal, coping, and social support as mediators of well-being in black and white family caregivers of patients with Alzheimer's disease. J Consult Clin Psychol 64:121–129, 1996

Hartley AA: Attention, in The Handbook of Aging and Cognition. Edited by Craik FIM, Salthouse TA. Hillsdale, NJ, Lawrence Erlbaum, 1992, pp 3–49

Hartley AA: Age differences in dual-task interference are localized to response-generation processes. Psychol Aging 16:47–54, 2001

Hartley AA, Kieley JM, Slabach EH: Age differences and similarities in the effects of cues and prompts. J Exp Psychol Hum Percept Perform 16:523–537, 1990

Haug H, Barmwater U, Eggers R, et al: Anatomical changes in aging brain: morphometric analysis of the human prosencephalon, in Neuropharmacology, Vol 21: Aging. Edited by Cervos-Navarro J, Sarkander HI. New York, Raven, 1983, pp 1–12

Hennessy CH, John R: American Indian family caregivers' perceptions of burden and needed support services. J Appl Gerontol 15:275–293, 1996

Herbst JH, McCrae RR, Costa PT Jr: Self-perceptions of stability and change in personality at midlife: the UNC Alumni Heart Study. Assessment 7:379–388, 2000

Hinrichsen GA, Ramirez M: Black and white dementia caregivers: a comparison of their adaptation, adjustment, and service utilization. Gerontologist 32:375–381, 1992

Hof PR, Bierer LM, Perl DP, et al: Evidence for early vulnerability of the medial and inferior aspects of the temporal lobe in an 82-year-old patient with preclinical signs of dementia: regional and laminar distribution of neurofibrillary tangles and senile plaques. Arch Neurol 49:946–953, 1992

Hooker K, Siegler IC: Separating apples from oranges in health ratings: perceived health includes psychological well-being. Behavior, Health, and Aging 2:81–92, 1992

Horn JL: The aging of human abilities, in Handbook of Developmental Psychology. Edited by Wolman BB. Englewood Cliffs, NJ, Prentice-Hall, 1982, pp 847–870

House JS, Landis K, Umberson D: Social relationships and health. Science 241:540–545, 1988

House JS, Kessler RC, Herzog AR, et al: Social stratification, age, and health, in Aging, Health Behaviors, and Health Outcomes. Edited by Schaie KW, Blazer D, House JS. Hillsdale, NJ, Lawrence Erlbaum, 1992, pp 1–32

Huettel SA, Singerman JD, McCarthy G: The effects of aging upon the hemodynamic response measured by functional MRI. Neuroimage 13:161–175, 2001

Hultsch DF, Dixon RA: Learning and memory in aging, in Handbook of the Psychology of Aging. Edited by Birren JE, Schaie KW. New York, Academic Press, 1990, pp 258–274

Huppert FA: Memory function in dementia and normal aging: dimension or dichotomy, in Dementia and Normal Aging. Edited by Huppert FA, Brayne C, Connor DO. New York, Cambridge University Press, 1994, pp 291–330

Idler E: Religious involvement and the health of the elderly: some hypotheses and an initial test. Social Forces 66:226–238, 1987

Ishii-Kuntz M: Intergenerational relationships among Chinese, Japanese, and Korean Americans. Family Relations 46:23–32, 1997

Ivnik RJ, Smith GE, Tangalos EG, et al: Wechsler Memory Scale: IQ-dependent norms for persons ages 65 to 97 years. Psychol Assess 3:156–161, 1991

Jeune B, Kannisto V: Emergence of centenarians and super-centenarians, in Longevity: To the Limits and Beyond. Edited by Robine J-M, Vaupel JW, Jeune B, et al. New York, Springer, 1997, pp 75–89

Kaszniak AW, Poon LW, Riege W: Assessing memory deficits: an information-processing approach, in Handbook for Clinical Memory Assessment of Older Adults. Edited by Poon LW. Washington, DC, American Psychological Association, 1986, pp 168–188

Katzman R, Aronson M, Fuld P, et al: Development of dementing illnesses in an 80-year-old volunteer cohort. Ann Neurol 25:317–324, 1989

Klisz D: Neuropsychological evaluation in older persons, in The Clinical Psychology of Aging. Edited by Storandt M, Siegler IC, Elias MF. New York, Plenum, 1978, pp 71–95

Knight BG, McCallum TJ: Heart rate reactivity and depression in African-American and White dementia caregivers: reporting bias or positive coping? Aging Ment Health 2:212–221, 1998

Knight B, Silverstein M, McCallum, et al: A sociocultural stress and coping model for mental health outcomes among African American caregivers in Southern California. J Gerontol B Psychol Sci Soc Sci 55B:P142–P150, 2000

Koenig HG, Siegler IC, George LK: Religious and non-religious coping: impact on adaptation in later life. J Relig Aging 5:73–94, 1989

Koss E, Haxby JV, DeCarli C, et al: Patterns of performance preservation and loss in healthy aging. Dev Neuropsychol 7:99–113, 1991

Kramer AF, Hahn S, McAuley E, et al: Exercise, aging, and cognition: healthy body, healthy mind, in Human Factors Interventions for Health Care of Older Adults. Mahwah, NJ, Lawrence Erlbaum, 2002, pp 91–120

Krause N, Van Tran T: Stress and religious involvement among older blacks. J Gerontol B Psychol Sci Soc Sci 44:S4–S13, 1989

Kray J, Lindenberger U: Adult age differences in task switching. Psychol Aging 15:126–147, 2000

Lawton MP, Kleban MH, Rajagopal D, et al: Dimensions of affective experience in three age groups. Psychol Aging 7:171–184, 1992

Lazarus RS: Coping with aging: individuality as a key to understanding, in Clinical Geropsychology. Edited by Nordhus IH, VandenBos GR, Berg S, et al. Washington, DC, American Psychological Association, 1998, pp 109–127

Lefley HP, Hatfield AG: Helping parental caregivers and mental health consumers cope with parental aging and loss. Psychiatr Serv 50:369–375, 1999

Lehr U: Centenarian—a contribution on longevity research. Z Gerontol 24:227–232, 1991

Levin J: Religion and health: is there an association, is it valid, and is it casual? Soc Sci Med 38:1475–1482, 1994

Levin J, Chatters L, Taylor R: Religious effects on health status and life satisfaction among Americans. J Gerontol B Psychol Sci Soc Sci 50B:S154–S163, 1995

Lezak MD: Neuropsychological Assessment, 2nd Edition. New York, Oxford University Press, 1983

Light LL: Memory and aging, in Memory. Edited by Bjork EL, Bjork RA. San Diego, CA, Academic Press, 1996, pp 443–490

Light E, Niederhe N, Lebowitz B (eds): Stress Effects on Family Caregivers of Alzheimer's Patients: Research and Interventions. New York, Springer, 1994

Lowenthal MF, Berkman PL, Beuler JA, et al: Aging and Mental Disorder in San Francisco. San Francisco, CA, Jossey-Bass, 1967

Madden DJ: Age-related slowing in the retrieval of information from long-term memory. J Gerontol 40:208–210, 1985

Madden DJ: Speed and timing of behavioral processes, in Handbook of the Psychology of Aging, 5th Edition. Edited by Birren JE, Schaie KW. San Diego, CA, Academic Press, 2001, pp 288–312

Madden DJ, Hoffman JM: Application of positron emission tomography to age-related cognitive changes, in Brain Imaging and Clinical Psychiatry. Edited by Krishnan KRR, Doraiswamy PM. New York, Marcel Dekker, 1997, pp 575–613

Madden DJ, Whiting WL: Age-related changes in visual attention, in Recent Advances in Psychology and Aging. Edited by Costa PT, Siegler IC. Amsterdam, the Netherlands, Elsevier (in press)

Madden DJ, Turkington TG, Coleman RE, et al: Adult age differences in regional cerebral blood flow during visual word identification: evidence from $H_2^{15}O$ PET. Neuroimage 3:127–142, 1996

Madden DJ, Gottlob LR, Allen PA: Adult age differences in visual search accuracy: attentional guidance and target detectability. Psychol Aging 14:683–694, 1999a

Madden DJ, Turkington TG, Provenzale JM, et al: Adult age differences in the functional neuroanatomy of verbal recognition memory. Hum Brain Mapp 7:115–135, 1999b

Madden DJ, Turkington TG, Provenzale JM, et al: Aging and attentional guidance during visual search: functional neuroanatomy by positron emission tomography. Psychol Aging 17:24–43, 2002

Manuck SB, Jennings R, Rabin BS, et al (eds): Behavior, Health and Aging. Mahwah, NJ, Lawrence Erlbaum, 2000

Martin P, Poon LW, Clayton GM, et al: Personality, life events and coping in the oldest-old. Int J Aging Hum Dev 34 (special issue 1):19–30, 1992

Matthews KA: A behavioral medicine perspective on aging and health, in The Psychology and the Aging Revolution. Edited by Qualls SH, Abeles R. Washington, DC, American Psychological Association, 2000, pp 197–205

Mayr U: Age differences in the selection of mental sets: the role of inhibition, stimulus ambiguity, and response-set overlap. Psychol Aging 16:96–109, 2001

McClelland JL, Rumelhart DE, the PDP Research Group: Parallel Distributed Processing: Explorations in the Microstructure of Cognition (Psychological and Biological Models Series, Vol 2). Cambridge, MA, MIT Press, 1986

McCrae RR, Costa PT Jr, Lima MPD, et al: Age differences in personality across the adult life span: parallels in five cultures. Dev Psychol 35:466–477, 1999

McCrae RR, Costa PT Jr, Ostendorf F, et al: Nature over nurture: temperament, personality, and lifespan development. J Pers Soc Psychol 78:173–186, 2000

McDonald K, Armstrong E: De-romanticizing Black intergenerational support: the questionable expectation of welfare reform. J Marriage Fam 63:213–223, 2001

McDowd JM, Shaw RJ: Attention and aging: a functional perspective, in The Handbook of Aging and Cognition, 2nd Edition. Edited by Craik FIM, Salthouse TA. Mahwah, NJ, Lawrence Erlbaum, 2000, pp 221–292

Miller KJ: Life satisfaction in older adults: the impact of social support and religious maturity. Dissertation Abstracts International—Section B: The Sciences and Engineering 59(6-B):3067, 1998

Mittenberg W, Seidenberg M, O'Leary DS, et al: Changes in cerebral functioning associated with normal aging. J Clin Exp Neuropsychol 11:918–933, 1989

Morris JC, McKeel DW, Storandt M, et al: Very mild Alzheimer's disease: informant-based clinical, psychometric, and pathological distinction from normal aging. Neurology 41:469–478, 1991

Mossey JM, Shapiro E: Self-rated health: a predictor of mortality among the elderly. Am J Public Health 72:800–808, 1982

Myerson J, Hale S, Wagstaff D, et al: The information loss model: a mathematical theory of age-related cognitive slowing. Psychol Rev 97:475–487, 1990

National Institute on Aging: Progress Report on Alzheimer's Disease (NIH Publ No 00-4859). Bethesda, MD, National Institutes of Health, 2000

Neighbors HW, Jackson JS, Bowman PJ, et al: Stress, coping, and black mental health: preliminary findings from a national study. Prevention and Human Services 2:5–29, 1983

Nkongho NO, Archbold PG: Reasons for caregiving in African American families. J Cult Divers 2:116–123, 1995

Parashos IA, Coffey CE: Anatomy of the aging brain, in Principles and Practice of Geriatric Psychiatry. Edited by Copeland JRM, Abou-Saleh MT, Blazer DG. New York, Wiley, 1994, pp 35–50

Patrick JH, Hayden JM: Neuroticism, coping strategies, and negative well-being among caregivers. Psychol Aging 14:273–283, 1999

Pederson NL, Reynolds CA: Stability and change in adult personality: genetic and environmental components. European Journal of Personality 12:365–386, 1998

Perls TT: Centenarians prove the compression of morbidity hypothesis, but what about the rest of us who are genetically less fortunate? Med Hypotheses 49:405–407, 1997

Peters E, Finucane ML, MacGregor DG, et al: The bearable lightness of aging: judgment and decision processes in older adults, in The Aging Mind: Opportunity in Cognitive Research. Edited by Stern PC, Carstensen LL. Washington, DC, National Academies Press, 2000, pp 144–165

Petersen RC, Smith G, Kokmen E, et al: Memory function in normal aging. Neurology 42:396–401, 1992

Picot S: Choice and social exchange theory and the rewards of Black American caregivers. J Natl Black Nurses Assoc 7:29–40, 1995

Plude DJ, Hoyer WJ: Age and the selectivity of visual information processing. Psychol Aging 1:4–10, 1986

Poon LW: Differences in human memory with aging: nature, causes and clinical implications, in Handbook of the Psychology of Aging. Edited by Birren JE, Schaie KW. New York, Van Nostrand Reinhold, 1985, pp 427–462

Poon LW (ed): Handbook for Clinical Memory Assessment of Older Adults. Washington, DC, American Psychological Association, 1986

Poon LW: Centenarians, in The Encyclopedia of Aging, 3rd Edition. Edited by Maddox GL, Atchley RC, Evans JG, et al. New York, Springer, 2001, pp 179–180

Poon LW, Fozard JL: Age and word frequency effects in continuous recognition memory. J Gerontol 35:77–86, 1980

Poon LW, Siegler IC: Psychological aspects of normal aging, in Comprehensive Review of Geriatric Psychiatry. Edited by Sadavoy J, Lazarus LW, Jarvik LF. Washington, DC, American Psychiatric Press, 1991, pp 117–145

Poon LW, Clayton GM, Martin P, et al: The Georgia Centenarian Study. Int J Aging Hum Dev 34:1–17, 1992a

Poon LW, Martin P, Clayton GM, et al: The influences of cognitive resources on adaptation and old age. Int J Aging Hum Dev 34:31–46, 1992b

Poon LW, Bramlett MA, Holtsberg PA, et al (eds): Who Will Survive to 105? Chicago, IL, Encyclopedia Brittanica, 1997

Rapoport SI: Positron emission tomography in Alzheimer's disease in relation to disease pathogenesis: a critical review. Cerebrovasc Brain Metab Review 3:297–335, 1991

Ravaglia G, Morini P, Forti P, et al: Anthropometric characteristics of healthy Italian nonagenarians and centenarians. Br J Nutr 77:9–17, 1997

Raz N: Aging of the brain and its impact on cognitive performance: integration of structural and functional findings, in The Handbook of Aging and Cognition, 2nd Edition. Edited by Craik FIM, Salthouse TA. Mahwah, NJ, Lawrence Erlbaum, 2000, pp 1–90

Raz N, Gunning FM, Head D, et al: Selective aging of the human cerebral cortex observed in vivo: differential vulnerability of the prefrontal gray matter. Cereb Cortex 7:268–282, 1997

Regius O, Beregi E, Klinger A: Verwandten-, angehörigen- und pflegerkontakte der hundertjahrigen in Ungarn [Extended family, immediate family and caregiver contacts of 100-year-old patients in Hungary]. Z Gerontol 27:456–458, 1994

Rook K: The evolution of social relationships in later adulthood, in Psychology and the Aging Revolution: How We Adapt to Longer Life. Edited by Qualls SH, Abeles N. Washington, DC, American Psychological Association, 2000, pp 173–191

Roschelle AR: No More Kin: Exploring Race, Class, and Gender in Family Networks. Thousand Oaks, CA, Sage Publications, 1997

Rosowsky E, Abrams RC, Zwirg RA: Personality Disorders in Older Adults. Mahwah, NJ, Lawrence Erlbaum, 1999

Rowe JW, Kahn RL: Successful Aging. New York, Pantheon Books, 1998

Rubin DC: Frontal-striatal circuits in cognitive aging: evidence for caudate involvement. Aging, Neuropsychology, and Cognition 6:241–259, 1999

Salthouse TA: Adult Cognition: An Experimental Psychology of Human Aging. New York, Springer-Verlag, 1982

Salthouse TA: Theoretical Perspectives on Cognitive Aging. Hillsdale, NJ, Lawrence Erlbaum, 1991

Salthouse TA: General and specific speed mediation of adult age differences in memory. J Gerontol B Psychol Sci Soc Sci 51B:P30–P42, 1996a

Salthouse TA: The processing-speed theory of adult age differences in cognition. Psychol Rev 103:403–428, 1996b

Salthouse TA: Pressing issues in cognitive aging, in Cognitive Aging: A Primer. Edited by Park DC, Schwart N. Philadelphia, PA, Psychology Press, 2000, pp 43–54

Salthouse TA, Becker JT: Independent effects of Alzheimer's disease on neuropsychological functioning. Neuropsychology 12:242–252, 1998

Salthouse TA, Fristoe N, Rhee SH: How localized are age-related effects on neuropsychological measures? Neuropsychology 10:272–285, 1996

Samuelsson SM, Alfredson BB, Hagberg B, et al: The Swedish Centenarian Study: a multidisciplinary study of five consecutive cohorts at the age of 100. Int J Aging Hum Dev 45:223–253, 1997

Schacter D: Implicit memory: history and current status. J Exp Psychol Learn Mem Cogn 13:501–518, 1987

Schaie KW: Intellectual development in adulthood, in Handbook of the Psychology of Aging, 3rd Edition. Edited by Birren JE, Schaie KW. New York, Academic Press, 1990, pp 291–309

Schaie KW, Schaie JP: Clinical assessment and aging, in The Handbook of the Psychology of Aging. Edited by Birren JE, Schaie KW. New York, Van Nostrand Reinhold, 1977, pp 692–723

Schmidt R, Fazekas F, Offenbacher H, et al: Neuropsychological correlates of MRI white-matter hyperintensities: a study of 150 normal volunteers. Neurology 43:2490–2494, 1993

Schulz R, Beach SR: Caregiving as a risk factor for mortality: the Caregiver Health Effects Study. JAMA 282:2215–2219, 1999

Seltzer MM, Greenberg JS, Krauss MW: A comparison of coping strategies of aging mothers of adults with mental illness or mental retardation. Psychol Aging 10:64–75, 1995

Siegler IC: The psychology of adult development and aging, in Handbook of Geriatric Psychiatry. Edited by Busse EW, Blazer DG. New York, Van Nostrand Reinhold, 1980, pp 169–221

Siegler IC: Developmental health psychology, in The Adult Years: Continuity and Change. Edited by Storandt MK, VandenBos GR. Washington, DC, American Psychological Association, 1989, pp 119–142

Siegler IC: Research paradigms in developmental health psychology—from theory to application: introduction to a special issue. J Gerontol 45:P113–P115, 1990

Siegler IC: Aging research and health: a status report, in Psychology and the Aging Revolution: How We Adapt to Long Life. Edited by Qualls SH, Abeles N. Washington, DC, American Psychological Association, 2000, pp 207–218

Siegler IC, Poon LW: The psychology of aging, in Geriatric Psychiatry. Edited by Busse EW, Blazer DG. Washington, DC, American Psychiatric Press, 1989, pp 163–201

Siegler IC, Welsh KA, Dawson DV, et al: Perceptions of personality change in patients evaluated for memory disorders. Alzheimer Dis Assoc Disord 5:240–250, 1991

Siegler IC, Peterson BL, Barefoot JC, et al: Using college alumni populations in epidemiologic research: the UNC Alumni Heart Study. J Clin Epidemiol 45:1243–1250, 1992

Siegler IC, Dawson DV, Welsh KA: Caregiver ratings of personality change in Alzheimer's disease patients: a replication. Psychol Aging 9:464–466, 1994

Siegler IC, Poon LW, Madden DJ, et al: Psychological aspects of normal aging, in The American Psychiatric Press Textbook of Geriatric Psychiatry, 2nd Edition. Edited by Busse EW, Blazer DG. Washington, DC, American Psychiatric Press, 1996, pp 105–127

Siegler IC, Bastian LA, Steffens DC, et al: Behavioral medicine and aging: middle age, aging and the oldest-old. J Consult Clin Psychol 70:843–851, 2002

Siegler IC, Bosworth HB, Elias MF: Adult development and aging in health psychology, in Comprehensive Handbook of Psychology, Vol 9: Health Psychology. Edited by Nezu AM, Nezu CM, Geller PA. New York, Wiley, 2003a, pp 487–510

Siegler IC, Bosworth HB, Poon LW: Disease, health and aging, in Comprehensive Handbook of Psychology, Vol 6: Developmental Psychology. Edited by Lerner RM, Easterbrooks MA, Mistri J. New York, Wiley, 2003b, pp 423–442

Smith TW, Kendall RC, Keefe FJ: Behavioral medicine and clinical health psychology: introduction to the special issue, a view from the decade of behavior. J Consult Clin Psychol 70:459–462, 2002

Spirduso WW: Reaction and movement time as a function of age and physical activity level. J Gerontol 30:435–440, 1975

Spirduso WW, Clifford P: Replication of age and physical activity effects on reaction and movement time. J Gerontol 33:26–30, 1978

Strong C: Stress and caring for elderly relatives: interpretations and coping strategies in an American Indian and White sample. Gerontologist 24:251–256, 1984

Taylor RJ, Chatters LM: Church-based informal support among elderly blacks. Gerontologist 26:637–642, 1986

Tulving E: Episodic and semantic memory, in Organization of Memory. Edited by Tulving E, Donaldson W. New York, Academic Press, 1972, pp 382–404

Vaillant GE: Aging Well: Surprising Guideposts to a Happier Life From the Landmark Harvard Study of Adult Development. Boston, MA, Little, Brown, 2002

Van Gorp WG, Mahler M: Subcortical features of normal aging, in Subcortical Dementia. Edited by Cummings JL. New York, Oxford University Press, 1990, pp 231–250

Van Gorp WG, Satz P, Mitrushina M: Neuropsychological processes associated with normal aging. Dev Neuropsychol 6:279–290, 1990

Vaupel JW, Carey JR, Christensen K, et al: Biodemographic trajectories of longevity. Science 280:855–859, 1998

Vitaliano PP, Scanlan JM, Siegler IC, et al: Coronary heart disease moderates the relationship of chronic stress with the metabolic syndrome. Health Psychol 17:520–529, 1998

Vitaliano PP, Scanlan JM, Zhang J, et al: A path model of chronic stress, the metabolic syndrome, and coronary heart disease. Psychosom Med 64:418–435, 2002

Waldstein SR: Health effects on cognitive aging, in The Aging Mind. Edited by Stern PC, Carstensen LL. Washington, DC, National Academy Press, 2000, pp 189–217

Wang H-X, Karp A, Winblad B, et al: Late-life engagement in social and leisure activities is associated with a decreased risk of dementia: a longitudinal study from the Kungsholmen Project. Am J Epidemiol 155:1081–1087, 2002

Waugh NC, Norman DA: Primary memory. Psychol Rev 72:89–104, 1965

Welleford EA, Harkins SW, Taylor JR: Personality change in dementia of the Alzheimer's type: relations to caregiver personality and burden. Exp Aging Res 21:295–314, 1995

Welsh KA, Hoffman JM: Positron emission tomography neuroimaging in dementia, in Handbook of Human Brain Function. Edited by Bigler E. New York, Plenum, 1996, pp 185–222

Welsh KA, Butters N, Hughes J, et al: Detection of abnormal memory in mild cases of Alzheimer's disease using CERAD neuropsychological measures. Arch Neurol 48:278–281, 1991

Welsh KA, Butters N, Mohs RC, et al: The Consortium to Establish a Registry of Alzheimer's Disease (CERAD), V: a normative study of the neuropsychological battery. Neurology 44:609–614, 1994

West RL: An application of prefrontal cortex function theory to cognitive aging. Psychol Bull 120:272–292, 1996

Whelihan WM, Lesher EL: Neuropsychological changes in frontal functions with aging. Dev Neuropsychol 1:371–380, 1985

Whitfield KE, Brandon DT, Wiggins SA: Sociocultural influences in genetic designs of aging: unexplored perspectives. Exp Aging Res (Special Issue) 28:391–405, 2002a

Whitfield KE, Weidner G, Clark R, et al: Sociodemographic diversity and behavioral medicine. J Consult Clin Psychol 70:463–481, 2002b

Williams RB: Hostility (and other psychosocial risk factors): effects on health and the potential for successful behavioral approaches to prevention and treatment, in Handbook of Psychology and Health. Edited by Baum A, Revenson TR, Singer JE. Hillsdale, NJ, Lawrence Erlbaum, 2000a, pp 661–668

Williams RB: Psychological factors, health, and disease: the impact of aging and the life cycle, in Behavior, Health, and Aging. Edited by Manuck SB, Jennings R, Rabin BS, et al. Hillsdale, NJ, Lawrence Erlbaum, 2000b, pp 135–151

Williams RB, Barefoot JC, Califf RM, et al: Prognostic importance of social and economic resources among medically treated patients with angiographically documented coronary artery disease. JAMA 267:520–524, 1992

Williams S, Dilworth-Anderson P: Systems of support in families who care for dependent African American elders. Gerontologist 42:224–236, 2002

Wilson-Ford V: Health-protective behaviors of rural black elderly women. Health Soc Work 17:28–36, 1992

Wingfield A, Stine-Morrow EAL: Language and speech, in The Handbook of Aging and Cognition, 2nd Edition. Edited by Craik FIM, Salthouse TA. Mahwah, NJ, Lawrence Erlbaum, 2000, pp 359–416

Wolfe JM: Visual search, in Attention. Edited by Pashler H. East Sussex, UK, Psychology Press, 1998, pp 13–73

Wood JB, Parham IA: Coping with perceived burden: ethnic and cultural issues in Alzheimer's family caregiving. J Appl Gerontol 9:325–339, 1990

Youn G, Knight BG, Jeong H, et al: Differences in famialism values and caregiving outcomes among Korean, Korean American, and White American caregivers. Psychol Aging 14:355–364, 1999

Zacks RT, Hasher L, Li KZH: Human memory, in The Handbook of Aging and Cognition, 2nd Edition. Edited by Craik FIM, Salthouse TA. Mahwah, NJ, Lawrence Erlbaum, 2000, pp 200–230

Zelinski EM, Crimmins E, Reynolds S, et al: Do medical conditions affect cognition in older adults? Health Psychol 17:504–512, 1998

CHAPTER 8

Social and Economic Factors Related to Psychiatric Disorders in Late Life

Linda K. George, Ph.D.

A comprehensive examination of geriatric psychiatry must include the perspectives of multiple disciplines. The authors of previous chapters addressed the physiological, neurological, sensory, and psychological changes that accompany the aging process. In this chapter, I examine the social and economic conditions of late life. (For the sake of convenience, henceforth the shorter term *social factors* will be used, although economic factors also are addressed.) Particular attention is paid to the ways that social conditions serve as risk factors for psychiatric disorders, as contingencies that affect the course and outcome of mental illness, and as determinants of mental health service utilization.

An adequate depiction of psychiatric disorders must include a dynamic perspective. The experience of psychiatric disorders varies over time as patients experience onset and remission of symptoms. Help seeking and the course of care also are longitudinal phenomena. The distinctive features of geriatric psychiatry are affected by additional dynamic processes. The aging process itself leads to intraindividual changes that can affect the risk of developing psychiatric disorders and the use of mental health services. In addition, the effects of social change—generating cohort differences—also must be examined; it can be documented that over the past decades, social and economic factors have changed substantially across cohorts entering and traversing late life. These cohort differences have important implications for generalizing results across cohorts and for using current knowledge to plan for the future.

Given the importance of age changes versus cohort differences in drawing conclusions about the role of social factors in geriatric psychiatry, these terms merit closer examination. *Age changes* are those changes in organisms that occur simply as a function of age. True age changes will be observed with considerable regularity across time and place because they are developmental. Most biological phenomena (as well as some psychological and social characteristics) that change with age appear to be driven by this kind of internal, developmental agenda. Other differences observed across age groups represent the effects of social changes that are external to the individual. The term *cohort* is used to refer to groups of people born at specific times—for example, the 1930 cohort consists of all persons born in 1930. Cohorts that experience different historical and environmental conditions often differ in ways that reflect those external conditions rather than developmental changes. Without longitudinal data from multiple cohorts, it is difficult to empirically distinguish between age changes and cohort differences. Moreover, some phenomena are affected by both age changes and cohort differences (see, for example, George et al. 1981).

Although it is difficult to separate age changes from cohort differences, this distinction is important for three reasons. First, the distinction is critical to attributions of

This work was supported by a grant from the John Templeton Foundation.

etiology or causality. In their pure forms, age changes reflect developmental phenomena, and cohort differences reflect social or environmental conditions. Second, the distinction is relevant to the generalizability of research findings. If a risk factor for psychiatric disorders changes with age, the observed pattern will be broadly applicable across cohorts. If a risk factor differs across age groups because of differences in environmental exposure, the effects of that risk factor may be cohort specific. Third, the distinction between age changes and cohort differences is important for the design of interventions. If levels of a risk factor differ substantially across cohorts, interventions can be targeted to the environmental conditions that place certain cohorts at greatest risk. If, instead, a risk factor changes with age, interventions must be targeted toward alteration of a developmental trajectory.

In this chapter, then, two dynamic phenomena are examined simultaneously. First, the processes underlying the occurrence of psychiatric disorders and mental health service utilization are addressed from a social perspective. Second, the degree to which social factors associated with psychiatric disorders and/or mental health service utilization either change with age or differ across cohorts is considered.

This chapter is organized in five sections. The first section focuses on social characteristics as risk factors for psychiatric disorders in later life. The social factors examined include demographic variables (such as race and gender), indicators of social integration (such as social roles and the availability of social support), socioeconomic status, and the experience of acute and chronic stress. The second section examines the degree to which exposure to social risk factors for psychiatric disorders changes with age and varies across cohorts. A central issue here is whether current cohorts of younger and middle-aged adults have experienced or will confront environmental conditions that place them at more or less risk

for psychiatric disorders compared with current cohorts of older adults. The third section focuses on the effect of social factors on the course and outcome of psychiatric disorders in later life. The central question of interest is whether social factors alter the probability or timing of recovery. The fourth section addresses social factors as determinants of mental health service use among older adults. An important distinction is made between help seeking (which reflects the decisions and behaviors of individuals needing mental health services) and provider behavior (i.e., how clinicians respond to older persons presenting with psychiatric problems). The final section of the chapter examines the effect of social and economic policies on older adults. These policies and programs have both direct effect—by affecting the likelihood of help seeking for psychiatric problems—and indirect effect—by affecting some social risk factors for mental illness, and thereby influencing the psychiatric status of the older population.

Social Risk Factors for Psychiatric Disorders

Theoretical Model

A consensual model of the precursors of psychiatric disorders has emerged in the literatures of the social science, epidemiological, and social psychiatry disciplines. The model remains vague in terms of specific operationalizations and statistical estimation; nonetheless, an overarching theoretical orientation has been forged. Table 8-1 presents the general conceptual model that emerges from previous research. It is a stage model in that each higher stage represents what are hypothesized to be increasingly proximate antecedents of psychiatric disorders.

TABLE 8–1. Stage model of the social precursors of psychiatric disorders

Stage	Name	Illustrative indicators
I	Demographic variables	Age, sex, race/ethnicity
II	Early events and achievements	Education, childhood traumas
III	Later events and achievements	Occupation, income, marital status, fertility
IV	Social integration	Personal attachments to social structure (e.g., religious participation, community roles), environmental context (e.g., neighborhood stability, economic climate)
V	Vulnerability and protective factors	Social support versus isolation, chronic stressors
VI	Provoking agents and coping efforts	Life events, coping strategies

The first stage consists of demographic variables that are associated with the risk of psychiatric disorders. Virtually all studies of social factors and psychiatric disorders include demographic factors, especially age, race, and sex. The causal mechanisms that underlie these relations are unclear, however. One suggested explanation is that demographic factors serve as proxies for more mechanistic social factors. For example, the greater prevalence of depressive symptoms reported by women compared with men may be due to gender differences in other risk factors such as marital status, income, and exposure to stress. Alternatively, demographic variables may serve as proxies for biological mechanisms. In this review, I emphasize the social meanings of demographic variables. However, possible biological mechanisms should not be overlooked. Indeed, most research emphasizes the multiple types of risk factors that are implicated in the etiology of psychiatric morbidity.

Stages II and III of the model represent events and achievements relevant to mental health outcomes that are distinguished primarily by their timing and recency. Stage II consists of relatively early experiences that are hypothesized to have persistent effects on an individual's vulnerability to psychiatric disorders. Examples of such experiences include childhood traumas (e.g., the early death or marital disruption of parents) and educational attainment. Stage III consists of later events and experiences, including family relationships and economic achievements. In most studies, Stage III indicators are based on the current statuses of individuals, reinforcing the temporal distinction between Stages II and III. It should be noted that Stage II risk factors need not be experiences that occurred during childhood or early adulthood; rather, any experiences that occurred before the time of measurement may be relevant. Again, causal interpretation of relations between risk factors and psychiatric outcomes is problematic. For example, some investigators view higher levels of education and income primarily as resources that facilitate effective coping; others view them as tapping exposure to environments (e.g., occupational and residential settings) that directly affect psychiatric status. Future research will need to address the specific mechanisms by which these factors affect mental health.

Stage IV consists of risk factors that represent dimensions of social integration. The term *social integration* has been used two ways in previous research. Some investigators define social integration at the individual level, referring to personal attachments to formal aspects of the social structure (religious affiliation and participation in organizations are two examples). Others define social integration at the aggregate level, referring to levels of sta-

bility and organization in the broader environments within which individuals function. In this chapter, I address social integration at both the individual and the aggregate level, although information is less plentiful for the latter. The rationale for examining social integration as a risk factor for psychiatric disorders rests on the assumptions that lack of social integration is psychologically stressful, impedes effective coping, or both.

Finally, Stages V and VI represent the classes of social risk factors that have received the greatest empirical attention. Vulnerability and protective factors refer to personal assets and liabilities that alter the probabilities of psychiatric problems. Chronic stressors are primary examples of vulnerability factors, and social support is a major illustration of a hypothesized protective factor. Provoking agents and coping efforts are more specific and proximate than vulnerability and protective factors. Life events have been the primary provoking agents examined in previous research and are viewed as sudden sources of stress that may be sufficiently severe to trigger the onset of psychiatric morbidity, especially in the presence of other risk factors. Coping efforts refer to the specific actions taken to confront a particular source of stress. Effective coping may either prevent stresses from generating negative mental health outcomes or minimize their effects. Stages V and VI are distinguished primarily on the basis of specificity and immediacy. For example, although life events and chronic stressors are both important because of the stresses they generate, life events are more discrete and bounded. Similarly, social support is viewed as a generalized resource for defusing stress, whereas coping efforts are specific to particular stressors.

The model in Table 8–1 should be viewed as a heuristic abstraction—as a useful way of summarizing trends in the literature on social risk factors for psychiatric disorders rather than as a model that has achieved consensus among investigators. Undoubtedly, some researchers would classify the social precursors of psychiatric morbidity in somewhat different categories. Moreover, most available studies do not include all the categories of risk factors included in this model. Nonetheless, most studies implicitly or explicitly adopt both the basic categories of risk factors and their ordering. Thus far, the conceptual framework depicted in Table 8–1 has been described in terms of direct effects—that is, the relationships, either bivariate or multivariate, between risk factors and psychiatric outcomes. An additional complexity is the possibility of interactive effects—that the effects of one risk factor are contingent on the presence or level of another risk factor.

In theory, any combination of risk factors may interact to alter the risk of psychiatric disorders. Evidence of such interactions is included in this chapter. I will use one illustration at this point to describe the potential importance of risk factor interactions. Because of the theoretical and empirical attention it has received, the interaction between life events and social support serves as the illustration. Some investigators propose that life events and social support exert independent effects on mental health outcomes, with life events increasing the risk of psychiatric disorders and social support reducing the risk. This is a hypothesis of direct effects. Other investigators suggest that social support buffers the effects of life events on psychiatric outcomes, maintaining that life events increase the risk of psychiatric disorders only (or primarily) among persons who lack adequate social support. This is an interactive hypothesis. Direct versus interactive effects are not mutually exclusive. It is possible, for example, that life events and social support directly affect mental health and that life events are especially damaging in the absence of social support. Thus, examination of the social precursors of psychiatric disorders includes consideration of not only multiple risk factors but also their interrelationships.

One limitation of the model presented in Table 8–1 should be noted. This model is based on research that examines social precursors of *nonorganic* mental disorders. For this reason, and because there are few studies of social risk factors for organic mental illness, this discussion is restricted to exploration of social risk factors for functional psychiatric disorders.

As presented here, there is nothing distinctively age related about the conceptual framework in Table 8–1, and this is a purposeful decision. This general conceptual model can be used to examine age/cohort differences in the relations between social risk factors and psychiatric disorders, age changes in those relations, and variability within the older population with regard to those relations. In this way, the distinctiveness of psychiatric disorders in later life can be empirically shown.

Methodological Issues

Measuring Psychiatric Disorders

Psychiatric disorders have been operationalized in a variety of ways. Two dimensions underlie most of this variability: 1) the use of diagnostic or symptom measures, and 2) the degree to which the measures tap general psychopathology or specific diagnostic categories. With regard to the first dimension, some instruments are designed to measure psychiatric disorders based on formal diagnostic criteria, typically one of the following nosological systems: DSM-III-R or DSM-IV and DSM-IV-TR (American Psychiatric Association 1987, 1994, 2000); Feighner diagnos-

tic criteria (Feighner et al. 1972); or Research Diagnostic Criteria (RDC; Spitzer et al. 1978). Other measures are symptom scales in which higher numbers of symptoms are assumed to represent more severe morbidity. Diagnostic and symptom measures can yield different conclusions. For example, several studies suggested that older people report more depressive symptoms, on average, than do middle-aged and younger adults but that the prevalence of major depression as a diagnosis is lower among older than among younger adults (Blazer et al. 1991; Henderson et al. 1993).

The second dimension applies primarily to symptom measures. Some scales include symptoms from a spectrum of disorders and generate measures of global psychopathology. Others measure symptoms within a single diagnostic category, such as depression or anxiety. The use of global psychopathology measures is problematic because some risk factors may be important for certain disorders but irrelevant to others. For example, there are substantial—and opposite—gender differences in the prevalence of alcohol abuse or dependence and depression, whereas gender differences are minimal for many other disorders (e.g., Kessler et al. 1994a).

Differences in measurement strategies, as well as in the specific assessment tools used, complicate cross-study comparisons. When studies reach inconsistent conclusions about the effects of a given risk factor, part of the variability in findings may be due to differences in measurement. On the other hand, when studies reach similar conclusions despite the use of different measurement strategies, confidence in those conclusions is increased.

Sample Composition

Sampling variability also accounts for some of the inconsistencies observed across studies. Not surprisingly, samples vary widely in size and composition. Small samples often result in statistical analyses that are "underpowered," and therefore meaningful relationships remain undetected. Compositional differences across samples affect the distributions of both psychiatric disorders and social risk factors. Consequently, sample size and composition must be taken into account when synthesizing research findings across studies.

The age compositions of the samples used in previous research are especially relevant to the discussion in this chapter. Some previous studies of the relations between social risk factors and psychiatric outcomes relied exclusively on data from older adults. More frequently, however, previous studies used data from samples covering much broader age ranges—typically, all adults age 18 and older. These two types of samples generate different, but valuable, information. Studies based on samples of older adults provide in-depth views of how social factors operate during later life. Investigators who use such designs cannot identify risk factor effects that are specific to old age, however. In contrast, data from age-heterogeneous samples can be used to determine 1) the role of age itself as a risk factor for psychiatric disorders and 2) whether other risk factors vary in direction or magnitude across age groups.

Complexity of Analyses

Differences in the types and complexity of the statistical techniques used across studies also complicate the task of synthesizing findings from previous research. Some studies provide only bivariate estimates of the relations between risk factors and psychiatric disorders. Although tantalizing, such studies are ultimately unsatisfying because it is not clear whether the observed relations are meaningful or spurious—that is, whether the relations will disappear in the face of statistical controls. Investigators increasingly recognize the importance of multivariate analyses in which the relations between risk factors and psychiatric outcomes are examined with potentially confounding and/or interrelated risk factors statistically controlled. Thus, I have paid primary attention in this chapter to findings from multivariate analyses.

Cross-Sectional Versus Longitudinal Studies

As noted previously, the onset and course of psychiatric disorders, as well as related help-seeking behaviors, are dynamic. Although the number and quality of longitudinal studies have increased in recent years, a large proportion of studies of social factors and psychiatric disorders are cross-sectional. Cross-sectional studies can be used to document the existence of hypothesized associations, but they cannot provide evidence of temporal order. Furthermore, cross-sectional data cannot provide information about the lag between exposure to a risk factor and the onset of mental illness. Evidence of temporal order and lagged effects can be obtained only from longitudinal data.

For the purposes of the discussion in this chapter, other kinds of longitudinal data also are needed. Specifically, information is needed about the extent to which exposure to social risk factors for psychiatric disorders changes with age and varies across cohorts. Fortunately, longitudinal data concerning these changes are quite plentiful. Throughout this chapter I have accorded major attention to results from longitudinal studies.

Evidence Bearing on the Theoretical Model

Evidence bearing on the model presented in Table 8–1 now can be extracted from previous research. Overall, the model receives considerable support, although the amount and quality of evidence vary widely across specific risk factors.

Demographic Variables

Age is related to the risk of psychiatric disorders, but the associations are complex and often inconsistent across studies. By using symptom scales measuring global psychiatric symptoms, a few studies have found higher levels of symptoms among older adults, but most have reported the absence of meaningful age differences. Evidence is most plentiful with regard to depressive symptoms. In studies based on age-heterogeneous samples, older adults—especially the very old—usually have reported levels of depressive symptoms equal to or higher than those reported by younger and middle-aged adults (Blazer et al. 1991; Mirowsky and Ross 1992). The results of studies of age differences within the older population are inconclusive. Most investigators have reported data showing that depressive symptoms are highest among the oldest old (Blazer et al. 1991; Mitchell et al. 1993), but at least one study showed a higher level of symptoms among the younger old (La Gory and Fitzpatrick 1992). In contrast, studies of psychiatric disorders (as opposed to symptom levels) report a lower prevalence among older than among younger adults for all nonorganic psychiatric disorders (for a review, see Robins and Regier 1991). These age differences are observed for both current and lifetime prevalence. The degree to which these age differences reflect cohort differences has not been definitively answered. Nonetheless, there is increasing consensus that there are significant cohort effects, as implied by the lower *lifetime* prevalence of depression among older adults. That is, it appears that every new generation has higher rates of depressive disorder than its predecessors (Burke et al. 1991; Kessler et al. 1994a; Levenson et al. 1998). The latter two studies reported similar patterns for alcohol abuse and dependence.

Evidence is also mixed concerning gender differences in psychiatric morbidity. Women report higher levels of psychiatric symptoms, especially depressive symptoms, than do men (Blazer et al. 1991; Jones-Webb and Snowden 1993; Kessler et al. 1994b). The results of studies based on diagnoses, however, suggest that global symptom scales mask considerable variation across specific disorders. Mood and somatic disorders are more prevalent among women, alcohol and substance abuse are more common among men, and schizophrenia and most anxiety disorders are unrelated to gender (Kessler et al. 1994a). Some evidence suggests that gender differences in depression may narrow substantially in later life (Chen et al. 2000). Henderson et al. (1993) found higher rates of depressive symptoms among older women than among older men but no gender difference in rates of major depressive disorder. Similarly, gender was not a significant predictor of the onset of major depression among older adults in a prospective United States study (George 1992). In a prospective study in Britain, however, Green et al. (1992) found a higher incidence of major depression among older women than among older men.

Evidence concerning the relation between race/ethnicity and psychiatric morbidity also is mixed. Race differences in depressive symptoms among the elderly are not clear-cut. For example, some investigators (Gallo et al. 1998; La Gory and Fitzpatrick 1992) reported a higher level of depressive symptoms among whites than among African Americans. In contrast, Blazer et al. (1991, 1998) reported no black-white differences in symptoms. Although evidence is scant, older Hispanics appear to report higher levels of depressive symptoms than do either whites or African Americans (Falcon and Tucker 2000). Race differences are rarely observed in studies based on diagnostic measures, with the exception of a higher prevalence of alcohol and drug abuse among nonwhites (Kessler et al. 1994a). This issue is further complicated by substantial race differences in education and income. Several authors have reported that bivariate relations between race and psychiatric morbidity disappear when socioeconomic status is statistically controlled (Blazer et al. 1991; Kubzansky et al. 2000; Williams et al. 1997).

Early Events and Achievements

Considerable evidence indicates that early events and achievements have persistent effects on psychiatric status throughout adulthood. Among indicators of socioeconomic status, education is most strongly related to psychiatric morbidity. (An advantage of examining education rather than income is the fact that education is less likely than income to be affected by mental illness; thus, even in cross-sectional studies, causal direction can be assumed with some confidence.) In general, high levels of psychiatric symptoms are strongly related to low levels of education. This pattern is observed in age-heterogeneous samples (Lynch et al. 1997; Mirowsky and Ross 2001) and studies of older adults (Kubzansky et al. 2000; La Gory and Fitzpatrick 1992; Mitchell et al. 1993). Some evi-

dence suggests that socioeconomic status in general, and education in particular, is a weaker predictor of psychiatric symptoms in late life than at younger ages (George 1992; Mirowsky and Ross 2001). Even when diagnostic measures are used, low education is generally recognized as a risk factor for psychiatric disorder (Robins and Regier 1991).

Although it is commonly assumed that childhood traumas place individuals at increased risk for psychiatric morbidity, it is only recently that this hypothesis has received strong empirical support. Evidence now shows that parental divorce or separation, parental problem drinking, childhood physical and/or sexual abuse, and childhood poverty are significant risk factors for a variety of psychiatric disorders during adulthood (Brown and Harris 1978; Greenfield et al. 1993; Kessler et al. 1997; Landerman et al. 1991; Molnar et al. 2001; Ross and Mirowsky 1999). Landerman and colleagues (1991) reported that childhood traumas also increase vulnerability to stressful life events during adulthood; this may be one of the mechanisms by which childhood problems exert persistent effects on adult mental health. Although studies to date have focused on age-heterogeneous samples, older adults were included in them.

Later Events and Achievements

Current and/or recent life conditions also are related to the risk of psychiatric disorder. Income and—to a lesser extent—occupation are related to psychiatric disorder, with low income and low occupational prestige increasing risk (Kessler et al. 1994a; Robins and Regier 1991). These relations are observed for both symptom scales and diagnostic measures. Although the relation between income and psychiatric morbidity is strong at the bivariate level, the effects of income are substantially reduced when educational attainment is statistically controlled. Retirement is obviously a common transition of later life—a transition that removes individuals from the occupational structure and results in substantial income loss. Nonetheless, no evidence indicates that retirement increases the risk of psychiatric disorders (Kim and Moen 2002; Midanik et al. 1995). This conclusion also is compatible with the lower prevalence of psychiatric disorders in later life. Thus, socioeconomic background appears to be a stronger predictor of psychiatric morbidity during late life than do retirement-related changes in economic status.

The relation between marital status and psychiatric disorders remains ambiguous despite considerable research. In general, marital status appears to be weakly associated with psychiatric morbidity, regardless of whether symptom scales or diagnostic measures are used (Robins and Regier 1991). In two studies of depression among community-dwelling older adults, the unmarried adults reported significantly more symptoms of depression than did the married adults (Blazer et al. 1991; Jones-Webb and Snowden 1993). Substantively, however, the differences in symptom levels were quite small. Two additional caveats should be observed. First, undesirable changes in marital status appear to have negative effects on mental health, especially in the few months immediately after marital disruption. However, changes in marital status are typically examined as stressful life events rather than as marital status changes. Second, the protective effects of marriage are confounded with measures of social support. Thus, in multivariate models, the effects of marital status are largely explained by stressful life events and social support.

Recently, Barrett (2000) examined the effects of marital *history* rather than marital status on psychiatric disorders. Marital history captures sources of heterogeneity that are ignored by measures of current marital status (e.g., among the currently married are individuals in first marriages as well as persons who have been married two or more times, and among the remarried, some previous marriages ended in divorce and others by widowhood). In general, Barrett found that marital history has significant effects on mental illness, over and above current marital status, but only for women. Regardless of the cause of the marital dissolution, remarried women were at significantly higher risk for depression than were women married only once. Not surprisingly, perhaps, women who had been widowed more than once were at greater risk for depression than were those widowed only once.

Evidence linking childbearing to psychiatric disorders is very limited. The few studies available suggest that psychiatric symptoms may be slightly higher among women caring for minor children than among their peers who are not responsible for child care (Kandel et al. 1985; Ross and Huber 1985). However, no evidence indicates that childbearing history is related to psychiatric status during later life. Indeed, children are a major source of social support for most older adults.

Social Integration

Although social integration is receiving increased attention, the research base remains small. The available evidence suggests that social integration may protect individuals from psychiatric disorders. At the individual level, participation in religion has received the most attention. A growing body of research suggests that church attendance

and participation in other religious activities are associated with a decreased risk of psychiatric morbidity, including alcohol abuse (Koenig et al. 1994; Neff and Husaini 1985), depression (Koenig et al. 1997; Mitchell et al. 1993), and anxiety disorders (Koenig et al. 1993a, 1993b). Moreover, the studies of anxiety disorders suggest that the effects of religious participation are somewhat stronger for older than for younger adults. Similar, albeit weaker, benefits are reported for participation in voluntary organizations (Grusky et al. 1985). Unfortunately, all previous studies in this area were based on cross-sectional data, so causal order remains problematic.

At the aggregate level, most studies have focused on dimensions of the environment such as degree of neighborhood stability; economic conditions, especially levels of unemployment; and neighborhood age or family structure. Overall, research results have been mixed, with some studies showing significant relations between disruptive environmental conditions and the prevalence of psychiatric disorders and other studies failing to do so. In one study of community-dwelling older adults, investigators examined the relations between selected environmental conditions and depressive symptoms (La Gory and Fitzpatrick 1992). Modest but significant relations were observed between depression and two environmental parameters: age density of the residential neighborhood and availability of public transportation. Older adults who had fewer age peers in their neighborhoods and/or who lacked access to transportation had higher levels of symptoms. In addition, an interaction was found between environmental variables and functional disability. The effects of disability on depression were stronger for persons who were disadvantaged on one or both of the environmental variables. The environmental variables were examined with other established predictors of depression (such as social support) statistically controlled.

Vulnerability and Protective Factors

Chronic stress has been the most frequently examined vulnerability factor. Several investigative teams have reported a robust relation between poverty and depressive symptoms in later life (Bruce and Hof 1994; La Gory and Fitzpatrick 1992)—an association also observed among all adults (Mirowsky and Ross 1999). Chronic illness likewise is a well-documented risk factor for psychiatric disorder in later life, especially for depression (Blazer et al. 1991; Husaini et al. 1991; Moldin et al. 1993; Roberts et al. 1997). In addition to chronic physical illnesses, an increased risk of depression during late life is associated with other health indicators, including cognitive impairment (Blazer et al. 1991), perceived poor health (Henderson et al. 1993), and disability (measured in terms of activities of daily living impairment) (Bruce 2001; Gurland et al. 1988; Oxman and Hull 2001; Mitchell et al. 1993). In cross-sectional studies, causal order is problematic for these health measures. Depression may be either a consequence or a cause of disability and perceptions of poor health. Cognitive impairment may be a part of the depressive episode rather than an independent phenomenon. At first glance, it might appear that chronic illness is not subject to these concerns. It is unlikely, for example, that depression can cause diabetes or cardiovascular disease. Although causal direction is less problematic, the etiological role of chronic illnesses in the onset of depression in later life remains unclear. For example, Moldin et al. (1993) reported equally high rates of comorbid physical illness and depression among younger and older adults. In a similar vein, George (1992) found that chronic illness was a strong predictor of the onset of a depressive episode for younger adults but not for middle-aged and older adults.

An extensive body of research indicates that caregiving for a mentally or physically ill elderly adult represents a chronic stressor that can lead to psychiatric problems. Many older adults have caregiving responsibilities—usually for spouses, but sometimes for very old parents or siblings. To date, research examining the effects of caregiver burden on psychiatric morbidity has focused on family caregivers of elderly adults with dementia. Studies suggest that 30%–50% of the caregivers of patients with dementia meet the criteria for a DSM-III or DSM-IV diagnosis of major depression (Schulz and Williamson 1991; Schulz et al. 1995; Song et al. 1997). Even larger proportions of caregivers have high levels of psychiatric symptoms, albeit below the thresholds for diagnosis.

The primary protective factor examined in previous research has been social support. There is consensus that social support is a multidimensional phenomenon. Most investigators recognize at least three major dimensions: 1) social network—the size and structure of the network of people available to provide support, 2) instrumental support—the specific tangible services provided by families and friends, and 3) perceptions of social support—subjective evaluations of satisfaction with the available support. Some investigators examine a fourth dimension: informational support, defined as the extent to which family and friends provide information that can be used when assessing options and confronting stress. The level of interaction with friends and family and the presence or absence of a confidant also have been addressed as indicators of social support.

Overwhelming evidence shows that social support protects individuals from psychiatric morbidity. Because of the large body of research supporting this conclusion, I restrict this discussion to studies of older adults. It should also be noted that the vast majority of these studies explore the effects of social support on depressive symptoms and disorder. The protective power of social support has been reported in numerous cross-sectional studies and a reassuring number of longitudinal investigations. Available evidence suggests that specific dimensions of social support may be differentially important in protecting against late-life depression. The relations between social network characteristics and depression have received the least support. Blazer et al. (1991) and Oxman and Hull (2001) found that older adults with smaller social networks reported more depressive symptoms; lack of a confidant also has been related to higher levels of symptoms (Hays et al. 1998; Oxman et al. 1992). Most studies, however, have failed to show significant relations between network size or structure and risk of depression. Levels of social interaction have consistently distinguished between depressed and nondepressed elders (Henderson et al. 1986; Oxman and Hull 1997; Oxman et al. 1992) but have not been shown to predict the onset of disorder. Some investigators have found that instrumental and informational support decreases the risk of depression, but these effects appear to be highly specific and dependent on the particular stressor under examination (Krause 1986; Mitchell et al. 1993). There is general consensus that perceptions of social support are most strongly related to depression—and, unlike other dimensions, this conclusion has strong support in both cross-sectional (Dimond et al. 1987; Krause 1986) and longitudinal studies (Brummett et al. 1998; George 1992; Holahan and Holahan 1987; Krause et al. 1989; Oxman and Hull 1997, 2001; Oxman et al. 1992).

The strong relations between perceived support and depression have raised interpretive questions. Henderson (1984), for example, worried that the dysphoria associated with depression might "contaminate" perceptions of social support among depressed persons. Several studies appear to resolve this concern, however. First, even in longitudinal studies, in which perceptions of social support are measured *before* the onset of depressive disorder, perceived support has had a significant protective effect (George 1992; Krause et al. 1989; Oxman et al. 1992). Second, other longitudinal studies have indicated that although perceived support significantly predicts the onset of depression, baseline levels of depression do not predict subsequent levels of support (Cronkite and Moos 1984; Krause et al. 1989). Thus, the dominant direction of causal influence appears to be from perceived support to depression rather than the reverse.

Information illuminating the relations between social support and psychiatric disorders other than depression among older adults is very meager. Several studies involving large proportions of older persons have indicated that the social networks of persons with schizophrenia are unusually small (Link et al. 1987). Grusky and colleagues (1985) reported that older persons with schizophrenia in the community have even smaller networks than do younger ones. Grusky et al. also found that the composition of the support networks of persons with schizophrenia differed, depending on illness severity. Persons with mild symptoms relied primarily on family members for social support. Individuals with severe symptoms relied primarily on nonfamily for assistance—usually formal service providers. In one study, researchers compared the social networks of older adults with and without late-onset alcohol problems. Dupree et al. (1984) found that those with alcohol problems had much smaller networks than did their peers. All of these studies were based on cross-sectional data; thus, causal order is unclear. In the one longitudinal study available, Hays and colleagues (1998) found that social support helped prevent the onset of a bipolar episode among older patients with a history of manic depression but was unrelated to first episodes of bipolar disorder in late life.

Provoking Agents and Coping Efforts

Life events are the major provoking agents implicated in the onset of psychiatric disorders. Two major strategies have been used to study the effects of life events: 1) studies of aggregated life events (summing the number of events that individuals experience in a given period); and 2) studies of specific life events (e.g., widowhood or retirement). The results of research based on both strategies suggest that life events—especially those that are perceived as negative—are strongly related to increased risk of both psychiatric symptoms and specific psychiatric disorders, especially depression, alcohol abuse, and generalized anxiety. These relations have been observed in both age-heterogeneous samples and samples of older adults; only the latter are referenced here (Cutrona et al. 1986; Dupree et al. 1984; George 1992; Hays et al. 1998; Lam et al. 1996; Lynch and George 2002; Neff and Husaini 1985—Cutrona et al. 1986; George 1992; and Lynch and George 2002 are longitudinal studies). With regard to specific events, bereavement has been shown to be a particularly strong predictor of depression in late life (Green et al. 1992; Surtees 1995).

Although the evidence is scant in volume, recent research suggests that cessation of driving also places older adults at increased risk for depressive symptoms and disorder (Fonda et al. 2001; Marottoli et al. 1997). It is interesting that it has taken nearly half a century of research to uncover that driving cessation is a stressful and consequential life event for older adults.

Both common sense and social science theory suggest that adequate coping will partially determine whether stress has negative effects on mental health. Scientific efforts to delineate the nature and effects of coping have been fraught with problems; valid methods for assessing coping effectiveness remain unavailable. Studying coping effects is particularly problematic because different stressors elicit, permit, and require different coping strategies. Limited evidence suggests that coping methods alter the probability that stress will have negative effects on mental health; some of that evidence is based on samples of older adults (Blanchard-Fields and Irion 1988; Freund and Baltes 1998). At this point, investigations of coping are uncommon. It is unlikely that major progress will be made unless and until advances in assessing coping effectiveness are realized.

Interactive Effects

Thus far, discussion of evidence bearing on the theoretical model in Table 8–1 has been restricted to main effects, both bivariate and multivariate. Three kinds of interactive effects also merit comment: the stress-buffering hypothesis, age-related interactions, and several interactions unrelated to age.

Stress-Buffering Hypothesis

Most studies support the stress-buffering hypothesis—that is, that stress has stronger negative effects on risk for psychiatric disorder in the absence of social support. This conclusion applies both to studies of age-heterogeneous samples and to research restricted to older adults. Virtually all studies to date have addressed the stress-buffering hypothesis with regard to depressive symptoms and disorders. Several studies, both cross-sectional and longitudinal, have suggested that life events are moderated by the effects of social support (Cutrona et al. 1986; Krause 1986). Social support also has been shown to buffer the effects of chronic financial strain (Krause 1987) and disability (Arling 1987) during later life. Considerable complexity underlies the moderating effects of social support on stress. For example, Krause (1986, 1987) showed that stress-buffering effects are observed 1) for some but not all dimensions of social support, 2) for some but not all kinds of specific stressors, and 3) for some but not all dimensions of depressed affect.

Age-Related Interactions

Determining whether age interacts with other social precursors of psychiatric disorder is the best strategy for identifying distinctive age differences in the onset of depression. Unfortunately, few investigators have examined age interactions in the risk factors for psychiatric disorders.

In perhaps the most comprehensive study to date, George (1992) explored age interactions of the predictors of the onset of major depression in a longitudinal study. Nine social factors were included in the study; six of them showed significant interactions with age. Three age groups were examined: young adults (ages 18–39), middle-aged adults (ages 40–64), and older adults (age 65 and older). The risk of onset of major depression was higher for women, African Americans, and urban residents—but all three of these relations were significant only among young adults. Lower level of education and the presence of chronic physical illness also increased the risk of depression only among younger adults. An interaction between marital status and age was shown to affect the risk of onset of major depression: being married was a significant protective factor only for the oldest respondents. Three risk factors did not interact with age. With other risk factors statistically controlled, income was unrelated to the risk of depression among all three age groups. In contrast, stressful life events and perceived social support were strongly related to risk of depression among all three age groups. Taken together, these findings suggest that the effects of social factors on the risk of depression tend to be weaker for older than for younger adults, although the strong effects of stress and social support on persons of all ages should not be overlooked.

Other Interactions

Some investigators have tested for gender and race interactions to better understand the role of these factors in psychiatric morbidity in later life. Husaini and colleagues (1991) used data from a sample of older African Americans and found that several social factors were associated with depression only among women: life events, level of social interaction, and perceived social support. Moldin et al. (1993) found that the effects of chronic physical illness on depression were significantly stronger for older women than for older men. Jones-Webb and Snowden (1993) used data from an age-heterogeneous sample and found that several risk factors for depression were differentially important for whites and African Americans. Higher socioeconomic status was a significant protective factor only for African Americans; in contrast, younger

age increased the risk of depression only among African Americans. Widowhood and unemployment increased the risk of depression only for whites. These findings require replication before firm conclusions can be drawn. It is clear, however, that increased attention should be paid to interactive effects in future research. Interactions provide a rigorous method for identifying the differential importance of social risk factors for specific subgroups of the older population.

Age Changes and Cohort Differences in Social Risk Factors

Thus far, we have considered one set of dynamics affecting psychiatric disorder in later life—the effect of social factors on the risk of mental illness. A second set of dynamics also must be considered: age changes and cohort differences that affect *exposure* to social risk factors for psychiatric morbidity. To the extent that exposure to risk factors varies with age or differs across cohorts, the proportion of the older population at risk for psychiatric disorders also varies. Thus, the six categories of social risk factors are reexamined, with a focus on age changes and cohort differences that affect their prevalence and distribution during later life.

Demographic Variables

Age and gender are largely irrelevant in this context because gender is a fixed characteristic and age changes are the focus of this discussion. Cohort differences in the age structure of society merit brief note, however. As is well documented, industrialized societies have been aging throughout this century because of increasing life expectancy and declining fertility—and it is predicted that this trend will continue well into the next century (U.S. Bureau of the Census 1999). Consequently, in the future, a larger proportion of the population of mentally ill individuals will consist of older adults. This does not mean that a larger proportion of the older population will experience mental illness—only that the number of mentally ill older adults will increase.

Race/ethnicity is a fixed characteristic. However, there are cohort differences in the ethnic compositions of societies. In the United States, current cohorts of older adults include substantial proportions of immigrants from Europe and Russia. Emigration from these countries declined precipitously after World War II, however, and future cohorts of elderly persons will differ in this regard. Currently, there is relatively little legal migration to the

United States, with most immigrants coming from Central America, South America, and the Far East. It is not clear how the size and composition of the immigrant population affect the prevalence of psychiatric disorders in later life.

Early Events and Achievements

Education typically is completed during early adulthood and does not change thereafter. There are substantial cohort differences in average levels of education, however. In comparison with their middle-aged and younger peers, current cohorts of older adults average relatively low levels of education (Schrammel 1998). Given the evidence (noted above) that education is negatively related to the prevalence of psychiatric disorders, higher levels of education may bode well for the mental health of future cohorts.

Childhood traumas become fixed experiences for individuals and do not change over time. Again, however, cohort differences are possible. Although there are few solid data on historical trends, cohort differences in the experience of specific childhood traumas are likely. Compared with their younger peers, current cohorts of older adults are more likely to have experienced parental death and severe poverty (because of the Great Depression) during childhood (George 1993). Conversely, current cohorts of young adults are substantially more likely to have experienced parental separation or divorce during childhood (Popenoe 1993). Children in recent cohorts also have confronted unprecedented rates of parental drug abuse (Robins and Regier 1991). The implications of these cohort differences for mental health during later life remain unclear.

Later Events and Achievements

As with education, occupational attainment and income levels are higher among younger than among older cohorts (Schrammel 1998). In light of the documented mental health benefits of higher socioeconomic status, future cohorts of older adults may be at lower risk for psychiatric disorders than are current cohorts. Family formation factors also differ substantially across cohorts. Compared with current cohorts of older adults, younger adults now are less likely to marry, more likely to marry for the first time at later ages, more likely to divorce, less likely to have children, and more likely to have fewer children (Popenoe 1993). These patterns generate major cohort differences in family size and structure. It is not clear whether or how these family changes will affect psychiatric outcomes during old age.

Social Integration

In American society, personal attachments to community structures tend to change with age. Participation in religious, civic, and other organizations peaks during late middle age and declines thereafter as a result of health and mobility problems (Cutler and Hendricks 2000). Consequently, formal social attachments typically decrease, albeit modestly, during later life. Data concerning cohort differences in personal attachments to social structure are rare. Some authors suggest a trend away from community participation (Bellah et al. 1985; Putman 2000). Data supporting that conclusion, however, are scant and of questionable quality. Moreover, even if this trend exists, its meaning is ambiguous. It may be, for example, that recent cohorts invest greater personal commitment in fewer community structures. However, firm data concern one facet of social integration: current cohorts of young and middle-aged adults attend religious services less frequently than have previous cohorts (Roof and McKinney 1987).

Conclusions about exposure to social disorganization at the aggregate level are difficult to draw because of the absence of data. Many would argue that increased rates of crime, technological change, and residential mobility signal increasing social disorganization that affects both current cohorts of older adults and the developmental histories of future cohorts of elderly. On the other hand, levels of financial security have increased steadily over the past century, resulting in a more materially secure population. Whatever the balance of these trends, substantial numbers of older adults are exposed to sources of social disorganization, including economic dislocations, residential mobility, and even "aging in place" in deteriorating neighborhoods.

Vulnerability and Protective Factors

Some chronic stressors are age related. Financial resources decrease and chronic illnesses increase during later life. Cohort differences also may operate. The economic climate of the larger society and the availability of income maintenance policies differ across time and can make financial strain more or less common during later life for specific cohorts. Similarly, medical advances affect both the health status of cohorts before old age and the ability to cure or manage chronic illnesses during later life. Policies that facilitate access to health care also affect the likelihood of impaired physical functioning during later life. Most evidence suggests that future cohorts will enter old age with better physical health and greater financial resources than their predecessors did. These trends should bode well for decreasing the risk of psychiatric disorders during later life among future cohorts.

Social networks tend both to decrease in size and to change in composition during later life (Antonucci 1990). These changes are largely a function of the death and impairment of age peers. Despite these changes, the vast majority of older adults is not socially isolated and reports adequate levels of emotional and instrumental assistance from family and friends. Cohort differences in the size and structure of support networks are likely. Social trends in family formation strongly suggest that older persons in the future will be less likely to have spouses, children, siblings, and extended kin (Popenoe 1993). It is possible, however, that nonfamilial relationships will compensate for these changes.

Provoking Agents and Coping Efforts

Considerable evidence indicates that age is related to the occurrence of life events. Compared with their younger peers, older adults average fewer life events overall but are more likely to experience specific types of life events, especially widowhood, deaths of other family members and friends, and illness onset (Turner et al. 1995). From a mental health perspective, these patterns have mixed implications. On the one hand, fewer life events should decrease the risk for psychiatric disorders. On the other hand, some events that are more common during later life are strongly related to psychiatric morbidity, especially depression. Neither empirical evidence nor theoretical speculation suggests major cohort differences in the frequency of life events during old age.

Information about the relation between age and coping efforts is slim and ambiguous. This reflects both the limited research base and the difficulties inherent in studying coping. At this point, there is no evidence of age-related declines or cohort differences in coping effectiveness. These conclusions, however, are based on an absence of data rather than on empirical evidence.

Social Factors That Affect Recovery From Psychiatric Disorders

Given that social factors are substantially implicated in the onset and prevalence of psychiatric disorders during later life, it is plausible to expect that such factors also might influence the course of illness and the timing of recovery. To understand the effects of social factors on recovery, longitudinal data are required, preferably with multiple measurements to provide an accurate picture of the dynamics of recovery and relapse. Fortunately, the number of studies of the course and outcome of psychiatric disorders has increased during the past few years. Limitations continue to characterize this research base, however. One problem is the limited scope of many studies. Many studies exclude older adults and/or social factors. The scope of disorders that have been studied is limited as well. Most studies examine depression, and a few focus on bipolar disorder or alcohol abuse; other disorders have not been studied. Finally, most studies ignore treatment variables, despite the obvious relevance of treatment quality to the likelihood of recovery.

Unipolar Depression and Bipolar Disorder

The results of most studies suggest that 40%–50% of depressed patients will recover from an episode of depression within the 1- to 3-year follow-up interval used in most investigations. Approximately half of the patients who recover will remain free of symptoms or below the diagnostic threshold for a major depressive episode. The remainder of the patients who recover will experience at least one relapse during the follow-up interval; a small proportion will cycle rapidly in and out of depressive episodes. Clearly, there is considerable variability in the prognosis and outcome of depressive disorder, and identification of factors that facilitate or impede recovery is an important research issue.

Whether the likelihood of recovery from a depressive episode is related to age remains unresolved. Most studies that compared older and younger depressed patients showed no age differences in the likelihood of recovery (Alexopoulos et al. 1996; Andrew et al. 1993; George et al. 1989; Hinrichsen and Hernandez 1993; Tuma 1996). Other studies have reported that older adults are less likely to recover than middle-aged and younger adults (Cole 1983; Hughes et al. 1992); these differences, although statistically significant, are relatively modest. Age at onset also may be important. For example, Alexopoulos et al. (1996) observed lower rates of recovery among depressed older adults experiencing their first episodes of depression than among those with a history of depressive episodes.

Gender has been studied as a potential predictor of recovery by multiple investigators. Most studies have shown that men are more likely than women to recover from an episode of depression (George et al. 1989; Hughes et al. 1992; Winokur et al. 1993). Again, however, results have been inconsistent. Most investigators have reported that gender is unrelated to recovery (Brugha et al. 1990a; Hinrichsen and Hernandez 1993; Zlotnick et al. 1996), and one study showed lower rates of recovery among older men than among older women (Baldwin and Jolley 1986).

Few studies have examined the role of socioeconomic status in recovery from depression. In the studies available, education—and, more broadly, socioeconomic status—did not affect the likelihood of recovery from depression (Andrew et al. 1993; George et al. 1989; Hinrichsen and Hernandez 1993). Despite the consistency of findings across studies, this issue requires additional attention. All of the studies cited here were based on clinical samples. Given that health care settings often serve patient populations that are relatively socially homogeneous, it is not clear that this relationship has received a compelling test.

The role of stress in facilitating or impeding recovery from depression has received considerable attention, although results are, again, not consistent. The effects of life events on the course and outcome of depression have been examined in six previous studies. In three of them, the occurrence of life events was associated with a decreased likelihood of recovery (Brugha et al. 1990a; Holahan and Moos 1991; Murphy 1983). In two of the studies, life events were unrelated to the likelihood of recovery (George et al. 1989; Hinrichsen and Hernandez 1993). Baldwin et al. (1993) suggested that the relation between life events and recovery from depression may be interactive rather than unidirectional. In their sample, life events reduced the likelihood of recovery among older patients without cerebral disease but not among those with cerebral disease. Investigators in two studies examined the effects of life events on recovery and relapse among patients with bipolar disorder. Again, the results were inconsistent. In one study, the occurrence of events increased the probability of relapse (Hunt et al. 1992); the other study showed no relation between life events and recovery or relapse (McPherson et al. 1993). McPherson and colleagues (1993) suggested that life events may be important in early episodes of bipolar disease but unimportant in later episodes, by which time the disease is less responsive to external factors. This hypothesis awaits empirical investigation.

Chronic stress has been explored in relation to recovery from depression in multiple studies. Chronic physical illness has been examined most frequently. Again, results have been mixed. Hinrichsen and Hernandez (1993) reported no relation between chronic illness and recovery from depression. In contrast, Baldwin and Jolley (1986) reported that chronic illness lowered the likelihood of re-

covery in their sample of older adults. Hughes et al. (1993) used data from a sample of middle-aged and older patients and reported that physical illness reduced recovery from depression among middle-aged subjects but not among older participants. Vieil and colleagues (1992) used a more comprehensive measure to study the relation between number of chronic stressors and recovery from depression. They found that higher levels of chronic stress were associated with reduced likelihood of recovery. In more recent studies, functional disability has been more frequently studied than physical illness as a chronic stressor. Evidence in these studies is consistent: rates of recovery from depression are lower among disabled older adults (Bosworth et al. 2002; Hays et al. 1997; Oxman and Hull 2001).

Social support has been the social factor most frequently studied in relation to recovery from depression during old age. However, the findings available do not translate into clear-cut conclusions. Some of the inconsistent findings undoubtedly reflect differences in sample composition. Additional complexity results from the fact that investigators have examined multiple facets of social support. It is helpful to begin with objective dimensions of social support and to then move to subjective perceptions of support quality.

Results are contradictory with regard to the relation between size of social network and probability of recovery from a depressive episode. Henderson and Moran (1983) observed no relation between network size and recovery from depression in their sample of community-dwelling adults. In contrast, in their sample of middle-aged and older depressed patients, George and colleagues (1989) found larger network size to be associated with poorer prognosis. The direction of this relation is counterintuitive and will be addressed shortly. Presence versus absence of a confidant also is a structural property of the social network. To date, no evidence shows that the presence of a confidant affects the likelihood of recovery from depression (Andrew et al. 1993; Murphy 1983). Marital status is another characteristic of the social network. Three previous studies have scrutinized the relation between marital status and recovery from depression. In two studies, marital status had no effect on recovery (Andrew et al. 1993; Hinrichsen and Hernandez 1993); in one study, married patients were less likely than unmarried patients to recover from an episode of depression (George et al. 1989). This result also is counterintuitive.

We believe that the surprising effects of social network size and marital status on recovery from depression reflect selectivity factors. In the community, undoubtedly most social networks and marital relationships are of high quality; consequently, having larger social networks and being married are likely to have positive effects on mental health. In clinical samples, however, patients likely disproportionately represent individuals whose social networks and marriages are problematic or of poor quality. If the quality of those relationships is poor, it is not surprising that their presence predicts a lower rather than a higher probability of recovery. Of course, when measures of quality are introduced, the focus is shifted from objective to subjective facets of social support.

Only one study has addressed the effects of levels of social interaction with network members and receipt of instrumental support on recovery from depression (George et al. 1989). Although both measures were significant in bivariate analyses (with higher levels of interaction promoting recovery and high levels of instrumental assistance impeding recovery), the relations were reduced to nonsignificance once the patients' perceptions of support were added in multivariate models.

Perceptions of support have received the most attention in previous studies of the course and outcome of depressive disorder. Again, results have been mixed. A few research teams have reported that perceptions of social support are unrelated to recovery (Andrew et al. 1993; Hinrichsen and Hernandez 1993; Hirschfeld et al. 1986). Most studies, however, have found that in prospective designs, perception of high-quality support significantly increases the likelihood of recovery (Blazer et al. 1992; Bosworth et al. 2002; Brugha et al. 1990b; George et al. 1989; Hays et al. 1997; Henderson and Moran 1983; Holahan and Moos 1991; Hughes et al. 1993; Oxman and Hull 2001; Sherbourne et al. 1995; Vieil et al. 1992). One study also reported that perceptions of support quality are positively related to recovery from bipolar disorder (Stefos et al. 1996).

Thus far, this discussion has focused on the direct effects of social factors on the course and outcome of depression. A few investigators also have examined the interactive effects of social factors on recovery. First, the stress-buffering hypothesis, positing that social support is more important among persons experiencing stressful life events than among those without such stress, has been tested in two studies. The findings in one study supported the stress-buffering hypothesis (Holahan and Moos 1991), whereas data from the other study did not (George et al. 1989). Second, social support has been shown to interact with other factors to affect the likelihood of recovery. George et al. (1989) found that perceived social support interacted with both age and gender, such that it was more important for middle-aged than for older adults and more important for men than for women.

One form of social integration, religious participation, has been shown to predict recovery from major depression (Koenig et al. 1998). Several dimensions of religious participation were examined: frequency of attending religious services, time devoted to private devotions (such as prayer and reading sacred texts), and intrinsic religious motivation (as opposed to participating for social rewards or escape from social pressures). Intrinsic religiosity was a strong predictor of recovery itself and of time until recovery. Service attendance and private devotions did not contribute explanatory power.

Recall from the discussion of social factors and the onset of depression that some investigators expressed concern that reports of perceived support by depressed persons may be contaminated by the dysphoria of their illness. This issue also has been raised with regard to the role of perceived support in recovery from depression (Henderson 1984). Results to date have failed to support the contamination hypothesis. First, as noted above, perceived support has been shown to interact significantly in one or more studies with life events, age, and gender. These complex interactions argue against the contamination hypothesis—it would be necessary to explain why the contamination disproportionately affected men, middle-aged adults, and persons who recently experienced stressful life events. Second, in studies in which bivariate correlations were reported, the relations between perceived support and severity of depressive symptoms were quite modest (typically $r = 0.2–0.3$), suggesting little overlap between the two concepts. Finally, two studies have reported that perceived support is more stable over time than is the presence of depressive symptoms (Blazer et al. 1992; Brugha et al. 1990a), thereby arguing against the position that they reflect the same underlying phenomenon.

Ideally, one would like to know about the relative efficacy of social factors compared with the clinical features of the illness episode in predicting recovery from depression. To date, researchers in four studies have made such "head-to-head" comparisons (Alexopoulos et al. 1996; Andrew et al. 1993; George et al. 1989; Hays et al. 1997). In all four studies, social factors were stronger predictors of outcome than were the clinical features of the index episode, although large proportions of variance remained unexplained. Stefos and colleagues (1996) reported the same results with regard to predictors of recovery from bipolar disorder. Examples of the clinical variables examined include previous episodes and hospitalizations, comorbid substance abuse, comorbid anxiety disorder, severity of symptoms at baseline, family history of disorder, and depressive subtype (e.g., melancholic vs. nonmelancholic).

Although firm conclusions about the relations between social factors and recovery are generally premature because of inconsistencies across studies, it is clear that social factors are implicated in the course and outcome of depression. Research efforts on these issues are increasing, but considerable additional attention is warranted.

Recovery From Alcohol Abuse or Dependence

Compared with the work that has been done concerning depression, the amount of research on the course and outcome of alcohol abuse and dependence has been very limited, and the studies available are quite dated. The available evidence suggests, however, that alcoholism is associated with a natural history considerably different from that observed with depression. Vaillant (1983) used extensive longitudinal data to describe three major patterns of alcohol-related disorders: 1) a consistent pattern of occasional abuse that does not lead to dependence, 2) an atypical pattern of early and massive alcohol misuse that leads to dependence during early adulthood, and 3) the major pattern, in which "social drinking" on a regular basis leads to persistent heavy drinking and eventual dependence. The population of older alcoholic patients contains two groups: 1) persons who developed alcoholism earlier in life and who continue alcohol abuse or dependence during old age and 2) late-onset alcoholic persons, for whom problem drinking emerged for the first time during late life (Helzer et al. 1991; Warheit and Auth 1985). Some investigators suggest that late-onset alcoholism is more strongly related to social risk factors than are early-onset alcohol problems (Dupree et al. 1984; Wattis 1983), but evidence for this assertion is scant.

A few researchers have investigated the possible role of social factors in the course of alcoholism, although most studies, unfortunately, are dated and/or rely on very small samples. Vaillant (1983) reported that social support and religious participation increased the probability of recovery from acute alcoholism, although these factors explain only a small proportion of the variance in illness duration. Similarly, Helzer et al. (1984) reported that social isolation—primarily, the absence of a spouse or confidant—was a predictor of longer acute episodes of alcoholism and, interestingly, that social isolation was more strongly predictive of recovery for older than for younger persons. Helzer and colleagues also reported that among older alcoholic persons, more favorable outcomes were associated with female gender, white race, and higher socioeconomic status. Other studies have supported the

conclusions that life events are related to poorer prognosis during later life (Finney et al. 1980; Wells-Parker et al. 1983) and that being married increases the likelihood of recovery, especially among older men (Bailey et al. 1965). Several investigators also have suggested that these social factors are more potent predictors of outcome for late-onset than for early-onset alcoholism (Abrahams and Patterson 1978–1979; Rosin and Glatt 1971; Schuckit et al. 1980). This topic clearly merits additional research.

Help Seeking for Psychiatric Disorders

Social factors have been shown to play a meaningful—albeit not fully understood—role in the onset and course of psychiatric disorders. They also are related both to the likelihood that individuals will seek help for psychiatric problems and to the source from which help is sought.

Mental Health Service Use

The primary theory underpinning research on health service use was developed by Ronald Andersen and colleagues (Andersen 1968; Andersen et al. 1975); it remains the dominant theory in the field (Andersen 1995). This simple yet highly useful theory posited that health service use is a function of three generic classes of antecedents: predisposing variables, enabling factors, and need factors. *Predisposing variables* are social and attitudinal variables (such as gender, age, educational level, and attitudes toward physicians) that predispose certain individuals to seek help from medical providers. *Enabling factors* are resources that facilitate health service use (e.g., income level and insurance coverage). *Need factors* are the signs and symptoms of disease and disability that can trigger the decision to seek health care. Andersen developed this theory to identify predictors of differential access to health care. The theory has been used more broadly, however, to examine the major predictors of health service use.

The Andersen model has been used primarily in studies of health service use for physical illnesses, both acute and chronic. However, it also has proven to be useful for understanding the role of social and economic factors in help seeking for psychiatric disorders. Those studies suggest that mental health treatments, especially in the mental health specialty sector, are viewed as more discretionary than are treatments for physical complaints both by the public and by administrators of reimbursement programs (e.g., insurance coverage is less likely to exist at all and is more limited for mental health treatments than for services sought for physical illness). And recent research confirms that this pattern has been stable for at least 25 years (Sturm and Sherbourne 2001). As one would hope in a health care system that strives for equity, need factors are the strongest predictors of service use for psychiatric disorders (Katz et al. 1997; Leaf et al. 1985). Nonetheless, predisposing and enabling factors are stronger predictors of service use for psychiatric disorders than they are for physical illnesses. Lower education and income levels, being a member of a racial or ethnic minority, being male, and being old are all associated with lower probability of receiving mental health treatment in the presence of psychiatric disorder (Katz et al. 1997; Leaf et al. 1985).

The relation between race and use of mental health services is especially troubling because race remains a significant predictor of service use after socioeconomic factors are taken into account. Research reinforces this fact. Padgett et al. (1994) examined patterns of mental health service use in a well-insured, nonpoor population—federal employees. No racial differences were found for inpatient psychiatric care. However, large differences in outpatient treatment between whites and African Americans were observed for adults of all ages and for the elderly in particular.

Interestingly, research on help seeking by older adults has identified an enabling factor that was omitted from the original Andersen model—that is, social support. Adding social support to the Andersen model requires that we address the interface between formal services provided by physicians and other professional providers and informal services provided by family and friends. Two competing hypotheses have been raised to explain the relation between formal and informal service use by impaired older adults (Noelker and Bass 1989). The first hypothesis suggests that formal services typically are used as substitutes for informal services. Thus, the *substitution hypothesis* posits that formal services will be used primarily by persons without informal sources of assistance. In contrast, the *supplementation hypothesis* posits that formal services are used most often to supplement the contributions of family and friends. Indeed, the supplementation hypothesis suggests that health professionals and informal providers complement and reinforce one another—for example, by working together to ensure the impaired older adult's maximum compliance with treatment plans. Tests of these competing hypotheses have seldom been performed with regard to mental health service use. The limited evidence available from research focused on physical illness primarily supports the supplementa-

tion hypothesis (Edelman and Hughes 1990; Murdock and Schwartz 1978; Noelker and Bass 1989; Smith 1985; Wan 1987), although some studies support the substitution hypothesis (Krause 1988). Given evidence that 1) mental health care is viewed as more discretionary than treatment for physical illness, and 2) the role of social support strongly affects the course and outcome of psychiatric disorders, investigation of these hypotheses in the context of mental health problems is a high-priority issue for future research. In the one study available, lack of social support increased volume of outpatient care among persons with high levels of psychiatric symptoms (Kouzis and Eaton 1998).

Another issue needs to be addressed with regard to predictors of mental health service use. As applied in previous research, the Andersen model has been used to predict both receipt of any medical care and volume of care received. However, recent evidence suggests that these indicators of service use must be examined separately with different models. The decision to seek or not seek treatment is largely in the control of the individual; thus, receipt of any care versus no care measures help seeking. In contrast, volume of treatment is largely determined by the physician or service provider. A study by Leaf and colleagues (1985) clearly showed the importance of this distinction. Although need factors were the strongest predictor of any care, they were not significant predictors of volume of care received. Similarly, women were more likely to seek care for psychiatric problems, but gender was unrelated to volume of care received. Interestingly, only age was a significant predictor of both receipt and volume of care. Both older (age 65 and older) and younger adults (aged 18–24) were less likely to seek mental health treatment than those aged 25–64, and when treatment was received, the older and younger adults obtained less care.

Although the Andersen model has dominated research on health service use, there are other useful theories. Two major alternatives are the *health belief models* (Strecher et al. 1997) and the *congruence theories* (Berkanovic and Telesky 1982). These theories focus on the beliefs, attitudes, and modes of symptom recognition and attribution that underlie decisions to seek medical care. Research based on these alternative theories adds a useful psychological and interpretive dimension to the social determinism of the Andersen model. In general, research based on these models is compatible with findings generated by use of the Andersen model. Of particular interest is the fact that the same subgroups found to be less likely to seek help in research based on the Andersen model (i.e., men, the old, and racial and ethnic minorities) are identified in research based on health belief and/or congruence models to be less likely to recognize symptoms, to make accurate attributions about their cause, and to believe that medical care would be beneficial (for a review, see Krause 1990).

Sector Choice for Treatment of Psychiatric Problems

It is widely recognized that the general medical sector provides the majority of care to persons with psychiatric disorders (Kessler et al. 1999; Regier et al. 1993). There also is considerable concern that mentally ill persons may receive lower quality care when treated in the general medical sector. These concerns are supported by evidence that general medical sector providers often 1) fail to identify psychiatric disorders; 2) fail to treat mental disorders, even when identified; and 3) do not provide the most efficacious treatments to the patients they treat (Gallo et al. 1999; Raue and Meyers 1997). Inappropriate use of psychotropic drugs is of particular concern, especially for older patients. Thus, it is important to understand the determinants of sector choice for treatment of psychiatric disorders.

Most older adults seeking outpatient care for mental health problems receive diagnoses and treatment in the general medical sector. George et al. (1988) examined data from three community samples and found that older adults were twice as likely to receive mental health treatments from general medical providers than from specialty mental health providers. Leaf et al. (1989) reported similar distributions across general medical and mental health sectors. Based on data from the National Ambulatory Medical Care Surveys (NAMCS), Schurman and co-workers (1985) reported that 80% of all older adults with primary or secondary psychiatric diagnoses received treatment by primary care physicians. Data from the 1989 and 1990 NAMCS indicated that both old and young adults were far less likely than the middle aged to receive mental health treatment from psychiatrists (Schappert 1993).

A major reason that most psychiatric disorders are treated in the general medical sector is that primary care physicians typically do not refer patients with psychiatric disorders to mental health professionals (Gallo et al. 1999). Schurman et al. (1985), for example, reported that primary care physicians refer only 5% of older patients with psychiatric problems to psychiatrists, although the most severely ill are the most likely to be referred. Rates of referral to mental health specialists were lower for older than for young and middle-aged patients. This pattern also has been observed in a health maintenance organization (HMO) setting in which psychiatrists

were located in the same building as the primary care physicians (Goldstrom et al. 1987).

As noted above, sector choice is important because evidence indicates that general medical providers treat psychiatric disorders differently than do mental health professionals. This issue is especially important because older adults are more likely than their younger peers to obtain mental health treatment in the general medical sector. Both the amount of time spent with patients and the types of treatments used differ between general medical and mental health providers. Schurman et al. (1985) reported that the average outpatient visit for treatment of psychiatric problems was 19.6 minutes for general medical providers compared with 44.3 minutes for mental health providers. The major factor accounting for this difference is that primary care physicians are unlikely to provide psychotherapy. Psychotherapy is provided in 96% of office visits to mental health professionals but in only 25% of visits to general medical providers (Schurman et al. 1985). In contrast, general medical providers are far more likely to prescribe psychotropic drugs than are mental health professionals. Schurman et al. reported that 78% of the office visits for mental health problems to primary care physicians included the prescription of psychotropic medications, as compared with 25% of the visits to mental health providers. Studies restricted to samples of older adults have found the same pattern. For example, Burns and Taube (1990) estimated that older adults with psychiatric disorders who are treated in the general medical sector are four times more likely to receive psychotropic drugs than to receive psychotherapy. Even more sobering are the results of another study: only 30% of the patients treated by mental health professionals obtained accurate psychotropic medication management (Young et al. 2001). This suggests serious medication mismanagement. Nonetheless, this rate is nearly twice as high as the rate of accurate psychotropic medication management (17%) observed among primary care providers.

Another barrier to use of mental health professionals by older adults with mental illness may be resistance by the older adults in need of care. Despite decades of public education, the stigma associated with mental illness and receiving care from mental health professionals remains a concern among many Americans (Link et al. 1997). And some evidence suggests that older adults are more concerned about stigma than are their younger peers (Sirey et al. 2001). This barrier is especially disconcerting in light of evidence that, in the abstract, older adults report that psychotherapy is greatly preferred over psychotropic medications for emotional problems (Landreville et al. 2001), and, as noted earlier, older adults are not likely to receive psychotherapy from their primary care physicians.

Public Policies and Programs

This chapter would not be complete without consideration of the role of public policies and programs. Public policies and programs are interventions. Not all public policies are intended to affect the risk of psychiatric disorder in later life or help seeking for such problems. Indeed, most policies and programs are intended to achieve very different goals. Nonetheless, because public policies and programs alter distributions of social and economic characteristics of the elderly, they frequently affect—either directly or indirectly—the prevalence and distribution of psychiatric disorders during later life.

In the United States, federal programs for the elderly are concentrated in two areas: income maintenance and health care financing. Social Security retirement benefits are the major income transfers to older Americans, but such income is augmented by other programs such as disability benefits and food stamps. Other policies ensure that older Americans are taxed at lower rates than their younger peers, permitting them to retain larger portions of their incomes. There is substantial heterogeneity in levels of income and assets among older adults. Nonetheless, on the whole, older Americans are less likely than are younger citizens to live in poverty (Crown 2001). As noted earlier, socioeconomic status is related both to the risk of psychiatric disorders in later life and to the likelihood that mental health services will be obtained. Thus, federal income maintenance programs undoubtedly affect the prevalence and distribution of psychiatric disorders in later life.

Medicare and Medicaid, the major public health care financing programs in the United States, were designed to serve the elderly and the poor, respectively. Medicare coverage is nearly universal among current cohorts of older adults, and a sizable minority of older Americans is covered by Medicaid. There is indisputable evidence that Medicare and Medicaid have increased accessibility to health services for older adults and the poor. Despite the beneficial effects of Medicare and Medicaid, mental health benefits—especially for Medicare—are much lower than those for physical illnesses. Indeed, even a change in the regulations that govern those programs can alter the availability and quality of health care.

Space limitations preclude a review of other, less universal policies and programs targeted in whole or in part toward older adults—programs ranging from veterans' benefits to senior centers to subsidized housing. All of these programs, as well as many others, however, have the potential to favorably affect risk factors for psychiatric disorders in later life and patterns of help seeking for mental health problems. Conversely, reductions in or elimination of these programs may increase risk factors for subgroups that are affected by the changes.

One issue emphasized throughout this chapter has been the degree to which risk factors vary across cohorts. Awareness of cohort differences is especially relevant for generalizing over time and anticipating future trends. The public policy arena, however, is one area in which speculation is very difficult because programs are often changed rapidly as a result of shifting political climates and priorities. Anticipation of the future is further complicated by the fact that the psychiatric status of future cohorts will be affected by the policies and programs to which they are exposed during earlier stages of the life course. Thus, we can only note that major policy changes have the potential to generate cohort differences in the prevalence and distribution of psychiatric disorders and in patterns of help seeking for mental health problems during later life.

Summary

Social and economic factors play complex and substantial roles in psychiatric disorders in later life. There is excellent evidence that some factors, such as stress and social support, are strongly related to the risk of psychiatric disorders in later life. For other potential risk factors, the links are less well documented, and additional research is needed. Evidence is accumulating that social factors also are implicated in both the course of and the likelihood of recovery from psychiatric disorders, although additional research is required to resolve the inconsistencies observed in previous studies. Social factors also are strongly related to the likelihood that older adults with psychiatric disorders will seek help for them and to the sources from whom treatment will be obtained. Federal income maintenance and health care financing programs directly affect distributions of social and economic risk factors and thus indirectly affect the prevalence and patterns of help seeking for psychiatric disorders in later life. The greatest and most interesting challenge in this area is monitoring the multiple dynamic processes that intersect and intertwine to affect the risk of experiencing psychiatric disorders, the likelihood of recovering from those illnesses, and the receipt of appropriate treatment for psychiatric disorders in later life.

References

Abrahams R, Patterson P: Psychological distress among community elderly: prevalence, characteristics, and implications for service. Int J Aging Hum Dev 9:1–19, 1978–1979

Alexopoulos GS, Meyers BS, Young RC, et al: Recovery in geriatric depression. Arch Gen Psychiatry 53:305–312, 1996

American Psychiatric Association: Diagnostic and Statistical Manual of Mental Disorders, 3rd Edition, Revised. Washington, DC, American Psychiatric Association, 1987

American Psychiatric Association: Diagnostic and Statistical Manual of Mental Disorders, 4th Edition. Washington, DC, American Psychiatric Association, 1994

American Psychiatric Association: Diagnostic and Statistical Manual of Mental Disorders, 4th Edition, Text Revision. Washington, DC, American Psychiatric Association, 2000

Andersen R: A Behavioral Model of 'Families' Use of Health Services. Chicago, IL, University of Chicago Center for Health Administration, 1968

Andersen RM: Revisiting the behavioral model and access to medical care: does it matter? J Health Soc Behav 36:1–10, 1995

Andersen R, Kravits J, Anderson O: Equity in Health Services. Cambridge, MA, Ballinger, 1975

Andrew B, Hawton K, Fagg J, et al: Do psychological factors influence outcome in severely depressed female psychiatric inpatients? Br J Psychiatry 163:747–754, 1993

Antonucci TC: Social supports and social relationships, in Handbook of Aging and the Social Sciences, 3rd Edition. Edited by Binstock RH, George LK. San Diego, CA, Academic Press, 1990, pp 205–227

Arling G: Strain, social support, and distress in old age. J Gerontol 42:107–113, 1987

Bailey M, Haberman P, Alksne H: The epidemiology of alcoholism in an urban residential area. Q J Stud Alcohol 26:19–40, 1965

Baldwin RC, Jolley DJ: The prognosis of depression in old age. Br J Psychiatry 149:574–583, 1986

Baldwin RC, Benbow SM, Marriott A, et al: Depression in old age—a reconsideration of cerebral disease in relation to outcome. Br J Psychiatry 163:82–90, 1993

Barrett AE: Marital trajectories and mental health. J Health Soc Behav 41:451–464, 2000

Bellah RN, Madsen R, Sullivan WM, et al: Habits of the Heart. Berkeley, University of California Press, 1985

Berkanovic E, Telesky C: Social networks, beliefs, and the decision to seek medical care: an analysis of congruent and incongruent patterns. Med Care 20:1018–1026, 1982

Blanchard-Fields F, Irion JC: The relation between locus of control and coping: age as a moderator variable. Psychol Aging 3:197–203, 1988

Blazer DG, Burchett B, Service C, et al: The association of age and depression among the elderly: an epidemiologic exploration. J Gerontol 46:M210–M215, 1991

Blazer DG, Hughes DC, George LK: Age and impaired subjective support: predictors of symptoms at one-year follow-up. J Nerv Ment Dis 180:172–178, 1992

Blazer DG, Landerman LR, Hays JC, et al: Symptoms of depression among community-dwelling elderly African-American and white older adults. Psychol Med 28:1311–1320, 1998

Bosworth HB, Hays JC, George LK, et al: Psychosocial and clinical predictors of unipolar depression outcome in older adults. Int J Geriatr Psychiatry 17:238–246, 2002

Brown GW, Harris T: Social Origins of Depression: A Study of Psychiatric Disorder in Women. London, Tavistock, 1978

Bruce ML: Depression and disability in late life: directions for future research. Am J Geriatr Psychiatry 9:99–101, 2001

Bruce ML, Hoff RA: Social and physical health factors for first-onset major depressive disorder in a community sample. Soc Psychiatry Psychiatr Epidemiol 29:165–171, 1994

Brugha TS, Bebbington PE, Sturt E, et al: The relation between life events and social support networks in a clinically depressed cohort. Soc Psychiatry Psychiatr Epidemiol 25:308–312, 1990a

Brugha TS, Bebbington PE, MacCarthy B, et al: Gender, social support, and recovery from depressive disorders: a prospective clinical study. Psychol Med 20:147–156, 1990b

Brummett BH, Babyak MA, Barefoot JC, et al: Social support and hostility as predictors of depressive symptoms in cardiac patients one month after hospitalization: a prospective study. Psychosom Med 60:707–713, 1998

Burke KC, Burke JD Jr, Rae DS, et al: Comparing age at onset of major depression and other psychiatric disorders by birth cohorts in five US community populations. Arch Gen Psychiatry 48:789–795, 1991

Burns B, Taube C: Mental health services in general medical care and in nursing homes, in Mental Health Policy for Older Americans: Protecting Minds at Risk. Edited by Fogel BS, Furino A, Gottlieb GL. Washington, DC, American Psychiatric Press, 1990, pp 63–84

Chen L, Eaton WW, Gallo JJ, et al: Understanding the heterogeneity of depression through the triad of symptoms, course and risk factors: a longitudinal, population-based study. J Affect Disord 59:1–11, 2000

Cole MG: Age, age of onset, and course of primary depression in the elderly. Can J Psychiatr 28:102–104, 1983

Cronkite RC, Moos RH: The role of predisposing and moderating factors in the stress-illness relationship. J Health Soc Behav 25:372–393, 1984

Crown W: Economic status of the elderly, in Handbook of Aging and the Social Sciences, 5th Edition. Edited by Binstock RH, George LK. San Diego, CA, Academic Press, 2001, pp 352–368

Cutler SJ, Hendricks J: Age differences in voluntary association memberships: fact or artifact? J Gerontol B Psychol Sci Soc Sci 55:S98–S107, 2000

Cutrona C, Russell D, Rose J: Social support and adaptation to stress by the elderly. Psychol Aging 1:47–54, 1986

Dimond M, Lund DA, Caserta MS: The role of social support in the first two years of bereavement in an elderly sample. Gerontologist 27:599–604, 1987

Dupree LW, Broskowski H, Schonfeld L: The Gerontology Alcohol Project: a behavioral treatment program for elderly alcohol abusers. Gerontologist 24:510–516, 1984

Edelman P, Hughes S: The impact of community care on provision of informal care to homebound elderly persons. J Gerontol 45:S74–S84, 1990

Falcon LM, Tucker KL: Prevalence and correlates of depressive symptoms among Hispanic elders in Massachusetts. J Gerontol B Psychol Sci Soc Sci 55:S108–S116, 2000

Feighner JP, Robins E, Guze SB, et al: Diagnostic criteria for use in psychiatric research. Arch Gen Psychiatry 26:57–63, 1972

Finney J, Moos R, Mewborn CR: Posttreatment experiences and treatment outcome of alcoholic patients six months and two years after hospitalization. J Consult Clin Psychol 48:17–29, 1980

Fonda SJ, Wallace RB, Herzog AR: Changes in driving patterns and worsening depressive symptoms among older adults. J Gerontol B Psychol Sci Soc Sci 56:S352–S364, 2001

Freund AM, Baltes PB: Selection, optimization, and compensation as strategies of life management: correlations with subjective indicators of successful aging. Psychol Aging 13:531–543, 1998

Gallo JJ, Cooper-Patrick L, Lesikar S: Depressive symptoms of whites and African Americans aged 60 years and older. J Gerontol B Psychol Sci Soc Sci 53:P277–P286, 1998

Gallo JJ, Ryan SD, Ford DE: Attitudes, knowledge, and behavior of family physicians regarding depression in late life. Arch Fam Med 8:249–256, 1999

George LK: Social factors and the onset and outcome of depression, in Aging, Health Behaviors, and Health Outcomes. Edited by Schaie KW, House JS, Blazer DG. Hillsdale, NJ, Lawrence Erlbaum, 1992, pp 137–159

George LK: Sociological perspectives on life transitions. Annu Rev Sociol 19:353–373, 1993

George LK, Siegler IC, Okun MA: Separating age, cohort, and time of measurement: analysis of variance or multiple regression. Exp Aging Res 7:297–314, 1981

George LK, Blazer DG, Winfield-Laird I, et al: Psychiatric disorders and mental health service use in later life: evidence from the Epidemiologic Catchment Area program, in Epidemiology and Aging. Edited by Brody J, Maddox GL. New York, Springer, 1988, pp 189–219

George LK, Blazer DG, Hughes DC, et al: Social support and the outcome of major depression. Br J Psychiatry 154:478–485, 1989

Goldstrom ID, Burns BJ, Kessler LG, et al: Mental health services use by elderly adults in a primary care setting. J Gerontol 42:147–153, 1987

Green BH, Copeland JRM, Dewey ME, et al: Risk factors for depression in elderly people: a prospective study. Acta Psychiatr Scand 86:213–217, 1992

Greenfield SF, Swartz MS, Landerman R, et al: Long-term psychosocial consequences of childhood exposure to parental problem drinking. Am J Psychiatry 150:608–613, 1993

Grusky O, Tierney K, Manderscheid RW, et al: Social bonding and community adjustment of chronically mentally ill adults. J Health Soc Behav 26:49–63, 1985

Gurland BJ, Wilder DE, Berkman C: Depression and disability in the elderly: reciprocal relations and changes with age. Int J Geriatr Psychiatry 3:163–179, 1988

Hays JC, Krishnan KR, George LK, et al: Psychosocial and physical correlates of chronic depression. Psychiatry Res 72:149–159, 1997

Hays JC, Landerman LR, George LK, et al: Social correlates of the dimensions of depression in the elderly. J Gerontol B Psychol Sci Soc Sci 53:P31–P39, 1998

Helzer JE, Carey KE, Miller RH: Predictors and correlates of recovery in older versus younger alcoholics, in Nature and Extent of Alcohol Problems Among the Elderly. Edited by Maddox G, Robins LN, Rosenberg N. Rockville, MD, National Institute on Alcohol Abuse and Alcoholism, 1984, pp 83–99

Helzer JE, Burnam A, McEvoy LT: Alcohol abuse and dependence, in Psychiatric Disorders in America. Edited by Robins LN, Regier DA. New York, Free Press, 1991, pp 81–115

Henderson AS: Interpreting the evidence on social support. Soc Psychiatry 19:49–52, 1984

Henderson AS, Moran PAP: Social relationships during the onset and remission of neurotic symptoms: a prospective community study. Br J Psychiatry 143:467–472, 1983

Henderson AS, Grayson DA, Scott R, et al: Social support, dementia, and depression among the elderly in the Hobart community. Psychol Med 16:379–390, 1986

Henderson AS, Jorm AF, MacKinnon A, et al: The prevalence of depressive disorders and the distribution of depressive symptoms in later life: a survey using draft ICD-10 and DSM-III-R. Psychol Med 23:719–729, 1993

Hinrichsen GA, Hernandez NA: Factors associated with recovery from and relapse into major depressive disorder in the elderly. Am J Psychiatry 150:1820–1825, 1993

Hirschfeld RMA, Klerman GL, Andreasen N, et al: Psychosocial predictors of chronicity in depressed patients. Br J Psychiatry 148:648–654, 1986

Holahan CK, Holahan CJ: Self-efficacy, social support, and depression in aging: a longitudinal analysis. J Gerontol 42:65–68, 1987

Holahan CJ, Moos RH: Life stressors, personal and social resources, and depression: a 4-year structural model. J Abnorm Psychol 100:31–38, 1991

Hughes DC, Turnbull JE, Blazer DG: Family history of psychiatric disorder and low self-confidence: predictors of depressive symptoms at 12-month follow-up. J Affect Disord 25:197–212, 1992

Hughes DC, DeMallie D, Blazer DG: Does age make a difference in the effects of physical health and social support on the outcome of a major depressive episode? Am J Psychiatry 150:728–733, 1993

Hunt N, Bruce-Jones W, Silverstone T: Life events and relapse in bipolar affective disorder. J Affect Disord 25:13–20, 1992

Husaini BA, Moore ST, Castor RS, et al: Social density, stressors, and depression: gender differences among the black elderly. J Gerontol 46:P236–P242, 1991

Jones-Webb RJ, Snowden LR: Symptoms of depression among blacks and whites. Am J Public Health 83:240–244, 1993

Kandel DB, Davies M, Rabers VH: The stressfulness of daily social roles for women: marital, occupational, and household roles. J Health Soc Behav 26:64–78, 1985

Katz SJ, Kessler RC, Frank RG, et al: Mental health use, morbidity, and socioeconomic status in the United States and Ontario. Inquiry 34:38–49, 1997

Kessler RC, McGonagle KA, Kinney AM, et al: Lifetime and 12-month prevalence of DSM-III-R psychiatric disorders in the United States: evidence from the National Comorbidity Survey. Arch Gen Psychiatry 51:8–19, 1994a

Kessler RC, McGonagle KA, Nelson CB, et al: Sex and depression in the National Comorbidity Survey, II: cohort effects. J Affect Disord 30:15–26, 1994b

Kessler RC, Davis CG, Kendler KS: Childhood adversity and adult psychiatric disorder in the US National Comorbidity Survey. Psychol Med 27:1101–1119, 1997

Kessler RC, Zhao S, Katz SJ, et al: Past-year use of outpatient services for psychiatric problems in the National Comorbidity Survey. Am J Psychiatry 156:115–123, 1999

Kim J, Moen P: Retirement transitions, gender, and psychological well-being: a life-course, ecological model. J Gerontol B Psychol Sci Soc Sci 57:P212–P222, 2002

Koenig HG, Ford SM, George LK, et al: Religion and anxiety disorder: an examination and comparison of associations in young, middle-aged, and elderly adults. J Anxiety Disord 7:321–342, 1993a

Koenig HG, George LK, Blazer DG, et al: The relationship between religion and anxiety in a sample of community-dwelling older adults. J Geriatr Psychiatry 26:65–93, 1993b

Koenig HG, George LK, Meador KG, et al: The relationship between religion and alcoholism in a sample of community-dwelling adults. Hosp Community Psychiatry 45:225–231, 1994

Koenig HG, Hays JC, George LK, et al: Modeling the cross-sectional relationships between religion, physical health, social support, and depressive symptoms. Am J Geriatr Psychiatry 5:131–144, 1997

Koenig HG, George LK, Peterson BL: Religiosity and remission of depression in medically ill older patients. Am J Psychiatry 155:536–542, 1998

Kouzis AC, Eaton WW: Absence of social networks, social support, and health services utilization. Psychol Med 28:1301–1310, 1998

Krause N: Social support, stress, and well-being among older adults. J Gerontol 41:512–519, 1986

Krause N: Chronic financial strain, locus of control, and depressive symptoms among older adults. Psychol Aging 2:375–382, 1987

Krause N: Stressful life events and physician utilization. J Gerontol 43:S53–S61, 1988

Krause N: Illness behavior in late life, in Handbook of Aging and the Social Sciences, 3rd Edition. Edited by Binstock RH, George LK. San Diego, CA, Academic Press, 1990, pp 228–244

Krause N, Liang J, Yatomi N: Satisfaction with social support and depressive symptoms: a panel analysis. Psychol Aging 4:88–97, 1989

Kubzansky LD, Berkman LF, Seeman TE: Social conditions and distress in elderly persons: findings from the MacArthur Studies of Successful Aging. J Gerontol B Psychol Sci Soc Sci 55:P238–P246, 2000

La Gory M, Fitzpatrick K: The effects of environmental context on elderly depression. Journal of Aging and Health 4:459–479, 1992

Lam DH, Green B, Power MJ, et al: Dependency, matching adversities, length of survival and relapse in major depression. J Affect Disord 37:81–90, 1996

Landerman R, George LK, Blazer DG: Adult vulnerability for psychiatric disorders: interactive effects of negative childhood experiences and recent stress. J Nerv Ment Dis 179:656–663, 1991

Landreville P, Landry J, Baillargeon L, et al: Older adults' acceptance of psychological and pharmacological treatments for depression. J Gerontol B Psychol Sci Soc Sci 56:P285–P291, 2001

Leaf PJ, Livingston MM, Tischler GL, et al: Contact with health professionals for treatment of psychiatric and emotional problems. Med Care 23:1322–1337, 1985

Leaf PJ, Bruce ML, Tischler GL, et al: Factors affecting the utilization of specialty and general medical mental health services. Med Care 26:9–26, 1989

Levenson MR, Aldwin CM, Spiro A III: Age, cohort, and period effects on alcohol consumption and problem drinking: findings from the Normative Aging Study. J Stud Alcohol 59:712–722, 1998

Link BG, Cullen FT, Frank J, et al: The social rejection of former mental patients: understanding why labels matter. Am J Sociol 92:1461–1500, 1987

Link BG, Struening E, Rahav M, et al: On stigma and its consequences: evidence from a longitudinal study of men with dual diagnoses of mental illness and substance abuse. J Health Soc Behav 38:117–190, 1997

Lynch SM, George LK: Interlocking trajectories of loss-related events and depressive symptoms among elders. J Gerontol B Psychol Sci Soc Sci 57:S117–S125, 2002

Lynch JW, Kaplan GA, Shema SJ: Cumulative impact of sustained economic hardship on physical, cognitive, psychological, and social functioning. N Engl J Med 337:1889–1895, 1997

Marottoli RA, Mendes de Leon CF, Glass TA, et al: Driving cessation and increased depressive symptoms: prospective evidence from the New Haven EPESE. J Am Geriatr Soc 45:202–206, 1997

McPherson H, Herbison P, Romans S: Life events and relapse in established bipolar affective disorder. Br J Psychiatry 163:381–385, 1993

Midanik LT, Soghikian K, Ransom LJ, et al: The effect of retirement on mental health and health behaviors: the Kaiser Permanente Retirement Study. J Gerontol B Psychol Sci Soc Sci 50:S59–S61, 1995

Mirowsky J, Ross CE: Age and depression. J Health Soc Behav 33:187–205, 1992

Mirowsky J, Ross CE: Economic hardship across the life course. American Sociological Review 64:548–569, 1999

Mirowsky J, Ross CE: Age and the effect of economic hardship on depression. J Health Soc Behav 42:132–150, 2001

Mitchell J, Mathews HF, Yesavage JA: A multidimensional examination of depression among the elderly. Research on Aging 15:198–219, 1993

Moldin SO, Scheftner WA, Rice JP, et al: Association between major depressive disorder and physical illness. Psychol Med 23:755–761, 1993

Molnar BE, Buka SL, Kessler RC: Child sexual abuse and subsequent psychopathology: results from the National Comorbidity Survey. Am J Public Health 91:753–760, 2001

Murdock SH, Schwartz DF: Family structure and the use of agency services: an examination of patterns among elderly native Americans. Gerontologist 18:475–481, 1978

Murphy E: The prognosis of depression in old age. Br J Psychiatry 142:111–119, 1983

Neff JA, Husaini BA: Stress-buffer properties of alcohol consumption: the role of urbanicity and religious identification. J Health Soc Behav 26:207–221, 1985

Noelker LS, Bass DM: Home care for elderly persons: linkages between formal and informal caregivers. J Gerontol 44:S63–S70, 1989

Oxman TE, Hull JG: Social support, depression, and activities of daily living in older heart surgery patients. J Gerontol B Psychol Sci Soc Sci 52:P1–P14, 1997

Oxman TE, Hull JG: Social support and treatment response in older depressed primary care patients. J Gerontol B Psychol Sci Soc Sci 56:P35–P45, 2001

Oxman TE, Berkman LF, Kasl S, et al: Social support and depressive symptoms in the elderly. Am J Epidemiol 135:356–368, 1992

Padgett DK, Patrick C, Burns BJ, et al: Ethnicity and the use of outpatient mental health services in a national insured population. Am J Public Health 84:222–226, 1994

Popenoe D: American family decline, 1960–1990: a review and appraisal. J Marriage Fam 55:527–555, 1993

Putman RD: Bowling Alone: The Collapse and Renewal of American Community. New York, Simon & Schuster, 2000

Raue PJ, Meyers BS: An overview of mental health services for the elderly. New Dir Ment Health Serv 76:3–12, 1997

Regier DA, Narrow WE, Rae DS, et al: The de facto U.S. mental and addictive disorders service system: Epidemiologic Catchment Area prospective 1-year prevalence rates of disorders and services. Arch Gen Psychiatry 50:85–94, 1993

Roberts RE, Kaplan GA, Shema SJ, et al: Prevalence and correlates of depression in an aging cohort: the Alameda County Study. J Gerontol B Psychol Sci Soc Sci 52:S252–S258, 1997

Robins LN, Regier DA (eds): Psychiatric Disorders in America. New York, Free Press, 1991

Roof WC, McKinney WC: American Mainline Religion. New Brunswick, NJ, Rutgers University Press, 1987

Rosin A, Glatt M: Alcohol excess in the elderly. Q J Stud Alcohol 32:53–59, 1971

Ross CE, Huber J: Hardship and depression. J Health Soc Behav 26:312–327, 1985

Ross CE, Mirowsky J: Parental divorce, life-course disruption, and adult depression. J Marriage Fam 61:1034–1045, 1999

Schappert SM: Office visits to psychiatrists: United States, 1989–1990. Advance Data From Vital Health Statistics 237, 1993

Schrammel K: Comparing the labor market success of young adults from two generations. Monthly Labor Review February:3–9, 1998

Schuckit MA, Atkinson JH, Miller PL, et al: A three-year follow-up of elderly alcoholics. J Clin Psychiatry 41:412–416, 1980

Schulz R, Williamson GM: A two-year longitudinal study of depression among Alzheimer's caregivers. Psychol Aging 6:569–578, 1991

Schulz R, O'Brien AT, Bookwala J, et al: Psychiatric and physical morbidity effects in Alzheimer's disease caregiving: prevalence, correlates, and causes. Gerontologist 35:771–791, 1995

Schurman RA, Kramer PD, Mitchell JB: The hidden mental health network. Arch Gen Psychiatry 42:89–94, 1985

Sherbourne CD, Hays RD, Wells KB: Personal and psychosocial risk factors for physical and mental health outcomes and course of depression among depressed patients. J Clin Consult Psychol 63:345–355, 1995

Sirey JA, Bruce ML, Alexopoulos GS, et al: Perceived stigma as a predictor of treatment discontinuation in young and old outpatients with depression. Am J Psychiatry 158:479–481, 2001

Smith K: Sex differences in benzodiazepine use among the elderly: effects of social support. Unpublished doctoral dissertation, Duke University, Durham, NC, 1985

Song LY, Biegel DE, Milligan SE: Predictors of depressive symptomatology among lower class caregivers of persons with chronic mental illness. Community Ment Health J 33:269–286, 1997

Spitzer RL, Endicott J, Robins E: Research Diagnostic Criteria (RDC) for a Selected Group of Functional Disorders, 3rd Edition. New York, New York State Psychiatric Institute, 1978

Stefos G, Bauwens F, Pardoen D, et al: Psychosocial predictors of major affective recurrences in bipolar disorder: a 4-year longitudinal study of patients on prophylactic treatment. Acta Psychiatr Scand 93:420–426, 1996

Strecher VJ, Champion VL, Rosenstock IM: The Health Belief Model and health behavior, in Handbook of Health Behavior Research, Vol 1: Personal and Social Determinants. Edited by Gochman DS. New York, Plenum, 1997, pp 71–91

Sturm R, Sherbourne CD: Are barriers to mental health and substance abuse care still rising? J Behav Health Serv Res 28:81–88, 2001

Surtees PG: In the shadow of adversity: the evolution and resolution of anxiety and depressive disorder. Br J Psychiatry 166:583–594, 1995

Tuma TA: Effect of age on the outcome of hospital treated depression. Br J Psychiatry 168:76–81, 1996

Turner RJ, Wheaton B, Lloyd D: The epidemiology of social stress. American Sociological Review 60:104–125, 1995

U.S. Bureau of the Census: World Population Profile: 1998 (WP/98). Washington, DC, U.S. Government Printing Office, 1999

Vaillant GE: The Natural History of Alcoholism. Cambridge, MA, Harvard University Press, 1983

Vieil HO, Kuhner C, Brill G, et al: Psychosocial correlates of clinical depression after psychiatric inpatient treatment: methodological issues and baseline differences between recovered and non-recovered patients. Psychol Med 22:415–427, 1992

Wan TH: Functionally disabled elderly: health status, social support, and use of health services. Research on Aging 9:61–78, 1987

Warheit GL, Auth JB: Epidemiology of alcohol abuse in adulthood, in Psychiatry, Vol 3. Edited by Cavenar JL. Philadelphia, PA, JB Lippincott, 1985, pp 512–537

Wattis JP: Alcohol and old people. Br J Psychiatry 143:306–307, 1983

Wells-Parker E, Miles S, Spencer B: Stress experiences and drinking histories of elderly drunken driving offenders. J Stud Alcohol 44:429–437, 1983

Williams DR, Yu Y, Jackson JS, et al: Racial difference in physical and mental health: socioeconomic status, stress, and discrimination. J Health Psychol 2:335–351, 1997

Winokur G, Coryell W, Keller M, et al: A prospective follow-up of patients with bipolar and primary unipolar affective disorder. Arch Gen Psychiatry 50:457–465, 1993

Young AS, Klap R, Sherbourne CD, et al: The quality of care for depressive and anxiety disorders in the United States. Arch Gen Psychiatry 58:55–61, 2001

Zlotnick C, Shea MT, Pikonis PA, et al: Gender, type of treatment, dysfunctional attitudes, social support, life events, and depressive symptoms over naturalistic follow-up. Am J Psychiatry 153:1021–1027, 1996

The Diagnostic
Interview in Late Life

The Psychiatric Interview of Older Adults

Dan G. Blazer, M.D., Ph.D.

The foundation of the diagnostic workup of the older adult experiencing a psychiatric disorder is the diagnostic interview. Unfortunately, in this age of increasing technology in the laboratory and standardization of interview techniques, the art of the clinical interview has suffered. In this chapter the core of the psychiatric interview, including history taking, assessment of the family, and the mental status examination, is reviewed. To supplement the clinical interview, structured interview schedules and rating scales that are of value in the assessment of older adults are described. Finally, techniques for communicating effectively with older adults are outlined.

History

The elements of a diagnostic workup of the elderly patient are presented in Table 9–1. To obtain historical information, the clinician should first interview the patient, if it is feasible. Then permission can be asked of the patient to interview family members. Members from at least two generations, if available for interview, can expand the perspective on the older adult's impairment. If the patient has difficulty in providing an accurate or understandable history, the clinician should concentrate especially on eliciting the symptoms or problems that the patient perceives as being most disabling, then fill the historical gap with data from the family.

Present Illness

DSM-IV and its text revision, DSM-IV-TR (American Psychiatric Association 1994, 2000), provide the clinician with a useful catalogue of symptoms and behaviors

TABLE 9–1. Diagnostic workup of the elderly patient

History

Symptoms—present episode, including onset, duration, and change in symptoms over time

Past history of medical and psychiatric disorders

Family history of depression, alcohol abuse/dependence, psychoses, and suicide

Physical examination

Evaluation of neurologic deficits, possible endocrine disorders, occult malignancy, cardiac dysfunction, and occult infections

Mental status examination

Disturbance of consciousness

Disturbance of mood and affect

Disturbance of motor behavior

Disturbance of perception (hallucinations, illusions)

Disturbance of cognition (delusions)

Disturbance of self-esteem and guilt

Suicidal ideation

Disturbance of memory and intelligence (memory, abstraction, calculation, language, and knowledge)

of psychiatric interest that are relevant to the diagnosis of the present illness. Symptoms are bits of data—the most visible part of the clinical picture and generally the part most easily agreed on among clinicians. Symptoms should be defined in such a way that, if clinicians each obtain equivalent information, minimal disagreement arises about the presence or absence of a symptom. The decision about whether those symptoms form a syndrome or derive from a particular etiology must be determined independently of the data collection on symptoms (see Chapter 2, "Demography and Epidemiology of Psychiatric Disorders in Late Life").

Even so, the clinical interaction may be confounded by bias when a clinician communicates with an older adult about psychiatric symptoms. As many insightful clinicians, such as Eisenberg (1977), have recognized, physicians diagnose and treat diseases—that is, abnormalities in the structure and function of body organs and systems. Patients have illnesses—experiences of disvalued changes in states of being and in social function. Disease and illness do not maintain a one-to-one relationship. Factors that determine who becomes a patient and who does not can be understood only by expanding horizons beyond symptoms. In other words, patienthood is a social state (Eisenberg and Kleinman 1981). During the process of becoming a patient, the older adult, usually with the advice of others, forms a self-diagnosis of his or her problem and makes a judgment about the degree of ill-being perceived. For some, illness is perceived when a specific discomfort is experienced. For others, illness reflects a general perception of physical or social alienation and despair. Given that few uniform, satisfactory definitions of illness (or ill-being) exist, it is not surprising that terms for wellness (or well-being) also mean different things to different people. The historical background and the values of the older adult in a social class and culture contribute to the formation of constructs regarding the nature of the problem, the cause, and the possibility for recovery.

For this reason, the clinician must take care to avoid accepting the patient's explanation for a given problem or set of problems. Statements such as "I guess I'm just getting old and there's nothing really to worry about" or "Most people slow down when they get to be my age" can lull the clinician into complacency about what may be a treatable psychiatric disorder. On the other hand, the advent of new and disturbing symptoms in an older adult between each office visit can exhaust the clinician's patience to the point at which adequate pursuit of the problem is derailed. For example, the older adult with hypochondria whose difficulty with awakenings during the night is increasing may insist that this symptom be treated with a sedative and plead with the clinician not to allow continual suffering. In the clinician's view, however, the symptom is a normal accompaniment of old age and therefore should be accepted. Distress over changes in functioning, such as sexual functioning, may overwhelm the older adult patient and, especially if the clinician is perceived as unconcerned, may precipitate self-medication or even a suicide attempt.

To prevent attitudinal biases when eliciting reports by the older adult (which may result in missing the symptoms and signs of a treatable psychiatric disorder), the clinician must include in the initial interview a review of the more important psychiatric symptoms in a relatively structured format. Common symptoms that should be reviewed include excessive weakness or lethargy; depressed mood or the blues; memory problems; difficulty concentrating; feelings of helplessness, hopelessness, and uselessness; isolation; suspicion of others; anxiety and agitation; sleep problems; and appetite problems. Critical symptoms that should be reviewed include the presence or absence of suicidal thoughts, profound anhedonia, impulsive behavior ("I can't control myself"), confusion, and delusions and hallucinations.

The review of symptoms is most valuable when it is considered in the context of symptom presentation. When did the symptoms begin? How long have they lasted? Has their severity changed over time? Are there physical or environmental events that precipitate the symptoms? What steps, if any, have been taken to try to correct the symptoms? Have any of these interventions proved successful? Do the symptoms vary during the day (diurnal variation)? Do they vary during the week or with seasons of the year? Do the symptoms form clusters— that is, are they associated with one another? Which symptoms appear ego-syntonic and which symptoms appear ego-dystonic? As symptoms are reviewed, a specific time frame facilitates focus on the present illness. Having a 1-month or 6-month window enables the patient to review symptoms and events temporally, an approach not usually taken by distressed elders, who tend to concentrate on immediate sufferings.

Critical to the assessment of the present illness is an assessment of function and change in function. The two parameters that are most important (and not included in usual assessments of physical and psychiatric illness) are social functioning and activities of daily living (ADLs). Questions should be asked about the social interaction of the older adult, such as the frequency of his or her visits outside the home, telephone calls, and visits from family and friends. Many scales have been developed to assess ADLs; however, in the interview the clinician can simply ask about ability to get around (for example, walk inside and outside the house), to perform certain physical activities independently (such as bathe, dress, shave, brush one's teeth, and pick out one's clothes) and to do instrumental activities (such as cook, keep one's bank account, shop, and drive).

Past History

Next, the clinician must review the past history of symptoms and episodes. The patient should be asked if he or she has had a similar episode or episodes in the past. How long did the episodes last? When did they occur? How many times in the patient's lifetime have such episodes occurred? Unfortunately, the older adult may not equate present distress with past episodes that are symptomatically similar, so the perspective of the family is especially valuable in the attempt to link current and past episodes. Other psychiatric and medical problems should be reviewed as well, especially medical illnesses that have led to hospitalization and the use of medication. Not infrequently, the older adult has experienced a major illness or trauma in childhood or as a younger adult, but he or she views this information as being of no relevance to the present episode and therefore dismisses it. Probes to elicit these data are essential. Older adults may ignore or even forget past psychiatric difficulties, especially if these difficulties were disguised. For example, mood swings in early or middle life may have occurred during periods of excessive and productive activity, episodes of excessive alcohol intake, or periods of vague, undiagnosed physical problems. Previous periods of overt disability in usual activities may flag those episodes. An older person sometimes becomes angry or irritated when the clinician continues to probe. Reassurance regarding the importance of obtaining this information will generally suffice, except when dealing with a patient who cannot tolerate the discomfort and distress, even for brief periods. Older persons who have chronic and moderately severe anxiety or a histrionic personality style, as well as distressed Alzheimer's patients, tolerate their symptoms poorly.

Family History

The distribution of psychiatric symptoms and illnesses in the family should be determined next. The older person with symptoms consistent with senile dementia or primary degenerative dementia is highly likely to have a family history of dementia. The genogram remains one of the best means for evaluating the distribution of mental illness and other relevant behaviors throughout the family tree. This genogram should include both of the parents, blood-related aunts and uncles, brothers and sisters, spouse(s), children, grandchildren, and great-grandchildren. A history should be obtained about institutionalization, significant memory problems in family members, hospitalization for a nervous breakdown or depressive disorder, suicide, alcohol abuse and dependence, electroconvulsive therapy, long-term residence in a mental health facility (and possibly a diagnosis of schizophrenia), and use of mental health services by family members (Blazer 1984).

Of relevance to the pharmacological treatment of certain disorders in older adults—especially depression—is the tendency of individuals in a family to respond therapeutically to the same pharmacological agent. If the older adult has a depressive disorder and biological relatives

have been treated effectively for depression, the clinician should determine what pharmacological agent was used to treat the depression. For example, a positive response to sertraline in a family member of the depressed older patient could make sertraline the drug of choice in treating that patient, assuming side effects are not at issue (Ayd 1975).

Mendlewicz and colleagues (1975) remind us that accurate genetic information can be better obtained when family members from more than one generation are interviewed. Many psychiatric disorders are characterized by a variety of symptoms, so asking the patient or one family member for a history of depression is insufficient. Research on the genetic expression of psychiatric disorders in families requires the psychiatric investigator to interview directly as many family members as possible to determine accurately the distribution of disorders throughout the family. Such detailed family assessment is not feasible for clinicians, yet a telephone call to a relative with permission from the patient may become a standard of clinical assessment as the genetics of psychiatric disorders are clarified.

Context

Psychiatric disorders occur in a biomedical and psychosocial context. The clinician, although he or she will of course determine what medical problems the patient has experienced, might overlook a variation in the relative contribution of these medical disorders to psychopathology. The psychosocial contribution to the onset and continuance of the problem is just as likely to be overlooked. Has the spouse of the older adult undergone a change? Are the middle-aged children managing high stress, such as caring for an emotionally disturbed child and the loss of employment simultaneously? Are the grandchildren placing emotional stress on the elderly patient, perhaps requesting money? Has the economic status of the older adult deteriorated? Has the availability of medical care changed? Although many psychiatric disorders are biologically driven, they do not occur in a psychosocial vacuum. Environmental precipitants remain important in the web of causation leading to the onset of an episode of emotional distress and are critical to the assessment of the older adult.

Medication History

Next, it is essential to evaluate the medication history of the older adult. A careful review of medications by the clinician is essential, although this may be done by a nurse or a physician's assistant. The clinician should ask the older person to bring in all pill bottles as well as a list of medications taken and the dosage schedule. A double check between the written schedule and the pill containers will frequently expose some discrepancy. Both prescription and over-the-counter drugs, such as laxatives and vitamins, should be recorded. The clinician can then identify the medications that are potentially critical in terms of drug-drug interactions and ask about them during subsequent visits.

Most elderly persons take a variety of medicines simultaneously, and the potential for drug-drug interaction is high. For example, concomitant use of fluoxetine and warfarin has been associated with an increase in the half-life of warfarin, which could lead to severe bruising (although this finding is not well documented). Some medications prescribed for older persons—such as the beta-blocker propranolol and the antihypertensive drug alpha-methyldopa—can exacerbate or produce depressive symptoms. Antianxiety agents and sedative-hypnotics can precipitate episodes of confusion and depression. Antidepressants, such as the tricyclics (TCAs), may adversely interact with other drugs, including the antihypertensive agent clonidine. Simultaneous administration of clonidine and a TCA may lead to poorly controlled episodes of hypertension with confusional episodes and possibly an exacerbation of vascular (multi-infarct) dementia. The physician, a nurse, a social worker, or a paraprofessional should carefully determine present and past medication use through a historical inventory and a review of the patient's medicine containers brought to the office.

Older persons are less likely than younger persons to abuse alcohol, but a careful history of alcohol intake is essential to the diagnostic workup. Older persons do not usually volunteer information about their alcohol intake, but they are generally forthcoming when asked about their drinking habits. Substance abuse beyond alcohol and prescription drugs is rare in older adults but not entirely absent.

Medical History

Given the high likelihood of comorbid medical problems associated with psychiatric disorders in late life, a comprehensive medical history is essential. Most older persons see a primary care physician fairly regularly (although decreasing payment by Medicare renders this assumption less accurate each year). The geriatric psychiatrist should obtain medical records, if possible. Major illnesses should be recorded. A brief phone call to the primary care physician can be extremely useful.

Family Assessment

Clinicians working with older adults must be equipped to evaluate the family—both its functionality and its potential as a resource for the older adult. Geriatric psychiatry, almost by definition, is family psychiatry. Just as an elevated white blood cell count is not pathognomonic for a particular infectious agent yet is critical to the diagnosis, the complaint that "my family no longer loves me" does not reveal the specific problems in the family yet does highlight the need to assess the potential of that family for providing care and support for the older adult (Blazer 1984). Determination of the nature of the family structure in interaction, the presence or absence of a crisis in the family, and the type and amount of support available to the older adult are the basic goals of a comprehensive diagnostic family workup.

The genogram detailing the distribution of illnesses across a family has already been described. A family tree review of individuals' roles in the family, as well as of members' availability to provide care to the older adult, is equally important. For clinical purposes, the family consists not only of individuals genetically related but also of those who have developed relationships and are living together as if they were related (Miller and Miller 1979). Many older adults, especially those who have been widowed, have close friendships that are virtually familial.

A primary goal of the clinician, as advocate for the psychiatrically disturbed older adult, is to facilitate family support for the elder during a time of disability. At least four parameters of support are important for the clinician to evaluate as the treatment plan evolves. These include 1) availability of family members to the older person over time; 2) the tangible services provided by the family to the disturbed older person; 3) the perception of family support by the older patient (and therefore the willingness of the patient to cooperate and accept support); and 4) tolerance by the family of specific behaviors that derive from the psychiatric disorder.

The clinician should ask the older person, "If you become ill, is there a family member who will take care of you for a short period of time?" Next, the availability of family members who can care for the older adult over an extended period can be determined. If a particular member is designated as the primary caregiver, plans for respite care should be discussed. Given the increased focus on short hospital stays and the documented higher levels of impairment on discharge, the availability of family members becomes essential to the effective care of the older adult after hospitalization for a psychiatric, or combined medical and psychiatric, disorder.

What specific, tangible services can be provided to the older adult by family members? Even the most devoted spouse can be limited in the delivery of certain services because he or she may not drive a car, and therefore cannot provide transportation, or is not physically strong enough to provide certain types of nursing care. Generic services of special importance in the support of the psychiatrically impaired older adult at home include transportation; nursing services (such as administering medications at home); physical therapy; checking on or continuous supervision of the patient; homemaker and household services; meal preparation; administrative, legal, and protective services; financial assistance; living quarters; and coordination of the delivery of services. These services have been termed generic because they can be defined in terms of their activities, regardless of who provides the service. Assessing the range and extent of service delivery by the family to the functionally impaired older person provides a convenient barometer of the economic, social, and emotional burdens placed on the family.

Regardless of the level of service provided by the family to the older person, if these services are to be effective, it is beneficial for the older person to perceive that he or she lives in a supportive environment. These intangible supports include the perception of a dependable network, participation or interaction in the network, a sense of belonging to the network, intimacy with network members, and a sense of usefulness to the family (Blazer and Kaplan 1983). Usefulness may be of less importance to some older adults who believe they have contributed to the family for many years and therefore deserve reciprocal services in their waning years. Unfortunately, family members, frequently stressed across generations, may not recognize this reciprocal responsibility.

Family tolerance of specific behaviors may not correlate with overall support. Every person has a level of tolerance for specific behaviors that are especially difficult. Sanford (1975) found that the following behaviors were tolerated by families of impaired older persons (in decreasing percentages): incontinence of urine (81%), personality conflicts (54%), falls (52%), physically aggressive behavior (44%), inability to walk unaided (33%), daytime wandering (33%), and sleep disturbance (16%). This frequency may appear counterintuitive, for incontinence is generally considered particularly aversive to family members. Yet the outcome of incontinence can be corrected easily enough. A few nights of no sleep, however, can easily extend family members beyond their capabilities for serving a parent, sibling, or spouse.

The Mental Status Examination

Physicians and other clinicians are at times hesitant to perform a structured mental status examination, fearing the effort will insult or irritate the patient or that the patients will view it as an unnecessary waste of time. Nevertheless, the mental status examination of the psychiatric patient in later life is central to the diagnostic workup.

Appearance may be determined by the psychiatric symptoms of the older person (e.g., the depressed patient may neglect grooming), cognitive status (e.g., the patient with dementia may not be able to match clothes or even put on clothes appropriately) and the environment of the patient (e.g., a nursing home patient may not be groomed as well as a patient living at home with a spouse).

Affect and mood can usually be assessed by observing the patient during the interview. Affect is the feeling tone that accompanies the patient's cognitive output (Linn 1980). Affect may fluctuate during the interview; however, the older person is more likely to demonstrate a constriction of affect. Mood, the state that underlies overt affect and is sustained over time, is usually apparent by the end of the interview. For example, the affect of a depressed older adult may not reach the degree of dysphoria seen in younger persons (as evidenced by crying spells or protestations of uncontrollable despair), yet the depressed mood is usually sustained and discernible from beginning to end.

Psychomotor activity may be agitated or retarded. Psychomotor retardation or underactivity is characteristic of major depression and severe schizophreniform symptoms, as well as of some variants of primary degenerative dementia. Psychiatrically impaired older persons, except some who have advanced dementia, are more likely to exhibit hyperactivity or agitation. Those who are depressed will appear uneasy, move their hands frequently, and have difficulty remaining seated through the interview. Patients with mild to moderate dementia, especially those with vascular dementia, will be easily distracted, rise from a seated position, and/or walk around the room or even out of the room. Pacing is often observed when the older adult is admitted to a hospital ward. Agitation can usually be distinguished from anxiety, for the agitated individual does not complain of a sense of impending doom or dread. In patients with psychomotor dysfunction, movement generally relieves the immediate discomfort, although it does not correct the underlying disturbance. Occasionally the older adult with motor retardation may actually be experiencing a disturbance in consciousness and may even reach an almost stuporous state. The patient may not be easily aroused, but when aroused, he or she will respond by grimacing or withdrawal.

Perception is the awareness of objects in relation to each other and follows stimulation of peripheral sense organs (Linn 1980). Disturbances of perception include hallucinations—that is, false sensory perceptions not associated with real or external stimuli. For example, a paranoid older person may perceive invasion of his or her house at night by individuals who disarrange belongings and abuse him or her sexually. Hallucinations often take the form of false auditory perceptions, false perceptions of movement or body sensation (such as palpitations), and false perceptions of smell, taste, and touch. The severely depressed older patient may have frank auditory hallucinations that condemn or encourage self-destructive behavior.

Disturbances in thought content are the most common disturbances of cognition noted in the psychotic older patient. The depressed patient often develops beliefs that are inconsistent with the objective information obtained from family members about the patient's abilities and social resources. In a series of studies, Meyers and co-workers (Meyers and Greenberg 1986; Meyers et al. 1985) found delusional depression to be more prevalent among older depressed patients than among middle-aged adults. Of 161 patients with endogenous depression, 72 (45%) were found to be delusional as determined by the Research Diagnostic Criteria (RDC; Spitzer et al. 1978). These delusions included beliefs such as "I've lost my mind," "My body is disintegrating," "I have an incurable illness," and "I have caused some great harm." Even after elderly persons recover from depression, they may still experience periodic recurrences of delusional thoughts, which can be most disturbing to an otherwise rational older adult. Older patients appear less likely to experience delusional remorse, guilt, or persecution.

Even if delusions are not obvious, preoccupation with a particular thought or idea is common among depressed elderly persons. Such preoccupation is closely associated with obsessional thinking or irresistible intrusion of thoughts into the conscious mind. Although the older adult rarely acts on these thoughts compulsively, the guilt-provoking or self-accusing thoughts may occasionally become so difficult to bear that the person considers, attempts, or succeeds in committing suicide.

Disturbances of thought progression accompany disturbances of content. Evaluation of the content and process of cognition may uncover disturbances such as problems with the structure of associations, the speed of associations, and the content of thought. Thinking is a goal-directed flow of ideas, symbols, and associations initiated in response to environmental stimuli, a perceived problem, or a task that requires progression to a logical or reality-based conclusion (Linn 1980). The compulsive or schizophrenic older adult may pathologically repeat the same word or idea in response to a variety of probes, as may the patient who has primary degenerative dementia. Some older adults with dementia exhibit circumstantiality—that is, the introduction of many apparently irrelevant details to cover a lack of clarity and memory problems. Interviews with patients who have this problem can be most frustrating because they proceed at such a slow pace. On other occasions, elderly patients may appear incoherent, with no logical connection to their thoughts, or they may produce irrelevant answers. The intrusion of thoughts from previous conversations into current conversation is a prime example of the disturbance in association found in patients with primary degenerative dementia (for example, Alzheimer's disease). This symptom is not typical of other dementias, such as the dementia of Huntington's disease. However, in the absence of dementia, even paranoid older adults do not generally demonstrate a significant disturbance in the structure of associations.

Suicidal thoughts are critical to the assessment of the psychiatrically impaired elderly patient. Although thoughts of death are common in late life, spontaneous revelations of suicidal thoughts are rare. A stepwise probe is the best means of assessing the presence of suicidal ideation (Blazer 1982). First, the clinician should ask the patient if he or she has ever thought that life was not worth living. If so, has the patient considered acting on that thought? If so, how would the patient attempt to inflict such harm? If definite plans are revealed, the clinician should probe to determine whether the implements for a suicide attempt are available. For example, if a patient has considered shooting himself, the clinician should ask, "Do you have a gun available and loaded at home?" Suicidal ideation in an older adult is always of concern, but intervention is necessary when suicide has been considered seriously and the implements are available.

Assessment of memory and cognitive status is most accurately performed through psychological testing. However, the psychiatric interview of the older adult must include a reasonable assessment. Although older adults may not complain of memory dysfunction, they are more likely than younger patients to have problems with memory, concentration, and intellect. There are brief, informal means of testing cognitive functioning that should be included in the diagnostic workup. The clinician proceeding through an evaluation of memory and intellect must also remember that poor performance may reflect psychic distress or a lack of education, as opposed to mental retardation or dementia. In addition, to rule out the potential confounding of agitation and anxiety, testing can be performed on more than one occasion.

Testing of memory is based on three essential processes: 1) registration (the ability to record an experience in the central nervous system); 2) retention (the persistence and permanence of a registered experience); and 3) recall (the ability to summon consciously the registered experience and report it) (Linn 1980). *Registration,* apart from recall, is difficult to evaluate directly. Occasionally, events or information that the older adult denies remembering will appear spontaneously during other parts of the interview. Registration usually is not impaired except in patients with one of the more severely dementing illnesses.

Retention, on the other hand, can be blocked by both psychic distress and brain dysfunction. Lack of retention is especially relevant to the unimportant data often asked for on a mental status examination. For example, requesting the older adult to remember three objects for 5 minutes will frequently reveal a deficit if the older adult has little motivation to attempt the task. Disturbances of recall can be tested directly in a number of ways. The most common are *tests of orientation* to time, place, person, and situation. Most persons continually orient themselves through radio, television, and reading material, as well as through conversations with others. Some elderly persons may be isolated through sensory impairment or lack of social contact; poor orientation in these patients may represent deficits in the physical and social environment rather than brain dysfunction. *Immediate recall* can be tested by asking the older person to repeat a word, phrase, or series of numbers, but it can also be tested in conjunction with cognitive skills by requesting that a word be spelled backward or that elements of a story be recalled.

During the mental status examination, intelligence can be assessed only superficially. Tests of simple arithmetic calculation and fund of knowledge, supplemented by portions of well-known psychiatric tests, are helpful. The classic test for calculation is to ask a patient to subtract 7 from 100 and to repeat this operation on the succession of remainders. Usually five calculations are sufficient to determine the ability of the older adult to complete this task. If the older adult fails the task, a less exacting test is to request the patient to subtract 3 from 20 and to repeat this operation on the succession of remainders until 0 is reached. These examinations must not be rushed, for older persons may not perform as well when they perceive time pressure. A capacity for *abstract thinking* is often tested by asking the patient to in-

terpret a well-known proverb, such as "A rolling stone gathers no moss." A more accurate test of abstraction, however, is classifying objects in a common category. For example, the elder is asked to state the similarity between an apple and a pear. Whereas naming objects from a category (such as fruits) is retained despite moderate and sometimes marked declines in cognition, the opposite process of classifying two different objects in a common category is not retained as well.

Rating Scales and Standardized Interviews

Rating scales and standardized or structured interviews have progressively been incorporated into the diagnostic assessment of the elderly psychiatric patient. Such rating procedures have increased in popularity as the need has increased for systematic, reproducible diagnoses for third-party carriers (part of the impetus for the dramatic change in nomenclature evidenced in DSM-IV) and for a standard means of assessing change in clinical status. A thorough review in this chapter of all instruments that are used is not possible. Therefore, selected instruments are presented and evaluated in this section, chosen either because they have special relevance to the geriatric patient or because they are widely used.

Cognitive Dysfunction and Dementia Schedules

A number of standardized assessment methods for delirium have emerged. Perhaps the best and the most easily used is the Confusion Assessment Method (CAM; Inouye 1990). This scale has incorporated DSM criteria for confusion into nine operationalized criteria, including acute onset (evidence of such onset), fluctuating course (behavior change during the day), inattention (trouble in focusing), disorganized thinking (presence of rambling or irrelevant conversations and illogical flow of ideas), and altered level of consciousness (rated from alert to comatose). Diagnosis requires both acute onset and fluctuating course, along with inattention and either disorganized thought or altered level of consciousness.

Two interviewer-administered cognitive screens for dementia have been popular in both clinical and community studies. The first is the Short Portable Mental Status Questionnaire (SPMSQ; Pfeiffer 1975), a derivative of the Mental Status Questionnaire developed by Kahn and colleagues (1960). The SPMSQ consists of 10 questions designed to assess orientation, memory, fund of knowledge, and calculation. For most community-dwelling older adults, two or fewer errors indicate intact functioning; three or four errors, mild impairment; five to seven errors, moderate impairment; and eight or more errors, severe impairment. The ease of administration of this instrument and its reliability as supported by accumulated epidemiological data make it useful for both clinical and community screens.

The Mini-Mental State Examination (Folstein et al. 1975) is a 30-item instrument that assesses orientation, registration, attention and calculation, recall, and language. It requires 5–10 minutes to administer and includes more items of clinical significance than does the SPMSQ. Seven to 12 errors suggest mild to moderate cognitive impairment and 13 or more errors severe impairment. This instrument is perhaps the most frequently used standardized screening instrument in clinical practice.

A number of clinical assessment procedures for dementia have emerged in recent years. The most widely used, and one of the first to appear, is the scale suggested by Blessed et al. (1968), usually referred to as the Blessed Dementia Index. In contrast to what can be gleaned by use of the screening scales described, clinical judgment is required in using the Blessed Dementia Index to assess changes in performance of everyday activities, such as handling money, household tasks, and shopping; changes in eating and dressing habits; changes in personality, interests, and drive; tests of information (orientation and recognition of persons); memory of past information, such as occupation, place of birth, and town where the individual worked; and concentration (calculation task). A score is assigned to each of these tasks, and a summary score is tabulated. The score has been shown to correlate well with the cerebral changes of primary degenerative dementia.

A more recent and comprehensive scale is the Alzheimer's Disease Assessment Scale (Rosen et al. 1984). This clinical rating scale includes ratings of spoken language, language comprehension, recall, ability to follow commands, word-finding difficulty in spontaneous speech, ability to name objects, constructional praxis, ideational praxis, orientation, word recall, word recognition, and a series of noncognitive behaviors, such as tearfulness, distractibility, depression, and motor activity.

A dementia scale for assessing the probability that dementia is secondary to multiple infarcts was suggested by Hachinski et al. (1975). In the study, cerebral blood flow in patients with primary degenerative dementia was compared with those who had multi-infarct dementia. Certain clinical features were determined to be more associated with multi-infarct dementia, and each of these

features was assigned a score. Those clinical features, along with their scores, are as follows: abrupt onset = 2, stepwise deterioration = 1, fluctuating course = 2, nocturnal confusion = 1, relative preservation of personality = 1, depression = 1, somatic complaints = 1, emotional incontinence = 1, history of hypertension = 1, history of strokes = 2, evidence of associated atherosclerosis = 1, focal neurological symptoms = 2, and focal neurological signs = 2. A score of 7 or greater was highly suggestive of multi-infarct dementia. However, given the frequent overlap of multiple small infarcts and primary degenerative dementia, as well as the difficulty of assessing these items effectively, most investigators have ceased to rely on the Hachinski scale for clinical use.

Depression Rating Scales

A number of self-rating depression scales have been used to screen for depression in patients at all stages of the life cycle; most of these scales have been studied in older populations. The Zung Self-Rating Depression Scale (Zung 1965) was the most widely used until recent years. The initial popularity of the Zung scale was probably due to the availability of data for persons throughout the life cycle, especially elderly persons (Zung 1967). Few randomly sampled community populations have been surveyed with the scale; therefore, a deficit exists in normative community standards. In this 20-item scale, each of the 20 symptoms is ranked from 0 ("none") to 3 ("all or about all the time"), according to severity. Most older adults can use the Zung scale, although the four choices may create problems for some elderly persons with mild cognitive impairment. Using the Zung scale, Freedman and colleagues (1982) found peak symptom levels in women ages 65–69 years and men ages 70–74 years.

The most widely used of the current instruments in community studies is the Center for Epidemiologic Studies Depression Scale (CES-D; Radloff 1977). This instrument, because of the normative population data available for it, has replaced the Zung scale in recent years as a common instrument for screening for depression. The CES-D scale is similar in format to the Zung scale. In a factor-analytic study of the CES-D in a community population, three factors were identified: enervation, positive affect, and interpersonal relationships (Ross and Mirowsky 1984). The disaggregation of these factors and the exploration of their interaction are significant steps forward in understanding the results derived from symptom scales such as the CES-D in older populations. For example, the enervation items (e.g., loss of interest, poor appetite) are more likely to be associated with a course of depressive episodes similar to that described for major depression with melancholia, and the positive-affect items more likely to be associated with life satisfaction scores.

A scale that has been widely used in clinical studies, although less studied in community populations, is the Beck Depression Inventory (BDI; Beck et al. 1961). The reliability of the BDI has been shown to be good in both depressed and nondepressed samples of older people (Gallagher et al. 1982). The instrument consists of 21 symptoms and attitudes, rated on a scale of 0 to 3 in terms of intensity. In another study by Gallagher et al. (1983), the BDI misclassified only 16.7% of subjects who had been diagnosed on the basis of the RDC as having major depression.

The Geriatric Depression Scale (GDS) was developed because the scales discussed above present problems for older persons who have difficulty in selecting one of four forced-response items (Yesavage et al. 1983). The GDS is a 30-item scale that permits patients to rate items as either present or absent; it includes questions about symptoms such as cognitive complaints, self-image, and losses. Items selected were thought to have relevance to late-life depression. The GDS has not been used extensively in community populations and is not as well standardized as the CES-D, but its yes/no format is preferred to the CES-D by many clinicians.

Of the interviewer-rated scales, the Hamilton Rating Scale for Depression (Ham-D; Hamilton 1960) is by far the most commonly used. The advantage of having ratings based on clinical judgment has made the Ham-D a popular instrument for rating outcome in clinical trials. For example, a reduction in the score to one-half the initial score or to a score below a certain value would indicate partial or complete recovery from an episode of depression.

A scale that has received considerable attention clinically, standardized in clinical but not community populations, is the Montgomery-Åsberg Rating Scale for Depression (Montgomery and Åsberg 1979). This scale follows the pattern of the Hamilton scale and concentrates on 10 symptoms of depression; the clinician rates each symptom on a scale of 0 to 6 (for a range of scores between 0 and 60). The symptoms include apparent sadness, reported sadness, inattention, reduced sleep, reduced appetite, concentration difficulties, lassitude, inability to feel, pessimistic thoughts, and suicidal thoughts. This scale, theoretically, is an improvement over the Hamilton scale in that it appears to better differentiate between responders and nonresponders to intervention for depression. The instrument does not include many somatic symptoms that tend to be more common in older adults, and therefore it may be of greater value in tracking the symp-

toms of depressive illness that would be expected to change with therapy.

General Assessment Scales

A number of general assessment scales of psychiatric status (occasionally combined with functioning in other areas) have been found to be useful in both community and clinical populations.

One of the more frequently used scales is the Global Assessment of Functioning Scale (GAF; American Psychiatric Association 2000). Using this scale, the rater makes a single rating, ranging from 0 to 100, that best describes—on the basis of his or her clinical judgment—the lowest level of the subject's functioning in the week before the rating. The scale has not been standardized for older adults, but its common use in psychiatric studies suggests the need for standardization. The scale was incorporated as Axis V in DSM-IV to measure overall functioning.

The Geriatric Mental State Schedule (Copeland et al. 1976), an adaptation of the Present State Exam (PSE; Wing et al. 1974) and the Psychiatric Status Schedule (Spitzer et al. 1968), is a semistructured interviewing guide that allows the rater to inventory symptoms associated with psychiatric disorders. More than 500 ratings are made on the basis of information obtained by a highly trained interviewer, who elicits reports of symptoms from the month preceding the evaluation. Data are computerized to derive psychiatric diagnoses (Copeland et al. 1986). The instrument measures depression, impaired memory, selected neurological symptoms such as aphasia, and disorientation.

The Comprehensive Assessment and Referral Evaluation (CARE; Gurland et al. 1977) is a hybridized assessment procedure developed for older adults. Dimensional scores are obtained in Memory–Disorientation, Depression–Anxiety, Immobility–Incapacity, Isolation, Physical–Perceptual Difficulty, and Poor Housing–Income. The goal of CARE is to provide a comprehensive assessment of the older adult that bridges the professional disciplines. The instrument has not been used extensively, although it has been used in cross-national studies. For example, Herbst and Humphrey (1980) used CARE in a study examining how hearing impairment relates to mental status. The investigators found a relationship between deafness and depression that was independent of age and socioeconomic status.

The Older Americans Resources and Services (OARS) Multidimensional Functional Assessment Questionnaire (Duke University Center for the Study of Aging and Human Development 1978), administered by a lay interviewer, produces functional impairment ratings in five dimensions: mental health, physical health, social functioning, economic functioning, and activities of daily living. In one community survey using OARS (Blazer 1978a), 13% of persons in the community were found to have mental health impairment. The OARS instrument was developed to integrate functional measures across a series of parameters relevant to older adults; it has been used widely in both community and clinical surveys. With the recent emphasis on discrete psychiatric disorders, however, the instrument has not been as widely used by mental health workers as it might otherwise have been.

Any discussion of clinical rating scales is not complete without a discussion of the Abnormal Involuntary Movement Scale (AIMS; National Institute of Mental Health 1975). There has been an increased incidence of tardive dyskinesia among older adults, coupled with the need for better documentation of this dreaded outcome of prolonged use of antipsychotic agents. Regular rating of patients on the AIMS by clinicians has therefore become essential to the practice of inpatient and outpatient geriatric psychiatry. The scale consists of seven movement disorders; the presence and severity of each is rated from "none" to "severe." Three items require a global judgment: severity of abnormal movements, incapacitation due to abnormal movements, and the patient's awareness of abnormal movements. Current problems with teeth or dentures are also assessed. Procedures are described to increase the reliability of this rating scale.

Structured Diagnostic Interviews

A number of structured interview schedules are now available for both clinical and community diagnosis. These interview schedules have allowed increased reliability of the identification of particular symptoms and psychiatric diagnoses. Unfortunately, if one adheres closely to the structured interview, the richness inherent in the unstructured interview tends to be lost. Comments made by the patient during the evaluation that could be used to trace relevant associations must be ignored to push through the interview schedule. Most of these interviews require more time than the traditional unstructured first session with the patient.

The oldest of the currently used interview schedules is the Present State Exam (PSE) (Wing et al. 1974). As noted above, the Geriatric Mental State Schedule is a variant of the PSE. The PSE is not an interview but a list of definitions of behaviors or symptoms of psychiatric interest, ranging from specific delusions to general changes in affect. The clinician scores whether the symptom is present, and a computer algorithm provides a diagnosis. Suggested questions for eliciting reports of the symptoms are available but not obligatory. Only 54 questions are required during the interview, although many additional probes are provided to track positive responses. The interview schedule provides an excellent education for many psychiatrists about the meaning of various symptoms relevant to work with older adults. Nevertheless, the focus on 1 month before the evaluation date and the association of the symptoms with the World Health Organization's International Classification of Diseases (ICD)—instead of the American Psychiatric Association's Diagnostic and Statistical Manual of Mental Disorders (DSM)—make the PSE less popular with American investigators.

The most frequently used instrument in the United States is the Structured Clinical Interview for DSM-IV (SCID; First et al. 1997). This instrument is easily adaptable to the RDC, DSM-IV, and DSM-IV-TR. Although specific questions are suggested for probing most areas of interest, the interviewer using the SCID has the flexibility to ask additional questions and can use any available data to assign a diagnosis. The interviewer must have clinical training but does not have to be a psychiatrist. Many of the symptoms may not be relevant to older adults (especially the extensive probes for psychotic symptoms), and the interview frequently takes 2½–3 hours to administer. Nevertheless, the experience gained by the clinician in using this instrument can contribute to a more effective clinical practice.

A relatively recent addition to the schedules available is the Diagnostic Interview Schedule (DIS; Robins et al. 1981). This highly structured, computer-scored interview, which can be administered by a lay interviewer, allows psychiatric diagnoses to be made according to DSM-IV criteria, Feighner criteria (Feighner et al. 1972), and RDC. The DIS questions probe for the presence or absence of symptoms or behaviors relevant to a series of psychiatric disorders, the severity of the symptoms, and the putative cause of the symptoms. Diagnoses of cognitive impairment, schizophrenia or schizophreniform disorder, major depression, generalized anxiety disorder, panic disorder, agoraphobia, obsessive-compulsive disorder, dysthymic disorder, somatization disorder, alcohol abuse and/or dependence, and other substance abuse and/or dependence can be made from Axis I of DSM-IV. A diagnosis of antisocial personality disorder (Axis II) can also be made. The instrument has proved reasonably reliable in clinic populations for both current and lifetime diagnoses.

The range of disorders probed by the DIS questions, coupled with the instrument's relative ease of administration (it generally takes 45–90 minutes to administer to an older adult), has made it popular for use in clinical studies. In addition, community-based comparative data are available on a large sample from the Epidemiologic Catchment Area study (Myers et al. 1984; Regier et al. 1984). The DIS can be supplemented with additional questions to probe for specific symptoms, such as melancholic symptoms and additional data on sleep disorders for depressed older adults. No problems have arisen when the instrument is used among older adults in the community. The memory decay that occurs in elderly persons in general is no more of a problem with this instrument than with others. Nevertheless, the DIS is of less value in the study of institutional populations and in reconstruction of lifetime history regardless of setting, because memory problems cannot be circumvented by clinical judgment. Supplementary data can be added to the instrument for developing a standardized diagnosis. A shortened version of the DIS, which has been used in recent epidemiological surveys, is the Composite International Diagnostic Interview (CIDI; World Health Organization 1989).

Effective Communication With the Older Adult

The clinician who works with the older adult should be cognizant of factors relating to both the patient and the clinician that may produce barriers to effective communication (Blazer 1978b). Many older persons experience a relatively high level of anxiety yet do not complain of this symptom. Stress deriving from a new situation, such as visiting a clinician's office or being interviewed in a hospital, may intensify such anxiety and subsequently impair effective communication. Perceptual problems, such as hearing and visual impairment, may exacerbate disorientation and complicate the communication of problems to the clinician. Elderly persons are more likely to withhold information than to hazard answers that may be incorrect—in other words, older persons tend to be more cautious. Elderly persons frequently take longer to respond to inquiries and resist the clinician who attempts to rush through the history-taking interview.

The elderly patient may perceive the physician unrealistically, on the basis of previous life experiences (that is, transference may occur). Although the older patient will sometimes accept the role of child, viewing the physician as parent, the patient is initially more likely to view the clinician as the idealized child who can provide reciprocal care to the previously capable but now impaired parent. Splitting between the physician and the children of the patient may subsequently occur. The clinician may perceive the older adult patient incorrectly because of fears of aging and death or because of previous negative experiences with his or her own parents. For a clinician to work effectively with older adults, these personal feelings should be discussed during training—and afterward.

Once physician and patient attitudes have been recognized and acknowledged, certain techniques have generally proved to be valuable in communicating with the elderly patient. These techniques should not be implemented indiscriminately, however, for the variation among the population of older adults is significant. First, the older person should be approached with respect. The clinician should knock before entering a patient's room and should greet the patient by surname (Mr. Jones, Mrs. Smith) rather than by a given name, unless the clinician also wishes to be addressed by a given name.

After taking a position near the older person—near enough to reach out and touch the patient—the clinician should speak clearly and slowly and use simple sentences in case the person's hearing is impaired. Because of hearing problems, older patients may understand conversation better over the telephone than in person. By placing the receiver against the mastoid bone, the patient with otosclerosis can take advantage of preserved bone conduction.

The interview should be paced so that the older person has enough time to respond to questions. Most elders are not uncomfortable with silence, because it gives them an opportunity to formulate their answers to questions and elaborate certain points they wish to emphasize. Nonverbal communication is frequently a key to effective communication with elderly persons, because they may be reticent about revealing affect verbally. The patient's changes in facial expression, gestures, postures, and long silences may provide clues to the clinician about issues that are unspoken.

One key to successful communication with an older adult is a willingness to continue working as a professional with that person. Older adults—possibly unlike some of their children and grandchildren—place a great deal of stress on loyalty and continuity. Most elderly patients do not require large amounts of time from clinicians, and those who are more demanding can usually be controlled through structure in the interview.

References

American Psychiatric Association: Diagnostic and Statistical Manual of Mental Disorders, 4th Edition. Washington, DC, American Psychiatric Association, 1994

American Psychiatric Association: Diagnostic and Statistical Manual of Mental Disorders, 4th Edition, Text Revision. Washington, DC, American Psychiatric Association, 2000

Ayd FJ: Treatment-resistant patients: a moral, legal and therapeutic challenge, in Rational Psychopharmacotherapy and the Right to Treatment. Edited by Ayd FJ. Baltimore, MD, Ayd Medical Communications, 1975

Beck AT, Ward CH, Mendelson M, et al: An inventory for measuring depression. Arch Gen Psychiatry 4:561–571, 1961

Blazer DG: The OARS Durham surveys: description and application, in Multidimensional Functional Assessment: The OARS Methodology—A Manual, 2nd Edition. Durham, NC, Duke University Center for the Study of Aging and Human Development, 1978a, pp 75–88

Blazer DG: Techniques for communicating with your elderly patient. Geriatrics 33:79–80, 83–84, 1978b

Blazer DG: Depression in Late Life. St Louis, MO, CV Mosby, 1982

Blazer DG: Evaluating the family of the elderly patient, in A Family Approach to Health Care in the Elderly. Edited by Blazer D, Siegler IC. Menlo Park, CA, Addison-Wesley, 1984, pp 13–32

Blazer DG, Kaplan BH: The assessment of social support in an elderly community population. Am J Soc Psychiatry 3:29–36, 1983

Blessed G, Tomlinson BE, Roth M: The association between quantitative measures of dementia and of senile change in the cerebral gray matter of elderly subjects. Br J Psychiatry 114:797–811, 1968

Copeland JRM, Kelleher MJ, Kellet JM, et al: A semi-structured clinical interview for the assessment and diagnosis of mental state in the elderly: the Geriatric Mental State Schedule. Psychol Med 6:439–449, 1976

Copeland JRM, Dewey ME, Griffiths-Jones HM, et al: A computerized psychiatric diagnostic system and case nomenclature for elderly subjects: GMS and AGECAT. Psychol Med 16:89–99, 1986

Duke University Center for the Study of Aging and Human Development: Multidimensional Functional Assessment: The OARS Methodology—A Manual, 2nd Edition. Durham, NC, Duke University Center for the Study of Aging and Human Development, 1978

Eisenberg L: Disease and illness: distinctions between professional and popular ideas of sickness. Cult Med Psychiatry 1:9–23, 1977

Eisenberg L, Kleinman A: Clinical social science, in The Relevance of Social Science for Medicine. Edited by Eisenberg L, Kleinman A. Boston, MA, D Reidel, 1981, pp 1–26

Feighner JP, Robins E, Guze SB, et al: Diagnostic criteria for use in psychiatric research. Arch Gen Psychiatry 26:57–63, 1972

First MB, Spitzer RL, Gibbon M: Structured Clinical Interview for DSM-IV. Washington, DC, American Psychiatric Press, 1997

Folstein MF, Folstein SE, McHugh PR: Mini-Mental State: a practical method for grading the cognitive state of patients for the clinician. J Psychiatr Res 12:189–198, 1975

Freedman N, Bucci W, Elkowitz E: Depression in a family practice elderly population. J Am Geriatr Soc 30:372–377, 1982

Gallagher D, Nies G, Thompson LW: Reliability of the Beck Depression Inventory with older adults. J Consult Clin Psychol 50:152–153, 1982

Gallagher D, Breckenridge J, Steinmetz J, et al: The Beck Depression Inventory and Research Diagnostic Criteria: congruence in an older population. J Consult Clin Psychol 51:945–946, 1983

Gurland B, Kuriansky J, Sharpe L, et al: The Comprehensive Assessment and Referral Evaluation (CARE)—rationale, development and reliability. Int J Aging Hum Dev 8:9–42, 1977

Hachinski VC, Iliff LD, Zilhka E, et al: Cerebral blood flow in dementia. Arch Neurol 32:632–637, 1975

Hamilton M: A rating scale for depression. J Neurol Neurosurg Psychiatry 23:56–62, 1960

Herbst KG, Humphrey C: Hearing impairment and mental state in the elderly living at home. BMJ 281:903–905, 1980

Inouye SK: Clarifying confusion: the confusion assessment method: a new method for detection of delirium. Ann Intern Med 113:941–950, 1990

Kahn RL, Goldfarb AI, Pollack M, et al: Brief objective measures for the determination of mental status in the aged. Am J Psychiatry 117:326–328, 1960

Linn L: Clinical manifestations of psychiatric disorders, in Comprehensive Textbook of Psychiatry, 3rd Edition, Vol 1. Edited by Kaplan HI, Freedman AM, Sadock BJ. Baltimore, MD, Williams and Wilkins, 1980, pp 990–1034

Mendlewicz J, Fleiss JL, Cataldo M, et al: Accuracy of the family history method in affective illness: comparison with direct interviews in family studies. Arch Gen Psychiatry 32:309–314, 1975

Meyers BS, Greenberg R: Late-life delusional depression. J Affect Disord 11:133–137, 1986

Meyers BS, Greenberg R, Varda M: Delusional depression in the elderly, in Treatment of Affective Disorders in the Elderly. Edited by Shamoian CA. Washington, DC, American Psychiatric Press, 1985, pp 37–63

Miller KT, Miller JL: The family as a system. Paper presented at the annual meeting of the American College of Psychiatrists, New York, February 1979

Montgomery SA, Åsberg M: A new depression scale designed to be sensitive to change. Br J Psychiatry 134:382–389, 1979

Myers JK, Weissman MM, Tischler GL, et al: Six-month prevalence of psychiatric disorders in three communities: 1980 to 1982. Arch Gen Psychiatry 41:959–967, 1984

National Institute of Mental Health: Development of a Dyskinetic Movement Scale (Publ No 4). Rockville, MD, National Institute of Mental Health, Psychopharmacology Research Branch, 1975

Pfeiffer E: A Short Portable Mental Status Questionnaire for the assessment of organic brain deficit in elderly patients. J Am Geriatr Soc 23:433–441, 1975

Radloff LS: The CES-D Scale: a self-report depression scale for research in the general population. Applied Psychological Measurement 1:385–401, 1977

Regier DA, Myers JK, Kramer M, et al: The NIMH Epidemiologic Catchment Area program: historical context, major objectives, and study population characteristics. Arch Gen Psychiatry 41:934–941, 1984

Robins LN, Helzer JE, Croughan J, et al: National Institute of Mental Health Diagnostic Interview Schedule: its history, characteristics, and validity. Arch Gen Psychiatry 38:381–389, 1981

Rosen WG, Mohs RC, Davis KL: A new rating scale for Alzheimer's disease. Am J Psychiatry 141:1356–1362, 1984

Ross CE, Mirowsky J: Components of depressed mood in married men and women: the CES-D. Am J Epidemiol 119:997–1004, 1984

Sanford JRA: Tolerance of debility in elderly dependents by supporters at home: its significance for hospital practice. BMJ 3:471–473, 1975

Spitzer RL, Endicott J, Cohen GM: Psychiatric Status Schedule, 2nd Edition. New York, New York State Department of Mental Hygiene, Evaluation Unit, Biometrics Research, 1968

Spitzer RL, Endicott J, Robins E: Research Diagnostic Criteria: rationale and reliability. Arch Gen Psychiatry 35:773–782, 1978

Wing JK, Cooper JE, Sartorius N: The Measurement and Classification of Psychiatric Symptoms. London, Cambridge University Press, 1974

World Health Organization: Composite International Diagnostic Interview. Geneva, Switzerland, World Health Organization, 1989

Yesavage JA, Brink TL, Rose TL, et al: Development and validation of a geriatric depression screening scale: a preliminary report. J Psychiatr Res 17:37–49, 1983

Zung WWK: A self-rating depression scale. Arch Gen Psychiatry 12:63–70, 1965

Zung WWK: Depression in the normal aged. Psychosomatics 8:287–292, 1967

CHAPTER 10

Use of the Laboratory in the Diagnostic Workup of Older Adults

Warren D. Taylor, M.D.

P. Murali Doraiswamy, M.D.

Laboratory testing is an essential component of the psychiatric evaluation in elderly individuals, who often present with comorbid medical illnesses. The laboratory does not replace the clinician; there is no test that is pathognomonic for a primary psychiatric illness. However, laboratory testing—although it cannot replace the clinical history and physical examination—does aid in the evaluation of comorbidities that complicate or contribute to a psychiatric diagnosis. It may even assist in identifying medical problems that mimic psychiatric illnesses, such as hypothyroidism masquerading as depression. To best use the laboratory, the clinician must be aware of the indications for and limitations of such tests.

There has been significant growth in available diagnostic tools. Progress in research and technology, particularly in imaging technology, advanced rapidly through the 1990s and into the early 2000s. We can expect similar advances in genetic testing and genetic medicine in the future. However, we must balance what we *can* do with what we *should* do, as guided by our clinical judgment, the relative risk to the patient, and the cost. Such decisions may be easy when considering a low-risk, inexpensive test such as urinalysis. The decision may be more difficult when considering a head computed tomography (CT) scan or magnetic resonance imaging (MRI), which are both much more costly. Genetic testing may carry great risks as well, such as effects on a patient's insurability or on the reproductive decisions of the patient's family. When all such risks have been considered, the deci-

sion to proceed with a test should be based on the clinical presentation and how the test results may change a treatment plan.

Because of space limitations, the following discussion of specific diagnostic tests is cursory and should not be considered an exhaustive review. We focus on tests currently used, as well as those being considered for clinical use. This chapter, we hope, will assist the clinician as he or she decides on laboratory tests appropriate for the individual patient and will provide adequate information for obtaining informed consent.

Serologic Tests

Basic clinical chemistry and hematologic screens are routine for all hospital admissions and many outpatient evaluations. Although the yield from these screens is low for identifying causes of psychiatric disorders such as anxiety or depression, the screens are critical to identifying previously undiagnosed or poorly controlled medical illnesses that may contribute to mental status changes. These screens are vital for the initial evaluation of dementia or delirium and should be considered in individuals with complicated medical histories. These tests should also be monitored when patients are taking medications that may result in dangerous abnormalities.

Fortunately, the tests are also low risk. For most of them, the only risk is that associated with the blood draw itself, which may include transient pain, bruising, and rarely bleeding or fainting. Such risks are reduced, but not eliminated, by skilled phlebotomists.

Hematologic Tests

A complete blood count (CBC) is a standard part of any evaluation. It screens for multiple problems, including infections and anemia. It also provides a platelet count, a value important to monitor in psychiatric medications associated with thrombocytopenia, such as divalproex sodium or carbamazepine. This concern is particularly important in elderly patients, because there is some evidence that the risk of drug-induced thrombocytopenia may increase with age (Trannel et al. 2001). Lithium, in contrast, may result in mild leukocytosis. Weekly or biweekly CBC testing is required for patients taking clozapine, because of the risk of agranulocytosis, and may be needed more frequently if the patient develops signs of infection.

Chemistry Tests

Most general chemistry panels have a variety of values that may be helpful in medical evaluations. Blood glucose values may reveal hyperinsulinemia and hypoglycemia, which may produce anxiety and weakness; more commonly it shows hyperglycemia, which may be associated with diabetes and result in lethargy, or in severe cases, delirium, diabetic coma, or ketoacidosis. It is critical for the diagnosis of diabetes, which can be diagnosed with 1) an overnight fasting glucose greater than 126 mg/dL, 2) a random plasma glucose greater than 200 mg/dL with symptoms of diabetes, or 3) an oral glucose tolerance test resulting in a plasma glucose greater than 200 mg/dL 2 hours after a 75-g glucose load (Dagogo-Jack 2001).

Kidney function tests are equally important. Blood urea nitrogen (BUN) and creatinine will be elevated in kidney failure and hypovolemic states such as dehydration. These tests also must be performed before initiating lithium therapy because of lithium's potential for nephrotoxicity. General chemistry panels also measure serum sodium and potassium. Hyponatremia has been reported with selective serotonin reuptake inhibitors (SSRIs), although not all investigators have found this result. Of all the electrolyte abnormalities, potassium disorders may be the most crucial to identify. They rarely cause psychiatric symptoms but may result in severe cardiac arrhythmias. Although calcium and magnesium levels are not always included in routine chemistry screens, it is also worthwhile to check these levels, because abnormal levels may result in paranoid ideation or frank psychosis. Any or all of these results may be abnormal in patients who are on hemodialysis.

Serologic Tests for Syphilis

Syphilis should be considered in any case of new-onset psychosis; the patient's being elderly does not exclude this disease from the differential. The Venereal Disease Research Laboratory (VDRL) and the rapid plasmin reagin (RPR) tests are screening tools for infection with *Treponema pallidum*, the cause of syphilis. These tests are unfortunately nonspecific; false-positive results may occur in acute infections and chronic illnesses such as systemic lupus erythematosus. More specific tests, the fluorescent treponemal antibody (FTA) and the microhemagglutination–*Treponema pallidum* (MHA-TP) may distinguish false-positive from true-positive results and may aid in diagnosing late syphilis when blood and even cerebrospinal fluid (CSF) reagin tests are negative.

Human Immunodeficiency Virus Testing

It is also important to consider testing for human immunodeficiency virus (HIV) infection. In 1996, the Centers for Disease Control and Prevention reported that 11% of all acquired immunodeficiency syndrome (AIDS) cases occurred in patients older than age 50 (Centers for Disease Control and Prevention 1998). Data from 1991 and 1996 show that the proportion of cases of HIV infection and AIDS related to blood products decreased by 1996 but that the age-related percentage of cases remained stable.

The diagnosis of AIDS in elderly persons is complicated; the disease has been described as the great imitator because its clinical presentation, as with syphilis, may mimic that of other diseases (Sabin 1987). AIDS may mimic not only medical illnesses but also neuropsychiatric disorders, and AIDS may result in dementia. Investigators have identified several differences between AIDS-related dementia and Alzheimer's disease (Table 10–1), but often the clinical distinction may be less clear.

There is no evidence that HIV treatment for elderly AIDS patients should be different from that for younger patients. It is thus the role of the geriatric psychiatrist to assist the internist by screening for risk factors—such as a history of sexually transmitted diseases, intravenous drug use, risky sexual behavior, or a history of blood transfusions—particularly if they occurred before the early 1990s. We recommend HIV testing in individuals with these risk factors or those who present with atypical neuropsychiatric symptoms. For patients for whom test-

TABLE 10–1. Differences between AIDS-related dementia and Alzheimer's disease

	AIDS-related dementia	Alzheimer's disease
Clinical presentation	Subcortical dementia preceded by subacute encephalitis Attention and concentration deficits common; aphasia and other cortical deficits uncommon Associated with physical complaints, including neuropathies, myelopathies, weight loss, and fatigue	Cortical dementia; no preceding encephalitis Attention and concentration deficits common; aphasia and other cortical deficits common Less commonly, directly associated with physical complaints
Progression	Rapid progression over months	Slower progression over years
Cerebrospinal fluid (CSF) analysis	Mild protein elevation May have mononuclear CSF pleocytosis	Not typically associated with CSF abnormalities
Treatment	No evidence for cholinesterase inhibitors Antiretroviral therapy may improve cognitive deficits	Cholinesterase inhibitors may result in improvement No role for antiretroviral therapy

Note. AIDS = acquired immunodeficiency syndrome. CSF = cerebrospinal fluid.
Source. Data summarized from multiple sources (Chiao et al. 1999; Sabin 1987; Wallace et al. 1993; Weiler et al. 1988).

ing is warranted, the geriatric psychiatrist will also play an important role in counseling the patient about the reasons behind testing, then providing further counseling as the test results become known.

Thyroid Function Tests

To understand the significance of thyroid test results, one must first understand the hormones themselves. Thyroxine, or T_4, is secreted by the thyroid and converted in many tissues to triiodothyronine, or T_3. Both T_4 and T_3 are reversibly bound to the plasma protein thyroxine-binding globulin (TBG), and only the small unbound fraction exerts its physiologic effects. Thyroid-stimulating hormone (TSH) increases production of T_4 from the thyroid, and high levels of T_4 act in a negative feedback loop to inhibit TSH production. Abnormal levels of T_4 or T_3 may result in psychological symptoms mimicking depression (low energy, fatigue) in hypothyroidism, and mimicking anxiety disorders or even psychosis in hyperthyroidism.

A serum TSH test is most commonly used as a screen for thyroid disease; it is an excellent screening test because of its high negative predictive value (Klee and Hay 1997). However, an abnormal TSH does not definitively diagnose thyroid disease; a physical examination and measurement of T_4, T_3, and TBG are required for a diagnosis. Many medications may result in increased TSH levels (amiodarone, estrogens) or decreased TSH levels (glucocorticoids, phenytoin) (Kaplan 1999).

Vitamin B$_{12}$, Folate, and Homocysteine

Measurement of serum vitamin B_{12} and folate levels is an integral part of the laboratory evaluation, as the prevalence of B_{12} deficiency increases with age: the deficiency is present in up to 15% of the elderly population (Stabler et al. 1997). B_{12} deficiency may have various clinical signs, including macrocytic anemia and neuropathy. Unfortunately, these clinical presentations are unreliable, because only a minority of individuals exhibit these manifestations.

B_{12} and folate deficiencies may result in neuropsychiatric disturbances, including depression, psychosis, and cognitive deficits. Studies in populations with dementia demonstrate that B_{12} deficiencies often result in delirium or disorientation (Carmel et al. 1995; Cunha et al. 1995). Deficits may also result in specific neuropsychological problems, including visuospatial and word fluency deficits (Wahlin et al. 2001) and even greater behavioral disturbances than are standard in patients with Alzheimer's disease (Meins et al. 2000). Supplementation may result in mild improvements in memory function and processing speed, particularly in individuals with mild to moderate levels of cognitive impairment, but individuals with severe dementia are unlikely to demonstrate significant cognitive improvement.

But B_{12} and folate levels may not tell the entire story: there is also considerable interest in homocysteine. Serum homocysteine levels may serve as a functional indicator of B$_{12}$ and folate status (Selhub et al. 2000), because vitamin B$_{12}$ is needed to convert homocysteine to methionine in one-carbon metabolism in brain tissue. Hyperhomocystinemia is prevalent in elderly persons, and high serum levels of homocysteine can be attributed to an inadequate supply of B$_{12}$ and folate, even in the presence of low normal serum levels (Selhub et al. 2000). High levels of homocysteine are further associated with increased risk of occlusive vascular disease, thrombosis, and stroke (Boushey et al. 1995). Hyperhomocystinemia is also associated with cognitive dysfunction (Leblhuber et al. 2000; Selhub et al. 2000), although not all authors found this association (Ravaglia et al. 2000). Fortunately, it appears that vitamin replacement can reduce plasma homocysteine levels and may also produce improvement in individuals with mild cognitive dysfunction, although individuals with severe dementia may show little improvement (Nilsson et al. 2000). Because hyperhomocystinemia may occur even in individuals with low normal serum B$_{12}$ levels, it is worthwhile to check for this complication and if present to treat with vitamin B$_{12}$.

Toxicology

When there is an acute change in an individual's mental status, an investigation of the cause of the change must include ingestion of a substance. This consideration is particularly important in individuals with a history of substance abuse or with a history of depression in which there is the risk of medication overdose. The consideration of substance-induced changes should therefore include not only illicit substances but also alcohol and prescription medications.

In circumstances when an individual is taking medications such as lithium, phenytoin, tricyclic antidepressants, or any medication that requires monitoring of blood levels, those levels should be checked. Toxic levels of many pharmacologic agents may cause a variety of psychiatric or life-threatening medical conditions. Likewise, levels for common over-the-counter medications such as acetaminophen and salicylates are available. Concomitantly, a serum alcohol level should also be drawn. Depending on the individual's history, even a negative result may be critical if there is the possibility of withdrawal. Finally, urine tests can show prescription medications, such as benzodiazepines, barbiturates, and opioids, and can also test for illicit substances such as cocaine and marijuana. Advanced age does not preclude addiction.

Urinalysis

Urinalysis is an inexpensive, noninvasive test that provides a large amount of information. It determines the urine's specific gravity, which may indicate dehydration, and also tests for glucose and ketones, important in the evaluation of diabetic patients.

In the elderly population, the most important use of the urinalysis may be as a screening tool for urinary tract infections (UTIs). A UTI is suggested by a microscopic examination showing high levels of white blood cells, bacteria, and possibly red blood cells. High numbers of epithelial cells make the results difficult to interpret, because they suggest contamination. A urine culture is a definitive means of diagnosing a UTI and will identify the infecting organism and its susceptibility to antimicrobial treatments.

Identification of a UTI is critical in the elderly population, particularly in those with dementia. Approximately 20% of the persons admitted from the community to a geropsychiatry unit may have a UTI, and in many cases it may result in a delirium; however, the condition improves with appropriate antibiotic treatment (Levkoff et al. 1991; Manepalli et al. 1990). As is true in all cases of delirium, a delirium from a UTI can result in confusion, disorientation, and increased agitation. Timely identification and treatment can improve outcomes and shorten or avoid hospitalizations.

Electrocardiography

Along with routine monitoring of vital signs, the electrocardiogram (ECG) is the most frequently used screen for cardiovascular disease. It provides a graphic representation of the heart's electrical activity, obtained via surface electrodes placed in specific locations on the patient's chest. This placement makes possible a graph of electrical activity from a variety of spatial perspectives. Very little risk is associated with the procedure.

In psychiatry, the most important roles of the ECG include screening for cardiovascular disease that may preclude the use of specific medications and monitoring for drug-induced electrocardiographic changes, either from standard doses or from overdose. Electrocardiographic changes associated with specific psychotropic medications are summarized in Table 10–2.

The tricyclic antidepressants (TCAs) are well known to be cardiotoxic in overdose; even at therapeutic doses, their use is considered unsafe in patients with cardiovascular disease, particularly ischemic disease (Roose 2000).

TABLE 10–2. Common electrocardiographic changes associated with psychotropic medications

Medication	Electrocardiographic change
Antipsychotics (typical or atypical agents)	Increased QTc interval Potential for torsades de pointes
β-blockers	Bradycardia
Lithium	Sick sinus syndrome Sinoatrial block
Tricyclic antidepressants	Increased PR, QRS, or QT interval AV block

Although the most common cardiovascular complication of TCAs is orthostatic hypotension (Glassman and Bigger 1981), TCAs have the same pharmacologic properties as type IA antiarrhythmics (such as quinidine and procainamide). TCAs slow conduction at the bundle of His; individuals with preexisting bundle branch block who take TCAs are at increased risk for AV block. Even therapeutic levels are associated with prolonged PR intervals and QRS complexes; these results may be more pronounced in elderly individuals as the incidence and severity of adverse drug reactions increase with age (Pollock 1999). If TCAs are used, baseline and frequent follow-up ECGs should be obtained.

Lithium may also result in electrocardiographic changes, and along with evaluations of thyroid and renal function, an ECG is recommended before the patient begins taking lithium and regularly while taking it. Lithium appears to most affect the sinus node, and even at therapeutic levels it may result in sick sinus syndrome or sinoatrial block, either of which may occur early or later in treatment. At higher levels, there have been reports of sinus arrest and asystole.

Antipsychotics also result in ECG changes; about 25% of individuals receiving antipsychotics exhibit ECG abnormalities (Thomas 1994). Although many of these changes have historically been considered benign, there is increased concern that prolongation of the QT interval (when corrected for heart rate, the QTc interval) may contribute to potentially fatal ventricular arrhythmias, particularly torsades de pointes. QTc prolongation in not a problem in itself but rather heralds the possibility of torsades or sudden death. QTc values are typically around 400 msec in duration; lower values are considered normal. Because the greater the duration, the greater the risk of torsades, 500 msec is frequently used as a cutoff (Glassman and Bigger 2001). It is important to note that other medications also affect the QTc interval and produce an additive effect when combined with an antipsychotic.

This phenomenon may be seen with almost any antipsychotic agent. The typical antipsychotic most associated with QTc prolongation is thioridazine, which in July 2000 received a black box warning in its package insert. Reports of torsades de pointes are also seen with pimozide and even "safe" agents such as haloperidol. Atypical antipsychotic agents also prolong QTc intervals to varying degrees. Ziprasidone appears to result in greater prolongation than other atypical antipsychotics, but less than thioridazine; olanzapine appears to have the least effect on QTc interval (Glassman and Bigger 2001). Unfortunately, there are currently concerns about QTc prolongation for all atypical antipsychotic agents.

Routine ECGs for all patients receiving antipsychotics are not currently recommended, but it is wise to be prudent. A careful history of cardiac illness, family history, and syncope should be obtained for all patients. ECGs should be considered more carefully in older individuals, particularly those with a history of cardiac illness and those receiving other medications that may affect the QTc interval.

The last consideration is medication overdose. With few exceptions, an ECG should always be obtained, even in cases where the medication used is not associated with arrhythmias. Obtaining an ECG is a reasonable choice because ECGs are easy to perform, noninvasive, and relatively inexpensive. ECGs are also important because some medications may affect heart rhythm in overdose when they would not do so at usual doses. Finally, it is not uncommon that suicidal patients do not report all the medications that they have used to overdose: suicide attempts may be impulsive, and patients who have an altered mental status may be unable to provide a complete report.

Imaging Studies

Plain film radiographs remain an integral piece of the diagnostic imaging performed today in geriatric psychiatry.

Such techniques are most commonly used to detect 1) lung pathology that may contribute to mental status changes and 2) bone fractures. Plain film radiographs are critical for individuals who have both severe dementia and either a recent history of falls or newly developed limb immobility.

Throughout the 1990s and the early 2000s, a number of new imaging techniques have greatly enhanced our diagnostic tools. These techniques are costly and therefore should be used only with good reasons for why they are needed and with knowledge of how specific findings may affect a patient's treatment plan. The following discussion focuses on commonly used structural imaging techniques: CT and MRI. Because the techniques are also discussed in other areas of the book, these sections focus on the scientific basis behind these tools and provide information to support their clinical use, particularly in brain imaging, and to facilitate informed consent.

This section does not discuss functional imaging techniques—those such as positron emission tomography (PET) and single photon emission computed tomography (SPECT) that play a role in examining brain metabolic rates or regional blood flow. At present, these imaging procedures have a limited clinical use and are primarily for research. PET imaging may prove to have a role in the clinical evaluation of dementia (Silverman et al. 2001), but it is still premature to recommend this modality for routine clinical practice.

Computed Tomography

CT, originally called computerized axial tomography (CAT), was introduced into clinical practice as "the ultimate X ray" in the 1970s. CT is a general term for several radiographic techniques resulting in the computer-assisted generation of a series of images showing slices of an organ or body region, such as the brain or the abdomen. The CT scanner uses a small X-ray device that rotates around the body region of interest in a fixed plane; these signals are sent to a computer that produces the corresponding cross-sectional slice for that plane. The computer can create sections in axial, coronal, and sagittal alignments. More recent advances in software and display systems have led to many useful clinical applications, including virtual CT colonoscopy or angiography.

When used to examine brain structure, CT can allow for the ready identification of many structures, although it does have limitations. By measuring differences in density, it can distinguish among CSF, blood, bone, gray matter, and white matter. The test is particularly useful for demonstrating bone abnormalities (such as skull frac-

tures), areas of hemorrhage (such as a subdural hematoma), and the mass effect of various lesions. It can also display atrophy or ventricular enlargement. However, because of surrounding bone, the test does not well visualize posterior fossa or brain stem structures.

A typical concern of patients is radiation exposure. Like other typical radiographic procedures, CT scans require the use of a limited amount of radiation; any given CT procedure results in a radiation exposure, but one that is well below government recommendations for individuals who work around radiation. However, these recommendations do not consider multiple CT scans (thus multiple radiation exposures) or CT studies that overlap scanned regions, a technique that increases the radiation dose (Nickoloff and Alderson 2001). CT imaging should be used when appropriate, but other assessment techniques that may result in lower radiation exposure should also be considered.

Magnetic Resonance Imaging

Whereas CT scanners rely on radiation, the MRI scanner creates a magnetic field that is 3,000–25,000 times the strength of the earth's natural magnetic field. The underlying principle behind MRI is that the nuclei of endogenous identifiable isotopes (such as hydrogen or phosphorus) behave like tiny spinning magnets. Strong magnetic fields alter this behavior, and an MRI scanner can identify the resultant change.

When a patient is put into the strong static magnetic field generated by the MRI scanner, his or her nuclei align parallel to the field. Because the nuclei are also spinning, they wobble randomly around the field; different molecules can be identified because their nuclei wobble at different frequencies. A second, oscillating magnetic field is then applied at a right angle to the first. This field affects only the nuclei that are in resonance with it—that is, the nuclei that wobble at the field's frequency. This second field forces those resonant nuclei to wobble in unison. When this field is deactivated, the nuclei return to their original positions, and the synchronized movement creates a voltage that can be measured and displayed. Measurements taken at various times during the procedure produce the different magnetic resonance images.

MRI has advantages and disadvantages compared with CT imaging. It produces higher-resolution images and can obtain good detail in regions that are poorly visualized on CT, such as the posterior fossa. Additionally, no radiation is involved. Unfortunately, the procedure is more grueling than CT: the patient must remain motionless for a longer period of time in a smaller, enclosed space. This requirement may be difficult for claustrophobic individuals. Additionally, the magnetic device must be housed in an area devoid of iron, and staff and patients must not carry or wear certain metals or have them embedded in their bodies. Moreover, MRI tends to be more costly than CT imaging in most institutions.

In the psychiatric workup of a geriatric patient, MRI should be considered for patients in whom the clinician suspects small lesions in regions difficult to visualize or for patients with demyelinating diseases such as multiple sclerosis. MRI can easily identify pathology in vascular dementia, although the findings in other types of dementia are less specific. Currently, the routine use of brain MRI in these patients is questionable, because findings are unlikely to affect treatment.

Electroencephalography

Electroencephalography is a technique in which scalp electrodes allow the measurement of cortical electrical activity. A skilled reader can interpret an electroencephalogram's (EEG's) waveforms to identify the presence of epileptic activity, the slowing of electrical activity, or a patient's sleep stage. It is most useful in a psychiatric evaluation of individuals with known or suspected seizure disorders. A history of brain injury or trauma with mental status changes or psychosis may be a particularly important indication for an electroencephalographic evaluation. Certain types of epilepsy, specifically temporal lobe epilepsy, are also associated with psychotic or manic symptoms. EEGs may also be used as part of a polysomnographic evaluation for sleep disturbances (see the following section, "Polysomnography").

For indications other than these, the use of EEGs in the psychiatric evaluation of elderly patients is limited. Electroencephalographic changes occur in both delirium and dementia, but these changes are not specific to a given diagnosis. In delirium, except that caused by alcohol or sedative-hypnotic withdrawal, electroencephalographic testing typically displays slowing of the posterior dominant rhythm and increased generalized slow-wave activity (Jacobson and Jerrier 2000). Electroencephalography has limited clinical use in this area because the diagnosis of delirium is typically made clinically, increased slow-wave activity is seen in other disorders, and the EEG provides minimal information about the causes of delirium.

Likewise, there are electroencephalographic changes in dementia; Alzheimer's disease results in multiple changes in electroencephalographic parameters (Kowalski et al. 2001; Stevens et al. 2001). The degree of change is corre-

lated with cognitive impairment (Kowalski et al. 2001). Various treatments, including cholinesterase inhibitors, may mitigate electroencephalographic changes in individuals with mild dementia (Kogan et al. 2001). This finding is not universal; there are also reports that worsening of the EEG does not always parallel clinical deterioration. However, significant negative correlations have been found between frontal theta activity and hippocampal volumes (Grunwald et al. 2001). Despite this and other research, electroencephalography has limited clinical utility in most dementing syndromes.

The exception may occur when Creutzfeldt-Jakob disease is a consideration in the differential diagnosis. Creutzfeldt-Jakob disease is a rare, rapidly progressive prion disease characterized by dementia and neurologic signs that may include gait disturbances and myoclonus. Electroencephalography may play an important role in diagnosing this disease: periodic sharp-wave complexes are strongly associated with Creutzfeldt-Jakob disease, with a sensitivity of 67% and a specificity of 86% (Steinhoff et al. 1996). However, although electroencephalography is an important diagnostic tool when considering Creutzfeldt-Jakob disease, it is important to remember that periodic sharp-wave complexes may also occur in Alzheimer's disease and dementia with Lewy bodies (Tschampa et al. 2001).

Polysomnography

Sleep disorders are a common problem in elderly persons. Although sleep disturbances are most often associated with psychiatric disorders such as dementia, delirium, and depression, the disturbances can exist without any other obvious psychiatric diagnoses. Fortunately, most metropolitan areas have diagnostic services for identifying and treating sleep complaints; their core diagnostic procedure is the polysomnogram.

The polysomnogram is an all-night procedure, and the full evaluation may require more than one night. It monitors cerebral and somatic functioning and has proved reliable and sensitive for recording the stages of sleep and concomitant physiological functioning. It incorporates three basic variables: the sleep EEG, the electro-oculogram (which measures eye motion), and the electromyogram (which measures air exchange and respiratory effort). Additional monitoring used in specific investigations includes hemoglobin oxygen saturation using pulse oximetry, an ECG, and electrodes placed over the anterior tibialis muscles to measure leg movement. Video recording of sleep behaviors and monitoring of penile tumescence may also be available.

For some evaluations, overnight stays in sleep laboratories, monitored by a technician, may-be necessary for collecting adequate data. The recent development of portable units now allows home monitoring or monitoring in a general hospital room. These units are compact and collect data by using scalp electrodes. Recordings are later evaluated by computer-assisted methods.

The polysomnogram, although essential for the evaluation of sleep disorders, is less useful in depression and dementia. These disorders do result in polysomnographic changes, but the polysomnogram contributes little toward an appropriate diagnosis or treatment decision. Many other psychiatric illnesses also have comorbid sleep complications, but a polysomnogram is not indicated in the majority of these cases. The polysomnogram should be reserved for patients in whom a specific sleep disorder is suspected or patients who have unexplained sleep disturbances in the absence of a primary psychiatric illness.

Genetic Testing

Genetic testing is at the forefront of a new wave of available laboratory tests. Research is currently investigating the genetic basis behind such diverse neuropsychiatric illnesses as dementia, narcolepsy, schizophrenia, and substance addiction. Similar research has already had success in Huntington's disease, an autosomal dominant disorder caused by a trinucleotide repeat; testing for the length of this repeat can predict whether an individual is susceptible to the illness. Understanding the genetic basis of diseases is critical not only for better diagnosis but also for better ability to tailor specific treatments to specific disorders.

Genetics in geriatric psychiatry is covered in more detail in Chapter 6, "Genetics." The brief section in this chapter serves as an introduction to genetic testing, including a discussion of a well-researched test examining for alleles of apolipoprotein E. Also included is a brief discussion of psychosocial concerns one must consider when ordering a genetic test.

APOE Testing

Extensive research has attempted to identify genetic markers for Alzheimer's disease. Mutations on chromosomes 1, 14, and 21 have been linked to rare forms of early-onset familial Alzheimer's disease; such findings may help counsel families in making decisions about pregnancies (Verlinsky et al. 2002). One of the most studied genes for Alzheimer's disease is *APOE*. This gene

encodes for an astrocyte-secreted plasma protein that is involved in cholesterol transport. Apolipoprotein E may also play a role in the regeneration of injured nerve tissue. There are three possible alleles (ε2, ε3, ε4) of the *APOE* gene that may be combined heterozygously (ε2/ ε3, ε2/ ε4, ε3/ ε4) or homozygously (ε2/ ε2, ε3/ ε3, ε4/ε4).

Multiple epidemiological studies have documented that the presence of the ε4 allele is a risk factor for Alzheimer's disease (Roses 1997). Additionally, the presence of ε4 alleles increases the specificity of the diagnosis of Alzheimer's disease. Despite these associations, the presence of an ε4 allele, even a homozygous ε4/ε4 genotype, is not diagnostic for Alzheimer's disease. Other causes of dementia would have to be explored as clinically indicated. *APOE* testing is not currently recommended to predict dementia risk in asymptomatic individuals.

Arguments against routine testing are lack of an effective treatment that modifies the disease course and lack of evidence that *APOE* status may influence current supportive treatments. Current treatments for cognitive dysfunction are limited to cholinesterase inhibitors, but response to these drugs is not dependent on *APOE* status. Although some evidence suggested that tacrine may be better for individuals who lack the ε4 allele than for those who have the ε4 allele (Farlow et al. 1998; Poirier et al. 1995; Sjogren et al. 2001), other studies using both tacrine and galantamine did not find such an association (Aerssens et al. 2001; McGowan et al. 1998; Raskind et al. 2000; Rigaud et al. 2000). Interpretation of these results are complicated for two reasons: individuals with specific genotypes who have dementia could experience different rates of progression of dementia, and the analyses were post hoc.

Ethical and Psychological Concerns

Genetic testing is more than a simple blood draw; its implications are farther ranging than the results of simple serum chemistry. Genetic testing is similar to HIV testing in that results may have significant psychological, social, and personal repercussions. For this reason, genetic testing should be considered only in the context of supportive counseling.

There has been considerable debate on the psychological repercussions of testing for Huntington's disease, because testing for this disorder has been available longer than for any other adult-onset genetic disease. Huntington's disease is therefore a useful model to consider. Testing can result in transient heightened anxiety and depression; in the long term, a positive test may result in hopelessness (Tibben et al. 1994). The test also has a significant impact on decisions to marry or bear children; although only the individual can decide how a test result may affect these decisions, he or she needs to be counseled about these considerations before taking the test.

Beyond personal and psychological concerns, there are also financial concerns. Genetic testing should be confidential. The inappropriate release of such information could result in job loss or lack of insurability. Medical and life insurance in particular could be exceedingly difficult to obtain if insurance agencies had access to the information. Again, these are issues that many who present for genetic testing may not consider.

But in the end, genetic testing is yet another tool at our disposal. It is a tool with much untapped potential. It also carries significant risks that are different from the risks associated with the other laboratory tests described in this chapter. As with the other procedures, clinicians must make sure that their patients or patients' families understand clearly not only the benefits but also the risks before they proceed.

References

Aerssens J, Raeymaekers P, Lilienfeld S, et al: apoE genotype: no influence on galantamine treatment efficacy nor on rate of cognitive decline in Alzheimer's disease. Dement Geriatr Cogn Disord 12:69–77, 2001

Boushey CJ, Beresford SAA, Omenn GS, et al: A quantitative assessment of plasma homocysteine as a risk factor for vascular disease: probable benefits of increasing folic acid intakes. JAMA 274:1049–1057, 1995

Carmel R, Gott PS, Waters CH, et al: The frequently low cobalamin levels in dementia usually signify treatable metabolic, neurologic and electrophysiologic abnormalities. Eur J Haematol 54: 245–253, 1995

Centers for Disease Control and Prevention: AIDS among persons aged >50 years—United States, 1991–1996. MMWR Morb Mortal Wkly Rep 47:21–27, 1998

Chiao EY, Ries KM, Sande MA: AIDS and the elderly. Clin Infect Dis 28:740–745, 1999

Cunha UG, Rocha FL, Peixoto JM, et al: Vitamin B12 deficiency and dementia. Int Psychogeriatr 7:85–88, 1995

Dagogo-Jack S: Diabetes mellitus and related disorders, in The Washington Manual of Medical Therapeutics. Edited by Ahya SN, Flood K, Paranjothi S. Philadelphia, Lippincott Williams & Wilkins, 2001, p 455

Farlow MR, Lahiri DK, Poirier J, et al: Treatment outcome of tacrine therapy depends on apoliprotein genotype and gender of the subjects with Alzheimer's disease. Neurology 50:669–677, 1998

Glassman AH, Bigger JT: Cardiovascular effects of therapeutic doses of tricyclic antidepressants: a review. Arch Gen Psychiatry 38:815–820, 1981

Glassman AH, Bigger JT: Antipsychotic drugs: prolonged QTc interval, torsade de pointes, and sudden death. Am J Psychiatry 158:1774–1782, 2001

Grunwald M, Busse F, Hensel A, et al: Correlation between clinical theta activity and hippocampal volumes in health, mild cognitive impairment, and dementia. J Clin Neurophysiol 18:178–184, 2001

Jacobson S, Jerrier H: EEG in delirium. Semin Clin Neuropsychiatry 5:86–92, 2000

Kaplan MM: Clinical perspectives in the diagnosis of thyroid disease. Clin Chem 45:1377–1383, 1999

Klee GG, Hay ID: Biochemical testing of thyroid function. Endocrinol Metab Clin North Am 26:763–775, 1997

Kogan EA, Korczyn AD, Virchovsky RG, et al: EEG changes during long-term treatment with donepezil in Alzheimer's disease patients. J Neural Transm 108:1167–1173, 2001

Kowalski JW, Gawel M, Pfeffer A, et al: The diagnostic value of EEG in Alzheimer disease: correlation with the severity of mental impairment. J Clin Neurophysiol 18:570–575, 2001

Leblhuber F, Walli J, Artner-Dworzak E, et al: Hyperhomocysteinemia in dementia. J Neural Transm 107:1469–1474, 2000

Levkoff S, Cleary P, Liptzin B, et al: Epidemiology of delirium: an overview of research issues and findings. Int Psychogeriatr 3:149–167, 1991

Manepalli J, Grossberg GT, Mueller C: Prevalence of delirium and urinary tract infection in a psychogeriatric unit. J Geriatr Psychiatry Neurol 3:198–202, 1990

McGowan SH, Wilcock GK, Scott M: Effect of gender and apolipoprotein E genotype on response to anticholinesterase therapy in Alzheimer's disease. Int J Geriatr Psychiatry 13:625–630, 1998

Meins W, Muller-Thomsen T, Meier-Baumgartner H-P: Subnormal serum vitamin B12 and behavioural and psychological symptoms in Alzheimer's disease. Int J Geriatr Psychiatry 15:415–418, 2000

Nickoloff EL, Alderson PO: Radiation exposures to patients from CT: reality, public perception, and policy. AJR Am J Roentgenol 177:285–287, 2001

Nilsson K, Gustafson L, Hultberg B: Improvement of cognitive functions after cobalamin/folate supplementation in elderly patients with dementia and elevated plasma homocysteine. Int J Geriatr Psychiatry 16:609–614, 2000

Poirier J, Delisle M-C, Quirion R, et al: Apolipoprotein E4 allele as a predictor of cholinergic deficits and treatment outcome in Alzheimer disease. Proc Natl Acad Sci USA 92:12260–12264, 1995

Pollock BG: Adverse reactions of antidepressants in elderly patients. J Clin Psychiatry 60:4–8, 1999

Raskind MA, Peskind ER, Wessel T, et al: Galantamine in AD: a 6-month randomized, placebo-controlled trial with a 6-month extension. Neurology 54:2261–2268, 2000

Ravaglia G, Forti P, Mailoi F, et al: Elevated plasma homocysteine levels in centenarians are not associated with cognitive impairment. Mech Ageing Dev 121:251–261, 2000

Rigaud AS, Traykov L, Caputo L, et al: The apolipoprotein E epsilon4 allele and response to tacrine therapy in Alzheimer's disease. Eur J Neurol 7:255–258, 2000

Roose SP: Considerations for the use of antidepressants in patients with cardiovascular disease. Am Heart J 140 (suppl 4):S84–S88, 2000

Roses AD: A model for susceptibility polymorphisms for complex diseases: apolipoprotein E and Alzheimer disease. Neurogenetics 1:3–11, 1997

Sabin TD: AIDS: the new "great imitator." J Am Geriatr Soc 35:460–464, 1987

Selhub J, Bagley LC, Miller J, et al: B vitamins, homocysteine, and neurocognitive function in the elderly. Am J Clin Nutr 71 (suppl):614S–620S, 2000

Silverman DH, Small GW, Chang CY, et al: Positron emission tomography in evaluation of dementia: regional brain metabolism and long-term outcome. JAMA 286:2120–2127, 2001

Sjogren M, Hesse C, Basun H, et al: Tacrine and rate of progression in Alzheimer's disease—relation of ApoE allele genotype. J Neural Transm 108:451–458, 2001

Stabler SP, Lindenbaum J, Allen RH: Vitamin B12 deficiency in the elderly: current dilemmas. Am J Clin Nutr 66:741–749, 1997

Steinhoff BJ, Racker S, Herrendorf G, et al: Accuracy and reliability of periodic sharp wave complexes in Creutzfeldt-Jakob disease. Arch Neurol 53:162–166, 1996

Stevens A, Kircher T, Nickola M, et al: Dynamic regulation of EEG power and coherence is lost early and globally in DAT. Eur Arch Psychiatry Clin Neurosci 251:199–204, 2001

Thomas SHL: Drugs, QT interval abnormalities, and ventricular arrhythmias. Adverse Drug React Toxicol Rev 13:77–102, 1994

Tibben A, Duivenvoorden HJ, Niermeijer MF, et al: Psychological effects of presymptomatic DNA testing for Huntington's disease in the Dutch program. Psychosom Med 56:562–532, 1994

Trannel TJ, Ahmed I, Goebert D: Occurrence of thrombocytopenia in psychiatric patients taking valproate. Am J Psychiatry 158:128–130, 2001

Tschampa HJ, Neumann M, Zerr I, et al: Patients with Alzheimer's disease and dementia with Lewy bodies mistaken for Creutzfeldt-Jakob disease. J Neurol Neurosurg Psychiatry 71:33–39, 2001

Verlinsky Y, Rechitsky S, Verlinsky O, et al: Preimplantation diagnosis for early onset Alzheimer disease caused by V717L mutation. JAMA 287:1018–1021, 2002

Wahlin T-BR, Wahlin A, Winblad B, et al: The influence of serum vitamin B12 and folate status on cognitive functioning in very old age. Biol Psychol 56:247–265, 2001

Wallace J, Paauw D, Spach D: HIV infection in older patients: when to expect the unexpected. Geriatrics 48:61–70, 1993

Weiler P, Mungas D, Pomerantz S: AIDS as a cause of dementia in the elderly. J Am Geriatr Soc 36:139–141, 1988

Neuropsychological Assessment of Dementia

Kathleen A. Welsh-Bohmer, Ph.D.

Deborah K. Attix, Ph.D.

Alzheimer's disease is by far the most common of the disorders of aging that cause dementia. The disorder affects nearly 10% of the population older than age 65 and was found to affect 25%–40% of individuals over age 85 (Breitner et al. 1999; Evans et al. 1991). Because of its slow and insidious onset, the early stages of the illness can be confused with relatively benign memory impairments that are associated with normal aging. The early symptomatic phase of Alzheimer's disease, now commonly referred to as mild cognitive impairment, can be indistinguishable on bedside clinical examination from normal aging, but the disease is more readily identified by means of detailed neuropsychological testing (Chen et al. 2001; Elias et al. 2000; B.J. Small et al. 2000; Tierney et al. 1996; Welsh et al. 1991) or with the aid of other diagnostic procedures, such as positron emission tomography (PET; Reiman et al. 1996; G.W. Small et al. 1995, 2000).

These and other medical advances in the care of dementia make the early identification of Alzheimer's disease and related disorders a health care imperative, with implications for both patient outcome and health care costs (Ernst and Hay 1994; Kawas and Brookmeyer 2001). The availability of treatments for Alzheimer's disease now permits medical intervention in this progressive disorder. Treatment in the early symptomatic phase offers the possibility of modifying disease onset and lessening disability (see Zandi and Breitner 2001 for review). At the broad societal level, identifying and treating Alzheimer's disease in its earliest stages of mild cognitive impairment and delaying further progression to fulminant disease can greatly reduce the prevalence of Alzhei-

mer's disease in the United States and lead to dramatic reductions in the total costs of care (Brookmeyer et al. 1998).

Neuropsychological assessment plays a central role in the diagnosis of early dementing disorders (Petersen et al. 2001) and in differentiation among the plethora of cognitive disorders that can interfere with functional ability and quality of life (Knopman et al. 2001). The neuropsychological assessment offers a sensitive, reliable, and noninvasive approach to early symptom verification as well as a potentially cost-effective means for managing patients with memory disorders (Welsh-Bohmer et al. 2003). The goals of this chapter are 1) to describe the instances in which neuropsychological assessment can be most useful in geriatric settings, 2) to detail the neuropsychological examination process, and 3) to summarize the neurobehavioral presentations of common disorders in geriatric practice, specifically the profiles of various dementias, normal aging, and depression.

Neuropsychological Assessment in Geriatric Settings

Central to the diagnosis of a dementing disorder in the elderly patient is determining the presence of disorders in memory and other cognitive processes, such as abstract thought, language, visuoperception, and personality (e.g., American Psychiatric Association 1987, 1994). The task of detecting symptoms is simplified to some extent in the advanced stages of brain disease; identifying dementing disorders is much more challenging for the clinician when the symptoms are far less obvious. Equally challenging is the clinical distinction between different forms of dementia that present in similar manners, such as Alzheimer's disease and frontotemporal dementia, described later in this chapter. The neuropsychological examination can assist the clinician in both situations. The neuropsychological evaluation permits an objective assessment of cognitive function by using standardized tests of a variety of cognitive abilities, including measures of intelligence; memory; attention and concentration; orientation to time, person, place, and situation; language; visuoperceptual functions; and sensory-motor ability. Interpreting test data is facilitated by normative standards for comparison and psychometric information, not only on test reliability and validity but also on the role of common modifying factors of performance—for example, age, education, and gender. Consideration is also given to the role of mood and personality variables.

In geriatric practice the neuropsychological evaluation is useful in four common situations, none of which are mutually exclusive. The first and by far the most frequent use of the evaluation is to assist in diagnosing a cognitive disorder. Specifically, the evaluation is used to verify the presence or absence of a cognitive syndrome (e.g., dementia) and to determine the likely differential diagnostic possibilities based on the behavioral profile (e.g., Alzheimer's disease vs. vascular dementia). Second, neuropsychological testing results are also commonly used as an objective baseline for tracking changes in mentation over time. These baselines are useful in clarifying diagnostic classifications of dementia due to Alzheimer's disease and similar disorders, in which the establishment of progression is essential. The neuropsychological examination in this context can also be used to monitor treatment response. A third common use is guiding clinical care decisions, including the determination of functional capacities and competency (see Koltai and Welsh-Bohmer 2000 for review). Issues typically confronted by a geriatric evaluation are ability to live independently, financial capacity, medication management, and driving safety. Finally, the neuropsychological evaluation can be used to guide appropriate therapeutic interventions. Identified cognitive strengths and weaknesses can be used for designing appropriate rehabilitation approaches, such as those involving compensatory strategies or psychotherapy (Koltai and Branch 1999).

The neuropsychological evaluation process itself can vary in form across clinical practices, depending in part on the populations typically served (e.g., Spanish speakers or native English speakers) and in part on the training emphasis of the neuropsychologist administering the exami-

nation. The approach can use a fixed battery or more flexible methods tailored to the referral issue. Regardless of the testing choices, there are standard features uniformly applied across neuropsychological settings to ensure that all testable areas of cognition are assessed (Lezak 1995). The evaluation typically begins with a diagnostic interview to identify the major referral issues and obvious symptoms. In this interview, a patient's language, behavioral organization, memory, mood, affect, and orientation to situation are observed in a naturalistic context. Generally, family members are separately interviewed (with the patient's consent) to determine changes in functional ability and to clarify historical and medical information. In the formal testing session, 10 central domains of cognition and behavior are generally assessed: orientation, intelligence, memory, attention and concentration, higher executive functions, language, visuoperception and spatial abilities, sensory-motor integration, mood, and personality. The tests commonly used to assess these functional domains are listed in Table 11–1. From the battery of tests, a profile of performance can be constructed, examined in reference to normative standards, and interpreted relative to the established behavioral profiles of known neurobehavioral syndromes.

Simplifying the geriatric assessment are a number of neuropsychological batteries designed for use with elderly persons and appropriate normative information. Among these are the Mattis Dementia Rating Scale (Mattis et al. 2002) and the neuropsychological battery from the Consortium to Establish a Registry for Alzheimer's Disease (CERAD; Morris et al. 1989). Both are relatively brief and are sensitive to early stages of Alzheimer's disease dementia. Additionally, the tests offer presentation formats, such as the use of large print and an oral format, to minimize the influences of sensory confounding (Welsh-Bohmer and Mohs 1997).

It must be emphasized that the neuropsychological examination is not simply a process of actuarial comparisons to normative tables. The neuropsychological evaluation, like other forms of clinical diagnosis, rests on an inferential process. The diagnosis is an iterative process that incorporates multiple sources of information to arrive at diagnostic impressions (Koltai and Welsh-Bohmer 2000). The psychologist must first assess the patient's likely premorbid ability in order to determine whether observed behaviors are newly acquired or reflect long-standing weaknesses. Once that determination has been made, impairments are assessed with consideration of potential confounding influences on performance, including the patient's motivation factors, extratest factors (such as interruptions), and other test behaviors that might interfere with optimal functioning (e.g., anxiety).

TABLE 11–1. Common neuropsychological tests used in geriatric assessment

Domain	Tests commonly used	References
Orientation/global mental status	Temporal Orientation Test Mini-Mental State Exam Alzheimer's Disease Assessment Scale—Cognitive (ADAS-COG)	Benton et al. (1964) Folstein et al. (1975) Mohs and Cohen (1988)
Intellect	Wechsler Adult Intelligence Scale, 3rd Edition (WAIS-III)	Wechsler (1997a)
Language	Multilingual Aphasia Examination Category Fluency Boston Naming Test	Benton and Hamsher (1983) Spreen and Strauss (1996) Kaplan et al. (1978)
Memory	Wechsler Memory Scale, 3rd Edition (WMS-III) California Verbal Learning Test—II Selective Reminding Test Consortium to Establish a Registry for Alzheimer's Disease (CERAD) Word List Memory Test Rey Auditory Verbal Learning Test	Wechsler (1997b) Delis et al. (1987) Buschke and Fuld (1974) Welsh-Bohmer and Mohs (1997) Ivnik et al. (1992)
Attention/concentration	Subtests from the WMS-III and WAIS-III	Lezak (1995)
Executive function	Trail Making Test Symbol Digit Modalities Test Short Category Test Wisconsin Card Sorting Test	Reitan (1958) Smith (1968) Wetzel and Boll (1987) Berg (1948)
Visuoperception	Benton Facial Recognition Test Judgment of Line Orientation Test Tests of constructional praxis	Benton et al. (1983) Benton et al. (1981) Lezak (1995)
Sensory-motor	Grooved Pegboard Test Finger Oscillation	Spreen and Straus (1996) Heaton et al. (1991)
Personality and mood	Minnesota Multiphasic Personality Inventory-2 (MMPI-2) Geriatric Depression Scale Beck Depression Inventory—II	Butcher et al (1989) Yesavage et al (1983) Beck et al (1996)

The interpretation of the likely medical and psychological contributions to the cognitive profile requires a good appreciation of brain-behavior organization. The neuropsychologist must consider whether the results make sense from a functional anatomical perspective and then analyze the profile to determine its conformity to known neurobehavioral syndromes, such as normal aging, mild cognitive impairment, Alzheimer's disease, and depression. Before final diagnostic determination, consideration is given to other data such as medical history, ancillary studies (including imaging data), and informants' report of functional change. The combined information more firmly supports the diagnosis of either normal aging or early dementia and improves diagnostic accuracy (Tschanz et al. 2000). In the next sections of this chapter we summarize the neuropsychology of normal aging and the differentiation of various forms of late-life dementia. We also consider in some detail the neuropsychology of geriatric depression and the contribution of mood disorders to the presentation of dementing disorders.

Neuropsychology of Normal Aging

By far the most common cause for cognitive change after age 50 is normal aging of the nervous system (Ebly et al. 1994). Compared to young adults, older individuals show selective losses in functions related to the speed and efficiency of information processing. Particularly vulnerable are memory retrieval abilities, attentional capacity, executive skills, and divergent thinking, such as working memory and multitasking (Cullum et al. 1990; Salthouse et al. 1996). On formal neuropsychological testing, memory measures involving delayed free recall are typically affected (Craik 1984), although not to the pronounced extent seen in Alzheimer's disease (Welsh et al. 1991). Unlike the patient with Alzheimer's disease, the older adult without the disease shows normal performance on other memory procedures, such as cued recall and delayed recognition. This profile of performance suggests that different mechanisms underlie the memory loss of aging and that of Alzheimer's disease. In Alzheimer's disease, it is suggested that the problem resides in the consolidation or storage of new information in long-term memory stores. In normal aging, the principal problem appears to be primarily the efficient accessing of recently stored information. Therefore, procedures providing structural support for recall (e.g., recognition) facilitate the retrieval process. Besides memory problems, older adults without dementing disorders also show some decrements compared to younger cohorts on tests of visuoperceptual, visuospatial, and constructional functions (Eslinger et al. 1985; Howieson et al. 1993; Koss et al. 1991). These modest declines can be illustrated by lower scores on tests involving visual analysis and integration, such as the Block Design subtest of the Wechsler Adult Intelligence Scale, 3rd Edition (WAIS-III; Wechsler 1997a) and similar tests involving visual integration. Performance on measures of executive control (e.g., the Trail Making Test; Reitan 1958), language retrieval (verbal fluency), and divided attention (e.g., the Digit Span test from WAIS-III; Wechsler 1997a) also tend to be lower in older groups than in their younger counterparts (Salthouse et al. 1996).

A number of explanations for age-related cognitive change have been suggested, none of which are mutually exclusive. All basically support the premise of a broad explanatory mechanism for age-related cognitive change rather than unique and specific changes in restricted cognitive domains. Speed of central processing has been one popular unifying notion, given that the majority of tasks affected in aging involve motor responses or reaction times (Salthouse 1985). This interpretation finds support from empirical studies using structural analytic methods to examine the relationship between age and a broad range of disparate cognitive tasks (Salthouse and Czaja 2000). The hypothesis about speed of processing may not, however, account for all ability differences due to age because some residual effects are still apparent after reduction of timing constraints (Klodin 1976; Satz et al. 1990). Another explanation posits that the profile of cognitive change in normal aging is the result of a loss in "fluid" abilities, skills that require novel problem solving and flexible thought (Botwinick 1977; Horn 1982). Well-rehearsed verbal abilities, so-called "crystallized" skills, by contrast, are less susceptible to age-associated change. More recent refinements of this hypothesis conceptualize normal aging as a selective vulnerability in frontal dysexecutive processes (Daigneault and Braun 1993; Mittenberg et al. 1989; Van Gorp et al. 1990). This notion is consistent with the behavioral difficulties observed, suggesting subtle impairments in integrative and retrieval functions, and is also supported by neuroimaging (Coffey et al. 1992; Gur et al. 1987; Langley and Madden 2000) and histopathological findings (Haug et al. 1983) within the frontal-subcortical brain connections. However, although the frontal hypothesis is conceptually appealing and capable of explaining much of the changes observed with aging, other work suggests that the deficits may not be localizable in their entirety to a single brain system (Salthouse et al. 1996). Research continues to identify the nature of the mechanisms that underlie age-related cognitive change and the association of these mechanisms with brain diseases common to aging, specifically Alzheimer's disease.

A significant problem in the interpretation of any of the earlier studies is that many did not routinely screen for nervous system disorders or operationalize their criteria for normal aging. These types of methodological variations between studies have resulted in large differences in subject samples and have left unclear the potential confounding influence of undetected medical or neurological problems. More recent normative studies in carefully constructed populations underscored the basic tenets of a broad-based change in efficiency of function. These studies also emphasized that age-related changes are modest and do not rise to the level of the impairment seen in dementia. To the clinician, this latter distinction is important. The discrimination between normal aging and dementia ultimately rests not only on the results of neuropsychological testing but on the careful documentation of functional decline. In normal aging, the cognitive losses described are annoying but not disabling. In dementia, the difficulties are more pronounced, even in the early stages, leading to functional changes and the need for accommodations in daily life.

Differentiation of Alzheimer's Dementia From Normal Aging

Alzheimer's disease is the leading cause of dementia in elderly persons (Katzman 1976). Alone or in combination with other nervous system disorders, Alzheimer's disease accounts for nearly 50% to 75% of all cases in Western countries (Ebly et al. 1995; Fratiglioni et al. 1999). The second most common cause of dementia, accounting for 15%–30% of cases, is vascular dementia, which includes disorders arising from either large- or small-vessel strokes (Lobo et al. 2000). Far less common are the frontal lobe disorders, which include the now well-recognized disorders of frontotemporal dementia, Pick's disease, and forms of progressive aphasia (Geldmacher and Whitehouse 1997). Lewy body dementia and related movement disorders of the basal ganglia—including Parkinson's disease, progressive supranuclear palsy, corticobasal degeneration, Huntington's disease, and multisystem atrophy—together account for 10% of the cases (Hanson et al. 1990). Rare illnesses, which are potentially reversible, include conditions such as hydrocephalus and metabolic disorders (e.g., Wilson's disease), which account for fewer than 5% of the cases of dementia (Savolainen et al. 1999). Exceptionally uncommon but serious infectious dementias, such as Creutzfeldt-Jakob disease, account for only 1 in 1.1 million cases (Holman et al. 1995).

The cognitive profiles of these various disorders overlap to some extent, but there are unique characteristics in many of the disorders that can be of diagnostic utility (see Table 11-2 for disease profiles). Alzheimer's disease dementia is the most highly investigated and best understood cognitive disorder. Its presentation is dominated by a pronounced impairment in recent-memory processing, which remains the most affected function of mentation in the majority of cases. This difficulty is now understood to arise from the selective involvement of the medial temporal lobe early in the illness (Braak and Braak 1991; Hyman et al. 1984), giving rise to impaired consolidation of newly learned information into the more permanent memory stores located across interconnected neocortical structures. On formal neuropsychological testing, the memory problem of Alzheimer's disease is manifest as a rapid forgetting of new information after very brief delays (5–10 minutes) (Welsh et al. 1991).

Patients in the mild prodrome of the illness, mild cognitive impairment, generally show only this isolated memory problem (see Petersen et al. 2001 for review). However, as the disease progresses, other areas of cognition are involved, reflecting the specific spread of neuropathological involvement to the lateral temporal areas, parietal cortex, and frontal neocortical areas (Welsh et al. 1992). Prototypical changes occur in expressive language, visuospatial function, higher executive controls, and semantic knowledge. At these latter stages of the illness, anomia with impaired semantic fluency (e.g., generation of names of animals) is generally seen on examination. Word search and circumlocution tendencies are common in conversational speech, whereas speech comprehension itself is better preserved, as are all other fundamental elements of communication (Bayles et al. 1989). Visuospatial problems become more prominent in later stages of the illness, resulting in dressing apraxia, difficulty in recognizing objects or people, and problems in performing familiar motor acts (Benke 1993). Subtle problems in spatial processing can occur early and may be detectable only on formal examination. The problem can be illuminated by tests of spatial judgment and visual organization (Rizzo et al. 2000). In everyday settings, the problem may manifest as

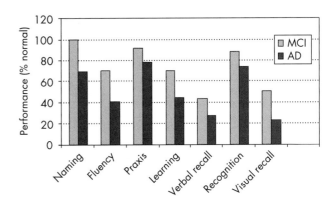

FIGURE 11–1. Profiles of neuropsychological test performance by patients with mild cognitive impairment and by patients with moderate Alzheimer's disease.

Bars indicate the performance of patients with mild cognitive impairment (n = 153; MCI in figure) and moderately impaired Alzheimer's disease patients (n = 277; AD in figure) on the subtests of the Consortium to Establish a Registry for Alzheimer's Disease (CERAD; Tariot 1996) neuropsychological battery, compared to the performance of normal elderly control subjects (n = 158) of similar age, sex, and education. The overall neuropsychological test performance of the Alzheimer's disease patients is well below that of both subjects with mild cognitive impairment and subjects experiencing normal aging. Patients with mild cognitive impairment perform at normal levels on naming and praxis. Learning and verbal fluency are mildly affected in this group, falling at 71% of normal. Memory is particularly affected in both Alzheimer's disease and mild cognitive impairment. Verbal recall on the CERAD Word List Memory test was 45% of normal in the sample with mild cognitive impairment and only 28% for the Alzheimer's disease patients. Visual memory was 51% of normal in mild cognitive impairment and 23% in Alzheimer's disease.

MCI = moderate cognitive impairment; AD = Alzheimer's disease.

Source. Data are derived from the Cache County Study of Memory sample (K. A. Welsh-Bohmer, unpublished).

intermittent topographical disorientation, leading to difficulties in finding familiar routes while driving (Rizzo et al. 1997). An example of the profound memory loss differentiating Alzheimer's disease and mild cognitive impairment from normal aging appears in Figure 11–1.

Vascular Dementia

The neuropsychological profile of vascular dementia differs in many respects from that of Alzheimer's disease, the main difference being the absence of the profound memory impairment classic in Alzheimer's disease (Tierney et al. 2001). Presentation varies according to the type and extent of the vascular disorder—multiple infarctions, a single strategic stroke, microvascular disease, cerebral hypoperfusion, hemorrhage, or combinations of these etiologies (Cohen et al. 2002). Multi-infarct

TABLE 11–2. Clinical cognitive syndromes and associated neuropsychological profiles

Cognitive syndrome and characteristics	Neuropsychological profile
Normal aging Subjective memory complaints Annoying but not disabling problems Frequent problems with name retrieval Minor difficulties in recalling detailed events	Impaired fluid abilities (novel problem solving) Deficiencies in memory retrieval Decreased general speed of processing Lowered performance on executive tasks and visuospatial skills/ visuomotor speed

Mild cognitive impairment
Subjective memory complaints
Noticeable change in memory as noted by informants
Clinical Dementia Rating score of 0.5 (mild, questionable
  dementia) (Hughes et al. 1982)
Problem is not disabling
	Memory performance 1.5 standard deviations below
	  age-matched peers
	Otherwise intact neurocognitive function
	Functional disorder limited to mild interference from the
	  memory difficulty

Alzheimer's disease Insidious onset Progressive impairment Prominent memory impairment Possible disorders: aphasia, apraxia, agnosia	Impaired memory consolidation with rapid forgetting Diminished executive skills Impaired semantic fluency and naming Impaired visuospatial analysis and praxis

Frontotemporal dementia
Prominent personality/behavioral change
Disinhibition or apathy
Impaired judgment, insight
Normal mental status initially
	Pronounced executive impairments
	  Cognitive inflexibility
	  Impaired sequencing
	  Perseverative, imitative, utilization behaviors
	    Poor use of feedback
	    Prone to interference
	Less obvious memory impairments

Lewy body dementia Fluctuations in alertness/acute confusional state Visual hallucinations Memory impairment Parkinsonian signs Neuroleptic sensitivity Falls resulting from orthostatic hypotension	Memory impairment of Alzheimer's disease but with some partial saving Pronounced apraxia, visuospatial difficulties Rapidly increasing quantifiable deficits in many cases
Vascular dementia Variation of symptoms with subtype Focality on examination Abrupt onset In multi-infarct dementia, stepwise progression	Language/memory retrieval difficulties common Benefit from structural support/cueing Asymmetric motor speed/dexterity Executive inefficiencies
Parkinson's disease dementia Extrapyramidal motor disturbance Gait dysfunction and frequent falls Bradykinesia Bradyphrenia	Slowed performance Retrieval memory deficit Executive deficiencies (slowed sequencing, impaired lexical fluency) Impaired fine motor speed (asymmetry common) Constructional deficits
Huntington's disease Early age at onset (midlife) Choreiform movements Dementia Bradyphrenia	Slowed performance Memory difficulty in retrieval Benefit from retrieval supports (recognition OK) Executive compromises Poor verbal fluency/preserved naming

TABLE 11–2. Clinical cognitive syndromes and associated neuropsychological profiles *(continued)*

Cognitive syndrome and characteristics	Neuropsychological profile
Progressive supranuclear palsy Extrapyramidal syndrome but no tremor Ophthalmic abnormalities (limited downgaze) Axial rigidity Pseudobulbar palsy Frequent falls	Mild dysexecutive symptoms: impaired sequencing, fluency, flexibility Motor slowing Memory weakness characterized as inefficiencies in storage and retrieval
Hydrocephalus Memory impairment Gait disturbance Incontinence	Slowed information processing Memory retrieval problems Benefit from retrieval supports
Creutzfeldt-Jakob disease Rare Typically, rapid onset and course Dementia with pyramidal and extrapyramidal signs Transient spikes on electroencephalogram	Rapidly evolving dementia Subtypes include a profile akin to Alzheimer's disease, or pronounced complex visuospatial disorder (Balint's syndrome)
Dementia of geriatric depression Affective disorder Psychomotor slowing Memory complaints Cognitive complaints linked temporally to the depressive disorder	Impaired performance on tasks involving effortful processing Impaired attention, concentration, sequencing, cognitive flexibility, and executive control Retrieval memory difficulty Memory improvement with cueing/recognition Behavioral tendencies to abandon tasks, poor motivation

dementia, arising from multiple large- and small-vessel strokes, demonstrates a pattern of multifocal impairments on testing that relates to the cerebral territories involved in the infarctions (Chui et al. 1992; Roman et al. 1993). In dementias attributable to diffuse small-vessel disease—with Binswanger's disease as the extreme end of the spectrum—test results follow a pattern reflecting the disruption in the dorsolateral prefrontal and subcortical circuitry (Kramer et al. 2002). Memory is involved, but deficits are often patchy in nature. Patients may show impaired recollection of some recent event but show a surprising memory of some other event occurring during the same time frame. On formal neuropsychological testing, the pattern shown in results of memory testing is one of inefficient acquisition of new information, leading to a flattened learning curve over repeating trials (Looi and Sachdev 1999; Padovani et al. 1995). Recall performance can be quite low—similar to Alzheimer's disease—but is typically without the rapid forgetting shown in Alzheimer's disease (Matsuda et al. 1998). The information acquired, though little, is generally retained; as a result, savings scores between a final learning trial and a later delayed recall trial are generally high. Finally, recognition improves dramatically with a recognition format, suggesting a primary difficulty in retrieval rather than in storage or consolidation of new information. Besides memory, dysexecutive functions are typically involved, leading to slowed sequencing, cognitive inflexibility, and decreased verbal fluency (Kertesz and Clydesdale 1994). Asymmetries in sensory-motor function and deficits in coordination are also frequently demonstrated.

Frontotemporal Dementia

Frontotemporal dementia refers to a heterogeneous group of neurodegenerative conditions that are now recognized as a major non–Alzheimer's disease dementia, although the exact prevalence of these conditions remains inconclusive (Hodges and Miller 2001). The neuropathological features of these groups of illnesses are disparate, but the histological changes and atrophy are uniformly confined to the frontal and anterior temporal cortices. From the outset, the disorders are clinically distinct from Alzheimer's disease and other forms of dementia. Typically, prominent early changes occur in behavior, personality, and/or language rather than impairments in memory and other aspects of cognition. As a consequence of impaired judgment and social inappropriateness, patients may have tremendous difficulties in their everyday lives, but on formal psychometric screening they may score entirely within normal limits. A number of investigations that have delineated the cognitive profile of these disorders (Pachana et al. 1996) indicate double dissociations between frontotemporal dementia and Alzheimer's disease. In Alzheimer's disease there is classic rapid forgetting; in frontotemporal dementia there is impairment in executive function. This dysexecutive syndrome is characterized by slowed information processing, cognitive rigidity, diminished abstract reasoning, poor response inhibition, and impaired planning and foresight. At the neurobehavioral level there are major changes in personality and general social decorum. Disinhibition or its converse, behavioral apathy and inertia, frequently occur. Patients' insight into their condition is also impaired, usually early in the course of the disorder—in contrast with Alzheimer's disease, in which insight is generally lost later in the dementia process. In fact, appreciation of memory and other symptoms may be quite acute early in Alzheimer's disease, and memory complaints may be a harbinger of the progressive disorder (Geerlings et al. 1999).

Clinically, the presentation of frontotemporal dementia varies considerably, owing in part to the distribution of pathological changes occurring in the frontal lobes (Jackson and Lowe 1996; McKhann et al. 2001; Snowden et al. 2002). At least three general subtypes of frontotemporal dementia are now recognized; classification is based on common features of clinical and neuropsychological presentation (Hodges 2001). These subtypes include a so-called frontal variant, a semantic variant, and a rare form involving mutism.

The frontal variant is primarily characterized by the changes in social behavior and personality previously described, reflecting the orbitofrontal (ventromedial) basis of the underlying pathology. Reduction in spontaneous speech is common and probably related to the extent of frontal/anterior cingulate involvement. Conventional neuropsychological tests are generally insensitive to detecting this type of disorder. Cognitive screening tests can often show no impairment until very late in the course of the illness. The most striking neuropsychological feature in this variant is poor planning and visuospatial organizational ability, which can be identified by performance on complex constructional tasks (e.g., the Rey-Osterrieth Complex Figure Test [Osterrieth 1944], the Block Design subtest of WAIS-III [Wechsler 1997a]), despite the individual's intact perceptual and spatial judgment abilities on tests in which organizational aspects are constrained. The diagnosis of frontotemporal dementia in these situations rests largely on the patient's history and the documentation of behavioral and personality change.

The semantic dementia variant of frontotemporal dementia is characterized by a progressive fluent aphasia in which there is a breakdown in the conceptual basis underlying language production and comprehension. Patients with this subtype complain of word loss and restriction in expressive vocabulary. Deficits on formal neuropsychological testing are characteristic in tests of semantic knowledge, both verbal (e.g., naming, category fluency) and nonverbal (e.g., Pyramids and Palm Trees test [Howard and Patterson 1992], judging semantic relatedness of pictures). Some patients with predominantly more right-hemisphere involvement may also have difficulty in face recognition or face naming. In imaging there is frequently asymmetric atrophy of the anterolateral temporal lobe, with sparing of medial temporal structures (e.g., hippocampus). It might be noted that cases of semantic dementia have often been included under the category of primary progressive aphasia, but current definitions of this disorder now suggest more heterogeneity in this entity, with fluent and nonfluent types (Weintraub et al. 1990).

The third and relatively rare variant of frontotemporal dementia is characterized by a nonfluent aphasia, which eventually progresses to behavioral inertia and frank mutism (Hodges 2001). Characteristically, the phonological and syntactic aspects of language are affected, but changes in behavior are rare. Patients with this variant of frontotemporal dementia present with speech dysfluency, phonological errors, and word-finding impairments. Memory for daily events is good, as are basic activities of daily living. On brain imaging, regional involvement includes the left perisylvian region, the insula, and the inferior frontal and superior temporal cortices. On postmortem examination, neuropathology is heterogeneous (Brun et al. 1994; Jackson and Lowe 1996). Approximately half the cases are Alzheimer's disease with atypical distribution of changes to the perisylvian regions; the other half have Pick's disease–like pathology (e.g., cortical thinning and gliosis) but almost invariably without the Pick bodies.

It should be underscored that the subtypes do not always present distinctly and that a combination of symptoms can occur. Other types of frontal lobe dementia also exist; they include presenile dementia associated with motor neuron disease, such as amyotrophic lateral sclerosis (ALS) with dementia. There are also a variety of degenerative conditions with secondary frontal lobe effects. Vascular conditions, such as subcortical ischemic vascular dementia or Binswanger's disease (mentioned previously), often present with frontal lobe impairments, which are probably secondary to the disruption of subcortical white matter pathways.

Huntington's Disease

Huntington's disease is a hereditary neurodegenerative disorder involving progressive chorea, dementia, and psychiatric disturbance. With onset typically in midlife, it is not easily confused with Alzheimer's disease dementia. However, the cognitive disorder in the condition is worth some consideration because it forms the prototype of the so-called subcortical dementias. This term is useful for classifying conditions such as Parkinson's disease, diffuse Lewy body dementia, progressive supranuclear palsy, and other conditions with primary neuropathological involvement of the extrapyramidal motor system (basal ganglia) and its connections.

The cognitive profile of Huntington's disease is one of retrieval problems with mild dysexecutive disturbances. In the early stages of the illness, the cognitive impairment of Huntington's disease is not as dramatic or as global as that seen in early-stage Alzheimer's disease (Butters et al. 1988). However, careful study of patients with preclinical Huntington's disease indicates that some cognitive decline is present well before the clinical onset of the disease (Jason et al. 1997; Kirkwood et al. 1999; Paulsen et al. 2001). Decrements in psychomotor speed, oculomotor functions, executive function, and motor skills have been shown to occur before the onset of clinically diagnostic Huntington's disease motor signs and to worsen as the illness progresses (Kirkwood et al. 1999; Paulsen et al. 2001). The deficits probably reflect early striatal neural loss and may also be related to the number of trinucleotide repeats present in the individual patient (Jason et al. 1997). The typical cognitive presentation of patients with manifest Huntington's disease involves a memory retrieval deficit and executive compromises. Such deficits reflect the neurobehavioral correlates of the neostriatal compromise and are manifest as inefficient and inconsistent memory and information processing. Whereas acquisition of new information may be roughly within expectations—suggesting adequate storage skills—free recall is typically compromised, and retrieval improves only with the provision of support through cues. Rapid sequencing, response inhibition, cognitive flexibility, and similar executive skills requiring rapid higher-level processing are typically also compromised.

Parkinson's Disease and Related Disorders

Cognition is commonly affected in Parkinson's disease but can be quite variable in both the nature and extent of symptoms. In some individuals the cognitive problems resemble normal aging somewhat; in others, dementia is manifest. Cognitive loss does not necessarily herald dementia. Typically, only 20%–40% of patients with Parkinson's disease are reported to have dementia (Cummings 1988; Friedman and Barcikowska 1994; Pillon et al. 1991; Reid 1992), and there is some evidence that younger age at onset is a risk factor for Parkinson's disease dementia (Friedman and Barcikowska 1994; Reid 1992).

In patients with idiopathic Parkinson's disease, cognitive changes are commonly noted as similar to those of Huntington's disease, probably reflecting the subcortical localization of the major neuropathology. However, carefully controlled investigations have shown that reduction of the cognitive profile of Parkinson's disease to a single "subcortical" subtype may be an oversimplification. As an example, memory impairments were seen in only half of the patients with Parkinson's disease examined in one study; the other half of the sample exhibited normal performance (Filoteo et al. 1997). Interestingly, only half of those with memory impairments showed performance consistent with what is typically observed in Huntington's disease; the remaining patients exhibited a memory profile more typically associated with Alzheimer's disease.

Part of the heterogeneity in presentation probably reflects an admixture of several similar syndromes that have overlapping but not identical pathological and neurochemical etiologies (Cummings 1988). Diffuse Lewy body dementia and the Lewy body variant of Alzheimer's disease are now recognized forms of dementia that share cognitive features common to Alzheimer's disease and Parkinson's disease. These disorders all show elements of rapid forgetting, albeit with some partial saving, and visuospatial disturbances (Hanson et al 1990; Salmon et al. 1996). Other conditions closely related to Parkinson's disease and diffuse Lewy body dementia include progressive supranuclear palsy, corticobasal degeneration, and multisystem atrophy. All these conditions are considered synucleinopathies, involving the pathological accumulation of the protein alpha-synuclein in midbrain structures of the nigrostriatal system. The prevailing features in these related conditions are parkinsonism, akinetic rigidity, and generalized slowing in motor movement/motor initiation and thought processes (bradykinesia and bradyphrenia, respectively).

When the overall level of dementia is controlled, some clinical differentiation between the similar conditions can be made; but the process of differential diagnosis should include, at a minimum, careful attention to the history of symptoms, the cognitive deficits manifest, and the presence or absence of defined behavioral impairments (Pillon et al. 1991). Making a solid differential diagnosis based solely on cognitive profile is difficult (Monza et al. 1998; Soliveri et al. 2000; Testa et al. 2001). Some differentiation, however, is possible. For example, cognitively impaired patients with Parkinson's disease can be differentiated from patients with Alzheimer's disease by the greater apathy observed in the former group and the memory impairment in the latter (Cahn-Weiner et al. 2002). Likewise, the neuropsychiatric profiles of the dementias of Alzheimer's disease and of Parkinson's disease differ (Aarsland et al. 2001). However, differentiating these disorders from each other requires integration of the clinical examination findings—which include both cognitive examination findings and behavioral ratings—with historical and ancillary data that include imaging.

Geriatric Depression and Mood Disorders

Among the most common uses of neuropsychological assessment in elderly persons are evaluating memory disorders and determining the role of depression. By itself, serious mood depression in elderly persons can result in disabling cognitive impairment, or what has been called the dementia of depression or pseudodementia (Breitner and Welsh 1995). The problem of geriatric depression is fairly common: some recent epidemiology-based studies suggested that 28% of elderly populations over age 65 exhibit prominent affective syndromes (Lyketsos et al. 2001). Depression also frequently co-occurs in the context of a range of medical disorders—including Alzheimer's disease, stroke, and Parkinson's disease—which complicates the diagnosis of these disorders and exacerbates the functional loss associated with each (Ballard et al. 1996; Krishnan 2000; Migliorelli et al. 1995; Reichman and Coyne 1995). Distinguishing between depression and other conditions in elderly patients can be challenging, but it can be assisted by a thorough screening of both depressive symptoms and cognitive status.

When such screening fails to give a clear picture of the contribution of depression to the cognitive picture, neuropsychological examination can help. To this end, it must be noted that depression in late life is clinically heterogeneous: some patients show severe cognitive disturbance, whereas others with seemingly equal levels of clinical depression show little cognitive impairment. This heterogeneity is influenced in part by the many disparate biological, medical, and social causes contributing to the depressive symptoms (Alexopoulos et al. 2002; Krishnan

1993), as well as a number of other factors, a few of which are premorbid personality disposition, severity of mood symptoms, medical comorbidities, and age (Boone et al. 1994, 1995).

Despite this heterogeneity, some distinctive neurocognitive and behavioral changes appear to be ascribable to the condition of late-life depression and are characteristic of a rather large subgroup of patients (Beats et al. 1996; Lockwood et al. 2002). In studies in which care was taken to restrict the study sample to cases of late-onset depression without psychotic symptoms and significant neurological comorbidities, a profile has emerged of cognitive, behavioral, and functional impairment that has been ascribed to disturbed function of the prefrontal cortical to striatal-pallidal-thalamic connections (Beats et al. 1996; Goodwin 1997; Lesser et al. 1996). Neurocognitively, the profile is one of a dysexecutive syndrome with impairments in planning, organization, initiation, sequencing, working memory, and behavioral shifting in response to feedback. Short-term memory and visuospatial skills are also disturbed, in part as a result of the attentional and organizational compromises. Behaviorally, the depression-dysexecutive syndrome of geriatric depressed patients is characterized by apathy and psychomotor retardation, as opposed to the prominent mood dysphoria of younger counterparts. On formal neuropsychological testing, geriatric depressed patients show impairments on tests sensitive to frontal lobe function. Difficulties can be readily seen on tests of selective and sustained attention, verbal fluency, inhibitory control, and set shifting (Boone et al. 1995; Lockwood et al. 2002). Memory is impaired in both acquisition and recall, leading to a profile characterized by a flattened learning curve and impaired free recall, after brief delays, of previously learned information (Hart et al. 1987). Recognition memory is better preserved but can be characterized by false-negative tendencies (i.e., not recognizing previous target material). The memory disturbance of depression is distinguished from that of Alzheimer's disease by the impaired acquisition and recognition elements in depression. In Alzheimer's disease, acquisition is relatively better preserved, whereas recognition is characterized by false-positive tendencies (i.e., recognizing foils incorrectly as previously presented targets). The profile of impairment in depression gives the impression of generalized cognitive inefficiency and suppression of performance. Other qualitative differences between the performance of these two groups may also be seen; depressed patients often have a heightened tendency to abandon effortful tests. Perseverative errors and intrusional tendencies, although common in patients with both disorders, are particularly common in depressed patients.

It is important to note that, even with treatment, not all the cognitive impairments associated with geriatric depression remit. In older patients, these continuing impairments may be due to the co-occurrence of another disease process, such as Alzheimer's disease or vascular dementia. Although far from conclusive, a number of studies have reported that depression in elderly persons exerts a discernible additional effect on cognition and functional independence and that depression may be a risk factor for later cognitive decline. Depression and cognitive status have both been independently related to the ability to perform basic activities of daily living and instrumental activities of daily living in Alzheimer's disease patients (Koltai and Branch 1999; McCue 1997; McCue et al. 1990). Additionally, depressed affect and severity of cognitive dysfunction appear to have an interactive or an additive effect on the performance of instrumental activities of daily living. Therefore, neuropsychological evaluation of elderly patients provides critical information about the nature of their cognitive failures and the extent to which their profile is suggestive of depression and dementia. This information has obvious implications for the diagnosis and management of these patients, regardless of whether all the cognitive change is reversible.

Conclusion

The neuropsychological evaluation is useful in the assessment of memory complaints in elderly patients. When considered in the context of the broader medical picture, the neuropsychological examination contributes significantly to the diagnosis of a broad class of dementing conditions—Alzheimer's disease, vascular dementia, Parkinson's disease–related dementias, and geriatric depression. Although not necessary in many instances, the neuropsychological examination has particular value in the early identification of brain diseases that might otherwise go undetected for some time. This early identification of neurodegenerative conditions allows the opportunity for intervention at a point in illness when such interventions are likely to be optimal (e.g., Zandi and Breitner 2001). Evaluation, as noted above, is also useful in identifying other conditions that may by themselves or in interaction with other neurological disorders cause excess disability. Depression is the most common example of such a problem, and vascular disorders are another example. The neuropsychological evaluation can be useful in identifying these potential comorbidities and others (e.g., sleep disturbance, substance abuse, medication interactions),

thereby highlighting potentially treatable conditions. Effective treatments initiated early in the disease or illness process offer the strong potential of delaying the onset of diseases, including progressive dementias, and thereby optimizing function and reducing associated health care costs (Kawas and Brookmeyer 2001; Mittelman et al. 1995).

It is also worth noting that the neuropsychological evaluation is often most useful in the exclusion of brain conditions. The results of a negative neuropsychological evaluation allow the opportunity to reassure concerned at-risk older adults, who might be considered the "worried well." The examination results can also be used as a baseline for tracking change over time and identifying problems as they emerge. Longitudinal follow-up in 12–18 months in individuals with normal or ambiguous examinations provides even more powerful information than evaluation at single time points alone. In the case of mild cognitive impairment, almost one third of patients will have converted to a diagnosis of Alzheimer's disease over this time frame (Petersen et al. 2001; Ritchie et al. 2001). Normal older adults generally show test-retest improvements over the same interval, assuming that no other comorbidities (e.g., depression) interfere at the later time point.

In summary, the neuropsychological evaluation provides a useful and cost-effective approach to the diagnosis and management of the growing geriatric population with memory complaints. Although a neuropsychological evaluation is not needed in the majority of patients with dementia cases in which symptoms are obvious and the diagnosis is secure, the evaluation can be enormously useful in more complex, less straightforward diagnostic situations, such as early Alzheimer's disease detection or geriatric depression. Because of its objective nature, the neuropsychological examination has strong applications in medical management, providing information about patients' capacities and deficits that is important to intervention approaches and to guiding future decision making about competency and safety.

References

Aarsland D, Cummings JL, Larsen JP: Neuropsychiatric differences between Parkinson's disease with dementia and Alzheimer's disease. Int J Geriatr Psychiatry 16:184–191, 2001

Alexopoulos GS, Kiosses DN, Klimstra S, et al: Clinical presentation of the "depression-executive dysfunction syndrome" of late life. Am J Geriatr Psychiatry 10:98–106, 2002

American Psychiatric Association: Diagnostic and Statistical Manual of Mental Disorders, 3rd Edition, Revised. Washington, DC, American Psychiatric Association, 1987

American Psychiatric Association: Diagnostic and Statistical Manual of Mental Disorders, 4th Edition. Washington, DC, American Psychiatric Association, 1994

Ballard C, Bannister C, Solis M, et al: The prevalence, associations and symptoms of depression amongst dementia sufferers. J Affect Disord 36:135–144, 1996

Bayles KA, Boone DR, Tomoeda CK, et al: Differentiating Alzheimer's patients from the normal elderly and stroke patients with aphasia. J Speech Hear Disord 54:74–87, 1989

Beats BC, Sahakian BJ, Levy R: Cognitive performance in tests sensitive to frontal lobe dysfunction in the elderly depressed. Psychol Med 26:591–603, 1996

Beck AT, Steer RA, Brown GK: Beck Depression Inventory, II. San Antonio, TX, The Psychological Corporation, 1996

Benke T: Two forms of apraxia in Alzheimer's disease. Cortex 29:715–725, 1993

Benton AL, Hamsher K de S: Multilingual Aphasia Examination. Iowa City, IA, AJA Associates, 1983

Benton AL, Van Allen MW, Fogel ML: Temporal orientation in cerebral disease. J Nerv Ment Dis 139:110–119, 1964

Benton AL, Eslinger PJ, Damasio AR: Normative observations on neuropsychological test performance in old age. J Clin Neuropsychol 3:33–42, 1981

Benton AL, Hamsher K de S, Varney NR, et al: Contributions to Neuropsychological Assessment. New York, Oxford University Press, 1983

Berg EA: A simple objective treatment for measuring flexibility in thinking. J Gen Psychol 39:15–22, 1948

Boone KB, Lesser I, Miller B, et al: Cognitive functioning in a mildly to moderately depressed geriatric sample: relationship to chronological age. J Neuropsychiatry Clin Neurosci 6:267–272, 1994

Boone KB, Lesser I, Miller B, et al: Cognitive functioning in older depressed outpatients: relationship of presence and severity of depression on neuropsychological test scores. Neuropsychology 9:390–398, 1995

Botwinick J: Intellectual abilities, in The Handbook of the Psychology of Aging. Edited by Birren JE, Schaie KW. New York, Van Nostrand Reinhold, 1977, pp 508–605

Braak H, Braak E: Neuropathological staging of Alzheimer-related changes. Acta Neuropathol (Berl) 82:239–259, 1991

Breitner JCS, Welsh KA: An approach to diagnosis and management of memory loss and other cognitive syndromes of aging. Psychiatr Serv 46:29–35, 1995

Breitner JC, Wyse BW, Anthony JC, et al: APOE-epsilon4 count predicts age when prevalence of AD increases, then declines: the Cache County Study. Neurology 53:321–331, 1999

Brookmeyer R, Gray S, Kawas S: Projections of Alzheimer's disease in the United States and the public health impact of delaying disease onset. Am J Public Health 88:1337–1342, 1998

Brun A, Englund B, Gustafson L, et al: Consensus statement: clinical and neuropathological criteria for frontotemporal dementia: the Lund and Manchester groups. J Neurol Neurosurg Psychiatry 57:416–418, 1994

Buschke H, Fuld PA: Evaluation of storage, retention and retrieval in disordered memory and learning. Neurology 24:1019–1025, 1974

Butcher JN, Dahlstrom WG, Graham JR, et al: Minnesota Multiphasic Personality-2 (MMPI-2): Manual for Administration and Scoring. Minneapolis, MN, University of Minnesota Press, 1989

Butters N, Salmon DP, Cullum MC, et al: Differentiation of amnesic and demented patients with the Wechsler Memory Scale—Revised. Clin Neuropsychol 2:133–148, 1988

Cahn-Weiner DA, Grace J, Ott BR, et al: Cognitive and behavioral features discriminate between Alzheimer's and Parkinson's disease. Neuropsychiatry Neuropsychol Behav Neurol 15:79–87, 2002

Chen P, Ratcliff G, Belle SH, et al: Patterns of cognitive decline in presymptomatic Alzheimer's disease: a prospective community study. Arch Gen Psychiatry 58:853–858, 2001

Chui HC, Victoroff JI, Margolin D, et al: Criteria for the diagnosis of ischemic vascular dementia proposed by the State of California Alzheimer's Disease Diagnostic and Treatment Centers. Neurology 42 (3, pt 1):473–480, 1992

Coffey CE, Wilkinson WE, Parashos IA, et al: Quantitative cerebral anatomy of the aging human brain: a cross-sectional study using magnetic resonance imaging. Neurology 43:527–536, 1992

Cohen RA, Paul RH, Ott BR, et al: The relationship of subcortical MRI hyperintensities and brain volume to cognitive function in vascular dementia. J Int Neuropsychol Soc 8:743–752, 2002

Craik FIM: Age differences in remembering, in Neuropsychology of Memory. Edited by Squire L, Butters N. New York, Guilford, 1984, pp 3–12

Cullum CM, Butters N, Troster AL, et al: Normal aging and forgetting rates on the Wechsler Memory Scale—Revised. Arch Clin Neuropsychol 5:23–30, 1990

Cummings JL: Intellectual impairment in Parkinson's disease: clinical, pathologic, and biochemical correlates. J Geriatr Psychiatry Neurol 1:24–36, 1988

Daigneault S, Braun CM: Working memory and the Self-Ordered Pointing Task: further evidence of early prefrontal decline in normal aging. J Clin Exp Neuropsychol 15:881–895, 1993

Delis DC, Kramer JH, Kaplan E, et al: California Verbal Learning Tests: Adult Version. San Antonio, TX, Psychological Corporation, 1987

Ebly EM, Parhad IM, Hogan DB, et al: Prevalence and types of dementia in the very old: results from the Canadian Study of Health and Aging. Neurology 44:1593–1600, 1994

Ebly EM, Hogan DB, Parhad IM: Cognitive impairment in the nondemented elderly: results from the Canadian Study of Health and Aging. Arch Neurol 52:612–619, 1995

Elias MF, Beiser A, Wolf PA, et al: The preclinical phase of Alzheimer disease: a 22-year prospective study of the Framingham Cohort. Arch Neurol 57:808–813, 2000

Ernst RL, Hay JW: The US economic and social costs of Alzheimer's disease revisited. Am J Public Health 84:1261–1264, 1994

Eslinger PJ, Damasio AR, Benton AL, et al: Neuropsychologic detection of abnormal mental decline in older persons. JAMA 253:670–674, 1985

Evans DA, Smith LA, Scherr PA, et al: Risk of death from Alzheimer's disease in a community population of older persons. Am J Epidemiol 134:403–412, 1991

Filoteo JV, Rilling LM, Cole B, et al: Variable memory profiles in Parkinson's disease. J Clin Exp Neuropsychol 19:878–888, 1997

Folstein MF, Folstein SE, McHugh PR: "Mini-mental state." J Psychiatr Res 12:189–198, 1975

Fratiglioni L, De Ronchi D, Aguero-Torres H: Worldwide prevalence and incidence of dementia. Drugs Aging 15:365–375, 1999

Friedman A, Barcikowska M: Dementia in Parkinson's disease. Dementia 5:12–16, 1994

Geerlings MI, Jonker C, Bouter LM, et al: Association between memory complaints and incident Alzheimer's disease in elderly people with normal baseline cognition. Am J Psychiatry 156:531–537, 1999

Geldmacher DS, Whitehouse PJ Jr: Differential diagnosis of Alzheimer's disease. Neurology 48 (5, suppl 6):S2–S9, 1997

Goodwin G.M: Neuropsychological and neuroimaging evidence for the involvement of the frontal lobes in depression. J Psychopharmacol 11:115–122, 1997

Gur RC, Gur RE, Obrist WD, et al: Age and regional cerebral blood flow at rest and during cognitive activity. Arch Gen Psychiatry 44:617–621, 1987

Hanson L, Salmon D, Galasko D, et al: The Lewy body variant of Alzheimer's disease: a clinical and pathological entity. Neurology 40:1–8, 1990

Hart RP, Kwentus JA, Taylor JR, et al: Rate of forgetting in dementia and depression. J Consult Clin Psychol 55:101–105, 1987

Haug H, Barmwater U, Eggers R, et al: Anatomical changes in aging brain: morphometric analysis of the human prosencephalon, in Neuropharmacology, Vol 21: Aging. Edited by Cervos-Navarro J, Sarkander HI. New York, Raven Press. pp 1–12, 1983

Heaton RK, Grant I, Matthews CG: Comprehensive Norms for an Expanded Halstead-Reitan Battery: Demographic Corrections, Research Findings and Clinical Applications. Odessa, FL: Psychological Assessment Resources, 1991

Hodges JR: Frontotemporal dementia (Picks disease). Clinical features and assessment. Neurology 56 (suppl):S6–S10, 2001

Hodges JR, Miller B: The classification, genetics and neuropathology of frontotemporal dementia. Introduction to the special topic papers: Part I. Neurocase 7 (1):31–35, 2001

Holman RC, Khan AS, Kent J, et al: Epidemiology of Creutzfeldt-Jakob disease in the United States 1979–1990: analysis of national mortality data. Neuroepidemiology 14:174–181, 1995

Horn J: The theory of fluid and crystallized intelligence in relation to concepts of cognitive psychology and aging in adulthood, in Aging and Cognitive Processes. Edited by Craik F, Trehub S. New York: Plenum, 1982, pp 237–278

Howard D, Patterson K: Pyramids and Palm Trees Manual. Thurston, Suffolk, England, Thames Valley Test Company, 1992

Howieson D, Holm L, Kaye J, et al: Neurologic function in the optimally healthy oldest old: neuropsychological evaluation. Neurology 43:1882–1886, 1993

Hughes CP, Berg L, Danziger WL, et al: A new clinical scale for the staging of dementia. Br J Psychiatry 140:566–572, 1982

Hyman BT, Van Horsen GW, Damasio AR, et al: Alzheimer's disease: cell-specific pathology isolates the hippocampal formation. Science 225:1168–1170, 1984

Ivnik RJ, Malec JF, Smith GE, et al: Mayo's older Americans normative studies: updated AVLT norms for ages 56–97. Clin Neuropsychol 6:83–104, 1992

Jackson M, Lowe J: The new neuropathology of degenerative frontotemporal dementias. Acta Neuropathologica 91:127–134, 1996

Jason GW, Suchowersky O, Pajurkova EM, et al: Cognitive manifestations of Huntington disease in relation to genetic structure and clinical onset. Arch Neurol 54:1081–1088, 1997

Kaplan EF, Goodglass H, Weintraub S: The Boston Naming Test, 2nd Edition. Philadelphia, PA, Lea and Febiger, 1978

Katzman R: The prevalence and malignancy of Alzheimer disease: a major killer (editorial). Arch Neurol 33:217–218, 1976

Kawas C, Brookmeyer R: Aging and the public health impact of dementia. N Engl J Med, 344:1160–1161, 2001

Kertesz A, Clydesdale S Neuropsychological deficits in vascular dementia vs Alzheimer's disease. Frontal lobe deficits prominent in vascular dementia. Arch Neurol 51:1226–1231, 1994

Kirkwood SC, Siemers E, Stout JC, et al: Longitudinal cognitive and motor changes among presymptomatic HD gene carriers. Arch Neurol 56:563–568, 1999

Klodin VM: The relationship of scoring treatment and age in perceptual-integrative performance. Exp Aging Res 2:303–313, 1976

Knopman DS, DeKosky ST, Cummings JL, et al: Practice parameter: diagnosis of dementia (an evidence based review). Report of the Quality Standards Subcommittee of the American Academy of Neurology. Neurology 56:1143–1153, 2001

Koltai DC, Branch LG: Cognitive and affective interventions to maximize abilities and adjustment in dementia. Annals of Psychiatry 7:241–255, 1999

Koltai DC, Welsh-Bohmer KA: Geriatric neuropsychological assessment, in Clinician's Guide to Neuropsychological Assessment, 2nd Edition. Edited by Vanderploeg RD. Mahwah, NJ, Lawrence Erlbaum, 2000, pp 383–415

Koss E, Haxby JV, DeCarli C, et al: Patterns of performance preservation and loss in healthy aging. Dev Neuropsychol 7:99–113, 1991

Kramer JH, Reed BR, Mungas D, et al: Executive dysfunction in subcortical ischaemic vascular disease. J Neurol Neurosurg Psychiatry 72:217–220, 2002

Krishnan KR: Neuroanatomic substrates of depression in the elderly. J Geriatr Psychiatry Neurol 6:39–58, 1993

Krishnan KR: Depression as a contributing factor in cerebrovascular disease. Am Heart J 140:70–76, 2000

Langley LK, Madden DJ: Functional neuroimaging of memory: implications for cognitive aging. Microsc Res Tech 51:75–84, 2000

Lesser IM, Boone KB, Mehringer CM, et al: Cognition and white matter hyperintensities in older depressed patients. Am J Psychiatry 153:1280–1287, 1996

Lezak MD: Neuropsychological assessment, 3rd Edition. New York, Oxford University Press, 1995

Lobo A, Launer LJ, Fratiglioni L, et al: Prevalence of dementia and major subtypes in Europe: a collaborative study of population-based cohorts. Neurologic Diseases in the Elderly Research Group. Neurology 54 (11, suppl 5):S4–S9, 2000

Lockwood KA, Alexopoulos GS, Van Gorp WG: Executive dysfunction in geriatric depression. Am J Psychiatry 159:1119–1126, 2002

Looi J, Sachdev PS: Differentiation of vascular dementia from AD on neuropsychological tests. Neurology 53:670–678, 1999

Lyketsos CG, Sheppard JM, Steinberg M, et al: Neuropsychiatric disturbance in Alzheimer's disease clusters into three groups: the Cache County study. Int J Geriatr Psychiatry 16:1043–1053, 2001

Matsuda O, Saito M, Sugishita M: Cognitive deficits of mild dementia: a comparison between dementia of the Alzheimer's type and vascular dementia. Psychiatry Clin Neurosci 52:87–91, 1998

Mattis S, Jurica PJ, Leitten CL: Dementia Rating Scale-2™ (DRS-2™): Professional Manual. Odessa, FL, Psychological Assessment Resources, 2002

McCue M: The relationship between neuropsychology and functional assessment in the elderly, in Handbook of Neuropsychology and Aging. Edited by Nussbaum P. New York, Plenum, 1997, pp 394–408

McCue M, Rogers J, Goldstein G: Relationships between neuropsychological and functional assessment in elderly neuropsychiatric patients. Rehabil Psychol 35:91–99, 1990

McKhann GM, Albert MS, Grossman M, et al: Clinical and pathological diagnosis of frontotemporal dementia: report of the Work Group on Frontotemporal Dementia and Pick's Disease. Arch Neurol 58:1803–1809, 2001

Migliorelli R, Teson A, Sabe L, et al: Prevalence and correlates of dysthymia and major depression among patients with Alzheimer's disease. Am J Psychiatry 152:37–44, 1995

Mittelman MS, Ferris SH, Shulman E, et al: Comprehensive support program: effect on depression in spouse-caregivers of AD patients. Gerontologist 35:792–802, 1995

Mittenberg W, Seidenberg M, O'Leary DS, et al: Changes in cerebral functioning associated with normal aging. J Clin Exp Neuropsychol 11:918–932, 1989

Mohs RC, Cohen L: Alzheimer's Disease Assessment Scale (ADAS). Psychopharmacol Bull 24:627–628, 1988

Monza D, Soliveri P, Radice D, et al: Cognitive dysfunction and impaired organization of complex motility in degenerative parkinsonism syndromes. Arch Neurol 55:372–378, 1998

Morris JC, Heyman A, Mohs RC, et al: The Consortium to Establish a Registry for Alzheimer's Disease (CERAD). Part I. Clinical and neuropsychological assessment of Alzheimer's disease. Neurology 39:1159–1165, 1989

Osterrieth PA: Le test de copie d'une figure complexe. Archives de Psychologie 30:206–356, 1944

Pachana NA, Boone KB, Miller BL, et al: Comparison of neuropsychological functioning in Alzheimer's disease and frontotemporal dementia. J Int Neuropsychol Soc 2:505–510, 1996

Padovani A, Di Piero V, Bragoni M, et al: Patterns of neuropsychological impairment in mild dementia: a comparison between Alzheimer's disease and multi-infarct dementia. Acta Neurol Scand 92:433–442, 1995

Paulsen JS, Zhao H, Stout J, et al, and the Huntington Study Group: Clinical markers of early disease in persons near onset of Huntington's disease. Neurology 57:658–662, 2001

Petersen RC, Smith GE, Waring SC, et al: Mild cognitive impairment: clinical characterization and outcome. Arch Neurol 56:303–308, 1999

Petersen RC, Stevens JC, Ganguli M, et al: Practice parameter: early detection of dementia: mild cognitive impairment (an evidence based review). Report of the Quality Standards Subcommittee of the American Academy of Neurology. Neurology 56:1133–1142, 2001

Pillon B, Dubois B, Agid Y: Severity and specificity of cognitive impairment in Alzheimer's, Huntington's, and Parkinson's diseases and progressive supranuclear palsy. Ann N Y Acad Sci 640:224–227, 1991

Reichman WE, Coyne AC: Depressive symptoms in Alzheimer's disease and multi-infarct dementia. J Geriatr Psychiatry Neurol 8:96–99, 1995

Reid WG: The evolution of dementia in idiopathic Parkinson's disease: neuropsychological and clinical evidence in support of subtypes. Int Psychogeriatr 4:147–160, 1992

Reiman EM, Caseli RJ, Yun LS, et al: Preclinical evidence of Alzheimer's disease in persons homozygous for the ε4 allele for apolipoprotein E. N Engl J Med 334:752–758, 1996

Reitan RM: Validity of the Trail Making Test as an indicator of organic brain damage. Percept Mot Skills 8:271–276, 1958

Ritchie K, Touchon J: Mild cognitive impairment: conceptual basis and current nosological status. Lancet 355:225–228, 2001

Ritchie K, Artero S, Touchon J: Classification criteria for mild cognitive impairment: a population-based validation study. Neurology 56:37–42, 2001

Rizzo M, Reinach S, McGehee D, et al: Simulated car crashes and crash predictors in drivers with Alzheimer disease. Arch Neurol 54:545–551, 1997

Rizzo M, Anderson SW, Dawson J, et al: Vision and cognition in Alzheimer's disease. Neuropsychologia 38:1157–1169, 2000

Roman GC, Tatemichi TK, Erkinjuntti T, et al: Vascular dementia: diagnostic criteria for research studies. Report of the NINDS-AIREN International Workshop. Neurology 43:250–260, 1993

Salmon DP, Galasko D, Hansen LA, et al: Neuropsychological deficits associated with diffuse Lewy body disease. Brain Cogn 31:148–165, 1996

Salthouse T: Speed of behavior and its implications for cognition, in Handbook for the Psychology of Aging, 2nd Edition. Edited by Birren JE, Shaie KW. New York, Van Nostrand Reinhold, 1985, pp 400–426

Salthouse TA, Czaja SJ: Structural constraints on process explanations in cognitive aging. Psychol Aging 15:44–55, 2000

Salthouse TA, Fristoe N, Rhee SH: How localized are age-related effects on neuropsychological measures? Neuropsychology 10:272–285, 1996

Satz P, Hynd GW, D'Elia L, et al: WAIS-R marker for accelerated aging and dementia, Alzheimer's type? Base rates of the Fuld formula in the WAIS-R standardization sample. J Clin Exp Neuropsychol 11:759–765, 1990

Savolainen S, Palijarvi L, Vapalahti M: Prevalence of Alzheimer's disease in patients investigated for presumed normal pressure hydrocephalus: a clinical and neuropathological study. Acta Neurochir (Wien)141:849–853, 1999

Small BJ, Fratiglioni L, Vittanen M., et al: The course of cognitive impairment in preclinical Alzheimer disease. Arch Neurol 57:839–844, 2000

Small GW, Mazziotta JC, Collins MT, et al: Apolipoprotein E type 4 allele and cerebral glucose metabolism in relatives at risk for familial Alzheimer disease. JAMA 273:942–947, 1995

Small GW, Ercoli LM, Silverman DH, et al: Cerebral metabolic and cognitive decline in persons at genetic risk for Alzheimer's disease. Proc Natl Acad Sci U S A 97:6037–6042, 2000

Smith A: The Symbol Digit Modalities Test: a neuropsychologic test for economic screening of learning and other cerebral disorders. Learning Disorders 3:83–91, 1968

Snowden JS, Neary D, Mann DM: Frontotemporal dementia. Br J Psychiatry 180:140–143, 2002

Soliveri P, Monza D, Paridi D, et al: Neuropsychological follow up in patients with Parkinson's disease, striatonigral degeneration type multisystem atrophy and progressive supranuclear palsy. J Neurol Neurosurg Psychiatry 69:313–318, 2000

Spreen O, Strauss E. A Compendium of Neuropsychological Tests: Administration, Norms, and Commentary, 2nd Edition. New York, Oxford University Press, 1996

Tariot PN: CERAD behavior rating scale for dementia. Int Psychogeriatr 8 (suppl3): 317–320, 1996

Testa D, Monza D, Ferrarini M, et al: Comparison of natural histories of progressive supranuclear palsy and multiple system atrophy. Neurol Sci 21:247–251, 2001

Tierney MC, Black SE, Szalai JP, et al: Recognition memory and verbal fluency differentiate probable Alzheimer disease from subcortical ischemic vascular dementia. Arch Neurol 58:1654–1659, 2001

Tierney MC, Szalai JP, Snow WG, et al: Prediction of probable Alzheimer's disease in memory impaired patients: a prospective longitudinal study. Neurology 46:661–665, 1996

Tschanz JT, Welsh-Bohmer KA, West N, et al: Identification of dementia cases derived from a neuropsychological algorithm: comparisons with clinically derived diagnoses. Neurology 54:1290–1296, 2000

Van Gorp WG, Mahler ME: Subcortical features of normal aging, in Subcortical Dementia. Edited by Cummings JL. New York, Oxford University Press, 231–250, 1990

Wechsler D: Wechsler Intelligence Scale, 3rd Edition, Manual. San Antonio, TX, Psychological Corporation, 1997a

Wechsler D: Wechsler Memory Scale, 3rd Edition, Manual. San Antonio, TX, Psychological Corporation, 1997b

Weintraub S, Rubin NP, Mesulam MM: Primary progressive aphasia: longitudinal course, profile and language features. Arch Neurol 47:1329–1335, 1990

Welsh K, Butters N, Hughes JP, et al: Detection of abnormal memory decline in mild Alzheimer's disease using CERAD neuropsychological measures. Arch Neurol 48:278–281, 1991

Welsh KA, Butters N, Hughes JP, et al: Detection and staging of dementia in Alzheimer's disease: use of the neuropsychological measures developed for the Consortium to Establish a Registry for Alzheimer's Disease (CERAD). Arch Neurol 49:448–452, 1992

Welsh-Bohmer KA, Mohs RC: Neuropsychological assessment of Alzheimer's disease. Neurology 49 (3 suppl 3): S11–S13, 1997

Welsh-Bohmer KA, Koltai DC, Mason DJ: The clinical utility of neuropsychological evaluation of patients with known or suspected dementia, in Demonstrating Utility and Cost Effectiveness in Clinical Neuropsychology. Edited by Prigatano G, Pliskin N. Philadelphia, PA, Psychology Press—Taylor and Francis Group, 2003, pp 177–200

Wetzel L, Boll TJ: Short Category Test, Booklet Format. Los Angeles, CA, Western Psychological Services, 1987

Yesavage J, Brink TL, Rose TL, et al: Development and validation of a geriatric depression scale: a preliminary report. J Psychiatr Res 17:37–49, 1983

Zandi PP, Breitner JC: Do NSAIDs prevent Alzheimer's disease? And, if so, why? The epidemiological evidence. Neurobiol Aging 22:811–817, 2001

PART

III

Psychiatric Disorders in Late Life

C H A P T E R   1 2

Cognitive Disorders

Murray A. Raskind, M.D.

Lauren T. Bonner, M.D.

Elaine R. Peskind, M.D.

The cognitive disorders are the most prevalent psychiatric disorders of later life. The predominant problem in these disorders is a clinically meaningful deficit in cognition that represents a decline from a previous level of functioning. The cognitive disorder focused on in this chapter is dementia; also discussed are delirium, amnestic disorder, alcoholic dementia, and Wernicke-Korsakoff syndrome. In this chapter, we attempt to use nomenclature that is consistent with DSM-IV-TR (American Psychiatric Association 2000).

Dementia is a syndrome of acquired impairment of memory and other cognitive functions caused by structural neuronal damage. Dementia is induced by a variety of specific diseases that damage and destroy neurons (e.g., Alzheimer's disease [AD], cerebrovascular disease). Delirium may either complicate dementia or impair cognition on its own. It is a syndrome of impaired attention and consciousness caused by disrupted brain physiology. Delirium results from a variety of specific disturbances that disrupt brain function (e.g., adverse effects of medications on the central nervous system [CNS], electrolyte imbalance). The presence of dementia lowers the threshold for delirium. Therefore, delirium commonly occurs in the setting of dementia (Levkoff et al. 1992; Marcantonio et al. 2000; Rahkonen et al. 2000).

Dementia is particularly costly to society, both in terms of financial resources dedicated to patient care and in terms of morbidity, mortality, and the stress that pa-

tients place on caregivers and the broader community. One-half of the beds in community long-term-care facilities are devoted to patients with dementia, most of whom have AD (Katzman 1986). The prevalence and burden of the cognitive disorders of later life will further increase as the proportion of elderly persons in the United States population increases over the next 50 years.

Dementia

Dementia is a syndrome—that is, a group of signs and symptoms that cluster together and are caused by a number of underlying diseases. These diseases produce neuronal loss or other structural brain damage. The central feature of dementia is acquired impairment of memory. In addition, at least one of the following cognitive deficits must be present: aphasia (language impairment secondary to disruption of brain function), apraxia (inability to perform complex motor activities despite intact motor abilities), agnosia (failure to recognize or identify objects despite intact sensory function), and disturbance in executive functions such as planning, organizing, sequencing, and abstracting. To meet formal criteria, the dementia must be severe enough to interfere with social or occupational functioning. Dementia resulting from any brain disorder has the aforementioned features in common.

Supported in part by the Department of Veterans Affairs, National Institute on Aging Alzheimer's Disease Research Center grant AG05316, and a minority faculty supplement to grant AG18644.

Clinical Features

Although all disorders causing dementia must produce acquired impairment of memory and impairment of other cognitive functions—impairments severe enough to interfere with daily activities—and must represent a substantial decline from a previous level of functioning, the specific dementia disorders have distinguishing features that reflect the nature of the underlying disease. Recognizing the likely disorder underlying dementia can have important treatment implications. Because AD is the most common dementia disorder of later life (Katzman 1976), the course of AD is often assumed to be the course of dementia in general. In fact, the course of AD is a relatively specific diagnostic feature of the disease (Khachaturian 1985; McKhann et al. 1984). The typical course of AD is one of insidious onset, with gradual but inexorable progression of cognitive deficits over a period ranging from 5 to 15 years or even longer. Other diseases causing dementia may have quite different clinical courses. For example, dementia due to head trauma has a sudden onset, and the course is stable or the patient may improve over time. Dementia due to anoxia (such as in older persons resuscitated not soon enough after cardiac arrest to prevent hypoxic brain damage) has a similar course. Vascular dementia can progress in a stepwise manner, reflecting new episodes of cerebral infarction, or can progress gradually in a manner indistinguishable from AD (Chui et al. 1992). In the case of persons with dementia due to alcohol use who subsequently abstain from alcohol, a substantial number show meaningful improvements in cognitive function (Victor and Adams 1971).

Differential Diagnosis

Dementia and Delirium

A common problem in the differential diagnosis of dementia is mistaking a delirium for dementia. An even more common problem is failing to recognize a delirium superimposed on an underlying dementia. Both delirium and dementia manifest as impairment in cognitive functions, but the two conditions differ in the pattern of deficits and the cognitive domains primarily involved. In at least the early and middle stages of dementia, the patient is alert and attentive, whereas in delirium the patient shows decreased attention to the environment and has an altered level of arousal. The delirious patient's cognitive deficits fluctuate, whereas those of the patient with dementia are usually stable. Unfortunately, in the more advanced stages of progressive dementia disorders of late life such as AD, attention is impaired. However, even in the late stages of AD, a fluctuating level of consciousness

is cause for concern—concern that a superimposed delirium may exist.

Dementia and Depression

A differential diagnostic problem that has received much attention is the differentiation of a major depressive episode from dementia in a cognitively impaired older person. Although the term *depressive pseudodementia* (Kiloh 1961) was justly criticized by Reifler (1982), the concept has some heuristic value. It is unusual for a major depressive episode to produce such severe cognitive impairment that distinction of the impairment from a specific dementia disorder such as AD is persistently difficult. However, depressive pseudodementia secondary to a primary major depressive episode does occur. It usually begins with dysphoric mood, loss of interest and pleasure, and other typical signs and symptoms of primary depression, with subsequent cognitive impairment. Furthermore, patients with depressive pseudodementia often have a history of primary affective disorder earlier in life. The clinical examination is helpful in this differential diagnostic problem. The patient with a primary depression is inattentive, excessively aroused (in agitated depression) or lethargic (in retarded depression), poorly motivated during a mental status examination, and frequently answers "I don't know" to questions probing cognitive function. Aphasia, apraxia, and anomia are not present in the patient with cognitive symptoms secondary to a primary depression. Depressive pseudodementia might be more accurately classified as depressive delirium, given that depression is a manifestation of disrupted brain physiology at the biochemical level and that impaired attention and level of arousal are prominent symptoms.

More common than depressive pseudodementia are depressive signs and symptoms complicating a preexisting dementia (Zubenko and Moossy 1988). Such depressive signs and symptoms, as well as a diagnosable major depressive episode, frequently complicate the clinical courses of vascular dementia and AD. Recent studies suggest that treatment of such major depressive episodes with selective serotonin reuptake inhibitors (SSRIs) and behavioral approaches is effective (see "Abnormalities of Brain Neurotransmitters").

Differentiating Specific Disorders Causing Dementia

The differential diagnosis of dementia does not end with the exclusion of delirium and depression. It is also important to make the diagnosis of a specific dementia disorder with as great a degree of certainty as possible, because prognosis varies among dementia disorders and there are specific treatments for several diseases causing dementia. The essential elements of the clinical evaluation of the older patient with acquired cognitive impairment are listed in Table 12–1. By far the most important part of the evaluation is a careful history, obtained not only from the patient (whose insight into and recollection of signs, symptoms, and clinical course are usually unreliable) but also from friends, relatives, or other persons familiar with the patient. A mental status examination focusing on the patient's level of awareness and attention, memory, calculation, language, praxis, visual-spatial skills, and executive functioning must be performed. Observation of the patient's affect during the examination usually is more helpful, in evaluating for depression, than the memory-impaired patient's subjective response to questions about his or her mood status in the recent past.

A physical examination—including a screening neurological evaluation, with special attention given to localizing neurological signs—is also essential. An inventory of current medications, both prescribed and over-the-counter, should routinely be taken in the evaluation, and a urine specimen should be obtained and analyzed for the presence of drugs if there is a question about the reliability of the drug history. This part of the evaluation is particularly important if the clinical picture suggests delirium. Behavioral toxicity associated with pharmacotherapy is the most common etiology of reversible delirium and behavioral impairments in the elderly patient (Larson et al. 1984). Serum electrolyte levels, blood urea nitrogen levels, and serum B_{12} levels should be measured and thyroid function tests (including a thyroid-stimulating hormone test) should be performed to rule out correctable causes of delirium and/or dementia. Early in their courses, both thyroid deficiency (Whybrow et al. 1969) and B_{12} deficiency (Lindenbaum et al. 1988; Strachan and Henderson 1965)

can manifest as a reversible delirium. However, if thyroid deficiency or B_{12} deficiency persists, neuronal loss and dementia ensue, and full recovery of cognitive function rarely occurs (Clarnette and Patterson 1994; Martin et al. 1992; Nilsson et al. 2000; Wang et al. 2001).

Diagnostic Neuroimaging

Although the routine inclusion of a computed tomography (CT) scan or magnetic resonance image of the brain in the evaluation of late-life cognitive impairment has been debated since Larson and colleagues' (1986) evaluation of the cost-effectiveness of these neuroimaging diagnostic procedures, they continue to be part of the standard diagnostic evaluation in most centers, particularly the evaluation of patients with early onset of cognitive impairment or with an atypical presentation. CT and magnetic resonance imaging can detect potentially treatable intracranial mass lesions such as tumors or subdural hematomas and can also suggest the presence of normal-pressure hydrocephalus (NPH). Although the presence of clearly defined infarcts revealed by CT or magnetic resonance imaging supports the diagnosis of vascular dementia or combined vascular dementia and AD (mixed dementia), the frequently observed periventricular hyperintensities on T2-weighted images obtained with high-resolution magnetic resonance scanners continue to be of unknown significance. These periventricular changes have not been clearly demonstrated to be attributable to "microvascular disease," and their usefulness in differential diagnosis remains unclear (Braffman et al. 1988; Chui et al. 1992; Fein et al. 1990; George et al. 1986). Finding a treatable subdural hematoma (Ishikawa et al. 2002), or the even rarer resectable benign intracranial neoplasm (Avery 1971), may be the most important reason for neuroimaging in the diagnostic evaluation of dementia.

TABLE 12–1. Evaluation of cognitive impairment in later life

History from patient and from relative or friend
Mental status examination
Physical examination, including neurological examination
Medication inventory and urinalysis
Head CT or MRI
Complete blood count
Serum VDRL test
Measurement of serum sodium, potassium, chloride, bicarbonate, and calcium levels
Measurement of serum blood urea nitrogen, creatinine, bilirubin, and albumin/globulin levels
Measurement of serum B_{12} level
Measurement of serum triiodothyronine, thyroxine, and thyroid-stimulating hormone levels
Brief cognitive test (e.g., Mini-Mental State Exam)

Note. CT = computed tomography; MRI = magnetic resonance imaging; VDRL = Venereal Disease Research Laboratory.

Cognition Evaluation

Use of a formal cognitive rating scale should be part of the standard evaluation of an older patient with acquired cognitive impairment. The Mini-Mental State Exam (MMSE; Folstein et al. 1975) is a brief and easily performed test that has proved to be widely useful. The MMSE permits the clinician to obtain data about orientation, registration and recall of information, attention, calculation, language, praxis, basic executive functioning, and visual-spatial skills. Although the MMSE is not designed for the differential diagnosis of the various specific dementia disorders, it provides a useful snapshot of overall cognitive function. Despite psychometric shortcomings, the MMSE has gained extremely wide acceptance as a means both of estimating cognitive function and of following changes in cognitive function over time. Longer cognitive evaluation instruments such as the Mattis Dementia Rating Scale (Mattis 1976) allow a more comprehensive evaluation of cognitive function and are useful if neuropsychological testing resources are available. The Mattis Dementia Rating Scale is a reliable instrument that correlates well with the functional capacity of patients with AD (Vitaliano et al. 1984). The Alzheimer's Disease Assessment Scale—Cognitive subscale (ADAS-Cog; Rosen et al. 1984) has been widely used in clinical trials of cognition-affecting drugs and allows reference of an individual patient's cognitive status to large published data sets from these studies.

Reversible Causes of Dementia

The search for reversible causes of cognitive impairment in the older patient must be actively continued. Unfortunately, such reversible disorders are the exception rather than the rule. Although early reports suggested that potentially correctable disorders causing cognitive impairment would be detected by a careful evaluation in up to 30% of patients with acquired cognitive loss (Fox et al. 1975; Freeman 1976; Victoratos et al. 1977), Larson and co-workers (1984) reported a more realistic yield of truly correctable disorders impairing cognitive function. These investigators conducted comprehensive outpatient diagnostic evaluations of patients with late-onset cognitive disorders. Of 107 unselected elderly outpatients referred for evaluation of global cognitive impairment of at least 3 months' duration, only 15 had potentially reversible disorders possibly related to their cognitive loss. Six patients with apparent cognitive loss secondary to adverse effects of medications formed the largest single group. Other potentially reversible causes of cognitive loss that were identified included hypothyroidism, subdural he-

matoma, and rheumatoid or lupus cerebrovasculitis. In only 3 of the 107 patients evaluated was there a proven reversible cause of cognitive loss, as demonstrated by return to normal cognitive function after treatment. One of these patients had a subdural hematoma, another had mixed-drug toxicity, and the third had rheumatoid cerebrovasculitis. Two of these 3 patients presented with only subtle and mild cognitive deficits. Furthermore, of the 13 patients in the series who were judged to have reversible cognitive deficits at intake evaluation and who were available for follow-up over a 2-year period, 3 of the 4 patients with hypothyroidism, 1 patient with subdural hematoma, and 4 of the 6 patients with behavioral toxicity associated with pharmacotherapy subsequently developed progressive cognitive deterioration consistent with AD.

The results of this study suggest that the most important parts of the diagnostic evaluation of a cognitively impaired older person are the attempt a) to delineate the specific disease causing dementia and b) to uncover the treatable or general medical and psychiatric disorders that may be exacerbating the cognitive deficits caused by a primary dementia disorder. However, clinicians should always keep in mind that unusual medically or surgically reversible disorders resembling dementia caused by a neurodegenerative disorder will occasionally present in a busy geriatric practice. Examples of such reversible disorders include frontal meningioma (Avery 1971), NPH (Adams et al. 1965), hypothyroidism (Larson et al. 1984), cerebrovasculitis (Larson et al. 1984), and subdural hematoma (Ishikawa et al. 2002). These disorders will be overlooked unless clinicians continue to carefully evaluate atypical presentations of cognitive impairment.

Specific Diseases Causing Dementia

Alzheimer's Disease

The majority of patients with late-life dementia of insidious onset and a progressive deteriorating course have AD (Katzman 1976). In DSM-IV-TR, the term *dementia of the Alzheimer's type* is used, but *Alzheimer's disease* is the much more generally accepted term for this devastating disease. Diagnostic criteria for AD are presented in Table 12–2. Technically, AD is a combined clinical and neuropathological diagnosis that can be made definitively only when a patient meeting antemortem clinical criteria for AD is found at postmortem examination to have the histopathological changes of AD (numerous neuritic plaques and neurofibrillary tangles in the hippocampus

---

TABLE 12–2. DSM-IV-TR diagnostic criteria for dementia of the Alzheimer's type

A. The development of multiple cognitive deficits manifested by both
   (1) memory impairment (impaired ability to learn new information or to recall previously learned information)
   (2) one (or more) of the following cognitive disturbances:
       (a) aphasia (language disturbance)
       (b) apraxia (impaired ability to carry out motor activities despite intact motor function)
       (c) agnosia (failure to recognize or identify objects despite intact sensory function)
       (d) disturbance in executive functioning (i.e., planning, organizing, sequencing, abstracting)

B. The cognitive deficits in Criteria A1 and A2 each cause significant impairment in social or occupational functioning and represent a significant decline from a previous level of functioning.

C. The course is characterized by gradual onset and continuing cognitive decline.

D. The cognitive deficits in Criteria A1 and A2 are not due to any of the following:
   (1) other central nervous system conditions that cause progressive deficits in memory and cognition (e.g., cerebrovascular disease, Parkinson's disease, Huntington's disease, subdural hematoma, normal-pressure hydrocephalus, brain tumor)
   (2) systemic conditions that are known to cause dementia (e.g., hypothyroidism, vitamin B_{12} or folic acid deficiency, niacin deficiency, hypercalcemia, neurosyphilis, HIV infection)
   (3) substance-induced conditions

E. The deficits do not occur exclusively during the course of a delirium.

F. The disturbance is not better accounted for by another Axis I disorder (e.g., Major Depressive Disorder, Schizophrenia).

Code based on presence or absence of a clinically significant behavioral disturbance:

   294.10 Without Behavioral Disturbance: if the cognitive disturbance is not accompanied by any clinically significant behavioral disturbance.
   294.11 With Behavioral Disturbance: if the cognitive disturbance is accompanied by a clinically significant behavioral disturbance (e.g., wandering, agitation).

Specify subtype:

   With Early Onset: if onset is at age 65 years or below
   With Late Onset: if onset is after age 65 years

Coding note: Also code 331.0 Alzheimer's disease on Axis III. Indicate other prominent clinical features related to the Alzheimer's disease on Axis I (e.g., 293.83 Mood Disorder Due to Alzheimer's Disease, With Depressive Features, and 310.1 Personality Change Due to Alzheimer's Disease, Aggressive Type).

---

and neocortex). A work group convened by the National Institute of Neurological Disorders and Stroke and by the Alzheimer's Disease and Related Disorders Association (now known as the Alzheimer's Association) developed the term *probable AD* to denote the condition of persons meeting antemortem clinical criteria for AD (McKhann et al. 1984).

A clinician of the 1960s would be mystified today at the emphasis placed on what was considered then to be a relatively uncommon "presenile" dementia disorder. That AD is now regarded as the most important neuropsychiatric disorder of later life would be difficult for the 1960s clinician to comprehend. This "epidemic" of AD can be attributed largely to increased knowledge of the etiology of dementia in later life. Before the landmark studies by Blessed et al. (1968), the large number of persons who developed dementia after age 65—"senile dementia"—were believed to have cerebrovascular insufficiency. Blessed et al. (1968) performed a careful neuro-

pathological and neurohistological study of senile dementia in elderly patients. In 70% of these patients, the only neuropathological lesions found were the neuritic plaques and neurofibrillary tangles described by Alzheimer in 1907 (Alzheimer 1907/1987) in his patient with early-onset dementia. Only in approximately 15% of patients with late-onset dementia could cognitive impairment be attributed to sequelae of cerebrovascular disease—specifically, infarcted brain tissue, which caused vascular dementia. Another 15% had neuropathology of both AD and vascular dementia. Multiple studies have confirmed that a dementia of insidious onset and with a gradually progressive course—whether beginning before or after age 65—is usually AD (Katzman 1986).

The likelihood that an antemortem diagnosis of AD by current DSM-IV-TR criteria or by National Institute of Neurological Disorders and Stroke–Alzheimer's Disease and Related Disorders Association criteria will be confirmed at postmortem examination is at least 85%

(Joachim et al. 1988; Morris et al. 1988; Tierney et al. 1988). This is an excellent rate of antemortem diagnostic accuracy, and it compares favorably with that for many common general medical disorders in which the high probability of an accurate antemortem clinical diagnosis is widely accepted. The clinician should not think that AD is a difficult diagnosis that can be made only after exclusion of a long list of both common and uncommon disorders with the potential to produce dementia. In an older person in whom dementia begins insidiously and progresses gradually but inexorably, the diagnostic plaques and tangles of AD are highly likely to be found at neuropathological examination. Diagnostic certainty is further enhanced if the patient has no history of stroke, alcoholism, preexistent Parkinson's disease, or poorly controlled hypertension.

Relatively recent studies have added new complexity to the specific diagnosis of late-life dementia. First, careful neuroimaging and neuropathological studies of predominantly old-old (mean age > 80 years) persons with dementia suggest that vascular lesions together with AD lesions commonly contribute to the clinical expression of dementia (i.e., mixed dementia) (Skoog et al. 1994; Snowdon et al. 1997). Second, more sensitive immunostains for Lewy bodies (the classic substantia nigra lesions of Parkinson's disease) have frequently revealed Lewy bodies in limbic brain and neocortex together with the plaques and tangles of AD—a condition called dementia with Lewy bodies (DLB) (Kotzbauer et al. 2001; McKeith et al. 1996; R.H. Perry et al. 1990). Mixed dementia and DLB are discussed more fully later in the chapter (see "Vascular Dementia" and "Dementia With Lewy Bodies").

Course

AD begins insidiously. Subtle difficulties in recent memory are almost always the first sign. Personality changes also occur early and manifest most often as apathy and loss of interest in persons and activities. Memory impairment gradually becomes more severe, and deficits in other cognitive domains—particularly executive functioning and visual-spatial skills—appear. Usually after several years of cognitive impairment, a fluent type of aphasia begins, characterized by difficulty in naming objects or choosing the right word to express an idea. Apraxia often occurs concurrently, and this loss of the ability to perform often routine motor activities, such as eating with utensils or dressing, places care burdens on the patient's family and other care providers. In the later stages of AD, many patients develop disrupted sleep-wake cycles; wander; have episodes of irritability, agita-

tion, and psychosis; and lose their ability to attend to personal care needs such as dressing, feeding, and personal hygiene. Motor signs, such as rigidity and myoclonic jerks and seizures, occur in subgroups of patients, particularly those with early-onset AD (i.e., beginning before age 70) (Risse et al. 1990a). The duration of the illness is rarely less than 5 years and may extend to more than 15 years.

Epidemiology

Prevalence studies suggest that approximately 5% of persons older than 65 years and 20% of persons older than 80 years have dementia severe enough to impair their ability to live independently (Mortimer 1983). It can be assumed that the majority of these persons have AD. The results of a classic study performed in East Boston, Massachusetts, suggest that the prevalence of AD in later life may be even higher (Evans et al. 1989). Evaluation of all noninstitutionalized persons age 65 or older in this geographically defined community of 32,000 individuals revealed an estimated AD prevalence rate of 10% among those older than 65 years and 47% among those older than 85 years. Even when data from persons with mild cognitive impairment were excluded, fully 8% of the individuals older than 65 years and 36% of those older than 85 years had moderate to severe cognitive impairment sufficient to limit their ability to live independently.

Pathogenesis and Pathophysiology

Attempts to understand basic mechanisms underlying AD have focused on several areas. One of these areas is the neurobiology of the formation and potential neurotoxic effects of the histopathological hallmarks of AD: neuritic plaques and neurofibrillary tangles (and their component proteins). In addition, studies have identified rare genetic mutations on chromosomes 1, 14, and 21 that cause AD in families with early-onset autosomal dominant heritable AD (Levy-Lahad et al. 1995; Mullan et al. 1992; Schellenberg et al. 1992; Sherrington et al. 1995). Also, a polymorphism has been identified in the *APOE* gene in which the ε4 allele increases the risk of AD in families with the more common late-onset sporadic AD (Corder et al. 1993). Epidemiologic studies continue to be conducted for the purpose of determining which environmental exposures or biologic variables have increased prevalence among persons with AD. An extensive discussion of these neurobiologic, genetic, and epidemiologic studies is beyond the scope of this chapter, but we will review some aspects of this research that are pertinent to a general understanding of AD.

Abnormalities of brain proteins β-amyloid and tau. Efforts in multiple laboratories have been directed toward understanding the possible role of β-amyloid (the major protein constituent of neuritic plaques) and the cytoskeleton protein tau (the major component of neurofibrillary tangles) in the pathogenesis of AD. β-Amyloid was first sequenced by Glenner and Wong (1984) from congophilic angiopathic deposits in postmortem brain tissue from patients with AD. β-Amyloid is a cleavage product of a normally expressed brain protein that is possibly involved in neuronal repair, amyloid precursor protein (APP) (Rosenberg 1993). The hypothesis that β-amyloid is involved in the pathogenesis of AD (Selkoe 2000) is supported by data from the rare families in whom point mutations in the *APP* gene on chromosome 21 (Mullan et al. 1992), the presenilin 1 gene on chromosome 14 (Schellenberg et al. 1992), and the presenilin 2 gene on chromosome 1 (Levy-Lahad et al. 1995) segregate with AD. Each of these mutations is associated with increased concentrations of β-amyloid (particularly the more neurotoxic β-amyloid 42).

The major constituent of neurofibrillary tangles is a hyperphosphorylated form of the microtubule-associated phosphoprotein tau. Several factors have increased interest in the protein chemistry of tau and tau's role in neuronal degeneration in AD. The correlation between the density of postmortem neurofibrillary tangles and antemortem cognitive deficits is more robust than that between neuritic plaques and cognitive deficits (Snowdon et al. 1997). Normal tau function enhances the formation and stability of intraneuronal microtubules. Dysfunctional tau, therefore, would disrupt critically important aspects of neuronal function. The tau in neurofibrillary tangles (and in the dystrophic neurites associated with senile plaques) is hyperphosphorylated (Mitchell et al. 2002). It appears that this hyperphosphorylation results from the failure of phosphatases to normally remove phosphate moieties from the tau molecule (Trojanowski and Lee 1995). Therefore, enhancing appropriate phosphatase activity is one potential AD therapeutic goal (Iqbal et al. 1999). That abnormal tau function can produce dementia in the absence of β-amyloid plaque deposition has been demonstrated convincingly in patients with familial frontotemporal dementia (FTD) (Sumi et al. 1992). In such patients, mutations in the tau gene on chromosome 17 are sufficient to produce dementia (Hutton et al. 1998; Poorkaj et al. 1998; Wilhelmsen et al. 1999), and deposits of β-amyloid are absent histologically.

Hypothalamic-pituitary-adrenal axis. It has been suggested that identification of the hypothalamic-pituitary-adrenal (HPA) axis changes that occur in patients with primary major depression would be helpful in the differential diagnosis of dementia and depression. Specifically, it was hypothesized that administration of the dexamethasone suppression test (DST) would be useful (McAllister et al. 1982; Rudorfer and Clayton 1981). Because resistance to suppression of the HPA axis by the potent synthetic glucocorticoid dexamethasone had been demonstrated in patients with a severe major depressive episode (Carroll et al. 1981), it was suggested that positive DST results—failure of a late-evening dose of dexamethasone to suppress plasma cortisol to below a predetermined level the following day—in a patient with acquired cognitive impairment and depressive signs and symptoms would favor the diagnosis of either primary major depressive episode or secondary major depressive episode complicating dementia. Unfortunately, it soon became apparent that such positive DST findings occurred as frequently in patients with AD uncomplicated by depression as in those with a primary major depressive episode (Raskind et al. 1982; Spar and Gerner 1982).

Although the demonstrations of increased HPA axis activity in AD (and in vascular dementia) negated the diagnostic utility of the DST, it remains possible that this neuroendocrine abnormality plays a role in the pathophysiology of AD. A growing body of evidence suggests that increased HPA axis activity in aging (Raskind et al. 1994)—a phenomenon that is exaggerated in patients with AD or vascular dementia (Balldin et al. 1983; Davis et al. 1986)—may lower the threshold for the neuronal loss of AD (Peskind et al. 2001; Sapolsky et al. 1987) (see "Abnormalities of Brain Neurotransmitters" following discussion of genetic risk factors below).

APOE ε4 genetic risk factor. Apolipoprotein E (apoE) has long been of interest to cardiologists for its involvement in cholesterol and lipid transport and for the effect of the genetic polymorphisms of *APOE* (*APOE* ε2, *APOE* ε3, and *APOE* ε4) on the risk of heart disease (Mahley and Huang 1999). Observations initially made at the Duke University Alzheimer's Disease Research Center (Corder et al. 1993) and repeatedly confirmed by many other investigators (Mahley and Huang 1999) demonstrated that *APOE* genotype has a major effect on the expression of AD. Specifically, the ε4 allele (the second most common *APOE* allele) clearly increases the risk of AD, and the ε2 allele (the least common allele) appears to decrease the risk of AD. It is important to recognize that presence of one or two ε4 alleles increases AD risk but is not causative of AD. Some persons carrying one or even two copies of the ε4 allele never develop AD, and many persons not carrying the ε4 allele do develop AD. In contrast, persons who carry the rare causative mutations for familial AD on chromosome 21 (in the *APP* gene), chromosome 14 (in the presenilin 1 gene), or chromosome 1 (in the presenilin 2 gene) will certainly develop AD if they live to the age of risk.

Despite intensive investigation, the mechanism by which the ε4 allele increases the risk of AD remains unclear. Differential effects of *APOE* alleles on β-amyloid deposition and on cytoskeletal stabilization are among the proposed mechanisms. Peskind et al. (2001) recently reported a potential mechanism for *APOE* genotype effects on AD risk that builds on the reported neurotoxic effect of high levels of cortisol (corticosterone in rodents) on hippocampal neurons (Sapolsky et al. 1987) and the aging-dependent effect of the ε4 allele to increase corticosterone concentrations in rodents (Raber et al. 2000). Peskind and colleagues (2001) measured cortisol concentrations in cerebrospinal fluid (CSF) of healthy older persons who had unimpaired cognition and of persons with AD. CSF cortisol levels varied by *APOE* genotype: subjects with the ε4 allele had higher CSF cortisol levels than did those homozygous for the ε3 allele, who in turn had higher CSF cortisol concentrations than did subjects with an ε2 allele. This pattern is consistent with the risk of AD that these alleles confer (Corder et al. 1993).

Abnormalities of brain neurotransmitters

Serotonin deficiency and SSRI treatment of depression. In patients with AD, there is a clear deficiency in brain serotonin systems, manifested by loss of serotonergic neurons in the brain stem raphe nuclei (Mann and Yates 1983; Yamamoto and Hirano 1985), decreased concentrations of serotonin and its metabolite in brain tissue (Arai et al. 1984; D'Amato et al. 1987) and CSF (Blennow et al. 1991; Volicer et al. 1985), and decreased serotonin receptor concentrations (Cross et al. 1984). This serotonin deficiency may be relevant to the pathophysiology and treatment of depressive signs and symptoms seen in some patients with AD. Scandinavian studies demonstrated that in persons with AD or vascular dementia, the selective serotonin reuptake inhibitor (SSRI) citalopram is more effective than placebo for signs and symptoms of depression as well as for anxiety and other nonpsychotic behavioral disturbances (Nyth et al. 1992). A preliminary study of sertraline therapy in AD patients with depression found that this SSRI reduced depression ratings more effectively than did placebo (Lyketsos et al. 2000). In these studies, SSRI adverse effects were uncommon. Although outcome data from well-designed treatment trials remain scant, SSRIs have become the

first choice for management of depressive signs and symptoms complicating AD. That nonpharmacological approaches can reduce depressive signs and symptoms in AD patients was confirmed by a trial in which behaviorally oriented psychotherapy effectively reduced depression in both AD patients and their caregivers (Teri 1994).

The norepinephrine system: compensatory upregulation may contribute to disruptive agitation. Another major neurotransmitter system affected in AD is the brain noradrenergic system. Studies of postmortem brain tissue have consistently demonstrated neuronal loss in the locus coeruleus (the major source of noradrenergic neurons innervating the CNS) in patients with AD (Bondareff et al. 1982; Mann et al. 1980; Tomlinson et al. 1981). Locus coeruleus neuronal loss at first suggests a brain noradrenergic deficiency in AD. On the other hand, studies measuring levels of both norepinephrine and its major metabolite, methoxyhydroxyphenylglycol (MHPG), in postmortem brain tissue have demonstrated an increased ratio of MHPG to norepinephrine in AD, suggesting increased norepinephrine turnover in locus coeruleus projection areas (Francis et al. 1985; Palmer et al. 1987; Winblad et al. 1982). Furthermore, norepinephrine and MHPG concentrations in CSF are normal or even increased in patients with AD, particularly in those who are in the later stages of the disease (Gibson et al. 1985; Raskind et al. 1984). An increased ratio of MHPG to locus coeruleus noradrenergic neuronal number in AD postmortem tissue suggests that compensatory upregulation of surviving locus coeruleus neurons might explain the above findings (Hoogendijk et al. 1999).

A recent study by Szot et al. (2000) using postmortem brain tissue supported that compensatory upregulation of locus coeruleus noradrenergic neurons occurs in AD and is associated with antemortem disruptive agitation. These investigators found increased messenger RNA expression for tyrosine hydroxylase (the rate-limiting synthetic enzyme for norepinephrine) in surviving locus coeruleus neurons in AD subjects with a history of disruptive agitation. Taken together with the finding of increased density of adrenergic postsynaptic receptors in AD subjects with antemortem aggressive behavior (Russo-Neustadt and Cotman 1997), these data suggest that enhanced responsiveness to brain noradrenergic outflow may contribute to the pathophysiology of disruptive agitation in AD. Support for this hypothesis in living AD patients was provided by Peskind et al. (1995), who demonstrated robust increases in CSF norepinephrine levels after yohimbine administration in both AD subjects and older subjects without dementia, but only AD subjects had meaningful increases in agitation ratings after CNS noradrenergic stimulation. These findings suggest that antagonism of locus coeruleus noradrenergic outflow with an α_2-adrenergic agonist (e.g., guanfacine, clonidine), blockade of postsynaptic β-adrenoceptors (e.g., with propranolol), or blockade of postsynaptic α_1-adrenoceptors (e.g., with prazosin) might relieve disruptive agitation in AD. Studies of these approaches are currently under way.

The presynaptic cholinergic deficit.   The search for abnormalities in brain neurotransmitter systems in AD that might be correctable by pharmacological treatment (that would result in subsequent symptomatic improvement) received impetus from the successful use of L-dopa to correct the brain dopamine deficiency in Parkinson's disease. That such a strategy might succeed in AD became plausible in the late 1970s with the discovery of a deficit in the brain presynaptic cholinergic system in postmortem brain tissue from patients with AD (Davies and Maloney 1976; E.K. Perry et al. 1978). This hypothesis regarding cholinergic deficiency received further support when Whitehouse and colleagues (1982) demonstrated extensive neuronal loss in the cholinergic nucleus basalis of Meynert in patients with AD. This basal forebrain magnicellular nucleus is the primary source of cholinergic projections to the neocortex and hippocampus. A brain presynaptic cholinergic deficit has also been demonstrated in vascular dementia (Erkinjuntti et al. 2002) and dementia with Lewy bodies (DLB) (E.K. Perry et al. 1994); see also "Dementia With Lewy Bodies" later in the chapter.

Advances in Therapeutics: Cholinesterase Inhibitors

A major step forward in AD therapeutics has been the demonstration that acetylcholinesterase inhibitors, which increase intrasynaptic acetylcholine levels, produce modest symptomatic improvement in AD and appear to slow symptomatic deterioration. Cholinesterase inhibitors have been demonstrated to be effective and are indicated for the mild to moderate stages of AD (usually defined arbitrarily as stages when the patient has an MMSE score of 10–24) (Farlow et al. 1992; Raskind et al. 2000; Rogers et al. 1998). These drugs improve cognitive function only modestly. They are best conceptualized as drugs that "stabilize" cognition, activities of daily living, and behavioral function and that slow clinical deterioration in AD. Stabilization of cognition and functioning for approximately 1 year has been demonstrated with both galantamine and donepezil (Raskind et al. 2000; Winblad et al. 2001). The fact that cholinesterase inhibitors are formally indicated for only the mild to moderate

stages of AD does not preclude their having positive effects in patients with more advanced disease; more severely impaired patients also seem to benefit from these agents (Feldman et al. 2001; Tariot et al. 2000). It also appears that cholinesterase inhibitors are effective in DLB (McKeith et al. 2000), vascular dementia, and mixed dementia (combined vascular dementia and AD) (Erkinjuntti et al. 2002). A consensus is emerging that cholinesterase inhibitor therapy should be started as soon as AD, DLB, vascular dementia, or mixed dementia becomes apparent and that treatment should be continued at least into moderately advanced stages of disease, provided the drug is well tolerated. The broadening spectrum of dementia disorders for which cholinesterase inhibitors are effective simplifies the differential diagnosis.

Tacrine was the first cholinesterase inhibitor demonstrated to be effective in AD (Knapp et al. 1994). However, hepatic toxicity has rendered this drug obsolete in AD treatment. Second-generation cholinesterase inhibitors have been shown to be as effective as tacrine and are free of hepatic toxicity. They are discussed here in the order of their introduction into clinical practice.

Donepezil was demonstrated to have positive effects on cognitive and overall function in several placebo-controlled trials involving AD patients with mild to moderate disease (Rogers and Friedhoff 1996; Rogers et al. 1998). Mean differences between active treatment and placebo approached 3 points on the Alzheimer's Disease Assessment Scale–Cognitive subscale (ADAS-Cog) in these multicenter studies. A northern European multicenter study compared donepezil and placebo, given for 12 months (Winblad et al. 2001). The condition of donepezil-treated patients remained significantly superior to the condition of patients who received placebo, and on average, scores on the MMSE did not significantly deteriorate from baseline. The 10-mg dose of donepezil administered once daily offers some advantage in terms of efficacy, but the 5-mg dose is also effective and is better tolerated. As is the case with all cholinesterase inhibitors, gastrointestinal symptoms—particularly nausea and vomiting (CNS cholinergic effects) and diarrhea (likely a peripheral cholinergic effect)—are the most frequent adverse effects (occurring in 10%–20% of patients given the 10-mg dose). Several recent studies demonstrated that donepezil is effective for maintaining levels of cognition and behavior in AD patients (including persons in long-term care) with dementia that is more severe than that of subjects who participated in the original Phase III trials (Feldman et al. 2001; Tariot et al. 2000). Donepezil may also be effective in vascular dementia (Pratt and Perdomo 2002). It remains the most frequently prescribed cholinesterase inhibitor.

Rivastigmine has been demonstrated to be more effective than placebo for maintaining cognitive function, global function, and activities of daily living in patients with AD. In multicenter placebo-controlled studies, there was approximately a 4-point difference on the ADAS-Cog between high-dose rivastigmine (6–12 mg/day) and placebo (Corey-Bloom 1998; Rösler et al. 1999). At these doses, gastrointestinal adverse effects such as nausea, vomiting, and diarrhea were relatively common (occurring in 40% of patients). In addition to inhibiting acetylcholinesterase, rivastigmine inhibits butyrylcholinesterase. The clinical meaningfulness of this latter effect remains to be determined, but butyrylcholinesterase appears to regulate brain acetylcholine levels in animal studies (Mesulam et al. 2002). Rivastigmine is the only cholinesterase inhibitor to have been compared with placebo in DLB. McKeith et al. 2000 found that rivastigmine was superior to placebo with regard to effects on cognitive deficits and on behavioral problems that are particularly prominent in DLB.

Galantamine is a reversible cholinesterase inhibitor that has the additional pharmacological effect of positively modulating nicotinic acetylcholine receptor responsiveness at an allosteric binding site (Maelicke et al. 2001). Because there is a prominent nicotinic cholinergic deficiency in AD (E.K. Perry et al. 1985), this additional action is potentially meaningful clinically. In large multicenter placebo-controlled trials (Raskind et al. 2000; Wilcock et al. 2000), galantamine was significantly superior to placebo in terms of effects on cognitive function, with an almost 4-point difference from placebo on the ADAS-Cog (Raskind et al. 2000). On average, ADAS-Cog scores of subjects who continued taking galantamine (24 mg/day) for an additional 6 months in an open extension of the United States study (Raskind et al. 2000) remained at the pretreatment baseline for the 1-year treatment trial, a finding that supports the concept of long-term symptomatic stabilization by galantamine. Activities of daily living, such as dressing and participating in activities, also remained stable for 12 months in patients receiving galantamine 24 mg/day for 1 year. AD subjects originally randomized to placebo for 6 months and then administered open-label galantamine failed to catch up with those who received galantamine for the entire 12 months. This finding is consistent with slowing of disease progression by galantamine therapy.

Similar long-term follow-up data suggesting slowed disease progression have emerged from studies of donepezil (Doody et al. 2001; Mohs et al. 2001) and rivastigmine (Farlow et al. 2000). In another multicenter placebo-controlled trial, patients randomized to either 16 or 24 mg of galantamine per day demonstrated better cognitive function and activities of daily living status than did AD patients randomized to placebo (Tariot et al. 2000). This study used a slow-dose titration schedule (increasing 8 mg every 4 weeks to a maximum of 24 mg/day), which minimized gastrointestinal adverse effects to a level comparable to that associated with administration of 10 mg of donepezil (10%–20%). In addition, galantamine decreased the emergence of behavioral problems as quantified by the Neuropsychiatric Inventory. Erkinjuntti et al. (2002) conducted a 6-month, multicenter, placebo-controlled study of galantamine in vascular dementia and mixed dementia. Galantamine was significantly superior to placebo with regard to effects on cognition, functioning, and behavior.

Other Approaches to Cognitive Enhancement

Vitamin E and selegiline. Oxidative damage may contribute to neuronal degeneration and death in AD (reviewed in Sano et al. 1997). On the basis of this putative pathogenic mechanism, drugs with antioxidant activity have been evaluated for their effects on both cognitive and functional decline. In a large multicenter trial, the National Institute on Aging–supported Alzheimer's Disease Cooperative Study evaluated two such drugs—vitamin E and selegiline—singly and in combination, in AD outpatients with moderately advanced disease (Sano et al. 1997). Both vitamin E and selegiline were more effective than placebo in delaying deterioration to functional end points that included nursing home placement, progression to severe dementia, and substantial loss of basic activities of daily living or death. The combination of vitamin E and selegiline was no more effective than either agent alone. Neither agent had beneficial effects on cognitive function per se. Given its low toxicity and low cost, vitamin E should be considered as a part of the regimen of persons with AD. The dose of vitamin E used in this study, 1,000 U given twice daily, was well tolerated.

Ginkgo biloba. Extracts of the leaf of the ginkgo biloba tree have been used in traditional Chinese medications and may have antioxidant as well as stimulant and antiinflammatory properties. In a multicenter, randomized, double-blind, placebo-controlled trial involving outpatients with AD or vascular dementia, a standardized extract of ginkgo biloba had small (less than half the effect of cholinesterase inhibitors) but statistically significant effects on cognitive function as measured by the ADAS-Cog (Le Bars et al. 1997). However, there was no effect on clinicians' ratings of global function. Interpreting the study results is difficult because the drop-out rate was very high (>50% in both groups) and because possible positive effects on mood that could have contributed to the slightly positive cognitive results were not reported. In a second multicenter, placebo-controlled study of ginkgo, involving persons with either AD, vascular dementia, or age-associated memory impairment, all of whom lived in Dutch homes for the elderly, results were negative. No significant differences were found in outcome measures between persons randomized to ginkgo and those randomized to placebo. Currently under way is a large, multicenter, National Institute on Aging–supported, AD prevention trial of ginkgo in healthy elderly subjects.

Estrogen replacement therapy.   Estrogens have neuroprotective effects in preclinical studies, and most (but not all) epidemiologic studies suggest that estrogen replacement therapy decreases the risk of AD in postmenopausal women (reviewed in Mulnard et al. 2000). A small placebo-controlled trial of estradiol in AD demonstrated positive effects on cognitive function (Asthana et al. 1999). However, a recently reported 1-year, multicenter, randomized placebo-controlled trial performed by the Alzheimer's Disease Cooperative Study demonstrated no benefit from treatment with Premarin (a preparation of mixed conjugated equine estrogens that is widely used clinically) in persons with AD (Mulnard et al. 2000). A similar negative result was achieved in a 16-week trial of Premarin in AD subjects (Henderson et al. 2000). Large placebo-controlled prevention studies are under way to determine whether administration of Premarin to cognitively intact postmenopausal women reduces the incidence of AD and age-associated memory impairment. The results of the trial conducted by Asthana et al. (1999) raise the possibility that transdermal estradiol may be more effective than Premarin in counteracting the pathophysiology of AD.

Nonsteroidal anti-inflammatory drugs (NSAIDs). Neuropathological data demonstrate an intense immune response associated with β-amyloid–containing neuritic plaques (McGeer and McGeer 1999; Wyss-Coray and Mucke 2000). This response raises the possibility that an autoimmunity-like phenomenon contributes to neuronal damage in AD. This hypothesis is supported by epidemiologic studies suggesting that NSAIDs decrease the risk of AD in cognitively intact older persons (Breitner and Zandi 2001; in t' Veld et al. 2001; McGeer et al. 1996). Unfortunately, a multicenter placebo-controlled trial of the anti-inflammatory steroid prednisone failed to demonstrate positive effects on cognition or disease progression in AD (Aisen et al. 2000). Similarly, a recently completed placebo-controlled trial of the standard NSAID

naproxen and the cyclooxygenase-2–specific NSAID rofecoxib yielded negative results (Thal 2002). However, the following hypothesis remains viable: NSAIDs reduce the risk of expression of AD in unaffected elders but the drugs are no longer effective after AD is clinically expressed (Breitner and Zandi 2001). Furthermore, the protective mechanism may not be the suppression of inflammation. A recent study demonstrated that the NSAIDs ibuprofen, indomethacin, and sulindac decreased β-amyloid production, whereas the NSAIDs naproxen, celecoxib, and rofecoxib did not (Weggen et al. 2001). A large-scale, prevention trial of naproxen and celecoxib in older healthy individuals is currently under way (Breitner and Zandi 2001). However, the recent preclinical demonstration that naproxen and celecoxib do not decrease β-amyloid production raises concern that the wrong NSAIDs may have been selected for evaluation.

Reducing β-amyloid generation.   Given the multiple levels of evidence supporting a pathogenic role of β-amyloid aggregation and deposition in the expression of AD (Selkoe 2000), substantial resources have been directed toward basic studies designed to develop approaches to reduce generation of β-amyloid from APP, its precursor protein molecule. APP has alternate cleavage pathways. Cleavage by the enzyme α-secretase occurs within the β-amyloid fragment, preventing β-amyloid production. In contrast, cleavage by the enzymes β-secretase (or BACE; β site APP cleavage enzyme) and then γ-secretase generates β-amyloid. With the recent identification of β-secretase and γ-secretase, which are necessary for the generation of β-amyloid (Selkoe 2000), opportunities now exist for inhibiting these enzymes in order to redirect APP metabolism toward nonamyloidogenic and presumably nonneurotoxic APP fragments. Protease inhibitors of β-secretase and γ-secretase are in the preclinical stages of development.

β-Amyloid immunization.   β-Amyloid immunization is a particularly novel approach to both preventing brain β-amyloid deposition and removing β-amyloid already deposited in the brain. Substantial enthusiasm has been generated for this approach as a potentially powerful AD therapeutic. In a transgenic mouse model in which an inserted human mutated amyloid precursor protein gene led to overexpression of APP and dense amyloid plaque deposition by age 18 months, immunization with β-amyloid 1–42 early in life prevented formation of amyloid plaques (Peskind et al. 2001). In addition, immunization of these mice in middle life resulted in dramatic reductions in the amyloid plaque deposition already present. Whether this approach will be applicable in humans remains to be seen. Unfortunately, an initial clinical trial of immunization with β-amyloid in AD patients was suspended after a substantial number of β-amyloid–vaccinated AD subjects developed meningitis. Passive immunization strategies currently being developed may prove less neurotoxic than the active vaccine.

Plasma homocysteine. An association between plasma homocysteine concentrations and AD has been demonstrated in several case-control studies. Homocysteine has adverse effects on the expression of atherosclerotic cerebrovascular disease and the in vitro neurotoxicity of β-amyloid, effects that provide clinical and neurobiologic rationale for a possible role of increased homocysteine levels in the pathogenesis of AD. Recent findings of the large prospective, observational Framingham study support a strong, graded association between total plasma homocysteine levels and the risk of dementia in general and AD specifically. A plasma homocysteine level in the highest quartile doubled the risk of AD. Because plasma homocysteine concentrations can be decreased by ingestion of folate, vitamin B_6, and vitamin B_{12}, a nutritional approach to treatment and prevention of AD using these vitamins has been proposed (Nilsson et al. 2001; van Asselt et al. 2001). A multicenter trial of this approach in persons with AD is underway, and prevention trials in cognitively healthy older persons are being planned.

Pharmacological Management of Disruptive Agitation

Disruptive agitation with or without psychotic delusions and hallucinations frequently complicates the more advanced stages of AD and commonly precipitates nursing home placement. Management of disruptive agitation was recently reviewed (Raskind and Barnes 2002). The typical antipsychotic drugs (e.g., haloperidol, thiothixene) are effective (albeit modestly) for disruptive agitation and psychosis in AD (Schneider 1993), but their pseudoparkinsonian adverse effects frequently prove troublesome. Because atypical antipsychotic drugs (e.g., risperidone, olanzapine, quetiapine) are at least as effective and are much less likely to produce pseudoparkinsonism, they have increasingly supplanted typical antipsychotics for managing disruptive agitation and psychosis in AD (Fernandez et al. 2002; Katz et al. 1999; Street et al. 2000). Risperidone (Katz et al. 1999) and olanzapine (Street et al. 2000) have been shown to be effective in placebo-controlled studies involving AD and/or vascular dementia patients with disruptive agitation or psychotic symptoms who are in long-term care. In these samples, 1 mg of risperidone per day or 5 mg of olanza-

pine per day provided the best balance of behavioral improvement and adverse effects.

Use of psychoactive drugs other than antipsychotics to treat AD patients for disruptive agitation is widespread, but the efficacy of these drugs has been poorly documented (Raskind and Peskind 2001). Anecdotal reports suggest possible efficacy of a broad range of compounds, including SSRIs, trazodone, valproate, carbamazepine, benzodiazepines, buspirone, and propranolol. The role of these compounds in the management of disruptive agitated behaviors complicating AD cannot be defined without well-designed, placebo-controlled outcome trials. A step in this direction was an Alzheimer's Disease Cooperative Study multicenter trial of haloperidol, trazodone, and placebo in community-dwelling AD outpatients with generally mild degrees of disruptive agitation and/or psychosis (Teri et al. 2000). Neither active agent was significantly superior to placebo.

Vascular Dementia

Even in the classic studies by Blessed et al. (1968) that established AD neuritic plaques and neurofibrillary tangles as the predominant neuropathology of late-onset dementia, a subgroup of patients (approximately 25%) were found to have cerebrovascular lesions (infarcts) as the apparent primary or contributing etiology of their dementia (Tomlinson et al. 1970). Recent studies have confirmed the importance of infarcts in the etiology of dementia in the demographic group most at risk for dementia: the old-old (persons older than 80 years) (Skoog et al. 1994; Snowdon et al. 1997). Pure vascular dementia (the multi-infarct dementia of DSM-III-R [American Psychiatric Association 1987]) is relatively uncommon, characterized by stepwise progression of patchy cognitive deterioration, focal neurological signs and symptoms (other than fluent aphasia and apraxia), and a history of inadequately controlled hypertension (Zubenko 1990). The DSM-IV-TR criteria for vascular dementia are presented in Table 12–3.

More frequently, dementia with a cerebrovascular contribution is mixed dementia—that is, progressive dementia with neuropathological findings of both cerebral infarcts and the plaques and neurofibrillary tangles of AD. Clinical-neuropathological correlation studies in community-based samples (in contrast to less representative samples derived from Alzheimer's disease center cohorts selected for antemortem characteristics) suggest that mixed dementia is more common than previously believed and may make up 10% to 30% of late-life dementia (Lim et al. 1999). It is often difficult to differen-

---

TABLE 12–3. DSM-IV-TR diagnostic criteria for vascular dementia

A. The development of multiple cognitive deficits manifested by both
  (1) memory impairment (impaired ability to learn new information or to recall previously learned information)
  (2) one (or more) of the following cognitive disturbances:
    (a) aphasia (language disturbance)
    (b) apraxia (impaired ability to carry out motor activities despite intact motor function)
    (c) agnosia (failure to recognize or identify objects despite intact sensory function)
    (d) disturbance in executive functioning (i.e., planning, organizing, sequencing, abstracting)

B. The cognitive deficits in Criteria A1 and A2 each cause significant impairment in social or occupational functioning and represent a significant decline from a previous level of functioning.

C. Focal neurological signs and symptoms (e.g., exaggeration of deep tendon reflexes, extensor plantar response, pseudobulbar palsy, gait abnormalities, weakness of an extremity) or laboratory evidence indicative of cerebrovascular disease (e.g., multiple infarctions involving cortex and underlying white matter) that are judged to be etiologically related to the disturbance.

D. The deficits do not occur exclusively during the course of a delirium.

Code based on predominant features:

  290.41 With Delirium: if delirium is superimposed on the dementia
  290.42 With Delusions: if delusions are the predominant feature
  290.43 With Depressed Mood: if depressed mood (including presentations that meet full symptom criteria for a Major Depressive Episode) is the predominant feature. A separate diagnosis of Mood Disorder Due to a General Medical Condition is not given.
  290.40 Uncomplicated: if none of the above predominates in the current clinical presentation

Specify if:

  With Behavioral Disturbance

Coding note: Also code cerebrovascular condition on Axis III.

---

tiate mixed dementia from pure AD clinically. Neuro-radiologic evidence of infarcts is helpful.

Snowdon et al. (1997) described a provocative relationship between cognitive function and both AD and cerebrovascular neuropathological lesions (studied post-mortem) in a carefully followed cohort of Catholic nun educators (mean age at death, 83 years) with similar life experiences and environments. Of 61 subjects meeting neuropathological criteria for AD, the 24 with infarcts had poorer cognitive function and a higher prevalence of dementia than did the 37 without infarcts. Infarcts in the basal ganglia, thalamus, or deep white matter were associated with an especially high prevalence and severity of dementia. Subjects with subcortical infarcts also had fewer postmortem AD lesions for a given amount of antemortem cognitive impairment than did subjects without subcortical infarcts. These findings suggest that infarcts lower the threshold for and increase the magnitude of dementia caused by AD.

Clinical differentiation of mixed dementia may be difficult, and this distinction appears to be increasingly irrelevant to the decision to prescribe a cholinesterase inhibitor. Galantamine was clearly demonstrated to be more effective than placebo in a large study involving persons with vascular dementia or mixed dementia (Erkin-

juntti et al. 2002). A preliminary report suggests that donepezil has similar efficacy (Pratt and Perdomo 2002).

Dementia With Lewy Bodies

Lewy bodies are synaptophysin-containing cytoplasmic inclusions that are the defining histologic lesions in the substantia nigra in Parkinson's disease. During the past 15 years, it has become clear that Lewy bodies outside the substantia nigra are present in a subgroup of patients with late-onset dementia who do not have clinically typical Parkinson's disease (Kosaka et al. 1988; Leverenz and Sumi 1986). Fluctuating cognitive function, visual hallucinations, and mild parkinsonism-like bradykinesia and rigidity (but rarely tremor) often present early in the disease course in these patients, who are now regarded as having dementia with Lewy bodies (DLB) (McKeith et al. 1996). Neuropathologically, these persons have Lewy bodies in limbic and neocortical areas, in addition to having modest amounts of the neuritic plaques and neurofibrillary tangles of AD. In unusual cases, diffuse forebrain Lewy bodies are the only demonstrable neuropathological lesions. To make matters more complex, a subgroup of persons with classic Parkinson's disease develop dementia in the later stages of the disease (Mayeux et al. 1988).

Several important features of DLB are relevant to pharmacological management. Treatment of the disturbing visual hallucinations, delusions, and agitation commonly expressed in the early stages of DLB is complicated by marked sensitivity to induction or exacerbation of extrapyramidal symptoms by typical antipsychotics such as haloperidol and even by atypical antipsychotics with some dopamine D_2 receptor affinity (e.g., risperidone and even olanzapine) (Graham et al. 1998). Use of an atypical antipsychotic with a very low incidence of extrapyramidal symptom induction, such as quetiapine or low-dose clozapine (Parkinson Study Group 1999), is a reasonable approach to treating psychotic symptoms in DLB. Another important feature of DLB is a substantial presynaptic cholinergic deficit, apparently even more profound than that in AD (E. K. Perry et al. 1994). A multicenter placebo-controlled trial of the cholinesterase inhibitor rivastigmine in patients with DLB demonstrated superiority of rivastigmine over placebo with regard to effects on both cognitive and behavioral symptoms (McKeith et al. 2000).

Dementia in Parkinson's Disease

The dementia that occurs in the later stages of Parkinson's disease is manifested by impaired memory and slowness of thinking. In general, language function and praxis are preserved, although aphasia and apraxia may occur (E. K. Perry et al. 1985). In an extensive review of the prevalence of dementia among patients with Parkinson's disease, Brown and Marsden (1984) conservatively estimated that some degree of dementia occurs in 20% of such patients. Mayeux and colleagues (1988), using standardized criteria for dementia and idiopathic Parkinson's disease, found a dementia prevalence of 11% among 339 patients with idiopathic Parkinson's disease. In this study, dementia was associated with older age, later onset of motor manifestations, more rapid progression of physical disability, and relatively poor response to L-dopa therapy. Regardless of the estimate of the prevalence of dementia in Parkinson's disease, dementia is clearly more common among such patients than among neurologically intact adults of the same age (Rajput et al. 1987). The difficult task of distinguishing between parkinsonian dementia and DLB in persons who develop dementia within a few years of developing parkinsonian motor signs is an area of ongoing investigation (Kotzbauer et al. 2001).

Frontotemporal Dementia

Frontotemporal dementia (FTD) is an evolving diagnostic category that includes a group of dementia disorders

with several clinical and neurobiologic features in common but also with substantial clinical and neuropathological variability. The diagnostic category includes Pick's disease, frontal lobe degeneration of non-Alzheimer type, amyotrophic sclerosis with frontal lobe degeneration linked to chromosome 17 (FTDP-17), and corticobasal degeneration. FTD typically presents with symptoms of frontal lobe dysfunction such as impaired judgment, perseveration, impulsivity, socially inappropriate behavior, and executive dysfunction. This frontal lobe syndrome (Neary and Snowden 1996) occurs early in the disease course (when memory is only mildly impaired) and can be mistaken for substance abuse, hypomania, or personality disorder. As the disease progresses, memory and speech become severely impaired, and full dementia develops. Although this clinical course commonly occurs in Pick's disease (the classically described form of FTD [Sjogren et al. 1952]), early symptoms often vary and can resemble those of AD, depression, or even schizophrenia. Brain neuroimaging may reveal frontal and anterior temporal atrophy, but neuroradiologic findings also can be variable.

Classically described Pick's disease is a progressive disorder of middle and late life that is often difficult to distinguish from AD (Heston et al. 1987). Although rare in most neuropathological series, it may have accounted for up to 5% of the cases of late-life progressive dementia that occurred in studies in Scandinavia (Sjogren et al. 1952) and Minnesota (Heston et al. 1987). The marked cholinergic deficit of AD does not appear to occur in Pick's disease (Wood et al. 1983). Frontotemporal atrophy and microscopic changes are present in Pick's disease; the latter include neuronal cell loss, gliosis, and the presence of massed cytoskeletal elements called Pick bodies. Although affective lability and excessive eating and other oral behaviors have been described in Pick's disease (Cummings and Duchen 1981), Heston et al. (1987) often could not easily clinically distinguish patients with Pick's disease from those with AD.

It is increasingly clear that abnormal function of the cytoskeletal protein tau ("taupathy") is a central feature of most forms of FTD (Wilhelmsen et al. 1999). In an FTDP-17 family in which tau inclusion bodies were morphologically and immunochemically indistinguishable from the neurofibrillary tangles of AD (Sumi et al. 1992), Poorkaj et al. (1998) found a causative mutation in the chromosome 17q21-22 region by sequencing the tau gene. Additional tau mutations were soon described by others (Hutton et al. 1998). Because these tau mutations demonstrated that tau dysfunction is sufficient to cause neurodegenerative dementia even in the absence of brain amyloid deposits such as neuritic plaques, there is increased interest in the role of tau abnormalities in the pathogenesis of the much more common dementia disorder, AD.

Dementia Due to Normal-Pressure Hydrocephalus

Normal-pressure hydrocephalus (NPH) was described by Adams et al. (1965) as an acquired disorder characterized by a triad of signs and symptoms—dementia, gait disturbance, and urinary incontinence associated with dilation of the cerebral ventricles—but with no evidence of persistently increased intracranial pressure. Although NPH is an unusual disorder, it is an important one to identify because of the potential for neurosurgical treatment and reversibility of the dementia and other symptoms. In most cases, the etiology of NPH is unclear, but previous subarachnoid hemorrhage or meningitis probably accounts for a sizable proportion of cases. A cerebroventricular shunting procedure can markedly improve cognitive function in some cases (Friedland 1989).

Clinical factors associated with a better postoperative outcome are the complete triad of signs and symptoms, with early gait disturbance; absence of gyral atrophy; and a known etiology (Hebb and Cusimano 2001; Thomasen et al. 1986). A factor associated with poor outcome is concomitant cerebrovascular disease (Boon et al. 1999). Despite these prognostic factors, it is difficult to predict which patients with NPH will respond well to a neurosurgical shunting approach and which will not. Interestingly, the presence of brain biopsy–determined AD histopathological changes and associated cognitive deficits did not substantially affect the outcome of a shunt procedure (Golomb et al. 2000). Drainage of 20–40 mL of CSF by lumbar puncture followed by transient clinical improvement may be an indication that the patient is likely to respond to neurosurgical intervention (Wikkelso et al. 1982). The cerebroventricular shunting procedure for NPH needs to be evaluated in controlled clinical trials. That such trials have not been done is understandable, given the invasive nature of this surgical procedure, but lack of such studies limits the ability to evaluate the therapeutic benefits of neurosurgical shunting for NPH (Clarfield 1989).

Dementia Due to Hypothyroidism or Vitamin B$_{12}$ Deficiency

Although early in their course, hypothyroidism and vitamin B$_{12}$ deficiency produce a syndrome more appropriately described as a delirium, persistent deficiencies result in neuronal loss and can produce a dementia that is irreversible. Hypothyroidism classically produces a cognitive syndrome of dementia accompanied by irritability, paranoid ideation, and depression. Unfortunately, it appears that once dementia is established, even aggressive thyroid replacement therapy does not result in a return to the patient's previous level of functioning (Larson et al. 1984). Vitamin B$_{12}$ deficiency can produce dementia even in the absence of anemia or megaloblastic bone marrow changes (Strachan and Henderson 1965). Anecdotal reports suggest that B$_{12}$ replacement in dementia that is apparently secondary to B$_{12}$ deficiency may produce some cognitive improvement (Gross et al. 1986; Rajan et al. 2002; Wieland 1986) but dementia persists. Lindenbaum et al. (1988) suggested that B$_{12}$ deficiency complicated by cognitive and other neuropsychiatric problems may be responsive to treatment with exogenous vitamin B$_{12}$. It is likely that observed improvement after B$_{12}$ treatment in older patients with dementia represents resolution of concomitant B$_{12}$-induced delirium (Nilsson et al. 2000). Increased plasma homocysteine levels may be involved in the pathophysiology of B$_{12}$-induced cognitive impairment (Wang et al. 2001), and increased plasma homocysteine concentrations may be a marker of response to treatment of B$_{12}$ deficiency in persons with dementia (Nilsson et al. 2001).

Dementia Due to Creutzfeldt-Jakob Disease

Creutzfeldt-Jakob disease is caused by a transmissible nonnucleic acid protein called a prion body. This rare disease, which affects multiple neurological systems, is characterized by a prolonged latency from exposure to expression of the disease (Prusiner and DeArmond 1990). It is rapidly fatal: death usually occurs within 2 years of the time symptoms first appear. It is rare in the elderly population, mainly occurring in persons in midlife. Dementia—an almost universal feature of this infection—is rapidly progressive and is accompanied by myoclonus, seizures, ataxia, rigidity, and other signs of widespread CNS involvement. Because AD patients (particularly those with early onset) may also demonstrate myoclonic jerks and seizures, the rapid clinical course and multiple motor system involvement that is characteristic of Creutzfeldt-Jakob disease help to differentiate between this transmissible disease (transmitted by direct contact with infected nervous system tissue) and nontransmissible AD (Mayeux et al. 1985; Risse et al. 1990b). Creutzfeldt-Jakob neurohistological changes include spongiform encephalopathy, neuronal loss, and gliosis.

Dementia Due to Neurosyphilis

Although neurosyphilis was once a common cause of dementia in later life, it has become almost unknown since the advent of widespread use of antibiotics. Given the recent increase in sexually transmitted diseases, however, neurosyphilis should be considered in the differential diagnosis of dementia. The latency from infection to development of paralytic dementia can be as long as 20 years. Considering that Venereal Disease Research Laboratory (VDRL) test results are negative in nearly one-third of patients with late syphilitic infection, the more sensitive fluorescent treponemal antibody absorption test is more likely to be diagnostic. Unfortunately, neurosyphilis may progress despite what appears to be adequate antibiotic therapy with ultra-high-dose penicillin (Wilner and Brody 1968).

Delirium

The criteria for delirium in DSM-IV-TR (Table 12–4) emphasize disturbance of consciousness, impairment of attention, and fluctuation over the course of the day. Delirium is due to disturbance of brain physiology, usually caused by a medical disorder or an ingested substance. In contrast, diseases that produce dementia cause neuronal damage and loss. One aspect of the new DSM-IV-TR criteria for delirium should be applied cautiously: the requirement that the disturbance must have developed over a short period, usually hours to days. In the elderly patient, a delirium secondary to drugs such as long-acting benzodiazepines or to illnesses such as renal failure may have a much longer prodromal period and an insidious onset. On the other hand, it is commendable that in DSM-IV-TR, brief duration is not specified as a criterion for delirium. In a careful study, Levkoff et al. (1992)

demonstrated that incident delirium in elderly persons hospitalized for medical or surgical reasons usually persists for months. Full resolution of symptoms of delirium in a short time was the exception rather than the rule in this study.

The disturbance in level of consciousness can range from reduced wakefulness or even stupor to severe insomnia and hyperarousal. Etiological factors for delirium are numerous and include systemic medical illnesses, toxic effects of both prescribed and nonprescribed medications, metabolic disorders, and a host of other illnesses and environmental stressors (e.g., intensive care unit syndrome) (see Table 12–5). Delirium due to withdrawal from alcohol (delirium tremens) and/or sedative-hypnotic drugs can occur in older persons, and denial of drug abuse is not restricted to the young.

Treatment of delirium should be directed toward correcting the underlying disorder when that disorder can be detected. Frequently, however, symptomatic treatment becomes necessary if disruptive behaviors such as agitation, delusions, hallucinations, or angry outbursts interfere with patient management or threaten the safety of the patient or others in the environment. Reassurance from a family member or a health care professional can sometimes be helpful in managing the manifestations of delirium; however, pharmacological intervention to resolve an acute crisis may be needed. Low doses of antipsychotic medication can be helpful. Delirium secondary to withdrawal from a CNS-depressive drug such as ethanol or a benzodiazepine should be treated with a cross-tolerant sedative-hypnotic drug. An episode of delirium often is the initial presentation of an underlying dementia. In a prospective 2-year study involving previously healthy, community-dwelling elderly individuals, 28 of 51 persons admitted to the hospital because of acute delirium were found to have an underlying dementia (Rahkonen et al. 2000).

TABLE 12–4. DSM-IV-TR diagnostic criteria for delirium due to a general medical condition

A. Disturbance of consciousness (i.e., reduced clarity of awareness of the environment) with reduced ability to focus, sustain, or shift attention.

B. A change in cognition (such as memory deficit, disorientation, language disturbance) or the development of a perceptual disturbance that is not better accounted for by a preexisting, established, or evolving dementia.

C. The disturbance develops over a short period of time (usually hours to days) and tends to fluctuate during the course of the day.

D. There is evidence from the history, physical examination, or laboratory findings that the disturbance is caused by the direct physiological consequences of a general medical condition.

Coding note: If delirium is superimposed on a preexisting Vascular Dementia, indicate the delirium by coding 290.41 Vascular Dementia, With Delirium.

Coding note: Include the name of the general medical condition on Axis I, e.g., 293.0 Delirium Due to Hepatic Encephalopathy; also code the general medical condition on Axis III.

TABLE 12–5.   Etiologies of delirium

Systemic illness
 Acquired immunodeficiency syndrome
 Burns and multiple trauma
 Congestive heart failure
 Hepatic insufficiency
 Infection
 Lupus erythematosus
 Pulmonary insufficiency
 Renal insufficiency
Metabolic disorders
 Hyperadrenocorticism
 Hypercalcemia
 Hypoadrenocorticism
 Hypoglycemia
 Hypothyroidism
Miscellaneous
 Intensive care unit syndrome
 Postoperative state (particularly cardiac surgery and cataract
  surgery)
 Withdrawal from alcohol, sedatives, hypnotics
Neurological disorders
 Cerebrovascular accident
 Head trauma
 Intracranial mass lesion
 Meningitis (acute and chronic)
 Neurosyphilis
 Seizure
 Subarachnoid hemorrhage
Pharmacological adverse effects
 Anticholinergic drugs
 Antiparkinsonian agents
 Antipsychotics (e.g., phenothiazines)
 Antispasmodics (e.g., belladonna)
 Bromide
 Cimetidine
 Corticosteroids
 Digitalis
 Sedatives, hypnotics
 Tricyclic antidepressants

Amnestic Disorder, Alcoholic Dementia, and Wernicke-Korsakoff Syndrome

The primary deficit in amnestic disorder is memory impairment manifested as the inability to learn new information or to recall previously learned information. Although acquired impairment of memory is a central feature of dementia, the diagnosis of amnestic disorder implies a much more discrete deficit that is limited—at least in terms of substantial impairment—to memory

function. Of course, careful neuropsychological evaluation often reveals deficits in other cognitive domains in persons who meet criteria for amnestic disorder.

The etiology of an amnestic disorder is usually damage to diencephalic and medial temporal lobe structures, which are important in memory function. Such damage can occur from head trauma, hypoxia, posterior cerebral artery distribution infarction, and herpes simplex encephalitis. However, the most common cause of amnestic disorder is alcoholism. The amnestic disorder caused by alcohol would be diagnosed, according to DSM-IV-TR criteria, as alcohol-induced persisting amnestic disorder. A synonymous term is *Korsakoff's psychosis*. The etiology of this disorder is often generally considered to be multiple episodes of Wernicke's encephalopathy caused by thiamine deficiency in the context of severe binge alcoholism, but direct neurotoxic effects of ethanol and its metabolite acetaldehyde (Charness 1993; Riley and Walker 1978) likely contribute to the pathogenesis of Wernicke-Korsakoff syndrome in many cases.

The diagnosis and definition of alcoholic dementia is a subject of continuing debate and controversy because there are no widely accepted standardized diagnostic or neuropathological criteria (Victor 1994). It is estimated that 10% of alcoholic individuals demonstrate permanent cognitive dysfunction (Charness 1993). Brains of alcoholic individuals exhibit atrophy of the cerebral and cerebellar cortex, corpus callosum, and deeper brain structures, including the mamillary bodies and hippocampus. Chronic alcohol users may have a number of cognitive deficits, depending on the affected brain regions. The common frontal lobe dysfunction in chronic alcohol users appears to be secondary to frontal cortical synapse loss (Brun and Andersson 2001). Presence of the ε4 allele of apoE may lower the threshold for alcoholic dementia (Muramatsu et al. 1997), particularly when cognitive deficits are broader than isolated memory loss.

The acute thiamine deficiency encephalopathy described by Wernicke is manifested by confusion, lateral gaze palsy, nystagmus, and ataxia. These clinical signs and symptoms reflect damage to brain areas adjacent to the third and fourth ventricles and in the medial temporal lobes. Thiamine is specifically therapeutic if administered promptly. This treatable cause of eventual amnestic disorder may be underdiagnosed. Of 51 patients showing the neuropathological stigmata of Wernicke's encephalopathy at postmortem examination, only 7 had received such a diagnosis antemortem (Harper 1979). Although it is widely believed that alcohol-induced amnestic disorder produces permanent cognitive deficits, the actual prognosis may not be so poor. Victor and Adams (1971) reported complete recovery in 21% of 104 patients, and some degree of recovery of cognitive function occurred in an additional 53% of patients who refrained from alcohol. This classic study suggests that alcohol-induced amnestic disorder is one of the most treatable of the cognitive disorders.

References

Adams RD, Fisher CM, Hakim S: Symptomatic occult hydrocephalus with normal cerebrospinal fluid pressure: a treatable syndrome. N Engl J Med 273:117–126, 1965

Aisen PS, Davis KL, Berg JD, et al: A randomized controlled trial of prednisone in Alzheimer's disease. Neurology 54:588–593, 2000

Alzheimer A: About a peculiar disease of the cerebral cortex (1907). Translated by Jarvik L, Greenson H. Alzheimer Dis Assoc Disord 1:7–8, 1987

American Psychiatric Association: Diagnostic and Statistical Manual of Mental Disorders, 3rd Edition, Revised. Washington, DC, American Psychiatric Association, 1987

American Psychiatric Association: Diagnostic and Statistical Manual of Mental Disorders, 4th Edition, Text Revision. Washington, DC, American Psychiatric Association, 2000

Arai H, Kosaka K, Iizuka R: Changes of biogenic amines and their metabolites in postmortem brains from patients with Alzheimer-type dementia. J Neurochem 43:388–393, 1984

Asthana S, Craft S, Baker LD, et al: Cognitive and neuroendocrine response to transdermal estrogen in postmenopausal women with Alzheimer's disease: results of a placebo-controlled, double-blind, pilot study. Psychoneuroendocrinology 24:657–677, 1999

Avery TL: Seven cases of frontal tumour with psychiatric presentation. Br J Psychiatry 119:19–23, 1971

Balldin J, Gottfries CG, Karlsson I, et al: Dexamethasone suppression test and serum prolactin in dementia disorders. Br J Psychiatry 143:277–281, 1983

Blennow KAH, Wallin A, Gottfries CG, et al: Significance of decreased lumbar CSF levels of HVA and 5-HIAA in Alzheimer's disease. Neurobiol Aging 13:107–113, 1991

Blessed G, Tomlinson BE, Roth M: The association between quantitative measures of dementia and of senile change in the cerebral gray matter of elderly subjects. Br J Psychiatry 114:797–811, 1968

Bondareff W, Mountjoy CQ, Roth M: Loss of neurons of origin of the adrenergic projection to cerebral cortex (nucleus locus ceruleus) in senile dementia. Neurology 32:164–168, 1982

Boon AJ, Tans JT, Delwel EJ, et al: The Dutch normal-pressure hydrocephalus study: the role of cerebrovascular disease. J Neurosurg 90:221–226, 1999

Braffman BH, Zimmerman RA, Trojanowski JQ, et al: Brain MR: pathologic correlation with gross and histopathology, 2: hyperintense white-matter foci in the elderly. Am J Radiol 151:559–566, 1988

Breitner JC, Zandi PP: Do nonsteroidal antiinflammatory drugs reduce the risk of Alzheimer's disease? N Engl J Med 345:1567–1568, 2001

Brown RG, Marsden CD: How common is dementia in Parkinson's disease? (editorial) Lancet 2:1262–1265, 1984

Brun A, Andersson J: Frontal dysfunction and frontal cortical synapse loss in alcoholism—the main cause of alcohol dementia? Dement Geriatr Cogn Disord 12:289–294, 2001

Carroll BJ, Feinberg M, Greden JF, et al: A specific laboratory test for the diagnosis of melancholia: standardization, validity, and clinical utility. Arch Gen Psychiatry 38:15–22, 1981

Charness ME: Brain lesions in alcoholics. Alcohol Clin Exp Res 17:2–11, 1993

Chui HC, Victoroff JI, Margolin D, et al: Criteria for the diagnosis of ischemic vascular dementia proposed by the State of California Alzheimer's Disease Diagnostic and Treatment Centers. Neurology 42:473–480, 1992

Clarfield AM: Normal-pressure hydrocephalus: saga or swamp? JAMA 262:2592–2593, 1989

Clarnette RM, Patterson CJ: Hypothyroidism: does treatment cure dementia? J Geriatr Psychiatry Neurol 7:23–27, 1994

Corder EH, Saunders AM, Strittmatter WJ, et al: Gene dose of apolipoprotein E type 4 allele and the risk of Alzheimer's disease in late onset families. Science 261:921–923, 1993

Corey-Bloom J, Anand R, Veach J: A randomized trial evaluating the efficacy and safety of ENA 713 (rivastigmine tartrate), a new acetylcholinesterase inhibitor, in patients with mild to moderately severe Alzheimer's disease. The ENA 713 B352 Study Group. International Journal of Geriatric Psychopharmacology 1:55–65, 1998

Cross AJ, Crow TJ, Ferrier IN, et al: Serotonin receptor changes in dementia of the Alzheimer type. J Neurochem 43:1574–1581, 1984

Cummings JL, Duchen LW: Kluver-Bucy syndrome in Pick's disease: clinical and pathologic correlations. Neurology 31:1415–1422, 1981

D'Amato RJ, Zweig RM, Whitehouse PJ, et al: Aminergic systems in Alzheimer's disease and Parkinson's disease. Ann Neurol 22:229–236, 1987

Davies P, Maloney AJ: Selective loss of central cholinergic neurons in Alzheimer's disease (letter). Lancet 2:1403, 1976

Davis KL, Davis BM, Greenwald BS, et al: Cortisol and Alzheimer's disease, I: basal studies. Am J Psychiatry 143:300–305, 1986

Doody RS, Geldmacher DS, Gordon B, et al: Open-label, multicenter, phase III extension study of the safety and efficacy of donepezil in patients with Alzheimer's disease. Arch Neurol 58:427–433, 2001

Erkinjuntti T, Kurz A, Gauthier S, et al: Efficacy of galantamine in probable vascular dementia and Alzheimer's disease combined with cerebrovascular disease: a randomised trial. Lancet 359:1283–1290, 2002

Evans IA, Funkenstein H, Albert MS, et al: Prevalence of Alzheimer's disease in a community population of older persons: higher than previously reported. JAMA 262:2551–2556, 1989

Farlow M, Gracon SI, Hershey LA, et al: A controlled trial of tacrine in Alzheimer's disease. The Tacrine Study Group. JAMA 268:2523–2529, 1992

Farlow M, Anand R, Messina J Jr, et al: A 52-week study of the efficacy of rivastigmine in patients with mild to moderately severe Alzheimer's disease. Eur Neurol 44:236–241, 2000

Fein G, Van Dyke C, Davenport L, et al: Preservation of normal cognitive functioning in elderly subjects with extensive white-matter lesions of long duration. Arch Gen Psychiatry 47:220–223, 1990

Feldman H, Gauthier S, Hecker J, et al: A 24-week, randomized, double-blind study of donepezil in moderate to severe Alzheimer's disease. Neurology 57:613–620, 2001

Fernandez HH, Trieschmann ME, Burke MA, et al: Quetiapine for psychosis in Parkinson's disease versus dementia with Lewy bodies. J Clin Psychiatry 63:513–515, 2002

Folstein MF, Folstein SE, McHugh PR: "Mini-mental state": a practical method for grading the cognitive state of patients for the clinician. J Psychiatr Res 12:189–198, 1975

Fox JH, Topel JL, Huckman MS: Dementia in the elderly: a search for treatable illnesses. J Gerontol 30:557–564, 1975

Francis PT, Palmer AM, Sims NR, et al: Neurochemical studies of early-onset Alzheimer's disease. Possible influence on treatment. N Engl J Med 313:7–11, 1985

Freeman FR: Evaluation of patients with progressive intellectual deterioration. Arch Neurol 33:658–659, 1976

Friedland RP: "Normal"-pressure hydrocephalus and the saga of the treatable dementias. JAMA 262:2577–2581, 1989

George AE, De Leon MJ, Kalnin A, et al: Leukoencephalopathy in normal and pathologic aging, II: MRI of brain lucencies. AJNR Am J Neuroradiol 7:567–570, 1986

Gibson CJ, Logue M, Growdon JH: CSF monoamine metabolite levels in Alzheimer's and Parkinson's disease. Arch Neurol 42:489–492, 1985

Glenner GG, Wong CW: Alzheimer's disease: initial report of the purification and characterization of a novel cerebrovascular amyloid protein. Biochem Biophys Res Commun 120:885–890, 1984

Golomb J, Wisoff J, Miller DC, et al: Alzheimer's disease comorbidity in normal pressure hydrocephalus: prevalence and shunt response. J Neurol Neurosurg Psychiatry 68:778–781, 2000

Graham JM, Sussman JD, Ford KS, et al: Olanzapine in the treatment of hallucinosis in idiopathic Parkinson's disease: a cautionary note. J Neurol Neurosurg Psychiatry 65:774–777, 1998

Gross JS, Weintraub NT, Neufeld RR, et al: Pernicious anemia in the demented patient without anemia or macrocytosis: a case for early recognition. J Am Geriatr Soc 34:612–614, 1986

Harper C: Wernicke's encephalopathy: a more common disease than realized. J Neurol Neurosurg Psychiatry 42:226–231, 1979

Hebb AO, Cusimano MD: Idiopathic normal pressure hydrocephalus: a systematic review of diagnosis and outcome. Neurosurgery 49:1166–1184, 2001

Henderson VW, Paganini-Hill A, Miller BL, et al: Estrogen for Alzheimer's disease in women: randomized, double-blind, placebo-controlled trial. Neurology 54:295–301, 2000

Heston LL, White JA, Mastri AR: Pick's disease: clinical genetics and natural history. Arch Gen Psychiatry 44:409–411, 1987

Hoogendijk WJ, Feenstra MG, Botterblom MH, et al: Increased activity of surviving locus ceruleus neurons in Alzheimer's disease. Ann Neurol 45:82–91, 1999

Hutton M, Lendon CL, Rizzu P: Association of missense and 5′-splice-site mutations in tau with the inherited dementia FTDP-17. Nature 393:702–705, 1998

in t' Veld BA, Ruitenberg A, Hofman A, et al: Nonsteroidal antiinflammatory drugs and the risk of Alzheimer's disease. N Engl J Med 345:1515–1521, 2001

Iqbal K, Alonso ADC, Gondal JA, et al: Inhibition of neurofibrillary degeneration: a rational and promising therapeutic target, in Alzheimer's Disease and Related Disorders: Etiology, Pathogenesis and Therapeutics. Edited by Iqbal K, Swaab DG, Winblad B, et al. Chicester, England, Wiley, 1999, pp 269–280

Ishikawa E, Yanaka K, Sugimoto K, et al: Reversible dementia in patients with chronic subdural hematomas. J Neurosurg 96:680–683, 2002

Joachim CL, Morris JH, Selkoe DJ: Clinically diagnosed Alzheimer's disease: autopsy results in 150 cases. Ann Neurol 24:50–56, 1988

Katz IR, Jeste DV, Mintzer JE, et al: Comparison of risperidone and placebo for psychosis and behavioral disturbances associated with dementia: a randomized, double-blind trial. Risperidone Study Group. J Clin Psychiatry 60:107–115, 1999

Katzman R: The prevalence and malignancy of Alzheimer disease: a major killer (editorial). Arch Neurol 33:217–218, 1976

Katzman R: Alzheimer's disease. N Engl J Med 314:964–973, 1986

Khachaturian ZS: Diagnosis of Alzheimer's disease. Arch Neurol 42:1097–1105, 1985

Kiloh LG: Pseudo-dementia. Acta Psychiatr Scand 37:336–351, 1961

Knapp MJ, Knopman DS, Solomon PR, et al: A 30-week randomized controlled trial of high-dose tacrine in patients with Alzheimer's disease. The Tacrine Study Group. JAMA 271:985–991, 1994

Kosaka K, Tsuchiya K, Yoshimura M: Lewy body disease with and without dementia: a clinicopathological study of 35 cases. Clin Neuropathol 7:299–305, 1988

Kotzbauer PT, Trojanowski JQ, Lee VM: Lewy body pathology in Alzheimer's disease. J Mol Neurosci 17:225–232, 2001

Larson EB, Reifler BV, Featherstone HJ, et al: Dementia in elderly outpatients: a prospective study. Ann Intern Med 100:417–423, 1984

Larson EB, Reifler BV, Sumi SM, et al: Diagnostic tests in the evaluation of dementia: a prospective study of 200 elderly outpatients. Arch Intern Med 146:1917–1922, 1986

Le Bars PL, Katz MM, Berman N, et al: A placebo-controlled, double-blind, randomized trial of an extract of *Ginkgo biloba* for dementia. North American EGb Study Group. JAMA 278:1327–1332, 1997

Leverenz J, Sumi SM: Parkinson's disease in patients with Alzheimer's disease. Arch Neurol 43:662–664, 1986

Levkoff SE, Evans DA, Liptzin B, et al: Delirium: the occurrence and persistence of symptoms among elderly hospitalized patients. Arch Intern Med 152:334–340, 1992

Levy-Lahad E, Wasco W, Poorkaj P, et al: Candidate gene for the chromosome 1 familial Alzheimer's disease locus. Science 269:973–976, 1995

Lim A, Tsuang D, Kukull W, et al: Clinico-neuropathological correlation of Alzheimer's disease in a community-based case series. J Am Geriatr Soc 47:564–569, 1999

Lindenbaum J, Healton EB, Savage DG, et al: Neuropsychiatric disorders caused by cobalamin deficiency in the absence of anemia or macrocytosis. N Engl J Med 318:1720–1728, 1988

Lyketsos CG, Sheppard JM, Steele CD, et al: Randomized, placebo-controlled, double-blind, clinical trial of sertraline in the treatment of depression complicating Alzheimer's disease: initial results from the Depression in Alzheimer's Disease study. Am J Psychiatry 157:1686–1689, 2000

Maelicke A, Samochocki M, Jostock R: Allosteric sensitization of nicotinic receptors by galantamine: a new treatment strategy for Alzheimer's disease. Biol Psychiatry 49:279–288, 2001

Mahley RW, Huang Y: Apolipoprotein E: from atherosclerosis to Alzheimer's disease and beyond. Curr Opin Lipidol 10:207–217, 1999

Mann DMA, Yates PO: Serotonin nerve cells in Alzheimer's disease. J Neurol Neurosurg Psychiatry 46:96–98, 1983

Mann DMA, Lincoln J, Yates PO, et al: Changes in the monoamine-containing neurones of the human CNS in senile dementia. Br J Psychiatry 136:533–541, 1980

Marcantonio ER, Flacker J, Michaels M, et al: Delirium is independently associated with poor functional recovery after hip fracture. J Am Geriatr Soc 48:618–624, 2000

Martin DC, Francis J, Protetch J, et al: Time dependence of cognitive recovery with cobalamin replacement: report of a pilot study. J Am Geriatr Soc 40:168–172, 1992

Mattis S: Mental status examination for organic mental syndrome in the elderly patient, in Geriatric Psychiatry: A Handbook for Psychiatrists and Primary Care Physicians. Edited by Bellack L, Karasu TB. New York, Grune & Stratton, 1976, pp 77–121

Mayeux R, Stern Y, Spanton S: Heterogeneity in dementia of the Alzheimer type: evidence of subgroups. Neurology 35:453–461, 1985

Mayeux R, Stern Y, Rosenstein R, et al: An estimate of the prevalence of dementia in idiopathic Parkinson's disease. Arch Neurol 45:260–262, 1988

McAllister TW, Ferrell RB, Price TRP, et al: The dexamethasone suppression test in two patients with severe depressive pseudodementia. Am J Psychiatry 139:479–481, 1982

McGeer EG, McGeer PL: Brain inflammation in Alzheimer disease and the therapeutic implications. Curr Pharm Des 5:821–836, 1999

McGeer PL, Shulzer M, McGeer EG: Arthritis and anti-inflammatory agents as possible protective factors for Alzheimer's disease: a review of 17 epidemiologic studies. Neurology 47:425–432, 1996

McKeith IG, Galasko D, Kosaka K, et al: Consensus guidelines for the clinical and pathologic diagnosis of dementia with Lewy bodies (DLB): report of the consortium on DLB international workshop. Neurology 47:1113–1124, 1996

McKeith I[G], Del Ser T, Spano P, et al: Efficacy of rivastigmine in dementia with Lewy bodies: a randomised, double-blind, placebo-controlled international study. Lancet 356:2031–2036, 2000

McKhann G, Drachman D, Folstein M, et al: Clinical diagnosis of Alzheimer's disease: report of the NINCDS-ADRDA Work Group under the auspices of Department of Health and Human Services Task Force on Alzheimer's disease. Neurology 34:939–944, 1984

Mesulam M-M, Guillozet A, Shaw P, et al: Acetylcholinesterase knockouts establish central cholinergic pathways and can use butyrylcholinesterase to hydrolyze acetylcholine. Neuroscience 110:627–639, 2002

Mitchell TW, Mufson EJ, Schneider JA, et al: Parahippocampal tau pathology in healthy aging, mild cognitive impairment, and early Alzheimer's disease. Ann Neurol 51:182–189, 2002

Mohs RC, Doody RS, Morris JC, et al: A 1-year, placebo-controlled preservation of function survival study of donepezil in AD patients. Neurology 57:481–488, 2001

Morris JC, McKeel DW, Fulling K, et al: Validation of clinical diagnostic criteria for Alzheimer's disease. Ann Neurol 24:17–22, 1988

Mortimer JA: Alzheimer's disease and senile dementia: prevalence and incidence, in Alzheimer's Disease: The Standard Reference. Edited by Reisberg B. New York, Free Press, 1983, pp 141–148

Mullan M, Crawford F, Axelman K, et al: A pathogenic mutation for probable Alzheimer's disease in the *APP* gene at the N-terminus of beta-amyloid. Nat Genet 1:345–347, 1992

Mulnard RA, Cotman CW, Kawas C, et al: Estrogen replacement therapy for treatment of mild to moderate Alzheimer disease: a randomized controlled trial. Alzheimer's Disease Cooperative Study. JAMA 283:1007–1015, 2000

Muramatsu T, Kato M, Matsui T, et al: Apolipoprotein E epsilon 4 allele distribution in Wernicke-Korsakoff syndrome with or without global intellectual deficits. J Neural Transm 104:913–920, 1997

Neary D, Snowden J: Fronto-temporal dementia: nosology, neuropsychology, and neuropathology. Brain Cogn 31:176–187, 1996

Nilsson K, Warkentin S, Hultberg B, et al: Treatment of cobalamin deficiency in dementia, evaluated clinically and with cerebral blood flow measurements. Aging (Milano) 12:199–207, 2000

Nilsson K, Gustafson L, Hultberg B: Improvement of cognitive functions after cobalamin/folate supplementation in elderly patients with dementia and elevated plasma homocysteine. Int J Geriatr Psychiatry 16:609–614, 2001

Nyth AL, Gottfries CG, Lyby K, et al: A controlled multicenter clinical study of citalopram and placebo in elderly depressed patients with and without concomitant dementia. Acta Psychiatr Scand 86:138–145, 1992

Palmer AM, Francis PT, Bowen DE, et al: Catecholaminergic neurones assessed ante-mortem in Alzheimer's disease. Brain Res 414:365–375, 1987

Parkinson Study Group: Low-dose clozapine for the treatment of drug-induced psychosis in Parkinson's disease. N Engl J Med 340:757–763, 1999

Perry EK, Tomlinson BE, Blessed G, et al: Correlation of cholinergic abnormalities with senile plaques and mental test scores in senile dementia. Br Med J 2:1457–1459, 1978

Perry EK, Curtis M, Dick DJ, et al: Cholinergic correlates of cognitive impairment in Parkinson's disease: comparisons with Alzheimer's disease. J Neurol Neurosurg Psychiatry 48:413–421, 1985

Perry EK, Haroutunian V, Davis KL: Neocortical cholinergic activities differentiate Lewy body dementia from classical Alzheimer's disease. Neuroreport 5:747–749, 1994

Perry RH, Irving D, Blessed G, et al: Senile dementia of Lewy body type. A clinically and neuropathologically distinct form of Lewy body dementia in the elderly. J Neurol Sci 95:119–139, 1990

Peskind ER, Wingerson D, Murray S, et al: Effects of Alzheimer's disease and normal aging on cerebrospinal fluid norepinephrine responses to yohimbine and clonidine. Arch Gen Psychiatry 52:774–782, 1995

Peskind ER, Wilkinson CW, Petrie EC, et al: Increased CSF cortisol in AD is a function of *APOE* genotype. Neurology 56:1094–1098, 2001

Poorkaj P, Bird TD, Wijsman E, et al: Tau is a candidate gene for chromosome 17 frontotemporal dementia. Ann Neurol 43:815–825, 1998

Pratt RD, Perdomo CA: Patient populations in clinical trials of the efficacy and tolerability of donepezil in patients with dementia and cerebrovascular disease ("vascular dementia"). The 308 Study Group. Paper presented at the 7th International Geneva/Springfield Symposium on Advances in Alzheimer Therapy, Geneva, Switzerland, April 4, 2002

Prusiner SB, DeArmond SJ: Prion diseases of the central nervous system. Monogr Pathol 32:86–122, 1990

Raber J, Akana SF, Bhatnagar S, et al: Hypothalamic-pituitary-adrenal dysfunction in *APOE* (-/-) mice: possible role in behavioral and metabolic alterations. J Neurosci 20:2064–2071, 2000

Rahkonen T, Luukkainen-Markkula R, Paanila S, et al: Delirium episode as a sign of undetected dementia among community dwelling elderly subjects: a 2 year follow up study. J Neurol Neurosurg Psychiatry 69:519–521, 2000

Rajan S, Wallace JI, Beresford SAA, et al: Screening for cobalamin deficiency in geriatric outpatients: prevalence and influence of synthetic cobalamin intake. J Am Geriatr Soc 50:624–630, 2002

Rajput AH, Offord K, Beard CM, et al: A case-control study of smoking habits, dementia, and other illnesses in idiopathic Parkinson's disease. Neurology 37:266–232, 1987

Raskind MA, Barnes RF: Alzheimer's disease: treatment of noncognitive behavioral abnormalities, in Psychopharmacology: The Fifth Generation of Progress. Edited by Davis K, Charney D, Coyle J, et al. New York, Lippincott Williams & Wilkins, 2002, pp 1253–1265

Raskind MA, Peskind ER: Treatment of noncognitive symptoms in Alzheimer's disease and other dementias, in Essentials of Clinical Psychopharmacology. Edited by Schatzberg AF, Nemeroff CB. Washington, DC, American Psychiatric Publishing, 2001, pp 447–457

Raskind MA, Peskind E, Rivard MR, et al: Dexamethasone suppression test and cortisol circadian rhythm in primary degenerative dementia. Am J Psychiatry 139:1468–1471, 1982

Raskind MA, Peskind ER, Halter JB, et al: Norepinephrine and MHPG levels in CSF and plasma in Alzheimer's disease. Arch Gen Psychiatry 41:343–346, 1984

Raskind MA, Peskind ER, Wilkinson CW: Hypothalamic-pituitary-adrenal axis regulation and human aging. Ann N Y Acad Sci 746:327–335, 1994

Raskind MA, Peskind ER, Wessel T, et al: Galantamine in AD: a 6-month randomized, placebo-controlled trial with a 6-month extension. The Galantamine USA-1 Study Group. Neurology 54:2261–2268, 2000

Reifler BV: Arguments for abandoning the term *pseudodementia*. J Am Geriatr Soc 30:665–668, 1982

Riley JN, Walker DW: Morphological alterations in hippocampus after long-term alcohol consumption in mice. Science 201:646–648, 1978

Risse SC, Lampe TH, Bird TD, et al: Myoclonus, seizures and rigidity in Alzheimer's disease. Alzheimer Dis Assoc Disord 4:217–225, 1990a

Risse SC, Raskind MA, Nochlin D, et al: Neuropathological findings in patients with clinical diagnoses of probable Alzheimer's disease. Am J Psychiatry 147:168–172, 1990b

Rogers SL, Friedhoff LT: The efficacy and safety of donepezil in patients with Alzheimer's disease: results of a US multicenter, randomized, double-blind, placebo-controlled trial. The Donepezil Study Group. Dementia 7:293–303, 1996

Rogers SL, Farlow MR, Doody RS, et al: A 24-week, double-blind, placebo-controlled trial of donepezil in patients with Alzheimer's disease. The Donepezil Study Group. Neurology 50:136–145, 1998

Rosen WG, Mohs RC, Davis KL: A new rating scale for Alzheimer's disease. Am J Psychiatry 141:1356–1364, 1984

Rosenberg RN: A causal role for amyloid in Alzheimer's disease: the end of the beginning. Neurology 43:851–856, 1993

Rösler M, Anand R, Cicin-Sain A, et al: Efficacy and safety of rivastigmine in patients with Alzheimer's disease: international randomised controlled trial. The B303 Exelon Study Group. BMJ 318:633–640, 1999

Rudorfer MV, Clayton PV: Depression, dementia and dexamethasone suppression (letter). Am J Psychiatry 138:701, 1981

Russo-Neustadt A, Cotman CW: Adrenergic receptors in Alzheimer's disease brain: selective increases in the cerebella of aggressive patients. J Neurosci 17:5573–5580, 1997

Sano M, Ernesto C, Thomas RG, et al: A controlled trial of selegiline, alpha-tocopherol, or both as treatment for Alzheimer's disease. The Alzheimer's Disease Cooperative Study. N Engl J Med 336:1216–1222, 1997

Sapolsky R, Armanini M, Packan D, et al: Stress and glucocorticoids in aging. Endocrinol Metab Clin North Am 16:965–980, 1987

Schellenberg GD, Bird T, Wijsman E, et al: Genetic linkage evidence for a familial Alzheimer's disease locus on chromosome 14. Science 258:668–671, 1992

Schneider LS: Efficacy of treatment for geropsychiatric patients with severe mental illness. Psychopharmacol Bull 29:501–524

Selkoe DJ: The origins of Alzheimer's disease: a is for amyloid. JAMA 283:1571–1577, 2000

Sherrington R, Rogaev EI, Liang Y, et al: Cloning of a gene bearing missense mutations in early onset familial Alzheimer's disease. Nature 375:754–760, 1995

Sjogren T, Sjogren H, Lindgren AGH: Morbus Alzheimer and Morbus Pick; a genetic, clinical and patho-anatomical study. Acta Psychiatr Neurol Scand 82:1–152, 1952

Skoog I, Nilsson L, Palmertz B, et al: A population-based study of dementia in 85-year-olds. N Engl J Med 328:153–158, 1994

Snowdon DA, Greiner LH, Mortimer JA, et al: Brain infarction and the clinical expression of Alzheimer disease. The Nun Study. JAMA 277:813–817, 1997

Spar JE, Gerner R: Does the dexamethasone suppression test distinguish dementia from depression? Am J Psychiatry 139:238–240, 1982

Strachan RW, Henderson JG: Psychiatric syndromes due to avitaminosis B_{12} with normal blood and bone marrow. Q J Med 34:303–317, 1965

Street JS, Clark WS, Gannon KS, et al: Olanzapine treatment of psychotic and behavioral symptoms in patients with Alzheimer's disease in nursing care facilities: a double-blind, randomized, placebo-controlled trial. The HGEU Study Group. Arch Gen Psychiatry 57:968–976, 2000

Sumi SM, Bird TD, Nochlin D, et al: Familial presenile dementia with psychosis associated with cortical neurofibrillary tangles and degeneration of the amygdala. Neurology 42:120–127, 1992

Szot P, Leverenz JB, Peskind ER, et al: Tyrosine hydroxylase and norepinephrine transporter mRNA expression in the locus coeruleus in Alzheimer's disease. Brain Res Mol Brain Res 84:135–140, 2000

Tariot PN, Solomon PR, Morris JC, et al: A 5-month, randomized, placebo-controlled trial of galantamine in AD. The Galantamine USA-10 Study Group. Neurology 54:2269–2276, 2000

Teri L: Behavioral treatment of depression in patients with dementia. Alzheimer Dis Assoc Disord 8 (suppl 3):66–74, 1994

Teri L, Logsdon RG, Peskind E, et al: Treatment of agitation in AD: a randomized, placebo-controlled clinical trial. Neurology 55:1271–1278, 2000

Thal L: No differences between rofecoxib, naproxen and placebo on clinical progression in Alzheimer's disease. Paper presented at the annual meeting of the American Academy of Neurology, Denver, CO, April 2002

Thomasen AM, Borgesen SE, Bruhn P, et al: Prognosis of dementia in normal-pressure hydrocephalus after a shunt operation. Ann Neurol 20:304–310, 1986

Tierney MC, Fisher RH, Lewis AJ, et al: The NINCDS-ADRDA Work Group criteria for the clinical diagnosis of probable Alzheimer's disease: a clinicopathologic study of 57 cases. Neurology 38:359–364, 1988

Tomlinson BE, Blessed G, Roth M: Observations on the brains of demented old people. J Neurol Sci 11:205–242, 1970

Tomlinson BE, Irving D, Blessed G: Cell loss in the locus coeruleus in senile dementia of Alzheimer type. J Neurol Sci 49:419–428, 1981

Trojanowski JQ, Lee VM: Phosphorylation of paired helical filament tau in Alzheimer's disease neurofibrillary lesions: focusing on phosphates. FASEB J 15:1570–1576, 1995

van Asselt DZ, Pasman JW, van Lier HJ, et al: Cobalamin supplementation improves cognitive and cerebral function in older, cobalamin-deficient persons. J Gerontol A Biol Sci Med Sci 56:M775–M779, 2001

Victor M: Alcoholic dementia. Can J Neurol Sci 21:88–99, 1994

Victor M, Adams RD: The Wernicke-Korsakoff Syndrome. Philadelphia, PA, FA Davis, 1971

Victoratos GC, Lonman JAR, Herzberg L: Neurological investigation of dementia. Br J Psychiatry 130:131–133, 1977

Vitaliano PP, Breen AR, Russo J, et al: The clinical utility of the dementia rating scale for assessing Alzheimer patients. J Chronic Dis 37:743–753, 1984

Volicer L, Direnfeld LK, Freedman M, et al: Serotonin and 5-hydroxyindoleacetic acid in CSF: differences in Parkinson's disease and dementia of the Alzheimer's type. Arch Neurol 42:127–129, 1985

Wang HX, Wahlin A, Basun H, et al: Vitamin B(12) and folate in relation to the development of Alzheimer's disease. Neurology 56:1188–1194, 2001

Weggen S, Eriksen JL, Das P, et al: A subset of NSAIDs lower amyloidogenic Abeta42 independently of cyclooxygenase activity. Nature 414:212–216, 2001

Whitehouse PJ, Price DL, Struble RG, et al: Alzheimer's disease and senile dementia: loss of neurons in the basal forebrain. Science 215:1237–1239, 1982

Whybrow PC, Prange AJ Jr, Treadway CR: Mental changes accompanying thyroid gland dysfunction. Arch Gen Psychiatry 20:48–63, 1969

Wieland RG: Vitamin B_{12} deficiency in the nonanemic elderly. J Am Geriatr Soc 34:618–619, 1986

Wikkelso C, Anderson H, Blomstrand C, et al: The clinical effect of lumbar puncture in normal-pressure hydrocephalus. J Neurol Neurosurg Psychiatry 45:64–69, 1982

Wilcock GK, Lilienfeld S, Gaens E: Efficacy and safety of galantamine in patients with mild to moderate Alzheimer's disease: multicentre randomised controlled trial. Galantamine International-1 Study Group. BMJ 321:1445–1449, 2000

Wilhelmsen KC, Clark LN, Miller BL, et al: Tau mutations in frontotemporal dementia. Dement Geriatr Cogn Disord 10:88–92, 1999

Wilner E, Brody JA: Prognosis of general paresis after treatment. Lancet 2:1370–1371, 1968

Winblad B, Adolfsson R, Carlsson A, et al: Biogenic amines in brains of patients with Alzheimer's disease, in Alzheimer's Disease: A Report of Progress. Edited by Corkin S. New York, Raven, 1982, pp 25–33

Winblad B, Engedal K, Soininen H: A 1-year, randomized, placebo-controlled study of donepezil in patients with mild to moderate AD. Neurology 57:489–495, 2001

Wood PL, Nair NP, Etienne P, et al: Lack of cholinergic deficit in the neocortex in Pick's disease. Prog Neuropsychopharmacol Biol Psychiatry 7:725–727, 1983

Wyss-Coray T, Mucke L: Ibuprofen, inflammation and Alzheimer disease. Nat Med 6:973–974, 2000

Yamamoto T, Hirano A: Nucleus raphe dorsalis in Alzheimer's disease: neurofibrillary tangles and loss of large neurons. Ann Neurol 17:573–577, 1985

Zubenko GS: Progression of illness in the differential diagnosis of primary depression. Am J Psychiatry 147:435–438, 1990

Zubenko GS, Moossy J: Major depression in primary dementia. Arch Neurol 45:1182–1186, 1988

C H A P T E R 1 3

Movement Disorders

Burton Scott, Ph.D., M.D.

$\mathbf{A}$s people age, a variety of movement disorders can either appear for the first time or progress after onset earlier in life. Arthritis, bursitis, tendonitis, and other non–central nervous system conditions can in some ways mimic neurological conditions by producing stooped posture and overall slowing of movement. In this chapter, I discuss central nervous system–based movement disorders that occur in elderly individuals and result in impaired or abnormal movement.

Movement disorders in the elderly population can be divided into *hypokinetic movement disorders* (in which the ability to move is decreased or impaired because of a neurological condition) and *hyperkinetic movement disorders* (in which there is excessive abnormal movement). Hypokinetic movement disorders encompass a variety of parkinsonian disorders, in which there is some combination of the following signs and symptoms: tremor at rest, rigidity, slowness of movement (bradykinesia), and balance difficulty (postural instability). These disorders include Parkinson's disease (PD) and several "Parkinson's plus" syndromes. Other gait disorders, such as normal-pressure hydrocephalus (NPH), are also included among the hypokinetic movement disorders. Hyperkinetic movement disorders include tremors, tics, dystonia, myoclonus, chorea, stereotypies, and other dyskinesias, including tardive dyskinesia and tardive dystonia. Tremor disorders are represented in both groups of movement disorders: tremor at rest is a cardinal feature of parkinsonism (a hypokinetic condition), and postural and kinetic tremor are features of essential tremor (ET; a hyperkinetic movement disorder).

Hypokinetic Movement Disorders

Parkinsonism

The term *parkinsonism* refers to a clinical condition that is characterized by some combination of resting tremor, rigidity, bradykinesia, and postural instability, but no specific etiology is inferred by the term. *Parkinson's disease* refers to levodopa-responsive, idiopathic parkinsonism associated with Lewy bodies and neuronal degeneration in the substantia nigra pars compacta. Secondary parkinsonism is parkinsonism due to other lesions of the basal ganglia, such as tumors, strokes (vascular parkinsonism), encephalitis, hypoxic or ischemic insult, and toxins (such as manganese, carbon monoxide, or carbon disulfide). NPH can cause a parkinsonian-like gait disorder, urinary incontinence, and dementia.

Parkinsonism is well known to be associated with use of dopamine receptor–blocking agents, including antipsychotic medications and antiemetics. Classic antipsychotic medications typically exhibit strong antagonism at dopamine D_2 receptors (Mendis et al. 1994), whereas the newer atypical antipsychotics have less affinity for dopamine D_2 receptors. The newer agents have fewer parkinsonian side effects but are not totally free of them (Chouinard et al. 1993). Based on clinical experience with PD patients who have levodopa-related psychosis, my colleagues and I have determined that, of these newer agents, risperidone has the greatest number of parkinsonian side effects, followed by olanzapine and then quetiapine. Clozapine exhibits a lower relative affinity for dopamine D_2 receptors compared with conventional antipsychotics (Meltzer 1992) and suppresses levodopa-related psychosis in PD while minimizing exacerbation of PD symptoms. Antiemetic agents such as metoclopramide, promethazine, and prochlorperazine can also produce parkinsonism as an acute side effect, and patients who take these medications for prolonged periods can develop tardive movement disorders. Older antidepressants that contain amitriptyline and a phenothiazine derivative also have side effects of parkinsonism and possibly tardive dyskinesia or tardive dystonia.

Parkinson's Disease

PD is a chronic, progressive, neurodegenerative illness that produces rigidity, slowness of movement (bradykinesia), postural instability, and, often, tremor at rest. It affects up to 1 million individuals in North America and is newly diagnosed in 20,000–50,000 patients each year. The prevalence of PD increases with age, with estimates of 1% at age 60 and up to 2.6% at age 85 or older (Mutch et al. 1986; Sutcliffe et al. 1985). PD results from progressive loss of dopamine-containing neurons in the substantia nigra pars compacta of the midbrain and is characterized pathologically by abnormal collections of proteins, called Lewy bodies, in the cytoplasm of degenerating neurons (Forno 1996; Golbe 1999). The diagnosis is made clinically (Gelb et al. 1999) because no laboratory test is diagnostic, and the diagnosis can be confirmed only at autopsy.

Other common clinical features of PD include hypomimia (masked facies or facial masking), micrographia (small handwriting), stooped posture, retropulsion, and shuffling and festinating gait. Symptoms typically begin gradually on one side of the body, and patients may ignore the initial symptoms when the nondominant arm is the arm affected first, particularly in the absence of tremor. The typical resting tremor in PD has a frequency of 4–6 Hz. When tremor occurs in the hand, it may have the classic pill-rolling appearance—that is, a combination of flexion-extension tremor of the fingers and thumb, giving the appearance of rolling a marble or pill between the thumb and fingertips. The resting tremor of PD typically attenuates at least transiently during voluntary movement of the affected extremity, such as when the patient picks up an object, and is to be distinguished from the postural, antigravity tremor observed in ET. Usually, treatment with levodopa, a precursor of the neurotransmitter dopamine, results in significant clinical benefit in PD.

PD can divided into two clinical forms: 1) tremor-dominant PD, in which tremor at rest is a prominent feature, and 2) postural instability and gait disorder, or akinetic PD, in which resting tremor is minimal, if present at all, and patients exhibit earlier balance difficulty. Both forms respond to levodopa treatment, at least initially; however, tremor-dominant PD tends to progress more slowly and thus has a more favorable prognosis than does akinetic PD.

The stiffness or rigidity of PD is detected clinically by testing for involuntary resistance to passive movement of the extremities. This resistance can manifest as lead-pipe rigidity—that is, a steady resistance to passive movement. In patients with resting tremor, the combination of rigidity and tremor results in cogwheel rigidity—that is, a jerky resistance to passive movement. In addition, active, voluntary movement of the contralateral extremity (synkinetic movement) can bring out subtle rigidity in an ipsilateral limb. For example, rapid, repetitive opening and closing of the contralateral hand in early PD may result in slightly increased tone in the ipsilateral arm; similarly, repetitive flexion-extension at the contralateral elbow can bring out abnormally increased tone in the ipsilateral leg in early PD.

Slowed movement, or bradykinesia, is tested in the clinic by observing the ease with which the patient performs repetitive movements such as tapping the index finger and thumb together, opening and closing the hand, twisting the hand clockwise and counterclockwise (like turning a doorknob), and tapping the heel on the ground. In a PD patient, the clinician looks for decreasing size of a repetitive movement. Micrographia can be a manifestation of bradykinesia. Early in PD, handwriting might be of normal size at the beginning of a sentence and then become progressively smaller by the end of the sentence.

Postural instability usually occurs later than the other clinical signs of PD and can be very disabling. Patients fall because of an inability to keep their feet under their center of gravity, and these patients exhibit retropulsion (inability to maintain balance when suddenly displaced backward) and anteropulsion (inability to maintain balance when suddenly displaced forward). Festination occurs in an upright, walking PD patient whose feet are lagging behind his or her center of gravity. This clinical sign manifests as rapid, tiny steps taken to keep from falling.

Onset of PD symptoms is usually recognized earlier in individuals with tremor-dominant PD, because even mild tremor is likely to bring a patient into clinic earlier. In patients with resting tremor, the tremor often increases with walking, and patients with early PD often exhibit decreased arm swing when walking. A reduction or absence of arm swing noticed by others may be the first indication of PD in a patient who does not have much resting tremor. Other patients may present with gradual loss of fine coordination of an extremity. The posture in a PD patient is often stooped, with flexion at the neck, upper back, shoulders, hips, and knees. The gait is typically narrow based and shuffling. Symptom onset is usually noticed earlier in patients affected first on the dominant side (i.e., the right hand in a right hand–dominant individual). By several years after onset of symptoms, it is expected that both sides of the body will be affected, although one side is often more affected than the other, even in chronic PD.

Medications used to treat PD can be divided into putative neuroprotective agents, drugs for treating symptoms (levodopa, dopamine agonists, others), and possible restorative agents (growth factors, neuroimmunophilins). There are no medications that clearly slow progression of PD and provide neuroprotection.

PD results from a deficiency of the neurotransmitter dopamine in the brain, and administration of levodopa (L-dopa), a precursor of dopamine, is the most effective treatment for PD symptoms. Thus, levodopa is the mainstay of therapeutic treatment in PD. Dopamine itself is not an effective medication in PD, because of its poor ability to cross the blood-brain barrier. However, levodopa effectively crosses the blood-brain barrier and is taken up by remaining dopaminergic neurons throughout the PD patient's brain, including the desired target—the substantia nigra. Levodopa is converted to dopamine within these neurons and is stored in synaptic vesicles for subsequent neurotransmission. In the United States, the usual formulation of levodopa (Sinemet) is a combination of levodopa and carbidopa, a peripheral decarboxylase inhibitor that reduces destruction of levodopa before it has a chance to cross the blood-brain barrier and reach the brain.

Selegiline is a relatively selective monoamine oxidase B inhibitor that delays the need for therapeutic treatment with levodopa in early PD by several months. However, selegiline's modest effect on parkinsonian symptoms appears to be due mostly to the drug's metabolism to an amphetamine-like metabolite that blocks synaptic dopamine reuptake, rather than to a true neuroprotective effect. Entacapone and tolcapone are catechol O-methyltransferase inhibitors that reduce the breakdown of levodopa before it reaches the brain, and these drugs may also slow the breakdown of dopamine in the brain. Because of rare, fulminant hepatotoxicity, tolcapone is not used much clinically. Anticholinergic medications (trihexyphenidyl, benztropine) are also commonly used to treat early PD symptoms. Amantadine, an antiviral medication with anticholinergic effects, produces mild improvement of parkinsonism early in the disease course, in part because of enhanced release of endogenous dopamine stores from the substantia nigra.

Dopamine agonists are useful adjuncts in the symptomatic treatment of PD. These agents act directly on dopamine receptors and are particularly useful in smoothing the therapeutic response to levodopa by reducing motor fluctuations ("on-off" phenomena) and by increasing the period of benefit obtained from each dose of levodopa. The side effects of dopamine agonists are similar to those of levodopa: hallucinations, dyskinesias (head bobbing and involuntary writhing or twisting movements of the extremities), and dystonia (muscle spasms) are most common. The dopamine agonists currently available in the

United States are bromocriptine, pergolide, pramipexole, and ropinirole.

Surgical treatment of PD includes 1) ablative surgery, in which destructive lesions are precisely placed in basal ganglia targets; 2) deep brain stimulator implantation, in which deep brain stimulation is applied to similar basal ganglia targets; and 3) potentially restorative procedures, such as transplantation of dopaminergic tissue (fetal tissue transplantation) (Lang and Lozano 1998a, 1998b). Ablative surgeries consist of thalamotomy, in which lesioning is performed at the ventral intermediate nucleus of the contralateral thalamus; pallidotomy, in which the target is the internal segment of the globus pallidus; and, less commonly, subthalamotomy, in which the target is the subthalamic nucleus. In deep brain stimulation, the neurosurgeon places a thin stimulating electrode at the target. The electrode is connected to an implantable pulse generator that can be adjusted to provide electrical pulses of sufficient energy and frequency to alter output from the targeted nuclei, thereby reducing contralateral PD symptoms. Potential restorative surgeries are exploring the use of dopaminergic tissue transplantation and introduction of growth factors, such as glial-derived neurotrophic factor (GDNF).

The differential diagnosis of PD includes a host of disorders that can mimic aspects of PD, including ET, drug-induced parkinsonism (see "Parkinsonism" at the beginning of this chapter), and other secondary parkinsonian syndromes (tumors and other mass lesions of the basal ganglia, vascular parkinsonism). Other disorders that can have parkinsonian features are NPH; primary gait ignition failure, which may represent early parkinsonism; and other atypical parkinsonian syndromes, such as progressive supranuclear palsy (PSP), multiple system atrophy, and cortical-basal ganglionic degeneration (or corticobasal degeneration); see "'Parkinson's Plus' Syndromes" discussed below.

Normal-Pressure Hydrocephalus (Communicating Hydrocephalus)

NPH, also known as communicating hydrocephalus, is more common in elderly persons and can be a cause of a progressive gait disorder in addition to urinary incontinence and memory decline. It is associated with a decrease in the rate of removal of cerebrospinal fluid (CSF) at the level of the arachnoid villi and superior sagittal sinus. NPH can develop after an episode of meningitis or a subarachnoid bleed but usually develops in the absence of these relatively rare conditions. Affected individuals may take small steps and exhibit a "magnetic gait," in which they experience difficulty lifting their feet to walk because of a sense that their feet are stuck to the ground. The triad of gait disorder, urinary incontinence, and memory loss suggests a diagnosis of NPH. Brain imaging demonstrates enlarged intraventricular spaces that are out of proportion to the size of the sulci. The diagnosis is supported by clinical improvement after a large-volume lumbar puncture or by observation of reversed CSF flow, identified by introducing a tracer into the CSF and performing cisternography to visualize the flow of tracer in the brain. Reduction of CSF during a single diagnostic lumbar puncture may not result in immediate clinical benefit. Placement of a lumbar drain for up to several days in the hospital may help determine whether the patient could benefit from surgical placement of a shunt to treat NPH.

"Parkinson's Plus" Syndromes

Progressive Supranuclear Palsy

PSP, or Steele-Richardson-Olszewski syndrome, features parkinsonism without prominent tremor, vertical gaze palsy, axial (midline) more than appendicular (arm and leg) rigidity, early postural instability, and poor response to levodopa (reviewed in Golbe and Davis 1993, Litvan 1998, and Litvan et al. 1996). The syndrome was first described by Steele, Richardson, and Olszewski in 1964. The Society for Progressive Supranuclear Palsy estimates that 20,000 people in the United States are affected with PSP—only 3,000–4,000 of whom have received a diagnosis—yielding an estimated known prevalence in the United States of 1.39 per 100,000. PSP is often associated with frequent falling, lack of eye contact, monotonous speech, sloppy eating, and slowed mentation (Jankovic et al. 1990). Patients may have a surprised or worried facial expression, with raised eyebrows resulting from bradykinesia and increased tone in facial musculature, and have difficulty opening their eyes because of eyelid apraxia (Jankovic 1984). There is early suppression of vertical optokinetic nystagmus and voluntary vertical saccades. Later in the illness, horizontal saccades and horizontal optokinetic nystagmus become suppressed. Impairment of voluntary downgaze is more specific to PSP, whereas impairment of voluntary upgaze is nonspecific in elderly individuals. As is expected with a supranuclear lesion, passive movement of the head can overcome the compromised voluntary eye movements in PSP.

PSP has an insidious onset, and often the first symptom is a decrease in postural stability, resulting in falls. The usual age at symptom onset is 55–70 years. Mean age at symptom onset is the early 60s (late 50s in PD). In PSP, the posture is upright and rigid, not stooped as in

PD, and the gait is typically stiff, with the legs extended at the knees, not flexed as in PD. In addition, PSP patients tend to pivot when turning, rather than exhibit en bloc shuffling as in PD.

Cognitive decline can begin in the first year of symptoms and may manifest as apathy, impaired abstract thinking, decreased verbal fluency, utilization or imitative behavior, and frontal release signs. Visual symptoms, including diplopia, blurry vision, burning eyes, and light sensitivity, appear in about 60% of cases during the first year, dysarthria in about 40% of cases, and bradykinesia in 20%.

Supranuclear gaze palsy has also been observed in other neurodegenerative disorders including diffuse Lewy body disease [dementia with Lewy bodies] (de Bruin et al. 1992), cortical-basal ganglionic degeneration (Gibb et al. 1990), and other parkinsonian syndromes. Atypical parkinsonian syndromes other than PSP may be suggested by a recent history of encephalitis, alien hand syndrome, cortical sensory deficits, focal frontal or temporoparietal atrophy, early cerebellar signs, early dysautonomia, severely asymmetric parkinsonism, or a relevant structural injury visualized by an imaging study.

Early in the course of PSP, visual pursuit may become saccadic (jerky), and voluntary saccades may become slow despite preserved range of extraocular movements. Saccades may become smaller or hypometric, and there may be decreased convergence of the eyes when they follow a target brought in toward the patient's nose. The ability to voluntarily suppress the vestibulo-ocular reflex during passive head movement decreases or disappears. Later, there is progression of eye-associated abnormalities, including slowing of eyelid opening and closing and slowing of eyelid saccades during attempted vertical gaze saccades. In addition, patients often lose the ability to suppress blinks in response to a bright light.

Another common eye-related sign seen in PSP is an excessive frequency or amplitude of square-wave jerks (small, involuntary, saccadic or jerky eye movements that intrude on ocular fixation). In addition, patients may have difficulty performing the antisaccade task, which involves looking rapidly in the direction opposite from a novel visual stimulus. A typical pattern in a patient with early PSP is to 1) make an increased number of errors while performing the antisaccade task, 2) exhibit hypometric saccades with normal latencies, and 3) exhibit impaired visual pursuit. Also, during vestibular and optokinetic nystagmus testing, initiation of the quick phase of nystagmus may be compromised, leading to tonic eye deviation to one side.

Another finding that supports a diagnosis of PSP is the presence of symmetric akinesia or rigidity, usually more in the proximal than distal portions of limbs. In contrast, akinesia or rigidity in PD is typically asymmetric at first, occurring initially on one side of the body, with the other side expected to become affected within a few years. Abnormal neck posture, especially retrocollis, is commonly seen in PSP, as are early dysphagia and dysarthria.

Unlike in PD, in PSP there is little or no response to levodopa therapy because of degeneration of secondary neurons downstream from dopaminergic substantia nigra pars compacta neurons. Response to other medical treatment is usually poor as well; however, some patients have at least a transient response to treatment with amantadine, carbidopa/levodopa (Sinemet), or dopamine agonists. There is no known effective neurosurgical intervention for PSP.

After symptom onset, the course of PSP is typically 5–10 years, and death may result from infections such as aspiration pneumonia or from complications of falls.

Neuropathology is the standard for certain diagnosis of PSP, which can be confused clinically with PD, cortical-basal ganglionic degeneration, multiple system atrophy (MSA), Alzheimer's disease, and dementia with Lewy bodies. Pathological changes in PSP include the development of neurofibrillary tangles and neuropil threads (filamentous structures in neuronal cytoplasm). Pathology is primarily found in the pallidum, subthalamic nucleus, substantia nigra, and pons. Abnormalities in tau protein, an important component of intracellular microtubules, have been implicated in some cases, and tau-positive astrocytes or astrocytic processes have been found in affected areas of the brain.

Multiple System Atrophy

MSA encompasses several "Parkinson's plus" conditions characterized by bilateral, symmetric parkinsonism that is poorly responsive to levodopa therapy, as well as absence or near absence of tremor (Quinn 1994; Shulman and Weiner 1997; Wenning et al. 1994). MSA is currently divided into two main clinical types: MSA-parkinsonism (MSA-P), in which parkinsonism is the main clinical feature; and MSA-cerebellar type (MSA-C), in which cerebellar ataxia is the main clinical feature. MSA-P represents about 80% of cases, MSA-C about 20%.

MSA-P encompasses conditions that were formerly diagnosed as striatonigral degeneration and Shy-Drager syndrome; these syndromes are no longer commonly used as separate diagnoses, and their symptoms are now included as part of MSA-P. Clinical features that may help distinguish striatonigral degeneration from other parkinsonian disorders include falls early in the illness, severe dysarthria and dysphonia, sleep apnea and excessive snor-

ing, anterocollis, respiratory stridor, and pyramidal signs (brisk reflexes and extensor plantar responses). In contrast, Shy-Drager syndrome was previously distinguished clinically by early autonomic impairment including orthostatic hypotension or syncope, impotence in males, and bowel and bladder dysfunction (Shy and Drager 1960). In MSA-P, parkinsonism and gait disturbance often develop later. In addition to neuronal degeneration in substantia nigra, putamen, and other nuclei, neuronal loss usually occurs in the intermediolateral columns of the spinal cord. Treatment of orthostatic symptoms includes liberalizing dietary salt, elevation of the head of the bed, and use of fludrocortisone, midodrine, and sometimes indomethacin and yohimbine. Although the clinical response to treatment is usually poor, trials of levodopa (up to 1,500 mg/day in divided doses) with or without a dopamine agonist (pergolide, pramipexole, ropinirole) are sometimes beneficial. The clinical course is approximately 10 years. Brain magnetic resonance imaging (MRI) may demonstrate decreased (dark) T2 signal laterally in the putamen of the basal ganglia (Kraft et al. 1999).

MSA-C, or sporadic olivopontocerebellar atrophy, often presents with gait ataxia. Other features that may develop are limb ataxia, breakdown of visual smooth pursuit, and cerebellar dysarthria (ataxic dysarthria). Autonomic dysfunction, parkinsonism, and pyramidal signs can also occur, but the cerebellar findings are usually most prominent. Brain MRI can demonstrate cerebellar and brain stem atrophy, particularly in the pons and medulla.

The neuropathology of MSA is significant for degeneration of the substantia nigra and putamen (striatum), with neuronal loss and iron deposition. Glial cytoplasmic inclusions, particularly in oligodendrocytes, are characteristic of all forms of MSA, and cell loss and gliosis can be found in the striatum, substantia nigra, locus coeruleus, pontine nuclei, middle cerebellar peduncles, Purkinje cells of the cerebellum, inferior olives, and the intermediolateral columns of the spinal cord. Lewy bodies and neurofibrillary tangles are not common in MSA.

Cortical-Basal Ganglionic Degeneration

Cortical-basal ganglionic degeneration (CBGD), also referred to as corticobasal degeneration, produces marked, asymmetric parkinsonism and dystonia (Litvan et al. 1997; Riley and Lang 2000; Schneider et al. 1997). Resting tremor is uncommon in this condition. CBGD can result in jerky (myoclonic), apraxic, rigid, akinetic movements and alien hand syndrome, in which one hand seems to have a "mind of its own" and seems no longer to belong to the patient. There may be early dementia, cortical sensory findings (such as hemineglect to double simultaneous tactile stimulation), or unilateral agraphesthesia (manifested as the inability to identify a number written on the palm of one's hand). Stimulus-sensitive myoclonus and action tremor may also be present. Response to levodopa therapy is poor, but administration of up to 1,500 mg/day in divided doses is sometimes of initial benefit. The disease course is typically 5–10 years from the time of symptom onset.

Neuropathological changes include swollen (ballooned) neurons, degeneration of substantia nigra and basal ganglia, and tau-positive inclusion bodies. Brain MRI often demonstrates asymmetric atrophy in posterior frontal and parietal cortex contralateral to the more affected side of the body (Savoiardo et al. 2000).

Frontotemporal Dementia and Parkinsonism Linked to Chromosome 17

In the degenerative condition called frontotemporal dementia and parkinsonism linked to chromosome 17 (FTDP-17), an insidious onset of behavioral or motor changes occurs. Typically in this disease, cognitive impairment leads to dementia, parkinsonism, nonfluent aphasia, a change in personality, and/or psychosis (Foster et al. 1997; Lund and Manchester Groups 1994). Onset is generally in the fifth decade of life and can be as late as the sixth decade. Duration is usually longer than 10 years but can be as short as 3 years. Behavioral changes range from aggressiveness to apathy and may include hyperorality, hyperphagia, obsessive stereotyped behavior, psychosis, delusions, and muteness. Motor findings can include parkinsonism, particularly rigidity, bradykinesia, and postural instability, but not resting tremor. Hyperreflexia, clonus, and extensor plantar responses may occur. Levodopa treatment produces no significant response. Autonomic function is spared early in the course until dementia becomes severe. Neuropsychological testing demonstrates disturbed executive functioning, with relative preservation of visual-spatial functioning, orientation, and memory until late in the disease course. Electroencephalographic findings are often normal until late in the disease, and functional imaging suggests frontal and anterior temporal hypoperfusion or hypometabolism.

Hyperkinetic Movement Disorders

Essential Tremor

Tremor is defined as a rhythmic oscillation across a joint resulting from involuntary, alternating activation of agonist and antagonist muscles. For example, tremor at the wrist results from alternating activation and relaxation of forearm flexor and extensor muscles.

ET is the most prevalent movement disorder among adults and the elderly, affecting up to 2% of the general population. The prevalence of ET increases with age, and in individuals older than 70 years, estimates of the prevalence of ET range up to more than 10%. Also called benign essential tremor and familial tremor, ET may not be benign and can result in severe impairment in activities of daily living in some affected individuals. ET manifests as postural and kinetic tremor of the arms and hands; the head and voice are often involved as well (reviewed in Jankovic 2000).

Postural tremor is tremor that appears when a posture is being held against gravity. This tremor is distinguished from the tremor at rest that is characteristic of tremor-dominant PD. Kinetic tremor is tremor that occurs with action or when approximating a target, such as during finger-to-nose testing. Kinetic tremor can be prominent and interfere with eating and drinking. Patients may need to use two hands to hold a cup or write. The tremor may interfere with bringing food to the mouth, holding a soupspoon, or carrying a tray.

The frequency of hand tremor in ET is typically 6–8 Hz; however, the tremor frequency may decrease with age (Bain et al. 2000). Progression may be more rapid in patients with age at onset of more than 60 years and in patients without head tremor. The tremor in ET is commonly symmetric in both upper extremities; however, one arm may be more involved than the other, and even unilateral tremor may occur. Patients may exhibit a "yes-yes," "no-no," or mixed head titubation and may have a tremulous voice as well. A key feature of ET, at least early on, is that the tremor is absent at rest, only occurring during action or when a posture is being held. Later in the course, some resting tremor may appear, but it is always less prominent than the postural or kinetic tremor. There is usually a clear family history of tremor, and often the tremor attenuates with alcohol use, a phenomenon that can contribute to development of alcoholism in susceptible individuals.

The mainstays of medical treatment for ET are propranolol therapy and primidone therapy. Deep brain stimulation targeting the ventral intermediate nucleus of the contralateral thalamus is sometimes helpful in medically refractory cases. Other tremor-related disorders seen in the elderly population include enhanced physiologic tremor (characterized by postural or kinetic tremor that is more prominent than normal physiologic tremor) and orthostatic tremor (a high-frequency, low-amplitude tremor that develops in the legs while the patient is standing still and responds to clonazepam therapy; Myers and Scott 2003).

Dystonia

Dystonia is a fairly common movement disorder that usually begins by middle age and may persist in elderly individuals (Scott 2000). In dystonia, involuntary muscle spasms result in bizarre, sustained postures. These postures initially occur during attempted voluntary movement and may persist at rest. Dystonia can be idiopathic (associated with no identifiable structural abnormality) or secondary (associated with a known structural lesion demonstrated by an imaging study) and can have a delayed onset, appearing after a previous injury (Scott and Jankovic 1996). Dystonia may be focal (affecting one body part), segmental (affecting two or more adjacent body parts), multifocal (affecting two or more nonadjacent body parts), generalized (affecting most of the body, including at least one leg), or hemidystonic (affecting one side of the body). Common examples of focal dystonia include writer's cramp (involuntary, sometimes painful cramping during attempted writing), blepharospasm (spasms resulting in increased, forceful blinking), spasmodic torticollis or cervical dystonia (a disorder in which there is sustained, involuntary twisting or turning of the neck), and oromandibular dystonia (muscle contractions producing involuntary grinding of the teeth or opening of the jaws during attempts to eat or talk). An example of segmental dystonia is craniofacial dystonia, in which both blepharospasm and jaw-closing spasms may occur. Hemidystonia most commonly results from a stroke or structural lesion, such as a mass in the contralateral basal ganglia, often in the putamen.

In an adult or an elderly person, dystonia tends to stay localized in the part of the body first affected, and it is less likely to affect other body parts. Medical treatments include administration of anticholinergic agents such as trihexyphenidyl; however, these medications are poorly tolerated by elderly patients. Other medications used are muscle relaxants such as baclofen and benzodiazepines such as clonazepam. The most effective treatment is often botulinum toxin injections. Dystonia can also be a tardive condition, like tardive dyskinesia (see below), in individuals exposed to dopamine receptor–blocking medications.

Tardive Movement Disorders

The term *tardive movement disorder* refers to hyperkinetic movements that develop in individuals with prolonged exposure to dopamine receptor–blocking medications such as phenothiazine-containing antiemetics and antipsychotic medications. Elderly women taking these medications appear to be most susceptible to tardive movement disorders. Tardive dyskinesia typically manifests as semivoluntary, repetitive oro-bucco-lingual movements. The movements often attenuate temporarily with concentration and typically disappear during sleep. The movements can also involve the head, face, and limbs and may appear choreiform, although they are often more stereotypic and repetitive than the more random movements of classic chorea. Tardive dyskinesia can affect muscles involved in breathing, resulting in respiratory dyskinesia. The term *tardive dystonia* refers to dystonic movements that are associated with chronic use of dopamine receptor–blocking agents and that are more difficult to treat. The sustained abnormal posturing of tardive dystonia can affect the neck in the form of retrocollis (backward displacement of the neck) and limb dystonia. *Akathisia* refers to inner restlessness in an individual treated with dopamine receptor–blocking agents. It manifests as constant squirming and fidgeting (when the person is sitting in a chair, for example).

Treatment for tardive movement disorders involves, whenever possible, first tapering the dose of the offending medication and then discontinuing the drug. Tetrabenazine, a dopamine-depleting agent available outside the United States, is often helpful in suppressing tardive movement disorders, particularly tardive dyskinesia. A newer, atypical antipsychotic medication such as quetiapine can be tried if tetrabenazine is not an option. Botulinum toxin injections are helpful in some patients with bothersome focal dyskinesias.

Chorea

The term *chorea* refers to involuntary, dancelike movements that consist of continuous, random, unpredictable, often twitchlike motions that flow from one body part to another. Chorea can be hard to distinguish from tardive dyskinesia in the absence of a complete history; however, movements in chorea are more random, and movements in tardive dyskinesia tend to be repetitive and stereotyped. Chorea can occur in elderly individuals in association with Huntington's disease, neuroacanthocytosis, overdose of drugs such as amphetamines or stimulants, alcohol intoxication, and metabolic abnormalities such as hyperthyroidism, hypo- or hypernatremia, hypo- or hyperglycemia, hypocalcemia, and hypomagnesemia. The term *hemiballismus* is applied to choreiform throwing or flinging movements affecting one side of the body, and this condition is often associated with a lesion of the contralateral subthalamic nucleus, most commonly due to a stroke. Therapy consists of treating any underlying toxic or metabolic condition and using tetrabenazine or an atypical antipsychotic such as quetiapine.

Tics

Tics are brief, repetitive, semivoluntary, jerklike movements. Vocal tics consist of audible vocalizations, and motor tics consist of rapid movements of the head, face, limbs, and other body parts. Tics can be simple or complex. They can usually be suppressed for a short time, but the patient often builds up an unpleasant sensation in the involved body part and experiences transient relief of the unpleasant sensation by performing the tic once again. The tic disorder—Gilles de la Tourette's syndrome, or Tourette's syndrome—begins in childhood but can persist in adults and the elderly. Tourette's syndrome is often associated with obsessive-compulsive disorder, which can be more disabling than the tics themselves. Other causes of tic disorders in elderly individuals include use of stimulants or other drugs, encephalitis, carbon monoxide poisoning, head trauma, and stroke. Treatments include administration of antipsychotic medications; however, the clinician must be aware of the associated risk of producing a tardive movement disorder, especially in elderly patients. Treatment with tetrabenazine or clonazepam is also helpful in some patients.

Myoclonus

The word *myoclonus* refers to sudden, jerklike or shocklike movements due to activation of affected muscles (positive myoclonus) or to sudden loss of activation of affected muscles (negative myoclonus). The movements are involuntary and can occur randomly or regularly. Myoclonus can arise from dysfunction at multiple levels of the central nervous system, from cortex to brain stem to spinal cord. For example, spinal inflammation from a dermatomal herpes infection (shingles) can result in focal myoclonus in the same dermatome. Negative myoclonus can manifest as asterixis (flapping movements of the hands when the arms are held outstretched with the wrists extended), as seen in hepatic failure. Also, disabling negative myoclonus affecting the legs and trunk on standing can be a consequence of hypoxic or ischemic brain stem injury in elderly patients. Benzodiazepines such as clonazepam, anticonvulsants such as levetiracetam, and piracetam are sometimes beneficial in the treatment of this condition.

Hemifacial Spasm

Hemifacial spasm is another movement disorder that occurs in the elderly population. The disorder consists of simultaneous, involuntary, rapid, jerklike movements of facial muscles on one side of the face. These movements are not painful. Typically, the patient experiences blinking of one eye and synchronous drawing up of the same side of the face. No sensory deficit on the affected side of the face should be present, because this disorder affects only the facial nerve (cranial nerve VII), which provides motor and not sensory innervation to the face. Hemifacial spasm appears to be caused by irritation of this facial nerve. The disorder is sometimes associated with an ectatic, tortuous basilar artery at the level of the pons in the brain stem. Physical contact between the basilar artery and the point where the facial nerve emerges from the pons is thought to produce aberrant, ephaptic nerve transmission in the facial nerve, resulting in transient activation of facial muscles on one side of the face. An ectatic basilar artery can be identified by brain MRI and magnetic resonance angiography (MRA). Anticonvulsants such as carbamazepine and phenytoin are sometimes helpful, and botulinum toxin injections are a common treatment. If medical treatment is insufficient, a neurosurgical procedure to insulate the facial nerve from the basilar artery can be considered.

Psychogenic Movement Disorders

Psychogenic movement disorders are diagnoses of exclusion and most commonly take the form of waxing and waning tremor, dystonia, or myoclonus that attenuates with distraction. The onset of these conditions is often abrupt, and it is often possible to identify periods of normal function between periods of dysfunction. Psychogenic tremor is characterized by tremor that speeds up or slows down in synchrony with repetitive movements of the opposite limb. The movements often respond to positive or negative suggestion, and successful treatment may involve intensive psychiatric or psychological intervention by professionals who are interested in these complex conditions.

Restless Legs Syndrome

Restless legs syndrome, which can occur in elderly persons, is characterized by unpleasant sensations in the legs when the individual is sitting or lying down, particularly when he or she is tired. The patient experiences creeping, crawling sensations under the skin of the calves, and these sensations attenuate only when the patient stands up and walks. No visible abnormal movement need be present, but the unpleasant leg sensations interfere with sleep and can be disabling for that reason. The condition sometimes results from renal failure or from iron deficiency anemia, in which case symptoms improve with successful treatment of the underlying medical condition. A sleep study (polysomnography) may identify periodic leg movements in sleep, which are commonly associated with restless legs syndrome. Use near bedtime of a dopamine agonist, clonazepam, levodopa, or, sometimes, a narcotic such as codeine may be beneficial. Prolonged use of levodopa, however, has been associated with eventual worsening of symptoms.

Conclusion

Movement disorders in the elderly population are to be distinguished from changes associated with normal aging, in which mobility may become somewhat more limited because of a lifetime of wear and tear on muscles, ligaments, bones, and joints. Normal aging includes some slowing of movement, aches and pains, and perhaps stooping. However, clinical experience permits distinguishing these phenomena of aging from neurodegenerative movement disorders. Excessive poverty of movement is indicative of a hypokinetic movement disorder such as PD or another parkinsonian condition. Development of a hyperkinetic movement disorder such as tremor, tics, chorea, or myoclonus cannot be attributed to normal aging and is worthy of further evaluation for the purpose of identifying an underlying, treatable condition.

References

Bain P, Brin M, Deuschl G, et al: Criteria for the diagnosis of essential tremor. Neurology 54:S7, 2000

Chouinard G, Jones B, Remington G, et al: Canadian multicenter placebo-controlled study of fixed doses of risperidone and haloperidol in the treatment of chronic schizophrenic patients. J Clin Psychopharmacol 13:25–40, 1993

de Bruin VMS, Lees AJ, Daniel SE: Diffuse Lewy body disease presenting with supranuclear gaze palsy, parkinsonism, and dementia: a case report. Mov Disord 7:355–358, 1992

Forno LS: Neuropathology of Parkinson's disease. J Neuropathol Exp Neurol 55:259–272, 1996

Foster NL, Wilhelmsen K, Sima AAF, et al: Frontotemporal dementia and parkinsonism linked to chromosome 17: a consensus conference. Participants of the Chromosome 17–Related Dementia Conference. Ann Neurol 41:706–715, 1997

Gelb DJ, Oliver E, Gilman S: Diagnostic criteria for Parkinson's disease. Arch Neurol 56:33–39, 1999

Gibb WRG, Luthert PJ, Marsden CD: Clinical and pathological features of corticobasal degeneration. Adv Neurol 53:51–54, 1990

Golbe LI: Alpha-synuclein and Parkinson's disease. Mov Disord 14:6–9, 1999

Golbe LI, Davis PH: Progressive supranuclear palsy, in Parkinson's Disease and Movement Disorders, 2nd Edition. Edited by Jankovic J, Tolosa E. Baltimore, MD, Williams & Wilkins, 1993, pp 145–161

Jankovic J: Progressive supranuclear palsy: clinical and pharmacologic update. Neurol Clin 2:473–486, 1984

Jankovic J: Essential tremor: clinical characteristics. Neurology 54:S21–S25, 2000

Jankovic J, Friedman DI, Pirozzolo FJ, et al: Progressive supranuclear palsy: motor, neurobehavioral, and neuro-ophthalmic findings. Adv Neurol 53:293–304, 1990

Kraft E, Schwarz J, Trenkwalder C, et al: The combination of hypointense and hyperintense signal changes on T2-weighted magnetic resonance sequences: a specific marker for multiple system atrophy? Arch Neurol 56:225–228, 1999

Lang AE, Lozano AM: Parkinson's disease. First of two parts. N Engl J Med 339:1044–1053, 1998a

Lang AE, Lozano AM: Parkinson's disease. Second of two parts. N Engl J Med 339:1130–1143, 1998b

Litvan I: Progressive supranuclear palsy revisited. Acta Neurol Scand 98:73–84, 1998

Litvan I, Agid Y, Calne D, et al: Clinical research criteria for the diagnosis of progressive supranuclear palsy (Steele-Richardson-Olszewski syndrome): report of the NINDS-SPSP international workshop. Neurology 47:1–9, 1996

Litvan I, Agid Y, Goetz C, et al: Accuracy of the clinical diagnosis of corticobasal degeneration: a clinicopathologic study. Neurology 48:119–125, 1997

Lund and Manchester Groups: Clinical and neuropathological criteria for frontotemporal dementia. J Neurol Neurosurg Psychiatry 57:416–418, 1994

Meltzer HY: The mechanism of action of clozapine in relation to its clinical advantages, in Novel Antipsychotic Drugs. Edited by Meltzer HY. New York, Raven, 1992, pp 1–13

Mendis T, Mohr E, George A, et al: Symptomatic relief from treatment-induced psychosis in Parkinson's disease: an open-label pilot study with remoxipride. Mov Disord 9:197–200, 1994

Mutch WJ, Dingwall-Fordyce I, Downie AW, et al: Parkinson's disease in a Scottish city. Br Med J (Clin Res Ed) 292:534–536, 1986

Myers BH, Scott BL: A case of combined orthostatic tremor and primary gait ignition failure. Clin Neurol Neurosurg 105:277–280, 2003

Quinn NP: Multiple system atrophy, in Movement Disorders 3 (Butterworth-Heinemann International Medical Reviews. Neurology 12). Edited by Marsden CD, Fahn S. Boston, MA, Butterworth-Heinemann, 1994, pp 262–281

Riley DE, Lang AE: Clinical diagnostic criteria, in Corticobasal Degeneration (Advances in Neurology, Vol 82). Edited by Litvan I, Goetz CG, Lang AE. Philadelphia, PA, Lippincott Williams & Wilkins, 2000, pp 29–34

Savoiardo M, Grisoli M, Girotti F: Magnetic resonance imaging in CBD, related atypical parkinsonian disorders, and dementias, in Corticobasal Degeneration (Advances in Neurology, Vol 82). Edited by Litvan I, Goetz CG, Lang AE. Philadelphia, PA, Lippincott Williams & Wilkins, 2000, pp 197–208

Schneider JA, Watts RL, Gearing M, et al: Corticobasal degeneration: neuropathologic and clinical heterogeneity. Neurology 48:959–969, 1997

Scott BL: Evaluation and treatment of dystonia. South Med J 93:746–751, 2000

Scott BL, Jankovic J: Delayed-onset progressive movement disorders after static brain lesions. Neurology 46:68–74, 1996

Shulman LM, Weiner WJ: Multiple-system atrophy, in Movement Disorders: Neurologic Principles and Practice. Edited by Watts RL, Koller WC. New York, McGraw-Hill, 1997, pp 297–306

Shy GM, Drager GA: A neurological syndrome associated with orthostatic hypotension. Arch Neurol 2:511–527, 1960

Steele JC, Richardson JC, Olszewski J: Progressive supranuclear palsy: a heterogeneous degeneration involving the brain stem, basal ganglia and cerebellum, with vertical gaze and pseudobulbar palsy, nuchal dystonia and dementia. Arch Neurol 10:333–359, 1964

Sutcliffe RL, Prior R, Mawby B, et al: Parkinson's disease in the district of the Northampton Health Authority, United Kingdom: a study of prevalence and disability. Acta Neurol Scand 72:363–379, 1985

Wenning GK, Ben Shlomo Y, Magalhaes M, et al: Clinical features and natural history of multiple system atrophy. An analysis of 100 cases. Brain 117:835–845, 1994

CHAPTER 14

Mood Disorders

Harold G. Koenig, M.D., M.H.Sc.

Dan G. Blazer, M.D., Ph.D.

The themes of aging and depression often coalesce. Frequent questions surrounding these themes include the following: Do persons become more depressed as they grow older? Does depression become more difficult to treat with increased age? Is depression more difficult to identify in the older adult? The answers to these questions rest in part with the definition of late-life depression. Depression in late life is not a unitary construct. Depending on how depression is defined, the answers to questions regarding late-life depression vary.

Depression can be construed in at least three ways, each of which has clinical relevance for older adults. First, depression can be viewed as a unitary phenomenon, with the various manifestations of depression forming a continuum. Sir Aubrey Lewis (1934) noted that the various classifications of depression are "nothing more than attempts to distinguish between acute and chronic, mild and severe" (p. 1). In more recent years, Kendell (1976) argued for the unitary view. Although the extremes of the continuum are different, precise boundaries can be found between these extremes. Depression symptom checklists, such as the Zung Self-Rating Depression Scale (Zung 1965), the Center for Epidemiologic Studies Depression Scale (CES-D; Radloff 1977), the Geriatric Depression Scale (Yesavage et al. 1983), and the Brief Depression Scale (Koenig et al. 1995), are therefore useful in determining the degree to which an individual suffers from depression in late life.

Most modern investigators, however, find it difficult to conceive of depression as phenomenologically homogeneous. A categorical approach, as exemplified in DSM-III-R (American Psychiatric Association 1987), DSM-IV (American Psychiatric Association 1994), and DSM-IV-TR (American Psychiatric Association 2000), has been of more interest to modern clinicians. If one views the af-

fective disorders as a group of distinct entities or independent syndromes, with each of the categories being mutually exclusive, diagnosis and management of depression are allied with the traditional medical model. Given the availability of excellent, but potentially dangerous, biological therapies, the categorical approach has been adopted by most geriatric psychiatrists. Specific therapies can be prescribed for distinct diagnostic entities. A radical overhaul has been suggested for the fifth edition of DSM, which is projected to be available in 2007 (McHugh 2001). In the new system, psychiatric disorders would be divided into four broad categories (disease, dimension, behavior, life story), and the focus would be more on the psychological or biological essence of disorders than on clinical appearance.

The third approach to the conceptualization of the depressed elder is a functional approach: when depressive symptoms become so severe that functioning is impaired, the case is considered worthy of clinical attention. Social functioning, especially the performance of role responsibilities, has been targeted as a critical variable in monitoring treatment. Examples of the functional approach can be found in many surveys of community subjects (Langner and Michael 1963; *Multidimensional Functional Assessment* 1978). Functioning is a critical element for family members, who do not view symptom remission alone as an essential marker of improvement but, rather, consider a return to social involvement and improved life satisfaction as critical signs. An older adult who sleeps better, has a better appetite, and ceases to be suicidal may be determined improved by the clinician but little improved by the family, if social isolation and disinterest in the social environment persist after appropriate therapy. The clinician can use Axis V of DSM-IV-TR to partially assess the effect of a disorder on social functioning.

The categorical approach to diagnosis—that is, a focus on Axis I of DSM-IV-TR—is adopted, for the most part, through the remainder of this chapter. Nevertheless, the reader should recognize that other constructs of depression must complement the categorical approach if it is to be effective in the diagnosis and treatment of older adults. Depressive symptoms that do not cluster in such a way that they fit the procrustean bed of a given diagnostic system may still be of clinical significance. Social and physical functioning, both during and after therapy, are at least as important in assessing the success of therapeutic intervention as is the remission of a series of symptoms.

There have been few changes in the categorization of major depression and other affective disorders in the transition from DSM-III-R to DSM-IV (and its text revision, DSM-IV-TR); where changes are relevant, we point them out.

Epidemiology of Late-Life Depression

Prevalence

General comments on the epidemiology of psychiatric disorders in late life are reported in Chapter 2, "Demography and Epidemiology of Psychiatric Disorders in Late Life." Using a community survey, investigators at Duke University Medical Center attempted to untangle the different subtypes of depression in late life (Blazer et al. 1987b). More than 1,300 older adults in urban and rural communities who were age 60 or older were screened for depressive symptomatology. Of the 27% reporting depressive symptoms, 19% had mild dysphoria only. Persons with symptomatic depression—that is, subjects with more severe depressive symptoms—made up 4% of the population. These individuals were primarily experiencing stressors, such as physical illness and stressful life events. Only 2% had a dysthymic disorder, and 0.8% were experiencing a current major depressive episode. No cases of current manic episode were identified. Finally, 1.2% had a mixed depression and anxiety syndrome. These data suggest that the traditional DSM-III-R depression categories do not apply to most depressed older adults in the community.

In a study involving psychiatric inpatients, subjects in midlife and subjects in late life were identified as experiencing a major depressive episode with melancholia (Blazer et al. 1987a). Criterion symptoms of depression and symptoms specifically associated with melancholic or endogenous depression did not differ across age groups. The syndrome of major depression with melan-

cholia is relatively common among older adults in inpatient settings and is easily enough recognized.

How does one reconcile these seemingly disparate results? *Depression in late life* remains a generic term that captures many constructs, some of which are well defined and others of which are ill defined. The burden of depression in the elderly, as indicated by the just-described frequency of significant depressive symptoms in community populations, is unquestioned. Many older persons with atypical presentations of depression do not meet criteria for major depression. Nevertheless, the usual reasons given for not identifying severe depression in an older adult in the clinical setting—pseudodementia, somatization, denial of depressive symptomatology, poor response to antidepressant medication, or masked depression—do not apply to most severely depressed elders, such as melancholic older adults. DSM-III-R and similar nomenclatures may therefore apply to some, but not all, depressive syndromes in late life.

Because of the association between medical illness and depression, many depressed elders may be either in acute-care settings or in nursing homes and thus be unavailable for (or be unable to participate in) community surveys. In contrast to low rates (1%) of major depression among older adults in the community, it has been estimated that depending on the diagnostic scheme, up to 21% of hospitalized elders fulfill criteria for a major depressive episode, and an additional 20%–25% have a minor depression (Koenig et al. 1997). Likewise, rates of major depression among elderly nursing home patients are even higher—exceeding 25% in some studies (Gerety et al. 1994).

Manic episodes in late life are uncommon but not unseen. In a study of 6-month prevalence of psychiatric disorders in three communities, no person older than 65 years, of more than 3,000 elders interviewed, was found to have a current manic episode (Myers et al. 1984). One reason for the very low prevalence in community populations may be the inability of structured instruments to identify the atypical presentation of manic episodes in elderly patients. When mania does occur, the syndrome may be so severe that the elder is hospitalized and therefore would not be located during a community inquiry. Alternatively, manic episodes in later life may present with a mixture of manic, dysphoric, and cognitive symptoms, with euphoria being less common (Post 1978). When mania is associated with significant changes in cognitive function—so-called manic delirium—it may be difficult to distinguish it from organic conditions or schizophrenia (Shulman 1986). Thus, manic episodes may present in an atypical manner that does not allow easy categorization, especially when they have been diagnosed using structured psychiatric interviews administered by lay interviewers, as in the Epidemiologic Catchment Area (ECA) surveys. Despite such considerations, however, the ECA surveys did diagnose bipolar disorder in 9.7% of nursing home patients, which suggests that this setting may have become a dumping ground for such patients (Weissman et al. 1991). In clinical settings, about 10%–25% of geriatric patients with mood disorder have bipolar disorder, and 3%–10% of all older psychiatric patients have this disorder (Wylie et al. 1999; Young and Klerman 1992). About 5% of all individuals admitted as geropsychiatry inpatients present with mania (Yassa et al. 1988).

Snapshot prevalence studies do not adequately represent late-life depression within the context of historical trends. The 20-year follow-up of the Midtown Manhattan Longitudinal Study illustrates the importance of cohort analysis (Srole and Fischer 1980). Nearly 700 of the original 1,660 adults, who were between ages 20 and 59 years at the time of the original study, were reinterviewed 20 years later using an identical instrument. This mental health impairment scale actually assessed primarily depressive symptomatology. Although in the assessments in both 1954 and 1974, the highest rates of mental health impairment were found among the elderly subjects (22% for the 50- to 59-year-olds, compared with 7% for the 20- to 29-year-olds in 1954), the prevalence of mental health impairment did not increase longitudinally with age. For example, from ages 50–59 years to ages 70–79 years, depression remained almost constant (22% in 1954 vs. 18% in 1974). How can these findings be explained? Cohort effects may influence the distribution of depressive symptoms across the life cycle more than may the effects of aging. The burden of depressive symptoms within a birth cohort may remain relatively constant throughout the life cycle.

Mortality

An additional parameter of late-life affective disorders is outcome. The epidemiology of suicide is discussed in Chapter 2, "Demography and Epidemiology of Psychiatric Disorders in Late Life." Examination of the association between depressive symptoms and all-cause mortality among older participants in the ECA study in North Carolina did not reveal a relationship between depressive symptoms and mortality when other known causes of mortality were included in a logistic analysis (Fredman et al. 1989). When age, activities of daily living, gender, and cognitive impairment were controlled, neither the diagnosis of major depression nor the accumulation of significant depressive symptoms at baseline predicted mortal-

ity 2 years after the initial interview in more than 1,600 community respondents at least 60 years old. However, in a more recent, 6-year follow-up of 764 community-dwelling women older than 65 years who were living in the Baltimore, Maryland, area, Fredman et al. (1999) found that the risk of death was 14.5% among women with CES-D scores of 0–1, 24%–28% among women with scores of 2–24, and 47% among those with scores greater than 24. After other variables were controlled, depressive symptoms were determined to be associated with increased mortality only among women in poor health.

In clinical populations, the findings have been more consistent. Murphy and colleagues (1988) examined all-cause mortality in a 4-year follow-up study involving 120 depressed elderly psychiatric inpatients, comparing them with 197 age- and gender-matched control subjects. Among the depressed women, mortality was twice the expected rate; among the men, it was three times the expected rate. Older men with physical health problems and depression were significantly more likely to die than were similarly aged, physically ill, nondepressed men. A study involving elderly veterans hospitalized with medical illness found a significantly higher mortality during hospitalization for 41 patients who were depressed, compared with 41 nondepressed patients matched for age, gender, and severity and type of medical illness (Koenig et al. 1989). Rovner and colleagues (1991) also found greater death rates among elderly nursing home patients with depression. Several recent studies involving medically ill elderly patients likewise found greater mortality among those with depression (Arfken et al. 1999; Covinsky et al. 1999; Black and Markides 1999).

These studies indicate higher rates of mortality for depressed elderly patients (men in particular) with concurrent physical health problems; in clinical samples, this relationship persisted after important covariates were controlled. The association between late-life depression and mortality is intuitively attractive, because older persons are thought to experience loss of meaningful roles and emotional support through retirement, death of friends or a spouse, decreased economic and material well-being, and increased isolation and loneliness (Atchley 1972; Fassler and Gavira 1978). When poor physical health compounds these age-related changes, depression may be particularly prone to affect health outcomes.

Prognosis

Until recently, long-term psychiatric follow-up investigations involving survivors of severe episodes of late-life depression were relatively scarce, given the frequency and clinical importance of the disorder. The typical course of major depression throughout the life cycle is remission and relapse. In patients who have a history of recurrent episodes, new episodes tend to be associated with similar symptoms and to last about as long as prior episodes. Classic studies of depression suggest that the duration of major depression throughout the life cycle is approximately 9 months if untreated (Dunner 1985). As individuals age, however, they may experience episodes more frequently, and these episodes can merge into a chronic condition.

Post (1972) argued that the episodes of depression in late life may last longer than at earlier stages of the life cycle. After observing 92 depressed elders for 3 years, he determined that only 26% completely recovered from their index episode, whereas 37% had further attacks with good recoveries and 37% experienced recurrent attacks on a baseline of chronic depression or remained continuously ill. Murphy and co-workers (Murphy (1983), observing 124 depressed elders for 1 year, found that 35% experienced a complete recovery, 19% recovered but later relapsed, 29% were continuously ill, and 17% either had dementia or died. Patients with delusional depression had particularly poor outcomes, with only 1 in 10 recovering. Recently, Denihan et al. (2000) followed 127 depressed community-dwelling elderly individuals for 3 years and found that 30% died, 34% had persistent or relapsing case-level depression, and 25% had other case- or sub-case-level mental illnesses. In that study, only 10% recovered completely by the end of the follow-up period.

Baldwin and Jolley (1986) followed 100 elderly psychiatric inpatients with severe unipolar depression for 3–8 years. Of these patients, 60% remained well throughout or had relapses with complete recovery, and only 7% had continuous depression. Likewise, in a direct comparison of middle-aged and elderly patients hospitalized for major depression, little difference was found between middle-aged and older adults in recovery (Blazer et al. 1992). Of the 44 older adults (at least 60 years old), 48% had not recovered from the depressive episode leading to hospitalization, 27% had recovered completely from the index episode but experienced a recurrence of another episode of major depression, and 25% had recovered completely without a recurrence. Of the 35 middle-aged patients, 46% had not recovered from the index episode, 45% had recovered completely but experienced a recurrence of another episode, and 9% had recovered completely and remained recovered. Significant depressive symptoms at the time of follow-up (a score of 16 or higher on the CES-D) were reported by 59% of the elderly subjects but only 43% of the middle-aged subjects.

These 1- to 2-year follow-up findings suggest that in terms of recovery and remission, older adults do not differ from their middle-aged counterparts. If they do recover, however, elders appear to experience residual depressive symptoms.

Cole et al. (1999) conducted a meta-analysis of 12 studies and estimated that 33% of the study subjects were well, 33% were depressed, and 21% had died by 24 months of follow-up. Physical illness, disability, cognitive impairment, and more severe depression were associated with worse outcomes. These studies involved depressed elderly persons living in the community and being seen by primary care physicians in outpatient settings. Lack of specialized psychiatric care may have been a factor in the poor prognosis of these groups.

Most clinicians and clinical investigators report that more than 70% of elderly patients with major depression who are treated with antidepressant medication (at an adequate dose for a sufficient time) recover from the index episode of depression. Reynolds and colleagues (1992) reported that treatment of physically healthy depressed elders with combined interpersonal psychotherapy and nortriptyline was associated with response rates nearing 80%. In a long-term outcome study of treatment-resistant depression in older adults, 47% of patients were clinically improved 15 months after treatment with an antidepressant or electroconvulsive therapy (ECT); at 4 years of follow-up, that percentage had increased to 71% (Stoudemire et al. 1993). These optimistic results are tempered by the fact that physical illness and impaired cognition may complicate both the course of depression and response to treatment (Baldwin and Jolley 1986; Cole 1983; Koenig et al. 1997; Murphy et al. 1988). Once an older patient has experienced one or more moderate to severe episodes of major depression, he or she may need to continue antidepressant therapy permanently, to minimize the risk of relapse (Greden 1993; Old Age Depression Interest Group 1993).

Persons with a dysthymic disorder (depressive neurosis) experience a more chronic course than do persons with major depression. By DSM-IV-TR definition, an individual's depressive symptoms must last at least 2 years for a dysthymic disorder diagnosis to be made. An undetermined percentage (as high as 4%–8%) of community-dwelling (and possibly institutionalized) elders experience moderately severe depressive symptoms for more than 2 years, although they report intermittent periods, lasting longer than a few days, of relative freedom from depressive symptoms. The severity of their symptoms is not great enough to meet the criteria for major depression, and the intermittent symptom-free periods disqualify them from the diagnosis of dysthymic disorder. Nevertheless, these individuals experience a chronic depression. Other older adults experience chronic depressions secondary to medical or even psychiatric disease—for example, alcoholism and anxiety disorders such as obsessive-compulsive disorder. Each of these disorders contributes to residual depression in ambulatory elderly individuals.

Factors associated with improved outcome in late-life depression include a history of recovery from previous episodes, a family history of depression, female gender, extroverted personality, current or recent employment, absence of substance abuse, no history of major psychiatric disorder, less severe depressive symptomatology, and absence of major life events and serious medical illness (Baldwin and Jolley 1986; Cole et al. 1999; Post 1972). The results of a number of studies suggest a relationship between social support during an index episode and outcome in psychological distress and depression. Intuition suggests that adequate support should enhance recovery from a severe or moderately severe psychiatric disorder such as major depression. In a study involving 493 community respondents, Holahan and Moos (1981) found that decreases in social support of family and in work environments were related to increases in psychological maladjustment over a 1-year follow-up period.

In a similar study, 104 inpatients with a diagnosis of major depression were followed for 1–2 years after their hospitalization (George et al. 1989). Fifty-three of these patients were age 60 or older. At follow-up, 33 reported that they had recovered from the index episode, and they scored lower than 10 on the CES-D. Subjects who reported an adequate social support network at the time of the index depressive episode were 2.3 times more likely to recover than those who reported an impaired social network (44% vs. 19%). In a multiple regression analysis, social support remained a predictor of recovery from major depression when age, gender, and the initial CES-D score were controlled. More recently, Dew and colleagues (1997) examined predictors of recovery over 18 weeks in 95 depressed persons at least 60 years old. These investigators found that higher levels of acute and chronic stressors, younger age at first depressive episode, endogenous depression, higher current anxiety, older current age, and poorer social supports predicted poorer responses.

Coping behavior may also affect the prognosis of late-life depression. One of the coping behaviors most commonly used by this generation of older adults is religious involvement. In a study involving 100 middle-aged or elderly adults, one-third of men and nearly two-thirds of women used religious cognitions or behaviors to help them cope with a stressful period (Koenig et al. 1988). A number of investigators have reported inverse associations between religious coping and depressive symptoms in older adults with or without medical illness (Braam et al. 1997b; Idler 1987; Koenig et al. 1992a; Pressman et al. 1990). A study involving 850 hospitalized medically ill elders found that those using religion to cope were less likely to be depressed and more likely to experience improvement in depressive symptoms over time (Koenig et al. 1992a). Religious involvement also appears to be a predictor of faster recovery from depression in both community-dwelling and clinical samples of older adults (Braam et al. 1997a; Koenig et al. 1998).

Personality pathology is another measurable phenomenon that is known to affect the outcome of major depression (Weissman et al. 1978). Unfortunately, there are no published reports of personality as a predictor of major depression outcome in elderly patients. In addition, studies with mixed-age samples have generally been confounded by the interaction of depressive symptomatology and personality variables at baseline assessment—that is, a depressed affect may influence the underlying personality. Given the stability of personality in late life, longitudinal studies of relationships between personality and both onset and outcome of major depression would be most helpful.

The outcome of bipolar disorder in elderly patients remains virtually unknown. In a long-term follow-up study involving 500 patients in Iowa, Winokur (1975) found a tendency for bipolar disorder to occur in clusters over time and speculated that early-onset bipolar illness may "burn itself out" in time. Shulman and Post (1980) studied elderly patients with bipolar disorder and found that only 8% had their first episode of mania before age 40. In a review of records of a small number of untreated patients with severe and prolonged bipolar disorder, Cutler and Post (1982) found a tendency toward more rapid recurrences late in the illness, with decreasing periods of normality. In other words, if bipolar disorder reemerges in the later years, the episodes of mania—or mania mixed with depression—may once again cluster, just as the disorder typically clusters at earlier periods of life. Most clinicians who have worked with patients with bipolar disorder in late life recognize the tendency of these disorders to recur frequently for a time, only to remit for an extended period.

Ameblas (1987) emphasized a relationship between life events and onset of mania, noting that stressful events were more likely to precede early-onset mania than late-onset mania. Likewise, Shulman (1989) stressed that increased cerebral vulnerability due to organic insults (stroke, head trauma, other brain insults) played a stronger role than life events in precipitating late-onset mania (a factor that may also play a role in treatment resistance). Young and Klerman (1992) emphasized the low rates of familial affective disorder and the increased frequency of certain diseases and drug use associated with late age at onset.

Controversy exists over whether age at onset of first manic episode affects response to treatment. Glasser and Rabins (1984) described no significant age-related differences in presentation or treatment response. Young and Falk (1989) reported that late-onset mania was associated with lower activity level, lower sexual drive, and less-disturbed thought processes; however, they also found that older age was associated with longer hospitalization, greater residual psychopathology, and poorer response to pharmacotherapy. Eastham et al. (1998) suggested that elderly patients with bipolar disorder often require lithium doses that are 25%–50% lower than those used in younger patients. Data on the use of valproic acid in elderly patients with this disorder are limited but encouraging. There is almost no information on the use of carbamazepine or other drugs in late-life bipolar disorder. ECT has been reported to be well tolerated and effective in the treatment of these patients (Eastham et al. 1998).

Risk Factors

The etiology of late-life affective disorders is undoubtedly multifactorial. Twin and family studies, along with studies focusing on molecular genetics, provide strong evidence for a heritable contribution to the etiology of major depression and bipolar disorder (Egeland et al. 1987; Slater and Cowie 1971). Evidence that these genetic factors weigh heavily in the etiology of bipolar disorders in late life is virtually nonexistent, although the biological nature of this disorder would suggest some genetic contribution. Evidence from studies of unipolar depression in late life suggests that the genetic contribution is weaker in late-life depression than in depression at earlier stages of the life cycle (Hopkinson 1964; Mendlewicz 1976; Schulz 1951). For example, Hopkinson (1964) found that the risk for immediate relatives of patients with onset of depression after age 50 was 8.3%, compared with 20.1% for relatives of patients with onset before age 50. Likewise, Stenstedt (1959) found that the risk of affective disorder among relatives of probands who became ill for the first time at age 60 or later was 4%–5%, higher than expected but lower than the risk among relatives of probands who developed bipolar disorder earlier in life.

Associated with the genetic predisposition for depression is the fact that major depression is more common in women (Myers et al. 1984). Most studies that consider the distribution of major depression across the life span confirm the persistence of the 2:1 ratio of women to men into late life. However, there is no evidence for a genetic predisposition—that is, a sex-linked mode of inheritance—that would favor women in the onset of major depression. Nevertheless, even in the best-controlled studies, the gender difference in the prevalence of the more severe depressions persists. The operable factor or factors persist into the later years. It is possible, however, that women are more likely to admit and complain about their dysphoric feelings than are men, who are more likely to deny feelings and instead act them out (such as through alcoholism or suicide).

Another contributing factor to late-life depression may be selective changes that occur in the activity and metabolism of neurotransmitters with aging. For example, D.S. Robinson et al. (1971) analyzed the concentrations of norepinephrine and serotonin in the hindbrains of 55 psychiatrically healthy subjects who died at various ages. Concentrations of both neurotransmitters decreased with age, but levels of the metabolite 5-hydroxyindoleacetic acid (5-HIAA) and the enzyme monoamine oxidase were found to increase with age.

Dysregulation of the hypothalamic-pituitary-adrenal (HPA) axis is also thought to contribute to a predisposition for depression. An association between increased cortisol concentrations and depression has been recognized for many years: there is an increase throughout the 24-hour circadian excretion of cortisol in depressed patients (Sachar 1975). This finding led Carroll et al. (1981) to propose the dexamethasone suppression test (DST) as a laboratory test for melancholic depression. In a large study involving men and women ages 20–78 years, Rosenbaum et al. (1984) found that 18% of persons older than 65 years were nonsuppressors of cortisol after administration of dexamethasone, compared with 9.1% of younger subjects. Whether this higher prevalence of nonsuppression reflects an increased propensity of older persons for dysregulation of the HPA axis, or whether it may result from difficulty in absorbing or metabolizing dexamethasone, remains to be discovered.

Dysregulation of the thyroid axis and of growth hormone release has also been implicated in the etiology of depression in later life. Blunted responses of thyroid-stimulating hormone (TSH) to thyrotropin-releasing hormone (TRH) are found in many healthy elderly subjects (Snyder and Utiger 1972) and in depressed patients (Targum et al. 1982). Secretion of growth hormone in elderly individuals occurs only during sleep and may cease altogether (Finkelstein et al. 1972). Drugs known to stimulate α-adrenoreceptors, such as clonidine, also affect the release of growth hormone, a response that has been shown to be blunted in patients with endogenous depression (Checkley et al. 1981).

Structural brain changes have also been found in geriatric patients with depression and in those with bipolar disorder. Alexopoulos and colleagues (1997) and Hickie and Scott (1998) reviewed the literature on vascular changes associated with geriatric depression and suggested that preventing these changes may help prevent this disorder. Disruption of prefrontal systems or their modulating pathways by single lesions or by an accumulation of lesions exceeding a threshold is hypothesized to be the central mechanism. However, Stewart and colleagues (2001) recently challenged the hypothesis that vascular disorders are a cause of late-life depression. In their study involving 287 community-based Caribbean-born adults ages 55–75 years, vascular risk factors were not associated with depression. Likewise, Lyness and colleagues (2000) found no association between cerebrovascular disease and depressive symptoms after controlling for medical illness burden in a sample of 247 older primary care patients followed for 1 year.

With regard to bipolar disorder, Young et al. (1999) completed brain computed tomography scans in 30 geriatric patients with mania and in 18 age-matched control subjects. Manic patients had significantly greater cortical sulcal widening and lateral ventricle–brain ratio scores compared with control subjects. Cortical sulcal widening was associated with age at illness onset and age at first manic episode.

Despite these numerous neurotransmitter, neuroendocrine, and structural changes that are common to old age and depressive illness, the relatively low prevalence of major depression and bipolar disorder in late life militates against the assumption that older persons are uniquely predisposed to melancholic or endogenous depression. Thus, protective factors yet to be discovered may also be operative in late life.

A relatively new putative contributor to the etiology of depressive disorders is desynchronization of circadian rhythms. The cyclicity of depressive disorders suggests an underlying disruption of the normal biochemical and physiological circadian rhythms. Vogel et al. (1980) noted that the clinical features of depression, especially insomnia and diurnal variation of mood, suggest abnormalities in biological rhythms. The disruption of the sleep cycle with age (though this is the only circadian rhythm known to be dramatically affected by age) suggests the possibility that circadian problems contribute to the etiology of depression in late life. As age increases, total sleep time gradually diminishes and sleep continuity decreases (Kupfer 1984; Ulrich et al. 1980). Endocrine secretion patterns, also associated with depression, are known to be less affected by the aging process (Lakatua et al. 1984).

Finally, social factors must be considered in the development of a risk model for depression in late life. Pfifer and Murrell (1986) examined the additive and interactive roles of six sociodemographic factors—three being from the domain of social resources and three being categories of life events—in the development of depressive symptoms. In a probability sample of more than 1,200 persons age 55 or older, 66 developed significant depressive symptoms (as measured by the CES-D) 6 months after an initial evaluation. Health and social support played both an additive and an interactive role in the onset of depressive symptoms, life events had weak effects, and sociodemographic factors did not contribute to depression onset. A weak support network in the presence of poor physical health placed older persons at an especially high risk for depressive symptoms. It must be recognized, however, that the occurrence of depressive symptoms is not analogous to the onset of a major depressive episode. Although the relationship between stressful life events and the onset of major depression across the life cycle has been established in a number of cross-sectional studies (Lloyd 1980), the relationship weakens when persons are studied longitudinally, as was observed in the study by Pfifer and Murrell (1986).

The interaction between social support and depression is more complex. Social support may contribute to the onset of major depression, it may contribute to the outcome of major depression, or it may be affected by depressive symptoms. By studying 331 community subjects selected at random, Blazer (1983) tested the hypothesis that a major depressive disorder contributes to a decline in social support. Impaired support was associated with the presence of major depressive disorder at baseline. Thirty months later, however, the surviving subjects whose social supports had improved were nearly three times more likely to have been depressed earlier than were subjects whose social supports did not improve. In other words, major depressive disorder was a significant predictor of improvement in supports at follow-up.

Diagnosis and Differential Diagnosis of Late-Life Affective Disorders

Four clinical entities listed under the mood disorders in DSM-IV-TR are relevant to depression in elderly patients: 1) bipolar I disorder (manic, depressed, and mixed) and bipolar II disorder; 2) major depressive disorder (single episode, recurrent, with or without melancholia, and with or without psychotic features); 3) dysthymic disorder; and 4) depressive disorder not otherwise specified (NOS), previously called atypical depression. Depressive symptoms are likewise present in other DSM-IV-TR disorders, such as bereavement, adjustment disorder with depressed mood, substance-induced mood disorder, and mood disorder due to a general medical condition. In still other psychiatric disorders, such as organic psychiatric disorders, paranoid disorders, sleep disorders, and hypochondriasis, depressive symptomatology is a central component of the clinical picture on occasion.

Bipolar Disorder

For a diagnosis of bipolar I disorder to be made, the patient must have experienced at least one manic episode. Bipolar II disorder involves recurrent episodes of major depression and at least one hypomanic episode (that does not meet the full criteria for a manic episode). For a diagnosis of manic episode to be made, at least three classic manic symptoms—such as overactivity, pressure of speech, distractibility, decreased sleep (without feeling a need for sleep), overspending, and grandiosity—must be present. Mood, however, can be either elevated or irritable and may be labile or mixed in the affective presentation (four of the aforementioned symptoms are required, however, if mood is only irritable).

Post (1978) found that most elderly patients with a bipolar disorder exhibited a depressive admixture with manic symptomatology. Spar et al. (1979) reported that manic elders are atypical in presentation, with dysphoric mood and denial of classic manic symptoms. As noted earlier, Shulman (1986) described the special problem of manic delirium. When an individual is experiencing a full-blown manic episode, cognitive function is difficult to test, yet perseverative behavior, catatonia-like symptoms, and even negativistic symptoms may emerge. The patient in manic delirium may demonstrate the delirium-like symptom of picking at imaginary objects. Differentiating a manic episode from an agitated depressive episode is often not possible without a thorough examination of the longitudinal course and therapeutic response to medications. In fact, more and more evidence suggests that mixed episodes (with both manic and depressive symptoms) may be the rule rather than the exception (American Psychiatric Association 2000, p. 363).

Major Depressive Disorder

First-onset episodes of major depression in late life are common and often go untreated for months or even years. For this reason, many investigators have suggested

that late-life depression is masked (Davies 1965; Lesse 1974; Salzman and Shader 1972). Some studies, however, suggest that older persons admit many feelings of sadness on self-rating scales for depression (Epstein 1976; Zung and Green 1972). In a study involving hospitalized patients with a diagnosis of major depressive episodes with melancholia, the criterion symptoms of depression and symptoms specifically associated with melancholia (or endogenous depression) did not differ between individuals in midlife and those in late life (Blazer et al. 1987a). Melancholic depression was relatively frequently identified in elderly patients and was symptomatically similar to that found in persons in middle age. Community surveys confirm that major depressive disorder is identified in elderly persons when usual case-finding methods are applied across the life cycle (Meyers et al. 1984). Nevertheless, there is still some concern, based on poor correlations between observer- and self-rated symptom scores, that elderly individuals (elderly African-American men, in particular) may conceal or deny symptoms on self-report (Koenig et al. 1992b). Thus, considerable effort at symptom elicitation may be required to obtain an accurate assessment.

Seasonal Affective Disorder

Variants of classic major depression also occur in elderly individuals. One such variant is seasonal affective disorder (Jacobsen et al. 1987). Diagnostic criteria for seasonal affective disorder include a history of depression fulfilling DSM-IV-TR criteria for major depression (as part of either major depressive disorder or bipolar disorder); a history of at least 2 consecutive years of fall or winter depressive episodes remitting in the spring or summer; and the absence of other major psychiatric disorders or psychosocial explanations for the seasonal mood changes. Light therapy, in which high-intensity light (10,000 lux) is used to approximate the visual experience of a sunny day (usually in the morning), and regular exposure to sunlight through walks in the late afternoon have proved to be of some value in the treatment of patients with these disorders. Recent studies suggest that institutionalized older adults with depression may be particularly responsive to light therapy (Sumaya et al. 2001).

Psychotic Depression

Late-onset psychotic depression deserves special attention. Meyers et al. (1984) studied the prevalence of delusions in 50 patients hospitalized for endogenous major depression. Depressed patients with illness onset at age 60 or later had delusions more frequently than did those with earlier onset. Individuals with delusional depression tended to be older and to respond to ECT, as opposed to tricyclic antidepressants (TCAs). Delusions of persecution or of having an incurable illness are more common than delusions associated with guilt. If guilt predominates the delusional picture, it usually involves some relatively trivial episode that occurred many years before the onset of the depressive episode, was forgotten over time, but is presently viewed as a major problem (Bridges 1986). For example, a one-time sexual liaison, forgotten or forgiven by the spouse, is resurrected by a patient with a fear of an ongoing venereal disease or cancer or is associated with chronic and severe pain. Nihilistic delusions (delusions of nothingness) may occur more commonly in late life. Focus on the abdomen is common in an elderly patient with a delusional or psychotic depression. Hallucinations are uncommon, however.

More recently, Thakur et al. (1999) compared the clinical, demographic, and social characteristics of psychotic and nonpsychotic depression in a tertiary care sample of 674 elderly and younger patients. In this study, younger age, psychomotor retardation, guilt, feelings of worthlessness, a history of delusions in the past, and increased suicidal ideation and intent were found more commonly in psychotic than in nonpsychotic patients, and these associations were largely confirmed when sociodemographic variables were controlled. Psychotic depression also tended to be associated with poor social support and, not surprisingly, bipolar illness. Cerebrovascular risk factors did not differ significantly between psychotic and nonpsychotic patients. The weakness of this study is that it dealt with hospitalized patients, not a population-based sample.

Dysthymic Disorder

Every clinician who has worked with elderly patients has observed significant and unremitting depressive symptoms associated with apparently psychosocial causes. Verwoerdt (1976) suggested that "reactive depressions" become more frequent with age (such as the depression associated with bereavement), whereas dysthymic disorder seems to be less frequent in the later part of the life cycle. However, community data suggest that the prevalence of dysthymic disorder in elderly persons is lower (but not dramatically lower) than the prevalence of major depression in this age group (Myers et al. 1984).

The psychological mechanisms of late-life dysthymic disorder usually do not include the classic mechanism of dysthymia—that is, self-reproach, guilt, and the turning inward of hostile feelings toward loss. Cath (1965) noted that manifest guilt in older persons is less prevalent, al-

though reaction to loss is a common factor. Busse et al. (1954) suggested that in elderly individuals, introjection is seldom a mechanism for developing depression. Instead, late-life depression is associated with a loss of self-esteem that results from the older adult's inability to satisfy needs and drives or to defend himself or herself against threats to security. Levin (1965) noted the role of restraint as a mechanism in the neurotic depressions of later life. Although sexual satisfaction and interest in sexuality continue to be important for the older adult, sexual drive, though persistent, may not at times be as easily mobilized into behavior. Restraint may derive from either physical problems or lack of an available partner.

Other investigators have emphasized the cultural factors that may contribute to a dysthymic disorder in late life. Wigdor (1980) noted that the major resources in today's culture lead to the development of habit patterns that emphasize activity and productivity—that is, Western society is an achievement-oriented society. With retirement from the workforce and cessation of parenting responsibilities, many older adults find that recognition, self-esteem, and confidence are withdrawn. These needs are not easily substituted. Erikson (1950) suggested that the primary developmental task for late life is the acquisition of integrity and that the means for achieving integrity is to resolve developmental crises that have persisted throughout the life cycle. In other words, striving for industry and generativity may continue to be important for the older adult. If the opportunities for realizing these productive urges are unavailable, or if the elder cannot reconcile previous generative disappointments, despair ensues.

Lazarus and Weinberg (1980), emphasizing the role of narcissistic pathology in the etiology of late-life depression, noted that narcissism may manifest itself in

> recurring depressions or defensive grandiosity in response to minor slights or disappointments, self-consciousness, overdependence on approval from others for maintenance of self-esteem, and the transitory periods of fragmentation and discohesiveness of the self. (p. 435)

Associated with the depressive symptoms are an over-concern with physical appearance, possessions, and past accomplishments, and the seeking of approval and reassurance from others.

In summary, although dysthymic disorders are no more common in late life than at other stages of the life cycle, late-life dysthymic disorders are to be expected, given the psychological tasks that older adults face and a social environment that may restrain and devalue elders. That elderly individuals maintain a sense of satisfaction and fulfillment despite these inevitable losses and responses from others is a testimony to the resilience of older adults and to the psychological integration that permits a mature completion of life's developmental tasks.

Some recent work suggests that dysthymic disorder in older persons may be different from that in younger persons. Devanand et al. (2000) examined 76 outpatients, age 60 or older, who had DSM-IV-TR dysthymic disorder. They found that less than one-third of patients had a diagnosable personality disorder. Personality disorder was associated with an earlier age at onset of depressive illness, a greater lifetime history of comorbid Axis I disorders, greater severity of depressive symptoms, and lower socioeconomic status. The most common personality disorders were the obsessive-compulsive and avoidant types—the personality disorders most commonly found in elderly patients with major depression. The late onset of dysthymia in many of the patients in the study, and the lack of psychiatric comorbidity, caused the authors to conclude that dysthymia in elderly individuals is different from dysthymia in younger persons.

Depressive Disorder Not Otherwise Specified

Another subtype of depression in elderly individuals is codified in DSM-IV-TR as depressive disorder NOS. This subtype of depression (called atypical depression in DSM-III [American Psychiatric Association 1980]) is more often intermittent and unexplained by psychosocial or clear biological factors. Two subcategories of depressive disorder NOS empirically capture the symptom pattern frequently seen by clinicians who work with depressed elders. First, the syndrome may fulfill the criteria for dysthymic disorder; however, there are intermittent periods of normal mood lasting more than a few months. The dysphoric older adult reports prolonged periods of depression, usually lasting for months but not extending for the entire 2 years required for a DSM-IV-TR diagnosis of dysthymic disorder. Other elders meet the second criterion for depressive disorder NOS: a brief episode of depression that does not meet the criteria for major depression and is apparently not a reaction to psychosocial stress (and therefore cannot be classified as an adjustment disorder). These episodes do not last the full 2 weeks required for a DSM-IV-TR diagnosis of major depressive disorder. Nevertheless, the symptoms can be moderately severe and most troubling to the older adult.

The possibility that pharmacological intervention will be effective in treating elders with depressive disorder NOS cannot be eliminated. Nevertheless, the difficulty in describing the heterogeneous phenomenology of the depressive syndromes in this category must be overcome if effective drug trials are to be implemented.

DSM-IV-TR includes the category "minor depressive disorder" in its appendix (American Psychiatric Association 2000, pp. 775–777). Minor depression is identical to major depressive disorder except that there are fewer symptoms (more than one but fewer than four additional symptoms besides depressed mood or anhedonia) and less impairment.

Bereavement

Bereavement is a universal human experience and therefore cannot properly be classified as a psychiatric disorder. Primary care physicians are likely to encounter the normal symptoms of grief, but these symptoms may be poorly recognized as such by the bereaved elder. Lindemann (1944), for example, suggested that the normal symptoms of bereavement include sensations of somatic distress such as tightness in the throat, shortness of breath, sighing respirations, lassitude, and loss of appetite. The bereaved are preoccupied with the image of the deceased and frequently can identify events about which they report guilt (often guilt at not having met the needs of the deceased). The grieving are often irritable and hostile and change their usual patterns of conduct. These behavior changes are disturbing to the family and include a pressure of speech, restlessness, an inability to sit still, and an inability to initiate and maintain usual activities. Pathological grief, in contrast, is delayed (an apparent denial of the loss) and/or distorted. Overactivity without a sense of loss, acquisition of symptoms of the last illness of the deceased, frank psychosomatic illness, an alteration of relationships with family and friends, hostility toward specific persons (not uncommonly, family members), and persistent loss of patterns of social interaction can be seen.

Uncomplicated bereavement is usually characterized by a symptom picture of major depression, yet the syndrome is recognized by the older adult as normal for the occasion and does not seriously interfere with necessary functioning. In DSM-IV-TR, the category of uncomplicated bereavement is designated for virtually all symptoms of depression experienced during the first 2 months after the loss, with the possible exception of extreme feelings of worthlessness or active suicidal ideation; any person exhibiting the full symptom picture of major depression at least 2 months after the death is considered to have a major depressive disorder warranting treatment (American Psychiatric Association 2000). For additional discussion of bereavement, see Chapter 19, "Bereavement and Adjustment Disorders."

Adjustment Disorder With Depressed Mood

Among the common presentations of depression in late life is depressed mood and expressions of hopelessness as a reaction to an identifiable stressor. The DSM-IV-TR category of adjustment disorder with depressed mood is reserved for those individuals who exhibit a maladaptive reaction to an identifiable stressor. The relationship of the syndrome to the stressful event is clear. Stressors for older adults include life events such as marital problems, difficulty with children, loss of a social role, and an ill-advised change of residence. Retirement is usually not a source of excessive stress for the older adult. Therefore, the onset of significant depressive symptomatology and withdrawal from activities after retirement may indicate a true adjustment disorder. Of much greater frequency, however, is the development of depressive symptomatology secondary to a physical illness. When an episode of depression accompanies a physical illness, and the level of symptoms dramatically exceeds the expected level, a diagnosis of either adjustment disorder or mood disorder due to a general medical condition is indicated.

Mood Disorder Due to a General Medical Condition

Called organic mood syndrome in DSM-III-R, the essential feature of mood disorder due to a general medical condition is a disturbance in mood resembling a major depressive episode caused by a specific organic factor. If that organic factor is a drug, alcohol, or another intoxicant, the syndrome is called substance-induced mood disorder. The toxic factors that most commonly cause depressive symptoms in older adults are medications. Agents frequently prescribed to older adults that can precipitate depressive symptoms include β-blockers, benzodiazepines, clonidine, reserpine, methyldopa, and even TCAs. Withdrawal of these agents produces a dramatic improvement in symptoms, although both patient and clinician may not associate these medications with the onset of the symptoms. Mild cognitive impairment is often observed in conjunction with the change in mood. Fearfulness, anxiety, irritability, and excessive somatic concerns may accompany the depressive symptoms as well.

Metabolic disorders induce appreciable depressive symptoms, and these are properly classified in the category of mood disorder due to a general medical condition. For example, hyperthyroidism and hypothyroidism are known to be associated with depressive features. These disorders are included in the discussion of physical illnesses that may contribute to a depressive episode (see "Depression and Medical Illness").

Depression and Medical Illness

Included in the category of mood disorder due to a general medical condition are depressive disorders that have been associated with a variety of physical illnesses, among them cardiovascular disease (Glassman and Shapiro 1998; Musselman et al. 1998), endocrine disturbances (Anderson et al. 2001), Parkinson's disease (Zesiewicz et al. 1999), stroke (Dam 2001), cancer (Spiegel 1996), chronic pain (Fifield et al. 1998), chronic fatigue syndrome (Kruesi et al. 1989), and fibromyalgia (Okifuji et al. 2000). As noted previously, depressive symptoms and disorders are common findings in surveys of general medical inpatients (Koenig et al. 1991, 1997; Schwab et al. 1965). Controversy continues over the degree to which acute or chronic medical illnesses cause depression because of direct physiological effects on the brain or because of a psychological reaction to the disability and other life changes evoked by these illnesses (Koenig 1991).

The association between depression and *hypothyroidism* has been well established (Pies 1997). Although the profoundly life-threatening symptoms of myxedema—stupor or coma—are rarely missed in diagnosis, less severe symptoms and signs are common with normal aging and major depression. These include constipation, cold intolerance, psychomotor retardation, decreased exercise tolerance, and cognitive changes, as well as flat affect. Laboratory evaluation will generally reveal decreased thyroxine and increased serum TSH concentrations. If these laboratory findings are obtained, intervention for the thyroid difficulty must precede intervention for the flat affect.

Depressive symptoms have also been associated with both the development and outcome of *cancer*. Early in modern medicine, Guy (1759) published his opinion that women with melancholia were more prone to develop breast cancer. Whitlock and Sisking (1979) studied 39 men and 90 women age 40 or older who had a primary diagnosis of depression. The subjects were followed for 28 months to 4 years. During the follow-up period, 9 men and 9 women died; 6 of these individuals died of cancer—a significantly higher number than would be expected. Depression may also result from a direct effect on the brain of neurohumoral substances released from the tumor (pancreatic cancer), or as a reaction to the diagnosis of cancer and the morbidity that ensues.

Physical functioning is highly correlated with depression in cancer patients. In one study (Bukberg et al.

1984), among patients with a Karnofsky score of 40 or less (that is, patients who were most disabled), almost 80% had major depression, whereas only 23% of those who scored 60 or better (that is, had moderate to good function) had major depression. Lower rates of depression (5%–13%) are found among ambulatory outpatients with cancer (Koenig and Blazer 1992). Many studies documenting high rates of depression in patients with cancer are controversial because they often involve patients referred for treatment of cancer, who may have more advanced or complicated illness. It is important that myths about depression and cancer be dispelled. One myth is that all cancer patients are depressed; another is that physicians should not bother to treat depression, because such patients should be depressed. In fact, when cancer patients become depressed, mortality may increase. With regard to hospitalized elders with cancer, at least one study has shown substantially higher mortality in cancer patients with major depression compared with nondepressed cancer patients (Koenig et al. 1989). Studies have also shown that "desire for hastened death" among terminally ill cancer patients is significantly increased among those who are depressed or feeling hopeless (Breitbart et al. 2000).

With regard to *cardiovascular disease* and depression, Schleifer and colleagues (1989) conducted structured psychiatric interviews of 283 patients (mean age, 64 years) admitted to the coronary care unit for myocardial infarction. The interviews were conducted using the Schedule for Affective Disorders and Schizophrenia 8–10 days after infarction and then again 3–4 months later. Initially, 45% met the diagnostic criteria for minor or major depression, including 18% with major depression. Three to 4 months later, 33% of patients continued to meet the criteria for depression, including 77% of those who had initially met the criteria for major depression. In another study, Frasure-Smith et al. (1993) followed 222 patients for 6 months after myocardial infarction; depression was a significant predictor of mortality (hazard ratio, 5.7; $P<0.001$), even after other relevant risk factors were controlled. In an extensive review of this literature, Glassman and Shapiro (1998) reported that 9 of 10 studies found increased cardiovascular mortality in depressed patients. Even when community-dwelling populations are examined and prospectively followed, the relationship between depression and cardiovascular mortality persists (after controlling for smoking and other risk factors).

The effect of physical illness on emotion can be more direct. Evidence is emerging that a neurology of depression exists, as noted in "Risk Factors" earlier in this chapter. The right hemisphere may be uniquely specialized for the perception, experience, and expression of emotion (Coffey 1987). Consistent differences have been observed in the emotional behavior of individuals who have had either left or right hemisphere stroke. A left-sided stroke may be associated with depressive and even catastrophic responses manifested as combinations of dysphoria, episodes of crying, despair, feelings of hopelessness, anger, and self-depreciation (Gainotti 1972; R.G. Robinson et al. 1990; Sackeim et al. 1982). A lesion of the right cerebral hemisphere is more often followed by a neutral, indifferent, or even euphoric response, with denial of deficits and social disinhibition. Although there are exceptions to the findings of these studies, the recognition that selective brain lesions may contribute to specific syndromes closely associated with the depressive disorders implies, in some cases, an anatomy of depression rather than generalized neurochemical abnormalities. Depression itself may also increase the subsequent risk of stroke through some poorly understood biological mechanism, as was recently reported (Jonas and Mussolino 2000).

Depression is a frequent accompaniment of *Parkinson's disease*, with prevalence rates ranging from 20% to 90%; Mayeux (1990) determined a rate of 50% after reviewing the medical records of 339 patients with the disease. In terms of the physical symptoms and signs of paralysis agitans, most older persons differ little from persons observed at earlier ages. The major problems encountered in treating an older adult with Parkinson's disease are secondary to either undue sensitivity to medications or the emotional state of the patient. The older adult with parkinsonism may become disoriented and aggressive and experience ideas of persecution. More commonly, the elder withdraws socially and expresses helplessness and hopelessness regarding the future and considerable anger regarding difficulties in adjusting doses of medication (Carter 1986). Slow movement, weakness, rigidity, and masked and unexpressive facial expressions suggest to the clinician the depressed affect associated with progression of Parkinson's disease. However, the appearance of depression may be more severe than the actual affect indicates. Clinicians must be judicious in determining the necessity of pharmacological intervention in a patient with Parkinson's disease.

Nevertheless, depression in patients with Parkinson's disease seldom disappears spontaneously, and many patients improve with treatment. Studies indicate that serotonin metabolism may be affected in depressed patients with Parkinson's disease (Mayeux 1990). Not only is there profound loss of dopamine-containing neurons in the substantia nigra, there is also cell loss in the serotonin pathway into the limbic and diencephalon areas in the nucleus of the dorsal raphe. Other work has shown decreased levels of serotonin metabolites (5-HIAA) in the cerebrospinal fluid of some depressed patients with Parkinson's disease, as well as genetic alterations in serotonin transporter expression in such patients (Mossner et al. 2001). Also, ECT has been shown to produce transient relief of both depression and motor symptoms in patients with Parkinson's disease. It is likely that the etiology of depression in these patients is multifactorial—dependent on the patient's premorbid personality characteristics, on the history of depression, on the degree of functional disability induced by the disease, and on biological changes in the brain that are induced by Parkinson's disease.

Vitamin B$_{12}$ (cobalamin) deficiency has long been associated with depressive symptoms. In a study involving 141 patients with neuropsychiatric abnormalities due to cobalamin deficiency, 28% of subjects had no anemia or macrocytosis at the time of initial evaluation (Lindenbaum et al. 1988). Characteristic features of cobalamin deficiency in these patients included a variety of neurological symptoms (neurosensory loss, ataxia, and memory loss) as well as weakness, fatigue, and depressive symptoms. Most of these patients were older than 65 years, and the distribution between men and women was equal. All but one of the patients in the study responded to cobalamin therapy, exhibiting improvement in neuropsychiatric symptoms, including depressed mood. Bell and colleagues (1991) compared B-complex vitamin status at time of admission in 20 geriatric and 16 young adult nonalcoholic inpatients with major depression. Twenty-eight percent of all subjects were deficient in B$_2$ (riboflavin), B$_6$ (pyridoxine), and/or B$_{12}$. None were deficient in B$_1$ (thiamine) or folate. Patients with psychotic depression had lower B$_{12}$ levels than did patients with nonpsychotic depression. Anemia and macrocytosis, however, should not be used to predict folate or B$_{12}$ deficiencies or refractoriness to antidepressants (Mischoulon et al. 2000); measurement of folate and B$_{12}$ levels should always be done when evaluating treatment refractoriness or ruling out deficiencies of these vitamins.

The association between *chronic pain* and depression has been established for many years (Blumer and Heilbronn 1982; Kraemlinger et al. 1983). The evidence for this association is based on the increased frequency of depression among patients with chronic pain and the frequent reports of pain by depressed patients, coupled with the high concurrence of biological markers for depression and markers for chronic pain. Krishnan et al. (1985) found that most items on a typical depression rating scale, such as the Hamilton Rating Scale for Depression (Hamilton 1960), did not discriminate patients with major depression from those with chronic low back pain.

Nevertheless, the items discriminated well between patients with and those without depression. In an attempt to unravel the relationship between chronic pain and depression, France et al. (1984) studied a group of 42 patients with chronic pain. These investigators found that 41% of those with major depression were nonsuppressors of cortisol in response to a challenge with dexamethasone, yet all patients without major depression had normal DST results. In general, chronic pain does not become more prevalent with aging, but many older persons do have specific and rather severe chronic pain syndromes, such as pain from cancer (Spiegel 1996) or severe arthritis (Fifield et al. 1998). The clinician must distinguish the patient with chronic pain from the individual with hypochondriasis (in which the relationship with depressive symptoms may be different).

Normal Aging

The differential diagnosis of late-life depression must include not only other psychiatric and physical disorders but also the changes of normal aging. Some investigators associate a depressed mood with aging. However, most longitudinal studies of depression and life satisfaction do not validate this assumption. Although Busse et al. (1954) found that elderly subjects were aware of more frequent and more annoying depressive periods than they had experienced earlier in life, only a small number admitted to severe and protracted periods of depression. Approximately 85% of the subjects in this study were able to trace the onset of these depressive episodes to specific stimuli. Epidemiologic data confirm that the frequency of severe late-life depression (major depression) is lower than at earlier stages of the life cycle (see Chapter 2, "Demography and Epidemiology of Psychiatric Disorders in Late Life").

Life satisfaction, morale, and adjustment were not found to decline in a 4-year longitudinal study of an elderly cohort (Palmore and Kivett 1977). Rather, life satisfaction is associated with health status, socioeconomic status, social participation, income, and living arrangements (Thomae 1980). Poor life satisfaction may be correlated with depressive symptoms, yet these two constructs must be considered independently. For example, severe clinical depression can occur within the context of satisfaction with one's life and adjustment to one's situation. On the other hand, dissatisfaction with life and demoralization may be manifested as poor self-esteem, feelings of helplessness and hopelessness, sadness, confused thinking, and so forth, yet never progress to the point at which the syndrome meets criteria for a psychiatric disorder. Rather, discouragement and dissatisfaction are typical of the elder who, as described by Frank (1973), "finds that he cannot meet the demands placed on him by the environment, and cannot extricate himself from his predicament" (p. 312).

The normal biological changes of aging may interact with depressive symptomatology as well. Older persons, for example, spend more time lying in bed at night either without attempting to sleep or unsuccessfully trying to sleep, and therefore complain of decreased sleep efficiency. Rapid eye movement (REM) sleep latency, a marker that has been associated with depression (see "Primary Sleep Disorder" later in this chapter), is also known to decrease slightly throughout life in both genders (Dement et al. 1982). Elderly persons are notorious for complaining of poor appetite and reduced food intake. Munro (1981) found that caloric intake decreases with aging. Poor dentition may contribute to decreased food intake as well. Taste acuity also lessens with increasing years (Schiffman and Pasternak 1979). Lethargy is another common complaint of older adults.

Organic Psychiatric Disorders

The psychiatric disorders that most commonly confound the differential diagnosis of depression are the organic psychiatric disorders: dementia, delirium, other cognitive disorders, and "mental disorders due to a general medical condition," according to DSM-IV-TR. Pseudodementia is a syndrome in which dementia is mimicked or caricatured by a functional psychiatric illness, most commonly depression (Wells 1979). Patients with pseudodementia respond on the mental status examination similarly to those with true degenerative brain disease. Although the condition is not rare among elderly persons, Kiloh (1961) reminded clinicians that the term *pseudodementia* is "purely descriptive and carries no diagnostic weight," and yet patients with pseudodementia are in danger of inaccurate diagnosis and therapeutic neglect. Wells (1979) distinguished depression presenting as pseudodementia from true dementia by the rapid onset of the cognitive problems in depression, the relatively short duration of symptoms, the consistent depressed mood associated with cognitive difficulties, and the tendency among depressed patients to highlight disabilities as opposed to concealing (or attempting to conceal) them. The depressed older adult is more likely to respond with "I don't know" on the mental status examination, whereas the elder with dementia is more likely to attempt answers or to attempt to deflect the questions. Cognitive impairment in depression fluctuates from one examination to another, whereas cognitive impairment in dementia is relatively stable.

Of greater clinical importance, however, is the frequent overlap of depressive symptoms and symptoms of the organic psychiatric disorders. Grinker et al. (1961) noted impaired recent memory in 21% and poor remote memory in 14% of subjects of all ages with depressive disorders. Reifler et al. (1982) studied 88 cognitively impaired elderly outpatients and found that depression was superimposed on dementia in 17 (19%). Patients with greater cognitive impairment exhibited fewer symptoms of depression. When treated with an antidepressant, patients responded with a remission of the depressive symptoms, but cognitive dysfunction persisted. Alexopoulos and colleagues (1993) followed 23 elderly depressed patients with "reversible dementia" and 34 depressed elders without dementia for an average of 34 months after treatment. Irreversible dementia developed significantly more often in the group with depression and reversible dementia (43%) than in the group with depression alone (12%). These researchers concluded that the combination of depression and reversible dementia in elderly patients often indicates the presence of an early dementing illness.

Work done specifically with Alzheimer's patients has shown a concurrent diagnosis of major depression in 20%–30% (Reifler et al. 1986). Both depressed and nondepressed Alzheimer's patients were treated with the relatively potent anticholinergic antidepressant imipramine; patients improved whether or not they were in the treatment group, and cognitive function did not decline (Reifler et al. 1989). Greenwald and colleagues (1989) reported that treatment of depressed elderly individuals with dementia and those without dementia resulted in an improvement of both depression and cognitive impairment.

The diagnostic problems may be more complex, however. Specifically, there may be actual cerebral changes in depression that contribute to the dementia-like syndromes seen in some depressed older adults (Thielman and Blazer 1986). When significant depressive symptoms are present, older adults may not spontaneously complain of difficulty with memory and concentration more frequently than persons at earlier stages of the life cycle, but the former do have more difficulty performing on mental status examinations (Blazer et al. 1986). There is some evidence that sleep studies can help differentiate normal aging, depression, and Alzheimer's disease. Dykierek and colleagues (1998) examined 35 patients with Alzheimer's disease, 39 depressed elderly patients, and 42 healthy older control subjects for two consecutive nights in the sleep laboratory. They found that nearly all REM sleep measures differentiated significantly between the three groups. REM density, rather than REM sleep latency, was particularly important in separating depressed elders from elders with dementia. Earlier, Brenner and colleagues

(1989) reported that waking electroencephalograms (EEGs) could help distinguish depressed elderly patients and those with pseudodementia (with few electroencephalographic abnormalities) from those with dementia (who often had EEGs that showed abnormalities, with approximately one-third of these patients having moderate or severe abnormalities).

Schizophrenia

Given the general propensity of older adults to exhibit more psychotic features during an episode of major depression, the appearance of an overt psychosis with delusional thinking suggests to many clinicians the onset of a major depressive episode. Paranoid ideation and delusions, however, may be evidence of a late-life schizophrenic disorder. Older adults with late-life schizophrenia-like symptoms generally do not become profoundly depressed. Rather, they are distressed and focus on a perceived hostile environment as the cause of all their difficulties. Although family members or physicians are often surprised to discover these symptoms, paranoid ideation and delusional thinking in a schizophrenia-like illness rarely begin suddenly. An inquiry into the history of the disorder uncovers gradual withdrawal, bizarre comments, and often elaborate preparations to ensure safety (such as multiple locks on the door, bars on the windows, or stockpiling of food). The source of threat gradually moves from outside to within (for example, there may be a perception of being sexually molested), yet the paranoid elder rarely has a sense of poor self-worth.

Primary Sleep Disorder

Idiopathic sleep problems are often accompanied by depressive symptoms. The normal changes in sleep that mimic depressive sleep problems are reviewed in Chapter 20, "Sleep and Circadian Rhythm Disorders." A number of sleep disorders also contribute to symptoms that mimic major depression. Delayed or advanced sleep phase syndrome—that is, the shift of the normal sleep cycle to later or earlier in the evening—is most disturbing to older persons who previously viewed their sleep as a habitual given. The elder who begins a night's sleep at 8:00 or 9:00 P.M. because of boredom or other conditions will awaken at 2:00 or 3:00 A.M. and thus complain of early-morning awakening. In addition, the anxiety inherent in awakening in a darkened home with no activity exacerbates the discomfort associated with a sleep phase syndrome.

Sleep apnea syndrome, which is more common with aging, may not be recognized by the older adult (especially if he or she lives alone; a spouse or sleeping partner cannot spend many nights with an apneic elder without recognizing that something is abnormal about the sleep pattern). However, the elder with sleep apnea typically only complains of lethargy and has vague concerns regarding sleep, including excessive sleep.

Hypochondriasis

Hypochondriasis is a frequent confounder in the differential diagnosis relating to the depressed older adult. Although the hypochondriacal elder may experience a depressed mood, the essential feature of hypochondriasis is an unrealistic interpretation of physical signs or sensations as abnormal, which in turn leads to a preoccupation with the fear or belief that one has a serious illness (American Psychiatric Association 1980). A number of investigators have found the prevalence of hypochondriacal symptoms to be increased among depressed elderly patients. de Alarcon (1964) noted that in a group of 152 patients with depression, 65% of the men and 62% of the women reported concomitant hypochondriacal symptoms, the most common being constipation. Nevertheless, caution should be used when attributing presumed hypochondriacal complaints to depression in older adults with medical illness. Other work suggests that among hospitalized medically ill patients, hypochondriacal and somatic complaints are equally common in depressed younger and depressed elderly patients when severity of medical illness is controlled (Koenig et al. 1993). Pincus et al. (1986) also found that symptoms of hypochondriasis measured using the Minnesota Multiphasic Personality Inventory could be attributed entirely to physical disease status, rather than to psychological status, in older patients with rheumatoid arthritis.

The concurrence of depressive and hypochondriacal symptoms may increase the risk of suicide. In de Alarcon's 1964 study, 24.8% of individuals with hypochondriacal symptoms attempted suicide, whereas only 7.3% of those without such symptoms did so. Hypochondriasis as a disorder differs from hypochondriacal symptoms. True hypochondriasis usually can be distinguished from depression by the duration of the episode (hypochondriasis usually persists from midlife on), the degree to which the patient appears to suffer from symptoms (depressed patients appear to suffer more), and the cyclicity of symptoms (cyclicity is atypical of hypochondriasis but typical of depression). The endogenously depressed older adult with many somatic complaints generally tolerates antidepressant medication as well as other elders do, whereas the hypochondriacal patient generally does not tolerate antidepressant medication because of the anticholinergic side effects (Blazer 1984).

Anxiety

Differentiation of depression from primary anxiety syndromes such as generalized anxiety disorder and adjustment disorder with anxiety is difficult because of the frequent coexistence of anxiety in late-life depression. Blazer and colleagues (1989) determined that early-morning anxiety was a symptom in nearly one-third of the elderly and middle-aged patients surveyed between 12 and 24 months after psychiatric admission for depression. Anxiety is a common symptom in persons with medical illness, especially cancer (Derogatis et al. 1983). Hopko et al. (2000) examined the coexistence of depressive symptoms (measured using the Beck Depression Inventory) in older patients with generalized anxiety disorder. Of all predictors, depressive symptoms accounted for the largest variance in clinician-rated anxiety symptoms, a finding that underscores the importance of evaluation for both syndromes. Anxiety as a primary disorder can usually be distinguished from primary depression by the time of symptom onset: anxiety precedes depressive symptoms. In addition, the patient with anxiety usually has a less depressed mood and more motor tension, autonomic hyperactivity, feelings of apprehension or worry, and hypervigilance.

Alcoholism

Alcoholism peaks in middle age and becomes less frequent in late life. Nevertheless, results of a recent study involving more than 10,000 older persons indicate that between 10% and 15% of elders fulfill criteria for definite or questionable alcohol abuse (Thomas and Rockwood 2001). Symptoms of alcoholism that may mimic depression include cognitive changes, disturbed sleep, chronic fatigue, weight loss, and suicidal thoughts. Alcohol abuse or dependence may also coexist with depression, and many elders with late-onset alcoholism may actually use alcohol as a form of self-medication for their depressive symptoms. However, a diagnosis of depression in an alcoholic patient should not be made until the patient has been sober for at least 2 weeks, because alcohol withdrawal may include dysphoria and other depressive symptoms.

Diagnostic Workup of the Depressed Older Adult

Of special importance in evaluating the depressed elder is assessment of the duration of the current depressive episode; the history of previous episodes; the history of drug and alcohol abuse; response to previous therapeutic interventions for the depressive illness; a family history of depression, suicide, and/or alcohol abuse; and the severity of the depressive symptoms. Establishing some indication of the risk of suicide is essential, for suicidal risk may determine the location of treatment. The physical examination must include a thorough neurological examination to determine whether soft neurological signs (e.g., frontal release signs) or laterality is present. Weight loss and psychomotor retardation in the depressed older adult may lead to a peroneal palsy, documented by electromyography and nerve conduction studies (Massey and Bullock 1978). Because the older adult is less occupied with physical activities and therefore tends to be sedentary, the peroneal nerve is subject to chronic trauma.

The laboratory workup of the depressed older adult should include a thyroid panel (triiodothyronine, thyroxine, and radioactive iodine uptake) and determination of TSH levels. If a supersensitive test is used, measurement of TSH levels can be relied on to detect both hypothyroidism and hyperthyroidism. TSH values between 5 and 10 μU/mL are suggestive of hypothyroidism, and those above 10 μU/mL are nearly diagnostic. TSH values below 1.0 μU/mL, and especially below 0.5 μU/mL, are suggestive of hyperthyroidism.

A blood screen enables the clinician to detect the presence of an anemia. However, at least one study has shown that red blood cell enlargement and abnormalities are not good predictors of deficits in vitamin B_{12} or folate (Mischoulon et al. 2000). Because both depressive and cognitive symptoms can result from deficits in vitamin B_{12} or folate, it is important to obtain levels of these vitamins.

Psychological testing can assist the clinician in distinguishing permanent from temporary cognitive deficits, as well as in identifying potential laterality of cognitive abnormalities. Nevertheless, in the midst of severe depressive illness, psychological testing may be of less value. Therefore, timing the use of psychological testing is essential to maximize the value of test results in clinical decision making.

Laboratory evaluation of depression has entered a new era. Depressive disorders that were once identified exclusively by clinical signs and symptoms can now be delineated by a combination of these signs and symptoms and biological markers. Although no true laboratory test is available for the diagnosis of major depression (or even the subtypes of major depression), use of the laboratory by clinicians as well as clinical investigators has increased dramatically.

The most used—and most debated—of these laboratory tests is the DST. On the basis of the recognized hyperactivity of the HPA axis in patients with depressive disorders, Carroll et al. (1981) suggested a modified DST as an aid in diagnosis of endogenous depression or melancholia. For the modified test, 1 mg of dexamethasone is administered at 11:00 P.M. The next day, blood samples are drawn at 4:00 P.M. and 11:00 P.M. for the determination of plasma cortisol levels. In the case of outpatients, only the 4:00 P.M. sample is drawn. An increased plasma concentration of cortisol in either of the blood samples signifies an abnormal, or positive, result. In most laboratories, the cutoff value for normal plasma cortisol concentrations after dexamethasone administration is 5 g/dL with competitive protein-binding assays. In the original study by Carroll and colleagues (1981), the test was nearly 50% sensitive and more than 90% specific for endogenous depression. Since the introduction of the DST, many investigators have replicated these results. Two factors have emerged from these investigations that bear attention, however. First, the DST may not be as specific as originally believed, given that persons with other psychiatric disorders also had positive DST results in these studies. In addition, a number of conditions may contribute to the production of false-positive results—conditions such as physical illness (Cushing's disease, diabetes mellitus), pregnancy, treatment with certain medications (barbiturates, meprobamate, phenytoin), low body weight, ongoing weight loss (which frequently accompanies depressive illness), and acute infectious illnesses with fever and dehydration.

The DST has been studied extensively in elderly populations. Magni et al. (1986) found a sensitivity of 73% for major depressive disorder among hospitalized depressed elders, with only 11% of the control subjects and 11% of the persons with dysthymic disorder having positive DST results. Jenike and Albert (1984) found that among persons with mild cognitive impairment secondary to Alzheimer's disease, the DST was useful in distinguishing depressed from nondepressed patients. However, when findings from subjects with more severe dementia were included in the analysis, the DST was determined to be less specific. Tourigny-Rivard et al. (1981) did not find that advanced age affected the overnight DST results in healthy adults, and they therefore suggested that the test would be equally useful for young and elderly persons. In general, however, investigators believe that nonsuppression after dexamethasone administration increases gradually with age, and thus the usefulness of the DST probably diminishes with increasing age, especially in persons older than 75 years. The test has not proved useful in differentiating depression in poststroke patients (Grober et al. 1991) or patients with chronic pain (Ward et al. 1992).

A second biologically related approach that has received increased attention is the use of sleep EEGs to identify depression. Generally, 2 nights of sleep recording are performed after patients have been drug free for 14 days, and mean data from the 2 nights are used for the study. REM density and REM sleep latency have both been proposed as potential markers for depression (Kupfer et al. 1978). Compared with control subjects, endogenously depressed patients appear to have increased sleep discontinuity (disruption of sleep architecture), reduced slow-wave sleep (Stages III and IV), shortened REM sleep latency (the time between the onset of sleep and the first REM period), and increased REM density (the ratio of the sum of eye movements to the duration of REM sleep). Trends in the sleep EEG that appear to mark endogenous depression are trends that often accompany normal aging. However, using sleep EEGs to study REM density and REM sleep latency in combination with other markers may help to increase the probability of identifying the more biologically derived depressive disorders.

Attention has been directed to platelet-binding density of tritiated imipramine as a marker of depressive illness. A number of reports have suggested that the maximal density of platelet imipramine binding sites is decreased in unmedicated subjects who have a unipolar affective disorder (Asarch et al. 1981; Briley et al. 1980). In contrast to the DST, which is associated with decreased specificity with aging, determining platelet-binding density of tritiated imipramine may actually be a more specific test for endogenous depression in elderly persons than in younger control subjects (Knight et al. 1986; Schneider et al. 1985). In a study by Knight and colleagues (1986), in which subjects between ages 35 and 50 years were compared with subjects at least 60 years old, the number of platelet tritiated imipramine binding sites was reduced in patients with major depression. Imipramine binding was particularly well correlated with depression in elderly patients, and it remained normal in subjects with other neuropsychiatric disorders, such as Alzheimer's disease and schizophrenia. More recent studies have not shown as strong a correlation with depression case identification or depression severity (Ellis et al. 1990). Even if it does prove useful diagnostically, imipramine binding has not been shown to change significantly during recovery from depression (Ellis et al. 1992).

Another marker that has been associated with depression throughout the life cycle is platelet monoamine oxidase activity. In a study by Schneider et al. (1986), platelet monoamine oxidase activity was found to be significantly higher in elderly depressed women than in gender- and age-comparable control subjects. There were no significant relationships between monoamine oxidase activity and duration of the current depressive episode, lifetime duration of the illness, or family history.

Another potential marker for biological depression is platelet α_2-adrenoceptors. This marker may also be of value in studying depression in late life, because neither binding capacity nor affinity of α_2-adrenoceptors on platelets is known to be correlated specifically with age (Buckley et al. 1986).

A more thoroughly studied marker that may have both diagnostic and therapeutic implications is blunted TSH response to TRH. TRH stimulates release of TSH from the anterior pituitary gland. The TRH test (measurement of serum TSH concentration after administration of TRH) has become a standard test in endocrinology. Administration of synthetic TRH challenges the anterior pituitary to respond. Differential response in the serum TSH levels may characterize disorders of the HPA axis. Although blunting of TSH response is not specific to depression, a number of studies have shown that TSH response is blunted in patients with depression (Gregoire et al. 1977; Loosen and Prange 1982). However, increasing age is also known to be associated with a blunted TSH response to TRH (Snyder and Utiger 1972). Because of this abnormality, supplemental thyroid has been prescribed to depressed persons, with occasional beneficial response. For example, liothyronine sodium, 25 g/day, could augment the therapeutic effects of traditional TCAs. This augmentation may be valuable in the treatment of some elders, because subclinical hypothyroidism occasionally contributes to depression in older adults. The first step, however, is a more thorough workup and the use of thyroid agents alone to determine whether the depressive symptoms are solely determined by hypothyroidism.

Given the ever-increasing list of potential markers—some that are to be investigated further, some that will be dropped from the list because they are not clinically useful—what is the best way for the clinician to integrate these markers into clinical practice? First, clinicians should recognize that the primary utility of such markers is in probing the biological contribution to depressive disorders of late life. None of these biochemical, neuroendocrinological, or circadian abnormalities yet qualifies as a biological marker for testing for a psychiatric disorder. They may never reach this status, because the etiology of late-life depression is multidetermined, with no clear evidence that one factor is necessary for symptoms to emerge. Nevertheless, these markers may be considered analogous to symptoms, in that they can be included in the data collected to increase the probability of delineat-

ing a real psychopathological entity that can be effectively treated and whose outcome can be predicted.

Treatment

Treatment of depression in late life is four-pronged, involving psychotherapy, pharmacotherapy, ECT, and family therapy. Because pharmacotherapy is covered in some detail in Chapter 24, "Psychopharmacology," we emphasize the remaining three therapeutic approaches here.

Psychotherapy

Cognitive-behavioral therapy is the only psychotherapy specifically designed to treat depression (Beck et al. 1979). Even the more recent technique of interpersonal therapy (Klerman et al. 1984) is primarily a cognitive-behavioral orientation to improving interpersonal relationships. The advantage of using cognitive-behavioral therapy in treating the older adult is that it is directive and time limited, usually involving between 10 and 25 sessions. Cognitive-behavioral therapy has been found to be effective in depressed elderly patients (Gallagher and Thompson 1982; Steuer et al. 1984) and in patients with chronic medical illnesses such as Type II diabetes (Lustman et al. 1998), heart disease (Kohn et al. 2000), and irritable bowel syndrome (Boyce et al. 2000). It may be particularly useful in patients who show only a partial response to antidepressant drug therapy (Scott et al. 2000).

The goal of behavioral and cognitive therapies is to change behavior and modes of thinking. This change is accomplished through behavioral interventions such as weekly activity schedules, mastery and pleasure logs, and graded task assignments. Cognitive approaches to restructuring negative cognitions or automatic thoughts include subjecting these cognitions to empirical reality testing, examining distortions (such as overgeneralizations, catastrophizing, and dichotomous thinking), and generating new ways of viewing one's life (Steuer et al. 1984). Depressed patients typically regard themselves and their present and future in somewhat idiosyncratic or negative ways. Such patients believe themselves inadequate or defective and believe that unpleasant experiences are caused by a problem with themselves and that they are therefore worthless, helpless, and hopeless. This cognitive triad leads the older adult to believe that he or she has a never-ending depression and that nothing pleasant will ever happen again. The cognitive model presupposes that these symptoms of depression are consequences of negative thinking patterns.

Thompson and colleagues (1987) randomly assigned 91 elders with major depression to cognitive therapy, behavioral therapy, or brief dynamic therapy (in which the importance of the patient-therapist relationship is stressed and realistic collaborative aspects of the therapeutic alliance are emphasized). Patients in each group underwent 16–20 sessions of therapy conducted by expert clinicians; 20 additional patients were assigned to a waiting-list control group. By the end of 6 weeks, 52% of the patients in therapy were in complete remission, and 18% showed significant improvement. All therapies were equally efficacious and superior to waiting for treatment.

Results of empirical studies (including the work of Gallagher and Thompson [1982], Steuer et al. [1984], and Thompson et al. [1987]) suggest that compared with control subjects, elders who engage in psychotherapy experience incremental improvement. Not only does the percentage of elders who respond to these treatments compare favorably with the percentage of younger subjects who respond, the degree of improvement appears equal to that obtained with medications, especially with milder forms of depression. Drug therapy is not appropriate for some elders, and cognitive, behavioral, and brief dynamic psychotherapy are viable alternatives. In addition, evidence has emerged that suggests that the long-term benefit of cognitive-behavioral therapy may be greater than that of pharmacotherapy, especially if the medications are discontinued during the first year of treatment.

Older adults who have minor depression or adjustment disorders, or who experience dysphoria because of losses of various types, often require less intensive forms of psychotherapy. Active listening and simple support may be sufficient to help distressed elders cope with their situation. Because religion is an important factor in the lives of many older adults, referral to a pastoral counselor may be particularly helpful and acceptable (Koenig and Weaver 1997).

Pharmacotherapy

TCAs remain the agents of choice for patients with more severe forms of major depression. Medications that are effective yet relatively free of side effects (especially cardiovascular effects) are preferred. In recent years, nortriptyline and desipramine have become the more popular medications for treating older adults with endogenous or melancholic major depression. However, doxepin remains a favorite among many practitioners. It is recommended that all elderly patients have an electrocardiogram (ECG) before initiation of treatment and again after therapeutic blood levels have been achieved. If the ECG shows a second-degree (or higher) block, a bifascicular bundle branch block, a left bundle branch block, or a QTc interval greater than 480 milliseconds, treatment with TCAs should not be initiated—or should be stopped, in patients taking these medications.

Experience with selective serotonin reuptake inhibitors (SSRIs) and bupropion has been growing in elderly patients (with or without medical illness). Venlafaxine (Staab and Evans 2000), paroxetine (Bump et al. 2001), fluoxetine (Heiligenstein et al. 1995; Judge et al. 2000), sertraline (Krishnan et al. 2001; Newhouse et al. 2000), and bupropion (Weihs et al. 2000) have been shown to be effective in geriatric depression. SSRIs have also proved effective in depressed older adults with stroke (Cole et al. 2001), vascular disease in general (Krishnan et al. 2001), or Alzheimer's disease (Lyketsos et al. 2000). These agents have become the drugs of first choice for mild to moderate forms of depression. Their lack of anticholinergic, orthostatic, and cardiac side effects; lack of sedation; and safety in overdose are important advantages in elderly patients. Nevertheless, for a significant number of older adults, the newer antidepressants cause other unacceptable effects, including excessive activation and disturbance of sleep, tremor, headache, significant gastrointestinal side effects, hyponatremia, and weight loss.

Antidepressant doses administered to persons in late life should be case specific but are generally lower than those given to persons in midlife. Starting therapeutic daily doses of SSRIs are as follows: sertraline, 12.5–50 mg; fluoxetine, 5–20 mg; paroxetine, 10–30 mg; venlafaxine, 37.5–200 mg (in divided doses); mirtazapine, 7.5–30 mg; and citalopram, 10–40 mg. Bupropion therapy should be initiated at 75 mg twice daily, with an increase to 150 mg twice daily (not to exceed 150 mg in a single dose). With regard to tricyclics, 25–50 mg of nortriptyline orally at bedtime or 25 mg of desipramine orally twice a day is frequently adequate for relieving depressive symptoms. Plasma levels of tricyclic medications can be helpful in determining dosing: nortriptyline levels between 50 and 150 ng/mL and desipramine levels greater than 125 ng/mL have been found to be therapeutic.

Trazodone and nefazodone are alternatives in patients who cannot tolerate tricyclics or one of the newer antidepressants. Trazodone has advantages over TCAs in that it is virtually free of anticholinergic effects, and it has advantages over the newer antidepressants in that it has strong sedative effects. Nevertheless, the drug is not without side effects, including excessive daytime sedation, priapism (occasionally), and significant orthostatic hypotension. The therapeutic daily dose of trazodone is

300 mg or more, an amount that many older patients cannot tolerate because of sedation. Nefazodone has fewer side effects than trazodone, but relatively high doses are required for efficacy, and sedation and impaired balance can be problems. For elderly patients with depression and significant anxiety, however, it may be useful.

Monoamine oxidase inhibitors (MAOIs) are another alternative to tricyclics and the newer antidepressants. It should be noted, if MAOIs are being considered because of intolerance of side effects of other antidepressants, that older adults usually do not tolerate MAOIs any better. If treatment with an MAOI is to follow treatment with an SSRI, a minimum of 1 or 2 weeks (for fluoxetine, 2–4 weeks) must elapse after discontinuation of SSRI therapy and before initiation of MAOI therapy, to avoid a serotonergic syndrome. If a patient's depression is severe and ECT is contemplated, use of an MAOI also precludes initiation of ECT until 10 days to 2 weeks after the drug is discontinued. Such a delay may seriously impede clinical management of the suicidal elder.

Some clinicians prescribe low morning doses of stimulant medications, such as 5 mg of methylphenidate, to improve mood in the apathetic older adult. The effectiveness of stimulants has not been conclusively demonstrated. Nevertheless, these agents are generally safe at low doses, and rarely does the clinician encounter an elder with a propensity to abuse stimulants or to become addicted when these drugs are given once daily.

For further details regarding psychopharmacological treatment of the older adult, see Chapter 24, "Psychopharmacology."

Electroconvulsive Therapy

ECT continues to be the most effective form of treatment for patients with more severe major depressive episodes (Scovern and Kilmann 1980). The induction of a seizure appears to be the factor that is effective in reversing a major depression. ECT was first established as a treatment in 1938, but it is not used as much as it was immediately after its development (Weiner 1982). Despite its effectiveness, ECT is not the first-line treatment of choice for a patient with major depression and should be prescribed only because other therapeutic modalities have been ineffective. ECT has been shown to be effective in selected individuals, primarily those who have major depression with melancholia, and especially those who have major depression with psychotic symptoms associated with agitation or withdrawal. Many older adults with such syndromes either do not respond to antidepressant medications or experience toxicity (usually postural hypotension) when taking antidepressants. The

presence of self-destructive behavior, such as a suicide attempt or refusal to eat, increases the necessity for intervening effectively; in such situations, ECT may be the treatment of choice.

If ECT is selected as an intervention, the clinician must first discuss in detail with the patient and the family the nature of the treatment and the reasons for this recommendation. Why is ECT necessary? What procedures will the patient undergo during a course of ECT? How many treatments can be expected, and how long will hospitalization continue? Can ECT be performed on an outpatient basis? What are the risks and side effects of ECT? What results, both immediate and long-term, can be expected? Even when the elderly patient is severely depressed, careful and thoughtful discussion with the patient and family will usually result in a willingness by the patient (often with encouragement from the family) to undergo the course of treatments. Once treatment is begun, fears of ECT usually remit.

The medical workup before ECT includes acquisition of a complete medical history, a physical examination, and consultation with a cardiologist if any cardiac abnormalities are recognized. Knowledge of a family history of a psychiatric disorder, of suicide, or of treatment with ECT is helpful in predicting response to treatment. Laboratory examination includes a complete blood count, a urinalysis, routine chemistries, chest and spinal X rays (the latter to document previous compression fractures), an ECG, and a computed tomography scan or magnetic resonance image (with computed tomography or magnetic resonance imaging [MRI] available, an EEG and a skull X ray are not routinely required). The presence of some abnormalities on magnetic resonance images does not militate against the use of ECT, however. For example, a series of older adults with major depression were found to have subcortical arteriosclerotic encephalopathy, demonstrated by MRI, but promptly improved after undergoing ECT (Coffey et al. 1987).

Before an older adult undergoes ECT, all medications should be withdrawn, if possible. As noted earlier (see "Pharmacotherapy"), any MAOI must be withdrawn 10 days to 2 weeks before the procedure, to prevent any toxic interactions with the anesthetic used during ECT. Reserpine and anticholinesterase drugs should also be withdrawn for at least 1 week. Lithium carbonate, TCAs, antipsychotics, and antianxiety agents (including sedative-hypnotics) are not absolutely contraindicated in patients who are to undergo ECT. Benzodiazepines, however, increase the seizure threshold and should be avoided. Generally, a short-acting barbiturate, such as chloral hydrate (500 mg orally at bedtime), is the most appropriate sedative-hypnotic, although chloral hydrate should not be given on the night preceding administration of ECT, if possible. Use of low-dose haloperidol or thiothixene is probably the most appropriate means of controlling severe agitation or psychotic symptoms.

The basic techniques for ECT are well described. Thirty minutes before treatment, an anticholinergic agent is administered intramuscularly to prevent complications of cardiac arrhythmias and aspiration. Directly before treatment, a short-acting anesthetic, such as thiopental or methohexital, is administered until an eyelash response is no longer present. Then a muscle relaxant, such as succinylcholine, is administered to prevent severe muscle contractions. Investigators are increasingly using unilateral electrode placement to the nondominant cerebral hemisphere, because evidence has accumulated that less confusion occurs after unilateral treatment than after bilateral treatment. Nevertheless, unilateral electrode placement does not preclude development of memory difficulties. (Some investigators question the efficacy of unilateral versus bilateral electrode placement, but bilateral electrode placement has not been clearly established as therapeutically superior to unilateral electrode placement.) The electrical stimulus is applied, and the seizure is monitored either by applying a tourniquet to one arm and observing the tonic and clonic movements in the extremity peripheral to the tourniquet or by direct electroencephalographic monitoring. Direct electroencephalographic monitoring is preferred, and a seizure lasting 25 seconds or more is required for optimal results.

Seizure duration varies with age. In a study involving 228 patients treated with ECT, Hinkle et al. (1986) found that of patients older than 60 years, a greater percentage were likely to have a seizure of 30 seconds or less. When ECT is repeated, use of caffeine may increase the likelihood of inducing a seizure without the necessity of restimulation using higher electrical parameters (which could lead to increased central nervous system toxicity).

ECT treatments are generally administered three times per week, and usually 6–12 treatments are necessary for adequate therapeutic response. A clear improvement is often noted after one of the treatments, with the patient reporting a remarkable improvement in mood and functioning. Two or three treatments are generally given after the ECT administration leading to improvement.

The risks and side effects of ECT in elderly patients are similar to those in the general population. Cardiovascular effects are of most concern and include premature ventricular contractions, ventricular arrhythmias, and transient systolic hypertension. Multiple monitoring during treatment decreases the (infrequent) risk of one of these side effects leading to permanent problems. Confusion and amnesia often result after a treatment, but the duration of this confusional episode is brief. Even with the use of unilateral nondominant treatment, however, some patients have prolonged memory difficulties. Headaches are a common symptom with ECT; they usually respond to nonnarcotic analgesics. Status epilepticus and vertebral compression fractures are some of the rare but more serious adverse effects. Compression fractures are a particular risk in older women because of the high incidence of osteoporosis in the postmenopausal population.

In terms of outcome, what can the clinician expect from the use of ECT in older adults? The overall success rate of ECT in patients who have not responded to drug therapy is usually 80% or greater, and there is no evidence that effectiveness is lower in older adults (Avery and Lubrano 1979). Wesner and Winokur (1989) examined the influence of age on the natural history of major depressive disorder and found that ECT reduced the rate of chronicity when it was used in patients age 40 or older but, surprisingly, not in those younger than 40 years.

A review of records of Medicare beneficiaries in the United States during 1987–1992 has suggested that use of ECT in elderly patients is increasing. Rosenbach and colleagues (1997) reported that the number of beneficiaries receiving ECT increased from 12,000 in 1987 to 15,560 in 1992—an increase of more than 20% (after calculations were adjusted for increased numbers of beneficiaries between 1987 and 1992). In a prospective, multisite study, Tew and colleagues (1999) compared characteristics and treatment outcomes of 133 adult (age 59 or younger), 63 young-old (ages 60–74 years), and 72 old-old (age 75 or older) patients treated with ECT for major depression. They found that patients less than 60 years old had a significantly lower rate of response to ECT (54%) than did young-old patients (73%) or old-old patients (67%). The investigators concluded that despite a higher level of physical illness and cognitive impairment, patients age 75 or older who had severe major depression tolerated ECT in a manner similar to the way in which younger patients tolerated the treatment, and the old-old patients demonstrated a similar or even better response. There is also evidence that ECT may be more effective and have fewer side effects than antidepressants when used to treat depression in old-old patients (Manly et al. 2000).

The relapse rate with no prophylactic intervention may exceed 50% in the year after a course of ECT. This relapse rate can be decreased if antidepressants or lithium carbonate is prescribed after the treatment. For some patients who exhibit a high likelihood of recurrence despite use of prophylactic medication, and/or who experience high toxicity and therefore cannot tolerate prophylactic medications, maintenance ECT may be necessary. For such patients, weekly or monthly treatments (usually on an outpatient basis) are prescribed, with careful monitoring of response and side effects. The combination of continuation ECT and antidepressant drug therapy has been shown to have greater efficacy than use of medications alone, following an effective course of ECT (Gagne et al. 2000).

Despite the effectiveness of ECT, few deny that treatment may lead to memory difficulties. In a study by Frith et al. (1983), 70 severely depressed patients were randomly assigned to eight real or sham ECT treatments and were divided according to the degree of recovery from depression afterward. Compared with nondepressed control subjects, the depressed patients were impaired on a wide range of tests of memory and concentration before treatment, but afterward performance on most tests improved. Real ECT induced impairments in concentration, short-term memory, and learning but significantly facilitated access to remote memories. At 6-month follow-up, all differences between real and sham ECT groups had disappeared.

Price and McAllister (1989) examined the efficacy of ECT in elderly depressed patients with dementia. Overall, the patients achieved an 86% response rate, with only 21% experiencing a significant worsening of cognition; the cognition problems were transient in most cases. Of particular importance is that 49% of the patients treated with ECT showed improvement in memory function after treatment. Likewise, Stoudemire et al. (1995) found that over time, ECT may lead to significant improvement in memory of cognitively impaired older adults with depression. Although data on the safety and efficacy of ECT in patients with concurrent medical illness derive primarily from retrospective studies involving psychiatric patients with stable disease, these data do support the use of ECT in patients with cardiovascular, neurological, endocrine, or metabolic conditions, as well as a variety of other conditions (Stoudemire et al. 1998). For more information on the efficacy and safety of ECT in patients with late-life depressions, see the comprehensive review by Greenberg (1997).

Family Therapy

The final component of therapy for the depressed elderly patient is work with the family. Not only may family dysfunction contribute to the depressive symptoms experienced by the older adult, but family support is critical to a successful outcome in the treatment of the depressed elder. A clinician must attend to 1) those members of the family who will be available to the elder, 2) the interaction between the older adult and family members and the interactions among other family members (both frequency and quality of interaction), 3) the overall family atmosphere, 4) family values regarding psychiatric disorders, 5) family support and tolerance of symptoms (such as expressions of wishing not to live), and 6) stressors encountered by the family other than the depression experienced by the elder (Blazer 1993).

Most depressed elders do not resist interaction between the clinician and family members. With the permission of the patient, the family should be instructed regarding the nature of the depressive disorder and the potential risks associated with depression in late life, especially suicide. Family members can assist the clinician in observing changes in behavior, such as an increase in discomfort (either physical or emotional), increased withdrawal and decreased verbalization, and preoccupation with medications or weapons. The family can assist by removing possible implements of suicide from places of easy access. The family can also take responsibility for administering medications to an older adult who is unreliable or whose potential for suicide is high.

Family members can benefit from simple instructions regarding how to communicate with the elderly depressed patient. Methods of responding to expressions of low self-esteem and pessimism, such as paraphrase and expression of understanding without a sense of responsibility to intervene, can be especially effective. Families can be taught, for example, to acknowledge to the patient: "I hear what you are saying, and I understand." Behavioral techniques for dealing with demanding or overly dependent elders can be taught to families as well. A depressed elder's demand for constant attention from a family member may necessitate "weaning" the patient from continued contact.

When the symptoms of depression become so severe that hospitalization is required, family members are valuable in facilitating hospitalization. Without a proper alliance between clinician and family, a family may be resistant to hospitalization and undermine attempts of the clinician to treat the older adult appropriately. It is usually necessary for the clinician to take responsibility for saying that hospitalization is essential—that the situation has reached the point at which the family has no choice. The clinician informs the patient—in the presence of the family—of the necessity of hospitalization, and the family in turn can support the clinician's position. In such a situation, the patient rarely resists hospitalization for long.

References

Alexopoulos GS, Meyers BS, Young RC, et al: The course of geriatric depression with "reversible dementia": a controlled study. Am J Psychiatry 150:1693–1699, 1993

Alexopoulos GS, Meyers BS, Young RC, et al: "Vascular depression" hypothesis. Arch Gen Psychiatry 54:915–922, 1997

Ameblas A: Life events and mania. Br J Psychiatry 150:235–240, 1987

American Psychiatric Association: Diagnostic and Statistical Manual of Mental Disorders, 3rd Edition. Washington, DC, American Psychiatric Association, 1980

American Psychiatric Association: Diagnostic and Statistical Manual of Mental Disorders, 3rd Edition, Revised. Washington, DC, American Psychiatric Association, 1987

American Psychiatric Association: Diagnostic and Statistical Manual of Mental Disorders, 4th Edition. Washington, DC, American Psychiatric Association, 1994

American Psychiatric Association: Diagnostic and Statistical Manual of Mental Disorders, 4th Edition, Text Revision. Washington, DC, American Psychiatric Association, 2000

Anderson RJ, Freedland KE, Clouse RE, et al: The prevalence of comorbid depression in adults with diabetes: a meta-analysis. Diabetes Care 24:1069–1078, 2001

Arfken CL, Lichtenberg PA, Tancer ME: Cognitive impairment and depression predict mortality in medically ill older adults. J Gerontol A Biol Sci Med Sci 54:M152–M156, 1999

Asarch KB, Shih JC, Kulsar A: Decreased 3H-imipramine binding in depressed males and females. Communications in Psychopharmacology 4:425–432, 1981

Atchley RC: Social Forces in Later Life. Belmont, CA, Wadsworth, 1972

Avery D, Lubrano A: Depression treated with imipramine and ECT: the DeCarolis study reconsidered. Am J Psychiatry 136:559–562, 1979

Baldwin JC, Jolley DJ: The prognosis of depression in old age. Br J Psychiatry 149:574–583, 1986

Beck AT, Rush AJ, Shaw BF, et al: Cognitive Therapy of Depression. New York, Guilford, 1979

Bell IR, Edman JS, Maroow FD, et al: B complex vitamin patterns in geriatric and young adult inpatients with major depression. J Am Geriatr Soc 39:252–257, 1991

Black SA, Markides KS: Depressive symptoms and mortality in older Mexican Americans. Ann Epidemiol 9:45–52, 1999

Blazer DG: Impact of late-life depression on the social network. Am J Psychiatry 140:162–166, 1983

Blazer DG: Hypochondriasis, in A Family Approach to Health Care in the Elderly. Edited by Blazer D, Siegler IC. Menlo Park, CA, Addison-Wesley, 1984, pp 140–156

Blazer DG: Depression in Late Life, 2nd Edition. St. Louis, MO, CV Mosby, 1993

Blazer DG, George LK, Landerman R: The phenomenology of late life depression, in Psychiatric Disorders in the Elderly. Edited by Bebbington PE, Jacoby R. London, Mental Health Foundation, 1986, pp 143–152

Blazer DG, Bachar JR, Hughes DC: Major depression with melancholia: a comparison of middle-aged and elderly adults. J Am Geriatr Soc 35:927–932, 1987a

Blazer DG, Hughes DC, George LK: The epidemiology of depression in an elderly community population. Gerontologist 27:281–287, 1987b

Blazer DG, Hughes DC, Fowler N: Anxiety as an outcome symptom of depression in elderly and middle-aged adults. Int J Geriatr Psychiatry 27:281–287, 1989

Blazer DG, Hughes DC, George LK: Age and impaired subjective support: predictors of symptoms at one-year follow-up. J Nerv Ment Dis 180:172–178, 1992

Blumer D, Heilbronn M: Chronic pain as a variant of depressive disease: the pain-prone disorder. J Nerv Ment Dis 170:381–394, 1982

Boyce P, Gilchrist J, Talley NJ, et al: Cognitive-behaviour therapy as a treatment for irritable bowel syndrome: a pilot study. Aust N Z J Psychiatry 34:300–309, 2000

Braam AW, Beekman ATF, Deeg DJH, et al: Religiosity as a protective or prognostic factor of depression in later life: results from a community survey in the Netherlands. Acta Psychiatr Scand 96:199–205, 1997a

Braam AW, Beekman ATF, van Tilburg TG, et al: Religious involvement and depression in older Dutch citizens. Soc Psychiatry Psychiatr Epidemiol 32:284–291, 1997b

Breitbart W, Rosenfeld B, Pessin H, et al: Depression, hopelessness, and desire for hastened death in terminally ill patients with cancer. JAMA 284:2907–2911, 2000

Brenner RP, Reynolds CF 3rd, Ulrich RF: EEG findings in depressive pseudodementia and dementia with secondary depression. Electroencephalogr Clin Neurophysiol 72:298–304, 1989

Bridges P: The drug treatment of depression in old age, in Affective Disorders in the Elderly. Edited by Murphy E. Edinburgh, Churchill Livingstone, 1986, pp 97–149

Briley MS, Raisman R, Sechter D, et al: [3H]-Imipramine binding in human platelets: a new biochemical parameter in depression. Neuropharmacology 19:1209–1210, 1980

Buckley C, Curtin D, Walsh T, et al: Aging and platelet alpha₂-adrenoceptors (letter). Br J Clin Pharmacol 21:721–722, 1986

Bukberg J, Penman D, Holland JC: Depression in hospitalized cancer patients. Psychosom Med 46:199–210, 1984

Bump GM, Mulsant BH, Pollock BG, et al: Paroxetine versus nortriptyline in the continuation and maintenance treatment of depression in the elderly. Depress Anxiety 13:38–44, 2001

Busse EW, Barnes RH, Silverman AJ, et al: Studies of the processes of aging, VI: factors that influence the psyche of elderly persons. Am J Psychiatry 110:897–903, 1954

Carroll BJ, Feinberg M, Greden JF, et al: A specific laboratory test for the diagnosis of melancholia: standardization, validation, and clinical utility. Arch Gen Psychiatry 38:15–22, 1981

Carter AB: The neurologic aspects of aging, in Clinical Geriatrics, 3rd Edition. Edited by Rossman I. Philadelphia, PA, JB Lippincott, 1986, pp 326–351

Cath SH: Some dynamics of middle and later years: a study in depletion and restitution, in Geriatric Psychiatry: Grief, Loss, and Emotional Disorders in the Aging Process. Edited by Berezin MA, Cath SH. New York, International Universities Press, 1965, pp 21–72

Checkley SA, Slade AP, Schur E: Growth hormone and other responses to clonidine in patients with endogenous depression. Br J Psychiatry 138:51–55, 1981

Coffey CE: Cerebral laterality and emotion: the neurology of depression. Compr Psychiatry 28:197–219, 1987

Coffey CE, Hinkle PE, Weiner RD, et al: Electroconvulsive therapy of depression in patients with white matter hyperintensity. Biol Psychiatry 22:626–629, 1987

Cole MG: Age, age of onset and course of primary depressive illness in the elderly. Can J Psychiatry 28:102–104, 1983

Cole MG, Bellavance F, Mansour A: Prognosis of depression in elderly community and primary care populations: a systematic review and meta-analysis. Am J Psychiatry 156:1182–1189, 1999

Cole MG, Elie LM, McCusker J, et al: Feasibility and effectiveness of treatments for post-stroke depression in elderly inpatients: systematic review. J Geriatr Psychiatry Neurol 14:37–41, 2001

Covinsky KE, Kahana E, Chin MH, et al: Depressive symptoms and 3-year mortality in older hospitalized medical patients. Ann Intern Med 130:563–569, 1999

Cutler NR, Post RM: Life course of illness in untreated manic-depressive patients. Compr Psychiatry 23:101–115, 1982

Dam H: Depression in stroke patients 7 years following stroke. Acta Psychiatr Scand 103:287–293, 2001

Davies BM: Depressive illness in the elderly patient. Postgrad Med 38:314–320, 1965

de Alarcon R: Hypochondriasis and depression in the aged. Gerontol Clin (Basel) 6:266–277, 1964

Dement WC, Miles LE, Carskadon MA: "White paper" on sleep and aging. J Am Geriatr Soc 30:25–50, 1982

Denihan A, Kirby M, Bruce I, et al: Three-year prognosis of depression in the community-dwelling elderly. Br J Psychiatry 176:453–457, 2000

Derogatis LR, Morrow GR, Fetting J, et al: The prevalence of psychiatric disorders among cancer patients. JAMA 249:751–757, 1983

Devanand DP, Turret N, Moody BJ, et al: Personality disorders in elderly patients with dysthymic disorder. Am J Geriatr Psychiatry 8:188–195, 2000

Dew MA, Reynolds CF III, Houck PR, et al: Temporal profiles of the course of depression during treatment: predictors of pathways toward recovery in the elderly. Arch Gen Psychiatry 54:1016–1024, 1997

Dunner DL: Affective disorder: clinical features, in Psychiatry, Vol 1. Edited by Michels R, Cavenar JO. Philadelphia, PA, JB Lippincott, 1985, pp 59–60

Dykierek P, Stadtmuller G, Schramm P, et al: The value of REM sleep parameters in differentiating Alzheimer's disease from old-age depression and normal aging. J Psychiatr Res 32:1–9, 1998

Eastham JH, Jeste DV, Young RC: Assessment and treatment of bipolar disorder in the elderly. Drugs Aging 12:205–224, 1998

Egeland JA, Gerhard DS, Pauls DL, et al: Bipolar affective disorders linked to DNA markers on chromosome 11. Nature 325:783–787, 1987

Ellis PM, McIntosh CJ, Beeston R, et al: Platelet tritiated imipramine binding in psychiatric patients: relationship to symptoms and severity of depression. Acta Psychiatr Scand 82:275–282, 1990

Ellis PM, Beeston R, McIntosh CJ, et al: Platelet 3H-imipramine binding during recovery from depression. Acta Psychiatr Scand 86:108–112, 1992

Epstein LJ: Depression in the elderly. J Gerontol 3:278–282, 1976

Erikson EH: Childhood and Society. New York, WW Norton, 1950

Fassler LB, Gavira M: Depression in old age. J Am Geriatr Soc 26:471–475, 1978

Fifield J, Tennen H, Reisine S, et al: Depression and the long-term risk of pain, fatigue, and disability in patients with rheumatoid arthritis. Arthritis Rheum 41:1851–1857, 1998

Finkelstein JW, Roffwarg HP, Boyar RM, et al: Age-related change in the twenty-four-hour spontaneous secretion of growth hormone. J Clin Endocrinol Metab 35:665–670, 1972

France RD, Krishnan KRR, Houpt JL, et al: Differentiation of depression from chronic pain with the dexamethasone suppression test and DSM-III. Am J Psychiatry 141:1577–1578, 1984

Frank JD: Persuasion and Healing. Baltimore, MD, Johns Hopkins University Press, 1973

Frasure-Smith N, Lesperance F, Talajic M: Depression following myocardial infarction: impact on 6-month survival. JAMA 270:1819–1825, 1993

Fredman L, Schoenbach VJ, Kaplan BH, et al: The association between depressive symptoms and mortality among older participants in the Epidemiologic Catchment Area–Piedmont Health Survey. J Gerontol 44:S149–S156, 1989

Fredman L, Magaziner J, Hebel JR, et al: Depressive symptoms and 6-year mortality among elderly community-dwelling women. Epidemiology 10:54–59, 1999

Frith CD, Stevens M, Johnstone EC, et al: Effects of ECT and depression on various aspects of memory. Br J Psychiatry 142:610–617, 1983

Gagne GG Jr, Furman MJ, Carpenter LL, et al: Efficacy of continuation ECT and antidepressant drugs compared to long-term antidepressants alone in depressed patients. Am J Psychiatry 157:1960–1965, 2000

Gainotti G: Emotional behavior and hemispheric side of the lesion. Cortex 8:41–55, 1972

Gallagher D, Thompson LW: Differential effectiveness of psychotherapies for the treatment of major depressive disorder in older adult patients. Psychotherapy: Theory, Research and Practice 19:42–49, 1982

George LK, Blazer DG, Hughes DC, et al: Social support and the outcome of major depression. Br J Psychiatry 154:478–485, 1989

Gerety MB, Williams JW Jr, Mulrow CD, et al: Performance of case-finding tools for depression in the nursing home: influence of clinical and functional characteristics and selection of optimal threshold scores. J Am Geriatr Soc 42:1103–1109, 1994

Glasser M, Rabins P: Mania in the elderly. Age Ageing 13:210–213, 1984

Glassman AH, Shapiro PA: Depression and the course of coronary artery disease. Am J Psychiatry 155:4–11, 1998

Greden JF: Antidepressant maintenance medications: when to discontinue and how to stop. J Clin Psychiatry 54 (suppl 8): 39–45, 1993

Greenberg RM: ECT in the elderly. New Dir Ment Health Serv 76:85–96, 1997

Greenwald BS, Kramer-Binsberg E, Marin DB, et al: Dementia with coexistent major depression. Am J Psychiatry 146:1472–1477, 1989

Gregoire F, Brauman H, de Buck R, et al: Hormone release in depressed patients before and after recovery. Psychoneuroendocrinology 2:303–312, 1977

Grinker RR, Miller J, Sabshin M, et al: The Phenomena of Depressions. New York, Harper & Row, 1961

Grober SE, Gordon WA, Sliwinski MJ, et al: Utility of the dexamethasone suppression test in the diagnosis of poststroke depression. Arch Phys Med Rehabil 72:1076–1079, 1991

Guy R: An Essay on Scirrhous Tumors and Cancer. London, J & A Churchill, 1979

Hamilton M: A rating scale for depression. J Neurol Neurosurg Psychiatry 23:56–62, 1960

Heiligenstein JH, Ware JE Jr, Beusterien KM, et al: Acute effects of fluoxetine versus placebo on functional health and well-being in late-life depression. International Psychogeriatrics 7 (suppl):125–137, 1995

Hickie I, Scott E: Late-onset depressive disorders: a preventable variant of cerebrovascular disease? Psychol Med 28:1007–1013, 1998

Hinkle P, Coffey CE, Weiner R, et al: ECT seizure duration varies with age. Paper presented at the annual meeting of the American Geriatrics Society, Chicago, IL, May 1986

Holahan CJ, Moos RH: Social support and psychological distress: a longitudinal analysis. J Abnorm Psychol 90:365–370, 1981

Hopkinson G: A genetic study of affective illness in patients over 50. Br J Psychiatry 110:244–254, 1964

Hopko DR, Bourland SL, Stanley MA, et al: Generalized anxiety disorder in older adults: examining the relation between clinician severity ratings and patient self-report measures. Depress Anxiety 12:217–225, 2000

Idler EL: Religious involvement and the health of the elderly: some hypotheses and an initial test. Social Forces 66:226–238, 1987

Jacobsen FM, Wehr TA, Sack DA, et al: Seasonal affective disorder: a review of the syndrome and its public health implications. Am J Public Health 77:57–60, 1987

Jenike MA, Albert MS: The dexamethasone suppression test in patients with presenile and senile dementia of the Alzheimer's type. J Am Geriatr Soc 32:441–444, 1984

Jonas BS, Mussolino ME: Symptoms of depression as a prospective risk factor for stroke. Psychosom Med 62:463–471, 2000

Judge R, Plewes JM, Kumar V, et al: Changes in energy during treatment of depression: an analysis of fluoxetine in double-blind, placebo-controlled trials. J Clin Psychopharmacol 20:666–672, 2000

Kendell RE: The classification of depressions: a review of contemporary confusion. Br J Psychiatry 129:15–28, 1976

Kiloh LG: Pseudo-dementia. Acta Psychiatr Scand 37:336–351, 1961

Klerman GL, Weissman MM, Rounsaville BJ, et al: Interpersonal Psychotherapy of Depression. New York, Basic Books, 1984

Knight DL, Krishnan KRR, Blazer DG, et al: Tritiated imipramine binding to platelets is markedly reduced in elderly depressed patients. Abstr Soc Neurosci 12:1251, 1986

Koenig HG: Treatment considerations for the depressed geriatric medical patient. Drugs Aging 1:266–278, 1991

Koenig HG, Blazer DG: Epidemiology of geriatric affective disorders. Clin Geriatr Med 8:235–251, 1992

Koenig HG, Weaver AJ: Counseling Troubled Older Adults: A Handbook for Pastors and Religious Caregivers. Nashville, TN, Abingdon, 1997

Koenig HG, George LK, Siegler IC: The use of religion and other emotion-regulating coping strategies among older adults. Gerontologist 28:303–310, 1988

Koenig HG, Shelp F, Goli V, et al: Survival and healthcare utilization in elderly medical inpatients with major depression. J Am Geriatr Soc 37:599–607, 1989

Koenig HG, Meador KG, Shelp F, et al: Depressive disorders in hospitalized medically ill patients: a comparison of young and elderly men. J Am Geriatr Soc 39:881–890, 1991

Koenig HG, Cohen HJ, Blazer DG, et al: Religious coping and depression in hospitalized medically ill older men. Am J Psychiatry 149:1693–1700, 1992a

Koenig HG, Meador KG, Goli V, et al: Self-rated depressive symptoms in medical inpatients: age and racial differences. Int J Psychiatry Med 22:11–31, 1992b

Koenig HG, Cohen HJ, Blazer DG, et al: Profile of depressive symptoms in younger and older medical inpatients with major depression. J Am Geriatr Soc 41:1169–1176, 1993

Koenig HG, Blumenthal J, Moore K: New version of brief depression scale (letter). J Am Geriatr Soc 43:1447, 1995

Koenig HG, George LK, Peterson BL, et al: Depression in medically ill hospitalized older adults: prevalence, correlates, and course of symptoms based on six diagnostic schemes. Am J Psychiatry 154:1376–1383, 1997

Koenig HG, George LK, Peterson BL: Religiosity and remission from depression in medically ill older patients. Am J Psychiatry 155:536–542, 1998

Kohn CS, Petrucci RJ, Baessler C, et al: The effect of psychological intervention on patients' long-term adjustment to the ICD: a prospective study. Pacing Clin Electrophysiol 23:450–456, 2000

Kraemlinger KG, Swanson DW, Maruta T: Are patients with chronic pain depressed? Am J Psychiatry 140:747–749, 1983

Krishnan KR, France RD, Pelton S, et al: Chronic pain and depression, I: classification of depression in chronic low back pain patients. Pain 22:279–287, 1985

Krishnan KR, Doraiswamy PM, Clary CM: Clinical and treatment response characteristics of late-life depression associated with vascular disease: a pooled analysis of two multicenter trials with sertraline. Prog Neuropsychopharmacol Biol Psychiatry 25:347–361, 2001

Kruesi MJ, Dale J, Straus SE: Psychiatric diagnoses in patients who have chronic fatigue syndrome. J Clin Psychiatry 40:53–56, 1989

Kupfer DJ: Neurophysiological "markers"—EEG sleep measures. J Psychiatr Res 18:467–495, 1984

Kupfer DJ, Foster FG, Coble P, et al: The application of EEG sleep for the differential diagnosis of affective disorders. Am J Psychiatry 135:69–74, 1978

Lakatua DJ, Nicolau GY, Bogdan C, et al: Circadian endocrine time structure in humans above 80 years of age. J Gerontol 39:648–654, 1984

Langner TS, Michael ST: Life Stress and Mental Health. Toronto, ON, Free Press of Glencoe, 1963

Lazarus LW, Weinberg J: Treatment in the ambulatory care setting, in Handbook of Geriatric Psychiatry. Edited by Busse EW, Blazer DG. New York, Van Nostrand Reinhold, 1980, pp 427–452

Lesse S: Masked Depression. New York, Jason Aronson, 1974

Levin S: Depression in the aged, in Geriatric Psychiatry: Grief, Loss, and Emotional Disorders in the Aging Process. Edited by Berezin MA, Cath SH. New York, International Universities Press, 1965, pp 203–225

Lewis AJ: Melancholia: a historical review. J Ment Sci 80:1 42, 1934

Lindemann E: Symptomatology and management of acute grief. Am J Psychiatry 101:141–148, 1944

Lindenbaum J, Healton EB, Savage DG, et al: Neuropsychiatric disorders caused by cobalamin deficiency in the absence of anemia or macrocytosis. N Engl J Med 318:1720–1728, 1988

Lloyd C: Life events and depressive disorder reviewed, I: events as predisposing factors. Arch Gen Psychiatry 37:529–535, 1980

Loosen PT, Prange AJ: Serum thyrotropin response to thyrotropin-releasing hormone in psychiatric patients: a review. Am J Psychiatry 139:405–416, 1982

Lustman PJ, Griffith LS, Freedland KE, et al: Cognitive behavior therapy for depression in type 2 diabetes mellitus. A randomized, controlled trial. Ann Intern Med 129:613–621, 1998

Lyketsos CG, Sheppard JM, Steele CD, et al: Randomized, placebo-controlled, double-blind clinical trial of sertraline in the treatment of depression complicating Alzheimer's disease: initial results from the Depression in Alzheimer's Disease study. Am J Psychiatry 157:1686–1689, 2000

Lyness JM, King DA, Conwell Y, et al: Cerebrovascular risk factors and 1-year depression outcome in older primary care patients. Am J Psychiatry 157:1499–1501, 2000

Magni G, Schifano F, De Leo D, et al: The dexamethasone suppression test in depressed and nondepressed geriatric medical inpatients. Acta Psychiatr Scand 73:511–514, 1986

Manly DT, Oakley SP Jr, Bloch RM: Electroconvulsive therapy in old-old patients. Am J Geriatr Psychiatry 8:232–236, 2000

Massey EW, Bullock R: Peroneal palsy in depression. J Clin Psychiatry 39:287, 291–292, 1978

Mayeux R: Depression in the patient with Parkinson's disease. J Clin Psychiatry 51 (suppl):20–23, 1990

McHugh PR: Beyond DSM-IV: from appearances to essences. Paper presented at the 154th annual meeting of the American Psychiatric Association, New Orleans, May 7, 2001

Mendlewicz J: The age factor in depressive illness: some genetic considerations. J Gerontol 31:300–303, 1976

Meyers BS, Kalayam B, Mei-Tal V: Late-onset delusional depression: a distinct clinical entity? J Clin Psychiatry 45:347–349, 1984

Mischoulon D, Burger JK, Spillmann MK, et al: Anemia and macrocytosis in the prediction of serum folate and vitamin B_{12} status, and treatment outcome in major depression. J Psychosom Res 49:183–187, 2000

Mossner R, Henneberg A, Schmitt A, et al: Allelic variation of serotonin transporter expression is associated with depression in Parkinson's disease. Mol Psychiatry 6:350–352, 2001

Multidimensional Functional Assessment: The OARS Methodology—A Manual, 2nd Edition. Durham, NC, Duke University Center for the Study of Aging and Human Development, 1978

Munro HN: Nutrition and aging. Br Med Bull 37:83–88, 1981

Murphy E: The prognosis of depression in old age. Br J Psychiatry 142:111–119, 1983

Murphy E, Smith R, Lindsay J, et al: Increased mortality rates in late-life depression. Br J Psychiatry 152:347–353, 1988

Musselman DL, Evans DL, Nemeroff CB: The relationship of depression to cardiovascular disease: epidemiology, biology, and treatment. Arch Gen Psychiatry 55:580–592, 1998

Myers JK, Weissman MM, Tischler GL, et al: Six-month prevalence of psychiatric disorders in three communities, 1980–1982. Arch Gen Psychiatry 41:959–967, 1984

Newhouse PA, Krishnan KR, Doraiswamy PM, et al: A double-blind comparison of sertraline and fluoxetine in depressed elderly outpatients. J Clin Psychiatry 61:559–568, 2000

Okifuji A, Turk DC, Sherman JJ: Evaluation of the relationship between depression and fibromyalgia syndrome: why aren't all patients depressed? J Rheumatol 27:212–219, 2000

Old Age Depression Interest Group: How long should the elderly take antidepressants? a double-blind placebo-controlled study of continuation/prophylaxis therapy with dothiepin. Br J Psychiatry 162:175–182, 1993

Palmore E, Kivett V: Change in life satisfaction: a longitudinal study of persons aged 46–70. J Gerontol 32:311–316, 1977

Pfifer JF, Murrell SA: Etiologic factors in the onset of depressive symptoms in older adults. J Abnorm Psychol 95:282–291, 1986

Pies RW: The diagnosis and treatment of subclinical hypothyroid states in depressed patients. Gen Hosp Psychiatry 19:344–354, 1997

Pincus T, Callahan LF, Bradley LA, et al: Elevated MMPI scores for hypochondriasis, depression, and hysteria in patients with rheumatoid arthritis reflect disease rather than psychological status. Arthritis Rheum 29:1456–1466, 1986

Post F: The management and nature of depressive illnesses in late life: a follow-through study. Br J Psychiatry 121:393–404, 1972

Post F: The functional psychoses, in Studies in Geriatric Psychiatry. Edited by Isaacs AD, Post F. New York, Wiley, 1978, pp 77–98

Pressman P, Lyons JS, Larson DB, et al: Religious belief, depression, and ambulation status in elderly women with broken hips. Am J Psychiatry 147:758–760, 1990

Price TRP, McAllister TW: Safety and efficacy of ECT in depressed patients with dementia: a review of clinical experience. Convulsive Therapy 5:61–74, 1989

Radloff LS: The CES-D scale: a self-report depression scale for research in the general population. Applied Psychological Measurement 1:385–401, 1977

Reifler BV, Larson E, Henley R: Coexistence of cognitive impairment and depression in geriatric outpatients. Am J Psychiatry 39:623–626, 1982

Reifler BV, Larson E, Teri L, et al: Dementia of the Alzheimer's type and depression. J Am Geriatr Soc 34:855–859, 1986

Reifler BV, Teri L, Raskind M, et al: Double-blind trial of imipramine in Alzheimer's disease patients with and without depression. Am J Psychiatry 146:45–49, 1989

Reynolds CF 3rd, Frank E, Perel JM, et al: Combined pharmacotherapy and psychotherapy in the acute and continuation treatment of elderly patients with recurrent major depression: a preliminary report. Am J Psychiatry 149:1687–1692, 1992

Robinson DS, Davis JM, Nies A, et al: Relation of sex and aging to monoamine oxidase activity of human brain, plasma, and platelets. Arch Gen Psychiatry 24:536–539, 1971

Robinson RG, Morris PLP, Fedoroff P: Depression and cerebrovascular disease. J Clin Psychiatry 51 (suppl 7):26–31, 1990

Rosenbach ML, Hermann RC, Dorwart RA: Use of electroconvulsive therapy in the Medicare population between 1987 and 1992. Psychiatr Serv 48:1537–1542, 1997

Rosenbaum AH, Schatzberg AF, MacLaughlin MS, et al: The dexamethasone suppression test in normal control subjects: comparison of two assays and effect of age. Am J Psychiatry 141:1550–1555, 1984

Rovner BW, German PS, Brant LJ, et al: Depression and mortality in nursing homes. JAMA 265:993–996, 1991

Sachar EJ: Neuroendocrine abnormalities in depressive illness, in Topics in Psychoendocrinology. Edited by Sachar EJ. New York, Grune & Stratton, 1975, pp 135–156

Sackeim HA, Greenberg MS, Weiman AL, et al: Hemispheric asymmetry in the expression of positive and negative emotions. Neurologic evidence. Arch Neurol 39:210–218, 1982

Salzman C, Shader RI: Responses to psychotropic drugs in the normal elderly, in Psychopharmacology in Aging. Edited by Eisdorfer C, Fann WE. New York, Plenum, 1972, pp 159–168

Schiffman S, Pasternak M: Decreased discrimination of food odors in the elderly. J Gerontol 34:73–79, 1979

Schleifer SJ, Macari-Hinson MM, Coyle DA, et al: The nature and course of depression following myocardial infarction. Arch Intern Med 149:1785–1789, 1989

Schneider LS, Severson JA, Sloane RB: Platelet 3H-imipramine binding in depressed elderly patients. Biol Psychiatry 20:1234–1237, 1985

Schneider LS, Severson JA, Pollock V, et al: Platelet monoamine oxidase activity in elderly depressed outpatients. Biol Psychiatry 21:1360–1364, 1986

Schulz B: Auszählungen in der Verwandtschaft von nach Erkrankungsalter und Geschlecht gruppierten Manisch-Depressiven. Arch Psychiatr Nervenkr 186:560–576, 1951

Schwab JJ, Clemmons RS, Bialow M, et al: A study of the somatic symptomatology of depression in medical inpatients. Psychosomatics 6:273–276, 1965

Scott J, Teasdale JD, Paykel ES, et al: Effects of cognitive therapy on psychological symptoms and social functioning in residual depression. Br J Psychiatry 177:440–446, 2000

Scovern AW, Kilmann PR: Status of electroconvulsive therapy: review of the outcome literature. Psychol Bull 87:260–303, 1980

Shulman KI: Mania in old age, in Affective Disorders in the Elderly. Edited by Murphy E. Edinburgh, Churchill Livingstone, 1986, pp 203–216

Shulman KI: The influence of age and aging on manic disorder. Int J Geriatr Psychiatry 4:63–65, 1989

Shulman KI, Post F: Bipolar affective disorder in old age. Br J Psychiatry 136:26–32, 1980

Slater E, Cowie V: The Genetics of Mental Disorder. London, Oxford University Press, 1971

Snyder PJ, Utiger RD: Response to thyrotropin releasing hormone (TRH) in normal man. J Clin Endocrinol Metab 34:380–385, 1972

Spar JE, Ford CV, Liston EH: Bipolar affective disorder in aged patients. J Clin Psychiatry 40:504–507, 1979

Spiegel D: Cancer and depression. Br J Psychiatry 169 (suppl):109–116, 1996

Srole L, Fischer AK: The Midtown Manhattan Longitudinal Study vs "The Mental Paradise Lost" doctrine: a controversy joined. Arch Gen Psychiatry 37:209–221, 1980

Staab JP, Evans DL: Efficacy of venlafaxine in geriatric depression. Depress Anxiety 12 (suppl 1):63–68, 2000

Stenstedt A: Involutional melancholia: an etiologic, clinical and social study of endogenous depression in later life, with special reference to genetic factors. Acta Psychiatr Neurol Scand 127 (suppl):5–71, 1959

Steuer JL, Mintz J, Hammen CL, et al: Cognitive-behavioral and psychodynamic group psychotherapy in treatment of geriatric depression. J Consult Clin Psychol 52:180–189, 1984

Stewart R, Prince M, Mann A, et al: Stroke, vascular risk factors and depression: cross-sectional study in a UK Caribbean-born population. Br J Psychiatry 178:23–28, 2001

Stoudemire A, Hill CD, Morris R, et al: Long-term outcome of treatment-resistant depression in older adults. Am J Psychiatry 150:1539–1540, 1993

Stoudemire A, Hill CD, Morris R, et al: Improvement in depression-related cognitive dysfunction following ECT. J Neuropsychiatry Clin Neurosci 7:31–34, 1995

Stoudemire A, Hill CD, Marquardt M, et al: Recovery and relapse in geriatric depression after treatment with antidepressants and ECT in a medical-psychiatric population. Gen Hosp Psychiatry 20:170–174, 1998

Sumaya IC, Rienzi BM, Deegan JF 2nd, et al: Bright light treatment decreases depression in institutionalized older adults: a placebo-controlled crossover study. J Gerontol 56:M356–M360, 2001

Targum SD, Sullivan AC, Byrnes SM: Neuroendocrine relationships in major depressive disorder. Am J Psychiatry 139:282–286, 1982

Tew JD Jr, Mulsant BH, Haskett RF, et al: Acute efficacy of ECT in the treatment of major depression in the old-old. Am J Psychiatry 156:1865–1870, 1999

Thakur M, Hays J, Krishnan KRR: Clinical, demographic and social characteristics of psychotic depression. Psychiatry Res 86:99–106, 1999

Thielman SB, Blazer DG: Depression and dementia, in Dementia in Old Age. Edited by Pitt B. Edinburgh, Churchill Livingstone, 1986, pp 251–264

Thomae H: Personality and adjustment to aging, in The Handbook of Aging and Mental Health. Edited by Birren J, Sloane RB. Englewood Cliffs, NJ, Prentice-Hall, 1980, pp 285–309

Thomas VS, Rockwood KJ: Alcohol abuse, cognitive impairment, and mortality among older people. J Am Geriatr Soc 49:415–420, 2001

Thompson LW, Gallagher D, Steinmetz-Breckenridge J: Comparative effectiveness of psychotherapies for depressed elders. J Consult Clin Psychol 55:385–390, 1987

Tourigny-Rivard M, Raskin DM, Rivard D: The dexamethasone suppression test in an elderly population. Biol Psychiatry 16:1177–1184, 1981

Ulrich RF, Shaw DH, Kupfer DJ: Effects of aging on EEG sleep in depression. Sleep 3:31–40, 1980

Verwoerdt A: Clinical Geropsychiatry. Baltimore, MD, Williams & Wilkins, 1976

Vogel GW, Vogel F, McAbee RS, et al: Improvement of depression by REM sleep deprivation: new findings and a theory. Arch Gen Psychiatry 37:247–253, 1980

Ward NG, Turner JA, Ready B, et al: Chronic pain, depression, and the dexamethasone suppression test. Pain 48:331–338, 1992

Weihs KL, Settle EC Jr, Batey SR, et al: Bupropion sustained release versus paroxetine for the treatment of depression in the elderly. J Clin Psychiatry 61:196–202, 2000

Weiner RD: The role of electroconvulsive therapy in the treatment of depression in the elderly. J Am Geriatr Soc 30:710–712, 1982

Weissman MM, Prusoff BA, Klerman GL: Personality and the prediction of long-term outcome in depression. Am J Psychiatry 135:797–800, 1978

Weissman MM, Bruce ML, Leaf PJ, et al: Affective disorders, in Psychiatric Disorders in America: The Epidemiologic Catchment Area Study. Edited by Robins LN, Regier DA. New York, Free Press, 1991, pp 53–80

Wells CE: Pseudodementia. Am J Psychiatry 136:895–900, 1979

Wesner RB, Winokur G: The influence of age on the natural history of unipolar depression when treated with electroconvulsive therapy. Eur Arch Psychiatry Neurol Sci 238:149–154, 1989

Whitlock FA, Sisking M: Depression and cancer: a follow-up study. Psychol Med 9:747–752, 1979

Wigdor BT: Drives and motivations with aging, in The Handbook of Aging and Mental Health. Edited by Birren JE, Sloane RB. Englewood Cliffs, NJ, Prentice-Hall, 1980, pp 245–261

Winokur G: The Iowa 500: heterogeneity and course in manic-depressive illness (bipolar). Compr Psychiatry 16:125–131, 1975

Wylie ME, Mulsant BH, Pollock BG: Age of onset in geriatric bipolar disorder: effects on clinical presentation and treatment outcomes in an inpatient sample. Am J Geriatr Psychiatry 7:77–83, 1999

Yassa R, Nair V, Nastase C, et al: Prevalence of bipolar disorder in a psychogeriatric population. J Affect Disord 14:197–201, 1988

Yesavage JA, Brink TL, Rose TL, et al: Development and validation of a geriatric depression screening scale: a preliminary report. J Psychiatr Res 17:37–49, 1983

Young RC, Falk JR: Age, manic psychopathology, and treatment response. Int J Geriatr Psychiatry 4:73–78, 1989

Young RC, Klerman GL: Mania in late life: focus on age at onset. Am J Psychiatry 149:867–876, 1992

Young RC, Nambudiri DE, Jain H, et al: Brain computed tomography in geriatric manic disorder. Biol Psychiatry 45:1063–1065, 1999

Zesiewicz TA, Gold M, Chari G, et al: Current issues in depression in Parkinson's disease. Am J Geriatr Psychiatry 7:110–118, 1999

Zung WWK: A self-rating depression scale. Arch Gen Psychiatry 12:63–70, 1965

Zung WWK, Green RL: Detection of affective disorders in the aged, in Psychopharmacology in Aging. Edited by Eisdorfer C, Fann WE. New York, Plenum, 1972, pp 213–224

Schizophrenia and Paranoid Disorders

Dilip V. Jeste, M.D.

Julie Loebach Wetherell, Ph.D.

Christian R. Dolder, Pharm.D., B.C.P.S.

Delusions, hallucinations, and other psychotic symptoms can accompany a number of conditions in late life. These symptoms may be more common than previously thought; a recent Swedish investigation found that the prevalence of any psychotic symptom in a population-based sample of 85-year-old individuals without dementia was 10.1%, with 6.9% experiencing hallucinations, 5.5% having delusions, and 6.9% experiencing paranoid ideation (Ostling and Skoog 2002). Some conditions that cause psychotic symptoms, such as delirium and substance-induced psychosis, are acute and tend to resolve when the underlying condition is treated. These conditions are discussed elsewhere in this volume. In this chapter, we review the epidemiology, presentation, and treatment of chronic late-life psychotic disorders not secondary to a mood disorder or a general medical condition other than dementia. Thus, we discuss early-onset schizophrenia, late-onset schizophrenia, very late onset schizophrenia-like psychosis (with onset after 60), delusional disorder, and psychosis of Alzheimer's disease (AD). We also address the risk factors for and the prevalence, course, prevention, and treatment of tardive dyskinesia (TD) in older patients.

Schizophrenia

Early-Onset Schizophrenia

Most individuals with schizophrenia develop the disease in the second or third decade of life (American Psychiat-

ric Association 2000). Although mortality rates in general, and suicide and homicide rates in particular, are higher among individuals with schizophrenia than in the general population (Hannerz et al. 2001; Hiroeh et al. 2001; Joukamaa et al. 2001), many patients with early-onset schizophrenia now live into older adulthood. Thus, approximately 80% of the older adults with schizophrenia typically have had an early onset of the disease and have a chronic course spanning several decades. The prevalence of schizophrenia among individuals ages 45–64 is approximately 0.6%, and prevalence estimates for elderly individuals range from 0.1% to 0.5% (Castle and Murray 1993; Copeland et al. 1998; Keith et al. 1991).

Longitudinal follow-up of schizophrenia patients indicates considerable heterogeneity of outcome. Approximately 20% of patients experience remission of both positive and negative symptoms (Ciompi 1980; Harding et al. 1987; Huber 1997). Another 20% experience worsening of symptoms, and the course in the remaining 60% remains largely unchanged (Belitsky and McGlashan 1993; Cohen 1990; Harvey et al. 1999). Initial deterioration usually occurs shortly after disease onset and is often limited to the first 5–10 years, followed by stability or even improvement of symptoms with aging. Factors associated with poorer prognosis for early-onset schizophrenia include chronicity, insidious onset, premorbid psychosocial or functional deficits, and prominent negative symptoms (Ram et al. 1992).

In one large sample of chronically institutionalized patients with schizophrenia, older age was associated with lower levels of positive symptoms and higher levels of negative symptoms (Davidson et al. 1995). Other investigations involving more representative outpatient samples have failed to find such a relationship between age and symptomatology (see, for example, Jeste et al. 1996).

Cognitive performance tends to remain stable, although it tends to be worse in patients with schizophrenia than in healthy older adults (Eyler Zorrilla et al. 2000; Heaton et al. 2001). Heaton and colleagues (2001) followed a large number of schizophrenia outpatients longitudinally for 6 months to 10 years and compared them with healthy subjects, using a comprehensive battery of neuropsychological measures. Schizophrenia patients had deficits relative to healthy subjects, particularly in the areas of learning, abstraction, and cognitive flexibility, but there was no evidence of cognitive deterioration over time. Eyler Zorrilla and colleagues (2000) compared a group of schizophrenia outpatients with healthy comparison subjects cross-sectionally using a dementia screening test and found that although cognitive performance seemed to worsen with aging, there were no age-related differences in the slope of cognitive decline between the two groups. Harvey and colleagues (1999) followed a group of chronically institutionalized older patients with schizophrenia longitudinally for 30 months and found a subset of approximately 30% who experienced a decline in cognitive and functional status; however, this sample was not representative of most community-dwelling elderly patients.

Level of functional impairment varies considerably among older adults with schizophrenia. Palmer and colleagues (2003) found that 30% of a group of older schizophrenic outpatients had been employed at least part-time since the onset of psychosis, 43% were current drivers, and 73% were living independently. In general, worse neuropsychological test performance, lower educational level, and negative symptoms, but not positive symptoms or depressed mood, are associated with poorer functional capacity in older outpatients with schizophrenia (Evans et al. 2003).

Late-Onset Schizophrenia

Some research, including work at our Advanced Center for Interventions and Services Research in Older People with Psychosis at the University of California, San Diego, has focused on patients whose schizophrenia symptoms began in mid- to late life. These individuals comprise a substantial minority of older schizophrenia patients. A literature review found that approximately 23% of patients with schizophrenia reportedly had an onset after age 40, with 3% being older than 60 years (Harris and

Jeste 1988). One investigation involving first-contact patients found that 29% of patients had an onset after age 44, with 12% reporting an onset after age 64 (Howard et al. 1993).

Historically, schizophrenia has been considered a disease of younger adulthood. Kraepelin (1919/1971) denoted schizophrenia *dementia praecox* to distinguish it from organic disorders arising in late life and to indicate a poor prognosis with progressive deterioration. However, in later years, Kraepelin observed that some cases arose for the first time in older age and that progressive decline was not a universal feature of the disease.

Subsequently, Bleuler (1943) described late-onset schizophrenia as being similar to early-onset schizophrenia but with an onset after age 40. Roth (1955) applied the term *late paraphrenia* to patients (primarily women) who had no family history of psychosis and whose symptoms (hallucinations, delusions, and sensory deficits) developed after age 65. The difference in family history implied a different etiology, raising the possibility of late-onset paraphrenia as a distinct disease entity from the more typical early-onset schizophrenia.

In DSM-I (American Psychiatric Association 1952) and DSM-II (American Psychiatric Association 1968) criteria for schizophrenia, age at onset was not specified. In DSM-III (American Psychiatric Association 1980), the diagnosis of schizophrenia was reserved for patients with an onset before age 45. Although DSM-III-R (American Psychiatric Association 1987) included a late-onset specifier for patients whose onset was at age 45 or later, in DSM-IV (American Psychiatric Association 1994) and its text revision, DSM-IV-TR (American Psychiatric Association 2000), age at onset is not specified.

The recent consensus statement by the International Late-Onset Schizophrenia Group suggested that schizophrenia with an onset after age 40 should be called late-onset schizophrenia and considered a subtype of schizophrenia rather than a related disorder (Howard et al. 2000). This decision was primarily based on evidence suggesting that schizophrenia with an onset in middle age is a neurodevelopmental disorder, rather than a neurodegenerative disorder, that shares more similarities than differences with schizophrenia with an earlier onset (Palmer et al. 2001).

Risk factors for and clinical presentation (including positive symptoms such as hallucinations, delusions, bizarre behavior, and thought disorder) of early-onset schizophrenia are similar to those associated with late-onset schizophrenia (Brodaty et al. 1999; Jeste et al. 1995b). The self-reported proportion of individuals with a family history of schizophrenia is similar among patients with early-onset schizophrenia and those with late-onset schizophrenia (10%–15%), and no consistent relationship has been found between age at onset and genetic risk of schizophrenia (Jeste et al. 1997b; Kendler et al. 1987). Levels of childhood maladjustment, measured retrospectively, were similar in late-onset and early-onset schizophrenia patients and higher than those in healthy subjects (Jeste et al. 1997b). Patients with late-onset schizophrenia show increased rates of minor physical anomalies relative to healthy subjects, and rates in the two groups of schizophrenia patients are comparable (Lohr et al. 1997).

Neuroimaging studies of patients with late-onset schizophrenia do not suggest the presence of strokes, tumors, or other abnormalities that could account for the development of schizophrenia in late life (Rivkin et al. 2000; Symonds et al. 1997), although nonspecific structural abnormalities such as enlarged ventricles and increased white matter hyperintensities may be more common in late- than in early-onset schizophrenia (Sachdev et al. 1999). In one preliminary study, magnetic resonance imaging showed a larger volume of thalamus in late-onset schizophrenia compared with early-onset schizophrenia (Corey-Bloom et al. 1995).

Long-term neuropsychological follow-up of a group of late-onset schizophrenia patients revealed no evidence of cognitive decline, again suggesting a neurodevelopmental rather than a neurodegenerative process (Palmer et al. 2003).

Early- and late-onset schizophrenia differ with regard to gender ratio, preponderance of the paranoid subtype, prevalence of negative symptoms, cognitive performance, and premorbid functioning. Individuals with an onset of schizophrenia in mid- to late life are predominantly women (Hafner et al. 1998; Jeste et al. 1997b). Estrogen may serve as an endogenous antipsychotic, masking schizophrenic symptoms in vulnerable women until after menopause (Seeman 1996). On the basis of this "estrogen hypothesis," researchers are investigating the efficacy of hormone replacement therapy as an adjunct treatment for postmenopausal women with psychosis (Kulkarni et al. 1996, 2001; Lindamer et al. 2001).

Data from our center suggest a higher prevalence of the paranoid subtype of schizophrenia among patients with late-onset schizophrenia (approximately 75%) relative to patients with early-onset schizophrenia (approximately 50%) (Jeste et al. 1997b). Patients with late-onset schizophrenia tend to have more auditory hallucinations or hallucinations with a running commentary, persecutory delusions with or without hallucinations, and organized delusions (Howard et al. 2000). Patients with late-onset schizophrenia have lower levels of negative symptoms on average (including affective blunting, alogia, avolition, and inattention) than patients with early-onset schizophrenia; however, late-onset schizophrenia patients

have higher levels of negative symptoms than normal subjects (Jeste et al. 1988, 1997b; Palmer et al. 2001).

On neuropsychological tests (after correction for age, education, and gender), patients with late-onset schizophrenia tend to demonstrate less impairment in learning, abstraction, and flexibility in thinking than patients with early-onset schizophrenia (Jeste et al. 1997b). A greater proportion of patients with late-onset schizophrenia have successful occupational and marital histories and generally higher premorbid functioning than do patients with early-onset schizophrenia. Finally, patients with late-onset schizophrenia typically require lower daily doses of antipsychotic medications compared with age-comparable patients with early-onset schizophrenia, although the general response to such medications is similar in both groups (Jeste et al. 1993, 1997b).

Sensory deficits, particularly hearing loss, are associated with psychotic symptoms in late life and have been proposed as a risk factor for late-onset schizophrenia (Howard et al. 1994; Raghuram et al. 1980). However, other data suggest that both early- and late-onset schizophrenia patients may be less likely than healthy older adults to receive appropriate correction of vision and hearing impairments (Prager and Jeste 1993). Thus, uncorrected sensory deficits may reflect poorer health care utilization by older psychotic patients and may not be a potential cause of psychosis in the elderly population.

Very Late Onset Schizophrenia-Like Psychosis

In its consensus statement, the International Late-Onset Schizophrenia Group proposed the diagnostic term *very late onset schizophrenia-like psychosis* for patients whose psychosis began after age 60 (Howard et al. 2000). Risk factors for and clinical features of early-onset schizophrenia, late-onset schizophrenia, and very late onset schizophrenia-like psychosis are compared in Table 15–1. Factors distinguishing patients with very late onset schizophrenia from "true" schizophrenia patients include a lower genetic load, less evidence of early childhood maladjustment, a relative lack of thought disorder and negative symptoms (including blunted affect), greater risk of TD, and evidence of a neurodegenerative rather than a neurodevelopmental process (Andreasen 1999; Howard et al. 1997).

Very late onset schizophrenia-like psychosis is a heterogeneous entity that has essentially replaced late paraphrenia as a catchall diagnostic category for late-life psychosis not due to schizophrenia. It includes conditions with etiologies as diverse as strokes, tumors, and other neurodegenerative changes. Clinical and research attention should be devoted to the presentation, cause, and

TABLE 15–1. Comparison of early-onset schizophrenia, late-onset schizophrenia, and very late onset schizophrenia-like psychosis

	Early-onset schizophrenia	Late-onset schizophrenia	Very late onset schizophrenia-like psychosis
Age at onset (years)	<40	~ 40–60 (middle age)	≥60 (late life)
Female preponderance	–	+	++
Negative symptoms	++	+	–
Minor physical anomalies	+	+	–
Neuropsychological impairment			
Learning	++	+	?++
Retention	–	–	?++
Progressive cognitive deterioration	–	–	++
Brain structure abnormalities (e.g., strokes, tumors)	–	–	++
Family history of schizophrenia	+	+	–
Early childhood maladjustment	+	+	–
Daily antipsychotic dose	Higher	Lower	Lower
Risk of tardive dyskinesia	+	+	++

Note. + = mildly present; ++ = strongly present; ?++ = probably strongly present, but few data exist; – = absent.
Source. Adapted from Palmer et al. 2001.

course of illness in patients who develop psychotic symptoms for the first time in old age.

Delusional Disorder

At least 6% of older adults have paranoid symptoms such as persecutory delusions, but most of these individuals have dementia (Christenson and Blazer 1984; Forsell and Henderson 1998; Henderson et al. 1998). The essential feature of a delusional disorder is a nonbizarre delusion (e.g., a persecutory, somatic, erotomanic, grandiose, or jealous delusion) without prominent auditory or visual hallucinations. Symptoms must be present for at least 1 month. When delusional disorder arises in late life, basic personality features are typically intact, and functioning outside the delusional sphere is preserved. Intellectual performance and occupational functioning are preserved, but social functioning is compromised. To make a diagnosis of delusional disorder, the clinician must rule out delirium, dementia, psychotic disorders due to general medical conditions or the use of a substance, schizophrenia, and mood disorders with psychotic features. The course of persecutory delusional disorder is typically chronic, but patients with other types of delusions may have partial remissions and relapses.

According to DSM-IV-TR, the prevalence of delusional disorder is 0.03% and is slightly higher among women than among men. The disorder typically first appears in middle to late adulthood; the average age at onset is 40–49 years for men and 60–69 years for women.

Risk factors for delusional disorder include a family history of schizophrenia or avoidant, paranoid, or schizoid personality disorder (Kendler and Davis 1981). Evidence supporting hearing loss as a risk factor for paranoia is mixed (Cooper and Curry 1976; Moore 1981). In one neuroimaging study, brain atrophy and white matter hyperintensities did not distinguish older psychotic patients with somatic delusions from those without such delusions (Rockwell et al. 1994). Evans and colleagues (1996) compared middle-aged and older patients with schizophrenia and delusional disorder and found no differences in neuropsychological impairment but discovered that more severe psychopathology was associated with delusional disorder. Finally, immigration and low socioeconomic status may be risk factors for delusional disorder (American Psychiatric Association 1994).

Psychosis of Alzheimer's Disease

Psychotic symptoms in elderly individuals may arise secondary to AD or other dementias. Systematic studies of psychosis in dementia have focused on AD because AD is the most common type of dementia in the elderly population, representing approximately 65%–70% of dementia cases (Cummings and Benson 1992). Approximately 35%–50% of AD patients manifest psychotic symptoms, typically in the middle stages of the disease (Cummings et al. 1987; Mendez et al. 1990; Wragg and Jeste 1989). In a large sample of patients with probable AD, the cumulative incidence of psychotic symptoms was 20% at 1 year, 36% at 2 years, 50% at 3 years, and 51% at 4 years (Paulsen et al. 2000). Delusions, especially of a persecutory nature, tend to be more common than hallucinations, the latter being more common in nursing homes and other institutional settings (Wragg and Jeste 1989). In one large naturalistic study of the course of psychotic symptoms in dementia, Devanand and colleagues (1997) found that hallucinations and paranoid delusions were more persistent than depressive symptoms but less prevalent and less persistent than behavioral disturbances, particularly agitation.

In Table 15–2, characteristics associated with psychosis of AD are compared with characteristics of schizophrenia in elderly patients (Jeste and Finkel 2000). The most common psychotic symptoms in AD are delusions (which tend to be paranoid, concrete, simple, and nonbizarre) and hallucinations (which are more frequently visual than auditory). Misidentification of caregivers is frequent, whereas schneiderian first rank symptoms, such as hearing a running commentary on one's actions or hearing multiple voices talking to one another, are rare (Burns et al. 1990). Delusions or hallucinations may need to be inferred from the patient's behavior because the patient may be unable to verbalize thoughts or perceptions owing to cognitive impairment, particularly in the later stages of the disease. Active suicidal ideation and past history of psychosis are rare. Because psychotic symptoms in patients with dementia tend to remit in the late stages of the disease, very long term maintenance therapy with antipsychotics is typically unnecessary. Finally, antipsychotic medication doses are lower for AD patients than for older adults with schizophrenia, and much lower than for younger adults.

AD patients with psychosis and those without psychosis differ in several important ways. Neuropsychologically, AD patients with psychosis show greater impairment in executive functioning and a more rapid cognitive decline (Jeste et al. 1992; Stern et al. 1994). Psychosis is associated with a greater prevalence of extrapyramidal signs in AD (Stern et al. 1994). Delusions in dementia have been associated with dysfunction in paralimbic areas of the frontotemporal cortex (Sultzer 1996). Neuropathologically, dementia patients with psychosis have shown increased neurodegenerative changes in the cortex, increased norepinephrine levels in subcortical regions, and reduced serotonin levels in both cortical and subcortical areas (Zubenko et al. 1991). In one study, AD patients with psychosis had much higher levels of tau protein in the entorhinal and temporal cortices than did nonpsychotic AD patients (Mukaetova-Ladinska et al. 1995).

TABLE 15–2. Comparison of psychosis of Alzheimer's disease with schizophrenia in older patients

	Psychosis of AD	Schizophrenia
Prevalence	35%–50% of AD patients	<1% of general population
Bizarre or complex delusions	Rare	Frequent
Misidentification of caregivers	Frequent	Rare
Common form of hallucinations	Visual	Auditory
Schneiderian first rank symptoms	Rare	Frequent
Active suicidal ideation	Rare	Frequent
Past history of psychosis	Rare	Very common
Eventual remission of psychosis	Frequent	Uncommon
Need for years of maintenance antipsychotic therapy	Uncommon	Very common
Usual optimal daily doses of commonly used atypical antipsychotics		
Risperidone	0.75–1.5 mg	1.5–2.5 mg
Olanzapine	2.5–7.5 mg	7.5–12.5 mg
Recommended adjunctive psychosocial treatment	Sensory enhancement, structured activities, social contact, behavior therapy[a]	Cognitive-behavioral therapy, social skills training[b]

Note. AD = Alzheimer's disease.
[a]Cohen-Mansfield 2001.
[b]Granholm et al. 2002; McQuaid et al. 2000.
Source. Adapted from Jeste and Finkel 2000.

Jeste and Finkel (2000) recommended specific diagnostic criteria for psychosis of AD in order to facilitate epidemiologic, clinical, and therapeutic research. These criteria include the presence of visual or auditory hallucinations or delusions, a primary diagnosis of AD, a chronology indicating that psychotic symptoms followed the onset of dementia, a duration of 1 month or longer, and severity significant enough to disrupt the patient's functioning. Criteria for schizophrenia, schizoaffective disorder, delusional disorder, or mood disorder with psychotic features should never have been met, the disturbance must not occur exclusively during the course of delirium, and the disturbance must not be better accounted for by another general medical condition or by physiological effects of a substance. Associated symptoms may include agitation; negative symptoms such as apathy, flattening of affect, avolition, or motor retardation; and depression (with depressed mood, insomnia or hypersomnia, feelings of worthlessness or excessive or inappropriate guilt, or recurrent thoughts of death).

Psychosis is also common in dementias such as those associated with Parkinson's disease and Lewy body disease. Visual hallucinations and secondary delusions are common in Lewy body disease, and vascular dementia may also be accompanied by delusions or hallucinations (Schneider 1999). Naimark et al. (1996) found psychotic symptoms in approximately one-third of a sample of Parkinson's disease patients, with hallucinations being more common than delusions. Because dopaminergic agents can increase the risk of psychotic symptoms, some of the psychotic symptoms may be iatrogenic. Such patients may show partial or total lack of insight and no other evidence of thought disorder.

Treatment

The modern era of pharmacological treatment for schizophrenia and related disorders began with the introduction of chlorpromazine in the early 1950s. Although this and other conventional agents were able to substantially improve the positive symptoms of schizophrenia (e.g., hallucinations and delusions), a number of treatment liabilities have been recognized over the years, such as movement disorders, sedation, orthostatic hypotension, and increased prolactin concentrations. Furthermore, these medications generally do not improve the negative symptoms of schizophrenia (e.g., amotivation, social withdrawal, blunted affect, and alogia) that also play an important role in the daily lives of patients with schizophrenia.

Atypical antipsychotic agents such as clozapine, risperidone, olanzapine, and quetiapine are the drugs of choice for older adults with psychotic symptoms and disorders. Because older adults are more susceptible to extrapyramidal symptoms, toxicity, and sedation, the saying "start low and go slow" applies to the use of these medications in older patients. Although there are few data on the use of these medications in older patients, these drugs have fewer extrapyramidal side effects and may be somewhat more effective against negative symptoms than conventional antipsychotics. These newer agents may also have some positive effect on cognitive deficits in schizophrenia.

Treatment of Schizophrenia and Delusional Disorder

Patients with late-onset schizophrenia respond well to low-dose antipsychotic medication, requiring approximately one-half the dose typically taken by older patients with early-onset schizophrenia and 25%–33% of the dose used in younger schizophrenic patients. Patients with psychosis secondary to dementia typically require even lower doses, approximately 15%–25% of the dose used by younger patients with psychosis. Maintenance pharmacotherapy is usually required for older schizophrenia patients because of the risk of relapse. Because psychosis of dementia frequently remits, it may be possible to taper medications after the psychotic episode has been resolved.

Generally, atypical antipsychotics carry a much lower risk of TD than do conventional antipsychotics. Clozapine therapy may be inappropriate because of the risk of leukopenia, agranulocytosis, and other side effects, such as orthostasis, sedation, and anticholinergic effects. The need for frequent blood sampling may also pose a problem for older patients. Risperidone in higher doses appears to carry a greater risk of extrapyramidal side effects. Other side effects of note include orthostatic hypotension, sedation, weight gain, and the risk of developing hyperglycemia and Type II diabetes (Allison et al. 1999; Jin et al. 2002; Wirshing et al. 1998).

Although antipsychotic medications can be efficacious in older patients with delusional disorder, some patients do not respond to treatment, and others have difficulty with adherence because of their delusional belief system.

Treatment of Psychosis of Alzheimer's Disease and Other Dementias

Atypical antipsychotics such as clozapine, risperidone, olanzapine, and quetiapine show promise as agents for treatment of patients with psychosis of dementia (Katz et al. 1999; Street et al. 2000). In a nursing home sample, 1- and 2-mg daily doses of risperidone were more effective than placebo in reducing psychotic symptoms and aggressive behavior, but the 2-mg dose was associated with a greater risk of extrapyramidal symptoms (Katz et al. 1999). Also in a nursing home setting, a placebo-controlled trial of olanzapine found that 5 mg/day was preferable to larger doses in treating AD-related psychosis and behavioral disturbances (Street et al. 2000).

Patients who have dementia with Lewy bodies or parkinsonian dementia are especially sensitive to side effects such as extrapyramidal symptoms and anticholinergic effects, so very low initial and target doses and very slow titration should be used to avoid adverse effects on motor symptoms (Stoppe et al. 1999). Clozapine has been shown to reduce symptoms and may improve tremor in some patients (Bonuccelli et al. 1997; Masand 2000). Trials of olanzapine for Parkinson's disease–related dementia have indicated improvement of psychotic symptoms (Graham et al. 1998; Wolters et al. 1996) but exacerbation of parkinsonian symptoms (Goetz et al. 2000; Wolters et al. 1996). Quetiapine appears to improve psychotic symptoms without worsening motor function (Yeung et al. 2000). Donepezil has also shown utility in treating paranoid and delusional ideation in patients who have dementia with Lewy bodies (Samuel et al. 2000).

Although conventional antipsychotics are reasonably effective in the treatment of psychosis of dementia, their side-effect profiles make them less desirable. The risk of extrapyramidal symptoms is higher among older patients than among younger patients (Jeste et al. 1999c). Moreover, the incidence of TD is higher among patients who begin taking conventional antipsychotics in old age than among similarly aged patients who began taking these medications at younger ages (Jeste et al. 1995b). More detailed information about TD in older patients is presented later in this chapter (see "Tardive Dyskinesia in Older Adults" below). Other side effects of antipsychotics include sedation, anticholinergic effects, cardiovascular effects (including orthostatic hypotension), parkinsonian reactions, and neuroleptic malignant syndrome. Careful monitoring for these side effects, as well as for involuntary abnormal movements, is recommended when working with psychotic dementia patients.

Psychosocial Treatment

Psychosocial treatment is a useful adjunct to pharmacological therapy. A supportive relationship with the treating physician can improve medication adherence and facilitate monitoring of symptoms, making hospitalization and other crises less likely. Enlisting the help of caregivers, family, neighbors, friends, and other community members may also facilitate the patient's care. Although research has not focused on older patients, social skills training and cognitive-behavioral therapy show promise with regard to reducing symptoms and improving functioning (Granholm et al. 2002; McQuaid et al. 2000).

Tardive Dyskinesia in Older Adults

TD is one of the most serious adverse effects of treatment with antipsychotics. This disorder, consisting of abnormal, involuntary movements, is generally caused by long-term treatment with antipsychotic medication. The movements are typically choreoathetoid in nature and principally involve the mouth, face, limbs, and trunk. In middle-aged and elderly patients, orofacial TD is twice as common as dyskinesias involving the limbs and trunk (Paulsen et al. 1996).

Incidence and Prevalence

TD is a side effect experienced by some patients receiving long-term treatment with antipsychotics. Yassa and Jeste (1992) reviewed 76 studies (published between 1960 and 1990) of the prevalence of TD. In a total population of roughly 40,000 patients, the overall prevalence of TD was 24.2%, although the prevalence was much higher in studies involving elderly patients treated with antipsychotics. Among young adults, the annual cumulative incidence of TD is 4%–5% (Kane et al. 1988), but the risk increases substantially with age and with increased antipsychotic exposure. Jeste and colleagues (1999c) evaluated 439 psychiatric patients (mean age, 65 years) and found that 28.8% met criteria for TD during the first 12 months of treatment with antipsychotics, 50.1% had TD by the end of 24 months of treatment, and 63.1% by the end of 36 months of treatment. The risk of severe TD has also been reported to be higher among older patients (Caligiuri et al. 1997).

Risk Factors

Although many studies have examined the risk factors for TD, an incomplete understanding remains. Aging appears to be the most important risk factor for TD (American Psychiatric Association 2000; Yassa and Jeste 1992). Although the mechanism of this increase is unclear, it may be due to pharmacokinetic changes in elderly individuals and to the tendency of the nigrostriatal system to degenerate with age (Jeste and Caligiuri 1993). Previous investigators found TD to be associated with early extrapyramidal symptoms (Chouinard et al. 1979; Saltz et al. 1991), alcohol abuse or dependence (Dixon et al. 1992; Olivera et al. 1990), and certain ethnicities (Glazer et al. 1994; Jeste et al. 1996; Lawson 1986). The presence of subtle, subclinical movement disorders at the beginning of antipsychotic treatment, assessed by sensitive instrumental procedures, also increases the risk of TD (Jeste et al. 1999b). Longer total exposure to typical antipsychotic agents has been associated with greater TD risk (Casey 1997), and within the elderly population, the cumulative amount of high-potency typical antipsychotics has been associated with higher TD risk (Jeste et al. 1995a).

The reduction of extrapyramidal symptoms and dyskinesia symptoms (as measured by rating scales) in short-term clinical trials of antipsychotics, along with the lower risk of extrapyramidal symptoms with the use of atypical agents, has led to the expectation that there is a reduced risk of TD during treatment with an atypical antipsychotic. Although more long-term prospective studies of the risk of TD with administration of atypical agents are needed, evidence supporting a reduced risk is emerging. The low risk of TD among clozapine-treated individuals has been reported (Kane et al. 1993), and a lower incidence of TD has also been reported in patients treated with risperidone (Chouinard et al. 1993; Jeste et al. 1999a, 1999b) or olanzapine (Tollefson et al. 1997).

Course and Outcome

TD may develop at any age and usually has an insidious onset. It may occur during exposure to antipsychotic medication or within 4 weeks of withdrawal from an oral antipsychotic (or within 8 weeks of withdrawal from a depot antipsychotic). Symptoms of TD can also increase transiently when a conventional antipsychotic is replaced by an atypical antipsychotic. For a diagnosis of TD to be made, the patient must have taken antipsychotics for at least 3 months (in older adults, only 1 month is necessary) (American Psychiatric Association 2000).

The most common features of TD are involuntary movements of the tongue, face, and neck muscles. The movements of TD are choreiform (rapid, jerky), athetoid (slow, sinuous), or rhythmic (stereotypical) (American Psychiatric Association 2000). The earliest symptoms typically involve buccolingual-masticatory movements. Less common are movements of the upper and lower extremities and trunk (Brandon et al. 1971; Edwards 1970; Guy et al. 1986). Involuntary movements of the muscle groups involved in breathing and swallowing are the least common.

Time is an important factor in the outcome of TD. One-third of TD patients experience remission within 3 months of discontinuation of antipsychotic medication, and approximately one-half have remission within 12–18 months of antipsychotic discontinuation (American Psychiatric Association 2000). In studies that followed patients for more than 5 years, TD seems to improve in one-half of the patients, with or without antipsychotic treatment (Kane et al. 1992). Elderly patients are reported to have lower rates of remission, especially if treatment with antipsychotics is continued. When TD patients are maintained with conventional antipsychotics, TD seems to be stable in 50%, worsen in 25%, and improve in the rest (American Psychiatric Association 2000; Kane et al. 1992).

Severe TD may lead to a number of physical and psychosocial problems. Severe oral dyskinesias may result in dental problems and ulcerations of the tongue, cheeks, and lips (Yassa and Jeste 1985). Swallowing disorders (Massengil and Nashold 1969) and respiratory disturbances (Ayd 1979; Casey and Rabins 1978; Jackson et al. 1980; Weiner et al. 1978) have also been reported. Disruptions of the normal activity of the esophagus may lead to gastrointestinal complications such as vomiting, dysphagia (Yassa and Jones 1985), and associated weight loss. Ballesteros et al. (2000) conducted a meta-analysis and concluded that severe TD is associated with increased mortality in psychiatric patients.

Treatment

Unfortunately, there are no consistently proven therapies for TD. Therefore, clinicians should focus on prevention of the disorder while regularly assessing patients for TD. Use of atypical antipsychotics, especially in elderly patients, is recommended because of the lower risk of TD associated with these drugs. In addition to initiating therapy with an atypical agent and switching to an atypical antipsychotic when feasible, clinicians should minimize antipsychotic use in all patients (Arana and Rosenbaum 2000).

Patients who develop TD while taking a conventional antipsychotic should take an atypical antipsychotic instead, because studies have shown that such a switch in medications can lead to improvements of TD symptoms. Clozapine has been shown to be effective in reducing TD in patients with existing TD (Kane et al. 1993; Lieberman et al. 1991; Simpson et al. 1978; Small et al. 1987); however, side effects such as agranulocytosis and anticholinergic effects limit its use. A beneficial effect of other atypical agents (i.e., risperidone and olanzapine) on preexisting TD has also been reported (Jeste et al. 1997a;

Littrell et al. 1998; Street et al. 2000). The reduced risk of TD associated with all atypical agents (when used at appropriate doses), and the possibility of improvement of existing TD symptoms when a typical antipsychotic is replaced by an atypical antipsychotic, supports the use of atypical agents as a preventive measure and as a therapeutic option for those who develop TD while taking a conventional antipsychotic.

The dosing of antipsychotics in elderly patients is an important consideration. Compared with younger patients, older adults often respond to lower doses of antipsychotics. Patients with dementia usually respond to a lower dose than do individuals with schizophrenia or other psychotic disorders. Not only should older patients begin with a low dose, but the maintenance dose should be as low as possible, even when atypical antipsychotics are used.

Numerous studies of various designs, though mostly small trials, have investigated many potential treatments for TD. One treatment that has demonstrated some efficacy has been the use of vitamin E. It has been proposed that antipsychotic treatment results in the production of free radicals that damage the neuronal components (Lohr and Jeste 1988), and thus an antioxidant such as vitamin E theoretically could improve the symptoms of TD. In a number of studies, vitamin E had a beneficial effect in patients with TD (Adler et al. 1993, 1998; Egan et al. 1992; Elkashef et al. 1990; Sajjad 1998; Shriqui et al. 1992). Although vitamin E is a possible agent for TD treatment and prophylaxis (Gardos 1999; Gupta et al. 1999), a recent multicenter, double-blind, placebo-controlled trial found no difference between vitamin E and placebo after 1 year of treatment of TD (Adler et al. 1999). Although study results are inconclusive, vitamin E may be a reasonably safe treatment option for patients with TD, especially in the early stages of the disorder.

Other agents have been studied, including calcium-channel blockers (i.e., diltiazem, verapamil, and nifedipine), clonazepam, and pyridoxine, but more studies are warranted (Gupta et al. 1999; Lerner et al. 2001). In a small, open-label trial by Caroff et al. (2001), addition of the cholinesterase inhibitor donepezil led to a significant improvement in mean total Abnormal Involuntary Movement Scale (AIMS) scores. It was thought that this type of agent might improve TD symptoms as a result of increased cholinergic synaptic transmission. Melatonin therapy has been studied as a possible treatment for TD. The antioxidant properties and dopamine attenuating activity of melatonin may lead to beneficial effects not only in the treatment but also in the prevention of TD. In a small, double-blind, placebo-controlled, crossover study,

melatonin was found to significantly improve mean AIMS scores in a group of patients with schizophrenia and TD (Shamir et al. 2001).

In summary, older patients treated with conventional antipsychotics are at high risk for TD. In light of the mounting evidence that atypical agents are associated with a reduced risk of extrapyramidal side effects and TD, strong consideration should be given to using an atypical antipsychotic when antipsychotic therapy in older patients is initiated. In the case of patients already taking a conventional agent, clinicians should strongly consider switching to an atypical antipsychotic, when feasible. Regardless of the type of antipsychotic, prescribing the lowest effective dose in elderly patients is critical.

References

Adler LA, Peselow E, Rotrosen J, et al: Vitamin E treatment of tardive dyskinesia. Am J Psychiatry 150:1405–1407, 1993

Adler LA, Edson R, Lavori P, et al: Long-term treatment effects of vitamin E for tardive dyskinesia. Biol Psychiatry 43:868–872, 1998

Adler LA, Rotrosen J, Edson R, et al: Vitamin E treatment for tardive dyskinesia. Veterans Affairs Cooperative Study #394 Study Group. Arch Gen Psychiatry 56:836–841, 1999

Allison DB, Mentore JL, Heo M, et al: Antipsychotic-induced weight gain: a comprehensive research synthesis. Am J Psychiatry 156:1686–1696, 1999

American Psychiatric Association: Diagnostic and Statistical Manual: Mental Disorders. Washington, DC, American Psychiatric Association, 1952

American Psychiatric Association: Diagnostic and Statistical Manual of Mental Disorders, 2nd Edition. Washington, DC, American Psychiatric Association, 1968

American Psychiatric Association: Diagnostic and Statistical Manual of Mental Disorders, 3rd Edition. Washington, DC, American Psychiatric Association, 1980

American Psychiatric Association: Diagnostic and Statistical Manual of Mental Disorders, 3rd Edition, Revised. Washington, DC, American Psychiatric Association, 1987

American Psychiatric Association: Diagnostic and Statistical Manual of Mental Disorders, 4th Edition. Washington, DC, American Psychiatric Association, 1994

American Psychiatric Association: Diagnostic and Statistical Manual of Mental Disorders, 4th Edition, Text Revision. Washington, DC, American Psychiatric Association, 2000

Andreasen NC: I don't believe in late onset schizophrenia, in Late-Onset Schizophrenia. Edited by Howard R, Rabins PV, Castle DJ. Philadelphia, PA, Wrightson Biomedical, 1999, pp 111–123

Arana GW, Rosenbaum JF: Handbook of Psychiatric Drug Therapy, 4th Edition. Philadelphia, PA, Lippincott Williams & Wilkins, 2000

Ayd FJ: Respiratory dyskinesias in patients with neuroleptic-induced extrapyramidal reaction. Int Drug Ther Newsl 14:1–4, 1979

Ballesteros J, Gonzalez-Pinto A, Bulbena A: Tardive dyskinesia associated with higher mortality in psychiatric patients: results of a meta-analysis of seven independent studies. J Clin Psychopharmacol 20:188–194, 2000

Belitsky R, McGlashan TH: The manifestations of schizophrenia in late life: a dearth of data. Schizophr Bull 19:683–685, 1993

Bleuler M: Die spätschizophrenen Krankheitsbilder. Fortschr Neurol Psychiatr Grenzgeb 15:259–290, 1943

Bonuccelli U, Ceravolo R, Salvetti S, et al: Clozapine in Parkinson's disease tremor. Effects of acute and chronic administration. Neurology 49:1587–1590, 1997

Brandon S, McClelland HA, Protheroe C: A study of facial dyskinesia in a mental hospital population. Br J Psychiatry 118:171–184, 1971

Brodaty H, Sachdev P, Rose N, et al: Schizophrenia with onset after age 50 years, 1: phenomenology and risk factors. Br J Psychiatry 175:410–415, 1999

Burns A, Jacoby R, Levy R: Psychiatric phenomena in Alzheimer's disease, I: disorders of thought content. Br J Psychiatry 157:72–76, 1990

Caligiuri MP, Lacro JP, Rockwell E, et al: Incidence and risk factors for severe tardive dyskinesia in older patients. Br J Psychiatry 171:148–153, 1997

Caroff SN, Campbell EC, Havey J, et al: Treatment of tardive dyskinesia with donepezil: a pilot study. J Clin Psychiatry 62:772–775, 2001

Casey DE: Will the new antipsychotics bring hope of reducing the risk of developing extrapyramidal syndromes and tardive dyskinesia? Int Clin Psychopharmacol 12:S19–S27, 1997

Casey DE, Rabins P: Tardive dyskinesia as a life-threatening illness. Am J Psychiatry 135:486–488, 1978

Castle DJ, Murray RM: The epidemiology of late-onset schizophrenia. Schizophr Bull 19:691–700, 1993

Chouinard G, Annable L, Ross-Chouinard A, et al: Factors related to tardive dyskinesia. Am J Psychiatry 136:79–82, 1979

Chouinard G, Jones B, Remington G, et al: A Canadian multicenter placebo-controlled study of fixed doses of risperidone and haloperidol in the treatment of chronic schizophrenic patients. J Clin Psychopharmacol 13:25–40, 1993

Christenson R, Blazer D: Epidemiology of persecutory ideation in an elderly population in the community. Am J Psychiatry 141:1088–1091, 1984

Ciompi L: Catamnestic long-term study on the course of life and aging of schizophrenics. Schizophr Bull 6:606–618, 1980

Cohen CI: Outcome of schizophrenia into later life: an overview. Gerontologist 30:790–797, 1990

Cohen-Mansfield J: Nonpharmacologic interventions for inappropriate behaviors in dementia: a review and critique. Am J Geriatr Psychiatry 9:361–381, 2001

Cooper AF, Curry AR: The pathology of deafness in the paranoid and affective psychoses of later life. J Psychosom Res 20:97–105, 1976

Copeland JRM, Dewey ME, Scott A, et al: Schizophrenia and delusional disorder in older age: community prevalence, incidence, comorbidity and outcome. Schizophr Bull 19:153–161, 1998

Corey-Bloom J, Jernigan T, Archibald S, et al: Quantitative magnetic resonance imaging of the brain in late-life schizophrenia. Am J Psychiatry 152:447–449, 1995

Cummings JL, Benson DF: Dementia: A Clinical Approach, 2nd Edition. Boston, MA, Butterworth-Heinemann, 1992

Cummings JL, Miller B, Hill MA, et al: Neuropsychiatric aspects of multi-infarct dementia and dementia of the Alzheimer type. Arch Neurol 44:389–393, 1987

Davidson M, Harvey PD, Powchik P, et al: Severity of symptoms in chronically institutionalized geriatric schizophrenic patients. Am J Psychiatry 152:197–207, 1995

Devanand DP, Jacobs DM, Tang MX, et al: The course of psychopathologic features in mild to moderate Alzheimer disease. Arch Gen Psychiatry 54:257–263, 1997

Dixon L, Weiden PJ, Haas G, et al: Increased tardive dyskinesia in alcohol-abusing schizophrenic patients. Compr Psychiatry 33:121–122, 1992

Edwards H: The significance of brain damage in persistent oral dyskinesia. Br J Psychiatry 116:271–275, 1970

Egan MF, Hyde TM, Albers GW, et al: Treatment of tardive dyskinesia with vitamin E. Am J Psychiatry 149:773–777, 1992

Elkashef AM, Ruskin PE, Bacher N, et al: Vitamin E in the treatment of tardive dyskinesia. Am J Psychiatry 147:505–506, 1990

Evans JD, Paulsen JS, Harris MJ, et al: A clinical and neuropsychological comparison of delusional disorder and schizophrenia. J Neuropsychiatry Clin Neurosci 8:281–286, 1996

Evans JD, Heaton RK, Paulsen JS, et al: The relationship of neuropsychological abilities to specific domains of functional capacity in older schizophrenia patients. Biol Psychiatry 53:422–430, 2003

Eyler Zorrilla LT, Heaton RK, McAdams LA, et al: Cross-sectional study of older outpatients with schizophrenia and healthy comparison subjects: no differences in age-related cognitive decline. Am J Psychiatry 157:1324–1326, 2000

Forsell Y, Henderson AS: Epidemiology of paranoid symptoms in an elderly population. Br J Psychiatry 172:429–432, 1998

Gardos G: Managing antipsychotic-induced tardive dyskinesia. Drug Saf 20:187–193, 1999

Glazer WM, Morgenstern H, Doucette J: Race and tardive dyskinesia among outpatients at a CMHC. Hosp Community Psychiatry 45:38–42, 1994

Goetz CG, Blasucci LM, Leurgans S, et al: Olanzapine and clozapine: comparative effects on motor function in hallucinating PD patients. Neurology 55:789–794, 2000

Graham JM, Sussman JD, Ford DS, et al: Olanzapine in the treatment of hallucinosis in idiopathic Parkinson's disease: a cautionary note. J Neurol Neurosurg Psychiatry 65:774–777, 1998

Granholm E, McQuaid JR, McClure FS, et al: A randomized controlled pilot study of cognitive behavioral social skills training for older patients with schizophrenia (letter). Schizophr Res 153:167–169, 2002

Gupta S, Mosnik D, Black DW, et al: Tardive dyskinesia: review of treatments past, present, and future. Ann Clin Psychiatry 11:257–266, 1999

Guy W, Ban TA, Wilson WH: The prevalence of abnormal involuntary movements among chronic schizophrenics. Int Clin Psychopharmacol 1:134–144, 1986

Hafner H, an der Heiden W, Behrens S, et al: Causes and consequences of the gender differences in age at onset of schizophrenia. Schizophr Bull 24:99–113, 1998

Hannerz H, Borga P, Borritz M: Life expectancies for individuals with psychiatric diagnoses. Public Health 115:328–337, 2001

Harding CM, Brooks GW, Ashikaga T, et al: Aging and social functioning in once-chronic schizophrenic patients 22–62 years after first admission: the Vermont story, in Schizophrenia and Aging. Edited by Miller NE, Cohen GD. New York, Guilford, 1987, pp 74–82

Harris MJ, Jeste DV: Late-onset schizophrenia: an overview. Schizophr Bull 14:39–55, 1988

Harvey PD, Silverman JM, Mohs RC, et al: Cognitive decline in late-life schizophrenia: a longitudinal study of geriatric chronically hospitalized patients. Biol Psychiatry 45:32–40, 1999

Heaton RK, Gladsjo JA, Palmer BW, et al: Stability and course of neuropsychological deficits in schizophrenia. Arch Gen Psychiatry 58:24–32, 2001

Henderson AS, Korten AE, Levings C, et al: Psychotic symptoms in the elderly: a prospective study in a population sample. Int J Geriatr Psychiatry 13:484–492, 1998

Hiroeh U, Appleby L, Mortensen PB, et al: Death by homicide, suicide, and other unnatural causes in people with mental illness: a population-based study. Lancet 358:2110–2112, 2001

Howard R, Castle D, Wessely S, et al: A comparative study of 470 cases of early and late-onset schizophrenia. Br J Psychiatry 163:352–357, 1993

Howard R, Almeida O, Levy R: Phenomenology, demography and diagnosis in late paraphrenia. Psychol Med 24:397–410, 1994

Howard R, Graham C, Sham P, et al: A controlled family study of late-onset non-affective psychosis (late paraphrenia). Br J Psychiatry 170:511–514, 1997

Howard R, Rabins PV, Seeman MV, et al: Late-onset schizophrenia and very-late-onset schizophrenia-like psychosis: an international consensus. Am J Psychiatry 157:172–178, 2000

Huber G: The heterogeneous course of schizophrenia. Schizophr Res 28:177–185, 1997

Jackson IV, Volavka J, James B, et al: The respiratory components of tardive dyskinesia. Biol Psychiatry 15:485–487, 1980

Jeste DV, Caligiuri MP: Tardive dyskinesia. Schizophr Bull 19:303–315, 1993

Jeste DV, Finkel SI: Psychosis of Alzheimer's disease and related dementias: diagnostic criteria for a distinct syndrome. Am J Geriatr Psychiatry 8:29–34, 2000

Jeste DV, Harris MJ, Pearlson GD, et al: Late-onset schizophrenia. Studying clinical validity. Psychiatr Clin North Am 11:1–13, 1988

Jeste DV, Wragg RE, Salmon DP, et al: Cognitive deficits of patients with Alzheimer's disease with and without delusions. Am J Psychiatry 149:184–189, 1992

Jeste DV, Lacro JP, Gilbert PL, et al: Treatment of late-life schizophrenia with neuroleptics. Schizophr Bull 19:817–830, 1993

Jeste DV, Caligiuri MP, Paulsen JS, et al: Risk of tardive dyskinesia in older patients: a prospective longitudinal study of 266 patients. Arch Gen Psychiatry 52:756–765, 1995a

Jeste DV, Harris MJ, Krull A, et al: Clinical and neuropsychological characteristics of patients with late-onset schizophrenia. Am J Psychiatry 152:722–730, 1995b

Jeste DV, Lindamer LA, Evans J, et al: Relationship of ethnicity and gender to schizophrenia and pharmacology of neuroleptics. Psychopharmacol Bull 32:243–251, 1996

Jeste DV, Klausner M, Brecher M, et al: A clinical evaluation of risperidone in the treatment of schizophrenia: a 10-week, open-label, multicenter trial involving 945 patients. Psychopharmacology (Berl) 131:239–247, 1997a

Jeste DV, Symonds LL, Harris MJ, et al: Nondementia nonpraecox dementia praecox? late-onset schizophrenia. Am J Geriatr Psychiatry 5:302–317, 1997b

Jeste DV, Lacro JP, Bailey A, et al: Lower incidence of tardive dyskinesia with risperidone compared with haloperidol in older patients. J Am Geriatr Soc 47:716–719, 1999a

Jeste DV, Lacro JP, Palmer B, et al: Incidence of tardive dyskinesia in early stages of low-dose treatment with typical neuroleptics in older patients. Am J Psychiatry 156:309–311, 1999b

Jeste DV, Rockwell E, Harris MJ, et al: Conventional vs. newer antipsychotics in elderly patients. Am J Geriatr Psychiatry 7:70–76, 1999c

Jin H, Meyer JM, Jeste DV: Phenomenology of and risk factors for new-onset diabetes mellitus and diabetic ketoacidosis associated with atypical antipsychotics: an analysis of 45 published cases. Ann Clin Psychiatry 14:59–64, 2002

Joukamaa M, Heliovaara M, Knekt P, et al: Mental disorders and cause-specific mortality. Br J Psychiatry 179:498–502, 2001

Kane JM, Woerner M, Lieberman J: Tardive dyskinesia: prevalence, incidence, and risk factors. J Clin Psychopharmacol 8:52S–56S, 1988

Kane JM, Jeste DV, Barnes TRE, et al: Tardive Dyskinesia: A Task Force Report of the American Psychiatric Association. Washington, DC, American Psychiatric Association, 1992

Kane JM, Woerner MG, Pollack S, et al: Does clozapine cause tardive dyskinesia? J Clin Psychiatry 54:327–330, 1993

Katz IR, Jeste DV, Mintzer JE, et al: Comparison of risperidone and placebo for psychosis and behavioral disturbances associated with dementia: a randomized, double-blind trial. J Clin Psychiatry 60:107–115, 1999

Keith SJ, Regier DA, Rae DS: Schizophrenic disorders, in Psychiatric Disorders in America: The Epidemiologic Catchment Area Study. Edited by Robins LN, Regier DA. New York, Free Press, 1991, pp 33–52

Kendler KS, Davis KL: The genetics and biochemistry of paranoid schizophrenia and other paranoid psychoses. Schizophr Bull 7:689–709, 1981

Kendler KS, Tsuang MT, Hays P: Age at onset in schizophrenia: a familial perspective. Arch Gen Psychiatry 44:881–890, 1987

Kraepelin E: Dementia Praecox and Paraphrenia (1919). Translated by Barclay RM. Huntington, NY, Krieger, 1971

Kulkarni J, de Castella A, Smith D, et al: A clinical trial of the effects of estrogen in acutely psychotic women. Schizophr Res 20:247–252, 1996

Kulkarni J, Riedel A, de Castella AR, et al: Estrogen—a potential treatment for schizophrenia. Schizophr Res 48:137–144, 2001

Lawson WB: Racial and ethnic factors in psychiatric research. Hosp Community Psychiatry 37:50–54, 1986

Lerner V, Miodownik C, Kaptsan A, et al: Vitamin B_6 in the treatment of tardive dyskinesia: a double-blind, placebo-controlled, crossover study. Am J Psychiatry 158:1511–1514, 2001

Lieberman JA, Saltz BL, Johns CA, et al: The effects of clozapine on tardive dyskinesia. Br J Psychiatry 158:503–510, 1991

Lindamer LA, Buse DC, Lohr JB, et al: Hormone replacement therapy in postmenopausal women with schizophrenia: positive effect on negative symptoms? Biol Psychiatry 49:47–51, 2001

Littrell KH, Johnson CG, Littrell S, et al: Marked reduction of tardive dyskinesia with olanzapine (letter). Arch Gen Psychiatry 55:279–280, 1998

Lohr JB, Jeste DV: Neuroleptic-induced movement disorders: tardive dyskinesia and other tardive syndromes, in Psychiatry, Revised Edition. Edited by Michels R, Cavenar JO Jr, Brodie NKH, et al. Philadelphia, PA, JB Lippincott, 1988, pp 1–17

Lohr JB, Alder M, Flynn K, et al: Minor physical anomalies in older patients with late-onset schizophrenia, early onset schizophrenia, depression, and Alzheimer's disease. Am J Geriatr Psychiatry 5:318–323, 1997

Masand PS: Atypical antipsychotics for elderly patients with neurodegenerative disorders and medical conditions. Psychiatric Annals 30:203–208, 2000

Massengil R Jr, Nashold B: A swallowing disorder denoted in tardive dyskinesia patients. Acta Otolaryngol 68:457–458, 1969

McQuaid JR, Granholm E, McClure FS, et al: Development of an integrated cognitive-behavioral and social skills training intervention for older patients with schizophrenia. J Psychother Pract Res 9:149–156, 2000

Mendez M, Martin R, Smyth KA, et al: Psychiatric symptoms associated with Alzheimer's disease. J Neuropsychiatry Clin Neurosci 2:28–33, 1990

Moore NC: Is paranoid illness associated with sensory defects in the elderly? J Psychosom Res 25:69–74, 1981

Mukaetova-Ladinska EB, Harrington CR, Xuereb J, et al: Biochemical, neuropathological, and clinical corrections of neurofibrillary degeneration in Alzheimer's disease, in Treating Alzheimer's and Other Dementias. Edited by Bergener M, Finkel SI. New York, Springer, 1995, pp 57–80

Naimark D, Jackson E, Rockwell E, et al: Psychotic symptoms in Parkinson's disease patients with dementia. J Am Geriatr Soc 44:296–299, 1996

Olivera AA, Kiefer MW, Manley NK: Tardive dyskinesia in psychiatric patients with substance use disorders. Am J Drug Alcohol Abuse 16:57–66, 1990

Ostling S, Skoog I: Psychotic symptoms and paranoid ideation in a nondemented population-based sample of the very old. Arch Gen Psychiatry 59:53–59, 2002

Palmer BW, McClure F, Jeste DV: Schizophrenia in late-life: findings challenge traditional concepts. Harv Rev Psychiatry 9:51–58, 2001

Palmer BW, Bondi MW, Twamley EW, et al: Are late-onset schizophrenia spectrum disorders neurodegenerative conditions? annual rates of change on two dementia measures. J Neuropsychiatry Clin Neurosci 15:45–52, 2003

Paulsen JS, Caligiuri MP, Palmer B, et al: Risk factors for orofacial and limbtruncal tardive dyskinesia in older patients: a prospective longitudinal study. Psychopharmacology (Berl) 123:307–314, 1996

Paulsen JS, Salmon DP, Thal LJ, et al: Incidence of and risk factors for hallucinations and delusions in patients with probable AD. Neurology 54:1965–1971, 2000

Prager S, Jeste DV: Sensory impairment in late-life schizophrenia. Schizophr Bull 19:755–772, 1993

Raghuram R, Keshavan MD, Channabasavanna SM: Musical hallucinations in a deaf middle-aged patient. J Clin Psychiatry 41:357, 1980

Ram R, Bromet EJ, Eaton WW, et al: The natural course of schizophrenia: a review of first-admission studies. Schizophr Bull 18:185–207, 1992

Rivkin P, Kraut M, Barta P, et al: White matter hyperintensity volume in late-onset and early onset schizophrenia. Int J Geriatr Psychiatry 15:1085–1089, 2000

Rockwell E, Krull AJ, Dimsdale J, et al: Late-onset psychosis with somatic delusions. Psychosomatics 35:66–72, 1994

Roth M: The natural history of mental disorder in old age. J Ment Sci 101:281–301, 1955

Sachdev P, Brodaty H, Rose N, et al: Schizophrenia with onset after age 50 years, 2: neurological, neuropsychological and MRI investigation. Br J Psychiatry 175:416–421, 1999

Sajjad SH: Vitamin E in the treatment of tardive dyskinesia: a preliminary study over 7 months at different doses. Int Clin Psychopharmacol 13:147–155, 1998

Saltz BL, Woerner MG, Kane JM, et al: Prospective study of tardive dyskinesia incidence in the elderly. JAMA 266:2402–2406, 1991

Samuel W, Caligiuri M, Galasko D, et al: Better cognitive and psychopathologic response to donepezil in patients prospectively diagnosed as dementia with Lewy bodies: a preliminary study. Int J Geriatr Psychiatry 15:794–802, 2000

Schneider LS: Pharmacologic management of psychosis in dementia. J Clin Psychiatry 60:54–60, 1999

Seeman MV: The role of estrogen in schizophrenia. J Psychiatry Neurosci 21:123–127, 1996

Shamir E, Barak Y, Shalman I, et al: Melatonin treatment for tardive dyskinesia: a double-blind, placebo-controlled, crossover study. Arch Gen Psychiatry 58:1049–1052, 2001

Shriqui CL, Bradwejn J, Annable L, et al: Vitamin E in the treatment of tardive dyskinesia: a double-blind placebo-controlled study. Am J Psychiatry 149:391–393, 1992

Simpson GM, Lee JM, Shrivastava RK: Clozapine in tardive dyskinesia. Psychopharmacology (Berl) 56:75–80, 1978

Small JG, Milstein V, Marhenke JD, et al: Treatment outcome with clozapine in tardive dyskinesia, neuroleptic sensitivity, and treatment-resistant psychosis. J Clin Psychiatry 48:263–267, 1987

Stern Y, Albert M, Brandt J, et al: Utility of extrapyramidal signs and psychosis as predictors of cognitive and functional decline, nursing home admission, and death in Alzheimer's disease: prospective analyses from the Predictors Study. Neurology 44:2300–2307, 1994

Stoppe G, Brandt CA, Staedt JH: Behavioural problems associated with dementia: the role of newer antipsychotics. Drugs Aging 14:41–54, 1999

Street JS, Tollefson GD, Tohen M, et al: Olanzapine for psychotic conditions in the elderly. Psychiatric Annals 30:191–196, 2000

Sultzer DL: Neuroimaging and the origin of psychiatric symptoms in dementia. Int Psychogeriatr 8 (suppl 3):239–243, 1996

Symonds LL, Olichney JM, Jernigan TL, et al: Lack of clinically significant gross structural abnormalities in MRIs of older patients with schizophrenia and related psychoses. J Neuropsychiatry Clin Neurosci 9:251–258, 1997

Tollefson GD, Beasley CM, Tran PV, et al: Olanzapine versus haloperidol in the treatment of schizophrenia and schizoaffective and schizophreniform disorders: results of an international collaborative trial. Am J Psychiatry 154:457–465, 1997

Weiner WJ, Goetz CG, Nausieda PA, et al: Respiratory dyskinesias: extrapyramidal dysfunction and dyspnea. Ann Intern Med 88:327–331, 1978

Wirshing DA, Spellberg BJ, Erhart SM, et al: Novel antipsychotics and new onset diabetes. Biol Psychiatry 44:778–783, 1998

Wolters EC, Jansen ENH, Tuynman-Qua HG, et al: Olanzapine in the treatment of dopaminomimetic psychosis in patients with Parkinson's disease. Neurology 47:1085–1087, 1996

Wragg R, Jeste DV: Overview of depression and psychosis in Alzheimer's disease. Am J Psychiatry 146:577–587, 1989

Yassa R, Jeste DV: Gender differences in tardive dyskinesia: a critical review of the literature. Schizophr Bull 18:701–715, 1992

Yassa R, Jones BD: Complications of tardive dyskinesia: a review. Psychosomatics 26:305–313, 1985

Yeung PP, Tariot PN, Schneider LS, et al: Quetiapine for elderly patients with psychotic disorders. Psychiatr Ann 30:197–201, 2000

Zubenko GS, Moossy J, Martinez AJ, et al: Neuropathologic and neurochemical correlates of psychosis in primary dementia. Arch Neurol 48:619–624, 1991

Anxiety and Panic Disorders

John L. Beyer, M.D.

Anxiety is commonly found in older adults but has received much less attention than mood disorders. The reason for this is unclear. Anxiety disorders as a group are the most common psychiatric conditions in the elderly (Blazer et al. 1991a), and the presence of these disorders may result in higher medical and psychiatric comorbidity (Lindesay et al. 1989).

Many people, including elderly people themselves, consider anxiety a natural response to aging. As aging occurs, so do concerns about changes in or losses of physical health, financial security, social support, and cognitive ability (Small 1997). In addition, older persons may have a real concern about their safety or become easily flustered when placed in unfamiliar situations (especially if they become disoriented). Thus they may choose not to participate in social situations (Blazer 1997).

It is remarkable that anxiety disorders appear to decrease with age. However, the effects of anxiety and anxiety disorders in older adults are often unrecognized and inadequately treated.

Epidemiology

The prevalence of anxiety disorders in the elderly has been a source of debate. Early studies generally found a high prevalence of anxiety symptoms in the elderly. Gurian et al. (1963) surveyed 2,460 community-dwelling adults for "cognitive anxiety" (worry, fear, nervousness) and "somatic anxiety" (shortness of breath, rapid heart rate). They found that cognitive anxiety was almost three times as common among persons age 65 or older than among those 21–44 years old; somatic anxiety occurred seven times as often. The investigators' combined estimate of the prevalence of clinically significant anxiety in the elderly subjects was 21.7%. These findings were substantiated by Gaitz and Scott (1972), who administered the same questionnaire to a community sample in Houston, Texas, and noted a similar rate of anxiety among older participants and a similar linear increase in somatic anxiety with increasing age. In 1984, Himmelfarb and Murrell reported that in a survey of more than 2,000 subjects in Kentucky, 17.1% of men age 55 or older and 21.5% of women age 55 or older experienced clinically significant levels of anxiety. Other clinical studies examining the rate of anxiety symptoms in elderly patients in primary care or family practices found that significant anxiety ranged from 5% to 30% (Oxman et al. 1987; Zung 1986).

The most extensive estimate of anxiety disorders in the elderly is from results of the Epidemiologic Catchment Area (ECA) study conducted in the early 1980s. In this study, more than 20,000 community-dwelling adults (at least 18 years old) at five sites in the United States were examined for psychiatric disorders using DSM-III (American Psychiatric Association 1980) criteria. The combined prevalence of phobia, panic disorder, and obsessive-compulsive disorder (OCD; the only anxiety disorders measured at all five sites) in people more than 65 years old was 5.5%. Among elderly subjects, anxiety disorders had the highest 1-year prevalence rate of any psychiatric diagnosis (Regier et al. 1990) (a finding consistent with that for all age populations sampled), but this rate was higher in the middle-aged group. Still, the number of elderly persons with anxiety disorders is significant, especially with regard to women older than 65 years, among whom the prevalence of any anxiety disorder (6.8%) was higher than that among men of any age.

DSM-IV-TR (American Psychiatric Association 2000) anxiety disorders are listed in Table 16–1.

TABLE 16–1. DSM-IV-TR anxiety disorders

Panic disorder
  With agoraphobia
  Without agoraphobia
Agoraphobia without history of panic disorder
Specific phobia
  Animal type
  Natural environment type
  Blood-injection-injury type
  Situational type
  Other type
Social phobia
Obsessive-compulsive disorder
Posttraumatic stress disorder
Acute stress disorder
Generalized anxiety disorder
Anxiety disorder due to a general medical condition
Substance-induced anxiety disorder

Diagnostic Classification and Phenomenology

Panic Disorder

A panic attack is an episode of intense fear or anxiety that is accompanied by multiple somatic and cognitive symptoms. During an attack, elderly individuals may complain that they feel as though they are having a heart attack or stroke and are going to die. Symptoms include palpitations or a pounding heart, sweating, tremulousness, shortness of breath, a choking sensation, chest pain, nausea, light-headedness, fear of dying or "going crazy," chills, and numbness and tingling in the extremities. The attack may quickly build to a peak intensity in 5–10 minutes and lasts anywhere from 5 to 30 minutes.

Having a panic attack and having panic disorder are not the same, however. Panic attacks may occur in a variety of anxiety disorders or medical conditions (such as hyperthyroidism) or as a response to certain medications or substances (such as caffeine). Whereas in panic disorder, panic attacks are recurrent and become the focus of the individual's fear. The presence of a strong desire to flee from the place where the attack is occurring (the fight-or-flight response) may lead to a pattern of avoiding places where the panic attacks occurred or where escape would be difficult if an attack recurred. This condition is called agoraphobia. Thus, patients may receive a diagnosis of panic disorder with or without agoraphobia.

Development of panic disorder in late life is relatively uncommon, but it does occur (Luchins and Rose 1989;

Sheikh and Cassidy 2000). Typically, however, elderly patients develop panic disorders earlier in life, and the symptoms continue throughout life. If the diagnosis is made in late life, frequently the disorder was missed previously (Sheikh et al. 1991). It is not uncommon for elderly adults to ascribe the symptoms to other causes, and the frequent waxing and waning of symptoms may make correct diagnosis difficult. When elderly persons do experience panic attacks, the symptoms are similar to those that occur in younger people. However, elderly individuals with late-onset panic attacks may have fewer symptoms and may do less to avoid the attacks (Sheikh et al. 1991).

Surprisingly, epidemiologic studies have found that panic disorder is uncommon in the elderly, compared with other age groups. The point prevalence for most studies is 0.3% or less (Bland et al. 1988; Lindesay et al. 1989; Manela et al. 1996). In the ECA study, the point prevalence among middle-aged subjects was 1.1%, whereas among those age 65 or older, the point prevalence was 0.4% (Regier et al. 1988). When lifetime prevalence was considered, 2% of persons ages 45–64 years met criteria for panic disorder, whereas only 0.3% of older persons met criteria. It is unclear whether this large difference in incidence represents a cohort effect. It has been suggested that the lifetime cases were underreported in the elderly group because the memory of anxiety symptoms deteriorated with age (Blazer 1997). Supporting this argument is the finding by Weissman et al. (1991), who evaluated depression in elderly persons and found that this group did significantly underreport lifetime symptoms of depression, compared with younger subjects.

Agoraphobia Without History of Panic Disorder

As mentioned earlier (see "Panic Disorder"), agoraphobia occurs when the focus of fear is on the occurrence of panic-like symptoms in public places or situations from which escape may be difficult if the symptoms occur. For elderly individuals, panic-like symptoms may include loss of bladder or bowel control or fear of fainting or falling and being unable to get up. The result is an avoidance of leaving home in order to escape potential embarrassment. It should be noted that elderly patients may indeed have realistic concerns that certain physical conditions necessitate assistance or have the potential for causing embarrassment. The diagnosis of agoraphobia should be made only when the fear or avoidance of public places is clearly in excess of what is usually associated with the patient's medical condition.

Specific Phobia

The main feature of specific phobias is the excessive and persistent fear of an object or situation (American Psychiatric Association 2000). These phobias are usually divided into four subtypes: fear of animals (such as fear of dogs or snakes), fear of natural events (such as fear of storms, heights, or water), fear of blood-injection-injury (such as fear triggered by seeing blood, experiencing an injury, or receiving medication by injection), and fear of situations (such as fear of driving, flying, crossing bridges, or being in enclosed spaces). Fears of animals and natural events are common during childhood and diminish with age. The blood-injection-injury subtype "is highly familial and is often characterized by a strong vasovagal response" (American Psychiatric Association 2000, p. 445). Situational phobias appear to be closely related to panic disorder. In these cases, the disorder is often chronic and persists in old age (Blazer et al. 1991b).

Social Phobia

Social phobia is a marked and persistent fear of social or performance situations in which embarrassment may occur. Individuals are afraid that others will judge them critically, and the phobic persons therefore avoid these situations. Examples of performance situations avoided include making a speech, eating in public, and using public restrooms. Elderly individuals with social phobia may avoid eating, drinking, or writing in public out of fear that others will notice their hands shaking because of tremor. The duration of social phobia is usually lifelong; however, the disorder fluctuates in severity and may even remit. For example, social phobia may diminish after a person with fear of dating marries, only to reemerge after the death of the spouse (American Psychiatric Association 2000).

Obsessive-Compulsive Disorder

"Obsessions are persistent ideas, thoughts, impulses, or images that are experienced as intrusive and inappropriate" (American Psychiatric Association 2000, p. 457). The individual senses that the content of the obsession is not the type of thought he or she would normally have, but the person also recognizes that it is his or her own thought and not one "inserted" from outside (American Psychiatric Association 2000). The usual obsessions are repeated thoughts about contamination, doubting, ordering, aggression, and sexual imagery (American Psychiatric Association 2000). Unlike what may occur in gener-

alized anxiety disorders (GADs), these thoughts are not just excessive anxiety about problems in the individual's life. Attempts to ignore or suppress the thoughts often increase the anxiety and lead to compulsions—repetitive behaviors done to reduce or prevent anxiety. Common compulsive activities include hand washing, checking behaviors, ordering, praying, counting, and repeating words or phrases.

In OCD, recurrent obsessions or compulsions become severe enough to cause significant distress or impairment of functioning. The individual usually knows that the obsessions or compulsions are excessive but feels unable to stop the behavior. In elderly patients, somatic concerns are common, involving repeated visits to the doctor for assurance. OCD usually begins in adolescence or early adulthood, with a gradual onset. The disorder usually has a waxing and waning course, and the kind of obsession or compulsive activity engaged in may change over time. About 15% of persons with the disorder have a progressive deterioration, whereas about 5% have episodic presentations, with minimal symptoms between episodes.

Point prevalence of OCD in elderly patients ranges from 0% to 1.5% (Bland et al. 1988; Copeland et al. 1987; Regier et al. 1988). Despite the low incidence, a review of cases from OCD clinics showed that approximately 5% of patients are older than 60 years (Jenike 1991; Kohn et al. 1997).

Posttraumatic Stress Disorder

In posttraumatic stress disorder (PTSD), the individual develops characteristic clusters of symptoms after exposure to a traumatic event that produced intense fear, helplessness, or horror. That event may be experienced directly; for example, the person may be the victim of a physical or sexual assault or of a crime, be involved in a motor vehicle accident, or receive a diagnosis of a life-threatening illness (American Psychiatric Association 2000). The trauma may also be experienced indirectly; for example, the individual may witness a traumatic accident or violent event or may learn about an unfortunate event occurring to a loved one, such as an unexpected death of a family member or close friend or a diagnosis of a life-threatening illness in a child.

The characteristic response of PTSD includes three clusters of symptoms. The first is *reexperiencing of the trauma*. The individual may have recurrent and intrusive memories or dreams of the trauma or may behave as though he or she were reliving the event at that moment. Alternatively, the trauma may be reexperienced when a person is exposed to symbols that remind him or her of it, symbols that produce intense distress or even physiological reactions.

The second cluster of symptoms involves *avoidance of stimuli* associated with the trauma. The individual may avoid thoughts, feelings, and conversations about the trauma or even avoid persons, places, or situations that remind him or her of the events. The person may also have amnesia related to significant parts of the trauma. Avoidance of emotions may also progress to diminished responsiveness or interest in activities, feelings of being detached or numb, or a sense of a foreshortened future.

The last cluster of symptoms is *persistent anxiety or increased arousal*. This may include difficulty falling asleep, hypervigilance, decreased concentration, exaggerated startle response, episodes of irritability, or anger outbursts.

PTSD may occur at any age and usually occurs immediately after the event (within the first 3 months). However, symptoms may also be delayed (they are considered delayed if they begin at least 6 months after the trauma). Often an acute stress disorder is first diagnosed (see "Acute Stress Disorder" below). Symptoms resolve in the first 3 months in 50% of patients, but many persons have symptoms for up to 5 years, or even until death (Flint 1999). The intensity or duration of symptoms is positively correlated with the severity of the trauma (Flint 1999).

Elderly individuals may be more likely than younger people to be victimized or to sustain life-threatening injuries, and thus new-onset PTSD may be more common than reported. However, there are no data on the prevalence of PTSD in the elderly population (Flint 1999). Most research involving elderly patients has focused on the effects of PTSD on survivors of the Holocaust or persons who were prisoners of war during World War II (Kuch and Cox 1992; Robinson et al. 1990; Sutker et al. 1993). Nearly half of the elderly Holocaust survivors studied met criteria for PTSD more than 40 years after the war (Kuch and Cox 1992). Approximately one-quarter of the former prisoners of war who were studied met criteria for PTSD more than 40 years after their release (Kluznik et al. 1986; Rosen et al. 1989).

Acute Stress Disorder

Acute stress disorder features symptoms similar to those of PTSD, except that the diagnosis of acute stress disorder is used when the symptoms of anxiety, dissociation, reexperiencing, avoidance, and hyperarousal occur for at least 2 days during the first month after the trauma. How-

ever, if symptoms are still significant after 4 weeks, the diagnosis of PTSD is made.

Generalized Anxiety Disorder

GAD is an excessive anxiousness or worry that occurs for most days over at least 6 months. In addition, the person may be restless, become fatigued easily, have difficulty concentrating, be irritable, have muscle tension, and have disturbed sleep. This anxiety interferes with the person's ability to function and may exceed the anxiety produced by the feared event. Common themes of a person's anxiety include job responsibilities, finances, health, misfortune to loved ones, and minor matters (such as excessive concern about chores or about being late). Most elderly patients with GAD report that for most of their lives, they have felt a nervousness that fluctuates according to the level of stress.

GAD is the second most common anxiety disorder in the elderly population (phobias are the most common). Point prevalence ranges from 0.7% to 7.1% (Blazer et al. 1991b; Copeland et al. 1987; Lindesay et al. 1989; Manela et al. 1996; Uhlenhuth et al. 1983). In the ECA study, the data regarding the presence of GAD (DSM-III definition) were obtained from three sites. The rate of GAD in elderly subjects was 2.2% (Blazer et al. 1991b), the median rate of all the studies mentioned (Flint 1999). Again, the frequency was lower than that among younger individuals and slightly higher among women than among men.

Anxiety Disorder Due to a General Medical Condition and Substance-Induced Anxiety Disorder

Anxiety symptoms are frequent manifestations of underlying disease or use of a medication or substance. To make this diagnosis, the physician must establish that the patient has a disease or has been exposed to a substance that could cause an anxiety response; in the latter case, the physician must also establish that the response is temporally related to the exposure. This diagnosis also is often considered when the features are atypical of a primary anxiety disorder (features such as an unusual age at onset or the absence of family history). A variety of medical conditions, drugs, and substances can cause anxiety symptoms (see Tables 16–2 and 16–3). Most late-onset panic attacks are associated with cardiovascular, gastrointestinal, and chronic pulmonary diseases (Hassan and Pollard 1994; Raj et al. 1995).

TABLE 16–2. Medical disorders associated with anxiety

Cardiac
  Angina
  Cardiac arrhythmias
  Congestive heart failure
  Hypertension
  Mitral valve prolapse
  Myocardial infarction
Endocrine
  Cushing's syndrome
  Hypoglycemia
  Hypo- or hyperparathyroidism
  Hypo- or hyperthyroidism
  Menopause
  Premenstrual syndrome
Neurological
  Cerebral arteriosclerosis
  Complex partial seizures
  Delirium
  Early dementia
  Huntington's disease
  Meniere's disease
  Migraine
  Multiple sclerosis
  Postconcussion syndrome
  Vestibular dysfunction
  Wilson's disease
Neoplastic
  Carcinoid syndrome
  Cerebral neoplasm
  Pheocromocytoma
Pulmonary
  Asthma
  Chronic obstructive pulmonary disease
  Hypoxic states
  Pulmonary embolism
Other
  Porphyria

TABLE 16–3. Medications and substances that can cause anxiety

Over-the-counter medications
  Caffeine
  Stimulants
Prescription medications
  Anticholinergics
  Psychostimulants (e.g., methylphenidate, amphetamine)
  Sedative-hypnotics (withdrawal)
  Steroids
  Sympathomimetics
Substances
  Alcohol
  Cocaine
  Hallucinogens
  Narcotics

Differential Diagnosis

Medical Illnesses

There is a complex interaction among anxiety, medical illness, and the medications used to treat these conditions (Flint 1999). First, the older adult may have the realistic worry about the effect and meaning of physical illness. Interestingly, the prevalence of anxiety disorders in the medically ill elderly population is lower than in young and middle-aged patients with medical illnesses (Cassem 1990; Magni and De Leo 1984), although even minor illness may have more consequences in an elderly person's life than in the life of a younger individual.

Second, anxiety may contribute to medical problems and complications. For example, people with high levels of anxiety are at higher risk for hypertension (Jonas et al. 1997), arrhythmias (Moser and Dracup 1996), and death from cardiovascular disease (Kawachi et al. 1994).

Third, medical illness may masquerade as anxiety symptoms. Listed in Table 16–2 are many medical illnesses in which anxiety is often a symptom. Conversely, many anxiety symptoms may masquerade as medical illness. This may be especially true in elderly patients, who tend to volunteer physical symptoms as emotional expressions. For example, of the top 25 symptoms that patients age 75 or older report to their physicians during routine office visits, many are symptoms of anxiety (such as dizziness, chest pain, shortness of breath, general weakness, tiredness, nervousness, palpitations, nausea, and urinary frequency) (White et al. 1986).

Finally, anxiety symptoms may be caused by the medications given to elderly persons to treat either physical or mental diseases. Table 16–3 is a partial list of medications whose package inserts include anxiety as a common side effect; also listed in the table are substances that commonly produce anxiety.

Comorbid Depression and Anxiety

Comorbid anxiety disorders appear to be quite common in depressed elderly individuals. Two small community studies found lower rates of comorbid GAD, phobic anxiety, and panic attacks in depressed elderly patients compared with younger groups (Ben-Arie et al. 1987; Livingston et al. 1997). However, Lenze et al. (2000) found that comorbid anxiety disorders had a relatively high rate of lifetime (35%) and current (23%) prevalence in depressed elderly patients. In addition, comorbid anxiety disorders were associated with a more severe presentation of depressive illness in elderly subjects. In another study, Alexopoulos (1990) determined that 38% of depressed elderly outpatients had at least one anxiety disorder. Parmelee et al. (1993) found that 65% of elderly nursing home residents displayed concurrent signs of anxiety.

Treatment

Nonpharmacological Treatment

Several cognitive and behavioral therapies have been demonstrated to be effective in treating anxiety disorders. Cognitive-behavioral therapy (CBT) has reliably been found to be effective for the panic disorders, GAD, social phobia, and PTSD. Exposure therapy has been found to be effective for specific phobias and compulsive behaviors. However, although the effectiveness of these therapies in younger adults has been relatively well established, no corresponding systematic studies involving older adults have been performed. Studies have suggested that these treatments should be efficacious in older adults. Steuer et al. (1984) looked at the use of CBT and psychodynamic therapies in depressed older adults and found that these therapies decreased not only the depression but also lowered the levels of anxiety. Swales et al. (1996) determined that CBT can be effective in older patients with panic disorder, while Stanley and Novy (2000) found this treatment to be effective in elderly subjects with GAD. There are also scattered case reports on the use of various psychotherapies in elderly patients.

Cognitive and behavioral therapies can be useful treatment alternatives in elderly patients, especially when medications must be avoided. However, other problems may hinder psychotherapeutic treatment in this age group, including severe physical limitations, cognitive impairments, and difficult access to care.

Pharmacological Treatment

A variety of medications have been used for the treatment of anxiety and anxiety disorders in elderly patients, but Zimmer and Gershon's (1991) conclusion that the "ideal geriatric anxiolytic has yet to be developed" (p. 294) still holds true. Choosing appropriate anxiolytic treatment for elderly patients poses several challenges. First, all medications have the potential for unwanted side effects. This is especially true when the drugs are taken by

elderly individuals, in whom age-related physical changes (such as changes in drug absorption, drug distribution, protein binding, cardiac output, hepatic metabolism, and renal clearance) and polypharmacy increase susceptibility to adverse reactions (Jenike 1989; Ouslander 1981; Thompson et al. 1983). In addition, changes in neurotransmitter and receptor function in the central nervous system may also increase sensitivity to psychotropic drugs (Salzman 1990).

Second, research on psychopharmacological treatment of elderly patients with anxiety disorders is limited. In a review of the literature, Krasucki et al. (1998) found few controlled clinical trials on anxiety disorders in elderly individuals. Therefore, decisions about treatment for elderly patients are usually extrapolations from findings of clinical studies involving younger, mixed-age, adult populations. Pearson (1998), summarizing the consensus from a National Institute of Mental Health workshop on late-life anxiety, noted three goals of research on anxiety in elderly patients: 1) achievement of consensus on the best approach to measuring and counting anxiety symptoms, syndromes, or disorders in late life, 2) improvement of knowledge of the differences between early- and later-onset anxiety disorders, and 3) performance of sufficient numbers of studies examining anxiety in older adults.

Because of the potential for drug side effects and the limited research on anxiety in elderly patients, effective treatment of anxiety in this age group is dependent on the physician's comprehensive assessment of the psychiatric, social, and medical conditions of the patient; a thorough review of the patient's drug history; and a thoughtful consideration of the multiple medication options.

Antidepressants

Selective serotonin reuptake inhibitors. Selective serotonin reuptake inhibitors (SSRIs) have become the mainstay of anxiety disorder treatment, for several reasons. First, various SSRIs have obtained U.S. Food and Drug Administration approval for use in the treatment of panic disorder, GAD, social phobia, and OCD in the general population. Fluoxetine has been shown to be effective in the treatment of depressed geriatric patients with agitation (Small 1997). Fluvoxamine and fluoxetine have been found to be effective for OCD in clinical trials that have included some elderly patients (Perse 1987; Tollefson et al. 1994; Wylie et al. 2000). Case studies have shown sertraline, paroxetine, venlafaxine, fluoxetine, citalopram, and fluvoxamine to be effective in social phobias and anxiety (Katzelnick et al. 1995; Kelsey 1995; Van Ameringen et al. 1993; van Vliet et al. 1994). SSRIs have also been successfully used to treat PTSD and specific phobias. Second, anxiety disorders and depressive disorders are frequently comorbid, and use of a single agent to treat both conditions decreases the rate of polypharmacy, a situation often occurring in elderly patients. Finally, the side-effect profiles of SSRIs are much more acceptable than those of many older medications.

Despite their preferred profiles, all SSRIs can cause side effects. The most common are nausea and diarrhea (which are usually dose dependent and time limited), changes in sexual arousal and performance, and decreases in appetite and weight (although weight gain has been associated with extended use). Some individuals report stimulating effects with administration of SSRIs that may produce tremor and jitteriness. Also, despite their being named for selective activity on the serotonin system, SSRIs may also affect other neurotransmitters. For example, paroxetine has some anticholinergic activity that may be more apparent in sensitive elderly patients.

Newer antidepressants. Other antidepressants are also being increasingly used for the treatment of anxiety in elderly individuals. Nefazodone has been reported to be effective in some depressed elderly patients with prominent anxiety symptoms (Small 1997). Its level of daytime sedation appears to be acceptable to elderly persons (van Laar et al. 1995), and the drug seems to have minimal anticholinergic or other side effects. Its more moderate serotonin reuptake inhibition may make it less likely than SSRIs to create agitation (Fawcett et al. 1995).

Venlafaxine, an antidepressant with both norepinephrine and serotonin activity, is increasingly being used to treat depression and anxiety in the general adult population (Silverstone and Ravindran 1999). Small increases in blood pressure may be seen at doses greater than 225 mg/day.

Mirtazapine is the first of a new class of antidepressants, the noradrenergic and specific serotonergic antidepressants. In trials of antidepressant treatment in the general adult population, mirtazapine has had beneficial effects on the concomitant symptoms of anxiety and sleep disturbances (Kasper et al. 1997). It has few anticholinergic, adrenergic, or serotonin-related adverse effects, but it can be sedating because of its antihistaminic effects. This drug may be a good choice for anxious elderly patients who are having difficulty sleeping or are losing weight.

Tricyclic antidepressants. Tricyclic antidepressants (TCAs) have been shown to be effective in treating a variety of anxiety states in elderly patients, such as mixed anxiety-depression states, panic disorder, OCD, and GAD (Crook 1982; Hershey and Kim 1988; Hoehn-Saric et al. 1988; Rickels et al. 1993; Rifkin et al. 1981). However, overall use of TCAs has decreased because of their significant side effects, their potential toxicity, and the emergence of other medications, such as SSRIs.

Common side effects are frequently caused by TCAs' effects on several receptor sites. α-Adrenergic blockade by TCAs may lead to significant orthostatic hypotension or cardiac conduction irregularities. Elderly patients are particularly susceptible to injury resulting from orthostatic decreases in blood pressure. Trazodone, a heterocyclic antidepressant, is sometimes used as a sedative or to treat agitation in patients with dementia, but postural hypotension, a side effect, may limit its use (Small 1997). Anticholinergic side effects of TCAs are dry mouth, blurred vision, constipation, urinary retention, and confusion or even psychosis. Confusion or psychosis may be particularly significant in patients with Alzheimer's disease or other disorders that impair memory. The major antihistaminic effects are sedation and weight gain. Secondary amine TCAs such as nortriptyline and desipramine are preferred for use in elderly patients because of the less intense anticholinergic and adrenergic side effects compared with tertiary amine TCAs. A baseline electrocardiogram is highly recommended before initiation of therapy, because TCAs can cause a prolonged QRS complex.

Monoamine oxidase inhibitors. Monoamine oxidase inhibitors have been effective in treating mixed anxiety-depression and panic disorder (Crook 1982; Hershey and Kim 1988), but they are rarely used today because of their potential side effects, the restrictive diet associated with use, and the availability of newer antidepressants. For elderly patients, the two most difficult possible side effects are orthostatic hypotension and acute hypertensive crisis due to drug-diet interactions. Phenelzine and tranylcypromine are thought to be the monoamine oxidase inhibitors of choice for elderly individuals (Schneider 1996). Older studies have even suggested that when used to treat anxiety, phenelzine may be more effective in elderly than in younger patients (Crook 1982) and may be just as well tolerated as nortriptyline (Georgotas et al. 1986).

Benzodiazepines

Since the 1960s, benzodiazepines have been the primary pharmacological agents for patients with situational anxiety, GAD, or panic disorder (Hayes and Dommisse 1987), but recommendations for first-line treatment of anxiety disorders are now changing to use of SSRIs. Still, benzodiazepines are frequently prescribed to elderly patients (American Psychiatric Association 1990), and epidemiologic data have suggested that they may be overused (Shorr and Robin 1994).

All benzodiazepines can cause impairment of cognition and motor function. The cognitive impairment may be severe enough to present as a pseudodementia, whereas motor impairment may cause falls and hip fractures. These effects are of special concern in elderly patients because benzodiazepines are so frequently used, and the adverse drug reactions have been noted to be almost twice as common in patients older than 70 years compared with patients age 40 or younger (Boston Collaborative Drug Surveillance Program 1973). Benzodiazepines may also cause a paradoxical reaction of restlessness, confusion, irritability, and even aggression. Outbursts of anger in elderly patients receiving benzodiazepines may actually be due to this disinhibition.

Benzodiazepines undergo two kinds of biotransformation: oxidation and glucuronide conjugation. Oxidative transformation occurs slowly, giving the drug a long half-life and producing many active metabolites. Conjugative transformation occurs rapidly, and the metabolic products are pharmacologically inactive. As a general rule, benzodiazepines that are inactivated by conjugation reactions appear to be less likely to interact with other medications. For example, cimetidine has been found to inhibit metabolism of benzodiazepines that require oxidation but not benzodiazepines inactivated by conjugation (such as lorazepam or oxazepam).

Elimination times of benzodiazepines vary in elderly individuals. Benzodiazepines with short half-lives are generally used to treat insomnia rather than daytime anxiety, but abrupt discontinuation of these drugs can produce rebound insomnia, and some benzodiazepines with short half-lives have been noted to cause confusion, agitation, and hallucinations in elderly persons (Shorr and Robin 1994). Benzodiazepines with long half-lives can significantly increase the risk of falls and hip fractures in elderly patients (Ray et al. 1989). For the most part, benzodiazepines with midrange half-lives and conjugation metabolism (such as lorazepam) are preferred for use in elderly patients because clearance is unaffected by aging and the drugs are less likely to accumulate and cause toxicity (American Psychiatric Association 1990).

Physiological dependence that may result in a withdrawal syndrome develops after 3–4 months of daily use (Salzman 1990). Withdrawal symptoms are likely to be more severe if therapy is discontinued abruptly or if the patient is receiving a short-half-life benzodiazepine or higher daily doses.

Buspirone

Buspirone, a novel antianxiety agent unrelated to benzodiazepines, has a high affinity for serotonin$_{1A}$. In addition, it enhances brain dopaminergic and noradrenergic activity (Eison and Temple 1986; Goa and Ward 1986). Research suggests that buspirone is effective in the treatment of GAD in elderly patients (Bohm et al. 1990; Napoliello 1986; Robinson et al. 1988; Singh and Beer 1988), but it does not appear to be effective for panic disorder (Sheehan et al. 1990). Some researchers suggest that buspirone therapy may be helpful in the treatment of mixed anxiety-depression symptoms or as an adjunct treatment for OCD.

For the most part, buspirone is well tolerated by elderly patients. Common side effects include nausea, headache, nervousness, dizziness, light-headedness, and fatigue. However, unlike benzodiazepines, buspirone does not appear to cause psychomotor impairment, dependence, withdrawal, or abuse (Banazak 1997). Furthermore, it does not interact with alcohol and other sedative drugs. Therefore, it may be of particular value for treating patients unable to tolerate the sedative effects of benzodiazepines, patients with respiratory illness (such as chronic obstructive pulmonary disease), or patients with a history of substance abuse (Steinberg 1994).

Two disadvantages of buspirone are the requirement of multiple daily doses and the lack of immediate effect. Buspirone's short half-life (averaging 2–3 hours) may necessitate administration up to three times a day (usually with meals). In addition, it may take from 1 to 3 weeks at therapeutic doses for the anxiolytic effect to begin. Some researchers have also suggested that the efficacy of buspirone may be reduced in patients previously treated with benzodiazepines (Schweizer et al. 1986).

Antipsychotics

Antipsychotics—especially the newer agents, such as olanzapine and risperidone—are frequently used in the treatment of severe agitation associated with psychosis, delirium, and dementia (Chou and Sussman 1988). More recently, antipsychotics have been used to treat refractory anxiety in dementia. However, the use of antipsychotics for the treatment of subjective anxiety states, especially in elderly patients, has never been systematically studied (Salzman 1991). Furthermore, adverse reactions such as sedation, extrapyramidal reactions, orthostatic hypotension, anticholinergic effects, and tardive dyskinesia can have devastating effects in elderly individuals. Therefore, antipsychotics are used sparingly in the treatment of anxiety disorders in elderly patients.

β-Blockers

β-Blockers have been shown to be effective in younger patients with somatic symptoms associated with GAD or performance (social) anxiety (Peet 1988). They have also been used in the treatment of aggression and agitation in patients with organic brain disease (Greendyke et al. 1986). However, the usefulness of β-blockers for treatment of anxiety in elderly persons is unknown (Sadavoy and LeClair 1997). Some researchers have suggested that propranolol in small doses (such as 5–10 mg one to four times a day) may be effective in elderly patients (Small 1997). However, β-blockers as a class should be avoided in patients with chronic obstructive pulmonary disease, congestive heart failure, heart block, insulin-dependent diabetes, severe renal disease, or peripheral vascular disease.

Antihistamines

Sedating antihistamines such as hydroxyzine and diphenhydramine are sometimes useful for treating anxiety or insomnia in elderly patients, but chronic use is rarely recommended, because these drugs are less effective than benzodiazepines and have significant anticholinergic side effects (Barbee and McLaulin 1990). They may be used in patients with mild symptoms, patients with severe chronic obstructive pulmonary disease, addiction-prone persons, alcoholic individuals, or patients in whom more traditional drugs are not effective (Rickels 1983).

References

Alexopoulos GS: Anxiety-depression syndromes in old age. Int J Geriatr Psychiatry 5:351–353, 1990

American Psychiatric Association: Diagnostic and Statistical Manual of Mental Disorders, 3rd Edition. Washington, DC, American Psychiatric Association, 1980

American Psychiatric Association: Benzodiazepine Dependence, Toxicity, and Abuse. Washington, DC, American Psychiatric Association, 1990

American Psychiatric Association: Diagnostic and Statistical Manual of Mental Disorders, 4th Edition, Text Revision. Washington, DC, American Psychiatric Association, 2000

Banazak DA: Anxiety disorders in elderly patients. J Am Board Fam Pract 10:280–289, 1997

Barbee JG, McLaulin JB: Anxiety disorders: diagnosis and pharmacotherapy in the elderly. Psychiatric Annals 20:439–445, 1990

Ben-Arie O, Swartz L, Dickman BJ: Depression in the elderly living in the community: its presentation and features. Br J Psychiatry 150:169–174, 1987

Bland RC, Newman SC, Orn H: Prevalence of psychiatric disorders in the elderly in Edmonton. Acta Psychiatr Scand Suppl 338:57–63, 1988

Blazer DG: Generalized anxiety disorder and panic disorder in the elderly: a review. Harv Rev Psychiatry 5:18–27, 1997

Blazer D[G], George LK, Hughes D: The epidemiology of anxiety disorders: an age comparison, in Anxiety in the Elderly: Treatment and Research. Edited by Salzman C, Lebowitz BD. New York, Springer, 1991a, pp 17–30

Blazer DG, Hughes D, George LK, et al: Generalized anxiety disorder, in Psychiatric Disorders in America: The Epidemiologic Catchment Area Study. Edited by Robins LN, Regier DA. New York, Free Press, 1991b, pp 180–203

Bohm C, Robinson DS, Gammans RE, et al: Buspirone therapy in anxious elderly patients: a controlled clinical trial. J Clin Psychopharmacol 10 (suppl 3):47S–51S, 1990

Boston Collaborative Drug Surveillance Program: Clinical depression of the central nervous system due to diazepam and chlordiazepoxide in relation to cigarette smoking and age. N Engl J Med 288:277–280, 1973

Cassem EH: Depression and anxiety secondary to medical illness. Psychiatr Clin North Am 13:597–612, 1990

Chou JCY, Sussman N: Neuroleptics in anxiety. Psychiatric Annals 18:172–175, 1988

Copeland JRM, Davidson IA, Dewey ME: The prevalence and outcome of anxious depression in elderly people aged 65 and over living in the community, in Anxious Depression: Assessment and Treatment. Edited by Racagni G, Smeraldi E. New York, Raven, 1987, pp 43–47

Crook T: Diagnosis and treatment of mixed anxiety-depression in the elderly. J Clin Psychiatry 43:35–43, 1982

Eison AS, Temple DL Jr: Buspirone: review of its pharmacology and current perspectives on its mechanism of action. Am J Med 80:1–9, 1986

Fawcett J, Marcus RN, Anton SF, et al: Response of anxiety and agitation symptoms during nefazodone treatment of major depression. J Clin Psychiatry 37:713–738, 1995

Flint AJ: Anxiety disorders in late life. Can Fam Physician 45:2672–2679, 1999

Gaitz CM, Scott J: Age and the measurement of mental health. J Health Soc Behav 13:55–67, 1972

Georgotas A, McCue RE, Hapworth W, et al: Comparative efficacy and safety of MAOIs versus TCAs in treating depression in the elderly. Biol Psychiatry 21:1155–1166, 1986

Goa KL, Ward A: Buspirone: a preliminary review of its pharmacologic properties and therapeutic efficacy as an anxiolytic. Drugs 32:114–129, 1986

Greendyke R, Kanter D, Schuster D, et al: Propranolol treatment of assaultive patients with organic brain disease: a double blind cross-over, placebo-controlled study. J Nerv Ment Dis 174:290–294, 1986

Gurian G, Vehoff J, Feld S: Americans View Their Mental Health. New York, Basic Books, 1963

Hassan R, Pollard CA: Late-life-onset panic disorder: clinical and demographic characteristics of a patient sample. J Geriatr Psychiatry Neurol 7:86–90, 1994

Hayes PE, Dommisse CS: Current concepts in clinical therapeutics: anxiety disorders, part 1. Clin Pharm 6:140–147, 1987

Hershey LA, Kim KY: Diagnosis and treatment of anxiety in the elderly. Ration Drug Ther 22:1–6, 1988

Himmelfarb S, Murrell SA: The prevalence and correlates of anxiety symptoms in older adults. J Psychol 116:159–167, 1984

Hoehn-Saric R, McLeod DR, Zimmerli WD: Differential effects of alprazolam and imipramine in generalized anxiety disorder: somatic vs. psychic symptoms. J Clin Psychiatry 49:293–301, 1988

Jenike MA: Geriatric Psychiatry and Psychopharmacology: A Clinical Approach. Chicago, IL, Year Book Medical, 1989, pp 248–271

Jenike MA: Geriatric obsessive-compulsive disorder. J Geriatr Psychiatry Neurol 4:34–39, 1991

Jonas BS, Franks P, Ingram DD: Are symptoms of anxiety and depression risk factors for hypertension? longitudinal evidence from the National Health and Nutrition Examination Survey I Epidemiologic Follow-up Study. Arch Fam Med 6:43–49, 1997

Kasper S, Przschek-Rieder N, Tauscher J, et al: A risk-benefit assessment of mirtazapine in the treatment of depression. Drug Saf 17:251–264, 1997

Katzelnick DJ, Kobak KA, Greist JH, et al: Sertraline for social phobia: a double-blind, placebo-controlled crossover study. Am J Psychiatry 152:1368–1371, 1995

Kawachi I, Sparrow D, Vokonas PS, et al: Symptoms of anxiety and risk of coronary heart disease. The Normative Aging Study. Circulation 90:2225–2229, 1994

Kelsey JE: Venlafaxine in social phobia. Psychopharmacol Bull 31:767–771, 1995

Kluznik JC, Speed N, Van Valkenburg C, et al: Forty-year follow-up of United States prisoners of war. Am J Psychiatry 143:1443–1446, 1986

Kohn R, Westlake RJ, Rasmussen SA, et al: Clinical features of obsessive-compulsive disorder in elderly patients. Am J Geriatr Psychiatry 5:211–215, 1997

Krasucki C, Howard R, Mann A: Anxiety and its treatment in the elderly. Int Psychogeriatr 11:25–45, 1998

Kuch K, Cox BJ: Symptoms of PTSD in 124 survivors of the Holocaust. Am J Psychiatry 149:337–340, 1992

Lenze EJ, Mulsant BH, Shear MK, et al: Comorbid anxiety disorders in depressed elderly patients. Am J Psychiatry 157:722–728, 2000

Lindesay J, Briggs K, Murphy E: The Guy's/Age Concern survey. Prevalence rates of cognitive impairment, depression and anxiety in an urban elderly community. Br J Psychiatry 155:317–329, 1989

Livingston G, Watkin V, Milne B, et al: The natural history of depression and the anxiety disorders in older people: the Islington community study. J Affect Disord 46:255–262, 1997

Luchins DJ, Rose RP: Late-life onset of panic disorder with agoraphobia in three patients. Am J Psychiatry 146:920–921, 1989

Magni G, De Leo D: Anxiety and depression in geriatric and adult medical inpatients: a comparison. Psychol Rep 55:607–612, 1984

Manela M, Katona C, Livingston G: How common are the anxiety disorders in old age? Int J Geriatr Psychiatry 11:65–70, 1996

Moser DK, Dracup K: Is anxiety early after myocardial infarction associated with subsequent ischemic and arrhythmic events? Psychosom Med 58:395–401, 1996

Napoliello MJ: An interim multicentre report on 677 anxious geriatric out-patients treated with buspirone. Br J Clin Pract 40:71–73, 1986

Ouslander JG: Drug therapy in the elderly. Ann Intern Med 95:711–722, 1981

Oxman TE, Barrett JE, Barrett J, et al: Psychiatric symptoms in the elderly in a primary care practice. Gen Hosp Psychiatry 9:167–173, 1987

Parmelee PA, Katz IR, Lawton MP: Anxiety and its association with depression among institutionalized elderly. Am J Geriatr Psychiatry 1:46–58, 1993

Pearson JL: Summary of a National Institute of Mental Health workshop on late-life anxiety. Psychopharmacol Bull 34:127–130, 1998

Peet M: The treatment of anxiety with beta-blocking drugs. Postgrad Med J 64 (suppl 2):45–49, 1988

Perse TL, Greist JH, Jefferson JW, et al: Fluvoxamine treatment of obsessive-compulsive disorder. Am J Psychiatry 144:1543–1548, 1987

Raj BA, Corvea MH, Dagon EM: The clinical characteristics of panic disorder in the elderly: a retrospective study. J Clin Psychiatry 54:150–155, 1993

Ray WA, Griffin MR, Downey W: Benzodiazepines of long and short elimination half-life and the risk of hip fracture. JAMA 262:3303–3306, 1989

Regier DA, Boyd JH, Burke JD Jr, et al: One-month prevalence of mental disorders in the United States. Based on five Epidemiologic Catchment Area sites. Arch Gen Psychiatry 45:977–986, 1988

Regier DA, Narrow WE, Rae DS: The epidemiology of anxiety disorders: the Epidemiologic Catchment Area (ECA) experience. J Psychiatr Res 24 (suppl 2):3–14, 1990

Rickels K: Nonbenzodiazepine anxiolytics: clinical usefulness. J Clin Psychiatry 44:38–43, 1983

Rickels K, Downing R, Schweizer E, et al: Antidepressants for the treatment of generalized anxiety disorder: a placebo-controlled comparison of imipramine, trazodone, and diazepam. Arch Gen Psychiatry 50:884–895, 1993

Rifkin A, Klein DF, Dillon D, et al: Blockade by imipramine or desipramine of panic induced by sodium lactate. Am J Psychiatry 138:676–677, 1981

Robinson D, Napoliello MJ, Schenk J: The safety and usefulness of buspirone as an anxiolytic drug in elderly versus young patients. Clin Ther 10:740–746, 1988

Robinson S, Rapaport J, Durst R, et al: The late effects of Nazi persecution among elderly Holocaust survivors. Acta Psychiatr Scand 82:311–315, 1990

Rosen J, Fields RB, Hand AM, et al: Concurrent posttraumatic stress disorder in psychogeriatric patients. J Geriatr Psychiatry Neurol 2:65–69, 1989

Sadavoy J, LeClair JK: Treatment of anxiety disorders in late life. Can J Psychiatry 42 (suppl 1):28S–34S, 1997

Salzman C: Practical considerations in the pharmacologic treatment of depression and anxiety in the elderly. J Clin Psychiatry 51 (suppl):40–43, 1990

Salzman C: Pharmacologic treatment of the anxious elderly patient, in Anxiety in the Elderly: Treatment and Research. Edited by Salzman C, Lebowitz BD. New York, Springer, 1991, pp 149–173

Schneider LS: Overview of generalized anxiety disorder in the elderly. J Clin Psychiatry 57 (suppl 7):34–45, 1996

Schweizer E, Rickels K, Lucki I: Resistance to the anti-anxiety effect of buspirone in patients with a history of benzodiazepine use. N Engl J Med 314:719–720, 1986

Sheehan DV, Raj AB, Sheehan KH, et al: Is buspirone effective for panic disorder? J Clin Psychopharmacol 10:3–11, 1990

Sheikh JI, Cassidy EL: Treatment of anxiety disorders in the elderly: issues and strategies. J Anxiety Disord 14:173–190, 2000

Sheikh JI, King RJ, Taylor CB: Comparative phenomenology of early onset versus late-onset panic attacks: a pilot study. Am J Psychiatry 148:1231–1233, 1991

Shorr RI, Robin DW: Rational use of benzodiazepines in the elderly. Drugs Aging 4:9–20, 1994

Silverstone PH, Ravindran A: Once-daily venlafaxine extended release (XR) compared with fluoxetine in outpatients with depression and anxiety. Venlafaxine XR 360 Study Group. J Clin Psychiatry 60:22–28, 1999

Singh AN, Beer M: A dose range–finding study of buspirone in geriatric patients with symptoms of anxiety (letter). J Clin Psychopharmacol 8:67–68, 1988

Small GW: Recognizing and treating anxiety in the elderly. J Clin Psychiatry 58 (suppl 3):41–47, 1997

Stanley MA, Novy DM: Cognitive-behavior therapy for generalized anxiety in late life: an evaluative overview. J Anxiety Disord 14:191–207, 2000

Steinberg JR: Anxiety in elderly patients: a comparison of azapirones and benzodiazepines. Drugs Aging 5:335–345, 1994

Steuer JL, Mintz J, Hammen CL, et al: Cognitive-behavioral and psychodynamic group psychotherapy in treatment of geriatric depression. J Consult Clin Psychol 52:180–189, 1984

Sutker PB, Allain AN Jr, Winstead DK: Psychopathology and psychiatric diagnoses of World War II Pacific theater prisoner of war survivors and combat veterans. Am J Psychiatry 150:240–245, 1993

Swales PJ, Solvin JF, Sheikh JI: Cognitive-behavioral therapy in older panic disorder patients. Am J Geriatr Psychiatry 4:46–60, 1996

Thompson TL II, Moran MG, Nies AS: Psychotropic drug use in the elderly. N Engl J Med 308:134–138, 1983

Tollefson GD, Rampey AH Jr, Potvin JH, et al: A multicenter investigation of fixed-dose fluoxetine in the treatment of obsessive-compulsive disorder. Arch Gen Psychiatry 51:559–567, 1994

Uhlenhuth EH, Balter MB, Mellinger GD, et al: Symptom checklist syndromes in the general population. Correlations with psychotherapeutic drug use. Arch Gen Psychiatry 40:1167–1173, 1983

Van Ameringen M, Mancini C, Streiner DL: Fluoxetine efficacy in social phobia. J Clin Psychiatry 54:27–32, 1993

van Laar MW, van Willigenburg AP, Volkerts ER: Acute and subchronic effects of nefazodone and imipramine on highway driving, cognitive functions, and daytime sleepiness in healthy adult and elderly subjects. J Clin Psychopharmacol 15:30–40, 1995

van Vliet IM, den Boer JA, Westenberg HG: Psychopharmacological treatment of social phobia: a double-blind placebo controlled study with fluvoxamine. Psychopharmacology (Berl) 115:128–134, 1994

Weissman MM, Bruce ML, Leaf PJ, et al: Affective disorders, in Psychiatric Disorders in America: The Epidemiologic Catchment Area Study. Edited by Robins LN, Regier DA. New York, Free Press, 1991, pp 53–80

White LR, Cartwright WS, Cornoni-Huntley J: Geriatric epidemiology. Annu Rev Gerontol Geriatr 6:215–311, 1986

Wylie ME, Miller MD, Shear MK, et al: Fluvoxamine pharmacotherapy of anxiety disorders in later life: preliminary open-trial data. J Geriatr Psychiatry Neurol 13:43–48, 2000

Zimmer B, Gershon S: The ideal late life anxiolytic, in Anxiety in the Elderly: Treatment and Research. Edited by Salzman C, Lebowitz BD. New York, Springer, 1991, pp 277–303, 1991

Zung WK: Prevalence of clinically significant anxiety in a family practice setting. Am J Psychiatry 143:1471–1472, 1986

Somatoform Disorders

Marc E. Agronin, M.D.

Somatoform disorders comprise a heterogeneous group of disorders in which physical symptoms or complaints without objective organic causes are present and in which there are strongly associated psychological factors. The seven somatoform disorders listed in DSM-IV-TR (American Psychiatric Association 2000) are somatization disorder, undifferentiated somatoform disorder, hypochondriasis, conversion disorder, pain disorder, body dysmorphic disorder (BDD), and somatoform disorder not otherwise specified. Older individuals with somatoform disorders are seen in all health care settings, where they frequently overuse medical services (Barsky 1979) and overburden general practitioners (Reid et al. 2001). They often come to the attention of a geriatric psychiatrist after another clinician has attempted unsuccessfully to resolve their physical symptoms. Somatoform disorders have not been well studied in late life, in part because many of the disorders tend to begin in early adulthood. In addition, somatoform symptoms in late life are often obscured by comorbid physical and psychiatric illnesses. In particular, somatoform disorders have been strongly associated with depression, anxiety, substance abuse, and personality disorders (Aigner and Bach 1999; Orenstein 1989; Otto et al. 2001; Polatin et al. 1993). Research involving older cohorts has usually focused on reported somatic symptoms rather than on specific diagnoses. Prevalence rates for somatoform disorders vary by diagnosis, but in general there are almost no data concerning older individuals.

Clinical Features

Somatoform symptoms are experienced by the affected individual as real physical sensations, pain, or discomfort, usually indistinguishable from symptoms of actual medical disorders and frequently coexisting with them. However, by definition, these symptoms do not have an established organic basis, despite the fact that they can lead to significant emotional distress and functional impairment. Associated psychological factors are presumed but not always apparent, and patients vary in their degree of insight into such factors.

In general, transient somatoform symptoms may be seen in 30%–50% of patients presenting to medical settings (Barsky et al. 1990; Busse 1993; Kellner 1985). When symptoms shift from representing transient expressions of somatic concern to representing more serious bodily preoccupation and impairment, and no organic cause emerges, a somatoform disorder becomes a more likely diagnosis. Somatoform disorders do not represent intentional, conscious attempts by patients to present factitious physical symptoms. Neither do they represent delusional thinking as found in psychotic states (although BDD can be associated with beliefs of delusional quality).

Patients are generally able to accept that their symptoms may be functional and have psychological roots (Martin and Yutzy 1994). Somatoform disorders differ from psychosomatic disorders, which are characterized by actual disease states with presumed psychological triggers. Instead, somatoform disorders involve a complex interaction between brain and body, in which the affected individual is unknowingly expressing psychological stress or conflict through the body. Not surprisingly, increased somatic symptoms and preoccupation with illness are often associated with anxiety and depression. It is possible that the underpinnings of these disorders, especially in late life, may be related to frontal lobe dysfunction (Flor-Henry et al. 1981).

Somatization Disorder

Somatization disorder is characterized by multiple physical complaints, in excess of what would be expected given the patient's history and examination findings. These complaints cannot be fully explained by medical workup and must include pain at four or more sites, as well as two gastrointestinal symptoms, one sexual symptom, and one pseudoneurological symptom (other than pain). Another term used in the literature for this disorder is *Briquet's syndrome* (Liskow et al. 1986; Orenstein 1989). Symptoms typically appear before age 30 and have usually persisted for years by the time of diagnosis. Somatization disorder is seen almost exclusively in women and may have a prevalence rate ranging from less than 1% to 3% (Faravelli et al. 1997; Martin and Yutzy 1994). High rates of the disorder have been noted among first-degree female relatives of affected individuals (Cloninger et al. 1986) and in certain medical conditions. For example, definite or probable somatization disorder was diagnosed in 42% of a sample of 50 medical outpatients with irritable bowel disease (Miller et al. 2001). Associated problems include drug abuse and dependence, depression and suicidality, and multiple and unnecessary medical treatments, including surgeries (Goodwin and Guze 1989).

Somatization disorder is a chronic psychiatric disorder, with the majority of individuals demonstrating consistent symptom patterns as they age (Cloninger et al. 1986; Goodwin and Guze 1989). A comparison study of symptoms in younger patients and older patients (>55 years old) found consistency (Pribor et al. 1994). The most difficult diagnostic feature to establish in elderly patients is the onset of symptoms before age 30, because such history can rarely be accurately determined. In addition, the presence of multiple physical symptoms in excess of what would be expected is a relative factor in late life, given the high incidence of comorbid illnesses. Cloninger (1986) suggested that symptoms of somatization disorder differ from those of true medical illness in that the former 1) involve multiple body systems simultaneously, 2) have an early onset and a chronic history without later development of pathognomonic symptoms of medical illness, and 3) are not associated with relevant physical or laboratory findings. These three principles may aid late-life diagnosis.

Undifferentiated Somatoform Disorder

In most elderly patients with somatoform symptoms, a diagnosis of undifferentiated somatoform disorder can be more easily made than a diagnosis of somatization disorder. Undifferentiated somatoform disorder is defined by the presence of one of more physical complaints, lasting at least 6 months, that cannot be fully explained by appropriate medical workup, and that result in considerable social, occupational, or functional impairment. Again, diagnosis is complicated in late life by the frequency of comorbid medical disorders. Determining whether the impairment is due to somatoform symptoms rather than comorbid medical disorders is difficult—and may be nearly impossible in the case of many debilitated elderly individuals. Prevalence rates for undifferentiated somatoform disorder have not been well established for any age group, although one community study in Italy found a rate of 13.8%—significantly higher than rates for every other somatoform disorder (Faravelli et al. 1997). Patients with chronic pain have been found to have quite high rates of undifferentiated somatoform disorder (Aigner and Bach 1999).

Hypochondriasis

Hypochondriasis is characterized by a preoccupation with fears of having a serious illness. These fears arise from misinterpretation of bodily symptoms, and the individual's preoccupation is resistant to medical evaluation and reassurance. Varying degrees of hypochondriacal symptoms are more common among individuals who are under stress due to medical illness in themselves or a relative or who have a history of serious illness, especially in childhood (Kellner 1987). Physical complaints tend to be based on common but transient symptoms that are viewed as portending a serious illness. In fact, most individuals have one or more somatic symptoms in any given week, and a small but not insignificant percentage of affected individuals and a higher percentage of somewhat neurotic individuals will develop mild anxiety with respect to such symptoms (Kellner 1987).

The line between normal somatic concern and hypochondriasis can be difficult to draw but depends on a pattern of dysfunctional behaviors that ultimately serve to increase anxiety and constrain medical treatment. Barsky (1979) suggested that underlying this pattern is a psychological state that tends to amplify bodily perceptions. Similar psychological states have been described in women who have fibromyalgia (McDermid et al. 1996), although without the behavioral patterns seen in hypochondriasis. In the person with hypochondriasis, it is the resultant conviction of having a disease that leads to a pattern of 1) anxious ruminations that one has a terrible illness and 2) repetitive medical consultations. The prevalence of hypochondriasis among medical outpatients is around 5% (Barsky 2001; Faravelli et al. 1997), and there is some debate regarding whether factors such as low education level, low socioeconomic status, and old age increase this rate (Barsky et al. 1991; Brink et al. 1981; Kellner 1986; Rief et al. 2001). Comorbid psychiatric disorders are common, especially major depression, panic disorder, and obsessive-compulsive disorder (Barsky et al. 1992).

Conversion Disorder

Conversion disorder is characterized by one or more motor or sensory deficits that cannot be fully explained by appropriate medical workup and that appear to be causally related to psychological factors. The diagnosis should specify whether the symptom or deficit is a motor or sensory one, involves a seizure, or entails a mixed presentation. As with other somatoform symptoms, however, the presence of true medical comorbidity can cloud the picture. The key to diagnosis of conversion symptoms is identification of the psychological conflict that seems to be prompting the symptom, but this approach requires in-depth psychotherapeutic investigation, which is not always feasible in older individuals.

Although conversion disorder has been reported in the elderly population (Weddington 1979), it is more common in young women, and the prevalence rate in the community is less than 1% (Cloninger 1986; Faravelli et al. 1997). Dula and DeNaples (1995) reviewed records of 42 patients who were seen in an emergency room and subsequently received a diagnosis of conversion disorder. Of these patients, 24 were women (average age, 33 years) and 18 were men (average age, 34 years). Comorbid diagnoses included substance abuse, chronic illness, head trauma, and previous conversion symptoms. Psychogenic nonepileptic seizures, sometimes referred to as pseudoseizures, represent one subtype of conversion symptoms. They are characterized by behavioral spells that mimic various forms of seizures but are not associated with electroencephalographic findings and have a presumed emotional etiology (Volow 1986). Nonepileptic seizures are more frequent in young women and are seen in 5%–20% of outpatients with epilepsy, often in combination with an actual seizure disorder (Chabolla et al. 1996).

Risk factors for conversion disorder include sexual abuse (Martin 1994), personality disorder, and other neurological illnesses (Ford and Folks 1985; Slater and Glithero 1965). Conversion disorder in late life is likely associated with an actual comorbid neurological disorder.

The prognosis is limited: in one sample, persistent symptoms were present in nearly 40% of subjects at 10-year follow-up (Mace and Trimble 1996).

Pain Disorder

Pain is the most common medical complaint in elderly persons, with pain due to musculoskeletal disease (e.g., osteoarthritis, back pain, headache) being the most common type of pain (Leveille et al. 2001). Close to 50% of elderly individuals have chronic pain, and the percentage approaches 70% for those in long-term care (Otis and McGeeney 2000). Persistent pain is associated with significant functional and social impairment (Scudds and Ostbye 2001), as well as comorbid psychiatric symptoms including depression, insomnia, and substance abuse. Pain assessment is often limited because of its dependence on subjective patient reports, which can be influenced by numerous confounding factors in late life, including dementia. Dementia may limit an individual's ability to verbalize pain, with the result that caregivers must rely on nonverbal behaviors. It has also been proposed that the pathological process in Alzheimer's disease may alter pain perception, perhaps by increasing the pain threshold (Scherder et al. 2001). Pharmacological treatment of pain, however, can lead to additional problems, due to medication side effects and drug-drug interactions.

In pain disorder, pain is the major focus of the clinical presentation, and psychological factors are believed to play critical roles in the onset, severity, exacerbation, or continuation of the pain. Diagnostic variants of pain disorder in DSM-IV-TR include pain disorder associated with psychological factors, a general medical condition, or both. Even when there are specific causes of pain, diagnosis hinges on identifying an overwhelming preoccupation with pain—a preoccupation sometimes involving a pattern of treatment resistance. The determination of such psychological factors is difficult, especially in late life, and the ensuing divisions between the relative roles of mind and body raise questions about diagnostic validity (Boland 2002).

This dilemma is illustrated by the overwhelming psychiatric comorbidity associated with both chronic pain and somatoform pain disorder. In a study involving individuals with chronic low back pain, 80% of subjects met criteria for at least one lifetime psychiatric disorder—including major depression, substance abuse, anxiety disorders, or personality disorders (Polatin et al. 1993)—usually with onset before the development of chronic pain. In another study involving individuals with chronic pain, 66% of the subjects (ages 18–65 years) met DSM-IV (American Psychiatric Association 1994) criteria for pain disorder (Aigner and Bach 1999). Of the patients with pain disorder, 22% had depression, 7% had hypochondriasis, 10% had somatization disorder, and more than 90% met criteria for undifferentiated somatoform disorder. Descriptions of pain characteristics did not differ between pain disorder associated with psychological factors and pain disorder due to both psychological factors and a general medical problem. Similar findings emerged from a study involving individuals with chronic headache (Okasha et al. 1999). In that study, somatoform pain disorder was diagnosed in more than 40% of individuals with no established organic etiology and in 20% of persons with an organic etiology. Personality disorders were diagnosed in 77% of members of the nonorganic-etiology group, compared with a rate of 24% in the organic-etiology group. Depressive disorders were also relatively common in the nonorganic-etiology group.

Body Dysmorphic Disorder

BDD is characterized by a preoccupation with an imagined or small defect in appearance. Common body parts that become the object of focus include facial features (e.g., the nose), breasts, and genitals. If there is an actual physical defect, this preoccupation greatly exceeds what would be expected. Affected individuals often spend considerable time engaging in repetitive behaviors such as looking at the body part in the mirror, touching or picking at it, and seeking reassurance from others regarding their concern (Phillips 1996). Symptoms tend to be chronic and often lead patients to make extraordinary attempts to deal with the imagined or slight defect, including unnecessary plastic surgery (Martin and Yutzy 1994). For this reason, BDD often presents to plastic surgeons long before coming to the attention of a psychiatrist. The disorder is commonly diagnosed in young adults and in women around the time of menopause, and it is often associated with comorbid depression, obsessive-compulsive behaviors, personality disorders, and even suicidality (Phillips 1998).

The estimated prevalence of BDD in women in the community is 0.7% (Faravelli et al. 1997; Otto et al. 2001). In a study involving 74 individuals with BDD, Phillips and McElroy (2000) found comorbid personality disorders in 57% of the sample; the most common personality disorders were avoidant (43% of patients with a personality disorder), dependent (15%), obsessive-com-

pulsive (14%), and paranoid (14%) personality disorders. In up to 50% of individuals with BDD, the somatic preoccupation may be delusional (Phillips 1998; Phillips et al. 1998). Although no prevalence figures for BDD in late life are available, such specific complaints are less common in older patients.

Somatoform Disorder Not Otherwise Specified

The diagnosis of somatoform disorder not otherwise specified is used when the patient has somatoform symptoms that do not meet the criteria for other somatoform disorders but that result in similar degrees of social, occupational, and functional impairment. Some somatoform presentations that fit this category are hypochondriacal symptoms of less than 6 months' duration; unexplained physical symptoms of less than 6 months' duration; and pseudocyesis, in which the false belief that one is pregnant is associated with objective (albeit false) symptoms of pregnancy.

Etiology

The causes of somatoform disorders are usually multifactorial and are often rooted in early developmental experiences and personality traits. For example, somatization and all somatoform disorders have been associated with the experience of serious illness early in life (Stuart and Noyes 1999), childhood abuse (Martin 1994; Walker et al. 1992), significant psychological stress (Hollifield et al. 1999; Ritsner et al. 2000), and the personality trait neuroticism (Affleck et al. 1992; Chaturvedi 1986; Costa and McCrae 1980; Phillips and McElroy 2000), which presents as a tendency to experience more negative emotions. As noted throughout the chapter, somatoform disorders are also highly associated with comorbid depression, anxiety and panic disorders, substance abuse, and personality disorders (Noyes et al. 2001). Somatization may be more common in women and in older individuals, although the prevalence of actual somatoform disorders has not been associated with increased age (with the exception of hypochondriasis). When present in late life, especially when the onset was recent, somatoform disorders may be associated with neuropsychological impairment and/or comorbid neurological illness (Sheehan and Banerjee 1999). These and other factors associated with an increased risk of somatoform disorders are listed in Table 17–1.

TABLE 17–1. Risk factors for somatoform disorders

Female gender
Childhood sexual abuse
Severe childhood abuse
Lower education level
Low socioeconomic status
Chronic medical illness
Chronic pain
Significant, persistent psychological stress
Psychiatric illness
    Other somatoform disorder
    Anxiety disorder
    Depressive disorder
    Substance abuse
    Personality disorder
Neuroticism
Alexithymia

Psychodynamic approaches suggest that somatoform disorders result from unconscious conflict in which intolerable impulses or affects are expressed through more tolerable somatic symptoms or complaints. The classic example of this phenomenon is found in conversion disorder, in which intolerable, unconscious impulses are converted into motor or sensory dysfunction. Freud first wrote about such a mechanism on the basis of his studies involving women who had what was then termed *hysteria* (Breuer and Freud 1893–1895/1955). Specifically, psychodynamic theory suggests that excessive and intolerable guilt or hostility are psychological sources of somatization—in particular, hypochondriasis (Barsky and Klerman 1983). In such cases, physical symptoms serve as a means of self-punishment for unacceptable unconscious impulses. Anger directed toward caregivers is indirectly expressed through distrust of and dissatisfaction with multiple physicians. Some researchers have suggested that underlying and complicating this psychodynamic rechannelization of anger or guilt is alexithymia, in which an individual has a relative inability to identify and express emotional states (Cox et al. 1994; Sriram et al. 1987). The experiencing and reporting of bodily sensations thus becomes a mode of emotional expression. Although alexithymia has long been postulated to play a role in both somatoform and psychosomatic illness, not all empirical research has supported the correlation of alexithymia with somatic complaints (Lundh and Simonsson-Sarnecki 2001).

In late life, somatoform disorders may represent a dysfunctional attempt to cope with accumulating physical and psychosocial losses, especially when these losses are associated with functional disability, anxiety, and depression. These include loss of or isolation from family, friends, and caregivers; loss of beauty and strength; financial setbacks; loss of independence; and loss of social role (e.g., as a result of retirement, the loss of a spouse, or occupational disability). The psychological distress and anxiety over such losses may be less threatening and more controllable when it is shifted to somatic complaints or symptoms. In turn, a sick role might be reinforced by increased social contacts and support. The presence of comorbid medical problems and the use of multiple medications may provide somatic symptoms around which psychological conflict can center. In long-term care, older individuals are faced with many additional overwhelming losses, and their own bodies often serve as the last bastion of control. Somatic preoccupation thus serves as a means of coping with stress, even though it is maladaptive and can result in excessive and unnecessary disability. It may also serve to mobilize and control resources and staff attention within the long-term-care environment.

Treatment

By definition, somatoform disorders present to clinicians with what appear to be legitimate somatic complaints of unknown physical etiology. It is only after repeated but fruitless workups, multiple and persistent complaints and requests, and sometimes angry and inappropriate reactions to treatment that clinicians begin to suspect a somatoform disorder. In some cases, the manner of presentation and the symptom complex are more immediately suggestive of a particular somatoform disorder. In any event, it is important for the clinician to remember that to the patient, the symptoms and complaints are quite real and disturbing. Even after workups have made it obvious that there are psychological factors involved, it is never wise to challenge the patient or suggest that the symptoms are "all in your mind." The typical response to such a suggestion is for the patient to seek additional opinions and medical tests, which in turn can perpetuate a cycle of somatization, in which underlying issues are never addressed.

Instead, the role of the physician must be to foster a supportive, consistent, and professional relationship with the affected individual. Such a relationship will provide reassurance as well as protect the patient from excessive and unnecessary medical visits and procedures. The clinician should focus on responding to individual complaints, perhaps with periodic but regularly scheduled appointments (Smith et al. 1986), and setting limits on workup and treatment, in a firm but empathic manner. This can be difficult to do when patients become demanding and attempt to consume excessive clinic time, but the clinician must endeavor to remain professional and to not personalize the situation or feel as though he or she were failing the patient. The clinician should focus on symptom reduction and rehabilitation and not attempt to force the patient to gain insight into the potential psychological nature of his or her symptoms (Kellner 1987).

It would obviously be hazardous for a clinician to diagnose a somatoform disorder prematurely, because underlying organic pathology might have eluded diagnosis. For example, multiple sclerosis, systemic lupus erythematosus, and acute intermittent porphyria often have complex presentations that elude initial diagnostic workup (Kellner 1987). Somatoform disorders may coexist with actual disease states; for example, many individuals with pseudoseizures also have a seizure disorder (Desai et al. 1982; Luther et al. 1982). Moene et al. (2000) found that slightly more than 10% of patients who received an initial diagnosis of conversion disorder actually had a true neurological disorder. This study finding is consistent with findings of other investigations (Mace and Trimble 1996). At the same time, it is important for the clinician to set limits on what he or she can offer and to make appropriate referrals to specialists and/or mental health clinicians.

The geriatric psychiatrist plays a more active role in addressing the somatoform disorder rather than simply the physical complaints. Unfortunately, most disorders tend to be lifelong. Therefore, the goal of treatment is not to cure the patient but to control symptoms. The clinician must form a therapeutic alliance through empathic listening and acknowledging of physical discomfort, without trivializing the somatic complaints. Sometimes an offer to review all available medical records can be a tangible way of conveying one's seriousness to the patient. Educating the patient about various symptom complexes and involving him or her in part of the decision making can be empowering for the patient, especially a patient with chronic pain (McDonald 1993).

Individual therapy that takes a psychodynamic approach will focus on helping the patient identify and then discuss psychological conflict and associated emotion. Cognitive-behavioral therapy will focus on identifying distorted thought patterns and anxiety triggers and replacing them with more realistic and adaptive strategies. For example, the somatic preoccupation seen in hypochondriasis and BDD can closely resemble symptoms of obsessive-compulsive disorder and may respond to techniques similar to those used in the latter disorder for ex-

tinguishing such thought patterns. In conversion disorder, hypnosis is sometimes used as both a diagnostic and therapeutic tool.

Pharmacotherapy is a central component of treatment for somatoform disorders. It can be targeted at a specific disorder or at underlying anxiety, depression, or thought patterns that appear delusional. Somatization disorder has been treated successfully with both antidepressants (Menza et al. 2001) and anticonvulsants or mood stabilizers (Garcia-Campayo and Sanz-Carrillo 2001). Hypochondriacal symptoms have responded to a variety of antidepressant medications—in particular, selective serotonin reuptake inhibitors—as well as to anxiolytics (Barsky 2001; Fallon et al. 1996; Oosterbaan et al. 2001). A meta-analysis of antidepressant therapy in pain disorder found that pharmacotherapy decreased pain intensity significantly more than placebo (Fishbain et al. 1998). Anticonvulsants have also been found to be useful in treating pain disorder, especially when the disorder is associated with a comorbid mood disorder (Maurer et al. 1999). BDD has responded well to antidepressant treatment (Phillips 1996; Phillips et al. 2002) and has also been treated with antipsychotics (Grant 2001; Phillips 1996). A study by Phillips et al. (2001) demonstrated a 60% response rate with selective serotonin reuptake inhibitors, a high relapse rate when medications were discontinued, and increased response with antidepressant augmentation. A double-blind, crossover study involving 29 patients with BDD found clomipramine to be superior to desipramine across a variety of symptomatic domains (Hollander et al. 1999). Even the delusional variant of BDD has been shown to respond to antidepressant treatment (Phillips et al. 1998).

The tendency of many psychiatrists to focus more on pharmacotherapy can become a trap with somatoform disorders, because the therapeutic relationship is such a key element. Given the chronic nature of somatoform symptoms, it is unlikely that pharmacotherapy will be a quick fix. When this narrow focus on treatment with medications fails to result in rapid control of symptoms, the patient may abandon the therapist for alternative treatment. Other patients may welcome such a focus because it keeps them from having to face underlying psychological issues. Instead, clinicians must be in it for the long haul and strike a balance between reasonable pharmacotherapy that targets specific symptoms of anxiety or depression and a supportive alliance in which the most appropriate therapy for the patient is used. If another clinician serves as the therapist, frequent communication between psychiatrist and therapist is necessary to coordinate treatment.

References

Affleck G, Tennen H, Urrows S, et al: Neuroticism and the pain-mood relation in rheumatoid arthritis: insights from a prospective daily study. J Consult Clin Psychol 60:119–126, 1992

Aigner M, Bach M: Clinical utility of DSM-IV pain disorder. Compr Psychiatry 40:353–357, 1999

American Psychiatric Association: Diagnostic and Statistical Manual of Mental Disorders, 4th Edition. Washington, DC, American Psychiatric Association, 1994

American Psychiatric Association: Diagnostic and Statistical Manual of Mental Disorders, 4th Edition, Text Revision. Washington, DC, American Psychiatric Association, 2000

Barsky AJ: Patients who amplify bodily sensations. Ann Intern Med 91:63–70, 1979

Barsky AJ: The patient with hypochondriasis. N Engl J Med 345:1395–1399, 2001

Barsky AJ, Klerman GL: Overview: hypochondriasis, bodily complaints, and somatic styles. Am J Psychiatry 149:273–283, 1983

Barsky AJ, Wyshak G, Klerman G: Transient hypochondriasis. Arch Gen Psychiatry 47:746–752, 1990

Barsky AJ, Frank C, Cleary P, et al: The relation between hypochondriasis and age. Am J Psychiatry 148:923–928, 1991

Barsky AJ, Wyshak G, Klerman G: Psychiatric comorbidity in DSM-III-R hypochondriasis. Arch Gen Psychiatry 49:101–108, 1992

Boland RJ: How could the validity of the DSM-IV pain disorder be improved in reference to the concept that it is supposed to identify? Curr Pain Headache Rep 6:23–29, 2002

Breuer J, Freud S: Studies on hysteria (1893–1895), in The Standard Edition of the Complete Psychological Works of Sigmund Freud, Vol 2. Translated and edited by Strachey J. London, Hogarth Press, 1955, pp 1–319

Brink T, Janakes C, Martinez N: Geriatric hypochondriasis: situational factors. J Am Geriatr Soc 29:37–39, 1981

Busse EW: Duke University Longitudinal Studies of Aging. J Gerontol 26:123–128, 1993

Chabolla DR, Krahn LE, So EL, et al: Psychogenic nonepileptic seizures. Mayo Clin Proc 71:493–500, 1996

Chaturvedi SK: Chronic idiopathic pain disorder. J Psychosom Res 30:199–203, 1986

Cloninger CR: Somatoform and dissociative disorders, in The Medical Basis of Psychiatry. Edited by Winokur G, Clayton PJ. Philadelphia, PA, WB Saunders, 1986, pp 123–151

Cloninger CR, Martin RL, Guze SB, et al: A prospective follow-up and family study of somatization in men and women. Am J Psychiatry 143:873–878, 1986

Costa PT Jr, McCrae RR: Somatic complaints in males as a function of age and neuroticism: a longitudinal analysis. J Behav Med 3:245–257, 1980

Cox BJ, Kuch K, Parker JD, et al: Alexithymia in somatoform disorder patients with chronic pain. J Psychosom Res 38:523–527, 1994

Desai BT, Porter RJ, Penry JK: Psychogenic seizures. A study of 42 attacks in six patients, with intensive monitoring. Arch Neurol 39:202–209, 1982

Dula DJ, DeNaples L: Emergency department presentation of patients with conversion disorder. Acad Emerg Med 2:120–123, 1995

Fallon BA, Schneier FR, Marshall R, et al: The pharmacotherapy of hypochondriasis. Psychopharmacol Bull 32:607–611, 1996

Faravelli C, Salvatori S, Galassi F, et al: Epidemiology of somatoform disorders: a community survey in Florence. Soc Psychiatry Psychiatr Epidemiol 32:24–29, 1997

Fishbain DA, Cutler RB, Rosomoff HL, et al: Do antidepressants have an analgesic effect in psychogenic pain and somatoform pain disorder? a meta-analysis. Psychosom Med 60:503–509, 1998

Flor-Henry P, Fromm-Auch D, Tapper M, et al: A neuropsychological study of the stable syndrome of hysteria. Biol Psychiatry 16:601–626, 1981

Ford CV, Folks DG: Conversion disorders: an overview. Psychosomatics 26:371–383, 1985

Garcia-Campayo J, Sanz-Carrillo C: Gabapentin for the treatment of patients with somatization disorder (letter). J Clin Psychiatry 62:474, 2001

Goodwin DW, Guze SB: Psychiatric Diagnosis, 4th Edition. New York, Oxford University Press, 1989

Grant JE: Successful treatment of nondelusional body dysmorphic disorder with olanzapine: a case report. J Clin Psychiatry 62:297–298, 2001

Hollander E, Allen A, Kwon J, et al: Clomipramine vs desipramine crossover trial in body dysmorphic disorder: selective efficacy of a serotonin reuptake inhibitor in imagined ugliness. Arch Gen Psychiatry 56:1033–1039, 1999

Hollifield M, Tuttle L, Paine S, et al: Hypochondriasis and somatization related to personality and attitudes towards self. Psychosomatics 40:387–395, 1999

Kellner R: Functional somatic symptoms and hypochondriasis: a survey of empirical studies. Arch Gen Psychiatry 42:821–833, 1985

Kellner R: Somatization and hypochondriasis. New York, Praeger, 1986

Kellner R: Hypochondriasis and somatization. JAMA 258:2718–2722, 1987

Leveille SG, Ling S, Hochberg MC, et al: Widespread musculoskeletal pain and the progression of disability in older disabled women. Ann Intern Med 135:1038–1046, 2001

Liskow B, Othmer E, Penick EC, et al: Is Briquet's syndrome a heterogeneous disorder? Am J Psychiatry 143:626–629, 1986

Lundh LG, Simonsson-Sarnecki M: Alexithymia, emotion, and somatic complaints. J Pers 69:483–510, 2001

Luther JS, McNamara JO, Carwile S, et al: Pseudoepileptic seizures: methods and video analysis to aid diagnosis. Ann Neurol 12:458–462, 1982

Mace CJ, Trimble MR: Ten-year prognosis of conversion disorder. Br J Psychiatry 169:282–288, 1996

Martin RL: Conversion disorder, proposed autonomic arousal disorder, and pseudocyesis, in DSM-IV Sourcebook, Vol 2. Edited by Widiger TA, Frances AJ, Pincus HA, et al. Washington, DC, American Psychiatric Association, 1994, pp 893–914

Martin RL, Yutzy SH: Somatoform disorders, in The American Psychiatric Press Textbook of Psychiatry, 2nd Edition. Edited by Hales RE, Yudofsky SC, Talbott JA. Washington, DC, American Psychiatric Press, 1994, pp 591–622

Maurer I, Volz HP, Sauer H: Gabapentin leads to remission of somatoform pain disorder with major depression. Pharmacopsychiatry 32:255–257, 1999

McDermid AJ, Rollman GB, McCain GA: Generalized hypervigilance in fibromyalgia: evidence of perceptual amplification. Pain 66:133–144, 1996

McDonald JS: Management of chronic pelvic pain. Obstet Gynecol Clin North Am 20:817–838, 1993

Menza M, Lauritano M, Allen L, et al: Treatment of somatization disorder with nefazodone: a prospective, open-label study. Ann Clin Psychiatry 13:153–158, 2001

Miller AR, North CS, Clouse RE, et al: The association of irritable bowel syndrome and somatization disorder. Ann Clin Psychiatry 13:25–30, 2001

Moene FC, Landberg EH, Hoogduin KA, et al: Organic syndromes diagnosed as conversion disorder: identification and frequency in a study of 85 patients. J Psychosom Res 49:7–12, 2000

Noyes R Jr, Langbehn DR, Happel RL, et al: Personality dysfunction among somatizing patients. Psychosomatics 42:320–329, 2001

Okasha A, Ismail MK, Khalil AH, et al: A psychiatric study of nonorganic chronic headache patients. Psychosomatics 40:233–238, 1999

Oosterbaan DB, van Balkom AJ, van Boeijen CA, et al: An open study of paroxetine in hypochondriasis. Prog Neuropsychopharmacol Biol Psychiatry 25:1023–1033, 2001

Orenstein H: Briquet's syndrome in association with depression and panic: a reconceptualization of Briquet's syndrome. Am J Psychiatry 146:334–338, 1989

Otis JAD, McGeeney B: Managing pain in the elderly. Clinical Geriatrics 8:48–62, 2000

Otto MW, Cohen WS, Harlow BL: Prevalence of body dysmorphic disorder in a community sample of women. Am J Psychiatry 158:2061–2063, 2001

Phillips KA: Body dysmorphic disorder: diagnosis and treatment of imagined ugliness. J Clin Psychiatry 57 (suppl 8):61–64, 1996

Phillips KA: Body dysmorphic disorder: clinical aspects and treatment strategies. Bull Menninger Clin 62:A33–A48, 1998

Phillips KA, McElroy SL: Personality disorders and traits in patients with body dysmorphic disorder. Compr Psychiatry 41:229–236, 2000

Phillips KA, Dwight MM, McElroy SL: Efficacy and safety of fluvoxamine in body dysmorphic disorder. J Clin Psychiatry 59:165–171, 1998

Phillips KA, Albertini RS, Siniscalchi JM, et al: Effectiveness of pharmacotherapy for body dysmorphic disorder: a chart-review study. J Clin Psychiatry 62:721–727, 2001

Phillips KA, Albertini RS, Rasmussen SA: A randomized placebo-controlled trial of fluoxetine in body dysmorphic disorder. Arch Gen Psychiatry 59:381–388, 2002

Polatin PB, Kinney RK, Gatchel RJ, et al: Psychiatric illness and chronic low-back pain. The mind and the spine—which goes first? Spine 18:66–71, 1993

Pribor EF, Smith DS, Yutzy SH: Somatization disorder in elderly patients. J Geriatr Psychiatry 2:109–117, 1994

Reid S, Whooley D, Crayford T, et al: Medically unexplained symptoms—GPs' attitudes towards their cause and management. Fam Pract 18:519–523, 2001

Rief W, Hessel A, Braehler E: Somatization symptoms and hypochondriacal features in the general population. Psychosom Med 63:595–602, 2001

Ritsner M, Ponizovsky A, Kurs R, et al: Somatization in an immigrant population in Israel: a community survey of prevalence, risk factors, and help-seeking behavior. Am J Psychiatry 157:385–392, 2000

Scherder E, Bouma A, Slaets J, et al: Repeated pain assessment in Alzheimer's disease. Dement Geriatr Cogn Disord 12:400–407, 2001

Scudds RJ, Ostbye T: Pain and pain-related interference with function in older Canadians: the Canadian Study of Health and Aging. Disabil Rehabil 23:654–664, 2001

Sheehan B, Banerjee S: Review: somatization in the elderly. Int J Geriatr Psychiatry 14:1044–1049, 1999

Slater ETO, Glithero E: A follow-up of patients diagnosed as suffering from "hysteria." J Psychosom Res 9:9–13, 1965

Smith GR Jr, Monson RA, Ray DC: Psychiatric consultation in somatization disorder: a randomized controlled study. N Engl J Med 314:1407–1413, 1986

Sriram TG, Chaturvedi SK, Gopinath PS, et al: Controlled study of alexithymia characteristics in patients with psychogenic pain disorder. Psychother Psychosom 47:11–17, 1987

Stuart S, Noyes R Jr: Attachment and interpersonal communication in somatization. Psychosomatics 40:34–43, 1999

Volow MR: Pseudoseizures: an overview. South Med J 79:600–607, 1986

Walker EA, Katon WJ, Hansom J, et al: Medical and psychiatric symptoms in women with childhood sexual abuse. Psychosom Med 54:658–664, 1992

Weddington WW: Conversion reaction in an 82 year old man. J Nerv Ment Dis 167:368–369, 1979

CHAPTER 18

Sexual Disorders

Marc E. Agronin, M.D.

Sexual issues and disorders have increasingly become a part of assessment and treatment by the geriatric psychiatrist, both in outpatient and in long-term care settings. This change is due in part to the fact that aging individuals are living longer and healthier lives and expect sexuality to continue to play an important role. The renewed interest in sexuality in late life has also been fueled by changing attitudes. The idea of sexuality in late life has often been denied or regarded with humor or even disgust. For many younger individuals, the idea of sexuality clashes with stereotypes of mom and dad or grandma and grandpa. The denial of sexuality in parents and grandparents then becomes the denial of sexuality in all older individuals. These defensive and distorted ways of thinking about sexuality in late life may lead many clinicians to view sexual dysfunction as a normal and untreatable part of aging. However, several factors have led to broadened perspectives on sexuality in late life. Certainly the sexual and feminist revolutions in the 1960s and 1970s shattered many stereotypes. In addition, the widespread use of hormone replacement therapy has allowed many women to maintain more vital and enjoyable sexual function well beyond menopause. For men, the advent of numerous treatments for erectile dysfunction (ED), a relatively common sexual dysfunction in late life, has also ensured the persistence of sexual function in later years. In particular, the discovery of oral erectogenic agents such as sildenafil (Viagra) has revolutionized the treatment of ED. The availability of sildenafil and the high-profile advertising campaign featuring former senator Bob Dole have made ED and sexuality in late life more common and comfortable topics of conversation. Images such as those portrayed through the advertising campaign also serve as a distinct contrast to the connotations of powerlessness and shame surrounding the term *impotence*. In turn, the destigmatization of ED has no doubt brought many older couples

in to treatment who otherwise might have suffered in silence and shame.

Sexual Behaviors in Late Life

Several major studies over the last 20 years have shown that a majority of individuals more than 60 years old continue to be sexually active, although with modest decreases in activity, determined in part by gender and the availability of partners. These studies have indicated that older men are more sexually active than older women and that individuals with steady partners are more active than single individuals. In general, sexual interest and activity in late life depend on the previous level of sexual activity; the availability, health, and sexual interest of the partner; and the individual's overall physical health (Comfort and Dial 1991, Kligman 1991).

One of the most recent studies of late-life sexuality was conducted by the American Association of Retired Persons and *Modern Maturity* (now *AARP The Magazine*) (Jacoby 2003). Using a mail survey, researchers gathered responses from 1,384 men and women age 45 years or older. The survey found that three-quarters of both men and women in the sample remained sexually active. Eighty-four percent of men and 78% of women ages 45–59 years had steady sexual partners, compared with 58% of men and 21% of women older than 75 years. In terms of frequency, 50% of individuals ages 45–59 years reported having sex at least once a week, compared with 30% of men and 24% of women ages 60–74 years. Of the respondents, the majority of men without partners said they masturbated, whereas more than 77% of women did not. The study also examined attitudes toward specific aspects of sexuality. Sixty percent of men and 35% of women said that sexual activity was important to their overall quality of life. Two-thirds of all respondents were extremely or somewhat satisfied with sex. Attitudes toward partners were generally favorable, with a majority of both genders describing their partners with terms that included "best friend," "kind and gentle," and "physically attractive." The study also found several generational differences in attitudes toward sex. Individuals older than 60 years were less likely than younger respondents to approve of oral sex, masturbation, and sex between unmarried partners.

Results of this study were consistent with findings of several earlier studies. Starr and Weiner (1981) found that 80% of men and women ages 60–91 years were sexually active, defined as having sex at least once a month. Marsiglio and Donnelly (1991) studied more than 800 married men and women age 60 years or older and found that more than 50% had sex at least monthly. The mean frequency for subjects between ages 60 and 75 years was 4.26 times per month; this frequency decreased to 2.75 times per month for those age 76 years or older. These figures can be compared with rates of sexual frequency among younger individuals (ages 19–59 years; $N = 3,432$) in an influential University of Chicago study (Michael et al. 1994). In that study, men had sex an average of 6.5 times per month; the average rate for women was 6.2 times per month. In a mail survey of 1,292 individuals ages 60–90 years, the National Council on the Aging (1998) found that 80% of respondents with sexual partners had sex at least once a month. By gender, 61% of men remained sexually active, compared with 37% of women. Eighty-five percent of women sought partners who were financially secure, whereas 79% of men sought partners who were interested in sex. Compared with women, men were twice as likely to want more sex than they were already having. Satisfaction with sex remained quite high in late life: 61% of respondents with partners indicated that sex was as physically satisfying as it was in their 40s. A sizable number of respondents attributed lower satisfaction to the fact that they or their partners had less physical desire, had a medical condition that interfered with sex, or took medications that reduced desire.

The Sexual Response Cycle and Aging

The effects of aging on sexual function must be viewed against the backdrop of normal adult sexual response. A four-stage model of the normal sexual response cycle was developed by sex researchers William Masters and Virginia Johnson (1966) from their pioneering work in human sexuality. The four-stage cycle illustrates the physi-

ological changes that take place in the body during sexual activity. These four stages are excitement or arousal, plateau, orgasm, and resolution. Kaplan (1974) and others (Snarch 1991; Zilbergeld and Ellison 1980) added a fifth stage, desire, to account for a psychological and physiological component of sexuality that underlies sexual response. In this later model, sexual response is not a linear process but rather a waxing and waning pattern of sexual arousal that may culminate in orgasm, depending on a host of factors. All these factors can be influenced by age-related changes in sexual function.

The first stage of the five-stage model, *desire*, involves physical and psychological urges to seek out and respond to sexual interaction. This drive is centered in the limbic system of the brain, particularly in the hypothalamus, and is stimulated in both sexes by testosterone. Desire is intimately linked to the physiological process of sexual *excitement* or *arousal* (the second stage); it is difficult for one to exist without the other. In both men and women, sexual arousal can be triggered by thoughts and fantasies or by direct physical stimulation. Autonomic nervous stimulation leads to predictable physiological responses, including increased muscle tone, increases in heart and respiratory rates, and increased blood flow to the genitals (vasocongestion). In men, these responses result in penile erection, whereas in women, they result in vaginal lubrication and swelling of breast and genital tissues, especially the clitoris. The relatively brief *plateau* stage is characterized by a sense of impending *orgasm* and is followed by orgasm and then a refractory period of relaxation called *resolution*. In both sexes, orgasm is characterized by euphoria associated with rhythmic contractions of genital muscles. In men, orgasm is brief and is accompanied by ejaculation. In women, orgasm tends to last longer and there may be multiple successive occurrences.

Normal aging produces several changes in the sexual response cycle (see Table 18–1). In women, the most significant changes occur during menopause, a 2- to 10-year period that usually ends in the early 50s. The decline and eventual cessation of ovarian estrogen production during menopause leads to important changes in sexual function, including atrophy of urogenital tissue (which increases the risk of urinary tract infections) and a decrease in vaginal size. Vaginal lubrication, vasocongestion, and erotic sensitivity of nipple, clitoral, and vulvar tissue are decreased during sexual excitement. As a result, sexual desire may decrease and sexual arousal may require more time. Sexual intercourse may be more uncomfortable because of reduced lubrication of vaginal and clitoral tissue, and orgasms may be felt as less intense. Up to 85% of menopausal women also experience symptoms such as

TABLE 18–1. Normal age-related changes in sexual function

Men

Testosterone production modestly decreases, with unpredictable effect on sexual function.

Sperm count changes minimally, but amount of functional sperm and rate of conception decrease.

There are no predictable changes in sexual desire (libido).

Increased tactile stimulation is needed for sexual arousal.

Erections take longer to achieve and are more difficult to sustain.

Penile rigidity decreases because of decreases in blood flow and smooth muscle relaxation.

Sensation of urgency during plateau stage is diminished.

Ejaculation is less forceful, with decreased ejaculate volume.

Refractory period increases by hours to days.

Women

During menopause, estrogen production decreases and eventually stops.

Sexual desire (libido) may decrease due in part to decreased testosterone levels.

Blood supply to pelvic region is reduced.

Vagina shortens and narrows. Vaginal mucosa is thinner and less lubricated.

During arousal, vaginal lubrication and swelling occur more slowly and are decreased.

Sexual arousal may take longer and may require increased stimulation.

During orgasm, strength and amount of vaginal contractions decrease.

Source.   Goodwin and Agronin 1997; Metz and Miner 1995; Spector et al. 1996.

hot flashes, headaches and neck aches, mood changes, and excess fatigue.

In most women, hormone replacement therapy reverses these age-associated changes in sexual function to a large degree. Estrogen can be administered orally or via a slow-release patch applied to the skin. Estrogen is often prescribed with progesterone to replicate previous hormone levels. In addition, estrogen cream can be applied directly to genital tissues to relieve irritation and enhance lubrication. Unfortunately, recent research findings have indicated a small but potentially unacceptable risk of breast and ovarian cancer associated with oral hormone replacement therapy (Lacey et al. 2002; Rossouw et al. 2002).

During menopause, women also experience decreases in testosterone production that lead to loss of libido (Sherwin et al. 1985), thinning of pubic hair, and decreased production of body oils that moisturize skin and hair. In addition, testosterone receptors in erogenous zones such as the nipples, vulva, and clitoris are less sensitized to sexual stimulation (Rako 1996).

Overall, the normal sexual changes in aging men occur gradually and tend to be more modest than the changes undergone by women (Metz and Miner 1995). Some researchers have wondered whether there is a male menopause, or "andropause." Research indicates, however, that testosterone levels in men do not decrease appreciably until after age 70 (Hoffman 2001) and that these decreases do not have any predictable negative effects on sexual desire or function (Metz and Miner 1995). Male fertility decreases moderately in later life. As men age, desire may involve less anticipatory physical arousal, and sexual arousal and orgasm may take longer to achieve. Older men require more physical stimulation to achieve erections, which tend to be less frequent, less durable, and less reliable. The volume of ejaculate during orgasm is decreased. However, there are no predictable decreases in physical pleasure. In older men, the resolution or refractory stage is much longer, lasting hours to days instead of minutes to hours as in younger men.

In both sexes, the effect of physiological changes in sexual function is mediated by a number of psychosocial factors. The more an individual knows about what constitutes normal age-associated changes in sexual function, the easier he or she may be able to accept these changes. For example, a man who does not understand the normal changes in erectile function may misinterpret them and believe that he has a sexual problem. Similarly, a woman may misinterpret vaginal dryness as an indication that she does not want to have sex. Such overreactions to normal changes can lead an individual to engage in less frequent or more limited sexual activity. Research has shown that a lack of information about changes in sexual function in later life can lead to excess fear and pain (Boyer and Boyer 1982).

Many older individuals also accept ageist stereotypes about sexuality, seeing their behaviors as inappropriate or potentially harmful, despite the individual's relatively normal sexual desire and capacity. Other individuals may lose self-confidence and feel less sexy, especially as they struggle to cope with age-associated changes in physical appearance, strength, and endurance. Such attitudinal barriers may be more damaging to sexuality than actual physiological changes (Starr and Weiner 1981).

The quality of an individual's relationship with a partner is also influential. Couples often have to adapt sexual technique and spend more time on foreplay to preserve previous levels of sexual function and enjoyment. Partners who are not able to work together may experience difficulty with sex and perhaps even sexual dysfunction. On the other hand, aging can also open many new possibilities for sexuality in later life. Partners may have more time to spend with each other once children have left home, or during retirement. For postmenopausal women, sex may be associated with a reduced level of anxiety, because of the impossibility of pregnancy.

Sexuality in Long-Term Care

Sexuality among residents in long-term care is stigmatized not only because the residents are elderly but also because they are no longer living independently and often have multiple medical and psychiatric problems, including cognitive impairment. As a result, both residents and staff tend to view sexuality in a negative manner. Residents often feel sexually unattractive and are pessimistic about whether sex would even be possible or enjoyable (Kaas 1978; Wasow and Loeb 1979). Not surprisingly, the rate of sexual activity is low in most nursing homes (Mulligan and Palguta 1987). For many residents, however, the desire for sexual relationships still exists. In a 1982 study involving 250 nursing home residents, White (1982) found that 91% had not been sexually active in the last month and 17% wanted to be sexually active but lacked privacy or a partner. Other common barriers to sexual activity among long-term-care residents include loss of interest, chronic illness, sexual dysfunction, and negative attitudes of staff (Richardson and Lazur 1995; Wasow and Loeb 1979).

When one or both members of a couple are living in a long-term-care facility, staff should consider residents' rights to sexual expression and accommodate the couple's privacy when appropriate. Mental health consultants can help remove barriers to sexual activity in long-term-care settings in several ways. A key to accomplishing this goal is educating staff about sexuality in late life so that stereotypes are dispelled. Such an education provides staff with an understanding of residents' rights to sexual expression and the role of sexuality in helping residents meet needs for intimacy and physical contact (Spector et al. 1996). By federal law, residents have the right to associate with and communicate privately with individuals of their own choosing (Federal Regulations 1990). Also, residents should be educated about sexuality in late life and about their sexual rights. One way to facilitate these educational goals for residents and staff in long-term-care settings is to develop and promote a policy on sexuality.

To carry out such a policy, clinical staff in long-term-care facilities should ensure that a sexual history is obtained during intake and routine nursing, medical, and mental health evaluations. These evaluations can also be used to assess residents' concerns and capacities with respect to sexual function and relationships. Long-term-care facilities must ensure adequate privacy for couples wishing to be intimate and must facilitate conjugal or home visits. To this end, facilities should provide private rooms for married couples or individuals with other partners, when feasible. Privacy can be increased with "Do Not Disturb" signs, locks on doors, and reminders to staff and residents to knock before entering a resident's room (Spector et al. 1996). Finally, facilities can provide beauty services such as hair styling and manicures (Richardson and Lazur 1995).

Sexual Dysfunction in Late Life

Although the majority of older individuals continue to engage in sexual activity, the prevalence of sexual dysfunction does increase with age (Spector et al. 1996). The DSM-IV-TR (American Psychiatric Association 2000) classification of sexual disorders is provided in Table 18–2. Erectile dysfunction (ED) is the most common form of sexual dysfunction in older men, affecting more than 50% of men ages 40–70 years and nearly 70% of men age 70 years or older (Althof and Seftel 1995; Feldman et al. 1994). In older women, the most common forms of sexual dysfunction include hypoactive sexual desire, inhibited orgasm, and dyspareunia (Bachmann and Leiblum 1991; Renshaw 1996). Unfortunately, physicians often fail to ask older patients about sexual function, perhaps because of the physicians' discomfort or acceptance of stereotypes. As a result, many older individuals endure treatable forms of sexual dysfunction and either are too ashamed to inquire about treatment or are ignorant or pessimistic about treatment. The geriatric psychiatrist can play a vital role in providing support, education, and treatment to such individuals.

Although medical and psychiatric problems and medication effects are usually the main causes of sexual dysfunction in late life, numerous psychological factors must be considered, including performance anxiety, the presence of another sexual disorder in one or both partners, fears of self-injury or death due to medical conditions (e.g., a history of myocardial infarction, shortness of breath), sensitivity to loss of personal appearance or control of bodily functions (e.g., incontinence), relationship problems, and life stress. The first occurrence of psychogenic sexual dysfunction often follows a stressful event such as the loss of a loved one, a divorce, a financial or occupational strain, or a major health scare. Such ma-

TABLE 18–2.   DSM-IV-TR classification of sexual dysfunction

Sexual desire disorders

Hypoactive sexual desire disorder: persistent or recurrent deficiency of sexual fantasies and desire for sex

Sexual aversion disorder: extreme aversion to and avoidance of genital sexual contact

Sexual arousal disorders

Female sexual arousal disorder: persistent or recurrent difficulty in achieving and/or maintaining vaginal swelling and lubrication during sexual activity

Male erectile disorder (impotence): persistent or recurrent inability to attain and/or maintain an erection adequate for sexual activity

Orgasmic disorders

Female or male orgasmic disorder: persistent or recurrent delay in or absence of orgasm in response to sexual stimulation

Premature ejaculation: persistent or recurrent uncontrollable, rapid ejaculation that occurs just before or shortly after penetration

Sexual pain disorders

Dyspareunia: recurrent or persistent genital pain associated with sexual intercourse

Vaginismus: recurrent or persistent involuntary spasm of vaginal muscles that limits or prohibits vaginal penetration

jor stresses may break sexual patterns and lead to uncertainty about how to resume sexual activity. As noted, the availability of partners is an acute issue for women, who outnumber men by more than two to one by age 85 years.

Medical and psychiatric disorders that are the most common causes of sexual dysfunction in geriatric patients are listed in Table 18–3. In both sexes, major risk factors for sexual dysfunction include diabetes mellitus, peripheral vascular disease, cancer, pulmonary disease, depression, stroke, dementia, Parkinson's disease, and substance abuse. These and other medical disorders exert both primary and secondary effects on sexual function. Examples of primary effects include impaired sexual arousal due to diabetic neuropathy and impaired genital vasocongestion due to peripheral vascular disease. Secondary effects such as fatigue, pain, and physical disability due to medical illness can make individuals feel less sexy and less confident in their sexual ability, which in turn can lead to hypoactive desire. Medications can also cause sexual dysfunction and can affect both men and women at any point in the sexual response cycle (Crenshaw and Goldberg 1996; Goodwin and Agronin 1997). The most common problematic medications include antihypertensives such as β-blockers and diuretics, antiandrogens, and many psychotropic medications (Gitlin 1994). Some of the medi-

cations most commonly associated with sexual dysfunction in late life are listed in Table 18–4.

TABLE 18–3.   Medical and psychiatric conditions commonly associated with sexual dysfunction in late life

Anxiety disorders (generalized anxiety disorder, obsessive-compulsive disorder, panic disorder)

Arthritis and other degenerative joint diseases

Atherosclerosis (peripheral vascular disease, cerebrovascular accident)

Cancer (especially urologic and genital cancers and their treatments)

Cardiac disease (coronary artery disease, congestive heart failure, myocardial infarction)

Chronic obstructive pulmonary disease

Chronic organ failure (renal, hepatic)

Dementia (e.g., Alzheimer's disease, vascular dementia)

Diabetes mellitus

Major depressive disorder and other mood disorders

Multiple sclerosis

Parkinson's disease

Prostate disease and prostate surgery

Schizophrenia and other chronic psychotic disorders

Substance abuse

TABLE 18–4.   Medications associated with sexual dysfunction in late life

α-Adrenergic blockers (prazosin, phentolamine)

Antiandrogens (leuprolide, ketoconazole)

Antidepressants (MAOIs, TCAs, SSRIs, venlafaxine)

Antihistamines

Antihypertensives (thiazide diuretics, β-blockers, ACE inhibitors, clonidine, spironolactone, calcium-channel blockers, reserpine)

Antipsychotics (conventional and atypical)

Benzodiazepines

Cancer chemotherapeutic agents

Cardiac medications (e.g., digoxin, amiodarone)

Corticosteroids

Disopyramide

L-Dopa

Histamine subtype 2 (H_2) receptor blockers

Mood stabilizers (lithium, valproic acid, carbamazepine)

Note.   ACE = angiotensin-converting enzyme; MAOI = monoamine oxidase inhibitor; SSRI = selective serotonin reuptake inhibitor; TCA = tricyclic antidepressant.

Source.   Goodwin and Agronin 1997; Kligman 1991.

Sexual dysfunction in late life is often comorbid with other psychiatric disorders. Symptoms range from transient dysfunction, present only during episodes of illness, to full-blown sexual disorders independent of the primary psychiatric disorder. Major depression often features loss of libido but may also be associated with inhibited arousal and ED. Symptomatic anxiety as well as anxiety and panic disorders are frequently associated with sexual dysfunction—in particular, sexual phobias and sexual aversion (Kaplan 1987). Unfortunately, many of the antidepressants used to treat mood or anxiety disorders can cause or exacerbate sexual dysfunction (see Table 18–4). ED, delayed or inhibited orgasm, and/or a decrease in desire is experienced by 10%–40% of men taking serotonin selective reuptake inhibitors (SSRIs) or tricyclic antidepressants (Segraves 1998). To a lesser extent, benzodiazepines have been associated with decreased sexual desire and ED, particularly when they are combined with lithium.

Schizophrenia and other psychotic disorders often involve sexual problems. Psychotic individuals with negative symptoms—such as social withdrawal or discomfort in the presence of others, apathy, and blunted affect—may have relatively little interest in sexual relationships. Psychotic patients with positive symptoms—such as delusions, hallucinations, and bizarre thought patterns—may have difficulty relating to others and interacting in sexually comfortable or appropriate ways. During periods of symptom remission, however, sexual relationships can be more appropriate. All antipsychotic medications can cause sexual dysfunction, usually in proportion to the dose (Crenshaw and Goldberg 1996; Gitlin 1994). Like antidepressant and anxiolytic medications, antipsychotics can decrease libido, interfere with sexual arousal, and inhibit erections, ejaculation, and orgasm.

Assessment

Evaluating sexual dysfunction in late life involves identifying the specific problem and then obtaining a comprehensive medical, psychiatric, and sexual history in order to identify potential causes, as well as potential pitfalls during treatment (Cheadle 1991). A comprehensive sexual history includes an individual's prior sexual experiences, current sexual functioning, and attitudes toward sexuality and toward any current partner. With older couples, interviewers must be able to identify relevant age-appropriate issues (Sbrocco et al. 1995). It is important to balance the need to gather sexual history with the responsibility to be sensitive to the fact that sexual data may be some of the most personal information that a patient will ever divulge. Finally, accurate assessment of sexual dysfunction in late life depends to a large degree on a comfortable and productive doctor–patient relationship, one in which the patient and his or her partner feel secure enough to disclose adequate history and the physician asks the right questions and has sufficient testing performed. Partner involvement is crucial to a successful outcome.

The medical workup for sexual dysfunction involves a physical examination, laboratory testing, and sometimes specialized diagnostic testing. The focus of the physical examination is on genital and urologic anatomy and function, and attempts are made to assess underlying vascular and neurological function. Laboratory testing typically involves examination of routine blood chemistry (e.g., blood count, electrolyte levels, glucose levels, lipid profile), testosterone and prolactin levels, thyroid function, and, in men, prostate-specific antigen levels. Specialized diagnostic tests for ED include nocturnal penile tumescence and rigidity testing (to determine whether natural erections occur during sleep) and penile duplex ultrasonography (to assess blood flow in the penis).

Treatment

Preservation and enhancement of sexual activity in geriatric patients requires recognition of and sensitivity to the fact that many of these individuals want and intend to continue with sex, despite changes in physical and sexual function. Once an evaluation is complete, both partners should be educated about normal and dysfunctional sexuality. This information helps to reassure the affected individual that he or she is not the only person with the particular problem, that the problem has specific causes, and that it can be treated. In addition, clinicians can help patients perceive sexuality as a form of physical and psychological intimacy and not solely as sexual intercourse. Providing such information to patients and discussing suggestions will build trust between the patient and the clinician, and this relationship will help the patient feel comfortable about seeking follow-up and being open about emotional reactions to the problem. Many treatments fail at this point, not because the treatments cannot work but because the patient and the clinician never establish a solid working relationship. Treatment can also fail when one partner refuses to cooperate with treatment or when problems within the couple's entire relationship become insurmountable.

Unique challenges are faced by couples in which one or both partners have a chronic medical illness or disability. These couples often need to shift their focus from intercourse to foreplay and to adapt sexual practices to account for physical limitations such as fatigue, loss of muscle strength, and pain (Schover and Jensen 1988).

Education is key. Organizations such as The American Cancer Society, the United Ostomy Organization, the National Jewish Center for Immunology and Respiratory Medicine, and others have published helpful guides to maintaining sexual function despite specific medical illnesses. Physicians should work to maximize both rehabilitative and palliative treatments—for example, making use of analgesics for pain, inhalers for shortness of breath, or physical therapy for joint immobility and muscle weakness. In addition, appropriate treatment of depression, anxiety, or psychosis can often lead to significant improvement in sexual function, assuming that the medications used to treat these disorders do not themselves cause problems. Some ways in which an older couple can enhance sexual function and cope with disability are outlined in Table 18–5.

TABLE 18–5. Ten ways to enhance sexual function in late life

1. Cultivate a positive attitude toward sexuality in later life.
2. Maintain optimal health and fitness. Avoid use of tobacco and excessive use of alcohol.
3. Maintain open and honest communication with your partner about how your sexual responsiveness has changed over time.
4. Focus on foreplay as much as on intercourse. Be open-minded about adapting sexual practices to your needs.
5. Maximize treatment of medical problems or disabilities that are interfering with sexual function. Consult a physician about any concerns regarding excess exertion during sex. To achieve adequate stamina, use appropriate exercise to build up strength and self-confidence.
6. *Before* sex, maximize treatment of symptoms that affect sex. For pain, consider taking a warm shower or bath, having a relaxing massage, or taking analgesics before sex. For shortness of breath, adapt sexual activity to minimize exertion and use prescribed inhalers ahead of time. Choose times of day for sex when pain is at a minimum.
7. If you are a woman, consider the use of estrogen cream, which can relieve vaginal dryness and improve vasocongestion in peri- or postmenopausal women. Tender genital or breast tissue may require more gentle stimulation, sometimes along with the use of an external lubricant.
8. Identify problematic medications and investigate alternative agents or strategies.
9. Avoid unrealistic expectations that sex must be the same as when you were younger.
10. Explore sexual positions that decrease exertion or account for equipment such as oxygen tanks or ostomy bags. Suggested positions for intercourse include lying side by side or sitting face-to-face.

Source. Butler and Lewis 1986; Goodwin and Agronin 1997.

When medication side effects impair sexual function, physicians can consider several options (Goodwin and Agronin 1997; Margolese and Assalian 1996). The first step is to continue administering the medication and wait for tolerance to develop; many side effects diminish or disappear after several weeks. If no change occurs, dose reduction can be tried. Simplifying the overall regimen might also be helpful, given that combinations of medications can cause more sexual side effects than each medication alone. For certain medications, such as antidepressants with short half-lives, a drug holiday in which administration of the medication is temporarily stopped for a day or two (such as for a weekend) can result in transient improvement in sexual function (Rothschild 1995). However, there is a risk of recurrence of psychiatric symptoms during this holiday. Ultimately, the clinician may have to consider replacing the medication with an agent that has less potential for sexual side effects. For example, the antidepressants bupropion (Walker et al. 1993), mirtazapine (Gelenberg et al. 2000), and nefazodone (Feiger et al. 1996) have not been associated with the degree of sexual dysfunction seen with tricyclic antidepressants and SSRIs. With regard to antipsychotic medications, more potent agents with less anticholinergic side effects may cause less dysfunction.

When sexual dysfunction is due to antidepressant medication, the clinician can also consider using antidotes to reverse sexual side effects (Gitlin 1994; Segraves 1998). Several antidotes include yohimbine, amantadine, cyproheptadine (which can also reverse the antidepressant effect of SSRIs), bethanecol, methylphenidate, buspirone, bromocriptine (for antipsychotic induced sexual dysfunction), and the antidepressants bupropion, nefazodone, mirtazapine, and trazodone. The oral erectogenic agent sildenafil has also been shown to reverse antidepressant-induced ED (Nurnberg et al. 1999). Depending on the chosen antidote for sexual side effects, the patient can take a dose anywhere from 30 to 60 minutes before anticipated sex and can take increasing doses until success is achieved. If intermittent use of an antidote does not work, a regularly scheduled daily dose should be considered.

If none of these strategies work, the clinician must consider the trade-off between the benefits of the original medication and the sexual side effects. For some individuals, stopping the medication poses too great a risk of recurrent psychiatric symptoms, and adequate alternatives may not exist. In this frustrating situation, affected individuals must choose between discontinuing a needed medication or coping with persistent sexual dysfunction.

Sex Therapy

In some older couples, sexual dysfunction has clear psychological roots; for example, sexual dysfunction often occurs in the context of a dysfunctional relationship. Sex therapy is always best done conjointly; both partners should be involved in therapy because both are an integral part of the problem and solution. Historically, a psychodynamic model was used in sex therapy to uncover underlying unconscious conflicts, but that approach is now viewed as less successful, and cognitive-behavioral techniques are used in current treatment models (Kaplan 1974, 1983; Rosen and Leiblum 1988). Brief supportive and educational counseling is a first step in treatment and can help dispel distorted and uninformed attitudes toward sexuality in general and toward a sexual problem in particular. Counseling can also help an individual or couple change sexual practices to resolve a problem. In other cases, more intensive couples therapy is needed to resolve long-standing relationship issues before work on a sexual problem can begin.

Sex therapy involves both cognitive and behavioral techniques, with an overall goal of building an association between relaxed and sensual physical intimacy and sexual relations. The same principles can be applied across the life span, with several refinements in late life. Using cognitive therapy techniques, the therapist attempts to change distorted cognitive attitudes toward sexual activity into more practical attitudes. For example, many men with ED find it difficult not to assume the role of spectator during sex—that is, not to watch themselves with their partners and be preoccupied with the status of their erections. This spectator role can increase anxiety and distract the man from concentrating on pleasurable sensations, with the result that ED is reinforced (Masters and Johnson 1970). To counter this, the man is taught to shift his mental focus from his erection to pleasurable aspects of the encounter (Kaplan 1974). ED may also be perpetuated by cognitive distortions such as catastrophizing, in which the man thinks that if he does not achieve an erection during sex, he will be rejected not only by his partner but by all women. Another common cognitive distortion is all-or-nothing thinking, in which the man thinks that he must achieve an instant erection during sex or else the whole thing is pointless. The problem with such unrealistic cognitive distortions is they often become self-fulfilling prophesies. The therapist helps the patient to gain insight into the negative effect of such thoughts and then to practice replacing them with more realistic and hopeful ones, sometimes even with positive assertions or affirmations of success (Goodwin and Agronin 1997).

Behavioral techniques used during sex therapy begin with exercises called *sensate focus*, in which a couple practices physical relaxation techniques during nonpressured sensual touching. Sensate focus helps to reduce performance anxiety and restore the natural flow of the sexual response cycle. Once the partners are able to feel relaxed and physically intimate together without sexual stimulation, they gradually progress to genital stimulation and then intercourse. Several adjustments in these exercises may be required for the older couple. For example, older patients with physical problems that involve some degree of disability may express concerns about being able to exert themselves adequately during sexual activity. The therapist might recommend one of several positions that minimize exertion, such as lying side by side or having one partner kneel on pillows and support himself or herself on a low bed. Other suggestions outlined in Table 18–5 might also apply. Such simple suggestions may remove some of the most anxiety-provoking barriers for an older couple, especially the common but unfounded belief that older persons lack the stamina or dexterity for sexual activity.

During sex therapy, the therapist continues to work with the couple on their relationship and tries to identify and confront resistance that inevitably arises during treatment. Such resistance to these seemingly innocuous exercises often reveals key problems in the relationship that are either causing the sexual dysfunction or impeding its treatment. Regardless of age, many couples find that sexual interest and pleasure reemerge and sexual function improves during sex therapy, allowing them to enjoy once again such a fundamental component of their relationship.

Erectile Dysfunction

ED is the most common sexual dysfunction in men. According to DSM-IV-TR, it is a disorder of sexual arousal characterized by the inability to achieve or sustain an erection that is adequate for sexual function. Historically, ED was seen as a psychological problem; however, now it is believed that in up to 80% of cases, ED is primarily caused by a problem with erectile physiology (Althof and Seftel 1995; Feldman et al. 1994). There are, however, important psychological components of ED in terms of both cause and effect. Many men equate erections with masculinity, potency, and vitality. As a result, ED in late life is often experienced by men as a harbinger of physical and sexual decline. Performance anxiety, stress, depression, and relationship problems can trigger or exacerbate ED. In turn, ED is associated with feelings of anger, anxiety, powerlessness, shame, and humiliation in front of one's partner. Recurrent ED can lead to depression.

The penis contains three cylindrical bodies: two corpora cavernosa lie atop the corpus spongiosum, which contains the urethra. These bodies contain spongy erectile tissue, composed of vascular spaces or sinusoids surrounded by smooth muscle. Erections occur when autonomic innervation leads to relaxation of cavernosal smooth muscle, allowing blood flow into the vascular spaces. This muscle relaxation is mediated by the release of the neurotransmitter nitric oxide, with subsequent activation of cyclic guanosine monophosphate (GMP). As the vascular spaces in the spongy erectile tissue expand, the penile veins that drain them are compressed against the surrounding collagenous sheath or tunica albuginea, preventing outflow. The erection subsides when smooth muscles surrounding the vascular spaces contract, mediated by the breakdown of cyclic GMP to GMP via phosphodiesterase 5. ED results from one of three physiological problems: 1) failure of erectile initiation because of psychological or neurological inhibition of nervous stimulation, 2) failure to attain penile arterial filling, or 3) failure to maintain penile veno-occlusion. The latter two causes are frequently associated with peripheral vascular disease, which in turn is associated with hypertension, hyperlipidemia, and tobacco use.

Treatment of ED in geriatric patients involves the same approaches as those used in younger men and has been revolutionized with the advent of oral erectogenic agents. Several major causes of ED are reversible and, if present, must be addressed before other treatments are considered. Hypogonadism with testosterone deficiency is a cause of ED in around 5% of cases. Testosterone is usually given topically, via a skin patch. This treatment should be avoided in men with a history of prostate or bladder cancer or with bladder outlet obstruction. Some men have ED as a result of vascular damage and may benefit from microsurgical revascularization. Peyronie's disease, characterized by scarring-caused curvature of the penis during erection, can also be treated, with resultant improvement in erectile function.

Penile intracavernosal self-injection was the first pharmacological treatment for ED. Injectable agents work by increasing smooth muscle relaxation and arterial dilatation in the penis. Two of the available agents (Caverject, Edex) are preparations of alprostadil, a synthetic form of prostaglandin E_1. Injection of these agents into the base of the penis 10–20 minutes before sex leads to erections in 70%–80% of men (Althof and Seftel 1995). Injection therapy with alprostadil has been associated with local pain, scar tissue formation with chronic use, and, rarely, priapism. Other injectable agents include vasoactive intestinal polypeptide, phentolamine, and papaverine, sometimes used in combination. Alprostadil is also available as a urethral suppository (MUSE; medicated urethral system for erection), the use of which can be associated with some penile discomfort and is rarely associated with hypotension (Padma-Nathan et al. 1997).

Sildenafil (Viagra) was the first oral erectogenic agent available for men with ED, followed by tadalafil (Cialis) and more recently vardenafil (Levitra). All three agents improve erectile function in men with both organic and psychogenic ED by serving as selective inhibitors of phosphodiesterase type 5 (PDE 5), the key enzyme found in penile erectile tissue. These PDE 5 inhibitors can be taken 30–60 minutes before anticipated sexual activity. Erections do not occur spontaneously on these medications but require adequate physical stimulation. The obvious advantages of PDE 5 inhibitors are ease of use and high rate of success in up to 70%–80% of affected men (Boolell et al. 1996; Porst et al. 2003a; Porst et al. 2003b). Potential side effects for these medications include headache, skin flushing, dizziness, gastrointestinal discomfort, blurred vision, and the potential for blood pressure decreases when combined with nitrates (e.g., sublingual nitroglycerin, isosorbide). In addition, the PDE 5 inhibitors should be used with caution in men with abnormal penile shape, a history of orthostatic hypotension, severe renal or hepatic disease, concomitant use of certain antiviral and antifungal medications, and diseases that increase the risk of priapism, such as sickle cell anemia, multiple myeloma, and leukemia.

Another type of oral erectogenic medication is sublingual apomorphine (Uprima), currently available outside the United States. It serves as a centrally active dopamine agonist and affects the area of the brain that causes erections (Segraves 2000). Apomorphine is rapidly absorbed and can help men achieve an erection in response to stimulation within 20–30 minutes. Potential side effects include nausea and the potential for hypotension and even syncope in a small percentage of users. Despite the efficacy of all oral erectogenic agents, it is important for older men to realize that these medications are not substitutes for poor sexual or marital relationships, and that these drugs can pose risks for men with brittle cardiovascular disease and/or for men seeking sexual exertion whose bodies are out of condition (Mobley and Baum 1999).

Two other important treatments for ED are the use of a vacuum constriction device and penile implants (Sison et al. 1997). Vacuum constriction devices restore erectile function by creating a vacuum (using a plastic tube placed over the penis and an attached pump) that causes blood flow into the penis. Once an erection is achieved, a ring is placed around the base of the penis to maintain rigidity, and the tube is removed. Although vacuum constriction devices are quite effective, their use requires some dexterity and can cause numbing, bruising, and delayed ejaculation (Dutta and Eid 1999). Penile implants are an effective but less frequently used treatment for ED. A number of penile implants are on the market, some of them semirigid and others consisting of inflatable tubes with implantable pumps (Evans 1998). Aside from the risks associated with surgery and the risks of infection, the main problem concerning these implants is mechanical failure, which occurs from 5% to 20% of the time (Lewis 1995). Penile implants can, however, be surgically repaired or reimplanted. Because surgical placement of an implant leads to destruction of erectile tissue, a prosthetic device will always be needed to achieve an erection.

Premature Ejaculation

Premature ejaculation is the most common sexual dysfunction in younger men, but its prevalence among older men is unknown (Althof 1995). Premature ejaculation is defined in DSM-IV-TR as persistent or recurrent uncontrollable, rapid ejaculation that occurs just before or shortly after penetration. Such rapid ejaculation usually prohibits adequate sexual intercourse. Historically, treatment involved psychotherapeutic and cognitive-behavioral techniques to slow down perception of sexual stimulation, as well as couples techniques in which the partner gently squeezes on the man's penis before penetration, to reduce sensation and stall ejaculation (Kaplan 1989). Treatment has changed significantly since the introduction of antidepressant medications (in particular, SSRIs) that can delay ejaculation without necessarily affecting erectile function (Mendels 1995; Waldinger et al. 1994).

Hypoactive Sexual Desire Disorder in Women

Hypoactive sexual desire is a significant sexual problem for women across the life span and involves multiple psychological and physical factors. In some older women, loss of libido results from a poor self-image—brought about by age-associated losses of physical strength and beauty—and from changes in sexual function due to cessation of estrogen production during menopause. An older woman's ability to see herself as a sexual being can be further eroded by exposure to negative societal attitudes and negative images of sexuality in late life. Unfortunately, many women internalize these distorted, ageist

beliefs. Treatment of low desire must begin with sex education and counseling to counter those psychological barriers. Estrogen replacement therapy may help improve sexual arousal and comfort, which in turn may lead to increased desire.

The critical physiological cause of low desire in women, however, appears to be the menopause-associated reduction in levels of free testosterone. Testosterone replacement therapy has been beneficial in women with hypoactive sexual desire (Basson 1999; Rako 1996), although side effects can include weight gain, virilization (e.g., growth of facial and chest hair, lowering of the voice), suppression of clotting factors, and even liver damage. These side effects can sometimes be prevented by using lower doses of testosterone, to avoid supraphysiological levels, and by avoiding the use of alkylated testosterone (Basson 1999).

Sildenafil therapy has also been studied in women with sexual dysfunction (hypoactive desire, orgasmic disorder, or dyspareunia) associated with female sexual arousal disorder, but though well tolerated, it did not lead to improvement (Basson et al. 2000).

Female Orgasmic Disorder

Orgasmic disorder is defined in DSM-IV-TR as persistent or recurrent delay or absence of orgasm after a normal sexual excitement phase. The disorder is common in younger women and is a relatively common form of sexual dysfunction in older women as well. Female orgasmic disorder is often comorbid with hypoactive desire, and many of the attitudinal barriers to resolution are the same in the two conditions. Many older women who have experienced inhibited orgasm for years resist seeking help, especially if they do not perceive inhibited orgasm as a problem or if it is not an issue in their relationship. Individual therapy involves relaxation techniques that incorporate sensual self-stimulation and masturbation, usually with the aid of a vibrator, to increase clitoral stimulation (Heiman and Lopiccolo 1976). Short-term group therapy can also be helpful, providing education and support (Barbach 1980). When orgasm can be achieved, sensate focus exercises can help to incorporate it into the couple's sexual relations.

Sexual Pain Disorders

The two female sexual pain disorders, dyspareunia and vaginismus, are grouped together in DSM-IV-TR but are two very different entities. Dyspareunia is recurrent pain that is associated with sexual intercourse. It is common in late life, especially after menopause. This disorder may be associated with a number of medical conditions that affect the genital region, including vulvitis, vulvodynia, and vulvar vestibulitis (Goodwin and Agronin 1997). Pain can also be associated with many pelvic disorders and can result from surgical or radiation treatment of gynecologic malignancies. Gynecologic examination should always be the first step, because treatment of the underlying condition can help reduce and perhaps resolve discomfort. Estrogen replacement therapy may be helpful for women with atrophic changes and decreased lubrication due to menopause. However, when dyspareunia is chronic, treatment can be challenging and should incorporate various methods of sex therapy. In older women, dyspareunia can significantly disrupt sexual relations, sometimes leading to abandonment of sex altogether. The goal of therapy may be to introduce the couple to sensual exercises (e.g., massage, foreplay, oral sex) that can substitute for sexual intercourse when pain is prohibitive.

Vaginismus occurs more commonly than suspected, and young women may present with the disorder when intercourse is first attempted. Without treatment, vaginismus can lead to an unconsummated marriage and avoidance of sexual relations throughout life. Treatment is almost always successful and involves both conjoint sex therapy and physical exercises in which the woman uses vaginal dilators in graduated sizes to extinguish the vaginal muscle contraction (Goodwin and Agronin 1997). No data are available on the disorder in late life. Presumably, a woman with vaginismus in late life has had the disorder since early adulthood.

Sexual Function and Dysfunction in Dementia

Sexuality continues to play an important role in the lives of many individuals with dementia, often by providing a nonverbal means of communication and intimacy. Depending on the degree of dementia, however, the ability to initiate sexual activity and sustain performance may be impaired. Agitation, disinhibition, and psychosis associated with dementia may give rise to sexually aggressive or inappropriate behaviors. Ethical issues also complicate sexuality associated with dementia. For example, one partner may not be fully competent to consent to sex, especially with another individual who has dementia (Haddad and Benbow 1993), or the nonaffected partner may seek to fulfill sexual needs outside the relationship. It is important to understand these issues when assessing and treating dementia patients and their caregivers. Unfortunately, health care professionals often fail to in-

quire about such issues, despite the frequency with which they affect couples (Duffy 1995).

Dementia affects sexuality in several ways. Sexual desire may remain strong and even increase, especially if inhibitions are reduced by cognitive impairment. As the dementia progresses, the cognitively intact partner may become concerned about whether the affected individual is truly consenting to sexual activity (Hanks 1992). The partner without dementia may also feel frustrated with a partner who does not always recognize him or her or who requests sex repeatedly because he or she cannot remember when they last had sex (Davies et al 1992; Redinbaugh et al. 1997). The cognitively intact partner's sexual desire may decrease because he or she views the dementia and associated changes in behavior and personality as a sexual turnoff. Partners may be further confused by conflicting feelings of love and fidelity for their spouses with dementia, and guilt over their desires for extramarital intimacy.

It is not surprising, then, that there is an overall decrease in sexual activity in affected couples. In one study, only 27% of couples with a partner affected by Alzheimer's disease were sexually active, compared with 82% of couples without dementia (Wright 1991). This decrease may also be attributed in part to sexual dysfunction associated with dementia. For example, cognitive impairment may reduce the capacity for paying attention during sex, as well as the ability to initiate and perform components of lovemaking (Duffy 1995; Redinbaugh et al. 1997). This impairment may explain why men with Alzheimer's disease have high rates of ED (more than 50% in one sample; Zeiss et al. 1990): they are unable to maintain a cognitive focus on physical and mental stimulation during sex. Such reasoning may also explain why inhibited orgasm (or anorgasmia) is common in women with dementia (Wright 1991). Few studies have examined sexual dysfunction in dementia, so the rates of specific sexual disorders in different types of dementia are not known.

Although the percentage of individuals with dementia who demonstrate sexually aggressive or inappropriate behaviors is relatively small, these persons tend to generate a disproportionate amount of anxiety for caregivers and to require a disproportionate amount of clinical attention from long-term-care staff. The problematic behaviors associated with dementia include inappropriate sexual comments or demands, hypersexual behaviors (e.g., repeated requests for sexual gratification, compulsive masturbation), disinhibition (e.g., exposing oneself, disrobing, or masturbating in public areas), and sexually aggressive behaviors (e.g., attempts to grope, fondle, or force sex on another person). In various studies, these behaviors were seen in 2%–7% of individuals with Alzheimer's disease (Burns et al. 1990; Kumar et al. 1988; Rabins et al. 1982), although these rates may be higher in institutionalized populations (Mayers 1994). For example, one study found that 25% of residents on a dementia unit engaged in sexually inappropriate behaviors (Hashmi et al. 2000). Because frontal and temporal regions of the brain are involved in behavioral control and inhibition, individuals with dementia affecting these areas of the brain may be particularly vulnerable to developing such inappropriate behaviors (Haddad and Benbow 1993; Lishman 1987; Raji et al. 2000). Other factors associated with inappropriate or hyperactive sexual behaviors include mania, psychosis, alcohol or drug abuse, stroke, head trauma (Hashmi et al. 2000), and use of L-dopa (Bowers et al. 1971).

When assessing an individual who has allegedly demonstrated problematic behaviors, it is critical to identify the context of the behaviors. For example, public disrobing or touching of genitals in public may not be due to sexual urges but may instead reflect underlying confusion, delirium, motor restlessness, or stereotypy associated with dementia. However, caregivers and long-term-care staff sometimes misinterpret innocuous behaviors as evidence of sexual disinhibition (Redinbaugh et al. 1997). A good example would be the aphasic individual with dementia who reaches out or grabs for attention while in his or her wheelchair, inadvertently hitting someone in the waist or chest area. The individual is simply reaching out for help from the height of his or her wheelchair, but the staff member who is touched in the groin or breast area may wrongly view this act as an act of sexual aggression. It is also important to recognize that even individuals with severe dementia have legitimate needs for physical stimulation and intimacy (Spector et al. 1996), and these persons may be reacting out of frustration and confusion because they lack the ability to communicate their needs verbally.

The geriatric psychiatrist must be able to address these challenging issues of sexuality in dementia. Regardless of the setting, individuals with dementia have a right to engage in sexual relationships if they still have the capacity to understand the nature of the relationship and provide reasonable consent. If the cognitively intact partner is concerned about the competence of his or her spouse to engage in sexual activity, a psychiatric or psychological consultation may shed light on the affected individual's understanding of the relationship. Lichtenberg and Strzepek (1990) proposed several questions to be answered in any interview geared toward determining an individual's capacity to consent to a sexual relationship: Does the individual know who is initiating sexual contact? Can the individual describe his or her preferred de-

gree of intimacy? Is the sexual activity consistent with the individual's previous beliefs and values? Can he or she say "no" to unwanted activity? Does the individual understand that a sexual relationship with someone other than his or her spouse may be temporary? Can the individual describe how he or she would react if the sexual relationship were to end? Responses to these questions will help determine the affected individual's awareness of the relationship, his or her ability to avoid coercion and exploitation, and his or her awareness of the possible risks.

One main purpose of psychological or psychiatric intervention is to provide education about sexuality to caregivers in the community and to staff in long-term-care settings. Such education will improve interpretation of and response to apparent inappropriate sexual behaviors. In addition, educational programs for long-term-care staff may foster attitudes that are more open-minded (White and Catania 1982).

Behavioral approaches for inappropriate sexual comments include setting verbal limits and directing the individual to a different topic. Staff and caregivers must be careful to avoid reinforcing inappropriate comments, such as by laughing at off-color jokes or teasing patients in a seductive manner in response to sexual comments. In the case of inappropriate or aggressive sexual advances, staff may need to physically remove the individual from the situation or keep him or her away from vulnerable individuals. Sometimes restrictive clothing (e.g., pants without zippers, pants with suspenders) can cut down on public displays of genitals, although caution must be used so that the individual is not inadvertently restrained. Because sexual advances may reflect unmet sexual needs, existing partners can be asked to consider providing more physical and perhaps sexual intimacy, the hope being that doing so will remove the drive to engage in inappropriate behaviors.

When behavioral approaches are insufficient, psychiatric consultation is needed to provide better control through pharmacotherapy. The choice of medication will depend on the nature and severity of the behaviors and on the presence of underlying psychopathology, if any. In general, however, much of sexual aggression can be viewed as any other form of agitation associated with dementia and can be treated accordingly. Thus, a variety of psychotropic agents—in particular, the atypical antipsychotics—may help treat both agitation (Tariot 1999) and sexual problems associated with dementia. Medications may also be used to treat specific underlying psychopathology. For example, overactive libido can sometimes be reduced through use of an antidepressant with sexual side effects, such as an SSRI or a tricyclic antidepressant (Raji et al. 2000; Segraves 1998), or through use of a β-blocker. If the inappropriate sexual behaviors are believed to reflect hypersexuality due to mania, use of an antipsychotic or a mood stabilizer is indicated. Another pharmacological strategy for decreasing libido and sexual aggression is use of hormone therapy. Estrogen has been shown to reduce aggression in men with dementia (Kyomen et al. 1999), a finding that may be applicable to sexually aggressive behaviors. Two steroid hormones with both progesterone and antiandrogen activity are medroxyprogesterone (MPA) and cyproterone acetate (CA). Medroxyprogesterone works by blocking synthesis of testosterone in the testes. Both agents have been shown to reduce sexually aggressive behaviors in individuals with dementia (Brown 1998; Cooper 1987; Nadal and Allgulander 1992). However, cyproterone acetate is available only in Europe. Side effects of both medroxyprogesterone and cyproterone include weight gain, glucose intolerance, and liver dysfunction.

References

Althof SE: Pharmacologic treatment of rapid ejaculation. Psychiatr Clin North Am 18:85–94, 1995

Althof SE, Seftel AD: The evaluation and management of erectile dysfunction. Psychiatr Clin North Am 18:171–192, 1995

American Psychiatric Association: Diagnostic and Statistical Manual of Mental Disorders, 4th Edition, Text Revision. Washington, DC, American Psychiatric Association, 2000

Bachmann GA, Leiblum SR: Sexuality in sexagenarian women. Maturitas 13:43–50, 1991

Barbach L: Women Discover Orgasm: A Therapist's Guide to a New Treatment Approach. New York, Free Press, 1980

Basson R: Androgen replacement for women. Can Fam Physician 45:2100–2107, 1999

Basson R, McInnes R, Smith MD, et al: Efficacy and safety of sildenafil in estrogenized women with sexual dysfunction associated with female sexual arousal disorder. Obstet Gynecol 95:S54, 2000

Boolell M, Gepi-Attee S, Gingell JC, et al: Sildenafil, a novel effective oral therapy for male erectile dysfunction. Br J Urol 78:257–261, 1996

Bowers MB, Woert MV, Davis L: Sexual behavior during L-dopa treatment for parkinsonism. Am J Psychiatry 127:1691–1693, 1971

Boyer G, Boyer J: Sexuality and aging. Nurs Clin North Am 17:421–427, 1982

Brown FW: Case report: sexual aggression in dementia. Annals of Long-Term Care 6:248–249, 1998

Burns A, Jacoby R, Levy R: Psychiatric phenomena in Alzheimer's disease, IV: disorders of behavior. Br J Psychiatry 157:86–94, 1990

Butler RN, Lewis MI: Love and Sex After 40: A Guide for Men and Women for Their Mid and Later Years. New York, Harper & Row, 1986

Cheadle MJ: The screening sexual history: getting to the problem. Clin Geriatr Med 7:9–13, 1991

Comfort A, Dial LK: Sexuality and aging: an overview. Clin Geriatr Med 7:1–7, 1991

Cooper AJ: Medroxyprogesterone acetate (MPA) treatment of sexual acting out in men suffering from dementia. J Clin Psychiatry 48:368–370, 1987

Crenshaw TL, Goldberg JP: Sexual Pharmacology: Drugs That Affect Sexual Function. New York, WW Norton, 1996

Davies HD, Zeiss A, Tinklenberg JR: 'Til death do us part: intimacy and sexuality in the marriages of Alzheimer's patients. J Psychosoc Nurs Ment Health Serv 30:5–10, 1992

Duffy LM: Sexual behavior and marital intimacy in Alzheimer's couples: a family theory perspective. Sex Disabil 13:239–254, 1995

Dutta TC, Eid JF: Vacuum constriction devices for erectile dysfunction: a long-term, prospective study of patients with mild, moderate, and severe dysfunction. Urology 54:891–893, 1999

Evans C: The use of penile prostheses in the treatment of impotence. Br J Urol 81:591–598, 1998

Federal Regulations, Code 42: The Patient's Bill of Rights. Chapter 4, Section 483, 1990

Feiger A, Kiev A, Shrivastava RK, et al: Nefazodone versus sertraline in outpatients with major depression: focus on efficacy, tolerability, and effects on sexual function and satisfaction. J Clin Psychiatry 57 (suppl 2):53–62, 1996

Feldman HA, Goldstein I, Hatzichristou DG, et al: Impotence and its medical and psychosocial correlates: results of the Massachusetts Male Aging Study. J Urol 151:54–61, 1994

Gelenberg AJ, McGahuey C, Laukes C, et al: Mirtazapine substitution in SSRI-induced sexual dysfunction. J Clin Psychiatry 61:356–360, 2000

Gitlin MJ: Psychotropic medications and their effects on sexual function: diagnosis, biology, and treatment approaches. J Clin Psychiatry 55:406–413, 1994

Goodwin AJ, Agronin ME: A Women's Guide to Overcoming Sexual Fear and Pain. Oakland, CA, New Harbinger, 1997

Haddad P, Benbow S: Sexual problems associated with dementia, part 2: aetiology, assessment and treatment. Int J Geriatr Psychiatry 8:631–637, 1993

Hanks N: The effects of Alzheimer's disease on the sexual attitudes and behaviors of married caregivers and their spouses. Sex Disabil 10:137–151, 1992

Hashmi FH, Krady AI, Qayum F, et al: Sexually disinhibited behavior in the cognitively impaired elderly. Clinical Geriatrics 8:61–68, 2000

Heiman L, Lopiccolo J: Becoming Orgasmic: A Sexual and Personal Growth Program for Women, Revised Edition. New York, Prentice-Hall, 1976

Hoffman AR: Should we treat the andropause (editorial)? Am J Med 111:322–323, 2001

Jacoby S: Great sex: what's age got to do with it? Modern Maturity (serial online) September/October 1999. Available at http: www.aarp.org/mmaturity/sept_oct99/greatsex.html. Accessed July 14, 2003.

Kaas MJ: Sexual expression of the elderly in nursing homes. Gerontologist 18:372–378, 1978

Kaplan HS: The New Sex Therapy. New York, Brunner/Mazel, 1974

Kaplan HS: The Evaluation of Sexual Disorders: Psychological and Medical Aspects. New York, Brunner/Mazel, 1983

Kaplan HS: Sexual Aversion, Sexual Phobias, and Panic Disorder. New York, Brunner/Mazel, 1987

Kaplan HS: Overcoming Premature Ejaculation. New York, Brunner/Mazel, 1989

Kligman EW: Office evaluation of sexual function and complaints. Clin Geriatr Med 7:15–39, 1991

Kumar A, Koss E, Metzler D, et al: Behavioral symptomatology in dementia of the Alzheimer type. Alzheimer Dis Assoc Disord 2:363–365, 1988

Kyomen HH, Satlin A, Hennen J, et al: Estrogen therapy and aggressive behavior in elderly patients with moderate-to-severe dementia. Am J Geriatr Psychiatry 7:339–348, 1999

Lacey JV Jr, Mink PJ, Lubin JH, et al: Menopausal hormone replacement therapy and risk of ovarian cancer. JAMA 288:334–341, 2002

Lewis RW: Long-term results of penile prosthetic implants. Urol Clin North Am 22:847–856, 1995

Lichtenberg PA, Strzepek DM: Assessments of institutionalized dementia patients' competencies to participate in intimate relationships. Gerontologist 30:117–120, 1990

Lishman WA: Cardinal psychological features of cerebral disorder, in Organic Psychiatry: The Psychological Consequences of Cerebral Disorder, 2nd Edition. Edited by Lishman WE. Oxford, Blackwell, 1987, pp 3–20

Margolese HC, Assalian P: Sexual side effects of antidepressants: a review. J Sex Marital Ther 22:209–224, 1996

Marsiglio W, Donnelly D: Sexual relations in later life: a national study of married persons. J Gerontol 46:S338–S344, 1991

Masters WH, Johnson VE: Human Sexual Response. Boston, MA, Little, Brown, 1966

Masters WH, Johnson VE: Human Sexual Inadequacy. Boston, MA, Little, Brown, 1970

Mayers KS: Sexuality and the patient with dementia. Sex Disabil 12:213–219, 1994

Mendels J: Sertraline for premature ejaculation (letter). J Clin Psychiatry 56:591, 1995

Metz ME, Miner MH: Male "menopause," aging, and sexual function: a review. Sex Disabil 13:287–307, 1995

Michael RT, Gagnon JH, Laumann EO, et al: Sex in America: A Definitive Survey. Boston, MA, Little, Brown, 1994

Mobley DF, Baum N: Sildenafil in elderly men: advice and caveats. Clinical Geriatrics 7:34–41, 1999

Mulligan T, Palguta RF Jr: Sexual interest, activity, and satisfaction among male nursing home residents. Arch Sex Behav 20:199–204, 1987

Nadal M, Allgulander S: Normalization of sexual behavior in a female with dementia after treatment with cyproterone. Int J Geriatr Psychiatry 8:265–267, 1992

National Council on the Aging: Healthy Sexuality and Vital Aging. Executive Summary. Washington, DC, National Council on the Aging, 1998

Nurnberg HG, Lauriello J, Hensley PL, et al: Sildenafil for iatrogenic serotonergic antidepressant medication–induced sexual dysfunction in 4 patients. J Clin Psychiatry 60:33–35, 1999

Padma-Nathan H, Hellstrom WJG, Kaiser FE, et al: Treatment of men with erectile dysfunction with transurethral alprostadil. Medicated Urethral System for Erection (MUSE) Study Group. N Engl J Med 336:1–7, 1997

Porst H, Padma-Nathan H, Giuliano F, et al: Efficacy of tadalafil for the treatment of erectile dysfunction at 24 and 36 hours after dosing: a randomized controlled trial. Urology 62:121–125, 2003a

Porst H, Young JM, Schmidt AC, et al: Efficacy and tolerability of vardenafil for treatment of erectile dysfunction in patient subgroups. Urology 62:519–523, 2003b

Rabins PV, Mace NL, Lucas MJ: The impact of dementia on the family. JAMA 248:333–335, 1982

Raji M, Liu D, Wallace D: Case report: sexual aggressiveness in a patient with dementia: sustained clinical response to citalopram. Annals of Long-Term Care 8:81–83, 2000

Rako S: The Hormone of Desire: The Truth About Sexuality, Menopause, and Testosterone. New York, Harmony Books, 1996

Redinbaugh EM, Zeiss AM, Davies HD, et al: Sexual behavior in men with dementing illnesses. Clinical Geriatrics 5:45–50, 1997

Renshaw D: Sexuality and Aging, in Comprehensive Review of Geriatric Psychiatry, 2nd Edition. Edited by Sadavoy J, Lazarus LW, Jarvik LF, et al. Washington, DC, American Psychiatric Press, 1996, pp 713–729

Richardson JP, Lazur A: Sexuality in the nursing home patient. Am Fam Physician 51:121–124, 1995

Rosen RC, Leiblum SR: Principles and Practice of Sex Therapy: Update for the 1990s. New York, Guilford, 1988

Rossouw JE, Anderson GL, Prentice RL, et al; Writing Group for the Women's Health Initiative Investigators: Risks and benefits of estrogen plus progestin in healthy postmenopausal women: principal results from the Women's Health Initiative randomized controlled trial. JAMA 288:321–333, 2002

Rothschild AJ: Selective serotonin reuptake inhibitor–induced sexual dysfunction: efficacy of a drug holiday. Am J Psychiatry 152:1514–1516, 1995

Sbrocco T, Weisberg BA, Barlow DH: Sexual dysfunction in the older adult: assessment of psychosocial factors. Sex Disabil 13:201–218, 1995

Schover LR, Jensen SB: Sexuality and Chronic Illness. New York, Guilford, 1988

Segraves RT: Antidepressant-induced sexual dysfunction. J Clin Psychiatry 59 (suppl 4):48–54, 1998

Segraves RT: New treatment for erectile dysfunction. Curr Psychiatry Rep 2:206–210, 2000

Sherwin BB, Gelfand MM, Brender W: Androgen enhances sexual motivation in females: a prospective, crossover study of sex steroid administration in the surgical menopause. Psychosom Med 47:339–351, 1985

Sison AS, Godschalk MF, Mulligan T: Erectile dysfunction in the elderly: treatment recommendations from the recent American Urological Association guidelines. Clinical Geriatrics 5:73–76, 1997

Snarch D: Constructing the Sexual Crucible: An Integration of Sexual and Marital Therapy. New York, WW Norton, 1991

Spector IP, Rosen RC, Leiblum SR: Sexuality, in Psychiatric Care in the Nursing Home. Edited by Reichman WE, Katz PR. New York, Oxford University Press, 1996, pp 133–150

Starr BD, Weiner MB: The Starr-Weiner Report on Sex and Sexuality in the Mature Years. New York, McGraw-Hill, 1981

Tariot PN: Treatment of agitation in dementia. J Clin Psychiatry 60 (suppl 8):11–20, 1999

Waldinger MD, Hengeveld MW, Zwinderman AH: Paroxetine treatment of premature ejaculation: a double-blind, randomized, placebo-controlled study. Am J Psychiatry 151:1377–1379, 1994

Walker PW, Cole JO, Gardner EA, et al: Improvement in fluoxetine-associated sexual dysfunction in patients switched to bupropion. J Clin Psychiatry 54:459–465, 1993

Wasow M, Loeb MB: Sexuality in nursing homes. J Am Geriatr Soc 27:73–79, 1979

White CB: Sexual interest, attitudes, knowledge, and sexual history in relation to sexual behavior in the institutionalized aged. Arch Sex Behav 11:11–21, 1982

White CB, Catania JA: Psychoeducational intervention for sexuality with the aged, family members of the aged, and people who work with the aged. Int J Aging Hum Dev 15:121–138, 1982

Wright LK: The impact of Alzheimer's disease on the marital relationship. Gerontologist 31:224–237, 1991

Zeiss AM, Davies HD, Wood M, et al: The incidence and correlates of erectile problems in patients with Alzheimer's disease. Arch Sex Behav 19:325–332, 1990

Zilbergeld B, Ellison C: Desire discrepancies and arousal problems in sex therapy, in Principles and Practice of Sex Therapy. Edited by Leiblum S, Pervin L. New York, Guilford, 1980, pp 65–101

Bereavement and Adjustment Disorders

Larry W. Thompson, Ph.D.

Joel L. Kaye, Ph.D.

Paulette C.Y. Tang, Ph.D.

Dolores Gallagher-Thompson, Ph.D., A.B.P.P.

In this chapter, we cover late-life bereavement in some depth, because the amount of conceptual and empirical research on this topic has substantially increased in the recent past. More is known about late-life bereavement than about the second topic covered in this chapter, adjustment disorders in the elderly population. A brief description of "normal grief" is presented along with issues such as what constitutes "abnormal grief," how grief manifests in older adults, and how it changes over time, as well as risk factors related to grief intensity. Finally, we review several interventions that have been found to be helpful, including cognitive-behavioral therapy. In the section on adjustment disorders, we review research and clinical data, along with information about how elderly persons tend to cope with stressful life events that are less threatening than the death of a loved one. Adjustment disorder is an important but often overlooked diagnosis in geriatric psychiatry, and it is hoped that continued focus on this topic will encourage relevant research and clinical investigation.

Late-Life Bereavement

Who Are the Elderly Bereaved?

The terms *bereavement* and *grief reaction* have been used to refer to any number of losses experienced by older adults. These losses include (but are not limited to) the death of a spouse, an adult child, another family member, or a close personal friend; divorce (Cain 1988); prolonged caregiving for a severely impaired relative (Bass et al. 1991); and a significant decline in one's own health, attractiveness, capabilities, opportunities, and so forth (Kalish 1987). When used in its narrowest sense, *bereavement* refers to the reaction or process that results after the death of someone close.

In the United States, the mean age at which widowhood or widowerhood takes place is 69 years for men and 66 years for women. Among persons age 65 or older, about 45% of women and 15% of men have lost a spouse (Federal Interagency Forum on Aging Related Statistics 2000). The mean duration of widowhood or widower-

This work was supported in part by grant R01-AG01959 from the National Institute on Aging and grants R01-MH36834 and R01-MH37196 from the National Institute of Mental Health.

hood is approximately 14 years for women versus only 7 years for men (U.S. Census Bureau 1984). These data, plus the fact that widowers are more likely to remarry after losing their wives, have often led to the interpretation that widowhood/widowerhood is a women's issue. However, research has shown that after the loss of a spouse, older men are at a higher risk for mortality than are women (see, for example, Thompson et al. 1984).

The rates of widowhood among persons age 65 or older are similar for whites and Hispanics and are slightly higher for African Americans (U.S. Census Bureau 1998). Given the prediction that the elderly population in each of these ethnic groups will increase considerably over the next 20 years (Federal Interagency Forum on Aging Related Statistics 2000), there is a clear need to understand how the processes of bereavement are mediated by cultural factors.

Theories About Adjustment to Permanent Losses

A number of theoretical perspectives have been developed to explain how people (of any age) respond to significant loss. Because reviewing all of the perspectives in depth is beyond the scope of this chapter, the interested reader is referred to comprehensive reviews by Osterweis et al. (1984) and, more recently, Stroebe and Schut (1999) and Stroebe et al. (2001). We will briefly mention major positions that reflect trends in the development of frameworks for describing the symptoms and process of grief.

From the classic work of Freud (1917[1915]/1957) ("Mourning and Melancholia") and Lindemann's (1944) study of acute grief, a theory of grief evolved in which the prime task of mourning was the gradual surrender of psychological attachment to the deceased individual so that new relationships could be formed. The mourning process was thought to involve specific tasks over a limited time, and if these tasks were not completed properly, psychopathology might result. In contrast, Bowlby (1961), in his attachment theory, emphasized that bereavement, as an involuntary separation from a loved one, gives rise to many forms of attachment behavior (such as separation anxiety and pining), the functions of which are not withdrawal from the lost object but reunion with it. The desire to reunite with or regain proximity to the deceased person, Bowlby (1961) predicted, would gradually dissipate through a series of stages, including shock, protest, despair, and, finally, breakage of the bond and adjustment to a new self.

Parkes (1972) and Horowitz (1976) proposed models that involve phases or stages of reaction to the death of a loved one (see Wortman and Silver 1987 for a review of stage models). The first phase begins at the time of the death and persists for several weeks. Shock and disbelief, combined with emotional numbness and cognitive confusion, characterize this period, and intense free-floating anxiety and sharp mood fluctuations occur as well. Specific somatic symptoms include sleeplessness, loss of appetite, and vague muscular aches and pains, and these symptoms lead to increased contact with primary care physicians and, commonly, requests for medication.

The second phase generally begins as the numbness and anxiety start to decrease—usually in about 4–6 weeks—and often lasts for the better part of a year. During this period, family and friends gradually become less available and often convey the message that the bereaved person should be getting on with life and should be getting over his or her grief, although the individual is far from ready to do so. It is only with increased time that the finality of the loss becomes more apparent to the bereaved person, and more of the sadness, anger, guilt, relief, and other strong emotions begin to surface, causing emotional lability and confusion. Specific symptoms such as frequent crying, chronic sleep disturbance, blue mood, poor appetite, low energy, feelings of fatigue, loss of interest in daily living, and problems with attention and concentration are common. Nevertheless, most individuals do not develop major depression, despite the fact that certain symptoms of grief and depression overlap.

Parkes (1972) referred to this second phase as a time of "yearning and protest," characterized by actual searching for the deceased individual in both behavioral and cognitive ways—for example, going to places frequented by the deceased person. Such endeavors bring momentary comfort and also, paradoxically, intensify feelings of grief. The bereaved person often wishes that the loved one would come in the door or be around the corner. Often, someone so similar to the lost loved one is seen that, for a moment, the survivor is certain it must be the deceased person. Auditory and visual hallucination-like experiences and "sense-of-presence" experiences are a common part of grieving. Bereaved persons may see the deceased individual sitting in his or her favorite chair, hear their names being called, or receive a message that all is well. These vivid experiences appear to be a normal part of grieving and have been documented in the clinical literature for more than 25 years. Rees (1971) provided an early perspective and Grimby (1993) reported more recent data on these cognitive phenomena, confirming that for most elderly persons, these illusions are a positive experience.

Other cognitive components of this period include frequent searching for the meaning of the death and for an explanation of why it occurred the way it did. Bereaved persons may frequently relive and recollect memories and scenes associated with the death, as if to confirm that the death has occurred and that it cannot be undone. Continuous emotional and social support are particularly important to continue during this period, although weathering this phase with the bereaved can be difficult for friends and family members (who may feel that they have heard the memories many times before).

The third and final phase of adaptation to loss involves identity reconstruction (Lopata 1975)—that is, gradual disengagement of some or most of the psychic energy that has been bound up with the deceased person and reinvestment of that energy into other relationships and activities. The length of this process is thought to depend on the centrality of roles that were lost as a result of the death or traumatic event, and on the amount and kind of new learning that must take place to develop a new sense of self. Lopata (1975) estimated that identity reconstruction takes at least a year. During this period, most of the troublesome somatic, cognitive, and behavioral symptoms tend to abate.

Although stage theories of adaptation have been widely accepted by health care professionals, little empirical evidence exists to support these theories. In fact, grief symptoms often do not abate in elderly widows and widowers, despite stage theory predictions (see, for example, Bierhals et al. 1995). To expect that grief will resolve or end is now considered erroneous by some theorists (Stroebe et al. 2001). Bereavement, as Rosenblatt (1996) contended, is a dynamic process that may continue for a number of years and even for the remainder of one's life. Also, bereaved individuals do not proceed from one clearly identifiable phase to another in an orderly fashion, a fact particularly true of older adults. Many elderly persons experience multiple losses, often without sufficient time in between to complete the grieving for one event before the next one occurs. Kastenbaum (1981) termed this "bereavement overload" and suggested that because of multiple losses, the process of grieving is likely to be significantly different and more complex among older individuals. Again, however, few empirical data exist.

In brief, one might best view these stages or phases of adaptation to loss in descriptive terms without oversimplify one's understanding of a very complicated phenomenon. As Shuchter and Zisook (1993) concluded, "grief's duration may be prolonged, at times even indefinite, and its intensity varies over time, from person to person, and from culture to culture. It cannot be understood from a static or linear perspective" (p. 43).

Some theories of grief also hold that experiencing a continuing bond with the deceased individual is symptomatic of psychological problems (e.g., Horowitz et al. 1980; Rando 1992–1993). However, evidence from empirical studies indicates otherwise. For example, drawing from findings by Parkes (1972) and Glick et al. (1974), Bowlby (1980) noted that at least half of the widows and widowers were still preoccupied with their deceased spouses and had a strong, persistent sense of presence of their deceased spouses 12 months after the loss. Stroebe and Stroebe (1989) found that not only did the widows and widowers maintain ties with their deceased spouses through sensing the presence of and searching for their deceased spouses, but they also actively reflected on past actions of their deceased spouses and used these actions as models for decision making and problem solving. Such data have led to a widespread consensus that bereaved persons do maintain an active, dynamic connection with the deceased individual and that a relatively continuous sense of grief does not necessarily reflect poor adjustment (Klass 1996; Reisman 2001; Rosenblatt 1996; Rosenblatt and Elde 1990; Silverman and Klass 1996). Nonetheless, a distinction has been made between adaptive and maladaptive continuing attachment, on the basis of the forms of the attachment. Maintaining abstract rather than concrete ties with the deceased person is suggestive of healthy adaptation (Pincus 1974). In a longitudinal study, Field and co-workers (1999) found that 7 months after the loss of a spouse, persons who comforted themselves using special possessions of the deceased spouse experienced more psychological distress and a smaller decrease in grief-specific symptoms over time than did persons who engaged in less searching behavior and were more inclined to maintain a bond with the deceased spouse through positive memories.

Another trend in bereavement theory has been to consider environmental changes and role adaptation along with individual emotional and psychological adjustments. For example, some bereavement models, such as that of Bowlby (1961, 1980), focus solely on intrapsychic processes, assuming specific but interdependent cognitive or psychological components that lead to detachment from the deceased person (e.g., being preoccupied with and remembering the deceased person, accepting the loss, making sense of the loss, and modifying one's assumptive world). In recent years, theorists have increasingly attended to the interpersonal and social processes involved in grieving. Many contemporary theorists now regard grieving as an ongoing effort not only at the individual but also at the collective level (i.e, societal, cultural) to adapt to and construct meaning of the loss (e.g., Neimeyer 1998).

Stroebe and Schut's (1999) dual-process model, an attempt to synthesize existing conceptualizations of the bereavement process, has been empirically validated (Richardson and Balaswamy 2001). Two types of bereavement-related stressors are distinguished in this model. First, *loss-oriented stressors* focus on the nature of the loss itself. Most clinical interventions have been developed for these stressors, which are manifested as emotional, behavioral, physiological, and cognitive symptoms. Second, *restoration-oriented stressors* refer to what an individual needs to deal with to adapt to the larger, objective environment. These stressors include facing changes in social and household roles, learning skills to perform tasks that the deceased individual used to take on, and developing new identities, such as changing from wife to widow. In spousal loss, the loss of the relationship is followed by the loss of company, feelings of loneliness, and the need to reorganize one's life, develop a new identity, and reestablish social networks (Stroebe and Schut 1999). In this dual-process model, both individual and cultural variations are thought to play important roles in the management of loss-oriented and restoration-oriented stressors (Stroebe and Schut 2001). Grief "tasks" usually have included confronting the loss, restructuring thoughts and memories about the deceased person, and emotionally withdrawing from (but not forgetting) the deceased person. Restoration tasks include accepting the changed world, spending time away from grieving, and developing new relationships and identities.

Stroebe and Schut's (1999) model also introduced the concepts of oscillation and "dosage" in bereavement. The idea behind these concepts is that the psychological mechanisms (such as denial, suppression of negative emotions, and inhibition of thoughts about the deceased individual) that are traditionally viewed as contributing to psychopathology are useful, provided that they do not occur in a persistent manner. When oscillation occurs often enough (as a result of repeated exposure), habituation may take place, and the bereaved individual may no longer need to confront or avoid the loss. The concept of dosage in bereavement is that there should not be a definitive period during which one engages relentlessly in mourning tasks; other interpersonal and environmental stressors need to be addressed as well.

Anticipatory Bereavement

Hospice and Palliative Care

Over the past decade, increasing research has been done on palliative care at the end of life and on hospice treatment approaches in the care of patients with terminal ill-

nesses. Hospice and other end-of-life settings are becoming increasingly common in the care of many elderly patients facing terminal illnesses. In 1998, approximately 3,100 hospice programs in the United States provided care for close to 540,000 people (Hospice Foundation of America 2003). The level of satisfaction with the overall care received in hospice or other palliative care settings is generally high (Medigovich et al. 1999; Ng and von Gunten 1998; Nolen-Hoeksema et al. 2000; Voltz et al. 1997; Wilkinson et al. 1999), and continued proliferation of these settings is likely, given the aging of the population.

Because of the particular focus of hospice on the emotional, interpersonal, and spiritual effects of terminal illness on patients and their loved ones, bereavement counseling is often an integral part of hospice care, both before and after a patient's death. Behaviors and issues involved in anticipatory bereavement are often brought up during such counseling. Although little research has been completed in this area, a recent survey of patients, family members, and physicians found that at least 90% believed that being free from anxiety, having someone who will listen, and saying good-bye to important people were very important at the end of life (Steinhauser et al. 2000). Despite the lack of replicated findings concerning effectiveness (Seale and Kelly 1997; Wrenn et al. 2001), bereavement counseling is advocated by leading hospice organizations and is legislated as a standard component of the Medicare hospice benefit (Hospice Care 2001). Although relatively few empirical studies have been conducted on the effects of hospice or palliative care versus more traditional types of care on bereavement outcomes (Berch 1999; Clukey 1997; Franco 1996; Gilbar 1998; Kramer 1997; Quigley and Schatz 1999; Ragow-O'Brien et al. 2000; Seale and Kelly 1997; Thornton 1998), initial findings suggest that enrollment in hospice, particularly in cases of painful illness and death, may affect bereavement adjustment in a positive manner (Ragow-O'Brien et al. 2000).

Anticipatory Mourning

The increase in hospice and palliative care treatment settings has increased the interest in anticipatory grief experienced by family members of dying patients. A number of studies suggest that a period of forewarning can have positive effects on the bereavement process (Kramer 1997; O'Bryant 1990–1991). In contrast, other studies suggest the presence of mediating factors of anticipatory grief, such as ties to homelands and neighborhood institutions (Ortiz et al. 1999), and the possibility that anticipatory work focusing on the impending death of a loved one would have negative effects or no effects on outcome after bereavement (Clayton et al. 1973; Lindemann 1944). In several thorough reviews of this literature, authors argued that differing ways of viewing and measuring anticipatory grief explain the confusing and contradictory findings (Evans 1994; Fulton et al. 1996; Rando 2000; Siegel and Weinstein 1983; Sweeting and Gilhooly 1990). To help reconcile differences and promote continued research, Rando (2000) introduced the term *anticipatory mourning,* a less restrictive phrase than *anticipatory grief.* Although complete agreement is lacking on the constructs and results pertaining to anticipatory mourning, available research suggests that continued efforts in this direction will be fruitful (Chapman and Pepler 1998; Gilliland and Fleming 1998; Sanders et al. 1979, 1985).

Cultural Variations in Bereavement Responses

Culture plays an important role in reactions to loss, the course of grieving, and outcomes of bereavement (Brown and Stoudemire 1983; Klass 1996; Wisocki and Skowron 2000). The manifestations, duration, and intensity of grief are likely to be culturally specific, and substantial individual and subcultural variations exist. From the literature describing cross-cultural and ethnic expressions after a death, it is clear that bereavement distress can be communicated and regulated through various pathways. Some theorists challenge the concept that grief is a universal emotional reaction to bereavement; they view death, loss, and grief as social constructs and grief as a cultural artifact that is shaped by the sociocultural environment (Corwin 1995; Neimeyer 1998; Rosenblatt 1993, 2001). At present, most of the work on cultural differences in bereavement is descriptive (Wisocki and Skowron 2000). Empirical studies on whether and how older adults in minority groups experience or cope with bereavement differently from Euro-Americans are virtually nonexistent. Most studies of cultural differences appear to focus exclusively on customs, rituals, and perceptions relating to appropriate expressions and behaviors concerning the death of a family member. It is not clear how these customs, rituals, and perceptions, which are considerably different from those in Anglo-Christian traditions, may regulate emotions and facilitate adaptive coping. Nevertheless, Romanoff and Terenzio (1998) suggested that rituals and funerals are a "condensed version of private, emotionally charged material" (p. 698) that enables emotions to be channeled and expressed and bereaved persons to transition from one social role to another.

In this chapter, we confine our interest to multicultural older adults living in the pluralistic United States

culture who have retained at least some aspects of their original culture of heritage. When a cultural or ethnic minority group migrates to a majority culture, some of the group's practices, values, and customs are expected to change, reflecting adaptation to the host culture. In the United States, the proportion of older adults of non-European ancestry is steadily increasing. Because reactions to death and the perceived meaning of death are likely to be different among different ethnic and cultural groups, care providers must become aware of their own cultural assumptions and biases about how grief should be experienced and managed and about what constitutes pathological grief. We suggest that to be sensitive to an older bereaved person, one should first learn how death is commonly perceived and dealt with in the bereaved person's culture of origin. To obtain such an understanding, one must inquire about 1) normative ways of expressing psychological pain resulting from death, 2) mourning practices and rituals, 3) beliefs regarding the degree of influence the deceased person continues to have on the bereaved person, and 4) how these beliefs potentially facilitate or hinder the process of coming to terms with the loss. For example, in the Western world, some people believe that death ends a spousal relationship, but some Chinese believe that death is only a temporary separation and that when the survivor dies, the couple are reunited.

Grief work. The concept of working through one's grief (Bowlby 1980; Freud 1917[1915]/1957; Lindemann 1944) or performing grief tasks (Worden 1991) may not be equally applicable to all cultures. The approach also lacks empirical support for its effectiveness in dealing with loss. Euro-American culture has generally conceptualized grief as more loss-oriented (Stroebe and Schut's [1999] dual-process model), and the focus has often been on individual manifestations of grief. In contrast, grief in other cultures may be associated with culturally sanctioned rituals, expressions, and meanings, which are shared within relationships.

The belief and meaning systems of a culture may have major implications for how individuals react to death and cope with bereavement. For many culturally mainstream Americans, death means the end of the relationship with the person, and a time for public and private expressions of grief follows (Shuchter and Zisook 1988). In other cultures, active ongoing interaction with a deceased family member (such as ancestor rituals like *sosen suhai* in Japan) is the norm rather than the exception (Goss and Klass 1997).

Outward emotional expressions of grief have been shown to be effective in helping bereaved individuals adjust in the mainstream culture (e.g., Mawson et al. 1981), but other cultures may view such expressions differently. For example, Tibetans believe that crying for the deceased person hinders that person's liberation or rebirth, and they believe that emotions should be channeled into spiritual practices for the deceased individual. Similarly, Buddhists often discourage open and intense statement of emotions (Goss and Klass 1997). Among the Navajo, excessive expression of emotions is not permitted (S.I. Miller and Schoenfeld 1973), and crying is considered inappropriate by some Indonesian Muslims (Wikan 1988).

Sometimes, denial of death is culturally appropriate (al-Adawi et al. 1997). Moreover, denial may lessen the anxiety associated with the enormous task of accepting the reality of loss and may be beneficial to the bereaved person (Janof-Bulman and Timko 1987; Stroebe 1992–1993). In fact, the concept of working through grief is foreign in many non-Western cultures, such as the Samoan culture (Ablon 1971), and a continuous relationship and continuous communication with the deceased individual are encouraged (al-Issa 1995).

Social support. Research has shown that perceived social support is vital to maintaining life satisfaction and reducing the risk of depression among elderly persons (e.g., Kogan et al 1995; Newsom and Schulz 1996). In theory, an older adult who belongs to a minority group and whose extensive network of family and friends has survived the challenges of emigration will be less likely to develop negative bereavement outcomes. Indeed, for persons from more collectivistic cultures in which extensive familial networking and familial support exist, mourning may not be so much an individual process as a grieving event for the entire extended family and even the community, such as among recent Mexican immigrants (Block 1998) and in the Rauto culture in Australia (Wisocki and Skowron 2000). Interventions may be designed to increase familial involvement so that grieving becomes a collaborative process for all family members (Nadeau 2001).

In one of the early multicultural studies done in the United States, Kalish and Reynolds (1981) found that African Americans had more exposure to persons who died violently (e.g., accidents, homicides, wars) than did Caucasian, Hispanic, and Japanese adults. Eisenbruch (1984) surmised that because blacks were less likely to die of old age than through violence, their belief systems, attachment patterns, and grief reactions might change so that the pain of separation through death could be better managed. As a consequence, African Americans may not seek help from health professionals to deal with their grief but may instead rely more on informal supports, such as their religion and church-based relationships. For

example, being able to summon emotional support from church members has been regarded as particularly helpful to African Americans during grieving (Rosenblatt 1993).

Japanese ancestor rituals, through which living persons are thought to be able to interact continually with the spirit of the deceased person (Klass 1996), are perhaps the most frequently documented culture-specific bereavement response among Asian groups. Similarly, for Chinese who follow the Taoist tradition, the deceased elderly individual is regarded as an ancestor who can bestow blessings on the surviving spouse and on younger generations. The deceased person's ashes (which are kept in an urn) and a photo of him or her are often placed on an altar at home. Incense is burned twice a day as a symbol of reverence, and food is offered on the altar to the deceased person. Among Chinese who ascribe to more traditional values, it is generally not acceptable to openly discuss either death or plans for death (Bowman and Singer 2001; Crain 1996), and grief is shared only within the family (Braun and Nichols 1997). It may therefore be difficult for health professionals to detect bereavement-related psychological problems in elderly Chinese persons, who may seem avoidant and appear to be somatizing. However, other groups may express bereavement-related emotions more freely and explicitly. Younoszai (1993) observed that most Mexicans perceive death as part of life, and the funeral, which everyone is expected to attend and which is typically organized according to orthodox Catholic practices, is a social event that brings the extended family together. Similarly, Block (1998) noted as a physician that Latinos, particularly first and second generations, value familial input when making treatment decisions, possess extensive social networks, place family interests before interests of the self, more readily accept death as unavoidable, and prefer a caring, personal approach to a scientific, matter-of-fact approach in the treatment process.

In summary, grief clearly is expressed in a variety of ways in different ethnic and cultural groups, and bereavement distress can be communicated and regulated through various pathways. Therefore, it is important to understand the cultural idioms of distress that are specific to a cultural or ethnic group and to consider how individuals from a particular culture or in a particular ethnic group may communicate distress idiosyncratically. Successful interventions with culturally diverse individuals require a knowledge of the nuances of the individual's unique history as well as consideration of the cultural beliefs, meaning systems, and rituals in both the minority group and the mainstream society.

Operational Definitions of "Normal" and "Abnormal" Grief

Given the wide variability in how people proceed through the grief process, how can one determine what is "normal" and what is not? As Shuchter and Zisook (1993) noted, such a determination is very difficult; they suggested that those who work in the field of bereavement and grief are still trying to validate and use this construct. In DSM-IV-TR (American Psychiatric Association 2000a), bereavement is in the V Code section, meaning it is a condition that may be the focus of attention or treatment but is not directly attributable to a psychiatric disorder. Uncomplicated bereavement is defined in DSM-IV-TR as follows:

> This category can be used when the focus of clinical attention is a reaction to the death of a loved one. As part of their reaction to the loss, some grieving individuals present with symptoms characteristic of a Major Depressive Episode (e.g., feelings of sadness and associated symptoms such as insomnia, poor appetite, and weight loss). The bereaved individual typically regards the depressed mood as "normal," although the person may seek professional help for relief of associated symptoms such as insomnia or anorexia. The duration and expression of "normal" bereavement vary considerably among different cultural groups. (American Psychiatric Association 2000a, pp. 740–741)

Differentiating between normal and complicated bereavement has not always been easy. In view of this, several specific symptoms that are not considered to be characteristic of a normal grief reaction are listed in DSM-IV-TR:

> These include 1) guilt about things other than actions taken or not taken by the survivor at the time of the death; 2) thoughts of death other than the survivor feeling that he or she would be better off dead or should have died with the deceased person; 3) morbid preoccupation with worthlessness; 4) marked psychomotor retardation; 5) prolonged and marked functional impairment; and 6) hallucinatory experiences other than thinking that he or she hears the voice of, or transiently sees the image of, the deceased person. (American Psychiatric Association 2000a, p. 741)

Definitional Problems and Issues

The absence of diagnostic criteria for "abnormal" grief and the lack of consensus or a gold standard regarding differentiating abnormal or complicated grief from normal grief, major depression, and other stress disorders have posed challenges for clinicians and researchers alike. Two sets of criteria have been proposed for identifying individ-

uals undergoing a complicated or traumatic bereavement. Horowitz et al. (1997) proposed criteria for "complicated grief disorder" that focus on two major areas: 1) *intrusive symptoms* (e.g., unbidden memories, strong spells of severe emotion related to the lost relationship, distressingly strong yearnings for the deceased) and 2) *signs of avoidance and failure to adapt* (e.g., feelings of emptiness or of being very much alone; avoidance of people, places, or activities that remind one of the deceased person; unusual levels of sleep disturbance; loss of interest in social, occupational, or recreational activities). These symptoms and signs need to be present for at least 14 months after the loss. Prigerson et al. (1999) proposed criteria for "traumatic grief" that focus on *separation distress* (e.g., yearning and searching for the deceased person, loneliness, intrusive thoughts about the deceased person) and *traumatic distress* (e.g., purposelessness; numbness or detachment; disbelief; feelings of meaninglessness; loss of a sense of trust, security, or control; excessive irritability, bitterness, or anger related to the death). These features must be present for at least 2 months. In addition to the time-frame difference (i.e., 2 months' duration versus presence at 14 months or thereafter), the criteria proposed by Prigerson et al. (1999) do not include symptoms of avoidance.

At present, it is not possible to state that one or the other set of criteria is superior or more valid in determining whether abnormal grief is present, but the development of such definitions will aid researchers in establishing constructs relevant for clinical and research purposes. However, given cultural variations in bereavement and the finding that continued attachment to the deceased individual is often viewed as comforting by the survivor and does not appear to interfere with subsequent adjustment (Wortman and Silver 1987), clinicians are encouraged to continue to ask questions about what constitutes normal and abnormal grief. We believe that the following two questions warrant further study: 1) Is it really necessary to substantially reduce one's attachment to a deceased individual in order to resolve one's grief? 2) Is it reasonable to expect a bereaved person to recover substantially within the "typical" span of 2 years, the duration most often used to demarcate a chronic grief reaction?

Thus, there still appears to be considerable divergence of opinion about what exactly constitutes a normal versus an abnormal grief reaction (at any age). Until data are accumulated to address this problem, it seems appropriate to continue the use of currently available (and evolving) diagnostic criteria, which clearly affirm that normal grief is not equivalent to the clinical syndrome of major depression, and which indicate specific symptoms to be evaluated to determine whether their presence and/or severity level suggests that a differential diagnosis is needed. The results of our own psychometric work in this regard—in which common self-report questionnaires were used to assess both depression and level of grief—generally support this position (Breckenridge et al. 1986; Gallagher-Thompson and Thompson 1994). Longitudinal studies can shed light on what might be considered a normal course of adaptation to spousal bereavement over a 2- to 3-year period.

Longitudinal Studies of Late-Life Bereavement

The National Institute on Aging has funded a number of longitudinal investigations of how older adults adapt to bereavement of various kinds, with an emphasis on death of a spouse. Preliminary results from several of these studies can be found in a book edited by Lund (1989), containing chapters by Lund, Caserta, and Dimond on their work predominantly with Mormon elders in Utah, along with chapters by Van Zandt and associates on rural bereaved elders and by Faletti and colleagues on predominantly Jewish elders in Miami, Florida. More recent reports of longitudinal studies can be found in a book edited by Stroebe and colleagues (1993).

For the most part, findings from these studies have been fairly consistent with regard to the kinds of symptoms that change over time, the rate of change that can be expected to occur, and the presence or absence of gender differences. When standard measures were used to determine outcomes such as depressed mood, anxiety, well-being, and level of grief, the most significant differences between bereaved and nonbereaved subjects have been found to occur 2–6 months after the spouse's death, a period in which increased levels of distress are common across a variety of measures. Typically, bereaved women reported more psychological distress than bereaved men, although this was not found in all studies (e.g., Lund et al. 1986). By 12 months postloss, levels of reported distress were no longer significantly different between bereaved and nonbereaved control subjects, although women's levels of distress generally remained higher (Harlow et al. 1991; Lund et al. 1989; Thompson et al. 1991). This finding suggests that considerable "recovery" on symptom-oriented measures was evident by the end of 1 year. However, despite a trend toward some reduction in the intensity of distress by 6 months postloss, many unpleasant symptoms were still present. Harlow and colleagues (1991) pointed out that symptoms have been reported to abate by 6 months but not to disappear.

One notable exception to these results regarding psychological distress measures concerns the level of grief reported by the bereaved individual over time. For example, in the study by Thompson and colleagues (1991), which used the Texas Revised Inventory of Grief (TRIG; Faschingbauer 1981) as the measure, elderly men and women had higher mean scores than the normative scores for experienced grief. This result occurred not only immediately after the spouse's death (2 months postloss) but also at 12 and 30 months postloss. Also, no gender differences were found on this measure, contrary to what was reported for other indices of psychological distress. Thompson et al. (1991) interpreted these findings as meaning that the level of grief remains high over at least a 30-month interval after a spouse's death and that the experience of grief is distinct from the experience of depressed mood and related symptoms, which lessen significantly over that same interval. In other words, depression and grief can be distinguished using brief self-report questionnaires, and one can anticipate that the former will abate considerably over time and that the latter may remain quite strong and still be considered normal for an older adult. These findings are consistent with earlier work by Zisook and Shuchter (1985, 1986), who also found that grief (as indexed by a continuing sense of attachment to the deceased person) was still strong, at times, even at 4 years postloss. Thus, *recovery* may be an unrealistic goal for older bereaved patients, particularly if the word *recovery* means that experiences such as still missing the deceased person and still fondly remembering the past are not to be tolerated. Most of this research has involved Caucasian elders; virtually no empirical data are available on the longitudinal effects of bereavement among diverse ethnic and cultural groups.

Risk Factors for Intensification of Grief

Grief has been characterized by many as not only a highly charged emotional state but also a significant risk factor for a wide range of negative outcomes, including mortality and major physical and mental health disturbances. On the other hand, some clinicians and researchers have been struck by the ability of many older adults to survive and cope quite well, overall, with the profound losses of old age. In their 10-year follow-up study of a national sample of bereaved men and women, McCrae and Costa (1993) found that the great majority of individuals showed considerable ability to adapt to this major life stress (although length of recovery seemed to vary considerably). Nevertheless, it seems important to attempt to identify elders who may be at risk for negative outcomes after spousal loss (for a thorough review, see Sanders 1993 and Stroebe et al. 2001). Several specific variables may result in more intense or difficult bereavement. These variables include the age and gender of the survivor, the mode of death, the presence of significant depression shortly after the death, self-esteem and perceived coping, prior relationship satisfaction, and social support. These variables are discussed in the following paragraphs. Strength of religious commitment and involvement, participation in culturally appropriate mourning rituals, and redistribution of roles within the family after the death may also have an impact on the grief process, although the literature is not clear on the relative contribution of these factors.

Some studies have shown that older persons adapt better than younger persons to the loss of a spouse. For example, Zisook and colleagues (1993) found that their oldest subjects demonstrated the most consistent improvement in distress levels over time. In contrast, Sable (1991), among others, found that older widows were more distressed throughout the first 3 years of bereavement than were their younger counterparts.

Older bereaved men who have lost their spouses are at high risk for death. In their review of both cross-sectional and longitudinal studies on this topic, Stroebe and Stroebe (1993) concluded that "the bereaved are indeed at higher risk of dying than are nonbereaved persons. Highest risk occurs in the weeks and months closest to loss, and men appear to be relatively more vulnerable than women" (p. 188). In an empirical study by Bowling (1988–1989), in which more than 500 elderly widows and widowers were followed for 6 years after their loss, men age 75 or older had excessive mortality compared with men of the same age in the general population. Bowling also found that certain additional variables, including low social contact, predicted mortality. Gallagher-Thompson and co-workers (1993) found that widowers who died within the first year of spousal bereavement had reported more often than survivors that their wives were their main confidants, and they had minimal involvement in activities with other persons after their wives' deaths.

Numerous studies have demonstrated that adaptation is more difficult when the death is violent (as in a homicide), stigmatized (as in the case of AIDS), or very unexpected or unanticipated. (For more detailed discussions of the clinical effects of these factors, see O'Neil 1989, Osterweis et al. 1984, Parkes and Weiss 1983, and Worden 1991.) Farberow and colleagues (1987) compared older adults whose spouses had died of natural causes with older adults whose spouses had committed suicide. They found that the effect of the suicide on the survivor was

not very notable during the early period of bereavement but became quite evident by the end of 1 year. Subjects whose spouses died of natural causes showed significant decreases in depression and other negative effects during the first year of bereavement, whereas subjects whose spouses committed suicide maintained high levels of depression and distress during most of the second year postloss. Both types of survivors seemed to manage their new roles and responsibilities adequately by 30 months postloss, despite the different patterns of emotional distress that they experienced in the interim. Thus, suicide does make the process of bereavement more psychologically stressful, particularly during the first year of bereavement. Farberow and colleagues (1992a) concluded that although most of the severe distress subsided over time, subjects experienced different courses and had varying remaining levels of distress after 30 months of bereavement.

Similar studies involving elders whose spouses (or other family members) were homicide victims have not been carried out, nor has much research been done on the effect of stigmatized deaths and/or very sudden deaths. However, Moss and colleagues (1993) did perform a careful study of impact of death of a mother on middle-aged daughters. These investigators found that relatively sudden deaths were associated with more intense grief than were deaths that occurred in a nursing home (in the latter case, presumably, individuals have time to prepare and say good-bye).

The presence of clinically significant symptoms of depression within the first 2 months after a spouse's death is a significant risk factor for poor outcome over time. Lund and co-workers (1993) found that intense negative emotions at 2 months postloss—such as a desire to die and frequent crying—were associated with poor coping 2 years later. Wortman and Silver (1989) reviewed a number of studies indicating that depression confounds successful resolution of grief. In our own work investigating the relationship between depression and later bereavement outcome (summarized in Gilewski et al. 1991), we found that individuals with self-reported depression in the moderate to severe range were at greatest risk for all other psychopathological symptoms, such as increased anxiety, hostility, interpersonal sensitivity, and other indices of global psychiatric distress. This result occurred whether their spouses had committed suicide or died of natural causes. However, subjects whose spouses had committed suicide and who were moderately to severely depressed at the outset had the highest mean score of any subgroup on the depression measure that was used, maintained higher mean levels of depression over time, and were more likely to score high on other distress measures. These data suggest that, again, the interaction of one or more risk factors may contribute to the greatest distress.

Several articles have suggested that bereaved elderly individuals with poor self-esteem and/or inadequate coping skills are at a greater risk for difficult bereavement. Johnson and colleagues (1986) conducted one of the few studies that directly addressed these variables in elders. As expected, individuals who, early in bereavement, reported themselves to be high in self-esteem and to be effective copers maintained a high self-esteem and remained effective copers throughout the first year of bereavement, whereas those who initially reported high stress levels generally had high levels of stress at subsequent times of measurement.

Satisfaction with the relationship, another variable that may complicate the grief process, has been widely addressed in the clinical literature (e.g., Parkes and Weiss 1983; Worden 1991), but there is little empirical research to support or refute the clinical lore. Only one relatively recent empirical study could be found that focused on the association between the bereaved elder's retrospective assessment of marital adjustment and subsequent self-reported levels of depression, and the results of the study were equivocal. Futterman and co-workers (1990) found that more positive ratings of marital satisfaction were made by bereaved subjects than by non-bereaved, currently married control subjects; and contrary to expectations, more positive ratings of satisfaction were associated with more severe depression. This pattern of results did not change significantly during the 2 years of the study, nor was it influenced by gender. The investigators suggested that idealization of the deceased spouse may occur and may affect satisfaction ratings, making it difficult to distinguish the true role of relationship satisfaction in later bereavement outcomes. Clearly, more research is needed in this area. Ideally, the quality of the relationship would be measured both before and after the spouse's death, to clarify how actual versus possibly idealized ratings might differentially affect the subsequent course of bereavement.

The role of social support is less ambiguous, overall. Since the publication of Cobb's seminal paper on the stress-buffering effects of social support (1976), such support has been widely recognized as a moderator of many kinds of life stress. In a comprehensive review of the role of social support in mitigating the effects of bereavement, Stylianos and Vachon (1993) made the point that social support should be viewed as a multidimensional process, including such aspects as the size, structure and quality of the network; types of support provided (and by whom); and the appraisal of the support.

Most studies have focused on only one aspect of support, although there is no single aspect that has been most frequently selected for study. With regard to late-life spousal bereavement, Dimond et al. (1987) found in their longitudinal study that the total size of the reported support network at baseline was positively correlated with perceived coping skills and life satisfaction at later times of measurement. They also found that the quality of the network was inversely related to later depression and was positively correlated with later measures of life satisfaction. Finally, through a series of multiple regression analyses, they found that several baseline social network factors made independent contributions to the variance accounted for in predicting depression at later times of measurement. This finding suggests that social support mitigates severe negative reactions to the loss of a spouse in older individuals.

Our own research involving individuals whose spouses had died of natural causes and individuals whose spouses had committed suicide also confirms and supports this position. In a series of analyses directly comparing these two groups, Farberow and colleagues (1992b) found that persons whose spouses committed suicide received significantly less emotional and practical support for their feelings of depression and grief than did persons whose spouses died of natural causes. This was particularly true about 6 months postloss. Also, individuals whose spouses committed suicide did not feel that they could confide in members of their network any more than did the non-bereaved comparison group. Gender differences were also noted: the bereaved women in both groups reported that they received more support overall compared with either group of bereaved men. The most common sources of support were other family members (particularly adult children), followed by friends and then siblings. Another significant difference concerned how social supports changed over time. The survivors of spouses who had natural deaths reported keeping roughly the same levels of feelings for the people in their network, whereas the feelings of the persons (especially men) whose spouses committed suicide fluctuated considerably over the 30 months. However, by the end point, both practical and emotional supports had increased among individuals whose spouses committed suicide and were more comparable to the levels reported by individuals whose spouses died of natural causes.

Taken together, these various studies suggest that certain risk factors, either singly or in combination, are associated with a more difficult subsequent grief process in elderly individuals. However, most of this research involved volunteer subjects, often from relatively advantaged socioeconomic backgrounds, who could see some benefit to themselves from being interviewed. Much remains to be learned about bereavement among elderly persons who are economically disadvantaged, are in poor health, or who have little or no family to rely on. In addition, more studies are needed on the interactive effect of several of these risk factors (particularly because they may change over time in relative intensity or salience to the individual), as well as on whether the same risk factors apply to bereavement due to other causes, such as divorce and death of a parent or an adult child. Clearly, more research is needed on risk factors among ethnically and culturally diverse elders.

Interventions for Late-Life Bereavement

Although the literature is not conclusive on many of the points discussed earlier in the chapter, considering the following questions is helpful when deciding whether some type of intervention is warranted: Does the symptom picture reflect normal grief, or does the grief appear to be complicated by clinical depression or some other psychiatric disorder? What risk factors seem to be present that would suggest that the individual may have a difficult grieving process ahead?

Treatment of Complicated Bereavement

If a clinical level of depression is present, that problem should be treated first, with medication and/or psychotherapy, so that it can resolve sufficiently to permit the grieving process to become the focus of attention when the patient is ready ("NIH Consensus Conference" 1992; Parkes and Weiss 1983; Raphael et al. 2001; Reynolds 1992). Reynolds (1992) stated, "Our clinical practice has been to intervene as early as 2 months, and certainly by 4 months, in the presence of clear syndromal major depression" (p. 50). Posttraumatic stress disorder, bereavement-related anxiety disorders, and subsyndromal depression are other common complications that require treatment (Reynolds et al. 1999; Schut et al. 1997). These conditions are particularly significant in older bereaved persons (Rosenzweig et al. 1997). Differentiation between normal and abnormal bereavement and other psychiatric disorders is vital to appropriate intervention choices (Raphael et al. 2001). Pharmacological treatments combined with psychotherapy appear to be more effective than either intervention alone in reducing depressive symptoms in the context of bereavement. For example, the late-life depression research group in Pittsburgh, Pennsylvania, tested the efficacy of nortriptyline therapy, interpersonal psychotherapy, and combined treatment in elderly patients with bereavement-related

major depression and reported that combined treatment was superior to either intervention alone, particularly among patients age 70 or older (M.D. Miller et al. 1997; Reynolds et al. 1999).

Various forms of individual and group psychotherapy have also been used to treat patients with complicated bereavement reactions. Findings regarding the effectiveness of both types of interventions have been mixed. (See Schut et al. 2001 for a review of clinical efficacy studies of individual and group interventions over the past 20 years.) Raphael and colleagues (1993) describe a variety of methods (including psychodynamic approaches, behavioral therapies, and cognitive therapies) for treating complex grief reactions, along with less intensive counseling techniques generally used in more normal grief reactions. Horowitz's (1976) time-limited psychodynamic therapy, for example, is a phase-oriented and personality-oriented approach to help patients work through their complex reactions to serious life events in 12 sessions. Techniques such as abreaction, clarification, and interpretation of defenses and affects are used in this approach to facilitate realistic appraisals of the implications of a death and to explore the effect of the loss of a relationship on the bereaved person's self-concept. This approach was empirically studied by Horowitz and colleagues (e.g., Horowitz et al. 1981, 1984; Windholz et al. 1985). (See Marmar et al. 1988 for a description of the application of this approach to older bereaved, depressed women.)

The effective use of a relatively brief, intensive, structured behavioral program, called guided mourning, to facilitate resolution of chronic grief was reported by Mawson and co-workers (1981), and these findings were replicated by Sireling and associates (1988). In this approach, 90-minute sessions are held three times weekly for 2 weeks, with subsequent less intense follow-up for 28 weeks. Patients are helped to repeatedly confront aspects of their loss so that they can relive painful memories and eventually diminish the negative effects associated with them.

Several forms of cognitive and cognitive-behavioral therapy have also been successfully used to treat patients with complex bereavement reactions. Viney's (1990) "personal construct" approach focuses on the description of core constructs that tend to be disrupted in intense grief, along with methods for reconstructing personal beliefs about oneself, to promote adaptation. Florsheim and Gallagher-Thompson (1990) described treatment of prolonged grief in a widower in his 70s that involved a blend of cognitive and behavioral techniques (such as challenging dysfunctional thoughts and teaching the patient to talk about his grief with his adult children). Other examples of the use of cognitive-behavioral methods to treat patients with complicated grief reactions can be found in an excellent conceptual chapter on this topic by Abrahms (1981) and in detailed case studies by Gantz et al. (1992) and Kaplan and Gallagher-Thompson (1995).

The Pittsburgh research group (Frank et al. 1997; Shear et al. 2001) developed a treatment for traumatic grief that involves principles similar to those featured in the treatment of posttraumatic stress disorder. The treatment for traumatic grief includes a series of cognitive-behavioral techniques such as imaginal exposure to the death scene; in vivo, graded exposure to avoided death-related circumstances; mindful breathing; and writing good-bye letters to the deceased person. Also integral to the treatment are homework assignments involving listening to tapes of imaginal exposure. The results were encouraging: complicated grief, anxiety, and depressive symptoms were significantly reduced, and patients who did not respond to interpersonal psychotherapy did respond to traumatic grief therapy.

One of the most comprehensive and clinically useful books on this topic was written by Worden (1991). He described various approaches that he developed for the treatment of grief, while distinguishing between grief counseling (for normal grief reactions) and grief therapy (for inhibited, chronic, or unresolved grief). His methods for grief therapy include reviving memories of the deceased person, along with facilitating the experiencing of a broad range of emotions to accompany these memories; helping the patient to acknowledge and deal with ambivalent feelings (to eventually achieve a balance); exploring and defusing "linking objects" (objects a mourner keeps to maintain a relationship with the deceased person); and helping the bereaved individual to say a final good-bye. Worden (1991) recommended specific modifications of this approach to help patients grieve particularly difficult losses, such as suicides and other forms of sudden death. He also integrated techniques such as psychodrama and role-playing, to intensify the emotional experience and provide the patient with options for working through the painful emotions.

Treatment of Normal Grief Reactions

Opinions differ regarding the use of medication to treat the unpleasant symptoms of depression (such as sleep and appetite problems) that typically accompany the first year of bereavement in patients experiencing a normal grief reaction. According to some psychiatrists and other health care providers, medication should be used sparingly and only briefly, if at all, because it is assumed that to recover adequately from grief, it is necessary to experience grief fully (e.g., Parkes 1972; Worden 1991).

Raphael et al. (2001) warned that in the case of bereavement without depression, prescribing antidepressants is not recommended. Others believe that the provider should intervene sooner rather than later, given the tendency of depressive symptoms to persist throughout the first year of spousal bereavement (see Reynolds 1992). Still others say that there is no empirical evidence that one must go through a difficult grieving process in order to resume one's life effectively, and therefore, pharmacological (and other) treatments for pain and suffering should be available to those who request them (Wortman and Silver 1987).

Currently, there are two well-recognized approaches for facilitating the experience (and expression) of normal grief. As noted in "Treatment of Complicated Bereavement" earlier in this chapter, Worden (1991) specified several methods of grief counseling for normal grief, including use of guided imagery to facilitate communication with the deceased person and use of symbols such as photos of the deceased person to evoke emotional expression. Worden was also noted for his conceptualization of mourning as four "tasks" that must be completed before grief can adequately resolve: accepting the reality of the loss, experiencing the pain of grief, adjusting to an environment in which the deceased individual is truly no longer there, and emotionally detaching oneself sufficiently from the deceased person to be able to resume a normal life. Bereaved persons are helped to accomplish these tasks through brief individual or group counseling, seen as adjunctive to their own psychological work on these issues. The effectiveness of grief therapy and counseling were reviewed in meta-analyses by Allumbaugh and Hoyt (1999), Former and Neimeyer (1999), and Kato and Mann (1999).

The majority of bereaved persons (particularly elders) do not seek professional assistance for their grief. Group counseling and self-help groups are much more widely used—that is, attending a support group specifically for bereaved persons has been the intervention most commonly recommended for and pursued by those experiencing an uncomplicated (but painful and lonely) bereavement. Lieberman (1993) conducted a thorough review of the relatively sparse literature on bereavement self-help groups. He described what are thought to be the basic curative factors in such groups, including a family-like atmosphere, encouragement of intense emotional expression, and sanction of development of a new self-image that reflects one's current status as an "I" rather than a "we." In contrast to the various forms of psychotherapy reviewed above in "Treatment of Complicated Bereavement," which tend to be relatively brief (or at least time limited), self-help groups encourage long-term involvement; as Lieberman (1993) pointed out, "membership is indeterminate and may persist far beyond professionally defined recovery" (p. 420). After reviewing the empirical data in support of this approach, Lieberman (1993) concluded that self-help groups for grieving persons (often groups with specific emphases, such as the "Compassionate Friends" self-help network for grieving parents) have been successfully used around the United States and that it is reasonable to expect that a large segment of the bereaved population can meet their social and psychological needs through this kind of intervention.

A final intervention that seems to us to hold promise, particularly for older men whose wives have died (and who are at risk for subsequent mortality), is one that proposes to help the bereaved person develop new affectional bonds to replace the major bond that was severed through death (Stoddard and Henry 1985). This approach is based on the assumption that most older men have only one strong emotional bond (i.e., with their wives); when that ends, the ensuing void must be filled with other affectional or emotional relationships, to protect against increased vulnerability to negative outcomes. This therapy consists of encouragement and support in turning social friendships into relationships that are emotionally fulfilling and not just socially gratifying. Although there is limited empirical support for this method at present, it is a conceptually appealing approach that warrants further investigation.

Finally, Prigerson and Jacobs (2001) suggested that for bereavement-related major depression, interventions should follow the practice guideline for depression (American Psychiatric Association 2000b), whereas for bereavement complications, use of selective serotonin reuptake inhibitors combined with cognitive-behavioral interventions is probably most effective. However, few empirical studies have focused on the efficacy of specific treatment programs.

Adjustment Disorders in Late Life

The diagnostic category of adjustment disorders has been underused in the assessment and treatment of older adults. DSM-IV-TR defines adjustment disorder as "a psychological response to an identifiable stressor or stressors that results in the development of clinically significant emotional or behavioral symptoms. The symptoms must develop within 3 months after the onset of the stressor(s)" (American Psychiatric Association 2000a, p. 679). Evidence of impairment in social or occupational functioning should be apparent during the reaction, or symptoms should be above and beyond what would be expected as a

normal reaction to a given stressor. This diagnosis is not applied if the symptom picture meets criteria for another specific disorder or if the reaction appears to be an exacerbation of another psychiatric disorder. If the stressor has a discrete beginning and end, it is assumed that this reaction will subside within a brief time after the stressor disappears. If the stressor is maintained for a long period, it is assumed that the individual will develop a more adaptive pattern of responding over time. By definition, an adjustment disorder must resolve within 6 months after the termination of the stressor. However, symptoms may persist longer if the stressor is chronic or has enduring consequences.

The specific type of adjustment disorder is coded according to the predominant symptom pattern (e.g., adjustment disorder with anxiety or depressed mood). The DSM-IV-TR criteria provide the opportunity to specify whether the adjustment disorder is acute (i.e., has persisted for less than 6 months) or chronic (has persisted for at least 6 months). This refinement might lead to an increase in diagnoses of adjustment disorders among the elderly, because in this population, stressors are frequently chronic and cumulative, and symptoms often persist longer than 6 months.

According to DSM-IV-TR, adjustment disorders are common, with prevalence rates between 2% and 8% in community samples of elderly individuals. However, very little attention has been focused on these disturbances in the literature. Certain authors have attributed this lack of attention to an "overelastic concept of 'depression'" (Casey et al. 2001), one that is not specific enough in its demarcations regarding the presence of depressive symptoms in the context of significant life stressors. The increase in stressors experienced by elderly persons might lead one to expect a greater proportion of adjustment disorders in this group. Another reason for the lack of emphasis in the clinical literature may be that many individuals with this disturbance may never have contact with the mental health system. Remedial assistance from the family or from institutions not connected with the health care system may facilitate quick recovery. Age stereotypes regarding emotional illness (Butler and Lewis 1982) may also discourage use of health care resources or may cause help-seeking efforts to be delayed until the disturbance becomes unbearably severe. This delay in seeking help increases the likelihood that the arbitrary period of 6 months will elapse, thereby excluding the individual from this diagnostic category.

However, an increasing number of studies have been focusing on this disorder, especially in medical populations who appear to be at a much higher risk for these disorders. Grossberg et al. (1990) determined that of 147 geriatric patients seen by psychiatrists in a 2-year period, 26% were diagnosed as having an adjustment disorder, with only the rate of affective disorder being higher (27%). Other investigators have found adjustment disorders to be common among patients with multiple sclerosis, cancer, or lupus and among patients receiving cardiac ventricular support or heart transplants (Cullivan et al. 1998; de Walden-Galuszko 1996; Harper et al. 1998; Hugo et al. 1996; Petrucci et al. 1999; Spiegel 1996; Sullivan et al. 1997). The finding by Strain and co-workers (1998) that 12% of patients referred to the psychiatry services of several teaching hospitals received a diagnosis of adjustment disorder further highlights the relevance of this diagnosis in medical settings and for elderly patients coping with medical illness and physical decline.

In an analysis of the literature on the epidemiology of depression, Blazer (1983) called attention to the possible importance of this diagnostic category. He noted that when self-report scales were used, the determined prevalence of depressive symptoms in community samples ranged from 10% to 45%, but the rate of clinical depression was substantially lower (around 2%–5%) when more stringent interview techniques of assessment were used. He concluded that the discrepancy could be accounted for in part by transient episodes of depressive symptoms accompanying bereavement or an adjustment reaction to other psychosocial stressors.

In more recent epidemiological studies, Blazer et al. (1987) identified a clinical subtype, referred to as symptomatic depression, which they suggested may apply to elderly individuals in the community who have adjustment disorder. However, Blazer and colleagues (1987) acknowledged that a definitive diagnosis could not be made on the basis of their data. The symptomatic depression subgroup constituted 4% of their community sample, but it is likely that even this proportion is an underestimate of the prevalence of the disorder.

Further evidence of the high prevalence of adjustment disorders among older patients was offered by Smith and colleagues (1998), who found that 29% of patients referred to a consultation-liaison service for depressive spectrum disorders received an accurate diagnosis of an adjustment disorder. Authors such as Blazer (1983) have provided compelling arguments for the utility of this diagnosis in working with elderly persons. Application of this diagnosis places the focus squarely on external stressors and the psychological and social resources available to the patient for coping with whatever unfortunate events might have occurred. Because age-related changes are likely in all these domains, this classification could be useful in many instances for the assessment and subsequent treatment of elderly patients.

With regard to external stressors, older people experience substantially more serious losses (Chiriboga and Cutler 1980; Lazarus and DeLongis 1983). For example, retirement often leads to loss of the work role; declining health can lead to a host of losses in physical and social functioning; and loss of loved ones and friends can occur not only through death but also through a move into a new environment, such as a retirement home. Although it is true that some of these losses cannot be avoided, many such losses are not unavoidable. In our own work with psychologically distressed elders, for example, we continue to be impressed with how often they underestimate the importance of their social network when making decisions about moving to a new situation during a time of transition. In many instances, had the significance of old friends and the difficulty of making new ones in a strange setting been given their proper due, the effect of loss of positive life aspects might have been mitigated. A similar story has been repeated many times with regard to retirement. With proper preparation, individuals can make retirement a transition from one work role to another rather than a loss of role, but all too often the potential hazard of this change is ignored.

The stress of such losses, however, may not be of primary importance; rather, how individuals cope with them may be the critical feature affecting health and well-being in elderly individuals (Billings and Moos 1981; Folkman et al. 1986). Greater acceptance of this position in the field has stimulated considerable interest in possible age differences in coping processes. Some authors have emphasized increased maturity with age in handling stressful situations (Vaillant 1977). Others have argued that age changes in coping behavior may be minimal but the kinds and severity of stressors encountered by elderly persons are more problematic, requiring different types of coping responses (Folkman et al. 1987; McCrae 1982).

There are clear indications that the coping strategies used by older individuals tend to differ from those used by younger individuals. Folkman et al. (1987) reported that in their study, younger persons used proportionately more active, interpersonal, problem-focused forms of coping, whereas the elderly individuals used intrapersonal, emotion-focused forms of coping involving distancing, acceptance of responsibility, and positive reappraisal. In another study, McCrae (1982) found that age differences in coping seemed to be due to the different kinds of stressors, but they also found that older individuals were generally less hostile in reaction to negative events and less likely to rely on escapist fantasy. Foster and Gallagher (1986) compared elderly depressed patients with nondepressed community volunteers matched for gender, age, and education and found that depressed patients were more likely to use emotional discharge than were those who were not depressed. Although no differences were found between the two groups in appraisal-focused and problem-focused coping, depressed patients rated all their strategies as significantly less helpful than did community participants.

The extent to which age-related changes in stressors, social support systems, and coping resources account for age differences in adjustment reactions is not clearly understood. However, the conceptual backdrop resulting from this line of research can provide clear direction for effective treatments of older patients with adjustment disorders. A logical first step would involve collaboration with patients to determine ways of neutralizing the stressful agents. Helping patients learn how to cope with negative events can also be immensely helpful, particularly with stressors that are not easily removed, such as chronic physical illness or drastic reductions in income. Such efforts will decrease the likelihood that a prolonged reaction to stress will lead to a more persistent and complicated psychiatric disorder. If stressors are left unchecked, the high frequency of losses and other negative events is likely to render successful adaptation much more difficult, particularly for elderly persons. The result could be a more severe disorder, requiring hospitalization and medical treatment. A frequent end point in this reaction to losses and negative events is a depressive episode.

Along these lines, the position advanced by George (1994) is clearly relevant. Recent emphasis on finding biological factors underlying psychiatric disorders may undermine the importance of external stressors in the development of some types of maladaptive behavior. Increased attention to the diagnostic classification of adjustment disorder, in both clinical and research settings, may correct any such trends by keeping the significance of negative events and poor coping behaviors in the foreground. For example, despite recent successes in identifying biological correlates of depression, considerable variance remains unexplained by such markers. This variance is understandable, given that depression is likely to be the final common pathway of several different causes. However, continued attempts to identify unique symptom patterns that occur in response to external stressors should lead to an improvement in the precision of differential diagnostic categories, along with their specific etiologies and associated treatment programs.

References

Ablon J: Bereavement in a Samoan community. Br J Med Psychol 44:329–337, 1971

Abrahms JL: Depression versus normal grief following the death of a significant other, in New Directions in Cognitive Therapy. Edited by Emery G, Hollon S, Bedrosian RC. New York, Guilford, 1981, pp 255–270

al-Adawi S, Burjorjee R, al-Issa I: Mu-Ghayeb: a culture-specific response to bereavement in Oman. Int J Soc Psychiatry 43:144–151, 1997

Allumbaugh DL, Hoyt WT: Effectiveness of grief therapy: a meta analysis. J Couns Psychol 46:370–380, 1999

American Psychiatric Association: Diagnostic and Statistical Manual of Mental Disorders, 4th Edition, Text Revision. Washington, DC, American Psychiatric Association, 2000a

American Psychiatric Association: Practice Guideline for the Treatment of Patients With Major Depressive Disorder, 2nd Edition. Washington, DC, American Psychiatric Association, 2000b

Bass DM, Bowman K, Noelker LS: The influence of caregiving and bereavement support on adjusting to an older relative's death. Gerontologist 31:32–42, 1991

Berch DG: Group treatment in a hospice bereavement program (abstract). Dissertation Abstracts International. Section B, The Sciences and Engineering 60:1289, 1999

Bierhals AJ, Prigerson HG, Fasiczka A, et al: Gender differences in complicated grief among the elderly. Omega (Westport) 32:303–317, 1995

Billings AG, Moos RH: The role of coping responses and social resources in attenuating the impact of stressful life events. J Behav Med 4:139–157, 1981

Blazer DG: The epidemiology of depression in late life, in Depression and Aging: Causes, Care and Consequences. Edited by Breslau L, Haug MR. New York, Springer, 1983, pp 30–50

Blazer DG, Hughes DC, George LK: The epidemiology of depression in an elderly community population. Gerontologist 27:281–287, 1987

Block JB: The meaning of death, in Healing Latinos: The Art of Cultural Competence in Medicine. Edited by Hayes-Bautista D, Chiprut R. Los Angeles, CA, Cedars-Sinai Health System, 1998, pp 79–85

Bowlby J: Processes of mourning. Int J Psychoanal 42:317–340, 1961

Bowlby J: Attachment and Loss, Vol 3: Loss: Sadness and Depression. London, Hogarth Press, 1980

Bowling A: Who dies after widow(er)hood? a discriminant analysis. Omega (Westport) 19:135–153, 1988–1989

Bowman KW, Singer PA: Chinese seniors' perspectives on end-of-life decisions. Soc Sci Med 53:455–464, 2001

Braun KL, Nichols R: Death and dying in four Asian American cultures: a descriptive study. Death Stud 21:327–359, 1997

Breckenridge J, Gallagher D, Thompson LW, et al: Characteristic depressive symptoms of bereaved elders. J Gerontol 41:163–168, 1986

Brown JT, Stoudemire GA: Normal and pathological grief. JAMA 250:378–383, 1983

Butler RN, Lewis MI: Aging and Mental Health, 3rd Edition. St. Louis, MO, CV Mosby, 1982

Cain BS: Divorce among elderly women: a growing social phenomenon. Soc Casework 69:563–568, 1988

Casey P, Dowrick C, Wilkenson G: Adjustment disorders: fault line in the psychiatric glossary. Br J Psychiatry 179:479–481, 2001

Chapman KJ, Pepler C: Coping, hope, and anticipatory grief in family members in palliative home care. Cancer Nurs 21:226–234, 1998

Chiriboga DA, Cutler L: Stress and adaptation: life span perspectives, in Aging in the 1980s. Edited by Poon L. Washington, DC, American Psychological Association, 1980, pp 347–362

Clayton P, Halikas J, Maurice W, et al: Anticipatory grief and widowhood. Br J Psychiatry 122:47–51, 1973

Clukey L: "Just be there!": the experience of anticipatory grief (abstract). Dissertation Abstracts International. Section B, The Sciences and Engineering 58:1208, 1997

Cobb S: Social support as a moderator of life stress. Psychosom Med 3:300–314, 1976

Corwin MD: Cultural issues in bereavement therapy: the social construction of mourning. In Session: Psychotherapy in Practice 1:23–41, 1995

Crain M: A cross-cultural study of beliefs, attitudes and values in Chinese-born American and non-Chinese frail homebound elderly. J Long Term Home Health Care 15:9–18, 1996

Cullivan R, Crown J, Walsh N: The use of psychotropic medication in patients referred to a psycho-oncology service. Psychooncology 7:301–306, 1998

de Walden-Galuszko K: Prevalence of psychological comorbidity in terminally ill cancer patients. Psychooncology 5:45–49, 1996

Dimond M, Lund DA, Caserta MS: The role of social support in the first two years of bereavement in an elderly sample. Gerontologist 27:599–604, 1987

Eisenbruch M: Cross-cultural aspects of bereavement, II: ethnic and cultural variations in the development of bereavement practices. Cult Med Psychiatry 8:315–347, 1984

Evans AJ: Anticipatory grief: a theoretical challenge. Palliat Med 8:159–165, 1994

Farberow NL, Gallagher DE, Gilewski MJ, et al: An examination of the early impact of bereavement on psychological distress in survivors of suicide. Gerontologist 27:592–598, 1987

Farberow NL, Gallagher-Thompson D, Gilewski M, et al: Changes in grief and mental health of bereaved spouses of older suicides. J Gerontol 47:P357–P366, 1992a

Farberow NL, Gallagher-Thompson D, Gilewski M, et al: The role of social supports in the bereavement process of surviving spouses of suicide and natural deaths. Suicide Life Threat Behav 22:107–124, 1992b

Faschingbauer TR: Texas Inventory of Grief—Revised Manual. Houston, TX, Honeycomb Publishing, 1981

Federal Interagency Forum on Aging Related Statistics: Older Americans 2000: Key Indicators of Well-Being. Washington, DC, Federal Interagency Forum on Aging Related Statistics, 2000

Field NP, Nichols C, Holen A, et al: The relation of continuing attachment to adjustment in conjugal bereavement. J Consult Clin Psychol 67:212–218, 1999

Florsheim M, Gallagher-Thompson D: Cognitive/behavioral treatment of atypical bereavement: a case study. Clin Gerontologist 10:73–76, 1990

Folkman S, Lazarus RS, Gruen RJ, et al: Appraisal, coping, health status, and psychological symptoms. J Pers Soc Psychol 50:571–579, 1986

Folkman S, Lazarus RS, Pimley S, et al: Age differences in stress and coping processes. Psychol Aging 2:171–184, 1987

Former B, Neimeyer RA: The effectiveness of grief counseling and therapy: a quantitative review. Paper presented at the annual meeting of the Association for Death Education and Counseling, San Antonio, TX, March 1999

Foster J, Gallagher D: An exploratory study comparing depressed and nondepressed elders' coping strategies. J Gerontol 41:91–93, 1986

Franco PC: The effect of caregiving during terminal illness on subsequent bereavement (abstract). Dissertation Abstracts International. Section B, The Sciences and Engineering 57:2219, 1996

Frank E, Prigerson HG, Shear MK, et al: Phenomenology and treatment of bereavement related distress in the elderly. Int Clin Psychopharmacol 12 (suppl 7):S25–S29, 1997

Freud S: Mourning and melancholia (1917[1915]), in The Standard Edition of the Complete Psychological Works of Sigmund Freud, Vol 14. Translated and edited by Strachey J. London, Hogarth Press, 1957, pp 237–260

Fulton G, Madden C, Minichiello V: The social construction of anticipatory grief. Soc Sci Med 43:1349–1358, 1996

Futterman A, Gallagher D, Thompson LW, et al: Retrospective assessment of marital adjustment and depression during the first 2 years of spousal bereavement. Psychol Aging 5:277–283, 1990

Gallagher-Thompson D, Thompson LW: Depression versus normal grief: similarities and differences in assessment and treatment. Paper presented at the annual meeting of the American Society on Aging, San Francisco, CA, March 19, 1994

Gallagher-Thompson D, Futterman A, Farberow N, et al: The impact of spousal bereavement on older widows and widowers, in Handbook of Bereavement. Edited by Stroebe MS, Stroebe W, Hansson R. Cambridge, UK, Cambridge University Press, 1993, pp 227–239

Gantz F, Gallagher D, Rodman J: Cognitive/behavioral facilitation of inhibited grief, in Comprehensive Casebook of Cognitive Therapy. Edited by Freeman A, Dattilio F. New York, Plenum, 1992, pp 201–207

George LK: Social factors and depression in late life, in Diagnosis and Treatment of Depression in Late Life: Results of the NIH Consensus Development Conference. Edited by Schneider LS, Reynolds CF III, Lebowitz BD, et al. Washington, DC, American Psychiatric Press, 1994, pp 131–153

Gilbar O: Length of cancer patients' stay at a hospice: does it affect psychological adjustment to the loss of the spouse? J Palliat Care 14:16–20, 1998

Gilewski MJ, Farberow NL, Gallagher DE, et al: Interaction of depression and bereavement on mental health in the elderly. Psychol Aging 6:67–75, 1991

Gilliland G, Fleming S: A comparison of spousal anticipatory grief and conventional grief. Death Stud 22:541–569, 1998

Glick IO, Weiss, RS, Parkes CM: The First Year of Bereavement. New York, Wiley, 1974

Goss RE, Klass D: Tibetan Buddhism and the resolution of grief: the Bardo-thodol for the dying and the grieving. Death Stud 21:377–395, 1997

Grimby A: Bereavement among elderly people: grief reactions, post-bereavement hallucinations, and quality of life. Acta Psychiatr Scand 87:72–80, 1993

Grossberg GT, Zimny GH, Nakra BR: Geriatric psychiatry consultations in a university hospital. Int Psychogeriatr 2:161–168, 1990

Harlow SD, Goldberg EL, Comstock GW: A longitudinal study of the prevalence of depressive symptomatology in elderly widowed and married women. Arch Gen Psychiatry 48:1065–1068, 1991

Harper RG, Chacko RC, Kotik-Harper D, et al: Detection of a psychiatric diagnosis in heart transplant candidates with the MBHI. J Clin Psychol Med Settings 5:187–198, 1998

Horowitz MJ: Stress Response Syndromes. New York, Jason Aronson, 1976

Horowitz MJ, Wilner N, Marmar C, et al: Pathological grief and the activation of latent self-images. Am J Psychiatry 137:1157–1162, 1980

Horowitz MJ, Krupnick J, Kaltreider N, et al: Initial response to parental death. Arch Gen Psychiatry 38:316–323, 1981

Horowitz MJ, Weiss DS, Kaltreider N, et al: Reactions to the death of a parent: results form patients and field subjects. J Nerv Ment Dis 172:383–392, 1984

Horowitz MJ, Siegel B, Holen A, et al: Diagnostic criteria for complicated grief disorder. Am J Psychiatry 154:904–910, 1997

Hospice Care, 42 CFR § 418.88 (2001)

Hospice Foundation of America: What is hospice? Available at http://www.hospicefoundation.org/what_is. Accessed July 21, 2003.

Hugo FJ, Halland AM, Spangenberg JJ, et al: DSM-III-R classification of psychiatric symptoms in systemic lupus erythematosus. Psychosomatics 37:262–269, 1996

al-Issa I: The illusion of reality or the reality of illusion. Hallucinations and culture. Br J Psychiatry 166:368–373, 1995

Janof-Bulman R, Timko C: Coping with traumatic life events: the role of denial in light of people's assumptive worlds, in Coping With Negative Life Events: Clinical and Social Psychological Perspectives. Edited by Snyder CR, Ford CE. New York, Plenum, 1987, pp 135–159

Johnson RJ, Lund DA, Dimond M: Stress, self-esteem, and coping during bereavement among the elderly. Soc Psychol Q 49:273–279, 1986

Kalish RA: Older people and grief. Generations 11:33–38, 1987

Kalish RA, Reynolds DK: Death and Ethnicity: A Psychocultural Study. New York, Baywood Publishing, 1981

Kaplan C, Gallagher-Thompson D: The treatment of clinical depression in caregivers of spouses with dementia. Journal of Cognitive Psychotherapy 9:35–44, 1995

Kastenbaum RJ: Death, Society, and Human Experience, 2nd Edition. St. Louis, MO, CV Mosby, 1981

Kato PM, Mann T: A synthesis of psychological interventions for the bereaved. Clin Psychol Rev 19:275–296, 1999

Klass D: Grief as an Eastern culture: Japanese ancestor worship, in Continuing Bonds: New Understandings of Grief (Series in Death Education, Aging, and Health Care, 0275-3510). Edited by Klass D, Silverman PR, Nickman SL. Washington, DC, Taylor & Francis, 1996, pp 59–70

Kogan ES, Van-Hasselt VB, Hersen M, et al: Relationship of depression, assertiveness, and social support in community-dwelling older adults. Journal of Clinical Geropsychology 1:157–163, 1995

Kramer D: How women relate to terminally ill husbands and their subsequent adjustment to bereavement. Omega (Westport) 34:93–106, 1997

Lazarus RS, DeLongis A: Psychological stress and coping in aging. Am Psychol 38:245–254, 1983

Lieberman MA: Bereavement self-help groups: a review of conceptual and methodological issues, in Handbook of Bereavement. Edited by Stroebe MS, Stroebe W, Hansson R. Cambridge, UK, Cambridge University Press, 1993, pp 411–426

Lindemann E: Symptomatology and management of acute grief. Am J Psychiatry 101:141–148, 1944

Lopata HZ: On widowhood: grief work and identity reconstruction. J Geriatr Psychiatry 8:41–55, 1975

Lund DA (ed): Older Bereaved Spouses. New York, Hemisphere, 1989

Lund DA, Caserta MS, Dimond MF: Gender differences through two years of bereavement among the elderly. Gerontologist 26:314–320, 1986

Lund DA, Caserta M, Dimond M: Impact of spousal bereavement on the subjective well-being of older adults, in Older Bereaved Spouses. Edited by Lund DA. New York, Hemisphere, 1989, pp 3–15

Lund DA, Caserta M, Dimond M: The course of spousal bereavement in later life, in Handbook of Bereavement. Edited by Stroebe MS, Stroebe W, Hansson R. Cambridge, UK, Cambridge University Press, 1993, pp 240–254

Marmar C, Horowitz MJ, Weiss DS, et al: A controlled trial of brief psychotherapy and mutual-help group treatment of conjugal bereavement. Am J Psychiatry 145:203–212, 1988

Mawson D, Marks IM, Ramm L, et al: Guided mourning for morbid grief: a controlled study. Br J Psychiatry 138:185–193, 1981

McCrae RR: Age differences in the use of coping mechanisms. J Gerontol 37:454–460, 1982

McCrae RR, Costa PT: Psychological resilience among widowed men and women: a 10-year follow-up of a national sample, in Handbook of Bereavement. Edited by Stroebe MS, Stroebe W, Hansson R. Cambridge, UK, Cambridge University Press, 1993, pp 196–207

Medigovich K, Porock D, Kristjanson LJ, et al: Predictors of family satisfaction with an Australian palliative home care service: a test of discrepancy theory. J Palliat Care 15:48–56, 1999

Miller MD, Wolfson L, Frank E, et al: Using interpersonal psychotherapy (IPT) in a combined psychotherapy/medication research protocol with depressed elders. A descriptive report with case vignettes. J Psychother Pract Res 7:47–55, 1997

Miller SI, Schoenfeld L: Grief in the Navajo: psychodynamics and culture. Int J Soc Psychiatry 19:187–191, 1973

Moss MS, Moss SZ, Rubinstein R, et al: Impact of elderly mother's death on middle age daughters. Int J Aging Hum Dev 37:1–22, 1993

Nadeau JW: Meaning making in family bereavement: a family systems approach, in Handbook of Bereavement Research: Consequences, Coping, and Care. Edited by Stroebe MS, Hansson RO, Stroebe W, et al. Washington, DC, American Psychological Association, 2001, pp 329–347

Neimeyer R: The Lessons of Loss: A Guide to Coping. Raleigh, NC, McGraw-Hill, 1998

Newsom JT, Schulz R: Social support as a mediator in the relation between functional status and quality of life in older adults. Psychol Aging 11:34–44, 1996

Ng K, von Gunten CF: Symptoms and attitudes of 100 consecutive patients admitted to an acute hospice/palliative care unit. J Pain Symptom Manage 16:307–316, 1998

NIH Consensus Conference. Diagnosis and treatment of depression in late life. JAMA 268:1018–1024, 1992

Nolen-Hoeksema S, Larson J, Bishop M: Predictors of family members' satisfaction with hospice. Hosp J 15:29–48, 2000

O'Bryant SL: Forewarning of a husband's death: does it make a difference for older widows? Omega (Westport) 22:227–239, 1990–1991

O'Neil M: Grief and bereavement in AIDS and aging. Generations 13:80–82, 1989

Ortiz A, Simmons J, Hinton WL: Locations of remorse and homelands of resilience: notes on grief and sense of loss of place of Latino and Irish-American caregivers of demented elders. Cult Med Psychiatry 23:477–500, 1999

Osterweis M, Solomon F, Green M (eds): Bereavement: Reactions, Consequences, and Care. Washington, DC, National Academy Press, 1984

Parkes CM: Bereavement: Studies of Grief in Adult Life. New York, International Universities Press, 1972

Parkes CM, Weiss RS: Recovery From Bereavement. New York, Basic Books, 1983

Petrucci R, Kushon D, Inkles R, et al: Cardiac ventricular support: considerations for psychiatry. Psychosomatics 40:298–303, 1999

Pincus L: Death and the Family. New York, Pantheon, 1974

Prigerson HG, Jacobs SC: Perspectives on care at the close of life. Caring for bereaved patients: "all the doctors just suddenly go." JAMA 286:1369–1376, 2001

Prigerson HG, Shear MK, Jacobs SC, et al: Consensus criteria for traumatic grief: a preliminary empirical test. Br J Psychiatry 174:67–73, 1999

Quigley DG, Schatz MS: Men and women and their responses in spousal bereavement. Hosp J 14:65–78, 1999

Ragow-O'Brien D, Hayslip B, Guarnaccia CA: The impact of hospice on attitudes toward funerals and subsequent bereavement adjustment. Omega (Westport) 41:291–305, 2000

Rando TA: The increasing prevalence of complicated mourning: the onslaught is just beginning. Omega (Westport) 26:43–59, 1992–1993

Rando TA: Anticipatory mourning: a review and critique of the literature, in Clinical Dimensions of Anticipatory Mourning. Edited by Rando TA. Champaign, IL, Research Press, 2000, pp 17–49

Raphael B, Middleton W, Martinek N, et al: Counseling and therapy of the bereaved, in Handbook of Bereavement. Edited by Stroebe MS, Stroebe W, Hansson R. Cambridge, UK, Cambridge University Press, 1993, pp 427–453

Raphael B, Minkov C, Dobson M: Psychotherapeutic and pharmacological intervention for bereaved persons, in Handbook of Bereavement Research: Consequences, Coping, and Care. Edited by Stroebe MS, Hansson RO, Stroebe W, et al. Washington, DC, American Psychological Association, 2001, pp 587–612

Rees WD: The hallucinations of widowhood. Br Med J 4:37–41, 1971

Reisman AS: Death of a spouse: illusory basic assumptions and continuation of bonds. Death Stud 25:445–460, 2001

Reynolds CF 3rd: Treatment of depression in special populations. J Clin Psychiatry 53 (suppl):45–53, 1992

Reynolds CF 3rd, Miller MD, Pasternak RE, et al: Treatment of bereavement-related major depressive episodes in later life: a controlled study of acute and continuation treatment with nortriptyline and interpersonal psychotherapy. Am J Psychiatry 156:202–208, 1999

Richardson VE, Balaswamy S: Coping with bereavement among elderly widowers. Omega (Westport) 43:129–144, 2001

Romanoff BD, Terenzio M: Rituals and the grieving process. Death Stud 22:697–711, 1998

Rosenblatt PC: Cross-cultural variation in the experience, statement, and understanding of grief, in Ethnic Variations in Dying, Death, and Grief: Diversity in Universality. Edited by Irish DP, Lundquist KF, Nelsen VJ. Washington, DC, Taylor & Francis, 1993, pp 13–19

Rosenblatt PC: Grief that does not end, in Continuing Bonds: New Understandings of Grief (Series in Death Education, Aging, and Health Care, 0275-3510). Edited by Klass D, Silverman PR, Nickman SL. Washington, DC, Taylor & Francis, 1996, pp 45–58

Rosenblatt PC, Elde C: Shared reminiscence about a deceased parent: implications for grief education and grief counseling. Fam Relat 39:206–210, 1990

Rosenzweig A, Prigerson H, Miller MD, et al: Bereavement and late-life depression: grief and its complications in the elderly. Annu Rev Med 48:421–428, 1997

Sable P: Attachment, loss of spouse, and grief in elderly adults. Omega (Westport) 23:129–142, 1991

Sanders CM: Risk factors in bereavement outcome, in Handbook of Bereavement. Edited by Stroebe MS, Stroebe W, Hansson R. Cambridge, UK, Cambridge University Press, 1993, pp 255–267

Sanders CM, Mauger PA, Strong PN Jr: A Manual for the Grief Experience Inventory. Tampa, University of South Florida, 1979

Sanders CM, Mauger PA, Strong PN Jr: A Manual for the Grief Experience Inventory. Palo Alto, CA, Consulting Psychologists Press, 1985

Schut HA, Stroebe MS, van den Bout J: Intervention for the bereaved: gender differences in the efficacy of two counselling programmes. Br J Clin Psychol 36:63–72, 1997

Schut H[A], Stroebe MS, van den Bout J, et al: The efficacy of bereavement interventions: determining who benefits, in Handbook of Bereavement Research: Consequences, Coping, and Care. Edited by Stroebe MS, Hansson RO, Stroebe W, et al. Washington, DC, American Psychological Association, 2001, pp 705–737

Seale C, Kelly M: A comparison of hospice and hospital care for the spouses of people who die. Palliat Med 11:101–106, 1997

Shear MK, Frank E, Foa E, et al: Traumatic grief treatment: a pilot study. Am J Psychiatry 158:1506–1508, 2001

Shuchter SR, Zisook S: Widowhood. The continuing relationship with the dead spouse. Bull Menninger Clin 52:269–279, 1988

Shuchter SR, Zisook S: The course of normal grief, in Handbook of Bereavement. Edited by Stroebe MS, Stroebe W, Hansson R. Cambridge, UK, Cambridge University Press, 1993, pp 23–43

Siegel K, Weinstein L: Anticipatory grief reconsidered. Journal of Psychosocial Oncology 1:61–72, 1983

Silverman PR, Klass D: Introduction: what's the problem? in Continuing Bonds: New Understandings of Grief (Series in Death Education, Aging, and Health Care, 0275-3510). Edited by Klass D, Silverman PR, Nickman SL. Washington, DC, Taylor & Francis, 1996, pp 3–27

Sireling L, Cohen D, Marks I: Guided mourning for morbid grief: a replication. Behav Ther 29:121–132, 1988

Smith GC, Clarke DM, Handrinos D, et al: Consultation-liaison psychiatrists' management of depression. Psychosomatics 39:244–252, 1998

Spiegel D: Cancer and depression. Br J Psychiatry 168:109–116, 1996

Steinhauser KE, Christakis NA, Clipp EC, et al: Factors considered important at the end of life by patients, family, physicians, and other care providers. JAMA 284:2476–2482, 2000

Strain JJ, Smith GC, Hammer JS, et al: Adjustment disorder: a multisite study of its utilization and interventions in the consultation-liaison psychiatry setting. Gen Hosp Psychiatry 20:139–149, 1998

Stoddard J, Henry JP: Affectional bonding and the impact of bereavement. Advances 2:19–28, 1985

Stroebe MS: Coping with bereavement: a review of the grief work hypothesis. Omega (Westport) 26:19–42, 1992–1993

Stroebe M[S], Schut H: The dual process model of coping with bereavement: rationale and description. Death Stud 23:197–224, 1999

Stroebe MS, Schut H: Models of coping with bereavement: a review, in Handbook of Bereavement Research: Consequences, Coping, and Care. Edited by Stroebe MS, Hansson RO, Stroebe W, et al. Washington, DC, American Psychological Association, 2001, pp 375–403

Stroebe M[S], Stroebe W: Who participates in bereavement research? a review and empirical study. Omega (Westport) 20:1–29, 1989

Stroebe MS, Stroebe W: The mortality of bereavement: a review, in Handbook of Bereavement. Edited by Stroebe MS, Stroebe W, Hansson R. Cambridge, UK, Cambridge University Press, 1993, pp 175–195

Stroebe MS, Stroebe W, Hansson R (eds): Handbook of Bereavement, Cambridge, UK, Cambridge University Press, 1993

Stroebe MS, Hansson RO, Stroebe W, et al: Introduction: concepts and issues in contemporary research on bereavement, in Handbook of Bereavement Research: Consequences, Coping, and Care. Edited by Stroebe MS, Hansson RO, Stroebe W, et al. Washington, DC, American Psychological Association, 2001, pp 3–22

Stylianos S, Vachon M: The role of social support in bereavement, in Handbook of Bereavement. Edited by Stroebe MS, Stroebe W, Hansson R. Cambridge, UK, Cambridge University Press, 1993, pp 397–410

Sullivan MJ, Mikail S, Weinshenker B: Coping with a diagnosis of multiple sclerosis. Can J Behav Sci 29:249–257, 1997

Sweeting HN, Gilhooly ML: Anticipatory grief: a review. Soc Sci Med 30:1073–1080, 1990

Thompson LW, Breckenridge JN, Gallagher D, et al: Effects of bereavement on self-perceptions of physical health in elderly widows and widowers. J Gerontol 39:309–314, 1984

Thompson LW, Gallagher-Thompson D, Futterman A, et al: The effects of late-life spousal bereavement over a 30-month interval. Psychol Aging 6:434–441, 1991

Thornton JCB: The hospice widow and grief resolution: perceived marital satisfaction and social support as factors influencing bereavement (abstract). Dissertation Abstracts International. Section B, The Sciences and Engineering 59:1337, 1998

U.S. Census Bureau: Demographic and socioeconomic aspects of aging in the United States (Current Population Reports, Series P-23, No 138). Washington, DC, U.S. Government Printing Office, 1984

U.S. Census Bureau: Current Population Survey Report. Marital and Living Arrangements: March 1998 (Update) (P20-514). Available at http://www.census.gov/prod/99pubs/p20-514u.pdf. Accessed November 3, 2003.

Vaillant GE: Adaptation to Life. Boston, MA, Little, Brown, 1977

Viney L: The construing widow: dislocation and adaptation in bereavement. Psychotherapy Patient 6:207–222, 1990

Voltz R, Akabayashi A, Reese C, et al: Organization and patients' perception of palliative care: a crosscultural comparison. Palliat Med 11:351–357, 1997

Wikan U: Bereavement and loss in two Muslim communities: Egypt and Bali compared. Soc Sci Med 27:451–460, 1988

Wilkinson EK, Salisbury C, Bosanquet N, et al: Patient and carer preference for, and satisfaction with, specialist models of palliative care: a systematic literature review. Palliat Med 13:197–216, 1999

Windholz MJ, Weiss DS, Horowitz MJ: An empirical study of the natural history of time-limited psychotherapy for stress response syndromes. Psychotherapy: Theory, Research, Practice, Training 22:547–554, 1985

Wisocki PA, Skowron J: The effects of gender and culture on adjustment to widowhood, in Handbook of Gender, Culture, and Health. Edited by Eisler RM, Hersen M. Mahwah, NJ, Erlbaum, 2000, pp 429–448

Worden JW: Grief Counseling and Grief Therapy, 2nd Edition. New York, Springer, 1991

Wortman C, Silver RC: Coping with irrevocable loss, in Cataclysms, Crises, and Catastrophes: Psychology in Action (The Master Lectures). Edited by VandenBos G, Bryant BK. Washington, DC, American Psychological Association, 1987, pp 185–235

Wortman C, Silver RC: The myths of coping with loss. J Consult Clin Psychol 57:349–357, 1989

Wrenn RL, Zylicz Z, Balk DE: Hospice care and the bereavement process in two countries: experience from the United States and the Netherlands. Illness, Crisis & Loss 9:173–189, 2001

Younoszai B: Mexican American perspectives related to death, in Ethnic Variations in Dying, Death, and Grief: Diversity in Universality. Edited by Irish DP, Lundquist KF, Nelsen VJ. Washington, DC, Taylor & Francis, 1993, pp 67–78

Zisook S, Shuchter SR: Time course of spousal bereavement. Gen Hosp Psychiatry 7:95–100, 1985

Zisook S, Shuchter SR: The first four years of widowhood. Psychiatr Ann 15:288–294, 1986

Zisook S, Shuchter SR, Sledge P, et al: Aging and bereavement. J Geriatr Psychiatry Neurol 6:137–143, 1993

CHAPTER 20

Sleep and Circadian Rhythm Disorders

Andrew D. Krystal, M.D., M.S.

Jack D. Edinger, Ph.D.

William K. Wohlgemuth, Ph.D.

Joseph M. Sharpe, M.D.

Sleep disorders are an important aspect of geriatric psychiatry. In the United States, more than half of non-institutionalized individuals older than 65 years report chronic sleep difficulties (Foley et al. 1995; "National Institutes of Health Consensus Development Conference Statement" 1991; Prinz et al. 1990). Sleep disturbances affect quality of life, increase the risk of accidents and falls, and, perhaps most importantly, are among the leading reasons for long-term-care placement (Pollack and Perlick 1991; Pollack et al. 1990; Sanford 1975). Working effectively with elderly individuals requires expertise in the diagnosis and treatment of sleep disorders.

Reviewing the basic nomenclature used to describe sleep disorders provides a first step in understanding sleep disorders in the elderly. The major disorders of sleep are typically divided into three groups: 1) difficulties in initiating and maintaining sleep (insomnias); 2) disorders of excessive daytime sleepiness; and 3) disorders of circadian rhythm. Insomnias are characterized by complaints of sustained difficulty in initiating or maintaining sleep and/or complaints of nonrestorative sleep, along with significant distress or impairment in daytime function (American Psychiatric Association 2000; American Sleep Disorders Association 1997). These disorders are frequently classified as either primary insomnia (in which no underlying psychiatric or medical disorder is associated with the condition) or secondary insomnia (in which a psychiatric or medical disorder is etiologically related to the sleep disturbance) (American Psychiatric Association 2000).

Disorders of excessive daytime sleepiness are characterized by persistent daytime sleepiness that causes significant distress or impairment in function (American Psychiatric Association 2000; American Sleep Disorders Association 1997). The most important disorders of excessive sleepiness are sleep apnea, periodic limb movement disorder (PLMD), and narcolepsy.

Circadian rhythm disorders manifest as a misalignment between an individual's sleep-wake cycle and the pattern that is desired or required (American Psychiatric Association 2000; American Sleep Disorders Association 1997). Affected individuals report that they cannot sleep at the times when sleep is desired, needed, or expected and that they fall asleep at times when wakefulness is desired, needed, or expected. The circadian rhythm is important for function because it is a cycle not only of sleep and wakefulness but also of many physiological processes and phenomena, including body temperature, alertness, cognitive performance, and hormone release (Czeisler et al. 1990; Folkard and Totterdell 1994; Minors et al. 1994).

Despite the variety and differing pathophysiologies of sleep disorders, the incidence of nearly all these disorders increases with age. The majority of age-related changes in sleep appear to stem from an increased incidence of sleep disturbances that lead to secondary sleep-related symptoms such as sleep apnea, PLMD, and medical and psychiatric disorders (Bliwise 1993; Foley et al. 1995; Gislason and Almqvist 1987; Prinz 1995; Prinz et al. 1990).

Yet evidence shows that in healthy elderly individuals without such disorders, changes in sleep and the circadian rhythm occur (Bliwise 1993; Foley et al. 1995; Gislason and Almqvist 1987; Prinz 1995; Prinz et al. 1990). Given that these changes are not necessarily associated with complaints of sleep disturbance or diminished daytime function, sleep and circadian rhythm disturbances may not be an inevitable consequence of aging. These factors provide some challenges for clinical care. One of these challenges is the need to use a different threshold for normality in elderly patients. Sleep attributes that are considered abnormal in a younger individual may not be associated with symptoms in an elderly person. Furthermore, clinical care of the elderly population requires a heightened awareness of and expertise in identifying underlying medical and psychiatric disorders.

Although these challenges can be formidable, they are not insurmountable. In this chapter, we first review the changes in sleep and circadian rhythm that occur in individuals without medical and psychiatric disorders. We then review the disorders that can cause disturbances of sleep and chronobiology and whose likelihood increases with age. Finally, we discuss evaluation and treatment of elderly individuals with a sleep complaint or suspected sleep-related dysfunction.

Influence of Aging on Sleep and Circadian Functions

Since the 1970s, extensive research has shown that marked changes in sleep and circadian rhythm accompany aging. Normative data derived from adults without complaints of sleep disturbance have implied that marked changes in the duration, continuity, and depth of nocturnal sleep accompany normal aging (Hirshkowitz et al. 1992). As shown in Figure 20–1, nocturnal sleep time steadily decreases across the life span, and nocturnal wake time increases, because of an increase in arousals. Accompanying these changes are marked reductions in Stage III and IV sleep (these stages are the deeper stages of non–rapid eye movement [REM] sleep). Although the clinical significance of these changes is unknown, they may relate to the reported reduction in subjective sleep quality and lowering of the arousal threshold with age (Riedel and Lichstein 1998; Zepelin et al. 1984).

The sleep-wake cycle appears to change significantly with age as well. The amplitudes of both the sleep-wake cycle and the 24-hour body temperature rhythm appear to decrease with aging (Bliwise 2000; Czeisler et al.

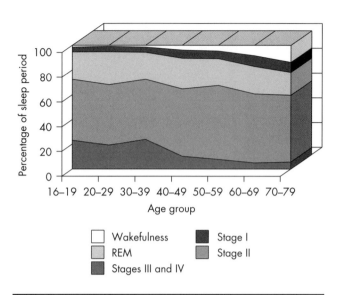

FIGURE 20–1. Sleep-stage distributions across age groups.

REM = rapid eye movement.

1999). Additionally, compared with younger age groups, older adults tend to awaken at an earlier phase (i.e., closer to the nadir of their 24-hour temperature rhythms), and they show a greater propensity to awaken during the later portions of their sleep episodes (Dijk et al. 1997; Duffy et al. 1998). Furthermore, multiple psychosocial changes that accompany aging may alter or eliminate important zeitgebers or time markers for the circadian system and promote the onset of sleep difficulties among older adults.

Disorders That Cause Sleep and Circadian Rhythm Disturbances

A number of medical and psychiatric conditions cause sleep difficulties and occur more frequently as age increases.

Primary Sleep Disorders

Sleep Apnea

In patients with sleep apnea, breathing ceases for periods of 10 seconds or more (Aldrich 2000), either because no effort is made to breathe (central sleep apnea) or because the oropharynx collapses during attempts to breathe (obstructive sleep apnea). The predominant type of sleep apnea seen in elderly individuals is obstructive sleep apnea (Ancoli-Israel et al. 1987). A number of studies suggest that the frequency of obstructive sleep apnea increases with age (Ancoli-Israel 1989; Ancoli-Israel et al. 1991; Dickel and Mosko 1990; Roehrs et al. 1983). Apnea generally causes excessive sleepiness, although mild to moderate apnea can be associated with insomnia. Referral to a sleep disorders specialist is required for diagnosis and treatment. The treatment of choice for obstructive sleep apnea is continuous positive airway pressure. This treatment involves blowing air through the nose at night to increase pressure within the upper airway, thereby preventing the collapse that leads to apnea. Some individuals (particularly those with anatomical anomalies predisposing them to apnea) are treated with upper airway surgery. Central sleep apnea is relatively rare, constituting 4%–10% of patients with apnea (White 2000). This disorder can occur due to a number of different pathophysiologies including any cause of waking alveolar hypoventilation, congestive heart failure, neurologic disorders, and nasal and upper airway obstruction. Therapy should be targeted to particular underlying process, though in many cases no such problem can be identified and CPAP is usually the first treatment attempted (White 2000).

Periodic Limb Movement Disorder and Restless Legs Syndrome

In periodic limb movement disorder (PLMD), repetitive muscular contractions occur during sleep; these contractions most commonly involve the legs and often cause sleep disturbances. When these events occur infrequently, they are not considered pathological, because they tend not to be associated with any symptoms (Roehrs et al. 1983). The frequency of these events is characterized in terms of the number of movements associated with arousal that occur per hour of sleep (the movement-arousal index). There is some debate about what movement-arousal index is abnormal. Thresholds ranging from 5 to 15 movements per hour have been suggested (Ancoli-Israel et al. 1991; Dickel and Mosko 1990). Some authors have suggested that a higher threshold for abnormality should be applied to elderly patients, who tend to be symptom free at movement-arousal indices typically associated with significant symptoms in younger individuals (Ancoli-Israel 1989). Perhaps even more relevant for those working with elderly patients is that PLMD, like sleep apnea, is more prevalent in the elderly population (Roehrs et al. 1983). Several studies indicate that clinically significant PLMD is seen in 30%–45% of adults age 60 years or older, compared with 5%–6% of all adults (Ancoli-Israel et al. 1991).

Individuals with PLMD may complain of leg kicks (most commonly noticed by the bed partner), cold feet,

excessive daytime sleepiness, and insomnia (Ancoli-Israel 1989; Ancoli-Israel et al. 1991; Roehrs et al. 1983). The insomnia may be characterized by difficulty in falling asleep or staying asleep (Ancoli-Israel 1989). Unfortunately, the presence of this disease is difficult to reliably predict based on the patient's history (Ancoli-Israel 1989; Dickel and Mosko 1990). Furthermore, a high level of confidence in the diagnosis is needed before institution of treatment, because treatment typically involves long-term use of medications that can have significant side effects (see "Pharmacological Treatment" later in this chapter). Therefore, when a history is suggestive of PLMD, standard practice is to make a referral for a polysomnogram for definitive diagnosis (Ancoli-Israel 1989). Polysomnography is also indicated when an individual has significant insomnia or hypersomnia that does not respond to usual treatment. Such a patient may have significant PLMD that was undetected when the patient's history was obtained.

Restless legs syndrome (RLS) is often associated with PLMD and is described as an uncomfortable feeling in the lower extremities that creates an irresistible urge to move. RLS occurs in 6% of the adult population and is present in up to 28% of patients older than 65 years (Clark 2001). Polysomnography is not needed for a diagnosis of RLS, which is made through history taking.

When compared in the general population, RLS is almost twice as prevalent in elderly women as elderly men. RLS, as well as PLMD, has been associated with anemia (O'Keeffe et al. 1994). In elderly patients, ferritin levels less than 45 µg/L have a positive correlation with an increased risk of RLS, and such patients often benefit from administration of supplemental iron (O'Keeffe et al. 1994). Also associated with PLMD and RLS are diabetes mellitus, pregnancy, iron deficiency anemia, and use of certain medications, including antidepressants (Bliwise et al. 1985). Workup to exclude these conditions is typically carried out before initiating medication treatment.

The same medications are effective for both RLS and PLMD. They include anticonvulsants, benzodiazepines, dopaminergic agonists, and opiates. Many practitioners use gabapentin and clonazepam as first-line agents because of the drugs' relatively favorable side-effect profiles; however, dopaminergic agonists appear to be the most effective medications. Opiates are typically reserved for patients who fail to respond to these other drugs. Because of the high prevalence of PLMD and RLS in the elderly population, the geriatric psychiatrist should be acquainted with the symptoms of PLMD and RLS. Effective treatment often significantly improves the quality of life of affected individuals.

Neuropsychiatric Disorders

Bereavement

Psychological factors that most commonly affect sleep in elderly persons are reactions to loss, such as loss of health or functional capacity, and reactions to the death of a friend or loved one. Although bereavement is normal, it is often associated with substantial sleep disturbance (American Psychiatric Association 2000). When bereavement is associated with more frequent intrusive thoughts and avoidance behaviors, there appears to be more sleep disturbance, predominantly in the form of difficulty in falling asleep (Hall et al. 1997). Bereavement and depression are closely linked, however. Depression is usually diagnosed only when symptoms have persisted for more than 2 months after a loss or when symptoms are severe, such as suicidal ideation, psychotic symptoms, malnutrition, or dehydration (American Psychiatric Association 2000). Antidepressant medication may be helpful. A short course of sedative-hypnotic therapy may provide substantial symptomatic relief. If this approach is taken, the medication should be tapered off when the other symptoms of bereavement diminish. Because the clinician will not know at the outset how long treatment will be needed, considerations related to longer-term treatment pertain (see "Pharmacological Treatment" later in this chapter). Also, even with a relatively short course (3–4 weeks) of treatment, rebound insomnia may occur. Therefore, the clinician should warn the patient of this possibility and wait at least several days after discontinuing the medication, so as to determine whether there is persistent insomnia. If all symptoms of bereavement have resolved except insomnia, cognitive-behavioral sleep therapy should be considered (see "Behavioral Treatment" later in this chapter). Grief counseling should also be considered.

Major Depression

Depression is a frequent cause of sleep disruption in individuals older than 60 years. Roughly 10%–15% of individuals older than 65 years experience clinically significant depressive symptoms (Hoch et al. 1989). The most frequent complaints in affected individuals are 1) a decrease in total sleep time and 2) waking earlier than desired. Daytime sleepiness may occur but is usually better characterized as fatigue.

Treatment of insomnia in individuals with major depression should always involve use of antidepressant medication. Administration of a sedating antidepressant is desirable for addressing the insomnia (see "Pharmacological Treatment" later in this chapter), but the drug may not be tolerated because of side effects. Whether to administer sedative-hypnotic medication along with a nonsedating antidepressant is a subject of debate. During treatment, the hope is that the insomnia will be short-lived and it will be possible to taper the sedative-hypnotic medication when other symptoms of depression begin to improve. (Issues related to tapering sedative-hypnotic medications are discussed above in "Bereavement.") Antidepressants may themselves cause sleep disturbance, necessitating longer-term therapy (Asnis et al. 1999). One study found that zolpidem 10 mg administered for 4 weeks to a nongeriatric population was highly effective and safe, with only 1 night of rebound insomnia after abrupt discontinuation (Asnis et al. 1999). Longer-term use for treatment of elderly patients has not been studied. In general, it is better to avoid use of sedative-hypnotic medication if possible and to consider behavioral therapy (see "Behavioral Treatment" later in this chapter). In many cases, however, sedative-hypnotic medication may be needed (see "Pharmacological Treatment" later in this chapter).

Alzheimer's Disease

Individuals with Alzheimer's disease have been found to experience an increased number of arousals and awakenings, to take more daytime naps, and to have a diminished amount of REM sleep and slow-wave sleep (Prinz et al. 1982). Individuals with dementia often experience evening or nocturnal agitation and confusion. This phenomenon, called sundowning, is among the leading reasons that individuals with dementia become institutionalized (Pollack and Perlick 1991; Pollack et al. 1990; Sanford 1975). The pathophysiology of sundowning is poorly understood. A number of features appear to increase the risk of sundowning, including greater dementia severity, pain, fecal impaction, malnutrition, polypharmacy, infections, REM sleep behavior disorder, PLMD, and environmental sleep disruptions (Bliwise 2000).

Treatment of sundowning should begin with an assessment for such conditions. If no causative condition can be found, or if attempts to eliminate the cause are unsuccessful, treatment should be instituted. Nonmedication management includes light therapy, elimination of daytime napping, and a structured activity program (Bliwise 2000). More research is needed to determine the efficacy of these interventions.

Medication management of sundowning is also an area in which more research is needed. Several studies have examined the use of benzodiazepines for the treatment of sleep problems in patients with Alzheimer's disease and sundowning, and these studies suggest that benzodiazepines are ineffective (Bliwise 2000). Atypical benzodiazepines (nonbenzodiazepine omega-1 benzodiazepine receptor agonists) have been prescribed to treat insomnia (see "Pharmacological Treatment" later in this chapter). Of the atypical benzodiazepines currently available in the United States to treat insomnia, zaleplon and zolpidem, only a preliminary study of zolpidem has been carried out, and the study findings suggest that it may have some efficacy (Shaw et al. 1992). Of all medications prescribed for sundowning, antipsychotic medications have the most evidence of efficacy (Bliwise 2000). Most studies involved older agents. Newer antipsychotics, such as risperidone, olanzapine, and quetiapine, have fewer side effects and are generally recommended (Bliwise 2000); however, studies of these medications are needed. Preliminary data suggest that melatonin may also have some utility. Clearly, more research is needed to address the highly important and difficult-to-treat problem of sleep disorders in patients with Alzheimer's disease.

Parkinson's Disease

Sleep complaints are noted in 60%–90% of individuals with Parkinson's disease (Trenkwalder 1998). The majority of Parkinson's disease patients with affected sleep experience difficulty in initiating and maintaining sleep, daytime fatigue, RLS, and an inability to turn over in bed. The last of these features was rated as the most troublesome symptom of sleep disturbance in a study by Lees et al. (1988). Another sleep problem seen in patients with Parkinson's disease is REM sleep behavior disorder, in which the patient acts out dreams because the paralysis that usually occurs during REM sleep is absent (Clarenbach 2000). Dopaminergic medications used to treat Parkinson's disease, such as carbidopa/levodopa, may contribute to sleep initiation problems and sleep difficulties in the first half of the night and may cause nightmares (Trenkwalder 1998). No study findings indicate how to manage sleep difficulties in patients with Parkinson's disease. The use of sedative-hypnotics and the use of tricyclic antidepressants have been described.

Medical Conditions

Pain

Pain is a central feature of many medical conditions that occur with increased frequency in elderly individuals; these conditions include arthritis, neuropathies, angina, reflux esophagitis, and peptic ulcer disease (Aldrich 2000).

Disruption of sleep is frequently noted in persons with significant pain (Pilowsky et al. 1985). Attempts to ameliorate the condition causing the pain should be the first step. When these attempts fail, treatment for the pain should be instituted. Often, combined behavioral and pharmacological treatment is needed. When treatment of the pain does not eliminate the sleeping difficulty, treatment for the insomnia should be instituted (see "Treatment of Insomnia" later in this chapter).

Chronic Obstructive Pulmonary Disease

Individuals with chronic obstructive pulmonary disease (COPD) have been found to have both subjective and objective evidence of disturbed sleep, but the degree of sleep disruption is unrelated to hypoxemia (Douglas 2000). Also, daytime sleepiness, which is seen in patients with sleep apnea, does not appear to occur. Polysomnography is not routinely indicated for individuals with COPD who have sleep difficulties (Connaughton et al. 1988), and the need for polysomnography in COPD patients should be determined in the same way that the need in other patients is determined. Sleep apnea appears to be no more common in persons with COPD than in the general population. Nocturnal oxygen may be needed in some patients; however, patients who tend to become most hypoxemic at night are patients who are most hypoxemic during the day (Connaughton et al. 1988). Oral theophyllines, which are frequently used in COPD treatment, are adenosine receptor antagonists and may have a sleep-disruptive effect (Douglas 2000). Also, patients with COPD should be instructed to avoid alcohol, which can exacerbate hypoxemia and promote other complications. Benzodiazepines should be used with great caution because they may increase inhibition of ventilatory responses and may worsen nocturnal hypoxemia (Douglas 2000). The effects of nonbenzodiazepine sedatives on COPD have not been determined, but these drugs should be used cautiously.

Cerebrovascular Disease

The sleep pathology associated with cerebrovascular disease depends on which areas of the brain are affected by the condition. Hypersomnia has been associated with lesions of the cephalad portions of the ascending reticular activating system, which includes the midbrain and paramedian region of the thalamus (the thalamic lesions most commonly occur in the dorsomedial nucleus, intralaminar nuclei, and centromedian nucleus) (Bassetti and Chervin 2000). Large lesions of the cerebral hemispheres and lesions of other regions such as the caudate and striatum have been less commonly associated with hypersomnia. Insomnia directly related to damage of specific areas of the brain is much less common than insomnia due to multifactorial complications of strokes or other medical or psychiatric conditions associated with an individual's cerebrovascular disease (Bassetti and Chervin 2000). Therefore, treatment should be directed toward these associated conditions.

Nocturia

The urge to urinate is an often overlooked cause of awakenings in the elderly population (Bliwise 2000). Surprisingly, it has been reported that nocturia (excessive urination at night) is the most common explanation given by elderly individuals for difficulty in maintaining sleep; 63%–72% of elderly persons cite nocturia as a reason for sleep maintenance problems (Middelkoop et al. 1996). Furthermore, several studies have documented the sleep disturbance caused by and daytime adverse effects of nocturia (Bliwise 2000). The most common causes of nocturia are conditions that increase in frequency with age: benign prostatic hypertrophy in men and decreased urethral resistance due to decreased estrogen levels in women (Bliwise 2000). Sleep apnea, which also increases in prevalence in the elderly population, can also lead to nocturia (Bliwise 2000). Thus, when evaluating elderly individuals with complaints of sleep maintenance, the clinician should assess for nocturia and the associated conditions that increase the risk of nocturia. If detected, this disorder can generally be effectively treated by addressing the underlying condition.

Menopause

Despite the enormous number of individuals with menopause-related sleep difficulties, there is a striking lack of research in this area (Krystal et al. 1998). Although little is known, there appears to be clear evidence that many women experience sleep disruption in association with vasomotor symptoms (night sweats, hot flushes, decreased urethral resistance often leading to nocturia) that are caused by decreased levels of circulating estrogen and progesterone (Bliwise 2000; Krystal et al. 1998). Several factors hinder elucidation of menopausal sleep disturbance. One is that many disorders that cause insomnia increase in frequency with age and are highly prevalent during the period in which women experience menopausal changes. Another factor is that although hormone replacement therapy is highly effective in ameliorating the vasomotor symptoms of menopause, the subjective reports of sleep disturbance often do not change (Krystal et

al. 1998). Although menopausal sleep disturbance is poorly understood, it has been suggested that behavioral conditioning occurs, just as is often the case with individuals who, having experienced insomnia during a period of high stress, continue to have insomnia after the stress has resolved (Krystal et al. 1998).

Given these considerations, elderly women with insomnia should be evaluated for underlying causes of sleep disturbance (e.g., medical and psychiatric conditions, primary sleep disorders), and it should be determined whether there is an association between changes in menstrual periods, vasomotor symptoms, and insomnia symptoms. If an association between insomnia and menopausal changes appears to exist, a trial of hormone replacement therapy could be considered. If hormone replacement therapy is contraindicated, or use of this treatment is not preferred, other treatments such as pharmacological management of insomnia or cognitive-behavioral sleep therapy should be considered (see discussions in "Pharmacological Treatment" and "Behavioral Treatment" later in this chapter). If hormone replacement therapy ameliorates vasomotor symptoms but insomnia complaints persist, behavioral therapy should be considered.

Loss of Hearing, Vision, and Mobility

Many elderly individuals experience decrements in hearing, vision, and mobility (e.g., walking, driving). These changes are due to a variety of medical conditions that increase in frequency with age. Changes in these vital functions can have a profound effect on sleep. Most frequently, this effect stems from a loss of activities in which the affected individual can engage. The person then takes unplanned naps or tries to sleep more than he or she is physiologically able to, in order to pass the time. The result is fragmentation of sleep and loss of circadian rhythmicity. Affected individuals report spending many frustrating hours awake in bed at night. Although this problem should be easily solved by increasing activity and developing new activity options, in practice, making these changes is difficult to achieve.

Evaluation of Individuals With Sleep-Related Complaints

The first step in evaluating a patient with sleep-related complaints is a comprehensive clinical evaluation. The patient should be carefully assessed for sleep disorders and for underlying medical, psychiatric, and environmental conditions. A physical examination should be performed if the history suggests a need for it. Several laboratory tests are available to the clinician, including overnight polysomnography and the Multiple Sleep Latency Test (MSLT). Subjective sleep logs and actigraphy can also be used. Each of these methods of assessment may be useful, depending on the nature of the complaint.

Polysomnography is the primary laboratory test in sleep medicine. It allows the determination of stages of sleep (wakefulness; Stage I, II, III, and IV sleep; and REM sleep) throughout the night, as well as monitoring of nocturnal breathing, movements, cardiac function, and brain function. Polysomnography is primarily used to evaluate for sleep apnea, PLMD, nocturnal seizures, and nocturnal medical or psychiatric events.

The MSLT is a daytime test in which the patient takes a series of four or five naps spaced 2 hours apart throughout the day. This test provides a physiological assessment of daytime sleepiness and is part of the assessment of narcolepsy.

A subjective sleep log can be useful, particularly in the assessment of complaints of insomnia and circadian rhythm disturbances. Each morning on awakening, for at least a week, the patient records information about the previous night's sleep. This information typically includes the time to bed, time to onset of sleep, number of awakenings during the night, length of awakenings, time of final awakening, rise time, quality of the night's sleep, and level of restedness. In addition, naps during the previous day and the use of sleep aids are recorded.

Actigraphy is an objective assessment of activity throughout the day and night. Patients wear an actometer, which is much like a wristwatch, 24 hours a day for several days. Data are typically recorded in 1-minute epochs and stored in the actometer's memory. The information is used to characterize the typical sleep-wake patterns and to determine the amount of wakefulness during the sleep period.

Choice of these methods is determined by the presenting complaint. For example, an individual complaining of excessive daytime sleepiness and snoring at night usually requires overnight polysomnography. Someone complaining of difficulty in staying asleep at night requires a sleep log assessment. An individual suspected of having narcolepsy requires polysomnography followed by an MSLT the next day. A person who complains of an inability to fall asleep until 3 A.M. and difficulty in awakening before noon may need actigraphy and a sleep log assessment.

To develop a diagnosis and a treatment plan, the clinician must combine the results of laboratory tests with the information obtained during the comprehensive evaluation. The treatment plan may include further testing, consultation, or institution of a treatment regimen.

Treatment of Insomnia

Although changes in sleep appear to be a part of aging, insomnia is not an inevitable consequence of aging. No treatment is needed to address the changes in sleep that normally occur. However, when individuals experience insomnia as defined in the chapter introduction, treatment should be instituted, because untreated insomnia is associated with significant morbidity and decreased quality of life (Gislason and Almqvist 1987; Zammit et al. 1999). Treatment of insomnia in elderly patients poses some particular challenges. We now discuss the two major types of treatment for insomnia: cognitive-behavioral therapy and pharmacological treatment. In this discussion, we focus on issues relevant to elderly patients.

Cognitive-Behavioral Therapy

Myriad lifestyle changes that accompany aging increase risks of insomnia among older adults (Morgan 2000). With aging comes the increased incidence of infirmities that lead to reduced activity levels and a general flattening of the sleep-wake activity rhythm. Retirement leads to increased vacant time and a loss of both routine and zeitgebers that regulate and stabilize the sleep-wake cycle. Retirement coupled with loss of a spouse may lead to dramatically reduced social contacts and increased boredom. Many individuals attempt to reduce hours of daytime boredom by daytime napping and by staying in bed longer during their nighttime sleep period. Such practices often lead to increased nocturnal wake time. Dysfunctional beliefs about sleep, such as "everyone should try to get 8 hours a night" and "older adults can do little to improve their sleep," may actually perpetuate sleep difficulties over time (Means and Edinger 2002; Morin et al. 1993). Nonpharmacological interventions that address these misconceptions and the sleep-disruptive habits they sustain are often useful for combating insomnia in older patients.

Currently, a range of behavioral interventions are available for treating these patients, including relaxation therapies, cognitive therapies, and treatments that target disruptive sleep habits. Among the more effective of these interventions is stimulus control therapy, developed by Bootzin (1972). This treatment is particularly useful for older adults who have fallen out of a normal sleep-wake routine and for those who compromise their nighttime sleep by excessive daytime napping. Stimulus control therapy addresses such problems by curtailing daytime napping and by enforcing a consistent sleep-wake schedule. In addition, this treatment enhances sleep-inducing qualities of the bedroom by eliminating sleep-incompatible behaviors in bed. The patient with insomnia is instructed to go to bed only when sleepy; establish a standard wake-up time; get out of bed whenever he or she is awake for more than 15–20 minutes; avoid reading, watching TV, eating, worrying, and engaging in other sleep-incompatible behaviors in the bed and bedroom; and refrain from daytime napping. This treatment has appeal because it is easily understood and usually can be outlined in one visit. However, follow-up visits are usually needed to assure compliance and achieve optimal success.

Because older adults appear to have a reduced homeostatic sleep drive (Dijk et al. 1997) as well as a propensity to spend excessive time in bed (Carskadon et al. 1982), measures are often needed to reduce the amount of time older patients with insomnia routinely allot for nocturnal sleep. Such a reduction is the aim of sleep restriction therapy (Spielman et al. 1987). Typically, this treatment begins with the patient maintaining a sleep log. After 2–3 weeks, the average total sleep time (TST) is calculated. Subsequently, an initial time-in-bed (TIB) prescription may be set either at the average TST or at a value equal to the average TST plus an amount of time that is deemed to represent normal nocturnal wakefulness (e.g., 30 minutes). However, unless evidence suggests that the individual has an unusually low sleep requirement, the initial TIB prescription is seldom set at less than 5 hours per night. The TIB prescription is increased by 15- to 20-minute increments after weeks in which the person with insomnia sleeps more than 85%–90% of the TIB, on average, and continues to report daytime sleepiness. Conversely, TIB is usually reduced by similar increments after weeks in which the individual sleeps less than 80% of the time spent in bed, on average. Because TIB adjustments are usually necessary, sleep restriction therapy typically entails an initial visit, when treatment instructions are given, and follow-up visits, when TIB prescriptions are altered.

Research suggests that stimulus control and sleep restriction therapies are more effective than most other nonpharmacological interventions (Morin et al. 1999; Murtagh and Greenwood 1995). Moreover, a recent meta-analytic comparison suggests that behavioral therapies compare favorably with hypnotic pharmacotherapies in terms of short-term treatment effects and, unlike hypnotics, have enduring benefits and few side effects (Smith et al. 2002). Recent clinical trials have also generally suggested that therapies combining stimulus control, sleep restriction, and cognitive strategies to alter dysfunctional, sleep-related beliefs hold particular promise for treatment of the sleep maintenance difficulties so

common in older age groups (Edinger et al. 2001; Morin et al. 1999). Given such findings, behavioral interventions should be included in treatment plans for older patients with insomnia, particularly when improper sleep scheduling and other lifestyle factors contribute to sleep complaints.

Pharmacological Treatment

The use of medications for the treatment of insomnia is controversial. Untreated insomnia is associated with significant adverse effects (Gislason and Almqvist 1987; Zammit et al. 1999), and medications rapidly and effectively treat this condition (Nowell et al. 1997). However, medications used to treat insomnia are associated with a number of limitations, including side effects, tolerance, physical dependence, and withdrawal symptoms (Nowell et al. 1997). Therefore, use of medications, particularly for more than 1 month at a time, should be avoided if possible ("Consensus Conference" 1984). In particular, other therapies should be the cornerstone of treatment for the 80% of individuals whose insomnia is due to an underlying medical or psychiatric condition (Kupfer and Reynolds 1997). In these patients, treatment should focus on the underlying condition. When aggressive management of the underlying condition is unsuccessful or the underlying condition cannot be eliminated, and when cognitive-behavioral therapy fails or is not indicated, use of a medication for treatment of the insomnia should be considered. In the 20% of patients with primary insomnia, drug therapy should be instituted if cognitive-behavioral therapy is unsuccessful, not indicated, or not preferred by the patient. Thus, the decision to prescribe medications for the treatment of insomnia should involve weighing the risks and benefits associated with medication management versus the risks and benefits of other options.

Once the decision has been made to use medications to treat insomnia, a number of factors should be considered. Different types of medications are used to treat insomnia. These drugs have different mechanisms of action and differ significantly in their attributes. The predominant medications include benzodiazepines, nonbenzodiazepine omega-1 receptor agonists (sometimes referred to as *atypical benzodiazepines*, the term used throughout this chapter), antidepressants, antihistamines (most commonly, diphenhydramine), and chloral hydrate.

Nearly all medications approved by the U.S. Food and Drug Administration (FDA) for the treatment of insomnia are related to benzodiazepine receptors. The efficacy of these medications has been demonstrated in a number of studies (Nowell et al. 1997). Currently, the

TABLE 20–1. Attributes of medications used to treat insomnia

	Half-life (hours)	Principal side effects
Benzodiazepines	2.9–74[a]	Motor and cognitive impairment
Zolpidem	2.6 ± 1	Motor and cognitive impairment (less than with benzodiazepine use)
Zaleplon	1	Motor and cognitive impairment (less than with benzodiazepine use)
Tricyclic antidepressants	12–43	Anticholinergic effects, weight gain, orthostatic hypotension, sexual dysfunction
Trazodone	11 ± 5	Orthostatic hypotension, priapism (rare)
Mirtazapine	20–40	Dry mouth, weight gain
Nefazodone	17 ± 6	Dry mouth, dizziness
Diphenhydramine	4 ± 2	Anticholinergic effects, motor impairment
Chloral hydrate	7 ± 3	Alcohol interaction, gastric irritation, motor and cognitive impairment, respiratory depression at high doses

[a]Benzodiazepine half-lives: flurazepam = 74 ± 24; diazepam = 43 ± 13; quazepam = 39; lorazepam = 14 ± 5; estazolam = 12 ± 12; temazepam = 11 ± 6; triazolam = 2.9 ± 1.
Source. Golden et al. 1998; Hobbs et al. 1996; Physicians' Desk Reference 2002; Potter et al. 1998.

most commonly prescribed medications are the atypical benzodiazepines. Although not FDA-approved for the treatment of insomnia, antidepressant medications have enjoyed a substantial increase in use since the mid-1980s—an increase that has coincided with a significant decrease in the use of benzodiazepines (Walsh and Engelhardt 1992). These statistics reflect a concern about tolerance of, withdrawal from, and the abuse potential of benzodiazepine-related medications, and in keeping with this concern, the FDA has thus far approved the use of these medications for only 1 month or less ("Consensus Conference" 1984). Besides withdrawal symptoms and abuse potential, other factors to be considered when choosing medications include half-life and side effects. Table 20–1 is a comparison of these factors by drug and drug class.

The fact that the most commonly prescribed medications, atypical benzodiazepines, have the shortest half-lives reflects an appreciation that the ideal sedative-hypnotic agent acts during the desired sleep period and has no effect after this period. Nearly all the older drugs have half-lives that suggest a much longer duration of action and the possibility of significant daytime impairment in some individuals. In particular, drugs such as flurazepam, diazepam, and quazepam may be useful for treating anxiety and depression because of their daytime effects after a bedtime dose, but these medications should not be used to treat insomnia except in unusual circumstances. Furthermore, problems with daytime impairment with these long-half-life medications are exacerbated in the elderly, who tend to metabolize drugs more slowly.

Of the medications most frequently used to treat insomnia, zaleplon has the shortest half-life, and therefore this drug is well suited for treating problems falling asleep. Because of its short half-life, zaleplon may also be useful in the middle of the night for individuals who sometimes wake up at that time (Stone et al. 2002). For some individuals, the half-life of zaleplon is too short to address their sleep difficulties. Although zolpidem has a longer half-life, it does not appear to have significant next-day effects in elderly patients; therefore, this medication can be used to treat both sleep initiation and sleep maintenance problems (Scharf et al. 1991). In individuals with severe early-morning awakening, zolpidem may have too short a duration of action, and an agent with a longer half life will be needed. The need for a longer-acting agent may be particularly likely with elderly individuals, who tend to be particularly prone to difficulty in staying asleep (see "Influence of Aging on Sleep and Circadian Functions" earlier in this chapter).

Medication-caused motor impairment is a particular concern in the elderly population. A risk of falls and associated fractures can occur 1) between the time of taking medication and getting into bed; 2) when the individual gets up in the middle of the night to use the bathroom (or for other reasons); and 3) the following day, in the case of long-half-life drugs. Indeed, several studies involving elderly subjects have indicated that use of benzodiazepines (particularly those with longer half-lives) significantly increases the risk of hip fracture (Ray et al. 1989; Wang et al. 2001a). For this reason, it is best to avoid prescribing benzodiazepines and any medication that causes motor impairment or, if use of such drugs is absolutely necessary, to prescribe as low a dose as possible, which will decrease the risk of falls. Zaleplon and zolpidem both appear to be associated with less risk of motor impairment compared with benzodiazepines, although one report notes an increased risk of hip fractures in elderly individuals taking zolpidem (Wang et al. 2001b). Furthermore, it is important to warn patients of the possibility of being unsteady on their feet when they are taking a medication that may cause this side effect; patients can then take precautions.

Similarly, many elderly individuals with insomnia have coexisting memory impairment that may be exacerbated by sedative-hypnotic medications. As a result, it is best to avoid using medications with memory impairment as a side effect, if possible, and to use the lowest dose possible in all circumstances. The anticholinergic effects of some antidepressants and diphenhydramine may also exacerbate memory difficulties, and these drugs are not tolerated well by elderly individuals prone to constipation and urinary retention.

Despite the FDA's approval of the use of sedative-hypnotic medications for periods of 1 month or less, longer-term treatment with medications is sometimes needed—for example, when an individual has chronic primary insomnia or has secondary insomnia and the underlying condition (assuming treatment of that condition does not ameliorate the insomnia) persists for longer than a month. The adverse effects of untreated insomnia (Gislason and Almqvist 1987; Zammit et al. 1999) have to be weighed against the problems associated with longer-term medication management of insomnia. The primary considerations are that 1) the risks of physical dependence and withdrawal symptoms increase as treatment increases and 2) exposure of individuals to side effects for a longer period increases the chances of an adverse event. When a decision has been made to implement longer-term medication management, atypical benzodiazepines and antidepressants are preferred, because fewer dependence and withdrawal problems are associated with their use. Antidepressants are best in this regard and may be useful when individuals can tolerate their side effects and do not experience the next-day effects that can occur because of the drugs' long half-lives.

In summary, medications may be needed for primary and secondary insomnia when other treatment options are not effective. In elderly patients, it is generally best to use short-half-life drugs; however, drugs with longer half-lives are sometimes needed if difficulty in staying asleep, a particular problem in the elderly population, is not adequately addressed. It is best to avoid using medications that cause motor and cognitive impairment, and

it is generally best to start with lower doses than used in nonelderly adults.

Conclusion

Management of sleep disorders in elderly patients is challenging. Although sleep disorders are not an inevitable consequence of aging, elderly persons are more prone to primary sleep disorders and medical and psychiatric conditions that cause sleep difficulties. Therefore, evaluation of a sleep complaint in an elderly individual should include a thorough workup to determine whether primary sleep pathology and associated psychiatric and medical disorders are present. Effective behavioral and medication treatments exist for treating sleep and circadian rhythm disorders in elderly patients, but these treatments have significant limitations. More research is needed to develop and assess nonmedication therapies that are effective in treating insomnia and normalizing the circadian rhythm. Particularly promising areas include cognitive-behavioral sleep therapy, exercise programs, and light therapy.

In addition, research to improve medication treatment is needed. Medications are needed that can help elderly individuals stay asleep and that do so without causing next-day sedation. Furthermore, medications are needed that do not cause motor or cognitive impairment or anticholinergic side effects and that are not associated with tolerance, dependence, or withdrawal problems. Although atypical benzodiazepines are improvements over benzodiazepines, controlled studies of the long-term safety and efficacy of the former are needed. Also, few studies of the efficacy and safety of antidepressants as sedative-hypnotics have been carried out; such studies are also needed. New sedative-hypnotic drugs under development include compounds that are unrelated to benzodiazepine receptors. Such compounds may be free of typical benzodiazepine effects, including motor and cognitive impairment, tolerance, dependence, and withdrawal symptoms.

Finally, a better understanding of sundowning is needed, as are more effective treatments for this common condition.

References

Aldrich MS: Cardinal manifestations of sleep disorders, in Principles and Practice of Sleep Medicine, 3rd Edition. Edited by Kryger MH, Roth T, Dement WC. Philadelphia, PA, WB Saunders, 2000, pp 526–534

American Psychiatric Association: Diagnostic and Statistical Manual of Mental Disorders, 4th Edition, Text Revision. Washington, DC, American Psychiatric Association, 2000

American Sleep Disorders Association: The International Classification of Sleep Disorders: Diagnostic and Coding Manual, Revised Edition. Rochester, MN, American Sleep Disorders Association, 1997

Ancoli-Israel S: Epidemiology of sleep disorders. Clin Geriatr Med 5:347–362, 1989

Ancoli-Israel S, Kripke DF, Mason W: Characteristics of obstructive and central sleep apnea in the elderly: an interim report. Biol Psychiatry 22:741–750, 1987

Ancoli-Israel S, Kripke DF, Klauber MR, et al: Periodic limb movements in sleep in community-dwelling elderly. Sleep 14:496–500, 1991

Asnis GM, Chakraburtty A, DuBoff EA: Zolpidem for persistent insomnia in SSRI-treated depressed patients. J Clin Psychiatry 60:668–676, 1999

Bassetti C, Chervin R: Cerebrovascular diseases, in Principles and Practice of Sleep Medicine, 3rd Edition. Edited by Kryger MH, Roth T, Dement WC. Philadelphia, PA, WB Saunders, 2000, pp 1072–1086

Bliwise DL: Sleep in normal aging and dementia. Sleep 16:40–81, 1993

Bliwise DL: Normal aging, in Principles and Practice of Sleep Medicine, 3rd Edition. Edited by Kryger MH, Roth T, Dement WC. Philadelphia, PA, WB Saunders, 2000, pp 26–42

Bliwise D[L], Petta D, Seidel W, et al: Periodic leg movements during sleep in the elderly. Arch Gerontol Geriatr 4:273–281, 1985

Bootzin RR: A stimulus control treatment for insomnia. Proc Am Psychol Assoc 7:395–396, 1972

Carskadon MA, Brown ED, Dement WC: Sleep fragmentation in the elderly: relationship to daytime sleep tendency. Neurobiol Aging 3:321–327, 1982

Clarenbach P: Parkinson's disease and sleep. J Neurol 247 (suppl 4):IV20–IV23, 2000

Clark MM: Restless legs syndrome. J Am Board Fam Pract 14:368–374, 2001

Connaughton JJ, Catterall JR, Elton RA, et al: Do sleep studies contribute to the management of patients with severe chronic obstructive pulmonary disease? Am Rev Respir Dis 138:341-344, 1988

Consensus Conference: Drugs and insomnia: the use of medications to promote sleep. JAMA 251:2410–2414, 1984

Czeisler CA, Johnson MP, Duffy JF, et al: Exposure to bright light and darkness to treat physiologic maladaptation to night work. N Engl J Med 322:1253–1259, 1990

Czeisler CA, Duffy JF, Shanahan TL, et al: Stability, precision, and near-24-hour period of the human circadian pacemaker. Science 284:2177–2181, 1999

Dickel MJ, Mosko SS: Morbidity cut-offs for sleep apnea and periodic leg movements in predicting subjective complaints in seniors. Sleep 13:155–166, 1990

Dijk DJ, Duffy JF, Riel E, et al: Altered interaction of circadian and homeostatic aspects of sleep propensity results in awakening at an earlier circadian phase in older people. J Sleep Res 26:710, 1997

Douglas NJ: Chronic obstructive pulmonary disease, in Principles and Practice of Sleep Medicine, 3rd Edition. Edited by Kryger MH, Roth T, Dement WC. Philadelphia, PA, WB Saunders, 2000, pp 965–975

Duffy JF, Dijk DJ, Klerman EB, et al: Later endogenous circadian temperature nadir relative to an earlier wake time in older people. Am J Physiol 275:R1478–R1487, 1998

Edinger JD, Wohlgemuth WK, Radtke RA, et al: Cognitive behavioral therapy for treatment of chronic primary insomnia: a randomized controlled trial. JAMA 285:1856–1864, 2001

Foley DJ, Monjan AA, Brown SL, et al: Sleep complaints among elderly persons: an epidemiologic study of three communities. Sleep 18:425–432, 1995

Folkard S, Totterdell P: "Time since sleep" and "body clock" components of alertness and cognition. Acta Psychiatr Belg 94:73–74, 1994

Gislason T, Almqvist M: Somatic diseases and sleep complaints. An epidemiological study of 3,201 Swedish men. Acta Med Scand 221:475–481, 1987

Golden RN, Dawkins K, Nicholas L, et al: Trazodone, nefazodone, bupropion, and mirtazapine, in Textbook of Psychopharmacology, 2nd Edition. Edited by Schatzberg AF, Nemeroff CB. Washington, DC, American Psychiatric Press, 1998, pp 251–269

Hall M, Buysse DJ, Dew MA, et al: Intrusive thoughts and avoidance behaviors are associated with sleep disturbances in bereavement-related depression. Depress Anxiety 6:106–112, 1997

Hirshkowitz M, Moore CA, Hamilton CR, et al: Polysomnography of adults and elderly: sleep architecture, respiration, and leg movement. J Clin Neurophysiol 9:56–62, 1992

Hobbs WR, Rall TW, Verdoorn TA: Hypnotics and sedatives; ethanol, in Goodman & Gilman's The Pharmacological Basis of Therapeutics, 9th Edition. Edited by Hardman JG, Limbird LE. New York, McGraw-Hill, 1996, pp 361–398

Hoch CC, Buysse DJ, Reynolds CF: Sleep and depression in late life. Clin Geriatr Med 5:259–272, 1989

Krystal AD, Edinger J, Wohlgemuth W, et al: Sleep in perimenopausal and post-menopausal women. Sleep Med Rev 2:243–253, 1998

Kupfer DJ, Reynolds CF III: Management of insomnia. N Engl J Med 336:341–346, 1997

Lees AJ, Blackburn NA, Campbell VL: The nighttime problems of Parkinson's disease. Clin Neuropharmacol 11:512–519, 1988

Means MK, Edinger JD: Behavioral treatment of insomnia. Expert Review of Neurotherapeutics 2:127–137, 2002

Middelkoop HA, Smilde-van den Doel DA, Neven AK, et al: Subjective sleep characteristics of 1,485 males and females aged 50–93: effects of sex and age and factors related to self-evaluated quality of sleep. J Gerontol A Biol Sci Med Sci 51:M108–M115, 1996

Minors DS, Waterhouse JM, Akerstedt T: The effect of the timing, quality, and quantity of sleep upon the depression (masking) of body temperature on an irregular sleep/wake schedule. J Sleep Res 3:45–51, 1994

Morgan K: Sleep and aging, in Treatment of Late-Life Insomnia. Edited by Lichstein KL, Morin CM. Thousand Oaks, CA, Sage, 2000, pp 3–36

Morin CM, Stone J, Trinkle D, et al: Dysfunctional beliefs and attitudes about sleep among older adults with and without insomnia complaints. Psychol Aging 8:463–467, 1993

Morin CM, Colecchi C, Stone J, et al: Behavioral and pharmacological therapies for late-life insomnia: a randomized controlled trial. JAMA 281:991–1035, 1999

Murtagh DR, Greenwood KM: Identifying effective psychological treatments for insomnia: a meta-analysis. J Consult Clin Psychol 63:79–89, 1995

National Institutes of Health Consensus Development Conference Statement: The treatment of sleep disorders in older people March 26–28, 1990. Sleep 14:169–177, 1991

Nowell PD, Mazumdar S, Buysse DJ, et al: Benzodiazepines and zolpidem for chronic insomnia: a meta-analysis of treatment efficacy. JAMA 278:2170–2177, 1997

O'Keeffe ST, Gavin K, Lavan JN: Iron status and restless legs syndrome in the elderly. Age Ageing 23:200–203, 1994

Physicians' Desk Reference, 56th Edition. Montvale, NJ, Medical Economics, 2002

Pilowsky I, Crettenden I, Townley M: Sleep disturbance in pain clinic patients. Pain 23:27–33, 1985

Pollack CP, Perlick D: Sleep problems and institutionalization of the elderly. J Geriatr Psychiatry Neurol 4:204–210, 1991

Pollack CP, Perlick D, Lisner JP, et al: Sleep problems in the community elderly as predictors of death and nursing home placement. J Community Health 15:123–135, 1990

Potter WZ, Manji HK, Rudorfer MV: Tricyclics and tetracyclics, in Textbook of Psychopharmacology, 2nd Edition. Edited by Schatzberg AF, Nemeroff CB. Washington, DC, American Psychiatric Press, 1998, pp 239–250

Prinz PN: Sleep and sleep disorders in older adults. J Clin Neurophysiol 12:139–146, 1995

Prinz PN, Peskind ER, Vitaliano PP, et al: Changes in the sleep and waking EEGs of nondemented and demented elderly subjects. J Am Geriatr Soc 30:86–93, 1982

Prinz PN, Vitiello MV, Raskind MA, et al: Geriatrics: sleep disorders and aging. N Engl J Med 323:520–526, 1990

Ray WA, Griffin MR, Downey W: Benzodiazepines of long and short elimination half-life and the risk of hip fracture. JAMA 262:3303–3307, 1989

Riedel BW, Lichstein KL: Objective sleep measures and subjective sleep satisfaction: how do older adults with insomnia define a good night's sleep? Psychol Aging 13:159–163, 1998

Roehrs T, Zorick F, Sicklesteel J, et al: Age-related sleep-wake disorders at a sleep disorder center. J Am Geriatr Soc 31:364–370, 1983

Sanford JRA: Tolerance of debility in elderly dependants by supporters at home: its significance for hospital practice. Br Med J 3:471–473, 1975

Scharf MB, Mayleben DW, Kaffeman M, et al: Dose response effects of zolpidem in normal geriatric subjects. J Clin Psychiatry 52:77–83, 1991

Shaw SH, Curson H, Coquelin JP: A double-blind comparative study of zolpidem and placebo in the treatment of insomnia in elderly psychiatric inpatients. J Int Med Res 20:150–161, 1992

Smith MT, Perlis ML, Park A, et al: Comparative meta-analysis of pharmacotherapy and behavior therapy for persistent insomnia. Am J Psychiatry 159:5–11, 2002

Spielman AJ, Saskin P, Thorpy MJ: Treatment of chronic insomnia by restriction of time in bed. Sleep 10:45–55, 1987

Stone BM, Turner C, Mills SL, et al: Noise-induced sleep maintenance insomnia: hypnotic and residual effects of zaleplon. Br J Clin Pharmacol 53:196–202, 2002

Trenkwalder C: Sleep dysfunction in Parkinson's disease. Clin Neurosci 5:107–114, 1998

Walsh JK, Engelhardt CL: Trends in the pharmacologic treatment of insomnia. J Clin Psychiatry 53:10–17, 1992

Wang PS, Bohn RL, Glynn RJ, et al: Hazardous benzodiazepine regimens in the elderly: effects of half-life, dosage, and duration on risk of hip fracture. Am J Psychiatry 158:892–898, 2001a

Wang PS, Bohn RL, Glynn RJ, et al: Zolpidem use and hip fractures in older people. J Am Geriatr Soc 49:1685–1690, 2001b

White DP: Central sleep apnea, in Principles and Practice of Sleep Medicine, 3rd Edition. Edited by Kryger MH, Roth T, Dement WC. Philadelphia, WB Saunders, 2000, pp 827–839

Zammit GK, Weiner J, Damato N, et al: Quality of life in people with insomnia. Sleep 22 (suppl 2):S379–S385, 1999

Zepelin H, McDonald CS, Zammit GK: Effects of age on auditory awakening thresholds. J Gerontol 39:294–300, 1984

Alcohol and Drug Problems

Dan G. Blazer, M.D., Ph.D.

The problems of alcohol and drug abuse in late life are closely related. Of the two, alcohol abuse is the more publicized but not necessarily the more prevalent. Misuse of both alcohol and drugs in the United States derives from the context of Western society. Primary care physicians and geriatric psychiatrists cannot diagnose or treat these disorders without appreciating the milieu from which they emerge and the factors that reinforce the behaviors.

Use of alcohol has a long and complex history in human societies (Maddox and Blazer 1985). Among the ancients, alcohol was described as the "water of life" and given magical, symbolic significance in religious and social ceremonies that marked transitions over the life course from birth to death. In other words, alcohol is such a domesticated drug—the recreational beverage of choice—that it is difficult to discuss alcohol as a potentially addictive substance like those "other drugs," such as cocaine. Yet clinicians are ambivalent about alcohol, and with good reason. Alcohol is associated with a wide range of personal and social problems across the life span. For example, intoxication is involved in an estimated 50% of all traffic fatalities.

Drug abuse must also be considered in the context of its culture. Neither illegal nor prescription drugs are perceived as recreational by the vast majority of older adults. Admitted drug abuse is a rare phenomenon in the older adult. Nevertheless, 25% of drugs and drug sundries consumed in this country are consumed by adults age 65 and older—2.5 times the proportion for the entire population. Older adults frequently have one or more chronic illnesses, and most of these individuals will take at least one prescription medication in any given year. Elderly people are comfortable taking medications, and many are skilled at detecting the optimal dose for certain types of subjective effects. They also recognize the nuances of side effects from one medication to another. The verita-

ble "pharmacy within the medicine cabinet" provides older persons with a wide selection of prescription and over-the-counter agents for treating a given malady. This fact, coupled with the decreased availability of primary medical care in some communities and the increased cost of such care, makes self-medication for physical and mental health problems a common occurrence. An inevitable outcome for older persons in an individualistic society, with multiple barriers to appropriate medical and psychiatric care, is the abuse of prescription and over-the-counter medications.

Both alcohol and drug problems confront clinicians who treat older adults. Occasionally, medication and alcohol misuse or abuse is the primary problem encountered. More often, however, this problem accompanies other disorders and complicates therapy. In this chapter, alcohol and drug problems are reviewed separately because, although these disorders undoubtedly overlap, each has unique characteristics and deserves separate attention.

Alcohol Abuse and Dependence

Investigation of alcohol abuse and dependence among older adults has increased in recent years. The reason for this attention is not a dramatic or even a persistent increase in rates of alcohol problems in the elderly. As reviewed elsewhere in this volume (see Chapter 2, "Demography and Epidemiology of Psychiatric Disorders in Late Life"), the current prevalence of alcohol abuse and dependence for persons ages 65 years and older ranges from 1.9% to 4.6% for men and from 0.1% to 0.7% for women (Myers et al. 1984). In other cultures, rates may be higher. For example, among men age 70 years and older in Sweden, 10% abused alcohol or were heavy drinkers (Mellstrom 1981). Although no differences were found among racial and ethnic groups in the Epidemiologic Catchment Area (ECA) studies (Myers et al. 1984), some studies suggested that rates are higher in older whites than in older African Americans (Ruchlin 1997). In the United States, even the lifetime prevalence of alcohol problems in older adults is lower than for younger persons in the population. This finding may partially be explained by cohort differences in drinking experiences and selective survival of more moderate drinkers. It is anticipated that with the increase of life expectancy rates and the aging of baby boomers, there will be an overall increase in alcohol problems among older adults, given the increase in alcohol problems throughout the population (Liberto et al. 1992). Another point to consider is the increased probability of alcohol-related problems in later life, even at lower levels of use. Saunders (1994) reported that 15% of men and 12% of women older than age 60 treated in primary care clinics drank in excess of the limits recommended by the National Institute on Alcohol Abuse and Alcoholism (NIAAA). The risk factors for alcohol abuse in elderly persons are similar to those for the general population—male gender, poor education, low income, and a history of other psychiatric disorders, especially depression. The comorbidity of alcohol problems and psychiatric illness in late life is 10%–15% (Finlaysen et al. 1988).

One explanation for the increased interest of clinicians in alcohol problems among elderly persons is that late life is perceived as a time of stressful events, such as retirement, widowhood, illness, and isolation. Alcohol use has traditionally been a culturally accepted strategy for stress reduction. With increased stress, older individuals may increase both their alcohol intake and their risk of alcohol-related problems. The decreased ability of the older adult to metabolize alcohol, coupled with concomitant medical problems, increases the risk of accidents, side effects, and overt toxicity. Alcohol abuse may first be noticed by family members as elderly persons become less capable of living alone. Discovery that a parent has a long history of alcohol intake may offend the social sensibilities of middle-aged children and grandchildren, who have held their parents and grandparents in high esteem (Maddox and Blazer 1985). The potential for alcohol problems to emerge in individuals who have maintained a relatively constant intake of alcohol over the majority of their adult lives will increase as more older adults reach their 80s and 90s, for alcohol toxicity can increase with the decreased ability to metabolize alcohol that occurs in late-late life.

Despite the scenario discussed in the last paragraph, the problem of alcohol abuse and dependence in late life, although serious, is not as severe as it is among young adults. Although the population at risk for late-life alcohol problems increases with each successive cohort ("the graying of the Western world"), the rate of increase has not been dramatic. In fact, most older persons living today were raised in a culture that included a strong tradition of temperance. In a national survey by Armor et al. (1977), 52% of elderly men and 68% of elderly women said they were abstainers. These percentages, however, are dropping and will continue to drop in cohorts entering late life in the twenty-first century. The increased percentage of users of alcohol does not necessarily suggest an increased percentage of those who abuse it, although increased per capita consumption is usually associated with an increase in the magnitude of abuse (Faris 1974).

Longitudinal studies of risk factors for alcohol problems in elderly persons are virtually nonexistent. Nevertheless, suggestive data from cross-sectional research may be informative in regard to potential etiological agents. For example, Glatt (1978) identified three precipitating factors in late-onset alcoholism: a habitual drinking pattern before late life, personality factors, and environmental factors. Personality characteristics that predispose to late-life drinking problems include anxiety and worry about one's social environment, such as loss of a loved one and loneliness. Personality factors appear to be less related to late-onset alcoholism than to an onset at earlier stages of the life cycle. Instead, alcohol problems in elderly individuals may precipitate stressful events such as marital discord and social isolation (especially from family). In their survey of alcohol abuse among elderly persons, Rathbone-McCuan et al. (1976) questioned 695 persons ages 55 years and older in Baltimore, Maryland. They found that older alcoholic individuals drank primarily to alleviate depression and to escape existing social problems. The older problem drinkers generally reported poorer health and had more physical problems than did the elderly normal drinkers. In addition, the older problem drinkers had more problems with finances and social isolation. Warheit and Auth (1984) found that, compared with a high-risk alcohol group of younger persons, those in a high-risk alcohol group who were ages 50 years and older were less likely to report difficulties in marital relationships and life satisfaction (although the trend was similar in the younger group).

Risk-factor studies of alcohol intake over time are relatively rare in the literature. Longitudinal studies for drinking patterns, however, are more common and provide insight into changing patterns of alcohol intake through the adult years. For example, more than 1,800 men ages 28–87 were studied for more than 10 years in the Veterans Administration's Normative Study of Aging

(Glynn et al. 1984). In this panel there was almost no change in mean alcohol consumption during the follow-up period. In addition, rates of problems with drinking did not decline over time. These data do not support the findings from previous cross-sectional studies that aging modifies drinking behaviors. Men in their 40s and 50s in 1973 were especially persistent in their alcohol intake over time. Gordon and Kannel (1983) found that participants in the Framingham Heart Study increased their alcohol consumption by more than 63% over a 20-year follow-up period (1952–1972). An increase in consumption from 1952 to 1972 is consistent with the stability in consumption reported in the Veterans Administration's normative aging study (Glynn et al. 1984) if one recognizes that both cohorts were influenced by a national trend toward increased alcohol use. That is, the tendency to decrease alcohol consumption with age may have been counterbalanced by social forces encouraging greater consumption.

In a follow-up of nearly 1,300 adults treated for moderately severe to severe alcohol problems, Helzer and colleagues (1984) found few age differences that predicted outcome. There was some evidence that among the survivors, older alcoholic individuals were less likely to experience persistent, severe problems. At the same time, all-cause mortality was higher for older adults, and alcohol-related mortality was similar for both young and elderly subjects. Among the predictors of continued alcoholism, social isolation was more strongly correlated in the older group than in the younger group. Organic brain syndrome was not associated with outcome for the younger sample, but its absence was associated with a good outcome for the older group. In summary, this sample of treated alcoholic patients followed for 6–10 years revealed a good outcome in a large proportion of the older subjects.

Pharmacological Properties of Alcohol

Ethyl alcohol (ethanol) is absorbed easily through the mucous membranes of the stomach, small intestine, and colon. Although peak blood levels are generally reached within 30–90 minutes after alcohol intake, complete absorption may take 2–6 hours. Many factors alter the rate of absorption, and some of these are age related. In general, alcohol absorption is as rapid in late life as it is at earlier stages of the life cycle. Most foods in the stomach retard absorption, especially milk and milk products. In contrast, because absorption from the small intestine is extremely rapid, patients who have undergone gastrectomy frequently complain that they quickly become intoxicated by small amounts of alcohol that would not

have been a problem before the operation (Garver 1984; Muehlberger 1958; Ritchie 1981).

Once absorbed, ethanol is distributed throughout the body, but not evenly. Alcohol is not distributed to fatty tissues (Garver 1984). Older adults have less total body water per unit mass, less extracellular fluid, and higher body fat. The net result is that a standard ingested dose of ethanol will result in a higher blood level in an older adult than in a younger adult because of the lower effective fluid volume for distribution (Wiberg et al. 1971), due in part to an increased proportion of lipid tissue with aging.

More than 90% of the alcohol that enters the body is completely oxidized. This process takes place in the liver, primarily under the influence of the hepatic enzyme alcohol dehydrogenase. There is no evidence that the activity of this enzyme decreases as a function of aging in humans (Garver 1984). At all ages, the metabolism of alcohol is slow and constant. Therefore, a definite limit must be placed on the amount of alcohol that is consumed in a given period; otherwise, intoxication or more serious consequences may result secondary to an accumulation of alcohol. The small amount of alcohol not oxidized may be either excreted in the urine (or other body fluids) or diffused into the alveolar air and exhaled. In other words, the body must process virtually all the alcohol ingested.

The process of alcohol metabolism can lead to secondary problems for the older adult. Gastric secretions are mediated psychically by alcohol, for alcohol is a very strong stimulus if enjoyed by the individual. The presence of alcohol in the stomach in concentrations of about 10% results in gastric secretions rich in acid but poor in pepsin (in contrast to the reflex secretion, which is rich in both). At stronger concentrations (40% or over), alcohol is directly irritating to the mucosa and may cause congestive hyperemia and inflammation. As a result, plasma protein may be lost into the gastrointestinal lumen, and erosive gastritis may ensue (Chowdhury et al. 1977; Ritchie 1981). Alcohol may also facilitate constipation if ingested habitually in moderate amounts. The mechanism is probably secondary to inadequate food intake and insufficient bulk. Diarrhea, on the other hand, may result from the irritant action of alcohol.

The oxidation of alcohol in the liver leads to a change in the ratio of nicotinamide adenine dinucleotide (NAD) to a relative increase in NAD's reduced form, nicotinamide adenine dinucleotide (NADH). This change, in turn, apparently enhances lipid synthesis by the liver. Alcohol may also indirectly promote the accumulation of fatty tissue in the liver. Acetylglycerophosphate increases in concentration with an accompanying stimulation of the esterification of fatty acids, which leads to a collection of fat in the liver (Kalant et al. 1980; Ritchie 1981). Accumulation of fat and an accompanying accumulation of protein may initially cause no difficulties, but eventually the process cannot be reversed, and the result is a progression to various stages of liver disease, especially cirrhosis. Alcoholic fatty liver and cirrhosis are diseases of middle and late life; these conditions are unlikely in persons who consume less than 80 g per day for 10–20 years.

Alcohol also exerts a diuretic effect on the kidneys. This effect appears to occur above and beyond the large amounts of fluids that chronic alcohol abusers usually ingest in alcoholic beverages. This diuresis may be secondary to a decrease in the release of antidiuretic hormone from the posterior pituitary. The relative increase in urine formation can be a problem, especially for elderly men whose urine flow is compromised by prostatic difficulties (Garver 1984; Ritchie 1981).

Although alcohol is popularly thought to be a sexual stimulant, chronic ingestion of alcohol often results in decreased sexual interest, if not impotence. The mechanism by which this effect occurs is a decrease in the release of luteinizing hormone from the anterior pituitary. The older adult who already believes that his or her sexual functioning is compromised may enter a vicious cycle by drinking to avoid the anxiety of decreased sexual performance, yet worsening the disability through alcohol intake.

Physical Consequences of Alcoholism in Later Life

When evaluating alcohol intake over time, the clinician must attend to the interaction between alcohol use and chronic or periodic illness in elderly patients. Although alcohol directly affects organ systems—alcohol increases cardiac rate and output secondary to its effect on cardiac muscle—the primary effect is cumulative. To illustrate this cumulative effect, consider the example of a person with chronic alcoholism who develops compromised hepatic functioning. This compromise in liver function may exacerbate osteomalacia secondary to decreased hepatic metabolism of vitamin D_3 to its more active 25-hydroxylated form.

Undernutrition that results from chronic alcohol intake, especially among those who use large amounts of alcohol over long periods (the "skid-row alcoholics"), commonly leads to cirrhosis. Cirrhosis is one of the eight leading causes of death among persons ages 65 years and older. Alcohol can damage the heart, resulting in alcohol-induced cardiomyopathies. In contrast, however, some investigators reported a reduction in coronary artery dis-

ease in subjects who drink moderate quantities of alcohol over time (Yano et al. 1977). This does not mean, however, that older persons should be advised to drink alcohol to prevent coronary heart disease.

Chronic effects of alcohol intake on the gastrointestinal tract are well known to clinicians who work with older adults. In general, persons with chronic alcoholism have a lower gastric basal acid output, a maximal acid output, and an increased likelihood of developing chronic atrophic gastritis. The preexisting atrophic gastritis that is common in elderly alcoholic individuals may facilitate the formation of gastric mucosal lesions, which lead to upper gastrointestinal bleeding. Absorption of both folic acid and vitamin B_{12} declines with chronic alcohol use. Because these substances are essential to cognitive functioning, their loss through malabsorption or through decreased dietary intake among elderly alcoholic persons may lead to cognitive and psychological impairment as well as the resultant anemias. Peripheral neuropathy may occur in as many as 45% of chronic alcoholic patients because of deficiency in thiamine and other B-complex vitamins.

Nutritional requirements do not change dramatically with aging, although older persons may require more protein (Gersovitz et al. 1982). Chronic alcoholism is associated with reduced intake of a number of nutrients, including protein. Protein malnutrition is manifested in individuals with alcoholism as muscle wasting, hypoproteinemia, and edema. Iron deficiency also occurs, but it is generally due to gastrointestinal blood loss rather than to decreased dietary intake or malabsorption. As noted above, older adults may be more subject to gastric lesions, which in turn may lead to chronic occult bleeding.

A concern equal in importance to the medical consequences of late-life alcohol use is the interaction of aging, alcohol, and dementia. Many investigators report chronic alcoholism to be associated with a variety of neuropsychological and cognitive deficits. Although chronic alcoholism does not appear to disrupt cognitive and neuropsychological functioning diffusely, specific clusters of cognitive functions are affected in the older alcoholic individual. Most investigators agree that intelligence remains relatively unaffected, but deficits are known to occur in memory and information processing. These deficits are similar to the impairment seen in patients suffering from alcoholic amnestic dementia (Wernicke-Korsakoff disease). Specifically, deficits most frequently found in alcoholic individuals are impaired performance in tasks involving visuospatial analysis, tactual spatial analysis, nonverbal abstraction, and set flexibility. Although recovery of many of these functions may occur with abstinence from alcohol, recovery rarely leads to complete remission of symptoms.

Alcohol produces a range of impairment—from the subtle cognitive difficulties that can affect nonalcoholic heavy drinkers, to progressively greater impairment in older adults who drink heavily over short periods of time, to the worst-case scenario of alcoholic amnestic dementia seen in those with long-term alcoholism. This chronic end-stage dementia is caused by thiamine deficiency as well as by the direct toxic effects of alcohol on brain tissue. Postmortem examination of the brains of persons with alcoholic amnestic dementia demonstrates widespread neuronal loss, especially in the frontal regions. Alcoholic patients also experience more rapid rates of cerebral atrophy and degeneration of the mammillary bodies. Clinically, the end stage of alcoholic dementia is characterized by relatively intact intellectual functioning associated with severe anterograde and retrograde amnesia. In contrast to patients with Alzheimer's disease, those with alcoholic dementia who abstain may exhibit stable or even improved short-term memory and motor performance over time.

To appreciate the scope of alcohol problems in the elderly population, the risk of death from alcohol use should be explored. In the 8-year outcome study described by Helzer et al. (1984), 24% of the 234 alcoholic subjects who were age 60 years or older at enrollment died before the study was completed, compared with 9% of the 1,048 alcoholic subjects younger than age 60. However, the proportion of subjects reported to have died of alcohol-related causes was similar for the younger and older alcoholic groups. Although data from death certificates leads to an underestimation of the overall number of deaths due to alcohol, that bias is consistent across age groups.

Nashold and Naor (1981) observed that reports of alcohol as the cause of death in Wisconsin increased markedly between 1963 and 1977. In the older age group, the majority of alcohol-related deaths were due to an underlying cause involving alcohol—for example, cirrhosis. In another study, Edwards and colleagues (1983) followed for 10 years 99 married men diagnosed as having alcoholism. The increase in risk over the expected deaths in this group was 2.68; 5 patients died by suicide or in circumstances suggesting suicide. Alcohol leads to an increased risk of mortality in middle life—thus limiting the number of alcoholic persons who survive to late life—but it is also associated with increasing mortality in late life. The causes of death among these individuals who drink chronically are varied and include suicide, accidents, cardiovascular and liver disease, and even cancer.

A number of parallels have been observed between the sleep characteristics in persons experiencing normal aging and in chronic alcoholic individuals who are abstinent. For example, the sleep of chronic alcoholic patients who have withdrawn from alcohol is characterized by decreased slow-wave sleep, interruptions of sleep, and decreased or interrupted periods of rapid eye movement (REM) sleep (Adamson and Burdick 1973). Prolonged abstinence from alcohol in middle life, however, will lead to improved sleep over time. In other words, the central nervous system (CNS) abnormalities produced by alcohol apparently reverse. The older person who uses alcohol as a sedative experiences an additional sleep problem. The relatively rapid metabolism of alcohol, in contrast to most sedative-hypnotics, may produce a rebound awakening at a point 3–4 hours into sleep. Even though the older adult using alcohol may fall asleep without difficulty, his or her sleep is disrupted during the night.

Given the relatively large number of prescription and nonprescription drugs used by older adults, the interaction of alcohol with these drugs is of special importance to elderly persons. The impairments produced by alcohol are augmented by drugs such as sedatives, anticonvulsants, antidepressants, major and minor tranquilizers, and analgesics (especially the opiates). Poor muscle coordination, impaired judgment, and slurred speech are common when these agents are used together. Other side effects are less frequent but can be equally serious. Older adults using oral hypoglycemic agents to treat adult-onset diabetes (type 2 diabetes mellitus) may experience unpleasant symptoms such as nausea and flushing, as do patients who combine disulfiram and alcohol use. Unpredictable fluctuations of plasma glucose concentrations are another potential adverse effect. The efficacy of some drugs, such as coumarin-type anticoagulants, is blocked by alcohol, because alcohol increases the metabolism of these drugs (Ritchie 1981). In contrast, plasma concentrations of alcohol are usually not changed by the use of other medications (Garver 1984).

Addiction, Tolerance, and Withdrawal

The most significant clinical problem faced by the clinician treating the older alcoholic individual is the potential for addiction and tolerance to the agent, with the concomitant problem of alcohol withdrawal. Because alcohol is a readily available addictive agent in Western society, it is usually the drug of choice for individuals who want to block unpleasant emotions with drugs.

Chronic use of high concentrations of alcohol will lead to addiction. Jaffe (1980) suggested that addiction can be defined operationally as "a behavioral pattern of drug use, characterized by overwhelming involvement with the use of a drug (compulsive use), the securing of its supply, and a high tendency to relapse after withdrawal" (p. 536). Older adults manifest their addiction when placed in a situation in which alcohol is not readily available. They may demonstrate increased anxiety and may pursue alcohol to decrease this anxiety. In addition, they experience sleep disturbance, nausea, and weakness, which are concomitants of a lowered blood alcohol level. Addiction is a unique problem for older adults, for at least two reasons. First, patterns of drinking have continued for many years (often from early or middle life), and lifelong habits are often not associated with problems of recent onset. In addition, the relatively "quiet" use of alcohol over the years desensitizes both the older adult and the family to the problems with alcohol (Pascarelli 1974; Schuckit 1977).

Akin to addiction is the potential for tolerance with chronic use of alcohol. Not only can older adults become tolerant to alcohol, but they may also become cross-tolerant to drugs similar to alcohol. Despite the potential for relatively normal function among alcoholic individuals (even when ethanol blood levels are relatively high), the heavy use of alcohol associated with tolerance continues to create irreversible changes in the liver, the gastrointestinal tract, and the CNS (Bosmann 1984). Cross-tolerance, especially to benzodiazepines, is of major clinical concern. Given that older adults are more likely to take benzodiazepines than are younger persons, the potential for abuse of both agents—separately or in combination—increases dramatically (Mellinger et al. 1978).

Symptoms following alcohol withdrawal are not appreciably different across the life cycle. Nevertheless, the older adult may manifest these symptoms, especially the more severe ones, for a longer period after acute cessation of alcohol intake. Initial symptoms include tremors, anxiety, nausea, vomiting, and perspiration. If the withdrawal syndrome is allowed to continue without intervention—either with a cross-tolerant drug (such as diazepam) or with reinstitution of alcohol—the tremulous state will peak within 1–2 days after the onset of the withdrawal syndrome. This tremulous peak is accompanied by hallucinations and, in severe cases, withdrawal seizures. Confusion, agitation, and disorientation mark the individual's level of consciousness. In the older adult with compromised health, the severity of this withdrawal syndrome is naturally greater (Bosmann 1984; Mello and Mendelson 1977).

Diagnostic Workup

Substance abuse problems in older adults are commonly missed. The Center for Substance Abuse Treatment's (CSAT's) Consensus Panel on Substance Abuse Among Older Adults (1998) recommends that every 60-year-old person should be screened for alcohol and prescription drug abuse as part of any routine physical examination. It is unusual for an older adult or a family member to present alcohol or drug use as a problem, and patient identification of a problem is unlikely to occur without prompting. The clinician is advised to assume that the patient drinks alcohol, and all questions related to the patient's alcohol use should be normalized as a routine and necessary part of every history and physical examination. The NIAAA guideline for older adults should be shared with the patient to help the patient conduct his or her own risk assessment and as a baseline to determine the need for a fuller evaluation. This guideline, as outlined in the Physician's Guide to Helping Patients with Alcohol Problems (National Institute on Alcohol Abuse and Alcoholism 1995), recommends no more than one drink per day and a maximum of two drinks on any drinking occasion. Symptoms of substance or alcohol abuse such as memory impairment, falls, or conflicts with family members may be misidentified as symptoms of aging. Presentation of these types of symptoms can be ideal opportunities to evaluate the patient's alcohol use.

The diagnostic workup of the older adult in whom an alcohol problem is suspected hinges on a comprehensive history. Detailed information should first be obtained from the patient on specifics of the drinking behavior. This information must be supplemented by family members, preferably from two generations. Unfortunately, some alcoholic older adults have virtually no family or other social network (the "skid-row alcoholics"), and historical information is therefore limited.

Questions that should be asked include the following: Does the elderly patient drink, and how often does he or she drink? Does he or she drink constantly? Is there a pattern of binge drinking? Elderly persons who suffer from chronic problems with alcohol are usually regular drinkers. Tolerance for binges decreases with age. A lifetime history of alcohol use provides a background for present patterns of use.

The CAGE questions (Ewing 1984) are commonly used for screening for alcohol problems:

Have you…

- **C**—…felt the need to **C**ut down on your drinking?
- **A**—…ever felt **A**nnoyed by criticism of your drinking?
- **G**—…had **G**uilty feelings about drinking?
- **E**—…ever taken a morning "**E**ye-opener"?

The CAGE questions are not as useful in screening older persons as they are in helping to identify alcohol problems among the younger population. Because older alcoholic individuals with a persistent drinking pattern over time tend to have problems with emergent physical and psychological symptoms, personal guilt or concern about drinking is less common. In fact, the older adult may not recognize the connection between new symptoms and drinking habits that have continued for decades. The Michigan Alcoholism Screening Test—Geriatric Version is a screening instrument specific to elderly persons that has particular utility in screening for alcoholism in older adults (Blow et al. 1992). The Alcohol Use Disorders Identification Test (AUDIT) is recommended by the CSAT Consensus Panel on Substance Abuse Among Older Adults as a tool for identifying problems among older members of ethnic minority groups (Center for Substance Abuse Treatment 1998).

Additional data to identify drinking problems in the elderly should be derived from the following categories: personal health, family health problems, interpersonal difficulties, and work difficulties (Ewing 1985). Patients should be asked about gastrointestinal symptoms such as nausea, vomiting, diarrhea, abdominal pain, and unexplained gastrointestinal hemorrhages. Neurological problems should be reviewed, including episodes of amnesia, headaches, and peripheral neuropathy. Falls, bruises, cuts, sprains, cigarette burns, skin diseases, and lack of attention to personal health often result from excessive alcohol use.

A thorough review of psychiatric symptoms is essential, including a detailed evaluation of cognitive status, history of major depression, symptoms of generalized anxiety, and psychotic symptoms (delusions and hallucinations). Paranoid ideation regarding relatives or friends is not uncommon in the older person who is severely alcoholic. It is critical to document suicidal ideation, given the elevated risk for suicide in both elderly and alcoholic populations.

A genetic predisposition to alcohol problems is less likely to be a contributing etiological factor in the elderly alcoholic patient—especially if the onset of significant drinking problems occurs later in life. Moreover, a history of alcohol abuse in the family of the older adult is also prone to bias, because complete historical information from alcoholic elderly patients regarding parents and siblings is usually difficult or impossible to obtain. A documented family history of psychiatric disorders (especially major depression and schizophrenia) or alcohol abuse or dependence is important nonetheless, and the clinician should search medical records in addition to interviewing the elderly alcoholic patient.

An indicator of emerging alcohol problems among older persons is concomitant problems in interpersonal relations. Although such problems occur most often in the marriage, they can also occur between the older adult and children or, occasionally, friends. Family problems may be the result of the drinking behavior (such as arguments over an appropriate amount to drink) or may result from symptoms of the alcohol abuse (such as paranoid ideation or cognitive difficulties).

During the physical examination of the older adult with alcoholism, the clinician should screen for medical problems that may exacerbate alcohol problems—or that may be exacerbated by chronic alcohol use—as well as for evidence of alcohol abuse, such as signs of neglect of personal hygiene. The neurological examination should be performed in detail, with attention directed to the evaluation of peripheral neuropathy. Traditional signs of chronic alcohol abuse, such as flushing of the face, injected conjunctiva, tremors, and malnutrition, may merge with normal signs of aging or poor health status.

If evidence of cognitive abnormalities emerges during the mental status examination (and it often does), further cognitive workup is indicated. The clinician should make every effort to keep the alcoholic older adult abstinent for 2–3 weeks before a detailed cognitive evaluation. Psychological tests may be threatening to the older adult who fears that deficits will appear that have been previously undetected. Baseline cognitive scores, however, can be especially important in monitoring the longitudinal progress of the patient, as well as in providing additional force to the clinical admonition to abstain from further alcohol use. For example, Parker et al. (1982) found that alcohol consumption above usual levels significantly increases problems with abstraction in formal testing.

Laboratory evaluation of the acutely alcoholic older adult should include thorough liver function evaluation—lactate dehydrogenase (LDH), serum glutamic-oxaloacetic transaminase (SGOT), serum glutamic-pyruvic transaminase (SGPT), and alkaline phosphatase. Given the potential for an electrolyte imbalance in this population, a screening chemistry is essential, with special attention to glucose. Low blood magnesium reflects a magnesium deficiency that may occur with alcohol use. Elevated serum and urine amylase suggest chronic pancreatitis. Alcoholic cardiomyopathy may be manifested on an electrocardiogram as frequent arrhythmias, especially atrial fibrillation.

Once the history, physical examination, and laboratory tests have been completed, the clinician should assign a diagnosis. Schuckit et al. (1985) reviewed the clinical implications of the diagnoses of alcohol abuse and dependence on the basis of DSM-III (American Psychiatric Association 1980). Ideally, a diagnostic system should provide etiological information, prognostic information, and information about response to treatment. Because etiological information is difficult to integrate into a diagnostic system—as is evidenced by the move away from etiology in DSM-III that was retained in subsequent editions of DSM—more emphasis has been placed on prognosis. When Schuckit and colleagues (1985) reviewed the clinical significance of the DSM-III distinction between men with diagnoses of either alcohol abuse or alcohol dependence, the authors found that the two groups were virtually identical. Subjects with alcohol dependence, however, took more drinks per drinking day and had more alcohol-related medical problems and past hospitalizations than those diagnosed as abusers. During the 1-year follow-up, those diagnosed as suffering from alcohol dependence were somewhat more likely to visit a public detoxification facility. Nevertheless, the authors did not support prognostic implications for the differentiation between alcohol abuse and alcohol dependence in alcoholic patients. These data should be considered within the context of the more dependent patterns of alcohol intake that emerge in late life.

Schuckit et al. (1985) also proposed that the criteria for alcohol dependence be changed to include more than just the accumulation of symptoms gathered retrospectively over the span of the alcoholic person's drinking behavior. Specifically, they suggested that more objective criteria be established for tolerance and withdrawal. Schuckit and colleagues' definition of tolerance requires a history of being able to function despite relatively high alcohol concentration—for example, walking or talking coherently in the presence of high blood alcohol levels. Their criteria for withdrawal are a hampered ability to work or to interact with peers or the necessity of medical intervention. In summary, the clinician should adapt the symptom presentations of alcohol abuse or dependence in elderly patients from DSM-IV (and its Text Revision, DSM-IV-TR; American Psychiatric Association 1994, 2000) to make these criteria more relevant to clinical management. Given reduced levels of tolerance and the diminished possibility that the older adult problem drinker will experience the common social, job, or legal consequences commonly associated with substance use disorders, a modified interpretation of the DSM-IV-TR criteria for substance use disorders for older adults should be considered. Documentation of these symptoms and signs, however, is critical regardless of the nomenclature used.

Intervention with the older adult alcoholic can be a challenging predicament. An array of motivational techniques and strategies have been developed and tested with positive results. Fleming et al. (1997) showed that 10%–30% of nondependent problem drinkers modified their drinking behaviors following a brief office-based intervention. Blow and Barry (2000) recently applied this model to adults with success. Prochaska et al. (1992) and Miller and Rollnick (1991) showed that motivational counseling directed toward a patient's readiness for change can lead the patient to accept the need for treatment. Miller and Sanchez (1994) developed the FRAMES model of intervention, providing the following schema for talking with patients about their abuse:

- Feedback about the person's use
- Responsibility of the patient to address the problem
- Advice with regard to what the patient might reasonably do
- Menu of options the patient has for addressing the problem
- Empathy directed to understanding the patient's ambivalence
- Self-efficacy of the patient to do something about the problem

Older adults will typically respond to an intervention approach that addresses substance use in the context of health and related issues. Establishing a controlled-drinking contract when clinically appropriate might be one way of leading patients to their own conclusions about the degree to which they have lost control of their ability to manage their alcohol use behavior. Providing an educational overview of the issue that includes a comparison of the patient's drinking with that of other older adults and with recommended guidelines (e.g., those of NIAAA, discussed earlier in this chapter) may be another useful way of awakening the patient's attention to the need to address the issue further. It is critical that the patient be duly informed of any intervention or treatment that he or she might receive and that an opportunity be given to establish a therapeutic partnership for change. Dictating terms and conditions regarding next steps may compromise the patient's likelihood of compliance. Including others such as family members, peer supports, social workers, and home health personnel in any educational and recommendation communications may prove helpful. It is critical that issues of stigma be addressed by ensuring a clinical presentation of the patient's circumstances. Acknowledging patient ambivalence and the challenges that exist with respect to any recommended behavior change is useful. Cultural issues that reinforce drinking behavior may need to be addressed. A direct and nonjudgmental but serious attitude will better ensure that the patient receives the correct message about the alcohol problem.

Treatment

According to Atkinson and Kofoed (1982), older adults respond to treatment the same as or better than younger adults. Most appropriate are specialized behavioral treatments for substance abuse that employ medical and community-based approaches directed to older adults. The treatment of the older patient with alcohol abuse or dependence must include biological, psychological, and psychotherapeutic interventions within the patient's social milieu, especially the family. The level of care for the older adult should be considered in the context of the patient's motivation, concerns about medical and/or psychiatric risks, and availability of community support. A useful guide in determining placement options might be *Patient Placement Criteria for the Treatment of Substance Related Disorders*, published by the American Society of Addiction Medicine (1996). Generally, the least intensive treatments should be considered first. However, if the older adult has acute intoxication that leads to a stuporous or comatose state, acute hospitalization must be instituted for withdrawal from alcohol and for institution of the therapeutic program (initially, pharmacological therapy). In milder cases of alcohol dependence, in which withdrawal is the first step, treatment may proceed in the outpatient setting. Outpatient withdrawal is possible only if the patient is highly motivated and is willing to allow open monitoring of the withdrawal program by the family, with frequent (often daily) contact with the clinician. In any case, the initial step in the treatment of alcoholism is to stop alcohol intake. Attempts to work over longer periods of time with the alcoholic individual who continues to drink are doomed to failure.

In the treatment of the older patient who is severely alcoholic, restoration of fluid and electrolyte balance during the initial phase of withdrawal is essential. Complaints of thirst and dry mucous membranes may delude the clinician into accepting a diagnosis of dehydration when, in fact, drying is resulting from alcohol expiration through the lungs. To avoid iatrogenic overhydration, the clinician should begin administration of 500–1,000 mL of a 5% normal saline solution while waiting for the results of the blood chemistry screen. Use of glucose solutions should be avoided; the older alcoholic patient may have subsisted on a diet high in carbohydrates, in addition to alcohol, which is metabolized almost entirely as a carbohydrate, and glucose solutions can lead to an iatrogenic increase in blood glucose to diabetic levels. Because of poor dietary nutritional intake, fluids should be supplemented with parenteral B vitamins. Individuals with chronic alcoholism, as noted above, may suffer from magnesium deficiency. Adding a deep intramuscular injection of magnesium at a dose of 0.10–0.15 mL/kg to the initial therapeutic regimen is an important adjunct to treatment (Blazer and Siegler 1984).

The next step in treatment is the institution of medications that are cross-tolerant with alcohol. Diazepam has been the drug of choice for managing patients in withdrawal because of its relatively extended half-life and cross-tolerance with alcohol. Initial doses depend on the patient's age and weight and the amount of alcohol consumed during the week before admission. Even with these data, however, doses must be carefully titrated during the first 24–48 hours of withdrawal. The usual starting dosage is between 5 mg and 15 mg every 6–12 hours until the delirium, agitation, and/or hallucinations are sufficiently decreased. If therapy proceeds on an outpatient basis, careful monitoring is necessary in order to ensure that alcohol is not added to the regimen of the benzodiazepine. After the first day, the diazepam dose can usually be decreased at a rate of approximately 20% per day. Other medium- to long-acting benzodiazepines—such as chlorazepate—can be used as well.

When an overt delirium emerges with seizures and hallucinations, diazepam is the anticonvulsant of choice because of its rapid onset of effect. An increase in memory problems, the onset of dysarthria, and the development of ataxia in the elderly patient indicate that drug intoxication has developed secondary to excessive medication or as a result of the synergistic effects of the drug with alcohol. When such intoxication occurs, the drug should be discontinued for 24–36 hours and the patient should be carefully observed for a recurrence of the withdrawal symptoms, the drug can then be reinstituted. If persistent signs and symptoms of withdrawal are seen longer than 3 days after the last known drink, the clinician should suspect dependence on minor tranquilizers or hypnotics as well as alcohol.

Some withdrawal programs in communities encourage withdrawal within a social setting based on social support in the absence of drug use (a detoxification center). Although some rehabilitation centers in hospitals may overuse medication, the severe effects of withdrawal, such as delirium tremens, should dissuade the clinician from routinely using alternative withdrawal settings, especially for the older adult.

After detoxification, the long-term goals of treatment become paramount in the treatment process. Although disulfiram has been used effectively in the treatment of chronic alcoholism to prevent continued use of alcohol, current thinking is that this medication may not be ideal for use in older adults because of the hazards of the alcohol-disulfiram interaction, as well as the toxicity of disulfiram itself (Center For Substance Abuse Treatment 1998). If this drug is used, a contract must be established between the patient and the physician plus at least one family member. A family member (or possibly the emergency department of a local hospital) should have the responsibility for administering the daily dose of disulfiram to the patient. The patient, in turn, must agree to take the tablet when offered. Both the patient and family members must be warned of the potential effects if alcohol is ingested while the patient is taking disulfiram. Acetaldehyde increases in the blood when ethanol and disulfiram are present concurrently, and this increase leads to the *acetaldehyde syndrome*—a flushing of the face, intense throbbing in the head and neck (which may develop into a pulsating headache), difficulty breathing, nausea, vomiting, sweating, thirst, chest pains, hypertension, vertigo, blurred vision, and confusion. These symptoms are outlined on the package insert provided by the manufacturer. There is no evidence that disulfiram is contraindicated in late life. Nevertheless, if the elderly patient's health status is compromised, the clinician must carefully weigh the benefits against the potential problems of prescribing disulfiram.

Of the other pharmacotherapies that might be considered, naltrexone (ReVia) is reported to reduce the frequency and severity of drinking relapses and is well tolerated by older adults (Center for Substance Abuse Treatment 1998). Other medications under investigation, such as acamprosate, are showing promising results in the support of the chronic alcoholic patient (Litten et al. 1996).

Therapeutic intervention with the family is essential. First, family members should be warned of the severe and potentially irreversible problems, especially memory problems, that alcohol can cause in the older adult. Most families are more concerned with the immediate effects of intoxication. If the older family member drinks silently without overt signs of intoxication, the behavior may be tolerated. The threshold for concern in the family must therefore be lowered through education. Patient, family, and clinician become a team as they seek to correct the problem. Family members may benefit from family education groups, multifamily therapy, and individual family therapy that might be offered through local outpatient substance abuse clinics. Participation in Al-Anon groups could be another place where family members could learn about alcoholism and establish adaptive ways to respond to the patient's recovery efforts or to relapses should they occur. Atkinson et al. (1993) found that married older alcoholics were more likely to comply with treatment if their spouses also became involved in the treatment process.

Specialized substance abuse treatment approaches may be of particular benefit to the older adult. Mainstreaming patients into treatment as usual may present particular challenges. Older adults will probably respond better to a nonconfrontational, informed approach. The key elements of effective treatment for the older adult are the involvement of family, the development of a viable community base of support, and counseling directed to dealing with issues such as depression, isolation, and boredom. Groups for older adults, if available, might be of particular benefit. Some evidence to date supports age-specific treatment approaches with regard to compliance and outcomes (Atkinson et al. 1993; Kashner et al. 1992; Kofoed et al. 1987; Thomas-Knight 1978). Kashner et al. (1992) showed that elderly patients in programs specific to their age group were 2.9 times more likely and 2.1 times more likely at 1 year to report abstinence than were patients in a mixed-age program.

Case management supports may need to be organized to ensure linkage with appropriate community resources. A patient's medical, psychiatric, and social needs must be met, because substance abuse treatment may be of limited benefit if other critical and related issues are not addressed. Patients with coexisting psychiatric disorders will benefit most from an integrated and coordinated approach to the treatment of the comorbidity. Issues related to housing, transportation, and meals may need to be considered for certain patients, who might require a higher level of care (such as a day treatment program) than is normally provided in traditional outpatient treatment. Age-specific settings such as senior centers, faith-based community areas such as houses of worship, and Veterans Affairs clinics may be ideal locations for offering specific group-based programs for the older adult patient. Ideally, these centers will be staffed with persons experienced and interested in working with older adults. It is critical that the specialized care concerns of this patient cohort be taken into account in the treatment planning process.

Self-help groups are essential to the long-term support of the abstinent alcoholic person. The Alcoholics Anonymous (AA) program has proved over many years to be effective in encouraging abstinence for individuals throughout the life cycle. Support groups provide social support coupled with appropriate pressure from peers who have experienced similar problems. AA is complementary to the authority of the clinician and must not be considered a threat to medical authority. AA meetings may be especially beneficial to the older alcoholic individual who is discouraged and lonely because of isolation and feelings of uselessness. Involvement in the group setting, coupled with a sense of helping others and interaction with younger persons, may reintegrate the sober elderly person into society. Ideally, the older adult will establish a relationship with his or her program sponsor, who can help ease the patient's transition into the AA community and serve as an ongoing resource and source of support to the older adult, particularly during the initial challenges of accepting the alcohol use as a problem.

However, many older persons resist the suggestion that they join a self-help group. Some reasons are that elderly persons continue to deny that they have a problem or that they believe themselves perfectly capable of correcting the problem alone. The self-sufficient attitude of the current elderly cohort is one reason that such beliefs are so persistent in the elderly. More commonly, the older adult feels no "fit" with the environment of such self-help groups. Thus, the cohort of elderly alcoholic persons in the latter part of the twentieth century did not experience recovery groups and self-help phenomena, unlike those persons who are reaching old age in the early years of the twenty-first century. Given these groups' frequent success, participation in self-help groups should be encouraged, but clinicians should not force the older adult to participate. In certain communities it is more likely that particular meetings exist that are more attractive to the neophyte older adult AA member: these will be more established, more traditional in structure, and more fully attended by long-standing members of the AA community.

Support from family members and the clinician, as well as integration into more traditional social environments, may accomplish the same purpose as self-help and support groups (Butler and Lewis 1977). In mobilizing coping resources, the social environment (acute and chronic stressors, social network resources), the health care system (availability of health care services such as medical intervention, behavioral therapy, and educational programs), and the coping strategies of the older patient can be woven into a unique matrix for a given elderly person. Such an integrated approach not only makes possible a more comprehensive evaluation of the diagnostic profile but also provides a framework on which successful treatment can be built. Intervention should target for change specific points within the system, but the intervention strategy should also reflect the clinician's continuing recognition that the entire system is interdependent.

Drug Abuse and Dependence

Drug abuse is usually associated with adolescents and young adults. Certainly the abuse of illicit drugs is un-

common in older adults. Nevertheless, the fact that drug abuse occurs among persons in later life must not be overlooked. The propensity of older adults to use prescription drugs inappropriately renders late life a period of high risk for the side effects of this misuse. Glantz (1981) suggested that the motivation for elderly persons to abuse drugs may be similar to the motivation for adolescents. Both must negotiate a period of uncertain and changing roles as well as changes in self-concept. Older persons face step-downs on the economic ladder and disadvantages in the employment market. Friends and relatives may not be as available because of distance, or may be removed by death. Although self-sufficiency continues to be a means of coping (adolescents and the elderly both strive for control), the ability of the impaired older adult to maintain self-reliance and independence is compromised. Drugs are easily available to both groups. The adolescent seeks illegal drugs on the street; the older adult obtains addictive drugs from local physicians. For example, Capel et al. (1972) discovered that the majority of drug-addicted persons who survive to late life continue their drug use via concealed habits, using substitute narcotics such as hydromorphone hydrochloride. Alcohol and barbiturates may be added to enhance the effects of this narcotic.

Even the progress from milder to more powerful drugs, frequently seen in the steps to addiction among adolescents, may have parallels among the elderly (Glantz 1981). Older persons begin taking mild analgesics and sedative-hypnotic agents but fail to obtain the relief they desire. Without realizing the danger of addiction, they progress to the use of narcotic analgesics for chronic pain problems and higher doses of tranquilizing and sedative-hypnotic agents. Once addiction and tolerance are established, older adults exhibit little initiative to reverse the problem. By obtaining medications from multiple physicians and borrowing medicines from family members, they feed their habit over time. Frequently, hospitalization uncovers the addiction, because withdrawal symptoms appear 3–4 days after admission to the hospital.

Problems deriving from excessive and inappropriate use of prescription and over-the-counter drugs are well documented in the geriatric literature. Law and Chalmers (1976) estimated that 85% of older persons living in the community and 95% of those residing in long-term-care facilities receive prescription drugs. In 1976, more than 12 prescriptions were written per person each year for persons ages 65 years and older (Lamy and Vestal 1976). Of drugs prescribed to older adults, 17%–23% are benzodiazepines (D'Archangelo 1993). Undoubtedly, such estimates would be even higher today.

Scope of the Problem

The frequency of excessive drug use in the elderly, especially the use of psychoactive drugs, is well documented. From a household survey of more than 2,000 people, Mellinger et al. (1978) reported that among persons older than age 60 years, 20% of women and 17% of men had regularly used psychoactive drugs during the year preceding the survey—rates higher than those for any other age group. In this age group, 11% of the men and 25% of the women had used a minor tranquilizer and/or a sedative at least once during the year preceding the survey—again, rates higher than those for any other age group. These rates may be declining in community samples, because rates of antianxiety and sedative-hypnotic use have decreased (Hanlon et al. 1992). Heightened public awareness of problems secondary to benzodiazepine use probably contributed to this decline.

A report from the National Medical Care Expenditure Survey (Rossiter 1983) documented that persons age 65 years and older were more likely than middle-age persons to have used pain relievers (25.9%) prescribed by a physician during the past year. Except for cardiovascular medications, analgesic and psychotherapeutic agents were the drugs used the most by older adults. In a review of nursing home prescribing habits, Ray et al. (1980) found that in 173 Tennessee nursing homes, 43% of the patients had received antipsychotic medications during the year preceding the survey, and 9% were chronic recipients—that is, they had received at least one dose daily for 365 days during the preceding year.

Christopher et al. (1978), reporting on 873 hospitalized persons in Dundee, Scotland, concluded that prescribing in this inpatient population was not excessive; an average of three medications was received at any given time. Patients on the geriatric ward were receiving the highest number of drugs. However, certain drug groups, especially the sedative-hypnotics, were prescribed excessively, with few attempts made to reduce the dose with patients' increasing age. The prevalence of hypnotic use ranged from more than 40% among the medical patients to more than 70% on the geriatric wards. In a survey involving 195 hospitalized persons over age 60 years, Salzman and van der Kolk (1980) found that one-third had received at least one psychotropic drug the day of the survey. Hypnotics were the most frequently prescribed drugs, with flurazepam as the drug of choice. The authors noted that each of the psychoactive drugs prescribed had potentially dangerous side effects and that the dosing did not reflect that the treating clinicians paid attention to the age of patients.

In the community, however, the evidence of significant abuse of illicit drugs in the elderly is remarkably absent. The best data available are those derived from the ECA studies. Myers et al. (1984) found no evidence of drug abuse in the age group 65 years and older at two of the three ECA sites surveyed and a prevalence of just 0.2% at the third site. More than 3,000 persons ages 65 years and older were interviewed for this survey. Regarding the lifetime prevalence of drug abuse or dependence, fewer than 0.1% of the subjects at these three ECA sites reported any such history (Robins et al. 1984). These studies are subject to bias, given the subjects' difficulty in recalling information regarding drug abuse and/or their denial of such use. Nevertheless, denial and selective recall are probably no more a problem for elderly persons than for persons at any other stage of life. What is more likely to contribute to the relatively low prevalence of current and lifetime drug abuse among elderly persons is a cohort effect (persons who were elderly in the 1980s were never heavy users of drugs) and selective mortality (persons from the present generation of older adults who used illicit medications did not survive to late life). However, community surveys that rely on household data may underestimate drug abuse, especially by failure to include homeless and transient persons.

Behavioral and Social Correlates

Many psychosocial factors contribute to the potential toxicity and addictive potential of both prescription and illicit drugs among the elderly population (Blazer 1983). Certain character traits of older adults contribute to increased drug use (Baldessarini 1977). The more passive older adult may use drugs prescribed by a number of physicians without question. Even "double prescribing," the prescription of the same drug by two or more physicians, can go unchallenged by the dependent elderly person. Addiction accrues over time without being noticed by the patient, family, or physician. Only when such a patient is admitted to the hospital for an unrelated disorder do the symptoms of addiction become apparent. Once hospitalized, passive older adults often fail to report the medications they were taking before hospitalization, expecting the physician to know how to manage their problem. The patients who appear most compliant could be the most prone to drug abuse in an outpatient medical or psychiatric practice.

In addition to character traits, the social setting surrounding the prescription of medications affects the patient's potential for abusing medications. Many psychosocial factors determine abuse of therapeutic drugs. Noncompliance, a most important factor in treating psychiatric disorders, usually does not contribute to drug abuse. Rather, older adults are more inclined not to take prescribed medications on schedule than to use prescribed drugs excessively. Blackwell (1973) estimated that up to 50% of patients do not take prescribed medications. The potential for addiction may be actualized, however, if the milieu for prescribing medications discourages communication between the older adult and the physician (Lamy 1980). Frequently, in the distracting and hurried environment of the physician's office, proper use of a medication is not communicated to older adults. Because older persons are hesitant to ask questions, they leave the office without understanding how a drug is to be used. To please the physician, they take the medication, but not at the dose required. The tendency for older persons to carry all their medications in one container increases the potential for confusion about when a particular drug should be taken. Intoxication from excessive use of the benzodiazepines is not uncommon under these circumstances.

The practice of sharing and swapping medications among older adults is not infrequent as a precipitant of abuse or dependence. Friends, roommates, or spouses can be treated by different physicians for similar problems. Through informal communication with one another regarding the effectiveness of individual drug therapies, the elderly person may mistakenly determine that a friend's physician has prescribed a better treatment than his or her own clinician. Because limited finances preclude obtaining a second opinion (or even an initial consultation), medications are informally shared. Through the additive effects of drugs, such as the sedative-hypnotics, evidence of addiction or abuse appears, often unexplained to the primary care physician. The diagnosis of the problem is further complicated because older adults are hesitant to reveal that they have obtained medications from another source.

Another contributor to problems of abuse is use of over-the-counter drugs. In Western societies, over-the-counter drugs are used even more often than prescription drugs. Chaiton et al. (1976) estimated that more than 50% of elderly persons responding to a community survey had used at least one over-the-counter drug during the 48 hours preceding the survey. Most of these persons had not consulted a physician about the use of the drug or its potential interaction with prescription drugs. The most commonly used the over-the-counter drugs are agents to improve sleep, to improve gastrointestinal symptoms such as constipation, and to relieve pain. The misuse of such drugs is likely to be associated with the use of multiple substances, insomnia, chronic pain, and relief from stress. The combination of nonprescription drugs that have anticholinergic effects (such as diphenhydramine) with prescribed antidepressants and/or phenothiazines can lead to anticholinergic toxicity or even a full-blown central anticholinergic syndrome.

"Do-something" prescribing is an iatrogenic contributor to drug abuse in elderly patients. The older adult who pays for a doctor's consultation expects a result—usually a prescription. The physician who writes a prescription also gains some assurance that he or she has upheld the patient–physician contract. Drugs prescribed under these circumstances are often not prescribed for specific target symptoms. Benzodiazepines, sedative-hypnotic agents, tricyclic antidepressants, and even neuroleptics become the drugs of choice because of the mistaken view that the drugs promote the general well-being of the patient. Not only do such prescribing practices reinforce a pattern of medical care that discourages the physician from talking with the older adult, but these practices also increase the likelihood of polypharmacy.

A variation on the theme of do-something prescribing that may contribute to drug addiction and/or abuse in elderly patients is defensive prescribing. Physicians who serve as medical directors of nursing homes or who have large consulting practices in long-term-care facilities are frequently called by nursing staff and even family members about patients' disturbing and uncontrollable physical or behavioral symptoms. Agitation and sleep problems are among those most commonly encountered by a stressed nursing staff. Against his or her better judgment, a physician may prescribe medications, not so much to alleviate a specific symptom in an older adult as to reassure staff and family members. Defensive prescribing is not an indictment of the care given by a physician, nursing staff, or family. Rather, it is a symptom of a difficult situation—the management of an acutely agitated and cognitively impaired older adult in a facility with limited personnel. Nevertheless, such prescribing practices must be recognized as major contributors to addiction and abuse in older adults.

Diagnostic Workup

The diagnostic workup of the older adult in whom a diagnosis of drug abuse or dependence is suspected is similar to the workup described in this chapter for those with suspected alcohol abuse and dependence. Many of the symptoms described earlier apply to prescription and nonprescription drug abuse as well. Although older adults may be seen after taking an overdose of a sedative, narcotic, or other agent, the most common presentations of drug misuse or abuse are symptoms of toxicity and/or withdrawal.

The benzodiazepines (both anxiolytics and sedative-hypnotics) are the most commonly prescribed drugs and are therefore the most likely to be abused. Symptoms characteristic of benzodiazepine toxicity include sedation, confusional states, "sundowning" (heightened agitation or frank delirium at night), ataxia, and even stupor or coma. The potential for a fatal overdose is low with these agents alone, but when benzodiazepines are combined with other agents, such as alcohol, this potential increases dramatically. Withdrawal symptoms, in contrast, may mimic the psychiatric disorder for which the drugs were originally prescribed. Anxiety and agitation, sleep problems, muscle cramps (especially in the legs), tremors, and perceptual distortions may emerge upon withdrawal. It is important to note the most serious withdrawal symptom: the onset of seizures.

Tricyclic antidepressants are frequently prescribed and may contribute to increased memory problems, confusion, and sedation. Confusion and even fugue states are described as occurring in the morning after an excessive nighttime dose of tricyclic antidepressants; these symptoms are frequently accompanied by postural hypotension and excessive lethargy. In a patient with bipolar disorder, successful use of an antidepressant to reverse depressive symptoms may later trigger an elevation in mood and an increase in activity. Even a frank manic episode with delusions and hallucinations can be precipitated by these drugs.

Lithium carbonate, a most effective drug in the treatment of manic-depressive illness, can be especially problematic for older adults. Symptoms including dizziness, ataxia, drowsiness, and confusion may occur when serum levels are below 1.0 mEq/L. Older persons do not tolerate lithium therapy as well as persons in middle life, and therefore the drug must be prescribed with extreme caution. Self-abuse with lithium is uncommon, but the desire of the clinician to obtain therapeutic effect in a patient who suffers from rapid-cycling bipolar disorder or unipolar recurrent depression augments the potential for lithium toxicity.

When these or other symptoms emerge, obtaining a thorough history from the patient and family (similar to that described earlier in the chapter for alcohol problems) is the next clinical step of importance. If the clinician questions the history provided by the patient, many laboratories provide a drug toxicity screen. Most of these laboratories can return results to the clinician within 6 hours. Specimens can be obtained from either urine or blood. Toxicity screens must be interpreted cautiously, for drugs are often cross-reactive to the probes used in the screen. Other ancillary laboratory procedures, such as electrophysiological tracing, cardiac monitoring, and radiologic examination (for problems deriving from drug use), can be obtained as well but are usually not required.

Treatment

Treatment approaches for drug abuse and dependence in the older adult are similar to those used for patients at other stages of the life cycle. Given that the older adult is frail, however, the clinician must be careful to err on the side of being conservative. Specifically, early hospitalization is indicated when evidence of abuse is present. For example, the older adult who chronically takes benzodiazepines and is found to be excessively lethargic should be hospitalized, despite the clinician's recognition of the cause of the problem and the family's insistence that the problem can be managed at home.

The immediate goal upon hospitalization is to remove the potential for acute toxicity from the medication. If drug ingestion is recent, gastric evacuation is indicated. In elderly patients, however, special care must be taken to avoid aspiration. Activated charcoal (30 g) has been recommended along with the lavage to absorb barbiturates, alcohol, and propoxyphene (Ellinwood et al. 1985). Once the clinician is convinced that the potential for acute toxicity has been removed, the patient should be transferred to a ward where close monitoring is possible. Electrocardiographic monitoring is often indicated for the first 24–48 hours. Monitoring of respiration, however, is of greatest importance, especially if the patient shows evidence of slow, rapid, or shallow breathing. When improvement does not ensue, peritoneal dialysis or hemodialysis may be indicated.

Once the patient has survived the immediate problems of overdose, the next challenge presented to the clinician is to manage withdrawal symptoms. Depending on the half-life of the drug, withdrawal may last from 6 hours to 8–10 days (the half-life of flurazepam, for example, may exceed 200 hours in an older adult). Support with the medication or a substitute drug is indicated during this period. At the same time, the clinician must begin educating the patient and family about the cause of the hospitalization and the need to change the outpatient drug therapy significantly in order to prevent the recurrence of such a problem. With most elderly persons, education and intervention during the course of an acute hospitalization for drug problems are effective. Older adults are often unaware of the potential problems of drug use and, when informed, are most happy to be free of the potential of future addiction or toxic reactions to a medication.

In some cases, however, the older adult will continue to seek medications, especially analgesics and benzodiazepine-like compounds. For these patients, careful outpatient monitoring and work with the family provide the best means of successfully achieving long-term abstinence from potentially abusable drugs. Because elderly persons tend to use the same pharmacy despite having multiple physicians, contact with the pharmacist can be especially helpful in monitoring drug use.

Behavioral interventions and treatments for older adults' drug abuse are complicated by the patients' ongoing medical needs to receive pharmacological treatment, as well as the assessed legitimacy of the drug use. Pain management with such patients can be a particularly complicated issue and is best assessed on an individual basis. Establishing a plan for managing the prescription of an analgesic is imperative, and a coordinated effort to communicate about the patient's medication-seeking behaviors must be established between physician, family members, and pharmacist. The use of alcohol in addition to the use and abuse of prescription and over-the-counter medications is a particular concern and one that requires vigilant monitoring and assessment.

References

Adamson J, Burdick JA: Sleep of dry alcoholics. Arch Gen Psychiatry 28:146–149, 1973

American Psychiatric Association: Diagnostic and Statistical Manual of Mental Disorders, 3rd Edition. Washington, DC, American Psychiatric Association, 1980

American Psychiatric Association: Diagnostic and Statistical Manual of Mental Disorders, 4th Edition. Washington, DC, American Psychiatric Association, 1994

American Psychiatric Association: Diagnostic and Statistical Manual of Mental Disorders, 4th Edition, Text Revision. Washington, DC, American Psychiatric Association, 2000

American Society of Addiction Medicine: Patient Placement Criteria for the Treatment of Substance-Related Disorders, 2nd Edition. Washington, DC, American Society of Addiction Medicine, 1996

Armor D, Johnston D, Pollich S, et al: Trends in U.S. Adult Drinking Practices. Santa Monica, CA, Rand Corporation, 1977

Atkinson RM, Kofoed LL: Alcohol and drug abuse in old age: a clinical perspective. Subst Alcohol Actions Misuse 3:353–368, 1982

Atkinson RM, Tolso RL, Turner JA: Factors affecting outpatient treatment compliance of older male problem drinkers. J Stud Alcohol 54:102–106, 1993

Baldessarini RJ: Chemotherapy in Psychiatry. Cambridge, MA, Harvard University Press, 1977

Blackwell B: Drug therapy: patient compliance. N Engl J Med 289:249–252, 1973

Blazer D: Drug management in the elderly, in Experimental and Clinical Interventions in Aging. Edited by Walker RF, Cooper RL. New York, Marcel Dekker, 1983, pp 343–354

Blazer D, Siegler IC: A Family Approach to Health Care in the Elderly. Menlo Park, CA, Addison-Wesley, 1984

Blow FC, Barry KL: Older patients with at-risk and problem drinking patterns: new developments in brief interventions. J Geriatr Psychiatry Neurol 13:115–123, 2000

Blow FC, Brower KJ, Schulenberg JE, et al: The Michigan Alcoholism Screening Test—Geriatric Version (MAST-G): a new elderly-specific screening instrument. Alcohol Clin Exp Res 16:372, 1992

Bosmann HB: Pharmacology of alcoholism in aging, in Alcoholism in the Elderly. Edited by Hartford JT, Samorajski T. New York, Raven, 1984, pp 161–174

Butler RN, Lewis MI: Aging and Mental Health: Positive Psychosocial Approaches, 2nd Edition. St. Louis, MO, CV Mosby, 1977

Capel WC, Goldsmith BM, Waddell KJ, et al: The aging narcotic addict: an increasing problem for the next decades. J Gerontol 27:102–106, 1972

Center for Substance Abuse Treatment: Substance Abuse Among Older Adults. Treatment Improvement Protocol (TIP) Series, No 26 (DHHS Publ No SMA 98-3179). Washington, DC, U.S. Government Printing Office, 1998

Chaiton A, Spitzer WO, Roberts RS, et al: Patterns of medical drug use: a community focus. Can Med Assoc J 114:33–37, 1976

Chowdhury AR, Malmud LS, Dinoso VP: Gastrointestinal plasma protein loss during ethanol ingestion. Gastroenterology 72:37–40, 1977

Christopher LJ, Ballinger BR, Shepherd AMM, et al: Drug-prescribing patterns in the elderly: a cross-sectional study of in-patients. Age Ageing 7:74–82, 1978

D'Archangelo E: Substance abuse in later life. Can Fam Physician 39:1986–1993, 1993

Edwards G, Oppenheimer E, Duckitt A, et al: What happens to alcoholics? Lancet 2:269–271, 1983

Ellinwood EH, Woody G, Krishnan RR: Treatment for drug abuse, in Psychiatry, Vol 2. Edited by Michels R, Cavenar JO. Philadelphia, PA, Lippincott, 1985, pp 1–12

Ewing JA: Detecting alcoholism: the CAGE questionnaire. JAMA 252:1905–1907, 1984

Ewing JA: Substance abuse: alcohol, in Psychiatry, Vol 2. Edited by Michels R, Cavenar JO. Philadelphia, PA, Lippincott, 1985

Faris D: The prevention of alcoholism and economic alcoholism. Prev Med 3:36–48, 1974

Finlaysen RE, Hunt RD, Davis LJ, et al: Alcoholism in elderly persons: a study of the psychiatric and psychosocial features of 216 inpatients. Mayo Clin Proc 63:761–768, 1988

Fleming MF, Barry KL, Manwell LB, et al: Brief physician advice for problem drinkers: a randomized controlled trial in community-based primary care practices. JAMA 277:1039–1045, 1997

Garver DL: Age effects on alcohol metabolism, in Alcoholism in the Elderly. Edited by Hartford JT, Samorajski T. New York, Raven, 1984, pp 153–160

Gersovitz M, Motio K, Munro HN, et al: Human protein requirements: assessment of the adequacy of the current recommended dietary allowance for dietary protein in elderly men and women. Am J Clin Nutr 35:6–14, 1982

Glantz M: Predictions of elderly drug abuse. J Psychoactive Drugs 13:117–126, 1981

Glatt MM: Experiences with elderly alcoholics in England. Alcoholism 2:23–26, 1978

Glynn RJ, Bouchard GR, Locastro JS, et al: Changes in alcohol consumption behaviors among men in the normative aging study, in Nature and Extent of Alcohol Problems Among the Elderly. Research Monograph No 14 (DHHS Publ No ADM 84-1321). Edited by Maddox G, Robins LN, Rosenberg N. Rockville, MD, National Institute on Alcohol Abuse and Alcoholism, 1984, pp 101–116

Gordon T, Kannel WB: Drinking and its relation to smoking, blood pressure, blood lipids and uric acid: the Framingham study. Arch Intern Med 143:1366–1374, 1983

Hanlon JT, Fillenbaum GG, Burchett B, et al: Drug-use patterns among black and nonblack community-dwelling elderly. Annals of Pharmacology 26:679–685, 1992

Helzer JE, Carey KE, Miller RH: Predictors and correlates of recovery in older versus younger alcoholics, in Nature and Extent of Alcohol Problems Among the Elderly. Research Monograph No 14 (DHHS Publ No ADM 84-1321). Edited by Maddox G, Robins LN, Rosenberg N. Rockville, MD, National Institute on Alcohol Abuse and Alcoholism, 1984, pp 83–100

Jaffe JH: Drug addiction and drug abuse, in The Pharmacological Basis of Therapeutics, 6th Edition. Edited by Gilman AG, Goodman LS, Gilman A. New York, Macmillan, 1980, pp 535–584

Kalant H, Kahnna JM, Israel Y: The alcohols, in Principles of Medical Pharmacology, 3rd Edition. Edited by Seemen P, Sellars V, Roschlau WH. Toronto, Canada, University of Toronto Press, 1980, pp 245–253

Kashner TM, Rodell DE, Ogden SR, et al: Outcomes and costs of two VA inpatient programs for older alcoholic patients. Hosp Community Psychiatry 43:985–989, 1992

Kofoed LL, Tolson RL, Atkinson RM, et al: Treatment compliance of older alcoholics: an elder-specific approach is superior to "mainstreaming." J Stud Alcohol 48:47–51, 1987

Lamy PP: Prescribing for the Elderly. Littleton, MA, PSG Publishing, 1980

Lamy PP, Vestal RE: Drug prescribing for the elderly. Hosp Pract (Off Ed) 11:111–118, 1976

Law R, Chalmers C: Medicines and elderly people: a general practice survey. Br Med J 1:565–568, 1976

Liberto JG, Oslin DW, Ruskin PE: Alcoholism in older persons: A review of the literature. Hosp Community Psychiatry 43:975–984, 1992

Litten RZ, Allen J, Fertig J: Pharmacotherapies for alcohol problems: a review of research with focus on developments since 1991. Alcohol Clin Exp Res 20:859–876, 1996

Maddox GL, Blazer DG: Alcohol and aging. Center Reports on Advances in Research (Duke University Center for the Study of Aging and Human Development) 8:1–6, 1985

Mellinger GD, Balter MB, Manheimer DI, et al: Psychic distress, life crisis, and use of psychotherapeutic medications: national household survey data. Arch Gen Psychiatry 35:1045–1052, 1978

Mello NK, Mendelson JH: Clinical aspects of alcohol dependence, in Drug Addiction, Vol 1: Morphine, Sedative/Hypnotic and Alcohol Dependence. Edited by Martin WR. Berlin, Springer, 1977, pp 613–666

Mellstrom D: Previous alcohol consumption and its consequences for aging, morbidity and mortality in men aged 70–75. Age Ageing 10:277–283, 1981

Miller WR, Rollnick S: Motivational Interviewing. New York, Guilford, 1991

Miller WR, Sanchez VC: Motivating young adults for treatment and lifestyle change, in Alcohol Use and Misuse by Young Adults. Edited by Howard GS, Nathan PE. South Bend, IN, University of Notre Dame Press, 1994

Muehlberger CW: The physiologic action of alcohol. JAMA 167:1840–1845, 1958

Myers JK, Weissman MM, Tischler GL, et al: Six-month prevalence of psychiatric disorders in three communities: 1980 to 1982. Arch Gen Psychiatry 41:959–967, 1984

Nashold RD, Naor EM: Alcohol-related deaths in Wisconsin: the impact of alcohol mortality. Am J Public Health 71:1237–1271, 1981

National Institute on Alcohol Abuse and Alcoholism: The Physician's Guide to Helping Patients With Alcohol Problems (NIH Publ No 95-3769). Rockville, MD, National Institute on Alcohol Abuse and Alcoholism, 1995

Parker ES, Parker DA, Brodie JA, et al: Cognitive patterns resembling premature aging in male social drinkers. Alcoholism 6:46–52, 1982

Pascarelli EF: Drug dependence: an age-old problem compounded by old age. Geriatrics 29:109–110, 1974

Prochaska JO, DiClemente CC, Norcross JC: In search of how people change: applications to addictive behaviors. Am Psychol 47:1102–1114, 1992

Rathbone-McCuan E, Lohn H, Levenson J, et al: Community Survey of Aged Alcoholics and Problem Drinkers. Final Project Report to DHEW (DHEW Grant No 1R18 AAD 1734–01). Baltimore, MD, Levindale Geriatric Research Center, June 1976

Ray WA, Federspiel CF, Schaffner W: A study of antipsychotic drug use in nursing homes: epidemiologic evidence suggesting misuse. Am J Public Health 70:485–491, 1980

Ritchie JN: The aliphatic alcohols, in The Pharmacological Basis of Therapeutics, 6th Edition. Edited by Gilman AG, Goodman LS, Gilman A. New York, Macmillan, 1980, pp 376–390

Robins LN, Helzer JE, Weissman MM, et al: Lifetime prevalence of specific psychiatric disorders in three sites. Arch Gen Psychiatry 41:949–958, 1984

Rossiter LF: Prescribed medicines: findings from the National Medical Care Expenditure Survey. Am J Public Health 73:1312–1315, 1983

Ruchlin HS: Prevalence and correlates of alcohol use among older adults. Prev Med 26(5 pt 1):651–657, 1997

Salzman C, van der Kolk B: Psychotropic drug prescriptions for elderly patients in a general hospital. J Am Geriatr Soc 28:18–22, 1980

Saunders PA: Epidemiology of alcohol problems and drinking patterns, in Principles and Practice of Geriatric Psychiatry. Edited by Copeland JR, Abou-Saleh MT, Blazer DG. New York, Wiley, 1994, pp. 801–805

Schuckit MA: Geriatric alcoholism and drug abuse. Gerontologist 17:168–174, 1977

Schuckit MA, Zisook S, Mortola J: Clinical implications of DSM-III diagnoses of alcohol abuse and alcohol dependence. Am J Psychiatry 142:1403–1408, 1985

Thomas-Knight R: Treating alcoholism among the aged: the effectiveness of a special treatment program for older problem drinkers. Diss Abstr Int 39:3000, 1978

Warheit GJ, Auth JB: The mental health and social correlates of alcohol use among differing life cycle groups, in Nature and Extent of Alcohol Problems Among the Elderly. Research Monograph No 14 (DHHS Publ No ADM 84-1321). Edited by Maddox G, Robins LN, Rosenberg N. Rockville, MD, National Institute on Alcohol Abuse and Alcoholism, 1984, pp 29–82

Wiberg GS, Samson JM, Maxwell WB, et al: Further studies on the acute toxicity of ethanol in young and old rats: relative importance of pulmonary excretion and total body water. Toxicol Appl Pharmacol 20:22–29, 1971

Yano K, Rhoads GG, Kajan A: Coffee, alcohol, and risk of coronary artery disease among Japanese men living in Hawaii. N Engl J Med 297:405–409, 1977

Personality Disorders

Thomas E. Oxman, M.D.
Richard B. Ferrell, M.D.

The diagnosis and treatment of personality disorders are relatively difficult and time intensive in comparison with those of many other psychiatric disorders. In elderly persons, these problems are confounded by a variety of additional issues, both negative and positive. The natural history of personality in later life is affected by the combination of increasing medical-neuropsychiatric comorbidity with ongoing normal psychosocial development.

With aging, the likelihood of multiple chronic diseases increases. The existence of comorbidity results in more functional impairment and requires adaptation (Besdine 1988; Blazer 2000). It can become more difficult to ascertain the primary cause of increased impairment and where best to focus therapeutic interventions. The risk of dementing disorders also increases dramatically in later life. A common feature of dementing disorders is a change in personality or an exacerbation of preexisting characteristics. Without longitudinal history it can be difficult to know whether such presentations are manifestations of a personality disorder, a dementing disorder, or both.

In contrast with these difficulties, it is not uncommon for geriatric psychiatrists to comment that they do not have to deal with problems of patients with personality disorders as much as do their general-psychiatry colleagues. Prevalence studies tend to support this observation. If these prevalence studies are valid, they can offer several explanations why personality disorders might fade with age. One that deserves attention is that of maturation, described in adult development theory and research.

Although general research in personality disorders has increased, there is a relative dearth with respect to elderly persons (Agronin and Maletta 2000). This lack is particularly clear in the area of treatment. Substantial evidence shows the negative effect of personality disorders

on the outcome of depressive disorders in elderly persons. Other than explaining poor outcomes, however, evidence on the methods and benefits of psychotherapy or pharmacotherapy for personality disorders in elderly persons remains limited. There is even less evidence on treatment and outcomes in nursing homes and general hospitals, the settings in which the geriatric psychiatrist is most likely to be called on to diagnose and treat personality disorders.

Definitions

Personality refers to an individual's habitual ways of relating to other people, interacting with the environment, and thinking about oneself (American Psychiatric Association 2000). To classify a problem as a personality disorder, DSM-IV (American Psychiatric Association 1994) and its Text Revision, DSM-IV-TR (American Psychiatric Association 2000), posit several necessary elements: a personality disorder is a pattern of experience and behavior that is noticeably different from cultural expectations. The pattern develops by early adulthood and is intractable and relatively stable across the life span. A personality disorder influences a wide range of both social and personal situations. As with all DSM-IV-TR disorders, a personality disorder results in significant distress or functional impairment. Finally, the enduring pattern must not be a manifestation of another mental disorder, a medical disorder, or use of a substance.

In treating elderly persons, ruling out manifestations of other disorders is particularly important because of the high prevalence of chronic medical disorders. When a change in personality occurs because of the comorbidity of another mental disorder, a medical disorder, or use of a substance, the DSM-IV-TR diagnosis of "personality change due to a general medical condition" is the appropriate diagnostic term. However, dementing disorders are also increasingly prevalent with age and are often associated with changes in personality. These changes may be totally unrelated to premorbid personality, as occurs in frontal lobe dementias (Lebert et al. 1995), or may be marked exaggerations of preexisting traits, as in Alzheimer's disease (Holst et al.1997; Niederehe and Oxman 1994). Because of the progressive pervasiveness of a dementing disorder, the DSM-IV-TR diagnosis of personality change due to a general medical condition does not apply. Although these issues are important in differential diagnosis, for the purposes of this chapter the discussion of personality disorder is focused more closely on conditions that meet DSM-IV-TR personality disorder criteria.

After making a global assessment of the presence or absence of a personality disorder based on the key features listed above, the next step is to identify a specific personality disorder or a personality cluster. Since 1980, DSM has categorized three different personality disorder clusters: A—odd, eccentric (including paranoid, schizoid, and schizotypal personality disorders); B—dramatic, erratic (including borderline, histrionic, narcissistic, and antisocial personality disorders); and C—anxious, fearful (including obsessive-compulsive, avoidant, and dependent personality disorders). The number of specific disorders has varied slightly over the past 20 years. Likewise, over the length of a life span often reaching 75–85 years, both personality and a personality disorder are likely to change somewhat; thus, attention to the identification of a cluster is particularly helpful. Because older patients with personality disorders commonly show symptoms of more than one personality disorder, diagnosis of a specific disorder is likely to be more difficult than in younger adults; thus, "personality disorder not otherwise specified" is a more common descriptive diagnosis for older patients.

Prevalence

The prevalence of personality disorders in the general population is less accurately known than that of Axis I disorders but is estimated at more than 10% for all ages (Agronin and Maletta 2000; Lenzenweger et al. 1997; Weissman 1990), a relatively high rate compared with many Axis I disorders. The prevalence of personality disorders in psychiatric settings is usually three to four times higher than that in the community, with frequent comorbidity of Axis I and Axis II disorders (Kunik et al. 1994; Zweig and Hillman 1999).

The prevalence of personality disorders in older persons is generally lower by about half than that in younger persons in the general population, i.e., 5%–10%. The prevalence in selected outpatient or inpatient samples of older persons can be as high as 25%–65% (Agbayewa 1996; Agronin and Maletta 2000; Ames and Molinari 1994; Camus et al. 1997; Cohen et al. 1994; Fogel and Westlake 1990; Kenan et al. 2000). In part, this lower prevalence appears to be due to a decline in severity over the years, especially of cluster B disorders (Black et al. 1995; Kenan et al. 2000; McGlashan 1986; Molinari et al. 1994; Robins et al. 1984; Snyder et al. 1985; Tyrer and Seiverwright 1988).

The association of personality disorders with depressive disorders in the elderly population is probably the single most reported comorbidity—especially cluster C (Abrams et al. 1994; Agbayewa 1996; Camus et al. 1997; Devanand et al. 2000; Fogel and Westlake 1990; Kunik et al. 1993), cluster B (Abrams et al. 2001; Sato et al. 1999; Vine and Steingart 1994), and personality disorder not otherwise specified (Kunik et al. 1993). The association is higher for early-onset than for late-onset depressive disorders (Abrams et al. 1994; Camus et al. 1997; Devanand et al. 2000; Fava et al. 1996). This association of personality disorders and depressive disorders is an important relationship because the presence of a personality disorder in the context of a depressive disorder complicates differential diagnosis and treatment planning. For depressive disorders, the worst outcomes occur among patients with comorbid personality disorders (Abrams et al. 2001; Brodaty et al. 1995; Thompson et al. 1988; Vine and Steingart 1994). Expectations about treatment outcomes with antidepressants, electroconvulsive therapy, or hospitalization are thus lowered, and decisions about the need for psychotherapy are increased. The relationship between personality disorder and depression may be etiological. That is, personality disorders predispose to the occurrence of depressive disorders (Abrams et al. 1994; Sato et al. 1999), or, alternatively, some chronic depression is the equivalent of a depressive disorder (Akiskal 1994, 2001).

The reports of lower prevalence of personality disorders in older persons have raised substantial controversy. There is some concern that the criteria for personality disorders used in earlier life may not adequately apply in later life (Abrams 1990; Kroessler 1990; Rosowsky and Gurian 1991), thus falsely lowering the prevalence in the elderly population. One suggested response is to modify the criteria for personality disorders in later life (Agronin and Maletta 2000). These arguments have some parallel to those positing that many DSM-IV-TR diagnostic criteria are age inappropriate for the elderly (Jeste et al. 1999).

Another suggested response is to adopt a dimensional approach. Personality researchers frequently use dimensional concepts relating to personality traits rather than the categorical language of disorders (American Psychiatric Association 2000; Costa and McCrae 1990; Eysenck 1998). Longitudinal studies found that personality traits (although not disorders) remained relatively stable over even 30-year periods (Bengston et al. 1985; Costa and McCrae 1988; Costa et al. 1987; Duggan et al. 1991; Schaie and Willis 1986). The exception to the clinical utility of a dimensional approach may be the hierarchy of defense mechanisms, included as an appendix in DSM-IV-TR. The clinical relevance of defense mechanisms is due to their being reversible and adaptive as well as pathological (Vaillant 1994). However, in this approach, even defense mechanisms thus become categorized as immature, intermediate, or mature. Finally, it can be noted that although a dimensional approach may improve description and identification, it is less clear how the approach would be used in treatment, other than to revert to a categorical approach that uses cutoff scores.

Rather than different criteria being needed for the elderly population, it is possible that the criteria are relevant but that at least some disorders, particularly those in cluster B, do improve with age (Kernberg 1984; Sadavoy and Fogel 1992; Solomon 1981; Tyrer and Seiverwright 1988). For example, older substance abusers showed lower levels of crime and drug use compared with when they were younger (Hanlon et al. 1990); and in general, the elderly are more law-abiding, with far fewer arrests (Harlow 1998). Thus, it is not inconsistent for older patients with personality disorders to exhibit fewer "high-energy" diagnostic criteria (e.g., lawbreaking, identity disturbance, promiscuity). Do these research results mean that a maturational change has occurred—or merely that the symptom displays are more subtle because of physical and institutional restrictions (Abrams 1990; Hillman et al. 1997; Rosowsky and Gurian 1991)? Although arguments for modified criteria may ultimately be valid, equal theory and evidence from adult development research at least support the current criteria and the resulting epidemiologic findings.

Adult Development

Erikson's concept of epigenesis is important in understanding how personality disorders might improve with age. Erikson was a strong proponent of the interaction of the psychosocial environment with development across the life span. Erikson's stage theory of late-life development (Erikson et al. 1986) proposed that the major developmental task of older age is to look back and seek meaning across the life span, rather than looking forward, as in previous developmental modes that are now in decline. The goal of this task as discussed by Erikson is to maintain more integrity than despair about one's life. In this process, as at previous life stages, each earlier life stage conflict must be reconciled and integrated with the current stage, allowing resolution of earlier conflicts. Persons with personality disorders might be expected to have greater difficulty in accomplishing this resolution than other individuals. However, this resolution is not an all-or-nothing phenomenon. The achievement of even some resolution may contribute to the mellowing of a personality disorder.

Vaillant provided empirical verification for Erikson's life stage concepts through longitudinal study of the maturation of defenses across the life span (Vaillant 2000, 2002; Vaillant and Milofsky 1980). Defenses are involuntary mental mechanisms for regulating the realities that persons are powerless to change. Vaillant and others (Haan 1977) have described a hierarchy of defenses from immature and maladaptive to mature and adaptive. Mature defenses include humor, altruism, sublimation, anticipation, and suppression. Mature and adaptive defenses synthesize and attenuate conflicts rather than distorting or denying them. Across several longitudinal studies that included privileged persons (Heath 1945), gifted persons (Terman 1925), and persons from the core inner city (Glueck and Glueck 1968), Vaillant established that mature defenses were more consistently identified primarily in Erikson's later developmental stages (Vaillant 1993; Vaillant and Drake 1985) and that, moreover, the development of these defenses was independent of education and social privilege (Vaillant 1993).

Events of psychological and social impact can reveal previously submerged difficulty. For example, the death of a spouse may unmask dependency problems. Retirement or bereavement may lead to narcissistic problems such as poor regulation of self-esteem and faulty adaptation to loss. However, experience—something that the elderly have more of than any other age group—may attenuate the impact of such later-life events, even for older persons with personality disorders. For example, in order to cope effectively with stress, persons must learn to recognize the difference between situations that can and cannot be changed and then must match the right coping skill with the right situation. Emotion-focused coping is employed when a situation cannot be changed, problem-focused coping when a situation can be changed. It is only through repeated experience that these skills develop (Ryff 1999). Although stressful situations certainly exacerbate the symptoms of personality disorders,

Neugarten (1970) pointed out how the meaning of stressful situations changes over time. We expect to experience the death of loved ones and our own declining health when we are older and have time to mentally rehearse how we will respond to these "on time" losses. When these losses occur "off time"—at earlier stages of life—the stress is usually experienced as much greater.

Consideration of this line of evidence should not minimize the impact of personality disorders or the need for some management of them in later life. Even if the prevalence of personality disorders truly does decline, there are still some elderly persons with continuing disorders that cause impairment to themselves and their environment. Consideration of adult development helps us understand how some persons with personality disorders may improve and to understand that this improvement is consistent with the epidemiologic findings of reduced psychopathology in later life. Equally important, adult developmental theory helps the clinician consider the positive aspects of development, even in persons with severe psychopathology (Erikson et al. 1986; Ryff 1999). Until the debate on the validity of the epidemiologic findings versus the criteria used to make those findings is more definitively settled, perhaps designations of personality disorder "in remission" or "in partial remission" would be a more appropriate and parsimonious way of addressing diagnoses of personality disorder in the elderly population.

Evaluation

Because personality disorders typically have a lifelong pattern, diagnosis generally requires greater historical and collateral information than for Axis I disorders. Complete understanding of the causes of signs and symptoms in geriatric psychiatry is a difficult accomplishment. The interplay of multiple etiologic factors is the rule, not the exception. The Structured Clinical Interview for DSM-IV Axis II Personality Disorders (SCID-II; First et al. 1997) and the Personality Disorders Examination (PDE; Loranger 1988) are semistructured interviews for personality disorders that can be used to guide a diagnostic interview and increase reliability. Historical information from medical records and from persons who have known a patient over a long period are still essential components of an accurate and valid diagnosis. The interview requires a longitudinal inquiry about various life stages to establish the historical presence of a personality disorder, even if not all current criteria are met. Several ancillary self-report instruments are available for initial screening

purposes—for example, the Millon Clinical Multiaxial Inventory—III (MCMI-III; Millon 1994), the Personality Diagnostic Questionnaire (PDQ-IV; Hyler et al. 1988), the Schedule for Nonadaptive and Adaptive Personality (Clark 1993), and the Wisconsin Personality Disorders Inventory (Klein et al. 1993). However, the results of these self-reports have a low concordance with the results of interview methods (Perry 1992), and their use is best established and tolerated in younger populations, not among elderly persons, in whom acquired brain disease is an increasing issue.

Geriatric psychiatrists are familiar with the phenomenon that acquired brain disease in later life appears to strengthen undesirable personality traits that were present, but less intense and conspicuous, in earlier adult life. However, if signs and symptoms of personality disorder were not present before the onset of dementing illness or brain injury, it is rational to assume that such illnesses play a causative role in the personality change. A reasonable approach to a diagnosis in geriatrics, as always, includes these elements: 1) careful and detailed review of the medical and psychosocial history, 2) mental status and physical examinations, with special attention to the neurologic examination, and 3) a screening laboratory examination—including, in some cases, brain imaging, an electroencephalogram, and neuropsychological tests.

In many instances, those most able to provide the historical information providing the best clues are family members. Whenever possible, their help should be sought concerning the older patient in whom personality disorder is suspected. Viewing the patient within the family context usually gives added depth of understanding to the clinical perspective.

Syndromes based on frontal lobe pathology that result in loss of normal executive function present some of the most difficult diagnostic challenges—especially if the onset of symptoms is subtle, the rate of progression is slow, and the main attributes of the premorbid personality are obscure. Patients with frontal or frontotemporal lobe disease may show good preservation of memory function. They are, however, prone to trouble with "mechanistic planning, verbal reasoning, or problem-solving" and "obeying the rules of interpersonal social behaviour, the experience of reward and punishment, and the interpretation of complex emotions" (Grafman and Litvan 1999, p. 1921).

These difficulties are similar to some of the problems experienced by many people with borderline, narcissistic, histrionic, paranoid, and antisocial personality disorders. Could one develop a later-life personality disorder de novo, without the presence of underlying brain disease or substance abuse? The answer is not definitively known, but the occurrence is probably rare. It is also possible that signs and symptoms of personality disorders can be quite evident in early adult life, then be diminished or quiescent in mid-adult life, and then reemerge under the stress of social losses or physical illness in later life (Rosowsky and Gurian 1992). The manifestations of personality disorders may vary in different parts of the life cycle. For example, in persons with borderline personality disorder, phenomena such as splitting, intense and unstable interpersonal relationships, impaired affective regulation, and extreme difficulty with control and regulation of anger often persist throughout the life cycle. Problems such as severe impulsivity, risky behavior, and self-mutilation tend to diminish with advancing age. However, other self-injurious behaviors may take their place. These include self-starvation, abuse of medicines, and noncompliance with medical treatment (Rosowsky and Gurian 1992). These behaviors may occur for other reasons, but their presence should at least alert the clinician to the possibility of borderline personality disorder. Late-onset obsessive-compulsive symptoms or traits are particularly likely to have a basis in brain disease.

Treatment Issues

Psychotherapy

In contrast to the unconscious maturation of defenses, the conscious alteration of personality is unusual. Although people are sometimes able to change patterns of behavior, attitudes, ways of thinking, and ways of feeling, changing the fundamental personality structure is extremely difficult. At the same time, it is possible and important to try to help patients avoid behavior that significantly harms them or others. Helping patients recognize and alter erroneous or distorted thinking is also important. Cognitive-behavioral or insight-oriented psychotherapy may significantly help older individuals who are functioning at higher levels and who are not otherwise seriously ill or incapacitated. For patients in psychiatric hospitals and for residents of group homes or nursing homes, intensive psychotherapy with a goal of changing lifelong maladaptive personality features is neither an available nor an indicated treatment modality. However, for such individuals, supportive and consistent psychotherapeutic contact can be of great benefit (Bienenfeld 1990).

As noted, psychotherapy of any type, either by itself or in combination with pharmacotherapy, with a goal of a global revision of maladaptive aspects of personality in later life, is unlikely to succeed. Individualized treatment targeting specific symptoms that discomfort, threaten, or endanger patients or their family or caregivers is far more realistic and likely to realize success—for example, behavioral management to minimize harm from impaired social judgment. It is important not to be rigid or negative about the psychotherapeutic potential of older patients. It is illness, not merely age, that limits or impairs the plasticity of the personality and the potential for self-change. Older patients are often impressive in their resilience, courage, open-mindedness, and willingness to try new ways of thinking and behaving—and those showing these characteristics include some individuals whose adaptation to life in earlier years was far from optimal. This observation is in keeping with Erikson's view of progressive development throughout life. Psychoanalytically oriented psychotherapy, cognitive-behavioral therapy, interpersonal therapy, dialectical behavior therapy, and other forms of psychotherapy all have their adherents and proponents (De Leo et al. 1999). All are probably helpful to certain individuals. The principal features of successful psychotherapy for geriatric patients are consistency, availability, empathic and respectful listening, flexibility, and open-mindedness on the part of the psychotherapist. These features are probably more important than a particular theoretical orientation.

Therapists who are not yet old themselves have a difficult challenge. They have no direct experience with or memory of being old (Rosowsky 1999). Some geriatric psychiatrists may be two full generations younger than their patients. Extraordinary empathy is required of these clinicians, but also of most practicing geriatric psychiatrists, who are usually caring for persons older than themselves.

Pharmacotherapy

A diagnosis of personality disorder should not preclude pharmacological treatment of concomitant psychiatric disorders such as affective illness or psychosis (Kunik et al. 1993). In fact, successful treatment of affective or psychotic symptoms may show that the symptoms were the result of these eminently treatable diseases, not entrenched maladaptive personality traits. Personality disorder, depressive illness, and acquired brain disease share overlapping symptom constellations: symptoms such as irritability, hostility, and uncooperativeness can derive from all three. Even the most perspicacious diagnostician may not be able to tease out a clear etiologic diagnosis for these difficult behavioral symptoms. In such cases, a treatment trial with antidepressant medicine is indicated.

Other symptoms—such as anger outbursts, apathy, and impaired social judgment—may also benefit from pharmacotherapy, particularly if the symptoms are acquired rather than being developmental, lifelong personality traits. Pharmacological treatment should be guided by systematic trials of pharmacotherapy for identified target symptom areas (affect, impulsivity/aggression, anxiety, thinking/psychosis), an assessment strategy (global rating or self-reports targeted to the symptom area), and a specified duration. Selective serotonin reuptake inhibitors and other newer antidepressant drugs, anticonvulsants, and atypical antipsychotic drugs, used alone or in combinations, may be useful in systematic trials for specified symptoms.

Caregiver Education

Education of caregivers is an important function of geriatric psychiatrists. Family members may be having great difficulty in dealing with unfamiliar negative, disinhibited, or inappropriate behavior. If an underlying medical or neurologic etiology can be discerned, caregivers can be reassured about the cause of the otherwise inexplicable changes in their relationship with their loved one. This reassurance helps reduce guilt, anxiety, and uncertainty in the family of the afflicted person.

Primary caregivers in nursing homes, who are usually overworked and underpaid, may not realize that much of the unpleasant behavior of patients that they encounter in their work is not under full volitional control. Uncooperativeness or angry outbursts may have the appearance of simple willfulness or intentionally oppositional behavior. Patients with long-standing personality disorders (as well as those with dementia, stroke, or other types of brain injury) typically have significant deficits in volitional capacity. Understanding this point does not necessarily make the care of these patients easier, but it does provide a perspective on behavior that is otherwise difficult to comprehend and tolerate.

Summary

Understanding of the causes of disordered personality development is far from adequate. Diagnosis, and especially treatment, of personality disorders in elderly patients is difficult. Understanding the relationship between lifelong development and acquired neuropsychiatric illness is an important diagnostic challenge. Geriatric psychiatrists must usually try to manage personality disorder symptoms and ameliorate their harmful effects

rather than attempting to cure the underlying disorder. Behavioral management, psychotherapy, pharmacotherapy, and caregiver support are the tools, which must be carefully used.

References

Abrams RC: Personality Disorders in the Elderly. Verwoerdt's Clinical Geropsychiatry, 3rd Edition. Edited by Bienenfeld D. Baltimore, Williams & Wilkins, 1990, pp 151–163

Abrams RC, Rosendahl E, Card C, et al: Personality disorder correlates of late and early onset depression. J Am Geriatr Soc 42:727–31, 1994

Abrams RC, Alexopoulos GS, Spielman LA, et al: Personality disorder symptoms predict declines in global functioning and quality of life in elderly depressed patients. Am J Geriatr Psychiatry 9:67–71, 2001

Agbayewa MO: Occurrence and effects of personality disorders in depression: are they the same in the old and young? [See comments.] Can J Psychiatry 41:223–226, 1996

Agronin ME, Maletta G: Personality disorders in late life: understanding and overcoming the gap in research. Am J Geriatr Psychiatry 8:4–18, 2000

Akiskal HS: Dysthymia: clinical and external validity. Acta Psychiatr Scand 383 (suppl):19–23, 1994

Akiskal HS: Dysthymia and cyclothymia in psychiatric practice a century after Kraepelin. J Affect Disord 62:17–31, 2001

Ames A, Molinari V: Prevalence of personality disorders in community-living elderly. J Geriatr Psychiatry Neurol 7: 189–194, 1994

American Psychiatric Association: Diagnostic and Statistical Manual of Mental Disorders, 4th Edition. Washington, DC, American Psychiatric Association, 1994

American Psychiatric Association: Diagnostic and Statistical Manual of Mental Disorders, 4th Edition, Text Revision. Washington, DC, American Psychiatric Association, 2000

Bengston V, Reedy M, Gordon C: Aging and self-conceptions: personality processes and social contexts, in Handbook of the Psychology of Aging. Edited by Birren JE, Schaie KW. New York, Van Nostrand Reinhold, 1985, pp 544–593

Besdine RW: Functional assessment in the elderly, in Geriatric Medicine, 2nd Edition. Edited by Rowe JW, Besdine RW. Boston, MA, Little, Brown, 1988, pp 37–51

Bienenfeld D: Verwoerdt's Clinical Geropsychiatry, 3rd Edition. Baltimore, MD, Williams & Wilkins, 1990

Black DW, Baumgard CH, Bell SE: The long-term outcome of antisocial personality disorder compared with depression, schizophrenia, and surgical conditions. Bull Am Acad Psychiatry Law 23:43–52, 1995

Blazer D: Psychiatry and the oldest old. Am J Psychiatry 157: 1915–1924, 2000

Brodaty H, Harris L, Peters K: A 16- to 45-year follow-up of 71 men with antisocial personality disorder. Compr Psychiatry 36:130–140, 1995

Camus V, De Mendonca Lima CA, Gaillard M, et al: Are personality disorders more frequent in early onset geriatric depression? J Affect Disord 46:297–302, 1997

Clark LA: Manual for the Schedule for Nonadaptive and Adaptive Personality (SNAP). Minneapolis, University of Minnesota Press, 1993

Cohen BJ, Nestadt G, Samuels JF, et al: Personality disorder in later life: a community study. Br J Psychiatry 165:493–499, 1994

Costa PT Jr, McCrae RR: Personality in adulthood: a six-year longitudinal study of self-reports and spouse ratings on the NEO Personality Inventory. J Pers Soc Psychol 54:853–863, 1988

Costa PT Jr, McCrae RR: Personality disorders and the five-factor model of personality. J Personal Disord 4:362–371, 1990

Costa PT Jr, Zonderman AB, McCrae RR, et al: Longitudinal analyses of psychological well-being in a national sample: stability of mean levels. J Gerontol 42:50–55, 1987

De Leo D, Scocco P, Meneghel G: Pharmacological and psychotherapeutic treatment of personality disorders in the elderly. Int Psychogeriatr 11:191–206, 1999

Devanand DP, Turret N, Moody BJ, et al: Personality disorders in elderly patients with dysthymic disorder. Am J Geriatr Psychiatry 8:188–195, 2000

Duggan CF, Shap P, Lee AS, et al: Does recurrent depression lead to a change in neuroticism? Psychol Med 21:985–990, 1991

Erikson EH, Erikson JM, Kivnick HQ: Vital Involvement in Old Age. New York, WW Norton, 1986

Eysenck HJ: Dimensions of Personality. New Brunswick, NJ, Transaction Publishers, 1998

Fava M, Alpert JE, Borus JS, et al: Patterns of personality disorder comorbidity in early-onset versus late-onset major depression. Am J Psychiatry 153:1308–1312, 1996

First MB, Gibbon M, Spitzer RL, et al: Structured Clinical Interview for DSM-IV Axis II Personality Disorders (SCID-II). Washington, DC, American Psychiatric Press, 1997

Fogel BS, Westlake R: Personality disorder diagnoses and age in inpatients with major depression. J Clin Psychiatry 51:232–235, 1990

Glueck S, Glueck E: Delinquents and Non-Delinquents in Perspective. Cambridge, MA, Harvard University Press, 1968

Grafman J, Litvan I: Importance of deficits in executive function. Lancet 354:1921–1922, 1999

Haan NA: Coping and Defending. San Francisco, CA, Jossey-Bass, 1977

Hanlon TE, Nurco DN, Kinlock TW, et al: Trends in criminal activity and drug use over an addiction career. Am J Drug Alcohol Abuse 16:223–238, 1990

Harlow CW: Special Report: Profile of Jail Inmates 1996 (Publ No NCJ 164620). Washington, DC, U.S. Department of Justice, 1998

Heath C: What People Are. Cambridge, MA, Harvard University Press, 1945

Hillman J, Stricker G, Zweig R: Clinical psychologists' judgment of older adult patients with character pathology: implications for practice. Professional Psychology: Research and Practice 28:179–183, 1997

Holst G, Hallberg IR, Gustafson L: The relationship of vocally disruptive behavior and previous personality in severely demented institutionalized patients. Arch Psychiatr Nurs 11:147–154, 1997

Hyler SE, Rieder RO, Williams JBW, et al: The Personality Diagnostic Questionnaire: development and preliminary results. J Personal Disord 2:229–237, 1988

Jeste DV, Alexopoulos GS, Bartels SJ, et al: Consensus statement on the upcoming crisis in geriatric mental health: research agenda for the next two decades. Arch Gen Psychiatry 56:848–853, 1999

Kenan MM, Kendjelic EM, Molinari VA, et al: Age-related differences in the frequency of personality disorders among inpatient veterans. Int J Geriatr Psychiatry 15:831–837, 2000

Kernberg O: Severe Personality Disorders: Psychotherapeutic Strategies. New Haven, CT, Yale University Press, 1984

Klein MH, Benjamin L, Rosenfelt R: The Wisconsin Personality Disorders Inventory. J Personal Disord 7:285–303, 1993

Kroessler D: Personality disorder in the elderly. Hosp Community Psychiatry 41:1325–1329, 1990

Kunik ME, Mulsant B, Rifai AH, et al: Personality disorders in elderly inpatients with major depression. Am J Geriatr Psychiatry 1:38–45, 1993

Kunik ME, Mulsant B, Rifai AH, et al: Diagnostic rate of comorbid personality disorder in elderly psychiatric inpatients. Am J Psychiatry 151:603–605, 1994

Lebert F, Pasquier F, Petit H: Personality traits and frontal lobe dementia. Int J Geriatr Psychiatry 10:1047–1049, 1995

Lenzenweger MF, Loranger AW, Korfine L, et al: Detecting personality disorders in a nonclinical population: Application for a two-stage procedure for case identification. Arch Gen Psychiatry 54:345–351, 1997

Loranger AW: Personality Disorders Examination (PDE) Manual. Yonkers, NY, DV Communications, 1988

McGlashan TH: The Chestnut Lodge follow-up study, III: long-term outcome of borderline personalities. Arch Gen Psychiatry 43:20–30, 1986

Millon T: Clinical Multiaxial Inventory—III (MCMI-III). Minneapolis, MN, National Computer Systems, 1994

Molinari V, Ames A, Essa M: Prevalence of personality disorders in two geropsychiatric inpatient units. J Geriatr Psychiatry Neurol 7:209–215, 1994

Neugarten BL: Adaptation and the life cycle. Journal of Geriatric Psychology 4:71–87, 1970

Niederehe GT, Oxman TE: The spectrum of dementias: construct and nosologic validity, in Dementia Presentations, Differential Diagnosis, and Nosology. Edited by Emery O, Oxman TE. Baltimore, MD, Johns Hopkins University Press, 1994

Perry JC: Problems and considerations in the valid assessment of personality disorders. Am J Psychiatry 149:1645–1653, 1992

Robins LN, Helzer JE, Weissman MM, et al: Lifetime prevalence of specific psychiatric disorders in three sites. Arch Gen Psychiatry 41:949–958, 1984

Rosowsky E: Personality disorders and the difficult nursing home resident, in Personality Disorders in Older Adults: Emerging Issues in Diagnosis and Treatment. Edited by Rosowsky E, Abrams RC. Mahwah, NJ, Lawrence Erlbaum, 1999, pp 257–274

Rosowsky E, Gurian B: Borderline personality disorder in late life. Int Psychogeriatr 3:39–52, 1991

Rosowsky E, Gurian B: Impact of borderline personality disorder in late life on systems of care. Hosp Community Psychiatry 43:386–389, 1992

Ryff CD: Psychology and aging, in Principles of Geriatric Medicine and Gerontology, 4th Edition. Edited by Hazzard WR, Blass JP, Ettinger WH, et al. New York, McGraw-Hill, 1999, pp 159–169

Sadavoy J, Fogel BS: Personality disorders in old age, in Handbook of Mental Health and Aging. Edited by Birren J, Sloane R, Cohen G. San Diego, CA, Academic Press, 1992, pp 433–462

Sato T, Sakado K, Uehara T, et al: Personality disorder comorbidity in early-onset versus late-onset major depression in Japan. J Nerv Ment Dis 187:237–242, 1999

Schaie KW, Willis S: Adult Development and Aging, 2nd Edition. Boston, MA, Little, Brown, 1986

Snyder S, Goodpaster WA, Pitts WM, et al: Demography of psychiatric patients with borderline traits. Psychopathology 18:38–49, 1985

Solomon K: Personality disorder in the elderly, in Personality Disorders: Diagnosis and Management, 2nd Edition. Edited by Lion JR. Baltimore, MD, Williams & Wilkins, 1981, pp 310–338

Terman LM: Genetic Studies of Genius, Vol 1: Mental and Physical Traits of a Thousand Gifted Children. Palo Alto, CA, Stanford University Press, 1925

Thompson LW, Gallagher D, Czirr R: Personality disorder and outcome in the treatment of late-life depression. J Geriatr Psychiatry 21:133–153, 1988

Tyrer P, Seiverwright H: Studies of outcome, in Personality Disorders: Diagnosis, Management and Course. Edited by Tyrer P. London, Wright, 1988, pp 119–136

Vaillant GE: The Wisdom of the Ego. Cambridge, MA, Harvard University Press, 1993

Vaillant GE: Ego mechanisms of defense and personality psychopathology. J Abnorm Psychol 130:44–50, 1994

Vaillant GE: Adaptive mental mechanisms: their role in a positive psychology. Am Psychol 55:89–98, 2000

Vaillant GE: Aging Well. Boston, MA, Little, Brown, 2002

Vaillant GE, Drake RE: Maturity of ego defenses in relation to DSM-III axis II personality disorder. Arch Gen Psychiatry 42:597–601, 1985

Vaillant GE, Milofsky E: Natural history of male psychological health, IX: empirical evidence for Erikson's model of the life cycle. Am J Psychiatry 137:1348–1359, 1980

Vine RG, Steingart AB: Personality disorder in the elderly depressed. Can J Psychiatry 39:392–398, 1994

Weissman M: The epidemiology of personality disorders: a 1990 update. J Personal Disord 7 (suppl):44–62, 1990

Zweig R, Hillman J: Personality disorders in adults: a review, in Emerging Issues in Diagnosis and Treatment: LEA Series in Personality and Clinical Psychology. Edited by Rosowsky E, Abrams RC. Mahwah, NJ, Lawrence Erlbaum, 1999, pp 31–53

Agitation and Suspiciousness

Lisa P. Gwyther, M.S.W.
David C. Steffens, M.D., M.H.S.

Suspiciousness and Paranoia

Psychiatrists working with older adults frequently encounter suspicious or paranoid behaviors, especially in patients with agitation. In fact, such ideation is not very uncommon in community populations of elderly adults. In a community study of elderly persons in San Francisco, 17% of the subjects reported that they were highly suspicious and 13% reported delusions (Lowenthal and Berkman 1967). Another study that included elderly persons in both urban and rural areas of North Carolina found that 4% of older adults experienced a sense of persecution by those around them (Christenson and Blazer 1984). Perceptions of a hostile social environment or ideas of persecution lead to greater stress, vigilance, and agitation among elderly persons, resulting in alienation from families and friends. Such individuals represent a challenge for clinicians who care for them.

Among suspicious or paranoid elderly persons, one group has long been recognized, particularly in Europe. The term *late-life paraphrenia* has been used to identify psychosis that has a late age at onset and to distinguish the condition from both chronic schizophrenia and dementia. Kraepelin used *paraphrenia* to classify a small group of patients who exhibited paranoid delusions and yet were able to maintain functioning in their social milieu for months or years. He observed that persons with paraphrenia were typically women, usually living alone. Although current DSM diagnostic nomenclature would classify many of those individuals as having delusional disorder, this late-life syndrome may be more complex. Sometimes paranoid ideation is accompanied by hallucinations. In addition, patients with this condition may have comorbid sensory deficits, especially visual or hear-

ing loss. Thus, although the condition may have features of delusional disorder, it may also have features and comorbidities that point to its being a different entity, perhaps along a continuum with schizophrenia. When the condition is accompanied by agitation, neuroleptics are usually the first-line treatment, although information is lacking on the effectiveness of this class of medications in delusional disorder. Caution with these medications is also warranted, given the increased sensitivity of elderly persons to neuroleptics (Soares and Gershon 1997).

Clearly, chronic paranoid schizophrenia persisting into late life is a major cause of suspiciousness and agitation in elderly persons. With accompanying functional decline and problematic behaviors occurring earlier in life in patients with schizophrenia, it is unusual for new cases of chronic schizophrenia to be diagnosed in elderly patients. Multimodal treatment—including neuroleptic medication, case management, and family education and involvement—is essential for ensuring adequate care. The occurrence of agitation in chronic paranoid schizophrenia patients is common and may indicate a need for an adjustment in neuroleptic dosing. However, new agitation arising in a previously stable older patient with schizophrenia may also indicate another problem, and clinicians need to be particularly attuned to the possibility of an acute medical problem. The medical causes of agitation discussed below for patients with dementia may also affect older patients with schizophrenia, who may require the same level of medical scrutiny.

Classic delusional disorder may occur at any age and is usually characterized by delusions centered on a single theme or series of connected themes. In elderly patients, delusions tend to be nonbizarre—for example, paranoid jealousy may be seen in individuals with a relatively intact premorbid personality (Yassa and Suranyi-Cadotte 1993).

Agitation may become an issue when such individuals are confronted by family or clinicians about their delusion. Data are lacking on treatment for this disorder. Neuroleptics, particularly pimozide, have been reported to be helpful for the delusion (Opler and Feinberg 1991), but behavioral intervention and nonneuroleptic medication may be better choices for sporadic agitation that may arise.

Diagnostic Approach to Patients With New Onset of Suspiciousness and Paranoia

As with most mental disorders, a careful psychiatric evaluation and history are key components of the initial approach to the suspicious or paranoid patient. Interviews of family members may be necessary for establishing a diagnosis, particularly if delusions and agitation are present. Part of the task of the clinician is to determine whether suspicious behavior is warranted. Older adults are occasionally abused or neglected; therefore, confronting family members about a patient's accusations of harm or neglect is often part of the assessment. If after such a confrontation the clinician is not convinced that the accusations are totally explained by the delusion, a social services agency or department should be requested to investigate further.

On the other hand, challenging the delusional patient is usually not recommended. It is important to seek an understanding of the patient's thought processes, so providing an atmosphere of acceptance (although not necessarily agreement) will allow the patient to express his or her beliefs and feelings. Reassurance should be provided in a manner conveying that although the clinician may not fully understand the whole situation, the goal is for the patient to feel better and more secure.

A laboratory workup is usually needed in new cases of paranoia to rule out an organic delusional syndrome. Blood chemistry, a complete blood count, and a thyroid profile should be obtained. If respiratory symptoms are present, a chest X ray may be needed. A computed tomography or magnetic resonance imaging brain scan may be indicated, especially if cognitive impairment or focal neurological findings are present. Because suspiciousness is often associated with sensory impairment, particularly visual and auditory deficits, audiometric and visual testing may identify potential areas for further intervention.

Treatment of paranoia may include neuroleptic medication, depending on the diagnosis, as discussed earlier in this chapter. (For a complete discussion of neuroleptics, please see Chapter 24, "Psychopharmacology.") Regardless of whether neuroleptics are prescribed, key compo-

nents of management of paranoia include reassurance for the patient, education for the family, and careful monitoring for development of agitation.

Agitation in Elderly Persons

Behavioral manifestations of dementia are common (Lyketsos et al. 2000) and represent major predictors of caregiver depression, burden, and stress across cultures (Chen et al. 2000; Gallicchio et al. 2002; Teri 1997). Anxiety and agitation, the most commonly cited psychiatric manifestations of dementia, can be as disruptive and painful for the person with dementia as they are for family caregivers. Disruptive or resistive behaviors resulting from anxiety and agitation increase the risk of harm to the affected individual and others (Chow and MacLean 2001; Tractenberg et al. 2001), and caregivers frequently become frightened, upset, or simply exhausted by the demands of caring for a family member with agitation.

Nonpharmacological Approaches

Nonpharmacological strategies are recommended as first-line approaches for the noncognitive manifestations of dementia. These approaches can be taught effectively to family and nonprofessional caregivers (Doody et al. 2001). Nonpharmacological approaches are most effective as adjuncts to pharmacotherapy, when pharmacotherapy is contraindicated, or when behaviors are obviously manifested in response to environmental or interpersonal triggers.

These strategies focus on changing the patient's activity, routines, and/or human, physical, and social environment to provide reassurance, appropriate stimulation, and security. As the person with dementia becomes less adaptable to change, the human and physical environment must adapt to him or her. Behavioral approaches generally include person-specific problem solving, enriched cues, adapted work or expressive activities, exercise, communication strategies, and caregiver skills training.

Key Messages for Families About Agitation in Dementia

Families of persons with dementia should be told directly that anxiety, suspiciousness, and restless agitation are common symptoms of brain disorders, even in the context of excellent, well-intentioned family care. At the same time, it is helpful to suggest that disruptive behaviors do not occur in a vacuum. Agitation has a person-specific situational context and meaning that may often, but not always, be understood. Agitated or even aggressive behavior is often beyond a dementia patient's control or intentionality. In fact, he or she may not be aware of agitation or a change in behavior.

Frequent or escalating agitation requires a prompt and multimodal response. Ignoring agitated or disruptive behaviors will not make them go away. Persons with dementia are most likely to be angry at what they perceive as an intolerable situation that no longer makes sense. For this reason it is wise for families not to take attacks or accusations personally. Families should also be reminded that persons with dementia are more likely to take out their frustration on those closest to them while appearing gracious and appropriate with strangers.

Families should be told that people with dementia generally can't "try harder." A corollary is that reasoning, arguing, coaxing, pleading, confronting, or punishing agitated persons may only escalate the distressing behavior. Families respond effectively if they understand that agitated people with dementia are likely to be scared and overwhelmed by disorientation and that they may forget appropriate public or private behavior. Agitation is frequently accompanied by a loss of impulse control that can result in uncharacteristic cursing, insensitivity, tactlessness, or sexually inappropriate behavior. Although people with dementia may seem insensitive to others' feelings, they are extremely sensitive to and will respond negatively to patronizing, angry, tense, rushed, or demanding nonverbal communication from family members.

Agitated persons with dementia generally respond well to calm, familiar settings with predictable routines and to requests tailored to their capacities, remaining strengths, and energy levels. Although Alzheimer's disease patients may appear to do less as a result of apathy, they can become fatigued from just trying to make sense of what is going on around them. Late-day fatigue or wearing out may explain some agitated behavior associated with "sundowning" (patients' becoming more confused, agitated, or psychotic in the late afternoon or early evening) and extremely exaggerated reactions to minor incidents. Furthermore, patients with mild to moderate Alzheimer's disease may resist activities they perceive as too difficult or too demeaning, in order to limit embarrassment or failure.

Questions to Guide Problem Solving for Agitation in Dementia

Consideration of the following nine questions can help pinpoint and resolve caregivers' problems with a patient's agitated behavior:

1. Which agitated, anxious, or resistive behaviors are most disruptive to family life at this point?
2. Describe the behavior. Is it harmful or does it cause distress to the person with dementia or to others? Can the family change expectations or increase tolerance for this change in the person as they knew him or her?
3. Is there any pattern, trigger, or time of day that sets off the behavior (e.g., a move, travel, hospitalization, or being asked to do a complex task)?
4. Does anything happen afterward that makes it worse (e.g., caregiver anger or abandonment or patient failure)?
5. Is the person uncomfortable (e.g., pain, hunger, thirst, constipation, full bladder, fatigue, infection, cold, fear, misperceived threats, difficult communication)?
6. Is the person looking for something familiar from the past (e.g., rummaging in drawers, searching for an outhouse or an old employer)?
7. Will a change in environment help (e.g., reduce number of people, confusion, stimuli, noise)?
8. Can the caregiver use familiar phrases to calm or reassure the person (e.g., "I'll get right on it"; "Ain't that the truth?"; "Even the Lord rested on Sundays")?
9. Can routines be changed or adapted to prevent future occurrences of the behavior (e.g., exercising early in the day, bathing less frequently, avoiding rush-hour shopping)?

Common Strategies That Reduce Agitation

Nonpharmacological strategies for reducing agitation usually involve redirection of the person's attention away from triggering events or contexts or distraction with offers of pleasant events specific to the person (going out for ice cream or a ride, listening to favorite music, or watching old videotapes). Other strategies include breaking down complex tasks into one-step guided directions, simplifying instructions, and allowing adequate rest or passive observation between stimulating activities. Environmental strategies include using labels, cues, or pictures; hazard-proofing the environment to reduce dangers of exploration or egress; removing guns or hazardous equipment; and using lighting or security objects to reduce nighttime confusion or daytime fear or uncertainty.

Communication Begins With Understanding

Families begin to communicate effectively when they can understand the experience and perspectives of people with dementia. With the current focus on early diagnosis and treatment of Alzheimer's disease, more individuals with insight who have new diagnoses of Alzheimer's disease are willing to provide direction. The following excerpts from a Canadian support group of patients with early-stage Alzheimer's disease can offer guidance to family caregivers:

> Please don't correct me. Remember, my feelings are intact and I get hurt easily. Try to ignore offhand remarks that I wouldn't have made in the past. If you focus on my mistakes, it just makes me feel worse. I may say something that is real to me but not factual to you. It is not a lie. Don't argue—it won't solve anything. (Snyder 2001, p. 2)

When a person with dementia is agitated, he or she may be thinking along the following lines (Gwyther 2000, p. 998):

> How dare you question me? I have always taken care of myself.
>
> I make sense—you and events don't.
>
> Your reality and reasoning wear me out.
>
> I am only protecting what is mine from those people—things keep disappearing.
>
> Can't you see this is not a good time? I'm overwhelmed and scared.

Communication Strategies to Reduce Agitation

First it is necessary to get the person's attention. Make sure vision and hearing are adequate or "tuned up." Use eye contact, call her by name in a clear adult tone, approach slowly from the side or front or crouch down at her level, and offer your hand, palm up. Listen, but do not feel compelled to talk constantly. Words are not as important as a calm tone, pleasant expression, and nondistracting environment (turn off the TV or turn down the radio). Use simple words, speak slowly, and give her time to process and respond. Repeat your words exactly, if necessary. Ask questions if you are unsure of her meaning. ("Am I getting closer to what you want?") Be patient—you may need to repeat to reassure her.

If frustration mounts, take a deep breath and suggest a better time to talk or another topic. Avoid popular expressions that may be ambiguous or vague, like "Don't go there," "NOT," or "bottom line." Use concrete subjects, names, and references. Avoid pronouns. Do not test or ask him if he remembers you. Use positive statements like "Let's go," rather than "Do you want to go now?" Explain what happens next, but wait until just before it will happen. Demonstrate or model so he can follow your lead. Use appropriate respectful humor or his favorite phrases ("See ya later, alligator"). It is always appropriate to make fun of yourself, especially if you forget. Smile, nod, gesture, or use photos when words fail.

Summary of Nonpharmacological Approaches

Families often want brief, concrete suggestions for dealing with agitation. The following format may be helpful (Alzheimer's Association 2001; Gwyther 2001):

DO—slow down, soothe the person, or structure the situation. Encourage and reinforce positive adaptations that work for the person ("I depend on my husband for brute strength in carrying those grocery bags"). Be extra gracious and polite. Back off and ask permission. Repeatedly reassure. Use visual and verbal cues and add light. Offer guided choices between two options. Avoid complex multistep directions or ambiguity. Distract with a favorite snack or ask for help with raking or another adult repetitive task. Increase time spent in pleasant activities like sitting in a porch glider at sunset. Offer security object, rest, or privacy after an upset. Limit caffeine and alcohol. Use comforting rituals like holding hands during grace, an afternoon tea break, checking the bird feeder, or a hand massage or manicure. Do for her what she can no longer comfortably do on her own. Join her in modified favorite activities—social, creative, or sports. Remove her from confusing, frustrating, or scary experiences like TV shows that she believes are happening to her.

DO NOT—raise your voice, take offense, corner, crowd, restrain, rush, criticize, ignore, confront, argue, reason, shame, blame, demand, lecture, condescend, moralize, force, explain, teach, show alarm, or make a sudden move out of the person's view.

SAY—May I help you? Do you have time to help me? Let's take a break now—we have earned it. You're safe here. I will get right on it. Everything is under control. I apologize (even if you didn't do it!). I'm sorry you are upset. I know it's hard. We're in this together. I will make sure those men can't get in here. Do what you can and I'll finish up. We're doing fine now.

Pharmacological/Medical Approaches

There are times when agitation warrants pharmacological intervention. Most clinicians view agitation as a condition manifested by excessive verbal and/or motor behavior. It is distinguished from aggression, which can also be verbal (e.g., cursing or threats) or physical (e.g., hitting, kicking, shoving objects or people). Agitation can escalate to aggression, so it is vital for the clinician to intervene early in approaching agitated patients. First, it becomes essential to determine the cause of agitation. Interventions are then directed at both treating the underlying cause and managing the agitation itself. Medical causes of agitation are shown in Table 23–1.

TABLE 23–1. Common medical causes of agitation in elderly persons

Medication
   Drug-drug interaction
   Accidental misuse
   CNS-toxic side effect
   Systemic disturbance (e.g., medication-induced electrolyte imbalance)
Urinary tract infection
Poor nutrition, decreased oral intake of food and fluid
Respiratory infection
Recent stroke
Occult head trauma if patient fell recently
Pain
Constipation
Alcohol/substance withdrawal
Chronic obstructive pulmonary disease

Agitation most commonly occurs in the context of delirium or dementia. These conditions will be discussed in depth below. Agitation can also be a feature of late-life depression. Although treatment of the underlying depression should also treat the agitation, the effects of antidepressant medications may not be apparent for several weeks. As stated above, it is usually best to consider nonpharmacological approaches to managing agitation. However, acute, severe, or escalating agitation may require medication such as a newer atypical neuroleptic or a benzodiazepine. Chronic treatment of agitation may require the clinician to consider other medications, including antidepressants and mood stabilizers. Choice of medication will depend on the setting and on the severity and chronicity of symptoms, as discussed below.

Agitation in the Context of Delirium

Delirium is a common disorder, with an estimated prevalence of 15%–50% among hospitalized elderly patients (Inouye 1998; Levkoff et al. 1991). Characterized by a disturbance of consciousness and a change in cognition, delirium typically has a rapid onset and runs a short course. The principal elements of the DSM-IV-TR diagnosis of delirium are 1) a disturbance of consciousness indicated by reduced awareness of the environment, along with diminished ability to focus, sustain, or shift attention, 2) a change in cognition (which may include deficits of memory, language, or orientation) or onset of a perceptual disturbance not better accounted for by a dementia, and 3) development of the condition over a short period, with a tendency to fluctuate during the course of the day (American Psychiatric Association 2000). DSM-IV-TR categorizes delirium by presumed etiology (including de-

lirium secondary to a medical condition, substance intoxication, and substance withdrawal), mixed or multiple etiologies, and uncertain etiology.

Delirium typically develops over hours to days and is provoked by certain medical illnesses, metabolic derangements, intoxications, and withdrawal states (Lipowski 1989). A prodromal period of subtle confusion, irritability, or psychomotor behavior change may precede the advent of the full syndrome. Confusion, intermittent clouding of sensorium or consciousness, and alterations in perception commonly occur, as do psychotic symptoms such as paranoia. Marked disturbances of the sleep cycle contribute to sundowning. Autonomic changes such as tachycardia and hypertension can also occur, particularly in the hyperactive form of delirium. Patients with this form often have increased irritability and startle responses and may be acutely sensitive to light and sound. In addition, delirious patients may experience profound shifts in mood and use rambling, illogical language while still having lucid intervals of relatively normal mental functioning. Although short-term memory may be disturbed, long-term memory is typically preserved. The syndrome usually runs a course of several days; however, the duration of illness is largely controlled by the course of the underlying condition that provoked the delirious episode.

Management of delirium is focused mainly on identifying and treating the underlying cause. However, the agitated delirious patient requires immediate attention, because the workup of the delirium may be impeded by agitated behavior, which may also put the patient and others at physical risk. Acute treatment of the agitation will probably require intramuscular or intravenous agents, typically benzodiazepines and neuroleptics. If there is no intravenous access, initial treatment with intramuscular lorazepam or haloperidol, alone or in combination, may be required. When intravenous access is established, these agents can also be used. Alternatives include other short-acting benzodiazepines such as midazolam or more sedating neuroleptics such as thiothixene. Use of intramuscular chlorpromazine should be avoided because of its effects on cardiovascular response, including orthostatic hypotension, which may occur should the patient try to stand up or get out of bed.

Agitation in the Context of Dementia

Agitation is a frequent behavioral symptom in dementia, with 24% of caregivers in one survey reporting agitation and/or aggression (Lyketsos et al. 2000). It occurs at some time in about half of all patients with dementia (Small et al. 1997). A person with dementia may become agitated throughout the day, intermittently through the day, or at specific times of day. For example, sundowning commonly occurs in dementia. One-fourth of inpatients with Alzheimer's disease were found on nursing evaluation to exhibit sundowning behavior (Little et al. 1995). Behaviors associated with agitation in patients who have dementia include aggression, combativeness, disinhibition, and hyperactivity. As with all behavioral problems, the first step in treatment is to identify the precipitants. Evaluation should include assessment for common systemic causes (e.g., infection, dehydration, constipation, and other illnesses) as well as changes in medication.

Pharmacological Treatment

If environmental measures are insufficient to control agitated or aggressive behavior, medication is usually needed. Guidelines for pharmacological treatment of agitation in elderly patients with dementia have been developed (Alexopoulos et al. 1998). High-potency neuroleptics (e.g., haloperidol) are effective for controlling acute agitation, especially when psychotic features are present (Small et al. 1997). Although there is no evidence to suggest that one neuroleptic agent is more effective than another, the atypical antipsychotics—clozapine (Clozaril), risperidone (Risperdal), olanzapine (Zyprexa), quetiapine (Seroquel), and ziprasidone (Geodon)—have a lesser frequency of extrapyramidal side effects (e.g., parkinsonism, tardive dyskinesia). These medications are particularly useful in agitated, psychotic patients with Parkinson's disease because their selective dopaminergic blockade does not interfere with dopamine's therapeutic effect on the basal ganglia. However, atypical antipsychotics are expensive, and most (with the exception of ziprasidone) are not currently available in injectable forms. Benzodiazepines can also be used to treat anxiety or infrequent agitation, but they are less effective than other agents for long-term treatment.

In general, when agitation is a consistent problem and neuroleptic treatment is required, we recommend starting with a low dose (e.g., 0.5 mg of haloperidol or 1 mg of risperidone) and administering it on a regular basis rather than attempting to treat specific episodes of agitation. Trying to treat a patient who is already agitated makes administering medication difficult, requires larger doses, and is likely to cause sedation and further clouding of thought.

The anticonvulsants carbamazepine and divalproex sodium (Depakote) are effective in treating behavioral disturbances in dementia and have a side-effect profile different from that of neuroleptics. In a double-blind study, Tariot and colleagues (1998) found that, compared with the placebo group, patients taking carbamazepine showed significant improvement in agitation and aggression. The

drug was well tolerated. The modal daily dose of carbamazepine was 300 mg, achieving a mean serum level of 5.3 μg/mL. One study has shown that carbamazepine may also be effective when added to neuroleptic therapy in patients with refractory agitation (Lemke 1995). Divalproex has also been shown to be an effective treatment for agitation in dementia (Narayan and Nelson 1997). In this study, the mean final divalproex dose was 1,650 mg/day, with a mean blood level of 64 μg/mL. Divalproex was well tolerated in this population except for reversible sedation in eight patients and transient worsening gait and confusion in one patient.

Other classes of drugs are useful for treating agitation. Antidepressants, especially selective serotonin reuptake inhibitors (SSRIs) and trazodone, are effective even in the absence of clear depressive symptoms. There is no established dose range for treatment of agitation with SSRIs, and in our experience the final doses used to achieve successful treatment of agitation have ranged widely. The acetylcholinesterase inhibitors, tacrine (Cognex), donepezil (Aricept), rivastigmine (Exelon), and galantamine (Reminyl), decrease agitation, possibly by stimulating attention and concentration (Levy et al. 1999). The beta-blocker propranolol hydrochloride (Inderal) inhibits impulsive behavior after frontal lobe injury and can be used to decrease agitation and aggressive behavior in dementia, but it may cause bradycardia and hypotension (Shankle et al. 1995).

The need for continued pharmacological treatment of agitation should be regularly reassessed. Generally, medication for agitation should not be viewed as long-term therapy. In one study, neuroleptic treatment was discontinued after agitation was successfully treated in nine patients with dementia (Borson and Raskind 1997). A placebo was then administered, and behavior was monitored for the next 6 weeks. Of the nine patients, eight did not need additional pharmacological treatment. Interestingly, five of the patients were less agitated after drug treatment was stopped.

However, some patients may require chronic medication treatment for agitation. In such cases, antidepressants, especially SSRIs, or anticonvulsants are the preferred treatments. Benzodiazepines and neuroleptics have obvious inherent risks when used chronically in elderly patients with dementia, and close monitoring for side effects (e.g., sedation and extrapyramidal side effects) is required. In the case of neuroleptics, agitated patients without an established psychotic illness must have clear documentation of previous failed trials of other medications and presence of severe agitated behavior. Such patients should have a trial period without the neuroleptic to determine whether ongoing use of the drug is needed.

References

Alexopoulos GS, Silver JM, Kahn DA, et al. (eds): Agitation in Older Persons with Dementia: A Postgraduate Medicine Special Report (The Expert Consensus Guideline Series). New York, McGraw-Hill, 1998

Alzheimer's Association: Fact Sheet: About Agitation and Alzheimer's Disease. Chicago, IL, Alzheimer's Association, 2001. Available at http://www.alz.org/ResourceCenter/ByType/FactSheets.htm (click on "Agitation"). Accessed October 7, 2003.

American Psychiatric Association: Diagnostic and Statistical Manual of Mental Disorders, 4th Edition, Text Revision. Washington, DC, American Psychiatric Association, 2000

Borson S, Raskind MA: Clinical features and pharmacologic treatment of behavioral symptoms of Alzheimer's disease. Neurology 48 (suppl 6):S17–S24, 1997

Chen JC, Borson S, Scanlan JM: Stage-specific prevalence of behavioral symptoms in Alzheimer's disease in a multi-ethnic community sample. Am J Geriatr Psychiatry 8:123–133, 2000

Chow TW, MacLean CH: Quality indicators for dementia in vulnerable community-dwelling and hospitalized elders. Ann Intern Med 135:668–676, 2001

Christenson R, Blazer D: Epidemiology of persecutory ideation in an elderly population in the community. Am J Psychiatry 141:1088–1091, 1984

Doody RS, Stevens JC, Beck C, et al: Practice Parameter: Management of Dementia (An Evidence-Based Review): Report of the Quality Standards Subcommittee of the American Academy of Neurology. Neurology 56:1154–1166, 2001

Gallicchio L, Siddiqui N, Langenberg P, et al: Gender differences in burden and depression among informal caregivers of demented elders in the community. Int J Geriatr Psychiatry 17:154–163, 2002

Gwyther L: Family issues in dementia: finding a new normal. Neurol Clin 18:993–1010, 2000

Gwyther L: Caring for People with Alzheimer's Disease: A Manual for Facility Staff. Washington, DC, American Health Care Association and Alzheimer's Association, 2001

Inouye SK: Delirium in hospitalized older patients. Clin Geriatr Med 14:745–764, 1998

Lemke MR: Effect of carbamazepine on agitation in Alzheimer's inpatients refractory to neuroleptics. J Clin Psychiatry 56:354–357, 1995

Levkoff S, Cleary P, Liptzin B, et al: Epidemiology of delirium: an overview of research issues and findings. Int Psychogeriatr 3:149–167, 1991

Levy ML, Cummings JL, Kahn-Rose R: Neuropsychiatric symptoms and cholinergic therapy for Alzheimer's disease. Gerontology 45 (suppl 1):15–22, 1999

Lipowski ZJ: Delirium in the elderly patient. N Engl J Med 320:578–582, 1989

Little JT, Satlin A, Sunderland T, et al: Sundown syndrome in severely demented patients with probable Alzheimer's disease. J Geriatr Psychiatry Neurol 8:103–106, 1995

Lowenthal MF, Berkman PL: Aging and Mental Disorders in San Francisco: A Social Psychiatry Study. San Francisco, CA, Jossey-Bass, 1967

Lyketsos CG, Steinberg M, Tschanz JT, et al: Mental and behavioral disturbances in dementia: findings from the Cache County Study on Memory in Aging. Am J Psychiatry 157:708–714, 2000

Narayan M, Nelson JC: Treatment of dementia with behavioral disturbance using divalproex or a combination of divalproex and a neuroleptic. J Clin Psychiatry 58:351–354, 1997

Opler LA, Feinberg SS: The role of pimozide in clinical psychiatry: a review. J Clin Psychiatry 52:221–233, 1991

Shankle WR, Nielson KA, Cotman CW: Low-dose propranolol reduces aggression and agitation resembling that associated with orbitofrontal dysfunction in elderly demented patients. Alzheimer Dis Assoc Disord 9:233–237, 1995

Small GW, Rabins PV, Barry PP, et al: Diagnosis and treatment of Alzheimer disease and related disorders: consensus statement of the American Association for Geriatric Psychiatry, the Alzheimer's Association, and the American Geriatrics Society. JAMA 278:1363–1371, 1997

Snyder L: Perspectives: A Newsletter For Individuals Diagnosed With Alzheimer's Disease. Alzheimer's Disease Research Center, University of California, San Diego, 2001, p 2

Soares JC, Gershon S: Therapeutic targets in late-life psychoses: review of concepts and critical issues. Schizophr Res 27:227–239, 1997

Tariot PN, Erb R, Podgorski CA, et al: Efficacy and tolerability of carbamazepine for agitation and aggression in dementia. Am J Psychiatry 155:54–61, 1998

Teri L: Behavior and caregiver burden: behavioral problems in patients with Alzheimer disease and its association with caregiver burden. Alzheimer Dis Assoc Disord 11 (suppl 4):S35–S38, 1997

Tractenberg RE, Garmst A, Weiner MF, et al: Frequency of behavioral symptoms characterizes agitation in Alzheimer's disease. Int J Geriatr Psychiatry 16:886–891, 2001

Yassa R, Suranyi-Cadotte B: Clinical characteristics of late-onset schizophrenia and delusional disorder. Schizophr Bull 19:701–707, 1993

Treatment of Psychiatric Disorders in Late Life

Psychopharmacology

Benoit H. Mulsant, M.D.

Bruce G. Pollock, M.D., Ph.D.

Pharmacological intervention in late life requires special care (DeVane and Pollock 1999). The elderly are more susceptible to drug-induced adverse events (Pollock 1999). Particularly troublesome among older persons are peripheral and central anticholinergic effects such as constipation, urinary retention, delirium, and cognitive dysfunction; antihistaminergic effects such as sedation; and antiadrenergic effects such as postural hypotension. In addition to interfering with basic activities, pronounced sedation and orthostatic hypotension pose a significant safety risk to elderly patients because they can lead to falls and fractures. This increased susceptibility to adverse effects is largely due to the pharmacokinetic and pharmacodynamic changes associated with aging: diminished glomerular filtration, changes in the density and activity of target receptors, reduced liver size and hepatic blood flow, and decreased cardiac output (Table 24–1). Illnesses that affect many elderly persons (e.g., diabetes) further diminish the processing and removal of medications from the body. In addition, polypharmacy and the associated risk of drug interactions add another level of complexity to the pharmacological treatment of older patients. Finally, poor adherence to treatment regimens—which can be due to impaired cognitive function, confusing drug regimens, or lack of motivation or insight associated with the psychiatric disorder being treated—is a significant obstacle to effective and safe pharmacological treatment.

Despite these challenges, psychiatric disorders can be successfully treated in late life with psychotropic drugs. During the 1990s, many new psychotropic drugs were shown to be effective and safe, resulting in improvement not only of psychiatric symptoms but also of physical health status, general functioning, and quality of life. To help clinicians face these challenges and to help them rationally select psychotropic medications for their older patients, in the remainder of this chapter we systematically summarize relevant data published in scientific journals as of June 2002 on the efficacy, tolerability, and safety of the major psychotropic drugs. Where it is available, we also present consensus expert opinion.

TABLE 24–1. Physiological changes in elderly persons associated with altered pharmacokinetics

Organ system	Change	Pharmacokinetic consequence
Circulatory system	Decreased concentration of plasma albumin and increased α_1-acid glycoprotein	Increased or decreased free concentration of drugs in plasma
Gastrointestinal tract	Decreased intestinal and splanchnic blood flow	Decreased rate of drug absorption
Kidney	Decreased glomerular filtration rate	Decreased renal clearance of active metabolites
Liver	Decreased liver size; decreased hepatic blood flow; variable effects on cytochrome P450 isozyme activity	Decreased hepatic clearance
Muscle	Decreased lean body mass and increased adipose tissue	Altered volume of distribution of lipid-soluble drugs leading to increased elimination half-life

Source. Adapted from Pollock BG: "Psychotropic Drugs and the Aging Patient." *Geriatrics* 53 (suppl 1):S20–S24, 1998.

Antidepressant Medications

Selective Serotonin Reuptake Inhibitors

The selective serotonin reuptake inhibitors (SSRIs) have now replaced tricyclic antidepressants (TCAs) and monoamine oxidase inhibitors (MAOIs) as first-line drugs for treating late-life depression (Alexopoulos et al. 2001). This change to SSRIs occurred because of their efficacy for both depressive and anxiety syndromes, their ease of use, and their safety and good tolerability. Citalopram, escitalopram, fluoxetine, paroxetine, and sertraline are approved in the United States for the treatment of depression. Although fluvoxamine is approved only for obsessive-compulsive disorder, the drug is also used to treat depression. As with most drugs, few clinical trials of SSRIs have been conducted under "real-life" geriatric sit-

uations (e.g., in long-term-care facilities) or in very old patients (Flint 1998; Schneider and Olin 1995). However, as of June 2002, close to 20 randomized, controlled trials of SSRIs in more than 3,000 geriatric patients with depression have been published (Table 24–2). Several controlled and open studies have also been conducted in special populations (Solai et al. 2001); a recent review of many of these trials concluded that SSRIs are efficacious, safe, and well tolerated in older patients, including those with dementia (Katona et al. 1998; Nyth and Gottfries 1990; Nyth et al. 1992; Olafsson et al. 1992; Taragano et al. 1997), cardiovascular disease (Roose 2000), cerebrovascular disease (Whyte and Mulsant 2002), stroke (Andersen et al. 1994; Robinson et al. 2000), or other medical conditions (Arranz and Ros 1997; Evans et al. 1997; Goodnick and Hernandez 2000; Trappler and Cohen 1998).

TABLE 24–2. Summary of randomized, controlled trials of SSRIs for treatment of geriatric depression

	Number of published trials and cumulative number of older participants	Dosages studied (mg/day)	Comments	References
Citalopram	4 $N = 669$	10–40	Citalopram was more efficacious than placebo and as efficacious as amitriptyline. Trials were conducted in depressed patients with stroke and in patients with dementia.	Andersen et al. 1994; Kyle et al. 1998; Nyth and Gottfries 1990; Nyth et al. 1992
Fluoxetine	8 $N = 1,103$	10–80	Fluoxetine was more efficacious than placebo and as efficacious as amitriptyline, doxepin, paroxetine, and sertraline. One trial was conducted in patients with dementia of the Alzheimer type.	Altamura et al. 1989; Doraiswamy et al. 2001; Evans et al. 1997; Feighner and Cohn 1985; Finkel et al. 1999; Schone and Ludwig 1993; Taragano et al. 1997; Tollefson et al. 1995
Fluvoxamine	3 $N = 185$	50–200	Fluvoxamine was more efficacious than placebo and as efficacious as dothiepin, imipramine, and mianserin.	Phanjoo et al. 1991; Rahman et al. 1991; Wakelin 1986
Paroxetine	5 $N = 846$	10–40	Paroxetine was as efficacious as amitriptyline, bupropion, clomipramine, doxepin, imipramine, fluoxetine, and nortriptyline. Trials included inpatients and patients with dementia or melancholic depression.	Dunner et al. 1992; Geretsegger et al. 1995; Guillibert et al. 1989; Katona et al. 1998; Mulsant et al. 1999, 2001b; Schone and Ludwig 1993
Sertraline	5 $N = 826$	50–200	Sertraline was as efficacious as amitriptyline, nortriptyline, and fluoxetine. Greater cognitive improvement occurred with sertraline than with nortriptyline or fluoxetine. Trials included long-term-care patients and patients with melancholic depression.	Bondareff et al. 2000; Cohn et al. 1990; Finkel et al. 1999; Newhouse et al. 2000; Oslin et al. 2000

Although a particular SSRI may have greater efficacy or be better tolerated in older persons than another SSRI, available data show that all available SSRIs have similar efficacy and tolerability in the treatment of depression in younger (Kroenke et al. 2001) and in older adults (Schneider and Olin 1995; Solai et al. 2001). However, experts favor the use of citalopram, escitalopram, or sertraline over fluvoxamine and fluoxetine (Alexopoulos et al. 2001; Mulsant et al. 2001a). This preference is in large part because of the favorable pharmacokinetic profiles of citalopram, escitalopram, and sertraline (Table 24–3), their lower potential for clinically significant drug interactions (Table 24–4), and data suggesting their superiority in terms of cognitive improvement (Furlan et al. 2001; Newhouse et al. 2000; Nyth and Gottfries 1990; Nyth et al. 1992). Fluoxetine, fluvoxamine, and paroxetine are more likely to be involved in significant drug interactions than are citalopram, escitalopram, and sertraline. In contrast to the other SSRIs, fluoxetine has an active metabolite with a half-life greater than 1 week. Although this very long half-life can be an advantage during discontinuation, it is a significant disadvantage if the patient experiences an adverse drug reaction (Druckenbrod and Mulsant 1994).

Several SSRIs—fluvoxamine, paroxetine, and sertraline—have well-established efficacy for anxiety disorders in younger adults (Nemeroff 2002). However, no published controlled trials and only one small open study (Wylie et al. 2000) support their efficacy in older patients with anxiety disorders. In the absence of such data, the use of SSRIs to treat geriatric anxiety disorders is mostly based on extrapolation from studies in younger adults and expert opinion (Lenze et al. 2002). By contrast, several published studies—including one randomized, placebo-controlled trial—suggest that SSRIs may be efficacious in the treatment of behavioral disturbances associated with dementia, including not only agitation and disinhibition but also delusions and hallucinations; in most of these trials, citalopram was the drug studied (Nyth and Gottfries 1990; Nyth et al. 1992; Pollock et al. 1997, 1999, 2002).

When SSRIs are prescribed to older patients, starting dosages are typically half the minimal efficacious dosage (see Table 24–3), and the dosage is usually doubled after 1 week. All the SSRIs can be administered in a single daily dose except for fluvoxamine, which should be given in two divided doses. Fluoxetine is usually taken in the morning, whereas citalopram and paroxetine are given at bedtime. Escitalopram and sertraline can be taken in the morning or in the evening. Although even the most frail older patients typically tolerate these drugs relatively well (Oslin et al. 2000), some patients experience some gastrointestinal distress (e.g., nausea) during the first few days of treatment. The syndrome of inappropriate secretion of antidiuretic hormone (SIADH) with significant hyponatremia is a rare but potentially dangerous adverse effect that is observed almost exclusively in the elderly (Fabian et al., in press; Woo and Smythe 1997). Patients who are taking diuretics seem to be at higher risk (Kirby and Ames 2001). SSRIs can also be associated with bradycardia and should be started with great cautions in patients with low heart rates (e.g., patients taking β-blockers). Even though SSRIs have been reported to be associated with extrapyramidal symptoms in some younger patients (Pies 1997), extrapyramidal symptoms surprisingly seem rare in older patients (Mamo et al. 2000) and SSRIs are well tolerated by most patients with Parkinson's disease (Richard and Kurlan 1997).

Other Newer Antidepressants

Only very limited controlled data support the efficacy and safety of bupropion, mirtazapine, nefazodone, and venlafaxine in older patients (Table 24–5). Nevertheless, due to their usually favorable side-effect profiles in younger

TABLE 24–3. Pharmacokinetic properties of selective serotonin reuptake inhibitors

	Half-life (days), including active metabolite(s)	Proportionality of dosage to plasma concentration	Risk of uncomfortable withdrawal symptoms	Age-related pharmacokinetic changes?	Efficacious dosage range in elderly (mg/day)[a]
Citalopram	1–3	Linear across therapeutic range	Low	Yes	20–40
Escitalopram	1–3	Linear across therapeutic range	Low	Yes	10–20
Fluoxetine	7–10	Nonlinear at higher dosages	Very low	Yes	20–40
Fluvoxamine	0.5–1	Nonlinear at higher dosages	Moderate	Yes	50–300
Paroxetine	1	Nonlinear at higher dosages	Moderate	Yes	20–40
Sertraline	1–3	Linear across therapeutic range	Low	No	50–200

[a]Starting dosage is typically half of the lower efficacious dosage; all the selective serotonin reuptake inhibitors can be administered in single daily doses except for fluvoxamine, which should be given in two divided doses.

TABLE 24–4. Newer antidepressants' inhibition of cytochrome P450 and potential for clinically significant drug-drug interaction

| | Cytochrome P450 | | | | Potential for clinically significant drug-drug interaction |
	1A2	2C9/2C19	2D6	3A4	
Bupropion	0	0	+	0	Low
Citalopram	+	0	+	0	Low
Escitalopram	+	0	+	0	Low
Fluoxetine	+	++	+++	++	High
Fluvoxamine	+++	+++	+	++	High
Mirtazapine	0	0	0	+	Low
Nefazodone	0	+	0	+++	High
Paroxetine	+	+	+++	+	Moderate
Sertraline	+	+	+	+	Low
Venlafaxine	0	0	0	0	Low

Note. 0 = minimal or no inhibition; + = mild inhibition; ++ = moderate inhibition; +++ = strong inhibition.
Source. Alderman et al. 2001; Belpaire et al. 1998; Brosen et al. 1993; Crewe et al. 1992; Ereshefsky and Dugan 2000; Gram et al. 1993; Greenblatt et al. 1998, 1999; Greene and Barbhaiya 1997; Iribarne et al. 1998; Jeppesen et al. 1996; Kashuba et al. 1998; Kobayashi et al. 1995; Pollock 1999; Preskorn and Magnus 1994, 1997; Rasmussen et al. 1998; Rickels et al. 1998; Solai et al. 1997, 2002; von Moltke et al. 1995, 2001; Weigmann et al. 2001.

patients and their various mechanisms of action, these drugs are the preferred alternatives in older patients who do not respond to or who cannot tolerate SSRIs (Alexopoulos et al. 2001). Still, recent controlled data suggesting that venlafaxine may be less safe than sertraline in a frail elderly population, without evidence for an increase in efficacy, suggest caution in the absence of systematic research (Oslin et al. 2003).

Bupropion

Published data supporting the safety and efficacy of bupropion in geriatric depression are limited to two small controlled trials (Branconnier et al. 1983; Doraiswamy et al. 2001; Weihs et al. 2000) (see Table 24–5) and one small open study (Steffens et al. 2001). Expert consensus favors the use of bupropion—alone or as an augmentation agent—in older depressed patients who have not responded to SSRIs or who cannot tolerate them (Alexopoulos et al. 2001). In particular, bupropion can be helpful for patients who complain of unbearable fatigue (Green 1997) or sexual dysfunction (Chengappa et al. 2001; Coleman et al. 2001; Croft et al. 1999; Labbate et al. 1997; Segraves et al. 2000). Although augmentation with bupropion has been reported to be helpful in younger and older patients who were partial

responders to SSRIs or venlafaxine (Bodkin et al. 1997; Spier 1998), the safety of this combination has not been established (see next paragraph).

In addition to the three small geriatric trials supporting its safety, controlled data on the use of bupropion in patients with heart disease (Kiev et al. 1994; Roose et al. 1991), in smokers (Chengappa et al. 2001; Tashkin et al. 2001), and in patients with neuropathic pain (Semenchuk et al. 2001) confirm clinical experience that bupropion is relatively well tolerated by medically ill patients. The most problematic adverse effects associated with bupropion are seizures, and bupropion is contraindicated in patients with preexisting seizure disorders or who are at risk for seizure disorders (e.g., poststroke patients). However, the sustained-release preparation of bupropion appears to be associated with a very low incidence of seizure, comparable to other antidepressants (Dunner et al. 1998). Bupropion has also been associated with the onset of psychosis in several case reports (Howard and Warnock 1999), and it is prudent to avoid this medication in psychotic patients or in patients at risk for the development of psychotic symptoms. The propensity of bupropion to induce psychosis in patients at risk has been attributed to its action on dopaminergic neurotransmission (Howard and Warnock 1999). The same mechanism has

TABLE 24–5. Summary of published randomized controlled trials of bupropion, mirtazapine, nefazodone, and venlafaxine for treatment of geriatric depression

	Number of published trials and cumulative number of older participants	Dosages studied (mg/day)	Comments	References
Bupropion	2 N = 163	100–450	Bupropion was as efficacious as imipramine and paroxetine.	Branconnier et al. 1983; Weihs et al. 2000
Mirtazapine	1 N = 115	15–45	Mirtazapine was as efficacious as low-dosage (30–90 mg/day) amitriptyline.	Hoyberg et al. 1996
Nefazodone	0	NA	NA	
Venlafaxine	3 N = 314	50–150	Venlafaxine was as efficacious and as well tolerated as dothiepin, was as efficacious as and better tolerated than clomipramine, and was more efficacious and better tolerated than trazodone. However, venlafaxine was as efficacious as, but less well tolerated and less safe than, sertraline.	Mahapatra and Hackett 1997; Oslin et al. 2003; Smeraldi et al. 1998

been hypothesized to underlie the association of bupropion with gait disturbance and falls in some patients (Joo et al. 2002; Szuba and Leuchter 1992). Although bupropion does not appear to inhibit cytochrome P450 and is therefore unlikely to cause drug interactions, it appears to be metabolized by the cytochrome P450 isoform 2B6 (Hesse et al. 2000), and adverse effects of bupropion such as seizures or gait disturbance may be more likely in patients who take drugs that can inhibit cytochrome P450 2B6, such as fluoxetine or paroxetine (Joo et al. 2002).

Mirtazapine

Even though mirtazapine has been shown to be efficacious in younger patients (Benkert et al. 2000; Fawcett and Barkin 1998; Guelfi et al. 2001), its efficacy has not yet been demonstrated in older patients (see Table 24–5). In the only published controlled trial of mirtazapine in geriatric depression (Hoyberg et al. 1996), its safety and tolerability were found to be comparable to those of amitriptyline, although the amitriptyline was administered at low dosages (30–90 mg/day) that would not usually be effective in treating depression. Consistent with the absence of controlled data, experts favor the use of mirtazapine as a third-line drug in older depressed patients who have not responded to or who are unable to tolerate SSRIs or venlafaxine (Alexopoulos et al. 2001).

The antidepressant activity of mirtazapine has been attributed to its blockade of α_2 autoreceptors, resulting in a direct enhancement of noradrenergic neurotransmission and an increase in synaptic levels of serotonin

(5-hydroxytryptamine [5-HT]), indirectly enhancing neurotransmission mediated by serotonin type 1A (5-HT$_{1A}$) receptors. In addition, like the antinausea drugs granisetron and ondansetron, mirtazapine inhibits the 5-HT$_2$ and 5-HT$_3$ serotonin receptors. Thus, mirtazapine could be particularly helpful for patients who do not tolerate SSRIs due to sexual dysfunction (Gelenberg et al. 2000; Montejo et al. 2001), tremor (Pact and Giduz 1999), or severe nausea (Pedersen and Klysner 1997). In one case series, mirtazapine was successfully used to treat depression in 19 mixed-age oncology patients who were receiving chemotherapy (Thompson 2000).

Due to its unique mechanism of action, mirtazapine can also been used in patients who have not responded to SSRIs (Gorman 1999), and in some cases it has been combined with SSRIs (Pedersen and Klysner 1997). However, such a combination should be used very cautiously because its safety has not been established and it has been associated with a serotonin syndrome in an older patient (Benazzi 1998).

Similarly, although mirtazapine has been used to treat depression in older patients with dementia (Raji and Brady 2001), its impact on cognition is not known and it has been associated with delirium (Bailer et al. 2000), possibly because of its antihistaminergic effect. The antihistaminergic effect of mirtazapine is most clearly linked to its propensity to commonly cause significant sedation and weight gain with lipid increase (Thompson 2000). Potentially more severe adverse effects of mirtazapine are neutropenia and even agranulocytosis (Hutchison 2001; Stimmel et al. 1997). Although these adverse effects appear to be very rare, they may occur more frequently in patients with compromised immune function (Stimmel et al. 1997).

Nefazodone

Given the absence of any controlled or open trials in geriatric depression, the data available on nefazodone in the elderly are limited to three publications. A pooled analysis of 250 older patients who participated in controlled trials suggested that nefazodone is safe and effective in these patients (Goldberg 1997). A small pharmacokinetic study showed that older persons metabolize nefazodone more slowly than younger patients and that geriatric dosages should be about 50% of the dosages used in younger adults (Barbhaiya et al. 1996). Finally, a cognitive study of a small group of healthy volunteers found that higher dosages of nefazodone (i.e., 200 mg twice daily) were associated with impairment of cognitive and memory functions (van Laar et al. 1995).

In the absence of data, it is not surprising that experts recommend the use of nefazodone as a third- or fourth-line drug after SSRIs, venlafaxine, bupropion, or mirtazapine (Alexopoulos et al. 2001). Furthermore, since the publication of these expert consensus guidelines, reports that the incidence of hepatic toxicity or even failure may be 10- to 30-fold higher with nefazodone than with other antidepressants have contributed to even further reduction of support for its use (Carvajal et al. 2002; Lucena et al. 1999). However, except for sedation, nefazodone is usually well tolerated (Robinson et al. 1996), and therefore it can be helpful in somatizers who complain of unbearable side effects with other antidepressants (Menza et al. 2001; Mulsant et al. 2001a; Sajatovic et al. 1999) or in patients who develop a sexual dysfunction with an SSRI that persists after switching to bupropion or mirtazapine (Ferguson et al. 2001; Montejo et al. 2001; Waldinger et al. 2001).

When nefazodone is prescribed, one needs to be mindful of potentially problematic drug interactions due to its strong inhibition of cytochrome P450 3A4, an isozyme responsible for the metabolism of the majority of drugs, including alprazolam, triazolam, carbamazepine, and cyclosporin (Alderman et al. 2001; Greene and Barbhaiya 1997; Rickels et al. 1998) (see Table 24–4).

Venlafaxine

Venlafaxine is the first available agent in a new class of dual-action antidepressants—that is, antidepressants that inhibit the reuptake of both serotonin and norepinephrine (Harvey et al. 2000). Its efficacy and safety in older patients have been established in two published randomized, controlled trials (Mahapatra and Hackett 1997; Smeraldi et al. 1998) (see Table 24–5) and four open series (Amore et al. 1997; Dahmen et al. 1999; Dierick 1996; Khan et al. 1995). Venlafaxine does not inhibit any of the major cytochrome P450 isoenzymes and thus has low potential for causing clinically significant drug interactions (see Table 24–4), making it an attractive choice for the treatment of geriatric depression (Staab and Evans 2000). However, venlafaxine is metabolized by cytochrome P450 2D6, and its concentration can increase markedly in genetically poor metabolizers and in patients who are treated with drugs that inhibit this isozyme (Benazzi 1999). Also, venlafaxine has been compared to sertraline in a randomized trial conducted under double-blind conditions in older nursing home residents. It was less well tolerated and less safe than sertraline without evidence for an increase in efficacy (Oslin et al. 2003).

Experts favor the use of venlafaxine as an alternative to SSRIs (Alexopoulos et al. 2001). Some trials conducted in younger patients suggest that venlafaxine may be particularly useful in patients with treatment-resistant depression (i.e., those who have not responded to an adequate trial of another agent) (de Montigny et al. 1999; Nierenberg et al. 1994; Thase et al. 2000). Furthermore, a meta-analysis of comparative studies conducted in younger depressed patients suggests that venlafaxine may also be more likely than SSRIs to produce remission (i.e., full resolution of depressive symptoms) as opposed to response (i.e., an improvement in depressive symptoms) (Entsuah et al. 2001; Thase et al. 2001). However, venlafaxine is one of the few newer antidepressants that exhibit a clear dose-response relationship (Kelsey 1996), and younger patients require higher dosages (225 mg/day or more) to obtain the benefits of its dual action (Harvey et al. 2000). Because the pharmacokinetics of venlafaxine are similar in younger and in older patients (Klamerus et al. 1996), geriatric patients may similarly require high doses, which are associated with some safety concerns (see below). Therefore, at present it seems prudent not to use venlafaxine as a first-line agent but to reserve it for those who do not respond to SSRIs (Alexopoulos et al. 2001; Mulsant et al. 2001a).

Venlafaxine can also be useful in the treatment of generalized anxiety disorder (Allgulander et al. 2001; Rickels et al. 2000) and of chronic pain syndromes (Barkin and Fawcett 2000; Kiayias et al. 2000; Schreiber et al. 1999) that are comorbid with depression or that present as primary problems. For the treatment of diabetic neuropathy and other pain syndromes, higher dosages (225 mg/day or more) of venlafaxine are usually needed because its antinociceptive effects seem to be mediated through its adrenergic action (Harvey et al. 2000; Schreiber et al. 1999).

Because, even at lower doses, venlafaxine inhibits the reuptake of serotonin, it shares the side-effect profile of SSRIs, including not only nausea, diarrhea, headaches, and excessive sweating but also SIADH and hyponatremia (Kirby and Ames 2001), sexual dysfunction (Montejo et al. 2001), serotonin syndrome (Graudins et al. 1998; McCue and Joseph 2001; Perry 2000), and withdrawal symptoms (Agelink et al. 1997; Fava et al. 1997). Although the extended-release preparation of venlafaxine seems to be associated with significantly fewer gastrointestinal side effects than the immediate-release preparation, use of the extended-release preparation does not seem to reduce the incidence or severity of withdrawal symptoms (Fava et al. 1997). In fact, it has been associated with the most severe and protracted antidepressant withdrawal syndromes that we have directly observed. In addition to these serotonergic side effects, venlafaxine has also been associated with adverse effects that can be linked to its action on the adrenergic system. Some are usually benign (e.g., dry mouth, transient agitation), but others can be problematic. In particular, treatment-emergent hypertension occurs in some older patients, generally in a dose-dependent fashion (Thase 1998; Zimmer et al. 1997). Even though it has also been used to safely treat a small series of older patients with poststroke depression (Dahmen et al. 1999), venlafaxine has also been associated with other cardiovascular adverse effects such as palpitations, arrhythmia, and acute ischemia (Lessard et al. 1999; Oslin et al. 2003; Reznik et al. 1999). Finally, adverse effects usually seen with TCAs and attributed to their anticholinergic effects have also been described, including constipation (Benazzi 1997), increased ocular pressure (Aragona and Inghilleri 1998), and urinary retention (Benazzi 1997).

Tricyclic Antidepressants and Monoamine Oxidase Inhibitors

TCAs and MAOIs have become third- and fourth-line drugs in the treatment of late-life depression because of their adverse effects and the special precautions their use in older patients entails (Mulsant et al. 2001a). The tertiary-amine TCAs—amitriptyline, clomipramine, doxepin, and imipramine—can cause significant orthostatic hypotension and anticholinergic effects, including cognitive impairment, and they should be avoided in the elderly (Beers 1997). MAOIs, now rarely used in older depressed patients, are discussed later in this section.

When one needs to use a TCA in an older patient, the secondary amines desipramine and nortriptyline are preferred because of their lower propensity to cause orthostasis and falls, their linear pharmacokinetics, and their more modest anticholinergic effects. Typically, the entire dose of desipramine or nortriptyline can be given at bedtime. The relatively narrow therapeutic index (i.e., the plasma level range separating efficacy and toxicity) of the secondary amines necessitates monitoring of plasma levels and electrocardiograms in older patients. After initiation of desipramine at 50 mg and nortriptyline at 25 mg, plasma levels can be obtained after 5–7 days and dosages adjusted linearly, targeting plasma levels of 200–400 ng/mL for desipramine and 50–150 ng/mL for nortriptyline. These narrow ranges may ensure efficacy while decreasing risks of cognitive toxicity and other side effects. Similar to the tertiary TCAs, desipramine and nortriptyline are type 1 antiarrhythmics: they have quinidine-like effects on cardiac conduction and should not be used in patients who have or are at risk for conduction defects (Roose et al. 1991).

Most anticholinergic side effects of desipramine or nortriptyline (e.g., dry mouth, constipation) resolve with time or else can usually be mitigated with symptomatic treatment (Mulsant et al. 1999; Rosen et al. 1993). However, TCAs have been associated with cognitive worsening (Reifler et al. 1989) and with more cognitive improvement than sertraline (Bondareff et al. 2000) or other SSRIs.

Even though they have been found to be efficacious in older depressed patients (Georgotas et al. 1986), MAOIs are now rarely used due to the significant hypotension that can be associated with their use and the risk of life-threatening hypertensive or serotonergic crises associated with dietary noncompliance or drug interactions. When MAOIs are used, phenelzine may be preferred to tranylcypromine because it has been more extensively studied in older patients (Georgotas et al. 1983, 1986). A typical starting dosage would be 15 mg/day with a target dosage of 45–90 mg/day in three divided doses. Patients need to be advised about dietary restrictions and should be instructed to inform any health providers (including pharmacists) that they are taking an MAOI.

Psychostimulants

The abuse of prescription amphetamine, which peaked in the 1970s, led to countervailing restrictions. Nonetheless, with the introduction of methylphenidate for childhood hyperkinesis, there was a resurgence of therapeutic interest in psychostimulants. Small double-blind trials suggest that methylphenidate is generally well tolerated and modestly efficacious for medically burdened depressed elders (Satel and Nelson 1989; Wallace and Kofoed

1995). Methylphenidate may also have specific utility in treating the apathy and anergia accompanying late-life depression or dementia (Kaplitz 1975). Nonetheless, caution is advised regarding the possible exacerbation of anxiety, psychosis, anorexia, and hypertension that may be associated with methylphenidate as well as its potential interactions with warfarin. Recently, interest has been renewed in using methylphenidate to augment antidepressant response to SSRIs (Lavretsky and Kumar 2001). Given that SSRIs may inhibit dopamine release, contributing to apathy in this population with diminished dopaminergic function, further exploration of methylphenidate as an augmenting agent is warranted. Experience with other dopaminergic medications—such as pemoline, piribedil, pramipexole, and ropinirole—in cognitively impaired elders has been more limited than experience with methylphenidate, but there have been encouraging reports (Eisdorfer et al. 1968; Nagaraja and Jayashree 2001; Ostow 2002). It should also be noted that paradoxically, sleepiness has been reported as a side effect in Parkinson's disease patients taking pramipexole and ropinirole (Etminan et al. 2001). The novel wakefulness-promoting agent modafinil, which appears to induce a calm alertness through nondopaminergic mechanisms, may also have utility in treating residual apathy and fatigue, but systematic geriatric data are currently nonexistent.

Antipsychotic Medications

Controlled data support that conventional antipsychotic drugs such as chlorpromazine, haloperidol, and perphenazine have a statistically significant but modest effect on the psychotic symptoms associated with dementia (Schneider et al. 1990). Uncontrolled data and clinical experience suggest that these drugs have efficacy for psychotic symptoms caused by other psychiatric disorders in late life such as schizophrenia, psychotic depression, and delirium (Mulsant and Gershon 1993). However, atypical antipsychotics have become the agents of choice for the treatment of psychotic symptoms of any etiology in all age groups (Collaborative Working Group on Clinical Trial Evaluations 1998). Although a relatively large number of trials comparing conventional and atypical antipsychotics in younger patients support this major shift in prescribing practice, only two such geriatric trials have been published. Both trials involved risperidone; one was a randomized study (Chan et al. 2001) and the other one was a switch study (Lane et al. 2002).

However, large case series (e.g., Frenchman and Prince 1997), expert opinion, and clinical experience strongly suggest that older patients are among those who may ben-

efit the most from this shift away from conventional antipsychotics (Condren and Cooney 2001; Glick et al. 2001; Jeste et al. 1999b; Lasser and Sunderland 1998; Salzman 2001; Tune 2001; Zaudig 2000). Indeed, the elderly are prone to developing extrapyramidal symptoms or tardive dyskinesia when treated with drugs that mainly block dopamine D_2 receptors (Caligiuri et al. 1999, 2000; Jeste et al. 1995; Pollock and Mulsant 1995; Saltz et al. 1989; Wirshing 2001). In turn, extrapyramidal symptoms are associated with cognitive impairment, decline in activities of daily living, and falls (with concomitant risk of hip fracture) (Larson et al. 1987; Tinetti et al. 1988). In a large pharmacoepidemiological study, conventional antipsychotics were also associated with a 2.4-fold increase in sudden cardiac death (Ray et al. 2001).

Except for two small randomized trials comparing risperidone and olanzapine to clozapine in patients with Parkinson's disease (Ellis et al. 2000; Goetz et al. 2000) (Table 24–6), there are not yet any controlled data comparing atypical antipsychotics in older patients (Schneider et al. 2001). The results of three naturalistic (i.e., nonrandomized) comparisons of risperidone with olanzapine are inconsistent (Edell and Tunis 2001; Madhusoodanan et al. 1999b; Verma et al. 2001). Therefore, the choice of a specific atypical antipsychotic to treat a specific patient should be guided by the strength of the available evidence relevant to the disorder being treated and, in the absence of such evidence, on the differing side-effect profiles of the six drugs currently available: clozapine, olanzapine, quetiapine, risperidone, aripiprazole, and ziprasidone.

Clozapine

Clozapine was the first antipsychotic referred to as being "atypical" due to its low likelihood of causing extrapyramidal symptoms. It is still considered the drug of choice for younger patients with treatment-refractory schizophrenia (Meltzer 1998), and one small case series suggests that it can be similarly helpful for the treatment of older patients with primary psychotic disorders that are refractory to other treatments (Sajatovic et al. 1997). A randomized, controlled trial comparing clozapine and chlorpromazine in older patients with schizophrenia (Howanitz et al. 1999) (see Table 24–6) and one large case series (Barak et al. 1999) also support the use of clozapine in moderate dosages (i.e., around 50–200 mg/day) in older patients with primary psychotic disorders. The strongest published geriatric studies of clozapine are focused on the treatment of drug-induced psychosis in patients with Parkinson's disease (Ellis et al. 2000; Goetz et al. 2000; Parkinson Study Group 1999;

TABLE 24–6. Summary of randomized, controlled trials of atypical antipsychotics in treatment of older patients with psychosis

	Number of published trials and cumulative number of older participants	Dosages studied (mg/day)	Comments	References
Aripiprazole	0	NA	NA	
Clozapine	5 $N = 133$	6.25–300	Clozapine was comparable to chlorpromazine in older patients with schizophrenia. Clozapine was more efficacious than placebo and olanzapine, and possibly comparable to risperidone, in patients with Parkinson's disease and DIP.	Ellis et al. 2000; Goetz et al. 2000; Howanitz et al. 1999; Parkinson Study Group 1999; Wolters et al. 1990
Olanzapine	2 $N = 221$	2.5–15	Low-dosage olanzapine was more efficacious than placebo in patients with BPSD and not as efficacious as (and more toxic than) clozapine in a small ($N = 15$) trial in patients with Parkinson's disease and DIP.	Goetz et al. 2000; Street et al. 2000
Quetiapine	0	NA	NA	
Risperidone	4 $N = 1037$	0.5–4	Low-dosage risperidone was more efficacious than placebo and as efficacious as low-dosage haloperidol in patients with BPSD and comparable to clozapine in a small ($N = 10$) trial in patients with Parkinson's disease and DIP.	Chan et al. 2001; De Deyn et al. 1999; Ellis et al. 2000; Katz et al. 1999
Ziprasidone	0	NA	NA	

Note. BPSD = behavioral and psychological symptoms in dementia; DIP = drug-induced psychosis.

Wolters et al. 1990) (see Table 24–6). The results of these studies suggest that clozapine at low dosages (12.5–50 mg/day) is the preferred treatment for this condition (Parkinson Study Group 1999). However, the use of clozapine in older patients is severely limited due to its significant hematologic, neurologic and cognitive, metabolic, and cardiac adverse effects (Alvir et al. 1993; Buckley and Sanders 2000; Centorrino et al. 2002; Hagg et al. 2001; Koller et al. 2001; Melkersson and Hulting 2001; Modai et al. 2000; Pollock and Mulsant 1995; Schuld et al. 2000; Sernyak et al. 2002; A.M. Walker et al. 1997).

Olanzapine

One published randomized, controlled trial involving 206 participants (Clark et al. 2001; Mintzer et al. 2001; Street et al. 2000) (see Table 24–5) and a few uncontrolled, open studies or large case series (Edell and Tunis 2001; Madhusoodanan et al. 1999b; Street et al. 2001; Verma et al. 2001) support the efficacy and safety of olanzapine in

the treatment of behavioral and psychological symptoms of dementia. However, in their study, Street and colleagues (2000) found an inverse dose-response relationship (i.e., patients receiving 15 mg/day had worse outcomes than patients receiving 5 mg/day), suggesting that higher dosages may be toxic in these patients (see below).

Uncontrolled data suggest that olanzapine is effective in the treatment of older patients with schizophrenia and other psychotic disorders (Madhusoodanan et al. 2000b; Sajatovic et al. 1998; Solomons and Geiger 2000).

Several randomized, controlled trials in younger patients have demonstrated that olanzapine is efficacious for the treatment of mania with or without psychotic features. Currently, olanzapine is the only atypical antipsychotic approved by the U.S. Food and Drug Administration (FDA) for the treatment of mania. Therefore, in the absence of any geriatric data, it should be the preferred atypical antipsychotic for older patients with mania. Some controlled and naturalistic data in younger patients suggest that olanzapine may also be useful in the treatment of psychotic depression (Konig et al. 2001; Narendran et al. 2001; Nelson et al. 2001) and treatment-refractory depression (Ghaemi et al. 2000; Rothschild et al. 1999; Shelton et al. 2001; Thase 2002), and it may have similar benefits in older patients.

The results of several small open trials and case series of olanzapine in the treatment of drug-induced psychosis in patients with Parkinson's disease or of psychosis in patients with Lewy body dementia have been inconsistent (Aarsland et al. 1999; Cummings et al. 2002; Friedman et al. 1998; Goetz et al. 2000; Marsh et al. 2001; Molho and Factor 1999; Onofrj et al. 2000; Sa and Lang 2001; Z. Walker et al. 1999; Wolters et al. 1996), with significant worsening seen in many patients (Goetz et al. 2000; Marsh et al. 2001; Molho and Factor 1999; Onofrj et al. 2000; Parkinson Study Group 1999; Z. Walker et al. 1999; Wolters et al. 1996). Therefore, great caution is needed if olanzapine is prescribed to parkinsonian patients.

Common side effects of olanzapine include sedation (Mouallem and Wolf 2001) and weight gain (Lindenmayer et al. 2001). Olanzapine has also been associated with significant increases in concentrations of glucose and lipids (Melkersson and Hulting 2001), which can occur even in the absence of weight gain but appear to be reversible on discontinuation of the drug (Lindenmayer et al. 2001). Extrapyramidal symptoms appear to be dose dependent and are rare at the dosages typically used in older patients (2.5–10 mg/day). Olanzapine has also been associated with significant electroencephalographic abnormalities (Centorrino et al. 2002; Schuld et al. 2000), and its strong blocking of the muscarinic receptor (Table 24–7) suggests that it can cause cognitive impairment (Byerly et al. 2001; Mulsant et al. 2003). This cognitive impairment is consistent with the decreased efficacy observed at higher dosages in older patients with dementia (Street et al. 2000). However, the mechanism of this potential toxicity is not clear (Beuzen et al. 1999; Byerly et al. 2001; Kennedy et al. 2001), and in two small case series olanzapine at low dosages was successfully used to treat delirium (Kim et al. 2001; Sipahimalani and Masand 1998).

Quetiapine

There are not yet any published controlled studies supporting the efficacy of quetiapine in the treatment of late-life psychoses. However, uncontrolled data suggest that it is safe and effective for these disorders (Madhusoodanan et al. 2000a; McManus et al. 1999; Tariot et al. 2000). The best geriatric data on quetiapine are from pa-

TABLE 24–7. Receptor blockade of atypical antipsychotics

	D_2	$5\text{-}HT_2$	M_1	α_2
Aripiprazole	*	++	0	+
Clozapine	+	++	++	+
Olanzapine	++	++	++	+
Quetiapine	+	++	0	++
Risperidone	+++	+++	0	++
Ziprasidone	++	++	0	+

Note. * = high affinity partial agonist; α_2 = alpha-adrenergic type 2; D_2 = dopamine type 2; $5\text{-}HT_2$ = 5-hydroxytryptamine (serotonin) type 2; M_1 = muscarinic type 1; 0 = none; + = minimal; ++ = intermediate; +++ = high.

tients with Parkinson's disease and drug-induced psychosis (Fernandez et al. 1999; Menza et al. 1999; Targum and Abbott 2000). In these patients at high risk for adverse effects, the overall efficacy and good tolerability of quetiapine suggest that it could be a useful alternative to clozapine. In addition, quetiapine lacks affinity for muscarinic receptors and does not produce electroencephalographic slowing (Centorrino et al. 2002), making it an attractive drug for older patients who have dementia or who are at risk for cognitive impairment (Byerly et al. 2001).

Risperidone

Of the six atypical antipsychotics currently available in the United States, risperidone has the most published geriatric data supporting its efficacy and safety for a variety of conditions. Three randomized, controlled trials involving more than 1,000 participants (Chan et al. 2001; Katz et al. 1999) (see Table 24–5) and more than 10 uncontrolled open studies or large case series (Frenchman and Prince 1997; Goldberg and Goldberg 1997; Herrmann et al. 1998; Irizarry et al. 1999; Laks et al. 2001; Lane et al. 2002; Lavretsky and Sultzer 1998; Negron and Reichman 2000; Rainer et al. 2001; Sajatovic et al. 1996; Verma et al. 2001; Zarate et al. 1997) support the efficacy and safety of risperidone at low dosages (0.5–1.5 mg/day) in the treatment of behavioral and psychological symptoms of dementia. Similarly, uncontrolled data suggest that risperidone is safe and effective in the treatment of older patients with schizophrenia and other psychotic disorders (Davidson et al. 2000; Furmaga et al. 1997; Kiraly et al. 1998; Madhusoodanan et al. 1999a; Sajatovic et al. 1999; Zarate et al. 1997).

Several small open trials of risperidone at low dosages in the treatment of drug-induced psychosis in patients with Parkinson's disease or of psychosis in patients with Lewy body dementia have had inconsistent results, with clear worsening of parkinsonian symptoms in some studies (Leopold 2000; Meco et al. 1997; Mohr et al. 2000; Rich et al. 1995; Workman et al. 1997). Therefore, risperidone should be used with great caution in the treatment of these disorders (Parkinson Study Group 1999). Although some naturalistic data in younger patients suggest that risperidone may also be useful in the treatment of younger patients with bipolar disorder, psychotic depression (Muller-Siecheneder et al. 1998; Ostroff and Nelson 1999), or treatment-refractory depression (Rubin and Arceneaux 2001), there are no relevant published geriatric data.

Commonly reported side effects of risperidone include hypotension on initiation of treatment and extrapyramidal symptoms (Davidson 2001). Extrapyramidal symptoms are dose dependent, and the threshold for extrapyramidal symptoms in the elderly is lower than in younger patients. Therefore, typical dosages for older patients should be between 0.5 and 2 mg/day. Risperidone causes only moderate electroencephalographic abnormalities (Centorrino et al. 2002), and it is rarely associated with cognitive impairment, probably because of its low affinity for muscarinic receptors (Byerly et al. 2001; Mulsant et al. 2003). Long-term follow-up has shown the risk of tardive dyskinesia associated with risperidone to be significantly lower than what is expected with conventional antipsychotics (Jeste et al. 1999a, 2000). Similarly, long-term use of risperidone has been associated with minimal weight gain (Barak 2002) and metabolic disturbances (Lindenmayer et al. 2001; Melkersson and Hulting 2001).

Aripiprazole and Ziprasidone

Aripiprazole and ziprasidone are the newest atypical antipsychotic drugs to become available in the United States. Based on both drugs' apparent minimal impact on glucose, lipids, and weight (Kingsbury et al. 2001; Potkin et al. 2003), and their lack of affinity for the muscarinic receptor (Byerly et al. 2001; Goodnick and Jerry 2002; see Table 24–7) and thus their low potential to cause cognitive impairment, aripiprazole and ziprasidone would appear to be attractive medications for older patients with psychosis. However, their use in older patients has been limited to a second-line treatment so far due to the almost total absence of geriatric data (Jeste et al. 2003; Wilner et al. 2000). In addition, some lingering concerns remain regarding the potential effects of ziprasidone on cardiac conduction in patients with preexisting cardiac disease.

Mood Stabilizers

As a class, mood stabilizers are high-risk medications for elderly patients. There is an absence of controlled studies and an abundance of concern regarding their potential toxicity, problematic side effects, and drug interactions. Lithium continues to be used for older patients with bipolar disorder and, less commonly, for antidepressant augmentation. Beyond their approved indications, anticonvulsants are often deployed in the management of agitation accompanying dementia as well as for bipolar illness. Despite the greater age-associated risks associated with lithium, recent data show that it is still used more commonly in elders with bipolar disorder than are the anticonvulsants (Umapathy et al. 2000). Currently, there is no consensus as to whether it is still appropriate to prescribe lithium as a first-line mood stabilizer for elders, nor is there agreement on the management of secondary mania (Snowdon 2000).

Lithium

Open and naturalistic trials suggest that lithium is efficacious in the acute treatment and prophylaxis of mania in older patients (Broadhead and Jacoby 1990; Eastham et al. 1998; Wylie et al. 1999). However, well-known physiological changes such as age-associated reductions in renal clearance and decreased total body water significantly affect the pharmacokinetics of lithium in older patients, increasing the risk of toxicity (Sproule et al. 2000). Moreover, specific medical comorbidities common in late life—such as renal dysfunction, hyponatremia, dehydration, and heart failure—also exacerbate the risk of toxicity (Oakley et al. 2001). Commonly used medications (e.g., thiazide diuretics, angiotensin-converting enzyme inhibitors, and nonsteroidal anti-inflammatory drugs) may precipitate toxicity by further diminishing the renal clearance of lithium. For all these reasons, older patients require lower dosages than younger patients to produce similar serum lithium levels.

More troubling is that elders are more sensitive to neurological side effects at lower lithium levels. There is speculation that this sensitivity is a consequence of increased permeability of the blood-brain barrier and perhaps more subtle changes in sodium-lithium countertransport (see Gangadhar et al. 1993). Whatever the underlying cause, neurotoxicity may be manifested as coarse tremor, slurred speech, ataxia, hyperreflexia, and muscle fasciculations. Cognitive impairment has been observed with levels well below 1 mEq/L, and frank delirium has been reported with serum levels as low as

1.5 mEq/L (Sproule et al. 2000). Consequently, older patients are typically treated with target levels of 0.4–0.8 mEq/L.

In addition to monthly or bimonthly lithium levels, electrolytes and the electrocardiogram should be checked regularly. Older patients also appear to be at higher risk for lithium-induced hypothyroidism and should have their thyroid-stimulating hormone concentration monitored at 6-month intervals. Lithium toxicity can be fatal and can produce persistent central nervous system impairment. Thus, lithium toxicity is a medical emergency that requires careful correction of fluid and electrolyte imbalances and that frequently requires administration of aminophylline and mannitol (or even hemodialysis) to increase lithium excretion.

Anticonvulsants

Anticonvulsants are increasingly being used as alternatives to lithium in the treatment of bipolar disorder and as alternatives to antipsychotics for the symptomatic management of agitation accompanying dementia. In general, side effects are more tolerable and less severe than those of lithium. In fact, pharmacoeconomic analyses comparing valproate and lithium in a nursing home population revealed that the minuscule acquisition costs of lithium were dramatically offset by an average expenditure of $2,875 more per patient for treatment of lithium-associated medical morbidities (Conney and Kaston 1999). Furthermore, there may be a subgroup of bipolar patients with dysphoria or rapid cycling who respond poorly to lithium but do well with anticonvulsants (Post et al. 1998). Similarly, given its putative etiology, mania associated with dementia and other neurological illness ("secondary mania") may respond preferentially to anticonvulsants (Shulman 1997).

Valproate

Valproate is a broad-spectrum anticonvulsant that has been approved in the United States for the treatment of acute mania. Small case series have suggested that valproic acid is relatively well tolerated by older bipolar patients (Kando et al. 1996; Noaghiul et al. 1998) and those with agitation in the context of dementia (Kunik et al. 1998). In addition, one placebo-controlled trial in 56 nursing home patients with agitation showed a modest benefit favoring valproate (Porsteinsson et al. 2001).

Sedation, nausea, weight gain, and hand tremors are common dose-related side effects. Mild stomach upset may be decreased by use of the enteric-coated divalproex salt. Thrombocytopenia is possible in more than half of

elderly patients treated with valproate and may ensue at lower total drug levels than in younger patients (Conley et al. 2001; Trannel et al. 2001). Also dose-related are reversible elevations in liver enzymes, occurring in 11% of patients, and transient elevations in blood ammonia levels, occurring in 21% of those receiving valproate (Davis et al. 1994). Although liver failure and pancreatitis are considered to be rare, their catastrophic consequences entail vigilance when prescribing valproate. Valproate has other metabolic effects of concern to aging patients, such as increases in bone turnover and reductions of serum folate, with concomitant elevations in plasma homocysteine concentrations (Kishi et al. 1997; Sato et al. 2001; Schwaninger et al. 1999).

The pharmacokinetics of valproate vary according to formulation, and valproic acid, divalproex sodium, and its extended-release preparation are not interchangeable. Valproate is principally metabolized by mitochondrial β-oxidation and secondarily by the cytochrome P450 system; typical half-lives are in the range of 5–16 hours and are not affected by aging alone. Concomitant administration of valproate will increase concentrations of phenobarbital, primidone, carbamazepine, diazepam, and lamotrigine. Conversely, concurrent administration of carbamazepine, lamotrigine, topiramate, and phenytoin may decrease levels of valproate, whereas fluoxetine and erythromycin may potentiate the effects of valproate. Changes in protein binding due to drug interactions are no longer considered clinically important beyond causing the misinterpretation of total (i.e., free and bound) drug levels (Benet and Hoener 2002). Valproate binding to plasma proteins is generally reduced in the elderly, suggesting that use of free drug levels may be preferable (Kodama et al. 2001). Toxicity may occur in patients with hypoalbuminemia despite total valproate concentrations within the usual therapeutic range (Gidal and Anderson 1998).

Carbamazepine

Carbamazepine has been reported to be effective for the acute treatment and prophylaxis of mania in younger patients (Post et al. 1998). In a placebo-controlled trial in 51 nursing home patients, carbamazepine was also found to be efficacious in treating agitation and aggression associated with dementia (Tariot et al. 1998). Carbamazepine is primarily eliminated by cytochrome P450 3A4, and its apparent clearance has been found to be reduced with aging (Bernus et al. 1997). Its interactions with other drugs are protean and complex. Carbamazepine concentrations are increased to potential toxicity by cytochrome P450 3A4 inhibitors such as macrolide antibiotics, antifungals, and some antidepressants (see Table 24–3). Cytochrome P450 3A4 inducers—such as phenobarbital, phenytoin, and carbamazepine itself—will lower concentrations of carbamazepine as well as concentrations of the many medically important drugs metabolized by this isoenzyme (Spina et al. 1996). Side effects of carbamazepine include nausea, dizziness, ataxia, and neutropenia. Older patients are at higher risk for drug-induced leukopenia and agranulocytosis as well as ataxia and, of course, drug interactions (Cates and Powers 1998). Oxcarbazepine, the 10-keto analog of carbamazepine, is a less potent cytochrome P450 3A4 inducer, and although studied in some small trials in bipolar patients, it has not been studied in dementia (Lima 2000).

Gabapentin

Although gabapentin is used in bipolar disorder, trials have not borne out its effectiveness and there are only anecdotal reports of its use in dementia (Letterman and Markowitz 1999; Pande et al. 2000). Nonetheless, it has a generally favorable side-effect profile and modest anxiolytic and analgesic effects, particularly for neuropathic pain. Gabapentin does not bind to plasma proteins and is not metabolized, being eliminated by renal excretion. In patients with renal impairment, neurological adverse effects such as ataxia, involuntary movements, disorganized thinking, excitation, and extreme sedation have been noted. Even in the absence of renal dysfunction, elderly patients may be prone to excessive sedation. Therefore, in the elderly, initial doses of 100 mg twice a day are more prudent than the 900 mg/day recommended as a starting dosage for younger patients with epilepsy.

Lamotrigine

Lamotrigine has recently been approved in the United States for the maintenance treatment of bipolar disorder to prevent mood episodes (depressive, manic, or mixed episodes). Randomized controlled trials in younger patients support that lamotrigine is more effective than placebo in treating bipolar depression (Calabrese et al. 1999b) and as effective as lithium in preventing both depressive and manic episodes (Bowden et al. 2003). Lamotrigine has also been found to be effective as monotherapy or as an adjunctive agent for the treatment of rapid-cycling and treatment-resistant bipolar disorder (Bowden et al. 1999; Calabrese et al. 1999a; Calabrese et al. 2000; Kusumakar and Yatham 1997; Passmore et al. 2003). One placebo-controlled trial suggests that lamotrigine may be useful as an augmenting agent in treatment-resistant depression (Barbosa et al. 2003).

There is only one small published case series of older patients with bipolar disorder treated with lamotrigine (Robillard and Conn 2002). However, controlled data in more than 200 older participants in epilepsy studies support that lamotrigine is relatively well tolerated by older patients (Brodie et al. 1999; Giorgi et al. 2001). In these studies, somnolence, rashes, and headaches were observed in a significant number of patients, but lamotrigine was better tolerated than carbamazepine or phenytoin. In contrast with many mood stabilizers and antidepressants, lamotrigine does not seem to be associated with weight gain (Morell et al. 2003).

In geriatric patients, rashes were the most common reason for study withdrawal, but they were less frequent with lamotrigine (3%) than with carbamazepine (19%) (Brodie et al. 1999). Severe rashes including Stevens-Johnson syndrome or toxic epidermal necrolysis have been observed in about 0.3% of adult patients (Messenheimer 1998). At the first sign of rash or other evidence of hypersensitivity (e.g., fever, lymphadenopathy), unless the signs are clearly not drug-related, lamotrigine should be discontinued and the patient should be evaluated. The incidence of rashes can be reduced by using a slower dose titration. Also, because valproate increases lamotrigine plasma concentration, the titration of lamotrigine needs to be slowed down and its target dosage needs to be halved in patients who are receiving valproate.

Anxiolytics

Social isolation, financial concerns, and declining intellectual and physical function may predispose elders to anxiety. New-onset anxiety is a frequent accompaniment of physical illness, depression, or medication side effects. The SSRIs and venlafaxine have displaced the long-acting benzodiazepines (e.g., diazepam) and medications with very short half-lives (e.g., alprazolam) as initial treatments for anxiety in late life, whereas the intermediate half-life benzodiazepine lorazepam and the nonbenzodiazepines (e.g., zaleplon, zolpidem) have become the most commonly used hypnotics.

Benzodiazepines and Nonbenzodiazepine Hypnotics

Detrimental effects of the benzodiazepines in elders frequently outweigh any short-term symptomatic relief that they may provide. Continuous benzodiazepine use increases the risk of falls, hip fractures, and cognitive impairment in elderly patients (Salzman et al. 1992; Sorock and Shimkin 1988). The popular nonbenzodiazepine zolpidem was found in a very large case-control study to double the risk of hip fracture, after controlling for age, gender, and medical conditions (Wang et al. 2001). Pharmacodynamically, controlling for drug concentration, benzodiazepines have been found to be more potent in older than in younger subjects (Reidenberg et al. 1978). Single small doses of diazepam, nitrazepam, and temazepam have caused significant impairment in memory and psychomotor performance in elderly subjects (Nikaido et al. 1990; Pomara et al. 1989).

Nevertheless, treatment with benzodiazepines may be indicated for a few weeks in the acute treatment of depression-related sleep disturbance when the primary pharmacotherapy is an antidepressant. Relative contraindications include heavy snoring (because it suggests sleep apnea), dementia (because such patients are at increased risk for daytime confusion, impairment in activities of daily living, and daytime sleepiness), and the use of other sedating medications or alcohol.

When benzodiazepines are used in the elderly, the compounds with long half-lives (clonazepam, diazepam, and flurazepam) should be avoided. It should also be remembered that several drugs with shorter half-lives (i.e., alprazolam, triazolam, midazolam, and the nonbenzodiazepines zaleplon and zolpidem) undergo phase 1 hepatic metabolism by cytochrome P450 3A4 that is subject to specific interactions and apparently age-associated decline (Freudenreich and Menza 2000; Greenblatt et al. 1991). Even in the absence of accumulation, sedatives with very short half-lives may cause difficulties such as increasing the likelihood that confused elders will awake in the middle of the night to stagger off to the bathroom. Oxazepam and lorazepam have acceptable half-lives that do not increase with age. These compounds are also not subject to drug interactions and have no active metabolites. Lorazepam is to be preferred, however for inducing sleep, because oxazepam has a relatively slow and erratic absorption. It is also useful to know that lorazepam is available in appropriately small doses (0.5-mg pills) and is the only benzodiazepine that is well absorbed intramuscularly.

Buspirone

The anxiolytic buspirone, a partial 5-HT$_{1A}$ agonist, may be beneficial for some anxious patients and appears to be well tolerated by the elderly without the sedation or addiction liability of the benzodiazepines (Robinson et al. 1988; Steinberg 1994). Buspirone may be helpful for elders with generalized anxiety disorder who are prone to falls, confusion, or chronic lung disease. Nonetheless, it is important to appreciate that buspirone may take several weeks to exert an anxiolytic effect; has no cross-tolerance with benzodiazepines; and may have side effects such as dizziness, headache, and nervousness (Strand et al. 1990). Unlike the SSRIs, buspirone is of limited use for panic or obsessive-compulsive disorders. Several case reports, open trials, and one small controlled study suggest that buspirone may be helpful in treating agitation in some demented patients (Cantillon et al. 1996). The pharmacokinetics of buspirone are not affected by age or gender, but coadministration with verapamil, diltiazem, erythromycin, or itraconazole will substantially increase buspirone concentrations, and overenthusiastic combinations with serotonergic medications may result in the serotonin syndrome (Mahmood and Sahajwalla 1999; Spigset and Adielsson 1997). Buspirone should be started at 5 mg three times a day and gradually increased by 5-mg increments every week to a maximum dosage of 60 mg/day.

TABLE 24–8. Cholinesterase inhibitors

Drug	Clearance	Dosing	Significant side effects	Pharmacodynamics
Donepezil	Half-life, 70–80 hr Cytochrome P450 3A4, 2D6	5–10 mg/day Start at 5 mg qhs	Mild nausea, diarrhea, agitation	Reversible acetylcholinesterase inhibition
Galantamine	Half-life, 7 hr Cytochrome P450 2D6, 3A4	8–24 mg/day divided bid Start at 4 mg bid	Moderate nausea, vomiting, diarrhea, anorexia, tremor, insomnia	Reversible acetylcholinesterase inhibition; nicotinic modulation may increase acetylcholine release
Rivastigmine	Half-life, 1.25 hr Renal	6–12 mg/day divided bid Start at 1.5 mg bid, retitrate if drug stopped	Severe nausea, vomiting, anorexia, weight loss, sweating, dizziness	Pseudoirreversible acetylcholinesterase inhibition, also butylcholinesterase inhibitions

Cognitive Enhancers

Cholinesterase Inhibitors

The four currently approved treatments for Alzheimer's disease in the United States—tacrine, donepezil, rivastigmine, and galantamine—are all acetylcholinesterase inhibitors (Table 24–8). The use of tacrine is no longer recommended because of its potential hepatotoxic effects. The principal side effects of these medications are concentration dependent and result from their peripheral cholinergic actions. With these side effects in mind, clinicians should be aware of the drugs' specific pathways of elimination and should be alert for potential pharmacokinetic drug interactions with cytochrome P450 2D6/3A4 inhibitors and cytochrome P450 3A4 inducers when prescribing donepezil and galantamine (Carrier 1999; Crismon 1998). Rivastigmine will be affected by renal function, and FDA warnings have emphasized the need for careful dose titration (and retitration if restarting) to prevent severe vomiting. Drugs with potent anticholinergic effects will of course directly antagonize the actions of cholinesterase inhibitors (Mulsant et al. 2003). The adverse cognitive effects of anticholinergic substances have been recognized for centuries (Feinberg 1993). Conversely and quite remarkably, physostigmine was an empirical treatment for dementia at least 8 years before Alzheimer's disease was described (Bellantonio and Kuchel 2002). The currently available cognitive enhancers have been demonstrated in controlled trials to result in modest improvements in cognition and function (Cummings 2000). Nonetheless, a rapid symptomatic deterioration occurs when these substances are discontinued, and no evidence suggests that they alter the underlying neuropathology of Alzheimer's disease or its eventual progression. In fact, there is speculation that acetylcholinesterase inhibition could actually accelerate neuronal loss (Kaufer and Soreq 1999). Therefore, before initiating anticholinesterase therapy it is imperative that comorbid depression be treated and that unnecessary anticholinergic medications be discontinued. In patients with diminished cognitive reserve, depression and even small anticholinergic effects can substantially impair cognition (Nebes et al. 1997).

NMDA Receptor Antagonist

Memantine, the first drug of this class, has recently been approved by the FDA for the treatment of moderate to severe Alzheimer disease. Evidence indicates that glutaminergic overstimulation may cause excitotoxic neuronal damage. As an uncompetitive antagonist with moderate affinity for NMDA receptors, memantine may attenuate neurotoxicity without interfering with glutamate's normal physiological actions. In patients with moderate to severe Alzheimer's disease, a daily dosage of 20 mg of memantine was well tolerated and significantly slowed the rate of deterioration compared with placebo in a 28-week U.S. multicenter trial (Reisberg et al. 2003). Importantly, a 6-month, placebo-controlled study in 401 donepezil-treated patients showed benefits of the combination therapy on cognition and activities of daily living relative to baseline (Tariot et al. 2003). In both studies, memantine was well tolerated at therapeutic doses, although it may cause confusion at higher doses. It does not appear to be implicated in drug-drug interactions, but it is excreted by the kidneys and its dosage may need to be reduced in patients with significant impairment in renal function.

References

Aarsland D, Larsen JP, Lim NG, et al: Olanzapine for psychosis in patients with Parkinson's disease with and without dementia. J Neuropsychiatry Clin Neurosci 11:392–394, 1999

Agelink MW, Zitzelsberger A, Klieser E: Withdrawal syndrome after discontinuation of venlafaxine. Am J Psychiatry 154:1473–1474, 1997

Alderman CP, Gebauer MG, Gilbert AL, et al: Possible interaction of zopiclone and nefazodone. Ann Pharmacother 35:1378–1380, 2001

Alexopoulos GS, Katz IR, Reynolds CF, et al (eds): Pharmacotherapy of Depressive Disorders in Older Patients: Expert Consensus Pocket Guide. White Plains, NY, Expert Knowledge System Press, 2001

Allgulander C, Hackett D, Salinas E: Venlafaxine extended release (ER) in the treatment of generalised anxiety disorder: twenty-four-week placebo-controlled dose-ranging study. Br J Psychiatry 179:15–22, 2001

Altamura AC, De Novellis F, Guercetti G, et al: Fluoxetine compared with amitriptyline in elderly depression: a controlled clinical trial. Int J Clin Pharmacol Res 9:391–396, 1989

Alvir JJ, Lieberman JA, Safferman AZ, et al: Clozapine-induced agranulocytosis: incidence and risk factors in the United States. N Engl J Med 329:162–167, 1993

Amore M, Ricci M, Zanardi R, et al: Long-term treatment of geropsychiatric depressed patients with venlafaxine. J Affect Disord 46:293–296, 1997

Andersen G, Vestergaard K, Lauritzen L: Effective treatment of poststroke depression with the selective serotonin reuptake inhibitor citalopram. Stroke 25:1099–1104, 1994

Aragona M, Inghilleri M: Increased ocular pressure in two patients with narrow angle glaucoma treated with venlafaxine. Clin Neuropharmacol 21:130–131, 1998

Arranz FJ, Ros S: Effects of comorbidity and polypharmacy on the clinical usefulness of sertraline in elderly depressed patients: an open multicentre study. J Affect Disord 46:285–291, 1997

Bailer U, Fischer P, Kufferle B, et al: Occurrence of mirtazapine-induced delirium in organic brain disorder. Int Clin Psychopharmacol 15:239–243, 2000

Barak Y: No weight gain among elderly schizophrenia patients after 1 year of risperidone treatment. J Clin Psychiatry 63:117–119, 2002

Barak Y, Wittenberg N, Naor S, et al: Clozapine in elderly psychiatric patients: tolerability, safety, and efficacy. Compr Psychiatry 40:320–325, 1999

Barbhaiya RH, Buch AB, Greene DS: A study of the effect of age and gender on the pharmacokinetics of nefazodone after single and multiple doses. J Clin Psychopharmacol 16:19–25, 1996

Barbosa L, Berk M, Vorster M: A double-blind, randomized, placebo-controlled trial of augmentation with lamotrigine or placebo in patients concomitantly treated with fluoxetine for resistant major depressive episodes. J Clin Psychiatry 64:403–407, 2003

Barkin RL, Fawcett J: The management challenges of chronic pain: the role of antidepressants. Am J Ther 7:31–47, 2000

Beers MH: Explicit criteria for determining potentially inappropriate medication use by the elderly. Arch Intern Med 157:1531–1536, 1997

Bellantonio S, Kuchel GA: Pharmacological approaches to cognitive deficits and incontinence (1899–2002): progress in geriatric care. Trends Pharmacol Sci 23:192–193, 2002

Belpaire FM, Wijnant P, Temmerman A, et al: The oxidative metabolism of metoprolol in human liver microsomes: inhibition by the selective serotonin reuptake inhibitors. Eur J Clin Pharmacol 54:261–264, 1998

Benazzi F: Urinary retention with venlafaxine-haloperidol combination. Pharmacopsychiatry 30:27, 1997

Benazzi F: Serotonin syndrome with mirtazapine-fluoxetine combination. Int J Geriatr Psychiatry 13:495–496, 1998

Benazzi F: Venlafaxine-fluoxetine interaction. J Clin Psychopharmacol 19:96–98, 1999

Benet LZ, Hoener B: Changes in plasma protein binding have little clinical relevance. Clin Pharmacol Ther 71:115–121, 2002

Benkert O, Szegedi A, Kohnen R: Mirtazapine compared with paroxetine in major depression. J Clin Psychiatry 61:656–663, 2000

Bernus I, Dickinson RG, Hooper WD: Anticonvulsant therapy in aged patients. Clinical pharmacokinetic considerations. Drugs Aging 10:278–289, 1997

Beuzen JN, Taylor N, Wesnes K, et al: A comparison of the effects of olanzapine, haloperidol and placebo on cognitive and psychomotor functions in healthy elderly volunteers. J Psychopharmacol 13:152–158, 1999

Bodkin JA, Lasser RA, Wines JD Jr, et al: Combining serotonin reuptake inhibitors and bupropion in partial responders to antidepressant monotherapy. J Clin Psychiatry 58:137–145, 1997

Bondareff W, Alpert M, Friedhoff AJ, et al: Comparison of sertraline and nortriptyline in the treatment of major depressive disorder in late life. Am J Psychiatry 157:729–736, 2000

Bowden CL, Calabrese JR, McElroy SL, et al: The efficacy of lamotrigine in rapid cycling and non-rapid cycling patients with bipolar disorder. Biol Psychiatry 45:953–958, 1999

Bowden CL, Calabrese JR, Sachs G, et al; Lamictal 606 Study Group: A placebo-controlled 18-month trial of lamotrigine and lithium maintenance treatment in recently manic or hypomanic patients with bipolar I disorder. Arch Gen Psychiatry 60:392–400, 2003

Branconnier RJ, Cole JO, Ghazvinian S, et al: Clinical pharmacology of bupropion and imipramine in elderly depressives. J Clin Psychiatry 44(5 pt 2):130–133, 1983

Broadhead J, Jacoby R: Mania in old age. A first prospective study. Int J Geriatr Psychiatry 5:215–222, 1990

Brodie MJ, Overstall PW, Giorgi L: Multicentre, double-blind, randomised comparison between lamotrigine and carbamazepine in elderly patients with newly diagnosed epilepsy. The UK Lamotrigine Elderly Study Group. Epilepsy Res 37:81–87, 1999

Brosen K, Skjelbo E, Rasmussen BB, et al: Fluvoxamine is a potent inhibitor of cytochrome P4501A2. Biochem Pharmacol 45:1211–1214, 1993

Buckley NA, Sanders P: Cardiovascular adverse effects of antipsychotic drugs. Drug Saf 23:215–228, 2000

Byerly MJ, Weber MT, Brooks DL, et al: Antipsychotic medications and the elderly: effects on cognition and implications for use. Drugs Aging 18:45–61, 2001

Calabrese JR, Bowden CL, McElroy SL, et al: Spectrum of activity of lamotrigine in treatment-refractory bipolar disorder. Am J Psychiatry 156:1019–1023, 1999a

Calabrese JR, Bowden CL, Sachs GS, et al: A double-blind placebo-controlled study of lamotrigine monotherapy in outpatients with bipolar I depression. Lamictal 602 Study Group. J Clin Psychiatry 60:79–88, 1999b

Calabrese JR, Suppes T, Bowden CL, et al: A double-blind, placebo-controlled, prophylaxis study of lamotrigine in rapid-cycling bipolar disorder. Lamictal 614 Study Group. J Clin Psychiatry 61:841–850, 2000

Caligiuri MP, Lacro JP, Jeste DV: Incidence and predictors of drug-induced parkinsonism in older psychiatric patients treated with very low doses of neuroleptics. J Clin Psychopharmacol 19:322–328, 1999

Caligiuri MR, Jeste DV, Lacro JP: Antipsychotic-induced movement disorders in the elderly: epidemiology and treatment recommendations. Drugs Aging 17:363–384, 2000

Cantillon M, Brunswick R, Molina D, et al: Buspirone vs. haloperidol: a double-blind trial for agitation in a nursing home population with Alzheimer's disease. Am J Geriatr Psychiatry 4:263–267, 1996

Carrier L: Donepezil and paroxetine: possible drug interaction. J Am Geriatr Soc 47:1037, 1999

Carvajal GP, Garcia D, Sanchez SA, et al: Hepatotoxicity associated with the new antidepressants. J Clin Psychiatry 63: 135–137, 2002

Cates M, Powers R: Concomitant rash and blood dyscrasias in geriatric psychiatry patients treated with carbamazepine. Ann Pharmacother 32:884–887, 1998

Centorrino F, Price BH, Tuttle M, et al: EEG abnormalities during treatment with typical and atypical antipsychotics. Am J Psychiatry 159:109–115, 2002

Chan WC, Lam LC, Choy CN, et al: A double-blind randomised comparison of risperidone and haloperidol in the treatment of behavioural and psychological symptoms in Chinese dementia patients. Int J Geriatr Psychiatry 16: 1156–1162, 2001

Chengappa KN, Kambhampati RK, Perkins K, et al: Bupropion sustained release as a smoking cessation treatment in remitted depressed patients maintained on treatment with selective serotonin reuptake inhibitor antidepressants. J Clin Psychiatry 62:503–508, 2001

Clark WS, Street JS, Feldman PD, et al: The effects of olanzapine in reducing the emergence of psychosis among nursing home patients with Alzheimer's disease. J Clin Psychiatry 62:34–40, 2001

Cohn CK, Shrivastava R, Mendels J, et al: Double-blind, multicenter comparison of sertraline and amitriptyline in elderly depressed patients. J Clin Psychiatry 51 (suppl B):28–33, 1990

Coleman CC, King BR, Bolden-Watson C, et al: A placebo-controlled comparison of the effects on sexual functioning of bupropion sustained release and fluoxetine. Clin Ther 23:1040–1058, 2001

Collaborative Working Group on Clinical Trial Evaluations: Treatment of special populations with the atypical antipsychotics. J Clin Psychiatry 59 (suppl 12):46–52, 1998

Condren RM, Cooney C: Use of drugs by old age psychiatrists in the treatment of psychotic and behavioural symptoms in patients with dementia. Aging Ment Health 5:235–241, 2001

Conley EL, Coley KC, Pollock BG, et al: Prevalence and risk of thrombocytopenia with valproic acid: experience at a psychiatric teaching hospital. Pharmacotherapy 21:1325–1330, 2001

Conney J, Kaston B: Pharmacoeconomic and health outcome comparison of lithium and divalproex in a VA geriatric nursing home population: influence of drug-related morbidity on total cost of treatment. Am J Manag Care 5:197–204, 1999

Crewe HK, Lennard MS, Tucker GT, et al: The effect of selective serotonin re-uptake inhibitors on cytochrome P4502D6 (CYP2D6) activity in human liver microsomes. Br J Clin Pharmacol 34:262–265, 1992

Crismon ML: Pharmacokinetics and drug interactions of cholinesterase inhibitors administered in Alzheimer's disease. Pharmacotherapy 18:47–54, 1998

Croft H, Settle E Jr, Houser T, et al: A placebo-controlled comparison of the antidepressant efficacy and effects on sexual functioning of sustained-release bupropion and sertraline. Clin Ther 21:643–658, 1999

Cummings JL: Cholinesterase inhibitors: a new class of psychotropic compounds. Am J Psychiatry 157:4–15, 2000

Cummings JL, Street J, Masterman D, et al: Efficacy of olanzapine in the treatment of psychosis in dementia with Lewy bodies. Dement Geriatr Cogn Disord 13(2):67–73, 2002

Dahmen N, Marx J, Hopf HC, et al: Therapy of early post-stroke depression with venlafaxine: safety, tolerability, and efficacy as determined in an open, uncontrolled clinical trial. Stroke 30:691–692, 1999

Davidson M: Long-term safety of risperidone. J Clin Psychiatry 62 (suppl 21):26–28, 2001.

Davidson M, Harvey PD, Vervarcke J, et al: A long-term, multicenter, open-label study of risperidone in elderly patients with psychosis. On behalf of the Risperidone Working Group. Int J Geriatr Psychiatry 15:506–514, 2000

Davis R, Peters DH, McTavish D: Valproic acid. A reappraisal of its pharmacological properties and clinical efficacy in epilepsy. Drugs 47:332–372, 1994

De Deyn PP, Rabheru K, Rasmussen A, et al: A randomized trial of risperidone, placebo, and haloperidol for behavioral symptoms of dementia. Neurology 53:946–955, 1999

de Montigny C, Silverstone PH, Debonnel G, et al: Venlafaxine in treatment-resistant major depression: a Canadian multicenter, open-label trial. J Clin Psychopharmacol 19:401–406, 1999

DeVane CL, Pollock BG: Pharmacokinetic considerations of antidepressant use in the elderly. J Clin Psychiatry 60 (suppl 20):38–44, 1999

Dierick M: An open-label evaluation of the long-term safety of oral venlafaxine in depressed elderly patients. Ann Clin Psychiatry 8:169–178, 1996

Doraiswamy PM, Khan ZM, Donahue RM, et al: Quality of life in geriatric depression: a comparison of remitters, partial responders, and nonresponders. Am J Geriatr Psychiatry 9:423–428, 2001

Druckenbrod R, Mulsant BH: Fluoxetine induced syndrome of inappropriate anti-diuretic hormone: a geriatric case report and a review of literature. J Geriatr Psychiatry Neurol 7: 254–256, 1994

Dunner DL, Cohn JB, Walshe TD, et al: Two combined, multicenter double-blind studies of paroxetine and doxepin in geriatric patients with major depression. J Clin Psychiatry 53 (suppl):57–60, 1992

Dunner DL, Zisook S, Billow AA, et al: A prospective safety surveillance study for bupropion sustained-release in the treatment of depression. J Clin Psychiatry 59:366–373, 1998

Eastham JH, Jeste DV, Young RC: Assessment and treatment of bipolar disorder in the elderly. Drugs Aging 12:205–224, 1998

Edell WS, Tunis SL: Antipsychotic treatment of behavioral and psychological symptoms of dementia in geropsychiatric inpatients. Am J Geriatr Psychiatry 9:289–297, 2001

Eisdorfer C, Conner JF, Wilkie FL: The effect of magnesium pemoline on cognition and behavior. J Gerontol 23:283–288, 1968

Ellis T, Cudkowicz ME, Sexton PM, et al: Clozapine and risperidone treatment of psychosis in Parkinson's disease. J Neuropsychiatry Clin Neurosci 12:364–369, 2000

Entsuah AR, Huang H, Thase ME: Response and remission rates in different subpopulations with major depressive disorder administered venlafaxine, selective serotonin reuptake inhibitors, or placebo. J Clin Psychiatry 62:869–877, 2001

Ereshefsky L, Dugan D: Review of the pharmacokinetics, pharmacogenetics, and drug interaction potential of antidepressants: focus on venlafaxine. Depress Anxiety 12 (suppl 1):30–44, 2000

Etminan M, Samii A, Takkouche B, et al: Increased risk of somnolence with the new dopamine agonists in patients with Parkinson's disease: a meta-analysis of randomised controlled trials. Drug Saf 24:863–868, 2001

Evans M, Hammond M, Wilson K, et al: Treatment of depression in the elderly: effect of physical illness on response. Int J Geriatr Psychiatry 12:1189–1194, 1997

Fabian TJ, Amico JA, Kroboth PD, et al: Paroxetine-induced hyponatremia in older adults: a twelve-week prospective study. Arch Intern Med (in press)

Fava M, Mulroy R, Alpert J, et al: Emergence of adverse events following discontinuation of treatment with extended-release venlafaxine. Am J Psychiatry 154:1760–1762, 1997

Fawcett J, Barkin RL: Review of the results from clinical studies on the efficacy, safety and tolerability of mirtazapine for the treatment of patients with major depression. J Affect Disord 51:267–285, 1998

Feighner JP, Cohn JB: Double-blind comparative trials of fluoxetine and doxepin in geriatric patients with major depressive disorder. J Clin Psychiatry 46(3 pt 2):20–25, 1985

Feinberg M: The problems of anticholinergic adverse effects in older patients. Drugs Aging 3:335–348, 1993

Ferguson JM, Shrivastava RK, Stahl SM, et al: Reemergence of sexual dysfunction in patients with major depressive disorder: double-blind comparison of nefazodone and sertraline. J Clin Psychiatry 62:24–29, 2001

Fernandez HH, Friedman JH, Jacques C, et al: Quetiapine for the treatment of drug-induced psychosis in Parkinson's disease. Mov Disord 14:484–487, 1999

Finkel SI, Richter EM, Clary CM, et al: Comparative efficacy of sertraline vs. fluoxetine in patients age 70 or over with major depression. Am J Geriatr Psychiatry 7:221–227, 1999

Flint AJ: Choosing appropriate antidepressant therapy in the elderly. A risk-benefit assessment of available agents. Drugs Aging 13:269–280, 1998

Frenchman IB, Prince T: Clinical experience with risperidone, haloperidol, and thioridazine for dementia-associated behavioral disturbances. Int Psychogeriatr 9:431–435, 1997

Freudenreich O, Menza M: Zolpidem-related delirium: a case report. J Clin Psychiatry 61:449–450, 2000

Friedman JH, Goldstein S, Jacques C: Substituting clozapine for olanzapine in psychiatrically stable Parkinson's disease patients: results of an open label pilot study. Clin Neuropharmacol 21:285–288, 1998

Furlan PM, Kallan MJ, Ten Have T, et al: Cognitive and psychomotor effects of paroxetine and sertraline on healthy elderly volunteers. Am J Geriatr Psychiatry 9:429–438, 2001

Furmaga KM, DeLeon OA, Sinha SB, et al: Psychosis in medical conditions: response to risperidone. Gen Hosp Psychiatry 19:223–228, 1997

Gangadhar BN, Subhash MN, Umapathy C, et al: Lithium toxicity at therapeutic serum levels. Br J Psychiatry 163:695, 1993

Gelenberg AJ, Laukes C, McGahuey C, et al: Mirtazapine substitution in SSRI-induced sexual dysfunction. J Clin Psychiatry 61:356–360, 2000

Georgotas A, Friedman E, McCarthy M, et al: Resistant geriatric depressions and therapeutic response to monoamine oxidase inhibitors. Biol Psychiatry 18:195–205, 1983

Georgotas A, McCue RE, Hapworth W, et al: Comparative efficacy and safety of MAOIs versus TCAs in treating depression in the elderly. Biol Psychiatry 21:1155–1166, 1986

Geretsegger C, Stuppaeck CH, Mair M, et al: Multicenter double blind study of paroxetine and amitriptyline in elderly depressed inpatients. Psychopharmacology (Berl) 119:277–281, 1995

Ghaemi SN, Cherry EL, Katzow JA, et al: Does olanzapine have antidepressant properties? A retrospective preliminary study. Bipolar Disord 2 (3 pt 1):196–199, 2000

Gidal B, Anderson G: Epilepsy in the elderly: special pharmacotherapeutic considerations. Consultant Pharmacist 1:62–74, 1998

Giorgi L, Gomez G, O'Neill F, et al: The tolerability of lamotrigine in elderly patients with epilepsy. Drugs Aging 18:621–630, 2001

Glick ID, Murray SR, Vasudevan P, et al: Treatment with atypical antipsychotics: new indications and new populations. J Psychiatr Res 35:187–191, 2001

Goetz CG, Blasucci LM, Leurgans S, et al: Olanzapine and clozapine: comparative effects on motor function in hallucinating PD patients. Neurology 55:789–794, 2000

Goldberg RJ: Antidepressant use in the elderly. Current status of nefazodone, venlafaxine and moclobemide. Drugs Aging 11:119–131, 1997

Goldberg RJ, Goldberg J: Risperidone for dementia-related disturbed behavior in nursing home residents: a clinical experience. Int Psychogeriatr 9:65–68, 1997

Goodnick PJ, Hernandez M: Treatment of depression in comorbid medical illness. Expert Opin Pharmacother 1:1367–1384, 2000

Goodnick PJ, Jerry JM: Aripiprazole: profile on efficacy and safety. Expert Opin Pharmacother 3:1773–1781, 2002

Gorman JM: Mirtazapine: clinical overview. J Clin Psychiatry 60 (suppl 17):9–13, 1999

Gram LF, Hansen MG, Sindrup SH, et al: Citalopram: interaction studies with levomepromazine, imipramine, and lithium. Ther Drug Monit 15:18–24, 1993

Graudins A, Stearman A, Chan B: Treatment of the serotonin syndrome with cyproheptadine. J Emerg Med 16:615–619, 1998

Green TR: Bupropion for SSRI-induced fatigue. J Clin Psychiatry 58:174, 1997

Greenblatt DJ, Harmatz JS, Shapiro L, et al: Sensitivity to triazolam in the elderly. N Engl J Med 324:1691–1698, 1991

Greenblatt DJ, von Moltke LL, Harmatz JS, et al: Drug interactions with newer antidepressants: role of human cytochromes P450. J Clin Psychiatry 59 (suppl 15):19–27, 1998

Greenblatt DJ, von Moltke LL, Harmatz JS, et al: Human cytochromes and some newer antidepressants: kinetics, metabolism, and drug interactions. J Clin Psychiatry 19 (suppl 1):23S–35S, 1999

Greene DS, Barbhaiya RH: Clinical pharmacokinetics of nefazodone. Clin Pharmacokinet 33:260–275, 1997

Guelfi JD, Ansseau M, Timmerman L, et al: Mirtazapine versus venlafaxine in hospitalized severely depressed patients with melancholic features. Mirtazapine-Venlafaxine Study Group. J Clin Psychopharmacol 21:425–431, 2001

Guillibert E, Pelicier Y, Archambault JC, et al: A double-blind, multicentre study of paroxetine versus clomipramine in depressed elderly patients. Acta Psychiatr Scand Suppl 350:132–134, 1989

Hagg S, Soderberg S, Ahren B, et al: Leptin concentrations are increased in subjects treated with clozapine or conventional antipsychotics. J Clin Psychiatry 62:843–848, 2001

Harvey AT, Rudolph RL, Preskorn SH: Evidence of the dual mechanisms of action of venlafaxine. Arch Gen Psychiatry 57:503–509, 2000

Herrmann N, Rivard MF, Flynn M, et al: Risperidone for the treatment of behavioral disturbances in dementia: a case series. J Neuropsychiatry Clin Neurosci 10:220–223, 1998

Hesse LM, Venkatakrishnan K, Court MH, et al: CYP2B6 mediates the in vitro hydroxylation of bupropion: potential drug interactions with other antidepressants. Drug Metab Dispos 28:1176–1183, 2000

Howanitz E, Pardo M, Smelson DA, et al: The efficacy and safety of clozapine versus chlorpromazine in geriatric schizophrenia. J Clin Psychiatry 60:41–44, 1999

Howard WT, Warnock JK: Bupropion-induced psychosis. Am J Psychiatry 156:2017–2018, 1999

Hoyberg OJ, Maragakis B, Mullin J, et al: A double-blind multicentre comparison of mirtazapine and amitriptyline in elderly depressed patients. Acta Psychiatr Scand 93:184–190, 1996

Hutchison LC: Mirtazapine and bone marrow suppression: a case report. J Am Geriatr Soc 49:1129–1130, 2001

Iribarne C, Picart D, Dreano Y, et al: In vitro interactions between fluoxetine or fluvoxamine and methadone or buprenorphine. Fundam Clin Pharmacol 12(2):194–199, 1998

Irizarry MC, Ghaemi SN, Lee-Cherry ER, et al: Risperidone treatment of behavioral disturbances in outpatients with dementia. J Neuropsychiatry Clin Neurosci 11:336–342, 1999

Jeppesen U, Gram L, Vistisen K: Dose-dependent inhibition of CYP1A2, CYP2C19, and CYP2D6 by citalopram, fluoxetine, fluvoxamine, and paroxetine. Eur J Clin Pharmacol 51:73–78, 1996

Jeste DV, Caligiuri MP, Paulsen JS, et al: Risk of tardive dyskinesia in older patients: a prospective longitudinal study of 266 outpatients. Arch Gen Psychiatry 52:756–765, 1995

Jeste DV, Lacro JP, Bailey A, et al: Lower incidence of tardive dyskinesia with risperidone compared with haloperidol in older patients. J Am Geriatr Soc 47:716–719, 1999a

Jeste DV, Rockwell E, Harris MJ, et al: Conventional vs. newer antipsychotics in elderly patients. Am J Geriatr Psychiatry 7:70–76, 1999b

Jeste DV, Okamoto A, Napolitano J, et al: Low incidence of persistent tardive dyskinesia in elderly patients with dementia treated with risperidone. Am J Psychiatry 157:1150–1155, 2000

Jeste DV, De Deyn P, Carson W, et al: Aripiprazole in dementia of the Alzheimer's type. J Am Geriatr Soc 51(suppl):543, 2003

Joo JH, Lenze EJ, Mulsant BH, et al: Risk factors for falls during treatment of late-life depression. J Clin Psychiatry 63:936–941, 2002

Kando JC, Tohen M, Castillo J, et al: The use of valproate in an elderly population with affective symptoms. J Clin Psychiatry 57:238–240, 1996

Kaplitz SE: Withdrawn, apathetic geriatric patients responsive to methylphenidate. J Am Geriatr Soc 23:271–276, 1975

Kashuba AD, Nafziger AN, Kearns GL, et al: Effect of fluvoxamine therapy on the activities of CYP1A2, CYP2D6, and CYP3A as determined by phenotyping. Clin Pharmacol Ther 64:257–268, 1998

Katona CLE, Hunter BN, Bray J: A double-blind comparison of the efficacy and safety of paroxetine and imipramine in the treatment of depression with dementia. Int J Geriatr Psychiatry 13:100–108, 1998

Katz IR, Jeste DV, Mintzer JE, et al: Comparison of risperidone and placebo for psychosis and behavioral disturbances associated with dementia: a randomized, double-blind trial. Risperidone Study Group. J Clin Psychiatry 60:107–115, 1999

Kaufer D, Soreq H: Tracking cholinergic pathways from psychological and chemical stressors to variable neurodeterioration paradigms. Curr Opin Neurol 12:739–743, 1999

Kelsey JE: Dose-response relationship with venlafaxine. J Clin Psychopharmacol 16 (3 suppl 2):21S–26S; discussion 26S–28S, 1996

Kennedy JS, Bymaster FP, Schuh L, et al: A current review of olanzapine's safety in the geriatric patient: from pre-clinical pharmacology to clinical data. Int J Geriatr Psychiatry 16 (suppl 1):S33–S61, 2001

Khan A, Rudolph R, Baumel B, et al: Venlafaxine in depressed geriatric outpatients: an open-label clinical study. Psychopharmacol Bull 31:753–758, 1995

Kiayias JA, Vlachou ED, Lakka-Papadodima E: Venlafaxine HCl in the treatment of painful peripheral diabetic neuropathy (comment). Diabetes Care 23:699, 2000

Kiev A, Masco HL, Wenger TL, et al: The cardiovascular effects of bupropion and nortriptyline in depressed outpatients. Ann Clin Psychiatry 6:107–115, 1994

Kim KS, Pae CU, Chae JH, et al: An open pilot trial of olanzapine for delirium in the Korean population. Psychiatry Clin Neurosci 55:515–519, 2001

Kingsbury SJ, Fayek M, Trufasiu D, et al: The apparent effects of ziprasidone on plasma lipids and glucose. J Clin Psychiatry 62:347–349, 2001

Kiraly SJ, Gibson RE, Ancill RJ, et al: Risperidone: treatment response in adult and geriatric patients. Int J Psychiatry Med 28:255–263, 1998

Kirby D, Ames D: Hyponatraemia and selective serotonin reuptake inhibitors in elderly patients. Int J Geriatr Psychiatry 16:484–493, 2001

Kishi T, Fujita N, Eguchi T, et al: Mechanism for reduction of serum folate by antiepileptic drugs during prolonged therapy. J Neurol Sci 145:109–112, 1997

Klamerus KJ, Parker VD, Rudolph RL, et al: Effects of age and gender on venlafaxine and O-desmethylvenlafaxine pharmacokinetics. Pharmacotherapy 16:915–923, 1996

Kobayashi K, Yamamoto T, Chiba K, et al: The effects of selective serotonin reuptake inhibitors and their metabolites on S-mephenytoin 4'-hydroxylase activity in human liver microsomes. Br J Clin Pharmacol 40:481–485, 1995

Kodama Y, Kodama H, Kuranari M, et al: Gender- or age-related binding characteristics of valproic acid to serum proteins in adult patients with epilepsy. Eur J Pharm Biopharm 52:57–63, 2001

Koller E, Schneider B, Bennett K, et al: Clozapine-associated diabetes. Am J Med 111:716–723, 2001

Konig F, von Hippel C, Petersdorff T, et al: First experiences in combination therapy using olanzapine with SSRIs (citalopram, paroxetine) in delusional depression. Neuropsychobiology 43:170–174, 2001

Kroenke K, West SL, Swindle R, et al: Similar effectiveness of paroxetine, fluoxetine, and sertraline in primary care: a randomized trial. JAMA 286:2947–2955, 2001

Kunik ME, Puryear L, Orengo CA, et al: The efficacy and tolerability of divalproex sodium in elderly demented patients with behavioral disturbances. Int J Geriatric Psychiatry 13:29–34, 1998

Kusumakar V, Yatham LN: An open study of lamotrigine in refractory bipolar depression. Psychiatry Res 72:145–148, 1997

Kyle CJ, Petersen HE, Overo KF: Comparison of the tolerability and efficacy of citalopram and amitriptyline in elderly depressed patients treated in general practice. Depress Anxiety 8:147–153, 1998

Labbate LA, Grimes JB, Hines A, et al: Bupropion treatment of serotonin reuptake antidepressant-associated sexual dysfunction. Ann Clin Psychiatry 9:241–245, 1997

Laks J, Engelhardt E, Marinho V, et al: Efficacy and safety of risperidone oral solution in agitation associated with dementia in the elderly. Arq Neuropsiquiatr 59:859–864, 2001

Lane HY, Chang YC, Su MH, et al: Shifting from haloperidol to risperidone for behavioral disturbances in dementia: safety, response predictors, and mood effects. J Clin Psychopharmacol 22:4–10, 2002

Larson EB, Kukull WA, Buchner D, et al: Adverse drug reactions associated with global cognitive impairment in elderly persons. Ann Intern Med 107:169–173, 1987

Lasser RA, Sunderland T: Newer psychotropic medication use in nursing home residents. J Am Geriatr Soc 46:202–207, 1998

Lavretsky H, Kumar A: Methylphenidate augmentation of citalopram in elderly depressed patients. Am J Geriatr Psychiatry 9:298–303, 2001

Lavretsky H, Sultzer D: A structured trial of risperidone for the treatment of agitation in dementia. Am J Geriatr Psychiatry 6:127–135, 1998

Lenze EJ, Mulsant BH, Shear MK, et al: Anxiety symptoms in elderly patients with depression: what is the best approach to treatment? Drugs Aging 19:753–760, 2002

Leopold NA: Risperidone treatment of drug-related psychosis in patients with parkinsonism. Mov Disord 15:301–304, 2000

Lessard E, Yessine MA, Hamelin BA, et al: Influence of CYP2D6 activity on the disposition and cardiovascular toxicity of the antidepressant agent venlafaxine in humans. Pharmacogenetics 9:435–443, 1999

Letterman L, Markowitz JS: Gabapentin: a review of published experience in the treatment of bipolar disorder and other psychiatric conditions. Pharmacotherapy 19:565–572, 1999

Lima JM: The new drugs and the strategies to manage epilepsy. Curr Pharm Des 6:873–878, 2000

Lindenmayer JP, Nathan AM, Smith RC: Hyperglycemia associated with the use of atypical antipsychotics. J Clin Psychiatry 62 (suppl 23):30–38, 2001

Lucena MI, Andrade RJ, Gomez-Outes A, et al: Acute liver failure after treatment with nefazodone. Dig Dis Sci 44:2577–2579, 1999

Madhusoodanan S, Brecher M, Brenner R, et al: Risperidone in the treatment of elderly patients with psychotic disorders. Am J Geriatr Psychiatry 7:132–138, 1999a

Madhusoodanan S, Suresh P, Brenner R, et al: Experience with the atypical antipsychotics—risperidone and olanzapine in the elderly. Ann Clin Psychiatry 11:113–118, 1999b

Madhusoodanan S, Brenner R, Alcantra A: Clinical experience with quetiapine in elderly patients with psychotic disorders. J Geriatr Psychiatry Neurol 13:28–32, 2000a

Madhusoodanan S, Brenner R, Suresh P, et al: Efficacy and tolerability of olanzapine in elderly patients with psychotic disorders: a prospective study. Ann Clin Psychiatry 12:11–18, 2000b

Mahapatra SN, Hackett D: A randomised, double-blind, parallel-group comparison of venlafaxine and dothiepin in geriatric patients with major depression. Int J Clin Pract 51:209–213, 1997

Mahmood I, Sahajwalla C: Clinical pharmacokinetics and pharmacodynamics of buspirone, an anxiolytic drug. Clin Pharmacokinet 36:277–287, 1999

Mamo DC, Sweet RA, Mulsant BH, et al : The effect of nortriptyline and paroxetine on extrapyramidal signs and symptoms: a prospective double-blind study in depressed elderly patients. Am J Geriatr Psychiatry 8:226–231, 2000

Marsh L, Lyketsos C, Reich SG: Olanzapine for the treatment of psychosis in patients with Parkinson's disease and dementia. Psychosomatics 42:477–481, 2001

McCue RE, Joseph M: Venlafaxine- and trazodone-induced serotonin syndrome. Am J Psychiatry 158:2088–2089, 2001

McManus DQ, Arvanitis LA, Kowalcyk BB: Quetiapine, a novel antipsychotic: experience in elderly patients with psychotic disorders. Seroquel Trial 48 Study Group. J Clin Psychiatry 60:292–298, 1999

Meco G, Alessandri A, Giustini P, et al: Risperidone in levodopa-induced psychosis in advanced Parkinson's disease: an open-label, long-term study. Mov Disord 12:610–612, 1997

Melkersson KI, Hulting AL: Insulin and leptin levels in patients with schizophrenia or related psychoses—a comparison between different antipsychotic agents. Psychopharmacology 154:205–212, 2001

Meltzer HY: Suicide in schizophrenia: risk factors and clozapine treatment. J Clin Psychiatry 59 (suppl 3):15–20, 1998

Menza MM, Palermo B, Mark M: Quetiapine as an alternative to clozapine in the treatment of dopamimetic psychosis in patients with Parkinson's disease. Ann Clin Psychiatry 11:141–144, 1999

Menza M, Lauritano M, Allen L, et al: Treatment of somatization disorder with nefazodone: a prospective, open-label study. Ann Clin Psychiatry 13:153–158, 2001

Messenheimer JA: Rash in adult and pediatric patients treated with lamotrigine. Can J Neurol Sci 25:S14–S18, 1998

Mintzer J, Faison W, Street JS, et al: Olanzapine in the treatment of anxiety symptoms due to Alzheimer's disease: a post hoc analysis. Int J Geriatr Psychiatry 16 (suppl 1): S71–S77, 2001

Modai I, Hirschmann S, Rava A, et al: Sudden death in patients receiving clozapine treatment: a preliminary investigation. J Clin Psychopharmacol 20:325–327, 2000

Mohr E, Mendis T, Hildebrand K, et al: Risperidone in the treatment of dopamine-induced psychosis in Parkinson's disease: an open pilot trial. Mov Disord 15:1230–1237, 2000

Molho ES, Factor SA: Worsening of motor features of parkinsonism with olanzapine. Mov Disord 14:1014–1016, 1999

Montejo AL, Llorca G, Izquierdo JA, et al: Incidence of sexual dysfunction associated with antidepressant agents: a prospective multicenter study of 1022 outpatients. Spanish Working Group for the Study of Psychotropic-Related Sexual Dysfunction. J Clin Psychiatry 62 (suppl 3):10–21, 2001

Morrell MJ, Isojarvi J, Taylor AE, et al: Higher androgens and weight gain with valproate compared with lamotrigine for epilepsy. Epilepsy Res 54:189–199, 2003

Mouallem M, Wolf I: Olanzapine-induced respiratory failure. Am J Geriatr Psychiatry 9:304–305, 2001

Muller-Siecheneder F, Muller MJ, Hillert A, et al: Risperidone versus haloperidol and amitriptyline in the treatment of patients with a combined psychotic and depressive syndrome. J Clin Psychopharmacology 18:111–120, 1998

Mulsant BH, Gershon S: Neuroleptics in the treatment of psychosis in late-life: a rational approach. Int J Geriatric Psychiatry 8:979–992, 1993

Mulsant BH, Pollock BG, Nebes RD, et al: A double-blind randomized comparison of nortriptyline and paroxetine in the treatment of late-life depression: 6-week outcome. J Clin Psychiatry 60 (suppl 20):16–20, 1999

Mulsant BH, Alexopoulos GS, Reynolds CF 3rd, et al: The PROSPECT Study Group. Pharmacological treatment of depression in older primary care patients: the PROSPECT algorithm. Int J Geriatr Psychiatry 16:585–592, 2001a

Mulsant BH, Pollock BG, Nebes R, et al: A twelve-week, double-blind, randomized comparison of nortriptyline and paroxetine in older depressed inpatients and outpatients. Am J Geriatr Psychiatry 9:406–414, 2001b

Mulsant BH, Pollock BG, Kirshner M, et al: Serum anticholinergic activity in a community-based sample of older adults: relationship with cognitive performance. Arch Gen Psychiatry 60:198–203, 2003

Nagaraja D, Jayashree S: Randomized study of the dopamine receptor agonist piribedil in the treatment of mild cognitive impairment. Am J Psychiatry 158:1517–1519, 2001

Narendran R, Young CM, Valenti AM, et al: Olanzapine therapy in treatment-resistant psychotic mood disorders: a long-term follow-up study. J Clin Psychiatry 62:509–516, 2001

Nebes RD, Pollock BG, Mulsant BH, et al: Low-level serum anticholinergicity as a source of baseline cognitive heterogeneity in geriatric depressed patients. Psychopharmacol Bull 33:715–719, 1997

Negron AE, Reichman WE: Risperidone in the treatment of patients with Alzheimer's disease with negative symptoms. Int Psychogeriatr 12:527–536, 2000

Nelson EB, Rielage E, Welge JA, et al: An open trial of olanzapine in the treatment of patients with psychotic depression. Ann Clin Psychiatry 13:147–151, 2001

Nemeroff CB: Comorbidity of mood and anxiety disorders: the rule, not the exception? Am J Psychiatry 159:3–4, 2002

Newhouse PA, Krishnan KR, Doraiswamy PM, et al: A double-blind comparison of sertraline and fluoxetine in depressed elderly outpatients. J Clin Psychiatry 61:559–568, 2000

Nierenberg AA, Feighner JP, Rudolph R, et al: Venlafaxine for treatment-resistant unipolar depression. J Clin Psychopharmacol 14:419–423, 1994

Nikaido AM, Ellinwood EH Jr, Heatherly DG, et al: Age-related increase in CNS sensitivity to benzodiazepines as assessed by task difficulty. Psychopharmacology 100:90–97, 1990

Noaghiul S, Narayan M, Nelson JC: Divalproex treatment of mania in elderly patients. Am J Geriatr Psychiatry 6:257–262, 1998

Nyth AL, Gottfries CG: The clinical efficacy of citalopram in treatment of emotional disturbances in dementia disorders. A Nordic multicentre study. Br J Psychiatry 157: 894–901, 1990

Nyth AL, Gottfries CG, Lyby K, et al: A controlled multicenter clinical study of citalopram and placebo in elderly depressed patients with and without concomitant dementia. Acta Psychiatr Scand 86:138–145, 1992

Oakley PW, Whyte IM, Carter GL: Lithium toxicity: an iatrogenic problem in susceptible individuals. Aust N Z J Psychiatry 35:833–840, 2001

Olafsson K, Jorgensen S, Jensen HV, et al: Fluvoxamine in the treatment of demented elderly patients: a double-blind, placebo-controlled study. Acta Psychiatr Scand 85:453–456, 1992

Onofrj M, Thomas A, Bonanni L, et al: Leucopenia induced by low dose clozapine in Parkinson's disease recedes shortly after drug withdrawal. Clinical case descriptions with commentary on switch-over to olanzapine. Neurol Sci 21:209–215, 2000

Oslin DW, Streim JE, Katz IR, et al: Heuristic comparison of sertraline with nortriptyline for the treatment of depression in frail elderly patients. Am J Geriatr Psychiatry 8: 141–149, 2000

Oslin DW, Ten Have TR, Streim JE, et al: Probing the safety of medications in the frail elderly: evidence from a randomized clinical trial of sertraline and venlafaxine in depressed nursing home residents. J Clin Psychiatry 64:875–882, 2003

Ostow M: Pramipexole for depression. Am J Psychiatry 159: 320–321, 2002

Ostroff RB, Nelson JC: Risperidone augmentation of selective serotonin reuptake inhibitors in major depression. J Clin Psychiatry 60:256–259, 1999

Pact V, Giduz T: Mirtazapine treats resting tremor, essential tremor, and levodopa-induced dyskinesias. Neurology 53: 1154, 1999

Pande AC, Crockatt JG, Janney C, et al: Gabapentin in bipolar disorder: a placebo-controlled trial of adjunctive therapy. Bipolar Disord 2 (3 pt 2):249–255, 2000

Parkinson Study Group: Low-dose clozapine for the treatment of drug-induced psychosis in Parkinson's disease. N Engl J Med 340:757–763, 1999

Passmore MJ, Garnham J, Duffy A, et al: Phenotypic spectra of bipolar disorder in responders to lithium versus lamotrigine. Bipolar Disord 5:110–114, 2003

Pedersen L, Klysner R: Antagonism of selective serotonin reuptake inhibitor-induced nausea by mirtazapine. Int Clin Psychopharmacol 12:59–60, 1997

Perry NK: Venlafaxine-induced serotonin syndrome with relapse following amitriptyline. Postgrad Med J 76:254–256, 2000

Phanjoo AL, Wonnacott S, Hodgson A: Double-blind comparative multicentre study of fluvoxamine and mianserin in the treatment of major depressive episode in elderly people. Acta Psychiatr Scand 83:476–479, 1991

Pies R: Must we now consider SRI's neuroleptics? J Clin Psycopharmacol 17:443–445, 1997

Pollock BG: Adverse reactions of antidepressants in elderly patients. J Clin Psychiatry 60 (suppl 20):4–8, 1999

Pollock BG, Mulsant BH: Antipsychotics in older patients: a safety perspective. Drugs Aging 6:312–323, 1995

Pollock BG, Mulsant BH, Sweet R, et al: An open pilot study of citalopram for behavioral disturbances of dementia. Am J Geriatr Psychiatry 5:70–78, 1997

Pollock BG, Rosen J, Mulsant BH: Antipsychotics and selective serotonin reuptake inhibitors for the treatment of behavioral disturbances in dementia of the Alzheimer type: a review of clinical data. Consultant Pharmacist 11:1251–1258, 1999

Pollock BG, Mulsant BH, Rosen J, et al: Comparison of citalopram, perphenazine, and placebo for the acute treatment of psychosis and behavioral disturbances in hospitalized, demented patients. Am J Psychiatry 159:460–465, 2002

Pomara N, Deptula D, Medel M, et al: Effects of diazepam on recall memory: relationship to aging, dose, and duration of treatment. Psychopharmacol Bull 25:144–148, 1989

Porsteinsson AP, Tariot PN, Erb R, et al: Placebo-controlled study of divalproex sodium for agitation in dementia. Am J Geriatr Psychiatry 9:58–66, 2001

Post RM, Frye MA, Denicoff KD, et al: Beyond lithium in the treatment of bipolar illness. Neuropsychopharmacology 19:206–219, 1998

Potkin SG, Saha AR, Kujawa MJ, et al: Aripiprazole, an antipsychotic with a novel mechanism of action, and schizoaffective disorder. Arch Gen Psychiatry 60:681–690, 2003

Preskorn SH, Magnus RD: Inhibition of hepatic P-450 isoenzymes by serotonin selective reuptake inhibitors: in vitro and in vivo findings and their implications for patient care. Psychopharmacol Bull 30:251–259, 1994

Preskorn SH, Alderman J, Greenblatt DJ, et al: Sertraline does not inhibit cytochrome P450 3A-mediated drug metabolism in vivo. Psychopharmacol Bull 33:659–665, 1997

Rahman MK, Akhtar MJ, Savla NC, et al: A double-blind, randomised comparison of fluvoxamine with dothiepin in the treatment of depression in elderly patients. Br J Clin Pract 45:255–258, 1991

Rainer MK, Masching AJ, Ertl MG, et al: Effect of risperidone on behavioral and psychological symptoms and cognitive function in dementia. J Clin Psychiatry 62:894–900, 2001

Raji MA, Brady SR: Mirtazapine for treatment of depression and comorbidities in Alzheimer disease. Ann Pharmacother 35:1024–1027, 2001

Rasmussen BB, Nielsen TL, Brosen K: Fluvoxamine is a potent inhibitor of the metabolism of caffeine in vitro. Pharmacol Toxicol 83:240–245, 1998

Ray WA, Meredith S, Thapa PB, et al: Antipsychotics and the risk of sudden cardiac death. Arch Gen Psychiatry 58:1161–1167, 2001

Reidenberg MM, Levy M, Warner H, et al: Relationship between diazepam dose, plasma level, age and central nervous system depression. Clin Pharmacol Ther 23:371–374, 1978

Reifler BV, Teri L, Raskind M: Double-blind trial of imipramine in Alzheimer's disease in patients with and without depression. Am J Psychiatry 146:45–49, 1989

Reisberg B, Doody R, Stoffler A, et al; Memantine Study Group: Memantine in moderate-to-severe Alzheimer's disease. N Engl J Med 348:1333–1341, 2003

Reznik I, Rosen Y, Rosen B: An acute ischaemic event associated with the use of venlafaxine: a case report and proposed pathophysiological mechanisms. J Psychopharmacol 13: 193–195, 1999

Rich SS, Friedman JH, Ott BR: Risperidone versus clozapine in the treatment of psychosis in six patients with Parkinson's disease and other akinetic-rigid syndromes. J Clin Psychiatry 56:556–559, 1995

Richard IH, Kurlan R: A survey of antidepressant drug use in Parkinson's disease. Parkinson Study Group. Neurology 49:1168–1170, 1997

Rickels K, Schweizer E, Case WG, et al: Nefazodone in major depression: adjunctive benzodiazepine therapy and tolerability. J Clin Psychopharmacol 18:145–153, 1998

Rickels K, Pollack MH, Sheehan DV, et al: Efficacy of extended-release venlafaxine in nondepressed outpatients with generalized anxiety disorder. Am J Psychiatry 157: 968–974, 2000

Robillard M, Conn DK: Lamotrigine use in geriatric patients with bipolar depression. Can J Psychiatry 47:767–770, 2002

Robinson D, Napoliello MJ, Schenck J: The safety and usefulness of buspirone as an anxiolytic drug in elderly versus young patients. Clin Ther 10:740–746, 1988

Robinson DS, Roberts DL, Smith JM, et al: The safety profile of nefazodone. J Clin Psychiatry 57 (suppl 2):31–38, 1996

Robinson R, Schultz S, Castillo C, et al: Nortriptyline versus fluoxetine in the treatment of depression and in short-term recovery after stroke: a placebo-controlled, double-blind study. Am J Psychiatry 157:351–359, 2000

Roose SP: Considerations for the use of antidepressants in patients with cardiovascular disease. Am Heart J 140 (4 suppl):84–88, 2000

Roose SP, Dalack GW, Glassman AH, et al: Cardiovascular effects of bupropion in depressed patients with heart disease. Am J Psychiatry 148:512–516, 1991

Rosen J, Sweet R, Pollock BG, et al: Nortriptyline in the hospitalized elderly: tolerance and side effect reduction. Psychopharmacol Bull 29:327–331, 1993

Rothschild AJ, Bates KS, Boehringer KL, et al: Olanzapine response in psychotic depression. J Clin Psychiatry 60:116–118, 1999

Rubin NJ, Arceneaux JM: Intractable depression or psychosis. Acta Psychiatr Scand 104:402–405, 2001

Sa DS, Lang AE: Olanzapine and clozapine: comparative effects on motor function in hallucinating PD patients. Neurology 57:747, 2001

Sajatovic M, Ramirez LF, Vernon L, et al: Outcome of risperidone therapy in elderly patients with chronic psychosis. Int J Psychiatry Med 26:309–317, 1996

Sajatovic M, Jaskiw G, Konicki PE, et al: Outcome of clozapine therapy for elderly patients with refractory primary psychosis. Int J Geriatr Psychiatry 12:553–558, 1997

Sajatovic M, Perez D, Brescan D, et al: Olanzapine therapy in elderly patients with schizophrenia. Psychopharmacol Bull 34:819–823, 1998

Sajatovic M, DiGiovanni S, Fuller M, et al: Nefazodone therapy in patients with treatment-resistant or treatment-intolerant depression and high psychiatric comorbidity. Clin Ther 21:733–740, 1999

Saltz BL, Kane JM, Woerner MG, et al: Prospective study of tardive dyskinesia in the elderly. Psychopharmacol Bull 25: 52–56, 1989

Salzman C: Treatment of the agitation of late-life psychosis and Alzheimer's disease. Eur Psychiatry 16 (suppl 1):25S–28S, 2001

Salzman C, Fisher J, Nobel K, et al: Cognitive improvement following benzodiazepine discontinuation in elderly nursing home residents. Int J Geriatr Psychiatry 7:89–93, 1992

Satel SL, Nelson JC: Stimulants in the treatment of depression: a critical overview. J Clin Psychiatry 50:241–249, 1989

Sato Y, Kondo I, Ishida S, et al: Decreased bone mass and increased bone turnover with valproate therapy in adults with epilepsy. Neurology 57:445–449, 2001

Schneider LS, Olin JT: Efficacy of acute treatment for geriatric depression. Int Psychogeriatr 7 (suppl):7–25, 1995

Schneider LS, Pollock VE, Lyness SA: A metaanalysis of controlled trials of neuroleptic treatment in dementia. J Am Geriatr Soc 38:553–563, 1990

Schneider LS, Tariot PN, Lyketsos CG, et al: National Institute of Mental Health Clinical Antipsychotic Trials of Intervention Effectiveness (CATIE): Alzheimer disease trial methodology. Am J Geriatr Psychiatry 9:346–360, 2001

Schone W, Ludwig M: A double-blind study of paroxetine compared with fluoxetine in geriatric patients with major depression. J Clin Psychopharmacol 13 (6 suppl 2):34S–39S, 1993

Schreiber S, Backer MM, Pick CG: The antinociceptive effect of venlafaxine in mice is mediated through opioid and adrenergic mechanisms. Neurosci Lett 273:85–88, 1999

Schuld A, Kuhn M, Haack M, et al: A comparison of the effects of clozapine and olanzapine on the EEG in patients with schizophrenia. Pharmacopsychiatry 33:109–111, 2000

Schwaninger M, Ringleb P, Winter R, et al: Elevated plasma concentrations of homocysteine in antiepileptic drug treatment. Epilepsia 40:345–350, 1999

Segraves RT, Kavoussi R, Hughes AR, et al: Evaluation of sexual functioning in depressed outpatients: a double-blind comparison of sustained-release bupropion and sertraline treatment. J Clin Psychopharmacol 20:122–128, 2000

Semenchuk MR, Sherman S, Davis B: Double-blind, randomized trial of bupropion SR for the treatment of neuropathic pain. Neurology 57:1583–1588, 2001

Sernyak MJ, Leslie DL, Alarcon RD, et al: Association of diabetes mellitus with use of atypical neuroleptics in the treatment of schizophrenia. Am J Psychiatry 159:561–566, 2002

Shelton RC, Tollefson GD, Tohen M, et al: A novel augmentation strategy for treating resistant major depression. Am J Psychiatry 158:131–134, 2001

Shulman KI: Disinhibition syndromes, secondary mania and bipolar disorder in old age. J Affect Disord 46:175–182, 1997

Sipahimalani A, Masand PS: Olanzapine in the treatment of delirium. Psychosomatics 39:422–430, 1998

Smeraldi E, Rizzo F, Crespi G: Double-blind, randomized study of venlafaxine, clomipramine and trazodone in geriatric patients with major depression. Primary Care Psychiatry 4:189–195, 1998

Snowdon J: The relevance of guidelines for treatment mania in old age. Int J Geriatr Psychiatry 15:779–783, 2000

Solai LK, Mulsant BH, Pollock BG, et al: Effect of sertraline on plasma nortriptyline levels in depressed elderly. J Clin Psychiatry, 58:440–443, 1997

Solai LK, Mulsant BH, Pollock BG: Selective serotonin reuptake inhibitors for late-life depression: a comparative review. Drugs Aging 18:355–368, 2001

Solai LK, Pollock BG, Mulsant BH, et al: Effect of nortriptyline and paroxetine on CYP2D6 activity in depressed elderly patients. J Clin Psychopharmacol 22:481–486, 2002

Solomons K, Geiger O: Olanzapine use in the elderly: a retrospective analysis. Can J Psychiatry 45:151–155, 2000

Sorock GS, Shimkin EE: Benzodiazepine sedatives and the risk of falling in a community-dwelling elderly cohort. Arch Intern Med 148:2441–2444, 1988

Spier SA: Use of bupropion with SRIs and venlafaxine. Depress Anxiety 7:73–75, 1998

Spigset O, Adielsson G: Combined serotonin syndrome and hyponatraemia caused by a citalopram-buspirone interaction. Int Clin Psychopharmacol 12:61–63, 1997

Spina E, Pisani F, Perucca E: Clinically significant pharmacokinetic drug interactions with carbamazepine. An update. Clin Pharmacokinet 31:198–214, 1996

Sproule BA, Hardy BG, Shulman KI: Differential pharmacokinetics of lithium in elderly patients. Drugs Aging 16:165–177, 2000

Staab JP, Evans DL: Efficacy of venlafaxine in geriatric depression. Depres Anxiety 12 (suppl 1):63–68, 2000

Steffens DC, Doraiswamy PM, McQuoid DR: Bupropion SR in the naturalistic treatment of elderly patients with major depression. Int J Geriatr Psychiatry 16:862–865, 2001

Steinberg JR: Anxiety in elderly patients. A comparison of azapirones and benzodiazepines. Drugs Aging 5:335–345, 1994

Stimmel GL, Dopheide JA, Stahl SM: Mirtazapine: an antidepressant with noradrenergic and specific serotonergic effects. Pharmacotherapy 17:10–21, 1997

Strand M, Hetta J, Rosen A, et al: A double-blind controlled trial in primary care patients with generalized anxiety: a comparison between buspirone and oxazepam. J Clin Psychiatry 51(suppl):40–45, 1990

Street JS, Clark WS, Gannon KS, et al: Olanzapine treatment of psychotic and behavioral symptoms in patients with Alzheimer disease in nursing care facilities: a double-blind, randomized, placebo-controlled trial. The HGEU Study Group. Arch Gen Psychiatry 57:968–976, 2000

Street JS, Clark WS, Kadam DL, et al: Long-term efficacy of olanzapine in the control of psychotic and behavioral symptoms in nursing home patients with Alzheimer's dementia. Int J Geriat Psychiatry 16 (suppl 1):S62–S70, 2001

Szuba MP, Leuchter AF: Falling backward in two elderly patients taking bupropion. J Clin Psychiatry 53:157–159, 1992

Taragano FE, Lyketsos CG, Mangone CA, et al: A double-blind, randomized, fixed-dose trial of fluoxetine vs. amitriptyline in the treatment of major depression complicating Alzheimer's disease. Psychosomatics 38:246–252, 1997

Targum SD, Abbott JL: Efficacy of quetiapine in Parkinson's patients with psychosis. J Clin Psychopharmacol 20:54–60, 2000

Tariot PN, Erb R, Podgorski CA, et al: Efficacy and tolerability of carbamazepine for agitation and aggression in dementia. Am J Psychiatry 155:54–61, 1998

Tariot PN, Salzman C, Yeung PP, et al: Long-Term use of quetiapine in elderly patients with psychotic disorders. Clin Ther 22:1068–1084, 2000

Tariot PN, Farlow MR, Grossberg G, et al: Memantine/donepezil dual therapy is superior to placebo/donepezil therapy for treatment of moderate to severe Alzheimer's disease (abstract). Int Psychogeriatr 15:289, 2003

Tashkin D, Kanner R, Bailey W, et al: Smoking cessation in patients with chronic obstructive pulmonary disease: a double-blind, placebo-controlled, randomised trial. Lancet 357:1571–1575, 2001

Thase ME: Effects of venlafaxine on blood pressure: a meta-analysis of original data from 3744 depressed patients. J Clin Psychiatry 59:502–508, 1998

Thase ME: What role do atypical antipsychotic drugs have in treatment-resistant depression? J Clin Psychiatry 63:95–103, 2002

Thase ME, Friedman ES, Howland RH: Venlafaxine and treatment-resistant depression. Depress Anxiety 12 (suppl 1):55–62, 2000

Thase ME, Entsuah AR, Rudolph RL: Remission rates during treatment with venlafaxine or selective serotonin reuptake inhibitors. Br J Psychiatry 178:234–241, 2001

Thompson DS: Mirtazapine for the treatment of depression and nausea in breast and gynecological oncology. Psychosomatics 41:356–359, 2000

Tinetti ME, Speechley M, Ginter SF: Risk factors for falls among elderly persons living in the community. N Engl J Med 319:1701–1707, 1988

Tollefson GD, Bosomworth JC, Heiligenstein JH, et al: A double-blind, placebo-controlled clinical trial of fluoxetine in geriatric patients with major depression. The Fluoxetine Collaborative Study Group. Int Psychogeriatr 7:89–104, 1995

Trannel TJ, Ahmed I, Goebert D: Occurrence of thrombocytopenia in psychiatric patients taking valproate. Am J Psychiatry 158:128–130, 2001

Trappler B, Cohen CI: Use of SSRIs in "very old" depressed nursing home residents. Am J Geriatr Psychiatry 6:83–89, 1998

Tune LE: Risperidone for the treatment of behavioral and psychological symptoms of dementia. J Clin Psychiatry 62 (suppl 21):29–32, 2001

Umapathy C, Mulsant BH, Pollock BG: Bipolar disorder in the elderly. Psychiatr Ann 30:473–480, 2000

van Laar MW, van Willigenburg AP, Volkerts ER: Acute and subchronic effects of nefazodone and imipramine on highway driving, cognitive functions, and daytime sleepiness in healthy adult and elderly subjects. J Clin Psychopharmacol 15:30–40, 1995

Verma S, Orengo CA, Kunik ME, et al: Tolerability and effectiveness of atypical antipsychotics in male geriatric inpatients. Int J Geriatr Psychiatry 16:223–227, 2001

von Moltke LL, Greenblatt DJ, Court MH, et al: Inhibition of alprazolam and desipramine hydroxylation in vitro by paroxetine and fluvoxamine: comparison with other selective serotonin reuptake inhibitor antidepressants. J Clin Psychopharmacol 15:125–131, 1995

von Moltke LL, Greenblatt DJ, Giancarlo GM, et al: Escitalopram (S-citalopram) and its metabolites in vitro: cytochromes mediating biotransformation, inhibitory effects, and comparison to R-citalopram. Drug Metab Dispos 29:1102–1109, 2001

Wakelin JS: Fluvoxamine in the treatment of the older depressed patient; double-blind, placebo-controlled data. Int Clin Psychopharmacol 1:221–230, 1986

Waldinger MD, Zwinderman AH, Olivier B: Antidepressants and ejaculation: a double-blind, randomized, placebo-controlled, fixed-dose study with paroxetine, sertraline, and nefazodone. J Clin Psychopharmacol 21:293–297, 2001

Walker AM, Lanza LL, Arellano F, et al: Mortality in current and former users of clozapine. Epidemiology 8:671–677, 1997

Walker Z, Grace J, Overshot R, et al: Olanzapine in dementia with Lewy bodies: a clinical study. Int J Geriatr Psychiatry 14:459–466, 1999

Wallace AE, Kofoed LL, West AN: Double-blind placebo-controlled trial of methylphenidate in older, depressed, medically ill patients. Am J Psychiatry 152:929–931, 1995

Wang PS, Bohn RL, Glynn RJ, et al: Zolpidem use and hip fractures in older people. J Am Geriatr Soc 49:1685–1690, 2001

Weigmann H, Gerek S, Zeisig A, et al: Fluvoxamine but not sertraline inhibits the metabolism of olanzapine: evidence from a therapeutic drug monitoring service. Ther Drug Monit 23:410–413, 2001

Weihs KL, Settle EC Jr, Batey SR, et al: Bupropion sustained release versus paroxetine for the treatment of depression in the elderly. J Clin Psychiatry 61:196–202, 2000

Whyte EM, Mulsant BH: Post-stroke depression: epidemiology, pathophysiology, and biological treatment. Biol Psychiatry 52:253–264, 2002

Wilner KD, Tensfeldt TG, Baris B, et al: Single- and multiple-dose pharmacokinetics of ziprasidone in healthy young and elderly volunteers. Br J Clin Pharmacol 49 (suppl 1):15S–20S, 2000

Wirshing WC: Movement disorders associated with neuroleptic treatment. J Clin Psychiatry 62 (suppl 21):15–18, 2001

Wolters EC, Hurwitz TA, Mak E, et al: Clozapine in the treatment of parkinsonian patients with dopaminomimetic psychosis. Neurology 40:832–834, 1990

Wolters EC, Jansen EN, Tuynman-Qua HG, et al: Olanzapine in the treatment of dopaminomimetic psychosis in patients with Parkinson's disease. Neurology 47:1085–1087, 1996

Woo MH, Smythe MA: Association of SIADH with selective serotonin reuptake inhibitors. Ann Pharmacother 31:108–110, 1997

Workman RH Jr, Orengo CA, Bakey AA, et al: The use of risperidone for psychosis and agitation in demented patients with Parkinson's disease. J Neuropsychiatry Clin Neurosci 9:594–597, 1997

Wylie ME, Mulsant BH, Pollock BG, et al: Age of onset in geriatric bipolar disorder: effects on clinical presentation and treatment outcomes in an inpatient sample. Am J Geriatr Psychiatry 7:77–83, 1999

Wylie ME, Miller MD, Shear MK, et al: Fluvoxamine pharmacotherapy of anxiety disorders in late life: preliminary open-trial data. J Geriatr Psychiatry Neurol 13:43–48, 2000

Zarate CA Jr, Baldessarini RJ, Siegel AJ, et al: Risperidone in the elderly: a pharmacoepidemiologic study. J Clin Psychiatry 58:311–317, 1997

Zaudig M: A risk-benefit assessment of risperidone for the treatment of behavioural and psychological symptoms in dementia. Drug Saf 23:183–195, 2000

Zimmer B, Kant R, Zeiler D, et al: Antidepressant efficacy and cardiovascular safety of venlafaxine in young vs old patients with comorbid medical disorders. Int J Psychiatry Med 27:353–364, 1997

Electroconvulsive Therapy

Richard D. Weiner, M.D., Ph.D.

Andrew D. Krystal, M.D., M.S.

Electroconvulsive therapy (ECT) involves the electrical induction of a series of seizures as a treatment for mental disorders, most notably major depression. This chapter covers the history of ECT; the extent to which it is used; indications; risks; the evaluation of patients for ECT; ECT technique; the use of ECT to alleviate episodes of illness (index ECT); management of patients after completion of the ECT course, including the use of ECT to prevent relapse (maintenance ECT); and finally, a brief discussion of what can be expected in the future of this treatment modality. Throughout, a particular focus is placed on the use of ECT in the elderly. With the mean age of individuals referred for ECT increasing, the importance of ECT in geriatric psychiatry continues to grow.

For general references on ECT, readers are referred to recent American Psychiatric Association recommendations (American Psychiatric Association 2001), as well as texts covering this subject matter by Abrams (2002) and Beyer and colleagues (1998). In addition, lay texts on the topic of ECT have been written by Fink (1999) and Endler (1990).

History

In 1935 the Hungarian neuropsychiatrist Ladislas von Meduna chemically induced seizures in a small series of schizophrenic patients (Fink 1984). His rationale for doing so was based on the hypothesis (later shown to be incorrect) that those with epilepsy had a reduced incidence of schizophrenia. Having achieved some partial success in therapeutic outcome, von Meduna's new convulsive therapy was greeted with great acclaim as a means to manage what had been an otherwise untreatable illness. When the use of pharmacoconvulsive ther-

apy spread to Italy shortly thereafter, another neuropsychiatrist, Ugo Cerletti, was impressed not only by the efficacy of this new treatment but also its technical difficulty (Endler 1988). From his work as an experimental epileptologist, Cerletti was aware of an electrical model of seizure induction that had been tried in animals. After some further experimentation, Cerletti and his assistant Lucio Bini were successful in treating one of their schizophrenic patients using electrical seizure induction. After more trials, electroconvulsive therapy rapidly replaced pharmacoconvulsive therapy throughout the world.

Although ECT was first used in the treatment of schizophrenia, clinicians soon realized that its highest therapeutic potency was in the mood disorders. The peak in ECT utilization was from the early 1940s through the mid-1950s, at which point the first effective antipsychotic and antidepressant medications came into clinical use. As would be expected, these new psychopharmacological agents obviated the need for ECT in many individuals with applicable disorders. However, trials comparing the antidepressant efficacy of ECT and these medications indicate that ECT remains the most rapid and effective means to induce remission (Weiner and Coffey 1988).

In the early days of ECT, there was considerable fear concerning the use of ECT in the elderly, largely because of the medical comorbidity that is often associated with this age group. The cardiovascular physiology of ECT was not well understood at the time, and more recent procedural innovations—such as oxygenation, muscular relaxation, general anesthesia, and physiological monitoring—had not yet been instituted. Instead, ECT during that period was accomplished in a distinctly nonmedical setting, often in psychiatrist's offices, without the presence of other medical staff or medical support resources.

As ECT methodology became more refined, however, practitioners became more willing to utilize it in previously underserved populations. Such use is particularly the case with the elderly, for whom ECT treatment has steadily grown in recent decades (Thompson et al. 1994). Thompson and colleagues reported that in 1986 approximately one-third of people receiving ECT were age 65 years or older. Since that time, the relative use of ECT in the elderly appears to have risen further. Rosenbach and coworkers (1997) observed a nationwide rise in ECT use from 4.2/10,000 to 5.1/10,000 among Medicare recipients between 1987 and 1992. In Texas, 48% of those treated with ECT during a 19-month period from 1993 to 1995 were at least age 65 years (Reid et al.1998). Similarly, using California data, Kramer (1999) reported an ECT treatment rate of 3.82/10,000 for individuals age 65 and above versus rates of 1.21/10,000 for those ages 45–64 and 0.48/10,000 for those ages 25–44.

There has been considerable speculation regarding the reasons for the growing use of ECT among the elderly. Some evidence shows that depressive episodes in this age group tend to be relatively more severe and also more resistant to medication, yet current data are not conclusive in this regard. In addition, elderly patients are more likely to be intolerant of medications. Although the lay press has sometimes asserted that increased use of ECT in the elderly may reflect a desire on the part of ECT practitioners to obtain Medicare reimbursement funding, existing low Medicare reimbursement rates make that argument less than credible. Instead, the available evidence indicates that ECT is used because it is safe, it works well, and it works rapidly.

Indications for ECT

Diagnostic Indications

The most common diagnostic indication for ECT is major depression (American Psychiatric Association 2001; Thompson et al. 1994). A significant body of literature not only supports the efficacy of ECT for major depression but suggests that it is the most rapid and effective treatment for this condition (Weiner and Krystal 2001). This literature includes a series of randomized, double-blind, placebo-controlled studies in which the placebo control was "sham ECT," whereby subjects received all aspects of a usual clinical ECT treatment except for the electrical stimulus (Brandon 1986). Evidence also suggests greater efficacy with ECT than with antidepressant medication in meta-analytical studies (Janicak et al. 1985); however, it should be noted that this type of analysis has not been carried out comparing ECT with newer antidepressant medications.

Regarding subtypes of depression, ECT appears to be effective in both melancholic and severe nonmelancholic depression (Sackeim and Rush 1995), as well as in bipolar and unipolar major depression (Weiner and Krystal 2001). In addition, it may be particularly effective in psychotic major depression (Sobin et al. 1996).

Although ECT is used more frequently for major depression than for other illnesses and the vast majority of ECT research studies have been carried out on this condition, evidence suggests that ECT has efficacy in a number of other mental disorders. A series of reports suggest that ECT has efficacy in the treatment of acute mania (Mukherjee et al. 1994; Small et al. 1988). In this regard, ECT has been reported to achieve a response rate as high as 80%, to have efficacy equal to that of lithium, and to have a significant advantage over lithium in patients who have not responded to lithium or antipsychotic medication. The relative efficacy of ECT compared with anticonvulsant antimanic agents has not yet been studied, nor do any systematic studies exist to indicate the utility of ECT in individuals with rapid-cycling bipolar disorder (Weiner and Krystal 2001).

Another disorder for which ECT appears to have efficacy is schizophrenia. Although ECT was first employed as a treatment for this condition, the superior response of patients with mood disorders was soon evident (Weiner and Krystal 2001). With the development of antipsychotic medications in the late 1950s, the use of ECT as a treatment for schizophrenia gradually declined. Still, a number of studies have suggested that antipsychotic medications and ECT have comparable efficacy (Fink and Sackeim 1996; Krueger and Sackeim 1995). In addition, more recent evidence suggests that for acute psychotic episodes, the combination of antipsychotic medications and ECT may have greater efficacy than either ECT or medications alone (Klapheke 1993; Sajatovic and Meltzer 1993). However, no evidence indicates that ECT has efficacy for the treatment of deficit or "negative" symptoms of schizophrenia (Weiner and Krystal 2001).

The presence of affective symptoms appears to increase the likelihood of response to ECT in those with schizophrenia. In this regard, case reports and case series suggest that individuals with schizoaffective disorder may respond better to ECT than those with schizophrenia (Fink and Sackeim 1996; Krueger and Sackeim 1995). Catatonia, which can be associated with both schizophrenia and mood disorders, is highly responsive to ECT (Krystal and Coffey 1997), even when this condition is associated with medical conditions such as systemic lupus erythematosus, uremia, hepatic encephalopathy, porphyria, and hyperparathyroidism (Fricchione et al. 1990; Rummans and Bassingthwaighte 1991).

Some evidence suggests that ECT may also be a useful treatment for Parkinson's disease when medication management fails or is not tolerated (Andersen et al. 1987; Kellner and Bernstein 1993; Krystal and Coffey 1997; Pritchett et al. 1994; Rasmussen and Abrams 1991). However, it should also be noted that patients with Parkinson's disease may be at increased risk for developing cognitive side effects and delirium with ECT (Figiel et al. 1991).

Response to ECT in the Elderly

Several prospective studies suggest that ECT is a highly effective treatment specifically for major depression in elderly individuals (O'Connor et al. 2001; Tew et al. 1999; Wesson et al. 1997). Furthermore, one study indicates that ECT has a significant impact on the course of major depression in the elderly, in terms of both efficacy and morbidity and mortality rates (Philibert et al. 1995). Also, evidence based on data from 584 subjects suggests that, if anything, the response to ECT increases with advancing age (Sackeim 1998). These data provide support for a role for ECT in the practice of geriatric psychiatry.

Continuation or Maintenance ECT

Although ECT is a highly effective treatment for a number of neuropsychiatric conditions, it is not a cure in the sense that it does not ensure that future episodes will not occur (Weiner and Krystal 2001; Weiner et al. 2000). As a result, it is important to institute some form of continuation or maintenance therapy (American Psychiatric Association 2001). This point is underscored by the findings from a recent study, which were that without receiving maintenance therapy, roughly 80% of patients successfully treated with ECT for major depression will relapse within 6 months (Sackeim et al. 2001). Most commonly, continuation or maintenance pharmacotherapy is instituted after a successful course of ECT. Nevertheless, prophylactic pharmacotherapy is not universally effective, and roughly 50%–60% of depressed patients will relapse within a year of the end of the ECT course when treated with typical continuation or maintenance pharmacotherapy (Sackeim et al. 1990, 2001). The relapse rate appears to be even higher among those whose depression was resistant to medication before the ECT course (Sackeim et al. 1990). One study suggests that, rather than single-agent therapy, more aggressive pharmacotherapy—specifically the combination of nortriptyline and lithium—is associated with a

decrease in the relapse rate to roughly 40% 6 months after ECT (Sackeim et al. 2001).

An alternative to continuation or maintenance pharmacotherapy is continuation or maintenance ECT. However, although a number of case series and retrospective reports suggest the efficacy of continuation or maintenance ECT, no controlled, randomized studies have yet been completed (see American Psychiatric Association 2001). At the present time, pharmacotherapy is usually instituted after a successful course of ECT unless at least one of the following conditions exists: 1) prophylactic pharmacotherapy has failed in the past; 2) the patient is intolerant of medications; 3) the patient has a medical illness that contraindicates medication management; or 4) the patient has a preference for prophylactic ECT (American Psychiatric Association 2001; Weiner and Krystal 2001).

Strategic Use of ECT

In general, the decision about whether to recommend ECT for a given patient should rest on a careful assessment of risks and benefits (American Psychiatric Association 2001). Even though ample evidence suggests that ECT is a highly effective treatment for a number of neuropsychiatric disorders, it is generally not used as a first-line treatment. However, first-line treatment with ECT should be considered when there is an urgent need for response in a patient with major depression or mania (American Psychiatric Association 2001; Quitkin et al. 1996). This situation typically occurs when the presenting condition threatens the life of the patient because of suicidality, malnutrition, dehydration, or inability to comply with treatment of a critical medical problem. In addition, the first-line use of ECT should be considered when, because of circumstances such as medical illness, ECT is deemed to be safer than pharmacotherapy (American Psychiatric Association 2001; Weiner et al. 2000). ECT should also be considered on a primary basis when a patient has an informed preference for ECT or when there has been a past preferential response to ECT in prior episodes (American Psychiatric Association 2001).

The secondary use of ECT is generally undertaken because of either a lack of response to pharmacotherapy or medication intolerance (American Psychiatric Association 2001). Unfortunately, there is no currently accepted definition for medication failure. Operationally, when making this decision, practitioners generally take into account the number of medications tried, the duration of treatment, the dosage administered, symptom severity, tolerance of pharmacotherapy, the expected risks associated with ECT, and patient preference (American Psychiatric Association 2001). In support of the use of ECT following medication failure are several studies indicating that a significant number of individuals respond to ECT after one or more failed trials of medication (Avery and Lubrano 1979; Paul et al. 1981; Prudic et al. 1996).

Risks of ECT and Its Use in Patients With Neurological and Medical Disorders

Because the decision about whether to pursue a course of ECT should involve an evaluation of both the expected risks and benefits of ECT, it is important to be able to carry out an assessment of the likelihood of potential adverse sequelae for each patient.

Mortality

Although it is difficult to accurately establish the mortality rate associated with any medical procedure, it has been estimated that the overall mortality rate with ECT is roughly 1 death per 80,000 treatments (American Psychiatric Association 2001). This relatively low mortality rate appears to be comparable to the risk of minor surgery and has been considered to be less than that associated with pharmacotherapy with tricyclic antidepressants (Sackeim 1998). Furthermore, some studies have suggested that depressed inpatients who receive ECT have a lower mortality rate after discharge than individuals who receive other types of treatment (Avery and Winokur 1976; Philibert et al. 1995). It is important to understand, however, that the likelihood of ECT-related death in high-risk populations—most commonly occurring in the elderly (see below)—can be substantially higher than that mentioned above. Still, even in such situations, the risk of undertaking ECT may be lower than the risk of not doing it.

Cognitive Side Effects

The most important side effect with ECT is cognitive dysfunction, which appears to be a key factor limiting the use of this treatment modality (American Psychiatric Association 2001). These side effects consist primarily of anterograde amnesia (difficulty retaining new information) and retrograde amnesia (difficulty recalling information learned in the past). Both anterograde and retrograde memory side

effects tend to most strongly affect information encountered during the period of time closest to the ECT treatment course. Anterograde amnesia typically resolves within a few weeks after the treatment course, whereas retrograde amnesia tends to resolve more slowly (American Psychiatric Association 2001; Weiner et al. 1986). Despite objective evidence that memory performance transiently decreases after ECT, some patients indicate that their memory function improves, likely a result of the lifting of depressive symptoms (American Psychiatric Association 2001; Weiner et al. 1986).

Both the degree and duration of objective and subjective memory side effects of ECT vary substantially among individuals who receive ECT. A number of research studies have identified factors that can affect objective memory side effects of ECT (American Psychiatric Association 2001). Bilateral placement of stimulus electrodes has been repeatedly shown to increase the risk of amnesia compared with unilateral ECT. In addition, greater risk is associated with higher stimulus intensity (compared with the seizure threshold), larger numbers of ECT treatments, higher dosages of barbiturate anesthetic, and less time between treatments. Furthermore, some patients—including those taking lithium and medications with anticholinergic properties, as well as those with preexisting cerebral disease—appear to be at increased risk of cognitive side effects (American Psychiatric Association 2001). Individuals with diseases affecting the basal ganglia and subcortical white matter may be at particular risk (Figiel et al. 1990).

Other Risks With ECT

It is important to identify individuals at risk for medical complications with ECT and to be aware of the modifications in ECT technique that may minimize risks. Elderly patients referred for ECT frequently have preexisting medical illnesses (Weiner and Krystal 2001). Although some such conditions appear to increase the risks of ECT (Weiner and Coffey 1988; Zielinski et al. 1993), none should be considered "absolute" contraindications to its use, given, as noted earlier, that risk is relative rather than absolute (Weiner et al. 2000; Weiner and Krystal 2001). The decision about whether to pursue a course of ECT should always involve a careful weighing of the risks and benefits of carrying out ECT with those of not using it. Conditions for which evidence suggests increased risks with ECT are discussed in the following subsections, as are modifications in ECT technique that may decrease these risks. Also covered are the central nervous system, cardiovascular, endocrinologic, metabolic, hematological, pulmonary, gastrointestinal, genitourinary, and musculoskeletal risks of ECT and the specific issue of adverse effects of ECT in the elderly.

Central Nervous System Disorders

The primary central nervous system (CNS) risks of ECT stem from the increase in intracranial and intravascular pressure that can occur with ECT seizures (Krystal and Coffey 1997). Despite these increases in pressure, the CNS complication rate is generally quite low. A number of CNS disorders leave individuals more vulnerable to increases in pressure than the general ECT population. These include the presence of any space-occupying CNS lesions such as tumors, subdural hematomas, intracranial arachnoid cysts, or normal-pressure hydrocephalus (Krystal and Coffey 1997). Patients with these conditions have been considered to be at increased risk for noncardiogenic pulmonary edema, cerebral edema, brain hemorrhage, and cerebral herniation (Krystal and Coffey 1997). Although space-occupying cerebral lesions were once considered an absolute contraindication to ECT, a number of reports describe successful ECT in individuals with these lesions. Those with small lesions without edema or a pretreatment elevation of intracranial pressure can usually be safely treated with ECT (Krystal and Coffey 1997). For the remainder of those with space-occupying CNS lesions, the risks may be diminished (although not removed) by pretreating with an antihypertensive agent, osmotic diuretics, and steroids and by employing hyperventilation during treatment.

The increase in intravascular pressure that occurs with ECT might be theoretically expected to lead to an increased risk of intracranial hemorrhage; however, such events are extremely rare (Krystal and Coffey 1997). Nonetheless, individuals with recent strokes, arteriovenous malformations, and aneurysms are considered to be at increased risk (Krystal and Coffey 1997). In two case series, involving a total of 34 patients who received ECT while recovering from strokes, no occurrences of hemorrhages or worsening of any stroke-associated deficits were reported (Currier et al. 1992; Murray et al. 1986). Still, the American Psychiatric Association (2001) recommends waiting as long as possible after a stroke before administering ECT. The use of antihypertensive agents should be considered to diminish the rise in intravascular pressure in patients with a history of hemorrhagic stroke; however, such prophylaxis may be counterproductive in individuals who have suffered cerebral ischemic events (American Psychiatric Association 2001).

Other adverse CNS conditions that can be associated with ECT include prolonged seizures (lasting longer than 3 minutes) and status epilepticus (a single seizure lasting at least 30 minutes, or more than one seizure in which consciousness is not regained during the interictal period) (American Psychiatric Association 2001). Prolonged seizures can lead to increased cognitive side effects, which can be minimized by rapidly administering antiepileptic drugs to terminate such events. It appears that the risk of both prolonged seizures and status epilepticus may be increased by some medications (including theophylline and lithium), as well as by medical conditions that lower the seizure threshold (such as hyponatremia), and also by the induction of multiple seizures in the same treatment session (American Psychiatric Association 2001).

As noted above, patients with preexisting cerebral disease may be particularly likely to experience problems with ECT-related amnesia. At times even frank delirium may occur. These risks, which appear to be most prominent in individuals with dementia or with basal ganglia disease, can be minimized by decreasing the frequency of treatments and using unilateral electrode placement.

Cardiovascular Disorders

Fluctuations in pulse and blood pressure that occur during ECT treatments may be associated with cardiovascular complications (Weiner et al. 2000). Immediately after the stimulus there is an increase in parasympathetic tone, which can lead to a sudden, but transient, decrease in heart rate, not uncommonly presenting as a brief period of asystole. The subsequent induced seizure, however, is associated with a sympathetic surge that markedly increases both blood pressure and heart rate. This sympathetic surge is then followed by a relative increase in parasympathetic tone as the induced seizure ends.

Despite these autonomic fluctuations, cardiovascular complications from ECT rarely occur in individuals without preexisting cardiovascular risk factors (Weiner et al. 2000). The risk is increased in those with recent myocardial infarction, uncompensated congestive heart failure, severe valvular disease, unstable aneurysms, unstable angina or active cardiac ischemia, uncontrolled hypertension, high-grade atrioventricular block, symptomatic ventricular arrhythmias, and supraventricular arrhythmias with uncontrolled ventricular rate (American Psychiatric Association 2001; Applegate 1997). For patients with these conditions, a consultation with a cardiologist is recommended to help with the risk-benefit analysis and to suggest treatment modifications that may decrease risks. It has been proposed that an assessment of functional cardiac status (such as a stress test) should be considered in 1) men younger than 60 and women under 70 with definite angina, 2) men older than 60 and women over 70 with probable angina, 3) all patients with angina and two risk factors for myocardial infarction, and 4) those with clinically significant extracardiac vascular disease (Applegate 1997). A finding of good functional status indicates that the risk is low; otherwise further cardiac evaluation is indicated.

Individuals with ischemic coronary artery disease are at risk for ischemia during both the periods of relative parasympathetic tone and the periods of increased sympathetic system tone (Weiner et al. 2000). When parasympathetic tone is increased, there is a risk of ischemia due to hypoperfusion; whereas when sympathetic activity rises, the increased cardiac workload can lead to complications. The risks of complications due to these factors can be decreased pharmacologically. β-Adrenergic blockers can be used to decrease cardiac workload, anticholinergic medications such as atropine can be used to decrease the occurrence and severity of bradycardia, and nitrates or calcium channel blockers may be used to decrease the risks of ischemia (Weiner et al. 2000). Typically, patients who are receiving medications for the treatment of coronary artery disease at the time of the referral for ECT are maintained on those medications throughout the ECT course, including administration before ECT on treatment days (Applegate 1997). Changes to the medication regimen or the addition of other medications to decrease the risks of complications should generally be considered in conjunction with a cardiologic consultant.

Patients with pathologies associated with low cardiac output such as heart failure or those with severe valvular disease are at particular risk during the sympathetic surge because of the increase in afterload and decreased diastolic filling time (Stern et al. 1997). Such patients should not be administered large volumes of fluid (Rayburn 1997). A number of medications have been suggested as means to decrease risks in these situations, including the use of β-adrenergic blockers, α-adrenergic blockers, nitrites, digitalis, and anticholinergic agents; however, all of these agents remain controversial (Weiner et al. 2000). There does not appear to be a single regimen that is optimal for all patients with these diseases, and the treatment plan should be individualized on the basis of risk-benefit considerations.

Arrhythmias may increase the risks of ECT. Bradyarrhythmias are typically best managed with atropine to prevent exacerbation during increases in parasympathetic tone. Because of the anticonvulsant effects of lidocaine, ventricular ectopy should be treated with other agents before the ECT treatment (Hood and Mecca 1983). There is a risk that individuals with atrial fibrillation may experience spontaneous cardioversion with ECT that can lead to an embolic event (Petrides and Fink

1996). As a result, consideration should be given to echocardiography (to rule out a mural thrombus) and the use of anticoagulants (Weiner et al. 2000).

Endocrinologic Disorders

The most commonly encountered endocrinologic disorder with ECT is diabetes mellitus. Patients with diabetes are more likely than other ECT patients to have problems stemming from the need to fast from midnight until the time of the ECT treatment. Insulin doses may need to be adjusted, and pretreatment intravenous glucose administration can be considered if indicated (Weiner et al. 2000).

In patients with hyperthyroidism and pheochromocytoma, β-adrenergic blockers are typically administered to prevent evoking a thyroid storm or hypertensive crisis, which can be elicited by the sympathetic surge (Weiner et al. 2000). In cases of pheochromocytoma, α-adrenergic and tyrosine hydroxylase blockers may be needed.

Metabolic Disorders

The metabolic problems that are of primary concern are hyperkalemia and hypokalemia, both of which may lead to cardiac arrhythmias. The former is of particular concern because of the transient rise in serum potassium caused by succinylcholine and the muscle activity that may occur during the induced seizures (Weiner et al. 2000). In individuals with hypokalemia, prolonged paralysis and associated apnea induced by succinylcholine may be seen. Although it is best to correct these conditions before administering ECT, in cases where correction is not possible, the use of paralytic agents other than succinylcholine should be considered.

Hematological Disorders

Thrombophlebitis carries with it the risk of embolism with ECT, a risk that is generally easily avoided with the use of anticoagulant medications. The use of warfarin has been recommended, with a goal of achieving an International Normalized Ratio (prothrombin time normalized to the laboratory control value) between 1.5 and 2.5 (Petrides and Fink 1996).

Pulmonary Disorders

Patients with asthma or chronic obstructive pulmonary disease have an increased risk of posttreatment bronchospasm, which should be mitigated by the use of bronchodilators (Weiner et al. 2000). Theophylline should be avoided if possible or the dose kept to a minimum because of an increased risk of prolonged seizures.

Gastrointestinal Disorders

Patients with gastroesophageal reflux are commonly encountered in the practice of ECT. Complications of aspiration may be diminished with the use of a pretreatment histamine-2 antagonist the night before and the morning of treatment (Weiner et al. 2000). To increase gastric emptying, pretreatment metoclopramide may be considered, and sodium citrate may also be used to neutralize the acidity of stomach contents. Although it has not been reported, fecal impaction has been mentioned as a risk factor for intestinal rupture with ECT (Weiner et al. 2000). Consequently, in patients referred for ECT, it is important to address constipation, which is particularly common in the elderly population.

Genitourinary Disorders

Similarly to fecal impaction, urinary retention could, in theory, lead to bladder rupture with ECT. As a result, it has been recommended that patients void before ECT, and urinary catheterization should be considered in those with significant obstruction or difficulty urinating (Weiner et al. 2000).

Musculoskeletal Disorders

Musculoskeletal conditions—such as osteoporosis, unstable fractures, and loose or damaged teeth—are common in the elderly and carry an increased risk of complications with ECT. Patients with osteoporosis or with recent or unstable fractures are at risk for bone damage during the induced convulsion. This risk can be addressed by using an increased dose of succinylcholine to ensure good neuromuscular relaxation. In extremely fragile individuals, even the muscle fasciculations that accompany the action of succinylcholine may be of concern, and therefore pretreatment with curare should be considered. The contraction of the jaw muscles that leads to teeth clenching cannot be diminished with the use of paralytic agents because it occurs by direct electrical stimulation of the muscle tissue and not via neuromuscular transmission. Therefore, the use of a mouth guard is always necessary. However, those with loose or damaged teeth may require customized devices, dental treatment, or tooth extraction before ECT.

Adverse Effects in the Elderly

Advanced age itself does not appear to increase the medical risks of ECT. As a group, however, the elderly have a higher frequency of comorbid medical and neurological conditions that increase the risks of treatment, as outlined above (Tomac et al. 1997). In addition, several studies have reported that the elderly tend to have greater and more prolonged cognitive impairment with ECT (see American Psychiatric Association 2001). As a result, in elderly patients, particularly those with preexisting cognitive impairment, modifications of treatment technique should be considered that will minimize cognitive side effects.

The greater frequency of comorbid medical and neurological disease in elderly persons also increases the risks associated with pharmacological management of their neuropsychiatric conditions. In some cases these risks can make pharmacological management extremely difficult and may lead to a referral for ECT. In this regard, Manly and colleagues (2000) compared the frequency of side effects associated with ECT and pharmacotherapy in a group of depressed patients older than age 75 years who were matched for age, sex, and diagnosis. These researchers reported that ECT resulted in fewer side effects (particularly cardiovascular and gastrointestinal) and greater efficacy than pharmacological management. This study underscores that ECT is a relatively safe treatment for the elderly and that in many cases it may be both the safest and most effective option.

Pre-ECT Evaluation

Basic Components of the Evaluation

Each pre-ECT evaluation should be carried out by an individual clinically privileged to administer ECT in conjunction with an anesthesia provider. This evaluation should include 1) a thorough psychiatric history and examination, including history of response to ECT and other treatments; 2) a medical history and examination, with special attention paid to cardiovascular, respiratory, neurological, and musculoskeletal systems; 3) a history of dental problems and examination for loose or missing teeth; and 4) a history of personal and family experiences with anesthesia (American Psychiatric Association 2001). Laboratory tests are generally performed, although there is no agreed-on routine set of tests to carry out in each case. The most commonly administered pre-ECT screening battery of tests includes a complete blood count, serum chemistry (including sodium and potassium), and electrocardiogram (American Psychiatric Association 2001). A chest radiograph is indicated in the setting of cardiovascular or pulmonary disease or where there is a history of smoking (American Psychiatric Association 2001; Weiner et al. 2000).

The decision about whether to pursue testing of cerebral function and structure (e.g., electroencephalogram and neuroradiological and neuropsychological assessment) should be made on an individual basis, guided by the history and examination. In addition, spinal radiographs should be considered in individuals with known or suspected spinal disease. Further testing or consultation should be considered when the nature or extent of a problem is uncertain, when the risks of ECT in the setting of the existing medical disease are unclear, or when there is uncertainty about how to modify ECT technique to decrease risks. In every case, the pre-ECT assessment should include an evaluation of the risks of cognitive impairment based on the considerations described above and the information obtained by history, examination, and testing. This evaluation should play a key role in recommendations about treatment technique in terms of electrode placement, treatment frequency, stimulus dosing, and medications that should be avoided.

Decision About Whether to Administer ECT

The decision about whether to recommend ECT should include a careful assessment of risks and benefits of ECT versus alternative treatments, based on the information obtained in the evaluation, as well as on the available literature. The starting point for this decision should be the psychiatric diagnosis. ECT should be seriously considered only when the patient has a condition for which there is evidence of ECT efficacy. For individuals with an ECT-responsive disease, a number of factors should be considered in developing a recommendation about ECT. These factors include the severity of the illness, the degree of refractoriness to other treatments, an assessment of the risks of ECT, and the patient's preference.

In conditions such as major depression, for which ECT is the most effective treatment known, the greater the severity of illness, the stronger the indication for ECT (Weiner and Krystal 2001). When psychosis is present or when there is a high degree of lethality because of suicidality, dehydration or malnutrition, or an inability of the patient to cooperate with necessary medical treatment, ECT is frequently the treatment of choice. Unfortunately, there are no proven guidelines for how to define treatment refractoriness in terms of medication dosage or duration or number of failed trials. Consequently, the choice of when to refer a patient for ECT on the basis of medication resistance or intolerance is generally based on factors such as symptom severity, the morbidity of the episode, and patient preference as much as it is on the characteristics of prior medication trials.

The assessment of risks based on the evaluation described above is an important part of the decision of whether to pursue ECT. The greater the perceived risk, the stronger the indication for ECT must be for a recommendation to be made. When the risks of ECT are assessed to be significantly life-threatening, it should be pursued only if the illness is so lethal that the risks of not pursuing ECT are assessed to be greater. As noted earlier, however, risk is a relative index.

Informed Consent

The collaborative aspect of decision making has been formalized as the legal doctrine of informed consent (American Psychiatric Association 2001). No patient with the capacity to give voluntary consent should be treated with ECT without their written, informed consent. Although there is no clear consensus about how to determine capacity to consent, it has generally been interpreted as evidence that the patient can understand information about the procedure and can act responsibly on the basis of this information (American Psychiatric Association 2001). The process of determining competency, the process for giving ECT involuntarily in cases of emergency, and the specific procedures regarding informed consent should be carried out as specified by applicable state statutes.

At a minimum, written consent should be obtained before a course of ECT, if an unusually large number of treatments become necessary, and before initiating continuation or maintenance ECT (American Psychiatric Association 2001). To adequately convey the risks and benefits, the consent form should include the following information: 1) a description of treatment alternatives; 2) a detailed description of how, when, and where ECT will be carried out; 3) a discussion of options regarding electrode placement; 4) the typical range of number of treatments; 5) a statement that there is no guarantee that the treatment will be successful; 6) a statement that continuation or maintenance treatment of some kind will be necessary; 7) discussion of the possible risks, including death, cardiac dysfunction, confusion, and memory impairment; 8) a statement that the consent also applies to emergency treatment that may be clinically necessary at times when the patient is unconscious; 9) a listing of patient requirements during the ECT course, such as taking nothing by mouth after midnight; 10) a statement that there has been an opportunity to ask questions and indication of who can be contacted with further questions; and 11) a statement that consent is voluntary and can be withdrawn at any time (American Psychiatric Association 2001).

Management of Medications

Each pre-ECT assessment should include an evaluation of the patient's medications and recommendations about how medications should be taken before and during the ECT course. Medications that are needed to decrease medical risks should be continued, but their dosing and timing of administration may need to be changed (American Psychiatric Association 2001). Similarly, orders should be written specifying dosage and timing of any medications that are to be added to decrease risks based on the pre-ECT evaluation. Other nonpsychotropic medications should be withheld until after the treatment on ECT days or—in the case of those that interfere with or increase the risks of ECT—should be discontinued.

Regarding the use of psychotropic medications during the ECT course, there are considerable differences of opinion and great variation in practice. The only situation in which compelling evidence exists for a potentiating effect of psychotropic medication on ECT is the use of antipsychotic agents in schizophrenic individuals (and inferentially in those with psychotic depression) (American Psychiatric Association 2001). The literature regarding the benefits of antidepressant medication as a means to augment the ECT response is unclear, although it does not appear that such a combination is associated with significantly increased risk. The primary reasons that have been given for the use of antidepressant medication augmentation are that it is difficult at times to accomplish drug withdrawal before instituting ECT, that there is a desire to decrease the risk of early relapse after ECT, and that "there is nothing to lose."

When possible, antidepressant medications should be chosen that have relatively fewer effects on cardiac function. Among the psychotropic medications that are best avoided or maintained at the lowest possible levels are 1) lithium—it may increase the risks for delirium or prolonged seizures; 2) benzodiazepines—their anticonvulsant properties may decrease efficacy (but can be reversed with flumazenil at the time of ECT) (Krystal et al. 1998); 3) antiepileptic drugs—their anticonvulsant properties may decrease efficacy, but they may be needed in those with epilepsy or with very brittle bipolar disorder (in which case they should be withheld the night before and the morning of treatment if possible); 5) bupropion and clozapine—they may increase the risk of prolonged seizures (the dosage should be kept at low to moderate levels).

ECT Technique

Inpatient Versus Outpatient Administration

Although ECT has traditionally been an inpatient treatment modality, a shift has occurred in recent years—much like the one that has occurred in the realm of surgical procedures—to offer it on an outpatient basis (American Psychiatric Association 2001). At present, inpatient ECT is reserved for situations in which the patient's psychiatric illness itself requires an inpatient level of care or where such a level is required to ensure that ECT can be safely administered (e.g., patients with high medical risk factors and no support system). These types of situations are particularly likely to occur with the elderly. Even when inpatient treatments are initially required, consideration should be given to switching to an outpatient mode when it is clinically feasible.

Anesthetic Considerations

ECT is a procedure involving general anesthesia. Airway management, administration of medications necessary for anesthesia, and handling of medical emergencies during and immediately following the ECT procedure are the responsibility of the anesthesia provider (American Psychiatric Association 2001). Appropriate medical backup should be present, particularly for high-risk cases.

The patient is ventilated by mask with 100% oxygen throughout the procedure, beginning at least a few minutes before anesthesia induction and lasting until a satisfactory level of spontaneous respiration is maintained during the postictal period. General anesthesia is usually provided by intravenous methohexital, typically 1 mg/kg (American Psychiatric Association 2001; Ding and White 2002). After loss of consciousness, the muscle relaxant succinylcholine is administered intravenously, again with a typical dosage of 1 mg/kg (American Psychiatric Association 2001). When the patient's muscles are relaxed (ascertainable by disappearance of relaxant-induced fasciculations and loss of deep tendon reflexes or twitch response to a peripheral nerve stimulator), the electrical stimulus can be delivered.

An anticholinergic medication, such as glycopyrrolate or atropine, may be administered before anesthesia to minimize the risk of stimulus-related asystole and the occurrence of postictal oral secretions. However, most practitioners use such agents selectively because they potentiate seizure-related tachycardia. β-Blocking medications (e.g., labetalol) are often used to minimize seizure-related hypertension and tachycardia when these effects are severe or when prophylaxis is indicated on the basis of preexisting cardiovascular disease. Again, it is best to use such agents selectively. When necessary, postictal agitation or delirium can be managed with the use of intravenous midazolam (1 mg) or haloperidol (2–5 mg), as well as by providing reassurance and maintaining a quiet, low-light environment for the postictal recovery process.

With the elderly, it is important to recognize that lower dosages of medications may be indicated because of altered metabolism or tolerance. On the other hand, under some circumstances (e.g., osteoporosis) higher doses may be necessary (in this case, of the relaxant agent).

Physiological Monitoring

In keeping with other procedures utilizing general anesthesia, vital signs and pulse oximetry are monitored throughout the procedure and during the immediate postictal period until stabilization occurs. After spontaneous respiration resumes and vital signs and oxygen saturation are trending toward baseline, the patient is moved to a postanesthesia care unit or area (previously referred to as a recovery room), where monitoring of vital signs and oxygenation continues.

Both the motor and electroencephalographic representations of seizure activity are monitored during ECT. To allow monitoring of the motor response in a patient whose muscles are relaxed, a blood pressure cuff is placed around the ankle and is inflated to approximately 200 mm Hg just before administration of the muscle relaxant. This action prevents muscle activity distal to the cuff from being suppressed during the seizure. Ictal electroencephalographic recordings are made, using recording leads placed on the head, in conjunction with amplification and display instrumentation built into the ECT device. It is recommended that two electroencephalographic channels be recorded so that seizure activity from both the left and right cerebral hemispheres can be monitored. Such recording can be accomplished by placing one pair of recording electrodes over the left prefrontal and left mastoid areas and the other pair over the homologous areas on the right.

Stimulus Electrode Placement

There are two major types of stimulus electrode placement: bilateral and unilateral nondominant (the right side for the great majority of individuals). Bilateral ECT involves placement of both stimulus electrodes over the frontotemporal regions, with the center of the electrode approximately 1 inch above the midpoint of a line transecting the external canthus of the eye and the tragus of the ear. The preferred type of unilateral nondominant placement involves location of one electrode over the right frontotemporal area (as above) and the other over the right centroparietal area, just to the right of the vertex of the scalp, a point defined by the intersection of lines between the inion and nasion and between the tragi of both ears.

There is significant controversy over the choice of stimulus electrode placement (American Psychiatric Association 2001). Although unilateral ECT appears to be effective in many patients as long as stimulus intensity is sufficient (see "Stimulus Dosing" below), some patients may preferentially respond to bilateral ECT. On the other hand, ECT-associated amnesia is greater with bilateral ECT. A reasonable practical trade-off is to use unilateral ECT initially, unless an urgent response is necessary, or the patient has shown a past preferential response to bilateral ECT, or he or she indicates a preference for bilateral ECT. Many attempts have been made to improve electrode placements to maximize efficacy and to minimize amnestic effects. A still-experimental recent development of this sort is bifrontal placement, in which the midpoints of the stimulus electrodes are placed 2 inches above the external canthus of each eye (Bailine et al. 2000).

The choice of stimulus electrode placement is particularly challenging in the elderly, in whom an urgent need for a rapid response is often present, yet in whom adverse cognitive effects are of more concern, especially in those who have preexisting cerebral impairment.

Stimulus Dosing

All contemporary ECT devices used in the United States utilize a bidirectional, constant-current, brief-pulse stimulus waveform. This waveform is more efficient than the older sine wave stimulus in inducing seizures and allows ECT to be administered with fewer adverse cognitive effects (Weiner et al. 1986). The paradigm for the choice of stimulus dose intensity, however, appears to be as controversial as the choice of electrode placement. The present disagreement centers on whether to dose with respect to an empirically determined seizure threshold estimate obtained at the first treatment (dose-titration technique) versus utilizing a formula based on factors such as age, gender, and electrode placement to make this decision (formula-based technique) (American Psychiatric Association 2001).

We have found that the dose-titration technique is better in that it offers a more precise means to determine the patient's seizure threshold (which can vary many-fold) and thereby allows the practitioner to more effectively control stimulus intensity (Coffey et al. 1995). In practice, seizure threshold is estimated at the first treatment by incrementally increasing the dose from a low level until a seizure is induced.

Regardless of dosing paradigm, compelling evidence suggests that stimulus intensity for unilateral ECT should be somewhere between 2.5 and 8 times seizure threshold (in terms of electrical charge), with the range reflecting current uncertainly as to the minimum dose necessary to optimize therapeutic outcome (McCall et al. 2000). In this regard, it is important to note that increasing stimulus intensity also increases the severity of ECT-associated memory impairment, although to a lesser degree than a switch to bilateral ECT. Stimulus intensity is less of an issue with bilateral ECT, in which a stimulus 1.5 times seizure threshold appears to be sufficient.

As alluded to above, seizure threshold is very much a function of age, with substantially higher thresholds being present in the elderly. This higher threshold leaves the elderly at greater risk for being unable to receive a stimulus of sufficient intensity, because the maximum output of ECT devices used in the United States is limited by U.S. Food and Drug Administration regulations (Krystal et al. 2000). The risk that the threshold will exceed the maximum available stimulus intensity is even greater late in the treatment course, because seizure threshold rises to a varying extent with the number of treatments. Research is now being directed toward further optimization of the stimulus waveform to obviate such difficulties.

Determination of Seizure Adequacy

ECT-induced seizures are identical to spontaneous grand mal seizures except that with ECT the motor response is attenuated pharmacologically. The electroencephalographic recording during ECT (ictal electroencephalogram) manifests the typical electroencephalographic features of a grand mal seizure, with chaotic polyspike activity marking the tonic portion of the seizure and repetitive polyspike and slow-wave discharges during the clonic component. During the immediate postictal period, a relative suppression (i.e., flattening) of electroencephalographic activity can typically be seen (Weiner et al. 1991).

Compelling evidence indicates that not all seizures are equally potent from a therapeutic perspective. With unilateral ECT, barely suprathreshold seizures—despite having identical durations as seizures from more moderately suprathreshold stimuli—are only minimally therapeutic

(Sackeim et al. 1993). Based on findings that seizures with higher stimulus intensity exhibit attributes such as higher amplitude, greater regularity in shape, and greater postictal electroencephalographic suppression (Krystal et al. 1995) and that such features are associated with the therapeutic response to ECT, a growing interest has developed in the possibility that electroencephalographically based stimulus dosing may one day be feasible. This type of innovation would be particularly attractive because it would allow practitioners a means to tailor the stimulus intensity to the minimum therapeutic dose for each individual and control for the variable rise in seizure threshold that occurs over the ECT course. Already, United States ECT device manufacturers have incorporated "seizure quality" features into their devices, although their utility for routine clinical usage remains to be established (see American Psychiatric Association 2001).

Frequency and Number of ECT Treatments

In the United States ECT is typically administered three times a week, with an index course usually lasting between 6 and 12 treatments, although more or fewer are sometimes necessary. The frequency of ECT may be reduced to twice a week or even once a week if amnesia or confusion becomes a major problem (American Psychiatric Association 2001). The decision about when to end the index ECT course depends on treatment outcome as well as the wishes of the consenter. In general, the treatments are stopped when a therapeutic plateau has occurred—that is, when the patient has reached a maximum level of response. If no substantial improvement occurs by the sixth treatment, consideration should be given to making changes in the ECT technique, such as switching stimulus electrode placement, increasing stimulus intensity, or discontinuing medications with anticonvulsant properties. If no response occurs after 8–10 treatments, alternative treatment modalities should be considered. At the present time, these modalities would generally involve combination pharmacotherapy utilizing multiple agents of different classes.

Maintenance Therapy

The conditions for which ECT is used are typically recurrent. The risk of relapse, particularly during the first 2–3 months, is extremely high, necessitating an aggressive program of maintenance treatment to minimize the likelihood of relapse. This maintenance treatment may be either pharmacological or in the form of continued ECT (at a greatly lowered frequency).

Pharmacological Maintenance Therapy

Pharmacological maintenance treatment is usually attempted after the initial index ECT course unless the patient indicates a strong preference for maintenance ECT. With major depression, evidence suggests that a combination of antidepressant and mood stabilizer may be more effective in maintaining remission than an antidepressant drug alone (Sackeim et al. 2001). Unfortunately, evidence shows that medication resistance during the index episode diminishes the likelihood of a sustained prophylactic effect (Sackeim et al. 1990). Maintenance pharmacotherapy following ECT treatment of mania or schizophrenia has not been well studied. In the absence of applicable data, an aggressive regimen of different drug classes should be considered.

Maintenance ECT

The high relapse rate following ECT, even with pharmacological maintenance therapy, has created renewed interest in the practice of maintenance ECT, which (until recently) has been relatively absent from the psychiatric literature. After a flurry of largely positive case-series reports (Rabheru and Persad 1997), a randomized trial of maintenance ECT versus pharmacotherapy in patients treated for major depression is currently under way.

Although there are no established guidelines for a maintenance ECT regimen, practitioners typically start with weekly treatments for 2–4 weeks, followed by another 1–2 months of biweekly treatments, followed by 3-week and then 4-week intervals. After 12 months, treatments are either stopped or continued at an even lower frequency. Although many maintenance ECT patients do well with such a regimen, others appear to require more frequent treatments or even supplementation with psychotropic medications. Others eventually relapse, leading to another index ECT course or a switch to alternative treatment modalities.

In terms of cognitive effects, maintenance ECT is significantly better tolerated than index ECT treatments, particularly if the interval between treatments is kept large. Still, some patients do have cumulative difficulties with amnesia, and these should be taken into account in treatment planning. Given the general good tolerance of maintenance ECT, there is no maximum lifetime number of ECT treatments.

Future of ECT

The use of ECT has persisted for more than 60 years, despite the development of many alternative treatment options. Still, its continued viability depends not only on innovations in alternative treatments but also on the continued optimization of ECT in terms of both efficacy and adverse effects. As noted above, research is under way to improve on the available options for both stimulus electrode placement and electrical stimulus parameters. Other work is being done to enable practitioners to better predict which patients might be ECT responders.

Future alternatives to ECT include not only new psychopharmacological agents but also new electromagnetic therapies such as transcranial magnetic stimulation, vagal nerve stimulation, and deep brain stimulation (George et al. 1999; Malone 2002; Marangell et al. 2002). Whether or not any of these new experimental techniques will partially or even fully replace ECT remains to be established. In the meantime, a clear role remains for ECT in the treatment of a variety of disorders, most notably major depression, for which the elderly are at a particularly high risk.

References

Abrams R: Electroconvulsive Therapy, 4th Edition. New York, Oxford University Press, 2002

American Psychiatric Association: The Practice of ECT: Recommendations for Treatment, Training, and Privileging. Washington, DC, American Psychiatric Press, 2001

Andersen K, Balldin J, Gottfries CG, et al: A double-blind evaluation of electroconvulsive therapy in Parkinson's disease with "on-off" phenomena. Acta Neurol Scand 76:191–199, 1987

Applegate RJ: Diagnosis and management of ischemic heart disease in the patient scheduled to undergo electroconvulsive therapy. Convuls Ther 13:128–144, 1997

Avery D, Lubrano A: Depression treated with imipramine and ECT: the DeCarolis study reconsidered. Am J Psychiatry 136:549–562, 1979

Avery D, Winokur G: Mortality in depressed patients treated with ECT and antidepressants. Arch Gen Psychiatry 33:1029–1037, 1976

Bailine SH, Rifkin A, Kayne E, et al: Comparison of bifrontal and bitemporal ECT for major depression. Am J Psychiatry 157:121–123, 2000

Beyer J, Weiner RD, Glenn MD: Practical Aspects of ECT: A Programmed Text, 2nd Edition. Washington, DC, American Psychiatric Press, 1998

Brandon S: Efficacy in depression: controlled trials. Psychopharmacol Bull 22:465–468, 1986

Coffey CE, Lucke J, Weiner RD, et al: Seizure threshold in electroconvulsive therapy, I: initial seizure threshold. Biol Psychiatry 37:713–720, 1995

Currier MB, Murray GB, Welch CC: ECT for post-stroke depression. J. Neuropsychiatry Clin Neurosci 4:140–144, 1992

Ding Z, White PF: Anesthesia for electroconvulsive therapy. Anesth Analg 94:1351–1364, 2002

Endler NS: The origins of electroconvulsive therapy. Convuls Ther 4:5–23, 1988

Endler NS: Holiday of Darkness, Revised. Toronto, Wall & Davis, 1990

Figiel GS, Coffey CE, Djang WT, et al: Brain magnetic resonance imaging findings in ECT-induced delirium. J Neuropsychiatry Clin Neurosci 2:53–58, 1990

Figiel GS, Hassen MA, Zorumski C, et al: ECT-induced delirium in depressed patients with Parkinson's disease. J Neuropsychiatry Clin Neurosci 3:405–411, 1991

Fink M: Meduna and the origins of convulsive therapy. Am J Psychiatry 141:1034–1041, 1984

Fink M: Electroshock: Restoring the Mind. New York, Oxford University Press, 1999

Fink M, Sackeim HA: Convulsive therapy in schizophrenia? Schizophr Bull 22:27–39, 1996

Fricchione GL, Kaufman LD, Gruber BL, et al: Electroconvulsive therapy and cyclophosphamide in combination for severe neuropsychiatric lupus with catatonia. Am J Med 88:442–443, 1990

George MS, Lisanby SH, Sackeim HA: TMS applications in psychiatry. Arch Gen Psychiatry 56:300–311, 1999

Hood DA, Mecca RS: Failure to initiate electroconvulsive seizures in a patient pretreated with lidocaine. Anesthesiology 58:379–381, 1983

Janicak PG, Davis JM, Gibbons RD, et al: Efficacy of ECT: a meta-analysis. Am J Psychiatry 142:297–302, 1985

Kellner CH, Bernstein JH: ECT as a treatment for neurologic illness, in The Clinical Science of Electroconvulsive Therapy. Edited by Coffey CE. Washington, DC, American Psychiatric Press, 1993, pp 183–210

Klapheke MM: Combining ECT and antipsychotic agents: benefits and risks. Convuls Ther 9:241–255, 1993

Kramer BA: Use of ECT in California, revisited: 1984–1994. J ECT 15:245–251, 1999

Krueger RB, Sackeim HA: Electroconvulsive therapy and schizophrenia, in Schizophrenia. Edited by Hirsch SR, Weinberger D. Oxford, UK, Blackwell, 1995, pp 503–545

Krystal AD, Coffey CE: Neuropsychiatric considerations in the use of electroconvulsive therapy. J Neuropsychiatry Clin Neurosci 9:283–292, 1997

Krystal AD, Weiner RD, Coffey CE: The ictal EEG as a marker of adequate stimulus intensity with unilateral ECT. J Neuropsychiatry Clin Neurosci 7:295–303, 1995

Krystal AD, Watts BV, Weiner RD, et al: The use of flumazenil in the anxious and benzodiazepine-dependent ECT patient. J ECT 14:5–14, 1998

Krystal AD, Dean MD, Weiner RD, et al: ECT stimulus intensity: are present ECT devices too limited? Am J Psychiatry 157:963–967, 2000

Malone D: The use of deep brain stimulation in psychiatric disorders (abstract). J ECT 18:62, 2002

Manly DT, Oakley SP Jr, Bloch RM: Electroconvulsive therapy in old-old patients. Am J Geriatr Psychiatry 8:232–236, 2000

Marangell LB, Rush AJ, George MS, et al: Vagus nerve stimulation (VNS) for major depressive episodes: one year outcomes. Biol Psychiatry 51:280–287, 2002

McCall WV, Reboussin DM, Weiner RD, et al: Titrated moderately suprathreshold vs fixed high-dose right unilateral electroconvulsive therapy: acute antidepressant and cognitive effects. Arch Gen Psychiatry 57:438–444, 2000

Mukherjee S, Sackeim HA, Schnur DB: Electroconvulsive therapy of acute mania episodes: a review of 50 years' experience. Am J Psychiatry 151:169–176, 1994

Murray GB, Shea V, Conn DK: ECT for post-stroke depression. J Clin Psychiatry 47:258–260, 1986

O'Connor MK, Knapp R, Husain M, et al: The influence of age on the response of major depression to electroconvulsive therapy: a C.O.R.E. Report. Am J Geriatr Psychiatry 9:382–390, 2001

Paul SM, Extein I, Calil HM, et al: Use of ECT with treatment-resistant depressed patients at the National Institute of Mental Health. Am J Psychiatry 138:486–489, 1981

Petrides G, Fink M: Atrial fibrillation, anticoagulation, and ECT. Convuls Ther 12:91–98, 1996

Philibert RA, Richards L, Lynch CF, et al: Effect of ECT on mortality and clinical outcome in geriatric unipolar depression. J Clin Psychiatry 56:390–394, 1995

Pritchett JT, Kellner CH, Coffey CE: Electroconvulsive therapy in geriatric neuropsychiatry, in Textbook of Geriatric Neuropsychiatry. Edited by Coffey CE, Cummings JL. Washington, DC, American Psychiatric Press, 1994, pp 633–659

Prudic J, Haskett RF, Mulsant B, et al: Resistance to antidepressant medications and short-term clinical response to ECT. Am J Psychiatry 153:985–992, 1996

Quitkin FM, McGrath PJ, Stewart JW, et al: Can the effects of antidepressants be observed in the first two weeks of treatment? Neuropsychopharmacology 15:390–394, 1996

Rabheru K, Persad E: A review of continuation and maintenance electroconvulsive therapy. Can J Psychiatry 42:476–484, 1997

Rasmussen K, Abrams R: Treatment of Parkinson's disease with electroconvulsive therapy. Psychiatr Clin North Am 14:925–933, 1991

Rayburn BK: ECT in patients with heart failure or valvular heart disease. Convuls Ther 13:145–156, 1997

Reid WH, Keller S, Leatherman M, et al: ECT in Texas: 19 months of mandatory reporting. J Clin Psychiatry 59:8–13, 1998

Rosenbach ML, Hermann RC, Dorwart RA: Use of electroconvulsive therapy in the Medicare population between 1987 and 1992. Psychiatr Serv 48:1537–1542, 1997

Rummans TA, Bassingthwaighte ME: Severe medical and neurologic complications associated with near-lethal catatonia treated with electroconvulsive therapy. Convuls Ther 7:121–124, 1991

Sackeim HA: The use of electroconvulsive therapy in late-life depression, in Clinical Geriatric Psychopharmacology, 3rd Edition. Edited by Salzman C. Baltimore, MD, Williams & Wilkins, 1998, pp 262–309

Sackeim HA, Rush AJ: Melancholia and response to ECT. Am J Psychiatry 152:1242–1243, 1995

Sackeim HA, Prudic J, Devanand DP, et al: The impact of medication resistance and continuation pharmacotherapy on relapse following response to electroconvulsive therapy in major depression. J Clin Psychopharmacol 10:96–104, 1990

Sackeim HA, Prudic J, Devanand DP, et al: Effects of stimulus intensity and electrode placement on the efficacy and cognitive effects of electroconvulsive therapy [see comments]. N Engl J Med 328:839–846, 1993

Sackeim HA, Haskett RF, Mulsant BH, et al: Continuation pharmacotherapy in the prevention of relapse following electroconvulsive therapy: a randomized controlled trial. JAMA 285:1299–1307, 2001

Sajatovic M, Meltzer HY: The effect of short-term electroconvulsive treatment plus neuroleptics in treatment-resistant schizophrenia and schizoaffective disorder. Convuls Ther 9:167–173, 1993

Small JG, Klapper MH, Kellams JJ, et al: Electroconvulsive treatment compared with lithium in the management of manic states. Arch Gen Psychiatry 45:727–732, 1988

Sobin C, Prudic J, Devanand DP, et al: Who responds to electroconvulsive therapy? a comparison of effective and ineffective forms of treatment. Br J Psychiatry 169:322–328, 1996

Stern L, Hirschmann S, Grunhaus L: ECT in patients with major depressive disorder and low cardiac output. Convuls Ther 13:68–73, 1997

Tew JD Jr, Mulsant BH, Haskett RF, et al: Acute efficacy of ECT in the treatment of major depression in the old-old. Am J Psychiatry 156:1865–1870, 1999

Thompson JW, Weiner RD, Myers CP: Use of ECT in the United States in 1975, 1980, 1986. Am J Psychiatry 151:1657–1661, 1994

Tomac TA, Rummans TA, Pileggi TS, et al: Safety and efficacy of electroconvulsive therapy in patients over age 85. Am J Geriatr Psychiatry 5:126–130, 1997

Weiner RD, Coffey CE: Indications for use of electroconvulsive therapy, in Review of Psychiatry, Vol 7. Edited by Frances AJ, Hales RE. Washington, DC, American Psychiatric Press, 1988, pp 458–481

Weiner RD, Krystal AD: Electroconvulsive therapy, in Treatments of Psychiatric Disorders, 3rd Edition. Edited by Gabbard GO, Rush AJ. Washington, DC, American Psychiatric Press, 2001, pp 1267–1293

Weiner RD, Rogers HJ, Davidson JR, et al: Effects of stimulus parameters on cognitive side effects. Ann N Y Acad Sci 462:315–325, 1986

Weiner RD, Coffey CE, Krystal AD: The monitoring and management of electrically induced seizures. Psychiatr Clin North Am 14:845–869, 1991

Weiner RD, Coffey CE, Krystal AD: Electroconvulsive therapy in the medical and neurologic patient, in Psychiatric Care of the Medical Patient, 2nd Edition. Edited by Stoudemire A, Fogel BS, Greenberg D. New York, Oxford University Press, 2000, pp 419–428

Wesson ML, Wilkinson AM, Anderson DN, et al: Does age predict the long-term outcome of depression treated with ECT? (a prospective study of the long-term outcome of ECT-treated depression with respect to age). Int J Geriatr Psychiatry 12:45–51, 1997

Zielinski RJ, Roose SP, Devanand DP, et al: Cardiovascular complications of ECT in depressed patients with cardiac disease. Am J Psychiatry 150:904–909, 1993

Diet, Nutrition, and Exercise

Robert J. Sullivan Jr., M.D., M.P.H.

The attainment of old age provides proof that an individual has consumed a diet sufficiently nutritious to support life for several decades—no mean feat in a period when the average human lifetime has achieved a length previously unknown in history. As age increases, lifelong eating habits need periodic reevaluation. Deterioration of the taste buds and in olfactory sensation makes some foods less palatable. Changes in living habits can result in altered dietary requirements. The onset of illness creates special dietary demands. Both elderly persons and those responsible for their care must be aware of potential problems with nutrition and diet to respond to the challenges of late life.

Exercise habits, like dietary patterns, are easily taken for granted. Most people are unaware how rapidly vigor declines with each hour of indolence until eventually the ability to respond to the demands of daily life is compromised. The gradual reduction in physical activity that typically accompanies aging is also accompanied by a diminution in appetite. Because balanced nutrient intake depends on consuming a variety of foods, nutrient deficits may follow a faltering intake.

A remarkable amount of disease and disability can be traced to diet and exercise habits. Analysis of death reports indicates that poor nutrition and inadequate exercise contribute to at least 300,000 deaths in the United States each year (McGinnis and Foege 1993). Among the maladies potentially controllable through improved diet and fitness are coronary artery disease, hypertension, stroke, diabetes, obesity, osteoporosis, certain cancers, cholelithiasis, hemorrhoids, hernias, constipation, irritable bowel syndrome, diverticulosis, and depression. Such problems are prevalent among older individuals and can be controlled through diet and exercise modification.

Nutrition

The science of nutrition involves the study of food intake to promote growth and to replace worn or injured tissues. Elderly individuals are vulnerable to nutrition problems as a result of health factors that are unique to their age. In this section, nutritional standards are explained and assessment techniques are presented.

Documenting Nutritional Status

Clinicians who care for older adults typically assess nutritional status by means of a diet history. Unfortunately, memory problems and inaccurate estimates of portion size limit the value of this approach. Standard height/weight tables, suitable for nutritional assessment in young and middle-aged individuals, are less reliable in the elderly because of reduced height associated with vertebral compression fractures, kyphosis, and spinal disc degeneration. Accordingly, geriatricians find value in documenting immune function and reserves of protein and fat as a means of verifying nutritional status.

Assessment of body protein stores involves two components. Although skill and experience are required, somatic protein stores can be measured by recording midarm circumference to assess muscle mass. Visceral protein stores are determined by measuring serum levels of various marker substances, of which serum hemoglobin and albumin are the most widely accepted.

Assessment of body fat stores permits determination of energy reserves. Water immersion is very accurate, but it requires a deep pool and is not well tolerated by patients. Bioelectric impedance measurements, commonly offered at health fairs and local fitness establishments, are easily performed and readily accepted but are not terribly accurate (Bussolotto et al. 1999). Tritium dilution and magnetic resonance imaging are accurate but are used primarily in research studies (Busetto et al. 2000). Dual-energy X-ray absorptiometry scanning is popular because of its accuracy, modest cost, and ready patient acceptance, although the equipment is not portable (Sergi et al. 1993). Measurement of waist and hip circumferences and skin-fold measurement by the use of calipers are easily done in the office or at the bedside and remain some of the most simple and effective tools for daily clinical work, although accuracy and precision are problematic (Ulijaszek and Kerr 1999).

Skin tests to ascertain T-lymphocyte activity are useful for assessing immune system function, *which declines with poor nutrition*. Intradermal injection of fungal antigens such as *Candida* or *Trichophyton*, to which virtually every healthy person is reactive, is commonly utilized. Fresh antigens for injection must be available, and interpretation of the test takes 48 hours. A total lymphocyte count below 1,500/mL is useful as evidence of an inadequate diet and can be quickly determined from routine blood counts (Bucci 1994).

For the majority of people, a diet history coupled with documentation of weight, triceps skin-fold thickness, midarm circumference, hemoglobin level, albumin level, and a total lymphocyte count will permit adequate evaluation of nutritional status. When applied to healthy elderly persons, these parameters are found to be in close agreement with national norms for all age groups (Burns et al. 1986), which suggests that when abnormalities occur, they present a true indication of malnutrition and are not simply changes related to aging.

Caloric Intake Profile Over a Lifetime

A fascinating series of studies of rats done more than six decades ago suggested that diet modification can prolong life (McCay et al. 1939). Spartan fare helped these rats to live longer. Total calorie limitation was more important than fat or protein limitation alone, and there could be no deficit of essential nutrients. The ideal program began with limitation in youth and extended throughout the life of the laboratory animal. The precise reason for improved longevity is not yet clear. From analysis of longitudinal study data in humans, it is apparent that low weight in the elderly is not necessarily beneficial, whereas obesity is a significant problem (Heiat et al. 2001). Higher body mass index values are associated with increased mortality rates (Calle et al. 1999).

Variation of Nutritional Needs With Age and Health

For most persons, growing old does not create a need for special diet supplements. Caloric needs vary with individual activity level and should be adjusted accordingly. Regular weight checks are the best means of monitoring the total caloric intake. A stable weight customarily signifies continuing good health.

With the onset of illness, nutritional demands can change dramatically. Most individuals have sufficient reserves to tide themselves over acute situations. With the sort of chronic illness typically encountered among elderly persons, specific attention may be needed to ensure adequate nutrition. Heart failure, lung failure, renal failure, chronic infection, and depression all result in weight loss, sometimes of substantial proportions. Studies in cancer patients have implicated humoral substances as being partially responsible for the anorexia that accompanies, and often precedes, overt clinical manifestations of neoplasia. Dementia is accompanied by weight loss, but the etiology of this process remains unknown (Barrett-Connor et al. 1996). The underlying mechanisms for appetite modulation need further elucidation so that clinicians may exert a greater influence on this vital function.

Nutrition is often compromised in the course of acute illness. Malnourishment has been found in elderly hospitalized patients at rates as high as 15% (Azad et al. 1999). Impaired wound healing and reduced immunocompetence have been attributed to malnutrition. Because of the frequency of nutrition problems among hospitalized patients, it is essential to record weight on admission and every 3 days thereafter. Laboratory tests to be followed include albumin levels and lymphocyte counts. Nutrition deprivation reaches critical proportions when a patient has been without substantial intake for a period of 10 days or suffers a weight loss exceeding 10% of baseline weight.

Diet

Building on the preceding discussion of nutrition, diet recommendations can be made for daily food consumption to achieve specific health goals. Diet adjustment falls within the tradition of primary, secondary, and tertiary preventive medicine. A well-proportioned diet can prevent the occurrence of malnutrition in the form of obesity or cachexia (primary prevention). In disease states such as iron deficiency, a diet supplement can cure an illness already present (secondary prevention). In diseases such as heart failure, dietary modification can control the course of an illness not otherwise curable by diet alone (tertiary prevention). The following discussion explores diet alternatives in sickness and in health.

Achieving an Adequate Diet

Although dietary habits of different cultures vary widely, people live to old age in many societies throughout the world. Studies of disease patterns show that dietary preferences affect the kinds of illness experienced by members of a population. Information gleaned from "natural experiments" has led to specific diet recommendations to capture the beneficial aspects of a particular cuisine. Each new generation has access to dietary alternatives that its predecessors could not have imagined. Throughout the twentieth century, developments made frozen foods, irradiated foods, hybrid vegetables, and fast foods readily available. Population mobility has encouraged the mingling of cultures, with the result that foods from many corners of the earth are widely known and appreciated. These trends yield expanded opportunities to achieve a healthful diet.

Barriers to an Adequate Diet

Throughout their lives, people seek to satisfy their basic needs of shelter, food, and security. At times, they encounter unforeseen difficulties in securing these necessities. In terms of diet, both major and minor events pose potentially threatening problems.

Social barriers are often cited as exerting an important influence on the diets of elderly persons. Inadequate financial reserves, poor housing, and limited benefit programs make pursuit of a balanced diet difficult. Lack of safety of public areas and excessive walking distance to food markets can present problems for residents living within major cities. Those living in rural areas experience similar isolation when the ability to drive is lost or when family members depart. The death of a spouse or housemate who had prepared meals may be a devastating blow. Without the means for getting food to the table, no one can consume a balanced diet.

Even when food is available, sensory changes can interfere with dietary intake. People who eat alone typically fail to prepare sophisticated or varied fare, with a resultant decline in food consumption volume and variety. Dental problems reduce the types of food that can be masticated (Fontijn-Tekamp et al. 1996). Vision limitations due to cataracts or glaucoma make food preparation and consumption problematic. Fear of soiling clothes with food or creating a messy table often leads vision-impaired individuals to withdraw from congregate meals, which

deprives them of social interactions. With increasing age, subtle shifts in gustatory senses occur. Disease or medication use can have a similar impact. Particularly distressing are the effects of dysosmia or dysgeusia (altered smell and taste), whereby common aromas or flavors are perceived as distinctly unpleasant (Schiffman 1997). Substantial changes in food preference are an inevitable consequence.

Medications can increase the need for specific dietary supplements. Trimethoprim and phenytoin are associated with increased need for vitamins D and K and folic acid. The use of barbiturates, cholestyramine, and aspirin calls for extra folic acid, iron, and vitamin C in the diet. Alcohol, neomycin, cholestyramine, and colchicine influence absorption of fat-soluble vitamins. The list goes on and on. Because nutrients are abundant in a normal diet, deficits induced by medication are rarely encountered. Individuals consuming a marginal diet will require attention to the nutritional demands created by each specific medical therapy.

Because it is chronic and progressive, altered anatomical function with age may induce subtle dietary changes. Atrophic gastritis, often clinically undetected, affects the absorption of several nutritional factors, with both reductions and elevations having been documented. Slowed intestinal transit time with aging is an important factor. Fortunately, in the absence of surgical alteration of the intestines to improve their integrity, elderly persons usually absorb sufficient nutrients to remain healthy, provided their diet contains a reasonable blend of needed components.

Diet as Preventive Therapy (Primary Prevention)

In some circumstances, diet modification is capable of alleviating disease, if not of outright cure. With the passage of time, more health problems can be expected to join the list, of which a few examples follow.

Dehydration

The elderly lose sensitivity to dehydration (Kenney and Chiu 2001), especially if they become demented or are being treated with diuretics. Therapy requires maintenance of sufficient water intake so that the body can perform normal adjustments to maintain renal integrity and electrolyte balance. A fluid intake of 2,900 mL/day is recommended (Kleiner 1999). Juice, coffee, tea, milk, and other liquids in the daily diet usually suffice to support normal bodily function without a need for attention to defined fluid intake goals.

Atherosclerosis

The value of a normal or low serum cholesterol level in reducing cardiovascular disease risk is well established (Fuster et al. 1992). Consuming dietary unsaturated oils (liquid at room temperature) in preference to saturated fats (solid at room temperature) contributes to cholesterol control (de Lorgeril et al. 1999; Rissanen et al. 2000). Emphasizing fish and grains in the diet can lead to stabilization and involution of atherosclerotic lesions (Harper and Jacobson 2001). Stroke, myocardial infarction, claudication, renal failure, visual decline, and other degenerative processes are favorably influenced in the bargain. Alcohol will raise the high-density lipoprotein ratio favorably if consumed in modest amounts of 2 ounces or less daily (Camargo et al. 1997).

Diverticulosis

Intraluminal recording devices have revealed that augmented dietary fiber intake reduces pressure within the colon and therefore contributes to a reduction in formation of diverticula. Epidemiological studies of populations known to consume high-fiber diets support this conclusion. For this reason, and for reasons mentioned elsewhere in this chapter, dietary fiber is now emphasized as a daily dietary constituent.

Cancer

Some diet components are known carcinogens, and others protect against cancer. Fiber in the diet may protect against cancer by several mechanisms. It speeds transit of fecal material through the body while it binds noxious elements, thus reducing gut contact time. The relatively low incidence of colon cancer in developing countries is explained in part by the high fiber content of primitive diets. High fiber consumption can cause problems for some people, however. Some minerals and drugs are bound by dietary fiber, thus reducing their absorption. Increased gas production resulting from bacterial action on gut fiber may be physically uncomfortable and socially inhibiting. Overall the advantages of increasing dietary fiber outweigh the problems (O'Keefe 1995).

Evidence suggests correlations between dietary constituents and cancer, although there is no unanimity of opinion about specific dietary modifications for cancer risk reduction. Factors such as smoking and environmental pollutants and carcinogens wield a much greater influence on cancer development than does diet. High insulin secretion associated with obesity has been linked to pancreatic cancer (Michaud et al. 2001), establishing yet another reason to maintain a normal weight. Consuming a diet high in saturated fat has been associated with an increased risk of colon cancer (Cummings and Bingham 1998) and prostate cancer (Kolonel et al. 1999), but not breast cancer (Velie et al. 2000). The interaction of nutrients with individual genetic factors contributes to the development or prevention of neoplasia. Understanding these complex relationships has implications for individual health that are the subject of current research (Rock et al. 2000). To date, a balanced diet that is rich in fruits and vegetables is considered more beneficial for cancer control than reliance on consumption of dietary supplements.

Diet as Therapeutic Intervention (Secondary Prevention)

In disease states that involve discrete nutrient deficits, it is sometimes possible to cure the condition by supplementing intake of the needed item.

Iron Deficiency

Iron is found in red meat and certain vegetables. Older persons typically maintain sufficient iron reserves through consumption of their normal diet. Acute blood loss such as that resulting from trauma, or chronic blood loss such as occurs with occult gastrointestinal bleeding, is a common reason for an iron deficit. Whenever depletion of iron stores is found, it is essential to seek a reason for blood loss. Once a diagnosis is made and effective treatment has returned the body to stability, an iron deficit can be treated by dietary supplements. The usual course of therapy returns iron stores to normal within 6 months.

Lactase Deficiency

Many adults gradually lose the ability to digest lactose, or milk sugar, as a result of the steady decline in intestinal lactase levels with each passing year. Lactase deficiency creates uncomfortable symptoms of gas production, diarrhea, and cramping within an hour or two of eating dairy products. The degree of lactase decline is variable, and some people must avoid all foods containing lactose.

Alleviation of symptoms from lactase deficiency is achieved with total elimination of milk products for a period of 3 days. A reintroduction of dairy foods will then delineate the level at which symptoms reappear. Acidophilus milk and yogurt contain bacteria that digest the lactose molecule, thus bypassing the need for endogenous lactase. Some cheeses are also low in lactose. Older persons typically find specific dairy products that can be consumed without discomfort.

Diet and Disease Control (Tertiary Prevention)

In certain disease states, nutritional changes can have a positive influence in controlling the impact or progression of a pathological process.

Osteoporosis

The cause of osteoporosis is unclear (Nordin et al. 1998). It is related to a complex interaction of vitamin D, calcium, and estrogen within the body, coupled with weight-bearing activity. Kyphosis, hip fractures, and collapse of spinal vertebrae are among the common sequelae of this disease, which is estimated to result in more than 70,000 fractures yearly. Very few people want to look old and bent, and so the search for a control of osteoporosis is driven by both cosmetic and medical considerations.

Dietary calcium deficiency among older persons is commonly found when community surveys of eating habits are undertaken. Because bones deficient in calcium are weak, logic suggests that calcium supplements could reduce the impact of osteoporosis. Some individuals experience adverse consequences from consuming calcium supplements. Intestinal discomfort is common, with symptoms of bloating or stomach pain. Constipation may develop, sometimes of major proportions. Absorption of excessive calcium can lead to the formation of renal stones. These side effects are perhaps acceptable if bone integrity is maintained in the bargain.

Fluoride supplements have been found to influence calcium balance favorably by creating an increase in bone density. Regrettably, new bone formed in response to fluoride intake is apparently brittle and may fail to improve weight-bearing ability or resistance to fracture (Riggs et al. 1990). Bisphosphonates are more effective than fluoride and enjoy widespread use with increasing evidence of success (Russell et al. 1999).

Glucose Regulation

Diabetics need multiple interventions to successfully control their disease, and one of the most important interventions involves diet. Achieving an ideal weight through enhanced physical activity and a reduction in total caloric intake is vitally important (Mokdad et al. 2001). Maintenance of blood sugar levels as close to normal as possible is essential to avoid microvascular deterioration. A Western dietary pattern is associated with a substantial increase in risk for the development of type 2 diabetes (van Dam et al. 2002), which can be prevented by changes in the lifestyle of high-risk subjects (Hu et al. 2001; Tuomilehto et al. 2001).

Vascular Volume Modification

In patients with heart failure and some forms of hypertension, an attempt is made to modify intravascular volume by limiting dietary sodium intake. Edema may be reduced and blood pressure normalized by this relatively simple intervention, particularly when combined with fruits, vegetables, whole grains, low-fat dairy products, and reduced saturated fats and sugars in the dietary approaches to stop hypertension (DASH) diet (Sacks et al. 2001). Unfortunately, sodium is often added to foods, and therefore salt intake is difficult to avoid. Many persons find that unsalted foods lack flavor and are therefore unappetizing. When salt intake cannot be lowered or proves ineffective, diuretic therapy may be necessary to improve the sodium balance.

In patients with renal failure who develop edema, sodium restriction may be harmful if it creates a reduction in vascular volume that leads to a loss of renal perfusion pressure. Such an illness requires skilled care with precise diet adjustment to optimize function.

Dementia

High serum homocysteine levels are a risk factor for atherosclerotic disease and dementia (Seshadri et al. 2002). Increasing the dietary intake of folic acid will reduce homocysteine levels, which may reduce the incidence of both diseases.

Stroke

Increasing the consumption of fruits and vegetables will reduce the risk of stroke (Joshipura et al. 1999). Prospective studies reveal that cruciferous and green leafy vegetables, as well as citrus fruits and juices, are protective.

Systemic Illness

Many illness conditions call for broad dietary interventions to stem a tide of adverse effects set in motion by the underlying pathological process. Systemic infections create metabolic demands at a time when the patient may not wish to eat. Stroke victims may be unable to swallow because of paralysis, confusion, or unconsciousness. Comprehensive diet augmentation can offset the demands of illness in these settings. Fortunately, food supplements are available that feature a balanced array of nutrients suitable for consumption as a beverage, for infusion through a feeding tube, or for infusion directly into a vein if required. Hospitals and long-term-care facility nutritionists are skilled at recognizing and treating deficits associated with dietary limitations imposed by ill health and at recommending solutions.

Specific Dietary Recommendations

Drawing on the preceding discussions, a number of dietary suggestions can be made for healthy individuals. Adjustments can then be made to meet the special requirements imposed by disease states.

Water

Most individuals need not be concerned with maintaining a specific level of water intake. The fluids consumed throughout the day suffice to meet normal needs. When the weather is warm, and during exertion, supplemental fluids are essential to offset losses from sweating. When body temperature rises in the presence of fever, additional fluids are also needed. Attention to urine volume and concentration can guide decisions regarding fluid supplements.

Calories

Calories from all sources should equal about 30 kcal/kg. Weight change is an excellent indication of success in caloric intake management. Too many calories consumed will yield an increase. Too few and weight drops. It should be noted that fat provides 9 cal/g, whereas protein and carbohydrates provide 4 cal/g. Shifting intake toward diets containing less fat and less refined sugars makes it easier to feel satisfied and still lose weight.

Protein

The daily protein intake should be approximately 12.5% of total calories. All bodily proteins are involved in sustaining structural and metabolic functions. Unlike fats and carbohydrates, the body maintains no protein reserves; therefore, a constant intake is required to replenish losses associated with normal tissue turnover. Protein deficits can be avoided through a balanced dietary intake. Meats can provide protein, along with vitamins and iron. Meat also includes the less desirable saturated fats and cholesterol, which can be minimized through broiling or grilling. Poultry with the skin removed before cooking is preferred as a dietary meat over beef, lamb, or pork. Eggs are a healthy source of protein that appears not to increase the risk of cardiovascular disease in healthy individuals (Hu et al. 1999b). Eating deep-water fish rich in omega-3 fatty acids will contribute to a significant reduction in the risk of myocardial infarction (Daviglus et al. 1997). Legumes such as beans, peas, and lentils are excellent protein source substitutes for meat products and receive insufficient attention in American diets. Consumption of high-protein diets will enhance renal blood flow and may contribute to renal deterioration (Pedrini et al. 1996). The value of high-protein, low-carbohydrate diets for purposes of weight loss is well established. However, the long-term consequences associated with chronic high fat intake are of great concern because of the potential increase in arteriosclerosis.

Fats and Oils

The consumption of fats and oils should be modest for two reasons. Because of their high caloric content, they contribute to obesity. A second reason for caution is the role played by fats in the development of arteriosclerosis. Animal-derived fats, including lard and dairy products, contribute to elevations in serum cholesterol. Plant-derived canola and olive oils are considered cardioprotective due to the presence of omega-3 fatty acids and alpha-linolenic acid. They are preferred for cooking over animal fats that were commonly used in the past. A diet with about 10% of calories as monounsaturated fat, 10% as polyunsaturated fat, and 10% saturated fat—and with less than 300 mg/day of cholesterol—is ideal. Individuals with a high risk of stroke or heart attack may benefit from a diet that is very low in fat content with emphasis on fruits, vegetables, and whole grains (Ornish et al. 1998), although such a diet will be difficult to sustain.

Carbohydrates

Carbohydrates—consisting of refined sugars and complex carbohydrates, starches, and fiber—complete the daily diet. Aside from lactose in milk and glycogen in meats, plants are the principal dietary sources of carbohydrates. Humans were originally vegetarian and appear to thrive when consuming diets high in plant fiber. Sugars provide energy and the components needed in nucleic acids, glycoproteins, and cell membranes. Complex carbohydrates provide dietary fiber. Emphasizing whole grains, fruits, and vegetables is better for health than a diet that is high in refined grains and sweets, which stimulate insulin production (Chandalia et al. 2000; Frost et al. 1999).

Alcohol is a carbohydrate. When consumed in moderation, alcoholic drinks appear to reduce the risk of arteriosclerosis (Camargo et al. 1997). Red wine appears to be no better than other alcoholic drinks in regard to protective effect.

Fiber

Dietary fiber includes cellules and fibrils of vegetable origin. Lignin and cellulose pass unchanged through the intestine, where they contribute to fecal bulk, retain fecal water, and shorten gut transit time. Gums, pectin, hemicelluloses, and mucilage from plant secretory cells represent the soluble portion of the fiber spectrum. Due to metabolism by intestinal bacteria, they do not contribute to fecal bulk. Although they are not absorbed as nutrients, these carbohydrate molecules exert numerous beneficial effects, as previously mentioned. Figs, prunes, raisins, and fresh fruits and vegetables are particularly rich sources of fiber and are recommended for daily consumption. Vegetarians, who necessarily consume substantial amounts of fiber daily, have excellent lipid profiles (Esselstyn 1999).

Minerals

Recommendations regarding the mineral content of the diet usually start with sodium. Humans function well with about a half-gram of sodium in the daily diet. For millions of years the human race survived with no salt added to foods. After the introduction of salt as a preservative more than 3,000 years ago, people acquired a taste preference for this mineral. Although salt preservation has been replaced with better methods, the typical daily American diet still contains 10 g of sodium or more (Roberts 2001). Such a high consumption is associated with the development of hypertension (Elliott et al. 1996). Fortunately, in the absence of disease, the body is capable of discarding excess sodium in the urine, where it does no harm. Persons with hypertension or heart failure are advised to restrict sodium intake.

Potassium supplements have proved helpful in treating those suffering from hypertension (Whelton et al. 1997). Persons with renal disease may need to limit potassium intake, and persons using diuretics may need supplemental potassium. Fortunately, most individuals do quite well at maintaining potassium levels through consumption of a balanced diet.

Iron is found in abundance in a balanced diet and is readily absorbed. In the absence of iron-loss disease, no supplemental sources are required.

Calcium intake for older men and women should be in the neighborhood of 1,500 mg/day, primarily from natural foods. A high intake sustained throughout life enhances bone strength (Dawson-Hughes et al. 1997) and may reduce the risk of stroke (Abbott et al. 1996). For most adults, the necessity of high calcium intake means consuming some dairy products daily. Calcium supplements are a necessary alternative for people who are unable to consume dairy products. Calcium citrate is used if achlorhydria is present.

The zinc content of a regular diet meets bodily requirements with ease. Zinc supplementation has been touted as a means to encourage wound healing for decu-

bitus ulcers and to stimulate immune cell function, although the effectiveness in patients who are not deficient remains unproven. If the dietary intake is balanced and adequate for maintenance of normal weight, especially when patients are using commercial liquid dietary supplements, zinc needs should be easily met without additional supplementation. Zinc supplementation has not been shown to reduce macular degeneration (Cho et al. 2001).

Iodine is needed for normal thyroid function. Commonly found in soil, iodine is consumed in adequate quantities with vegetables and fruits. Where the soil is depleted of iodine, supplementation is necessary. Because iodized salt is widely available, iodine depletion is now virtually nonexistent throughout the United States.

Selenium is sometimes recommended for supplementation, although deficits are extremely rare. It is toxic at high doses, and research data to date indicate that satisfactory levels are contained in a balanced diet.

Other trace elements—including magnesium, copper, chromium, silicon, manganese, and cobalt—are readily available in a mixed diet that includes fruits and vegetables. Supplemental tablets with these elements are not currently recommended for those in good health. Alcoholics may become depleted of magnesium if hunger is constantly assuaged by drink rather than a nutritious diet, and supplements may be required to replenish body stores.

Vitamins

Most vitamins that are necessary for the maintenance of metabolism are readily found in the food of a balanced diet. Although vitamin supplements are often recommended to alleviate fatigue or malaise, there is little likelihood that a significant improvement will be appreciated at intake beyond the minimum daily requirements. This has not stopped the widespread promotion of vitamin supplements at numerous retail outlets.

Vitamin A is the second most popular vitamin purchased as a specific supplement. It is used particularly for its antioxidant properties, assumed to be valuable in lowering the risk for cancer and cardiovascular disease. The closely related compound beta-carotene *may increase cancer risk and is not recommended as a supplement* (Alpha Tocopherol, Beta Carotene Cancer Prevention Study Group 1994). Sufficient quantities of vitamin A to meet nutritional needs are present in dark-colored fruits, yellow vegetables, meats, fish, and dairy products. Although excessive carotene consumption does not result in toxic effects, vitamin A itself can cause adverse effects when taken in large quantities. Long-term intake of high levels may contribute to hip fracture in women (Feskanich et al. 2002).

Individual components of the vitamin B group are often sold in drug and nutrition stores in combination or individual formulations. Vitamin B_{12} and folic acid are among the best-known of this collection. Folic acid supplementation may retard the development of colon cancer (Giovannucci et al. 1998). Low folate levels are associated with elevated homocysteine levels, which is correlated with increased risk for cardiovascular disease (Robinson et al. 1998). Routine vitamin fortification of foods with folic acid and cyanocobalamin will have a major epidemiological benefit for primary and secondary prevention of heart disease (Tice et al. 2001). A balanced diet has more than adequate resources to meet dietary minimums of the vitamin B group for most individuals. Alcoholics may require folic acid supplements when their drinking habit interferes with an adequate dietary intake. Up to 30% of elderly individuals develop atrophic gastritis with a decline in intrinsic factor. The ensuing deficit in vitamin B_{12} absorption requires replacement with intramuscular injections or concentrated oral supplements.

Vitamin C has been in the headlines for years, ever since Dr. Linus Pauling promoted it as a cold remedy. Although a reduction in cold frequency was never proved, vitamin C remains the top-selling vitamin on the retail market. The major dietary source is citrus fruits and tomatoes. Regrettably, overuse of this vitamin has toxic effects. It has the potential to create renal oxalate stones and can cause diarrhea and vitamin B_{12} absorption difficulties when used to excess. Recent advances in understanding the role of antioxidants in the aging process may alter the appreciation of the role of this vitamin. Vitamin C may be protective due to its influence on immune mechanisms, inhibition of nitrosamine formation in the stomach, and antioxidative effects, although long-term intervention studies proving this point remain to be published. Reliance on a balanced diet alone is sufficient for maintenance of needed tissue levels.

Vitamin D is synthesized in the body wherever sunlight is available. As little as 15 minutes of sun exposure twice weekly is enough to meet bodily demands. Dietary sources are meat, fish, and fortified milk. Elderly persons typically have low sunlight exposure and low absorption. Oral supplementation with 400 units of vitamin D daily is sufficient between ages 50 and 70, with 800 units daily recommended for those older than 70. Amounts in excess of that level may contribute to the formation of renal stones.

Vitamin E is known to serve as an intracellular antioxidant and may prove to be protective against cancer. Dietary sources include vegetable and seed oils. High-dose therapy with vitamin E does not appear to reduce the incidence of cardiovascular disease among those at high risk (Heart Outcomes Prevention Evaluation Study Investigators 2000). Vitamin E is found in adequate amounts in a regular diet, and supplements have no proven value.

Elderly persons who do not eat a balanced diet may benefit from a daily multivitamin tablet containing the U.S. Department of Agriculture (USDA) Recommended Daily Allowance of vitamins (Willett and Stampfer 2001). Use of high-dose vitamin supplements should be discouraged. In addition, 1,500 mg of calcium is recommended. All vitamin and mineral supplements should be considered as complementing a balanced diet and never as a replacement (Chernoff 2001).

Summary

Correlation of dietary variations with disease patterns among different cultures is providing new insights regarding components of diets that yield the greatest benefit for disease prevention and therapy. Regular consumption of fruits and vegetables appears to be particularly important, yet less than a third of Americans consume the USDA–recommended levels. Incorporating a quality diet into daily life will pay long-term dividends in terms of overall health and a reduction in mortality rate (Kant et al. 2000; Stampfer et al. 2000).

Exercise

Exercise receives insufficient attention regarding its potential contribution to a healthy life. Exercise is a subcategory of physical activity that is planned, structured, repetitive, and purposive (Caspersen et al. 1985). If regularly done, it contributes to the development of physical fitness, which is defined as the ability to carry out daily tasks with vigor and alertness, without undue fatigue, and with ample energy to enjoy leisure-time pursuits and meet unforeseen emergencies (President's Council on Physical Fitness and Sports 1971). Another advantage of physical activity is that the associated enhanced metabolic rate permits increased food consumption, creating the opportunity to increase the intake of essential nutrients (Astrand 1992). The following subsections explore the value of (and the problems associated with) an exercise program.

Correlation of Age and Inactivity

There is a remarkable similarity between growing old and being inactive (Bortz 1982). When forced to be immobile, the human body will quickly lose vigor and begin to look old. Balance becomes unsteady, and strength declines in those who withdraw from an active lifestyle. This apparent correlation between aging and inactivity is remarkable. The value of such an observation lies in the potential opportunity to recover lost function. Although one can never reclaim lost youth, with physical conditioning one can regain the vigor of bygone days.

Etiology of Inactivity

When the opportunity arises to participate in fitness programs, older persons are less likely than more youthful persons to accept the challenge. Several reasons for this reluctance are postulated, as outlined below.

Lack of Knowledge Regarding the Value of Exercise and Perception of Discomfort

In the modern era, the concept of exercise as an enjoyable pastime was eclipsed by images of painful exertion or competitive endeavors. However, more recent changes in the understanding of physical conditioning have altered that image. It is now appropriate for persons of all ages and both sexes to exercise at a level that suits their interests and needs. Sport and competition are available if desired, along with multiple noncompetitive options that are valuable for maintaining fitness. Unfortunately, many elderly people have not embraced this new perception of exercise. Only 15% of adults engage in regular vigorous physical activity, and 60% report no regular or sustained leisure-time activity at all (U.S. Public Health Service 1996). As many as 12% of deaths each year in the Unites States can be attributed to a sedentary lifestyle (Pate et al. 1995).

Fear of Injury

Among the concerns voiced by older persons when contemplating an exercise program are fears of muscle injury or of falling and possibly sustaining a bone fracture. Many worry about triggering a heart attack if they exert themselves. The key to avoiding such risks is to engage in fitness activities that are within limits imposed by disease, disuse, or inherited conditions. Virtually everyone can engage in a properly tailored fitness program with the confidence that no harm will occur. Pre-exercise evaluation by a physician will delineate the limits that an individual should observe. Within those limits, regular exercise will maintain physical capacity, yielding significantly improved resources for participation in the activities of daily life.

Lack of Time

A lack of time to participate in exercise activities is frequently cited as a critical factor by those contemplating participation in fitness programs (Godin et al. 1985). Before retirement, work demands may indeed impose time restrictions. After retirement, even with involvement in numerous activities, most individuals have sufficient flexibility that they can establish their own priorities and place exercise among the items they consider essential, should they choose to do so.

Lack of Access to Resources

One problem to be resolved by all individuals who are interested in a physical conditioning program is access to suitable resources. The cost of membership at an exercise facility, the distance from home to the facility, the presence of exercise periods specifically dedicated to older members at the facility, and companionship while exercising are important considerations that affect participation.

Fortunately, there are many alternatives to a facility-centered exercise program. Often, one can make use of resources close at hand to accomplish similar physical development. Brisk walking is an effective, inexpensive, and enjoyable exercise of proven value (Manson et al. 1999) that can be done in the immediate home environment with good compliance (Pereira et al. 1998). In-home exercise equipment is available in a huge variety of price ranges and fitness training types. The value of modest exercise extends into late life (Hakim et al. 1998; Wannamethee et al. 1998) and is as effective as formal exercise programs in improving fitness, blood pressure, and body composition (Andersen et al. 1999; Dunn et al. 1999).

Lack of Interest in Exercise

Unfortunately, a large number of persons simply lack the motivation to maintain fitness. Physical inactivity among the elderly is not unique to modern Western society and may represent a cross-cultural phenomenon. Because exercise programs are voluntary, people who join them are self-selected as perceiving significant value in the undertaking, and studies utilizing such groups are subject to bias. To minimize participant dropout rates and maximize attendance, emphasis on companionship among the participants and close attention to graded advancements of effort is helpful. Inclusion of an education component, with attention to the special needs of smokers or obese patients, is also beneficial.

Types of Activity

Components of exercise programs have evolved over a number of years and continue to change as research indicates special value for particular aspects. Flexibility, strength, and endurance are the three elements around which any program is built. Although an individual exercise may target only one of these elements, there is considerable overlap in the end result. Thus, a weight-lifting program designed to build strength also produces enhanced endurance and flexibility.

Limbering and Flexibility

First among the activities that any individual should do at the start of an exercise session are limbering and warm-up exercises, followed by gentle stretching and flexing. The goal is to prepare ligaments and muscles for the strengthening and endurance activities to follow. Injuries are much less likely to occur if a proper warm-up is undertaken.

Limbering and warm-up exercises can be done in any open space. Chair exercises are available for those incapable of standing because of balance problems or weakness. Floor mats are useful, because many of the activities require lying on one's side or back. When available, a pool with water at chest height is a great asset for flexibility training. The maintenance of flexibility has daily value for activities such as donning clothes, trimming toenails, and attending to personal hygiene.

Strength

Physical conditioning programs traditionally emphasize the development of specific muscle groups for a particular sport or event. The same concept applies to conditioning programs for life. An individual must have sufficient strength to carry out daily activities. Muscle cells developed in youth persist throughout life, representing banked reserves waiting to be used. Muscle strength is developed by contraposing muscle contraction against resistance. Weight lifting is the traditional method used for this purpose. Machines have been devised that permit every muscle group in the body to be selectively laden with the ideal load to encourage maximum development. Resistance devices using hydraulic pistons are available in which the load can be adjusted by twisting a dial. Hydraulic apparatuses can resist motion in two directions, thereby speeding reciprocal muscle development in one exercise effort.

Homegrown alternatives to professional weight-lifting equipment are legion. Sacks filled with sand, strips of rubber tubing, and water-filled bags lifted by ropes on pulleys fastened to doors are but a few of the ingenious ways to provide resistance for muscle development. Vigorous walking or regular stair climbing are remarkably effective, inexpensive, and available methods to encourage musculoskeletal development.

Endurance

The third part of a fitness program involves enhancement of the cardiovascular system to improve endurance. *Aerobic conditioning* is the term used to describe training that requires an individual to stay within limits that permit inhaled oxygen to fully supply the needs of the body during exercise. The body responds by increasing its efficiency of oxygen transport and use from the lungs to each individual cell component. Improved oxygen use permits extended periods of muscle activity without fatigue. This aspect of physical conditioning is quantified by measuring oxygen consumption during maximal exercise exertion.

The endurance and strength aspects of conditioning are distinct. One has only to compare the physiques of a long-distance runner and a wrestler to see the archetypes of these two concepts. Most elderly individuals will benefit more from a runner type of program than from a wrestler approach, although both have value.

Activity Initiation

Initiating a fitness program after years of inconsistent exertion involves some thoughtful planning to avoid injuries to the musculoskeletal or cardiovascular system. Physical limitations must be identified, specific exercises selected, monitoring parameters chosen, and exertion ranges established. Regular reassessment is needed so that the program can be upgraded in response to progress by the participant.

Injury Risk Assessment

The checkup before exercise should focus on identifying medical conditions that will be affected by exercise. Endocrine, cardiovascular, orthopedic, and neurological conditions are of prime interest. Diabetics may require adjustment in their glycemic control regimen, because exercise will decrease the need for insulin. The circulatory system checkup focuses on adequate cardiac and peripheral circulatory reserves. Orthopedic conditions and physical deformities are worthy of attention if they will impose limits on exertion. Lung disease and asthma may reduce ventilation during exertion. Neurological disease can alter balance, coordination, or muscle use. Dementia that precludes the understanding of exercise limits will require that an escort be available to provide guidance. Medication review will document pharmaceuticals capable of altering performance indicators. For example, β-blocking medications will lower pulse rates, which must be taken into account in establishing a proper training range for the pulse.

Fitness Assessment

Initial evaluation should assess the applicant's ability to participate in established workout routines and should identify any need for special attention. The standard for determining fitness is the exercise tolerance test (ETT), conducted on a treadmill or bicycle ergometer. Although baseline ETT data will provide a satisfying measure of progress for the participant, the tests are expensive and are rarely required for community exercise programs. The ETT has little value for predicting adverse cardiac events (Hollenberg et al. 1998), which has led some experts to suggest that it be omitted in favor of simpler measures (Gill et al. 2000; Pollock et al. 2000). Timed walking studies or Activity Readiness Questionnaires (Shephard 2000) suffice to establish exercise recommendations. Individuals choosing to exercise at home typically have no prior assessment, and the overwhelming majority of them experience no harm. The requirement for prior assessment should not stand in the way of initiating a modest exercise program. The hazards of exercise are minor in relation to the value received.

Program Organization

The value of group versus solo exercise programs is the subject of some debate. Exercising by oneself yields the maximum versatility in terms of scheduling and privacy, with generally good results. Group exercise programs are widely available at fitness centers, community agencies such as the YMCA/YWCA, and city recreation departments. The majority of these programs cater to persons with no known physical impediments. Some programs are tailored exclusively to the special needs of those recovering from an illness such as myocardial infarction. All supervised programs incorporate many weeks of gradually increasing exertion with careful observation for untoward events. During this time, the participant is taught principles of safe and effective exercise that can be applied throughout the remainder of the participant's life.

Many people skip the evaluation and plunge into a self-designed exercise program without hesitation. The majority do very well with this approach, especially when they take note of signals that their bodies convey about exercise limits. An ideal program includes a 5-minute limbering and warm-up period, followed by a 30-minute exercise period during which the heart rate is kept in a target training range previously determined as ideal. This is followed by a cool-down period for an additional 10 minutes. Each part of this sequence is important for safe and effective exercise. Ideally, the exercise program should be repeated a minimum of 3 days a week. Daily is even better (Pollock et al. 1998).

One aspect of exercise that is often misunderstood is the tremendous value that accrues at submaximal exertion levels. One need not punish the body to vastly improve physical performance. A person should be comfortable at all times and should be easily able to converse while exercising. Most important of all, the person should enjoy the process.

Benefits of Exercise

The benefits of exercise are believed to reach beyond the simple enhancement of muscle performance. Self-image and emotional stability are enhanced as well (Blumenthal et al. 1999). Whereas weight control is facilitated by an increase in caloric consumption related to exercise, obesity is ultimately determined by food intake. Nutrition can be enhanced by physical exertion, provided that an increased caloric intake is associated with greater variety in the diet. Weight-bearing activity improves bone calcium metabolism and strength. Control of hypertension and diabetes may be favorably affected by even mild activity such as walking (Hu et al. 1999a). The amount of exercise determines the magnitude of improvement in the high-density lipoprotein cholesterol level (Williams 1997). Maintaining physical activity will cut the risk of coronary disease almost in half (Berlin and Colditz 1990) and will protect against stroke (Hu et al. 2000).

Virtually all who partake in regular exercise programs report an improved ability to manage their activities of daily living. They are less dependent on motorized resources such as elevators or automobiles and can participate in more activities without fatigue. Immediate benefits are evident in the increased distances walked by those who have claudication (Gardner et al. 2000) and the reduction of depression symptoms (Singh et al. 2001). Moreover, they are delighted to find that former vigor can be successfully recalled.

Hazards of Exercise

The majority of older persons experience few problems as they undertake exercise as part of a fitness program. The benefits are assumed to outweigh the risks, provided that appropriate limits are set and cautious advances are undertaken.

Of greatest concern is the possibility of sudden death due to rupture of arteriosclerotic plaques with platelet activation induced by exercise (Bartsch 1999; Burke et al. 1999). However, cardiac arrest is a rare event, and exercise incorporated in leisure-time activity has been shown to reduce the risk of sudden death (Albert et al. 2000; Lemaitre et al. 1999). When a careful physical evaluation has been done in advance and the patient cooperates by observing established limits, there is little likelihood that exercise will constitute a significant risk. In the long run, there will be a risk reduction resulting from the program.

The risk of musculoskeletal injuries can be kept to a minimum by attending to proper warm-up routines, using good equipment during the workout, and avoiding overexertion.

Osteoarthritis flares are a constant concern. Research suggests that exercise can reduce pain and disability (van Baar et al. 1999) and may delay or prevent the need for surgical intervention (Deyle et al. 2000). Tai chi and pool exercises with motion against water resistance are remarkably effective and safe for arthritic patients (Hartman et al. 2000). When arthritis flares do occur, rest and anti-inflammatory medications are recommended. Restarting exercise later with altered routines may protect fragile joints.

Osteoporosis presents significant risks for the elderly patient. Falls of any nature can lead to fractures, particularly of the hip and wrist. Vertebral collapse can be terribly painful. When fractures occur, cessation of exercise is required until healing is complete. In most cases, reinstitution of exercise is then appropriate, and weight-bearing activity will strengthen bone. Some particularly fragile persons must limit exercise to a pool, where falls are impossible and stress is greatly reduced.

Thermal condition during exercise requires attention, because older persons often fail to appreciate extremes of heat or cold. Avoiding outside exercise in freezing weather is essential. Warm clothing is needed whenever the temperature is below 60°F. Temperatures above 80°F are likewise troublesome, especially if the humidity is high. Brisk walking in shopping malls has become popular because malls offer year-round stable temperatures, an interesting environment, solid footing, and the availability of help if problems occur.

Fatigue may be a complaint of the exercise program participant and usually represents an overly vigorous approach to physical exertion. However, close watch must be kept for congestive heart failure or other medical conditions that have become unbalanced and are manifesting as systemic complaints. Prior screening of exercise candidates should exclude those whose medical status is too precarious to undertake an active fitness program. Maintaining the target intensity of 60%–70% of maximal heart rate minimizes the risks. Within this range, comfortable, safe, and effective programs can be created to keep most participants feeling far younger than their chronological age would suggest.

Conclusion

Intensive efforts are under way to find the optimal nutritional elements that will reduce the likelihood of developing disease throughout life. At this time, a number of trends are worth following, of which limitation of fat intake and regular consumption of fiber seem to have the greatest value. Provided that individuals are able to eat a balanced diet, their nutritional status should maintain itself with no need for supplementation. Supplements, if used at all, should include only calcium. With disease states, special attention to nutrition is essential for recovery or control. Numerous helpful diet modifications can be prescribed that may control illness with little or no need for medications.

Physical exertion, when enjoyed as part of an ongoing fitness program, can make older persons feel and act younger than their chronological years. Health care professionals are strongly encouraged to promote a less sedentary lifestyle for their older patients (Christmas and Andersen 2000). The benefits associated with regular exercise and physical activity contribute to a healthier independent lifestyle, greatly improving the functional capacity and quality of life for older adults (Mazzeo et al. 1998). Care is necessary when initiating any activity change, but experience has shown that reserves from early life can be recalled to active service without undue hardship. The improvement in activities of daily living and the potential for expanding one's resources for dealing with stress or illness make exercise an attractive element in a program of health promotion or maintenance.

References

Abbott RD, Curb JD, Rodriguez BL, et al: Effect of dietary calcium and milk consumption on risk of thromboembolic stroke in older middle-aged men: the Honolulu Heart Program. Stroke 27:813–818, 1996

Albert CM, Mittleman MA, Chae CU, et al: Triggering of sudden death from cardiac causes by vigorous exertion. N Engl J Med 343:1355–1361, 2000

Alpha Tocopherol, Beta Carotene Cancer Prevention Study Group: The effect of vitamin E and beta carotene on the incidence of lung cancer and other cancers in male smokers. N Engl J Med 330:1029–1035, 1994

Andersen RE, Wadden TA, Bartlett SJ, et al: Effects of lifestyle activity vs structured aerobic exercise in obese women: a randomized trial. JAMA 281:335–340, 1999

Astrand PO: Physical activity and fitness. Am J Clin Nutr 55:1231S–1236S, 1992

Azad N, Murphy J, Amos SS, et al: Nutrition survey in an elderly population following admission to a tertiary care hospital. CMAJ 161:511–515, 1999

Barrett-Connor E, Edelstein SL, Corey-Bloom J, et al: Weight loss precedes dementia in community-dwelling older adults. J Am Geriatr Soc 44:1147–1152, 1996

Bartsch P: Platelet activation with exercise and risk of cardiac events. Lancet 354:1747–1748, 1999

Berlin JA, Colditz GA: A meta-analysis of physical activity in the prevention of coronary heart disease. Am J Epidemiol 132:612–628, 1990

Blumenthal JA, Babyak MA, Moore KA, et al: Effects of exercise training on older patients with major depression. Arch Intern Med 159:2349–2356, 1999

Bortz WM: Disuse and aging. JAMA 248:1203–1208, 1982

Bucci LR: A functional analytical technique for monitoring nutrient status and repletion, part 2: validation. Am Clin Lab 13:25–27, 1994

Burke AP, Farb A, Malcom GT, et al: Plaque rupture and sudden death related to exertion in men with coronary artery disease. JAMA 281:921–926, 1999

Burns R, Nichols L, Calkins E, et al: Nutritional assessment of community-living well elderly. J Am Geriatr Soc 34:781–786, 1986

Busetto L, Tregnaghi A, Bussolotto M, et al: Visceral fat loss evaluated by total body magnetic resonance imaging in obese women operated with laparascopic adjustable silicone gastric banding. Int J Obes Relat Metab Disord 24:60–69, 2000

Bussolotto M, Ceccon A, Sergi G, et al: Assessment of body composition in elderly: accuracy of bioelectrical impedance analysis. Gerontology 45:39–43, 1999

Calle EE, Thun MJ, Petrelli JM, et al: Body-mass index and mortality in a prospective cohort of U.S. adults. N Engl J Med 341:1097–1105, 1999

Camargo CA Jr, Hennekens CH, Gaziano JM, et al: Prospective study of moderate alcohol consumption and mortality in U.S. male physicians. Arch Intern Med 157:79–85, 1997

Caspersen CJ, Powell KE, Christenson GM: Physical activity, exercise, and physical fitness: definitions and distinctions for health-related research. Public Health Rep 100:126–131, 1985

Chandalia M, Garg A, Lutjohann D, et al: Beneficial effects of high dietary fiber intake in patients with type 2 diabetes mellitus. N Engl J Med 342:1392–1398, 2000

Chernoff R: Nutrition and health promotion in older adults. J Gerontol A Biol Sci Med Sci 56 Spec No 2(2):47–53, 2001

Cho E, Stampfer MJ, Seddon JM, et al: Prospective study of zinc intake and the risk of age-related macular degeneration. Ann Epidemiol 11:328–336, 2001

Christmas C, Andersen RA: Exercise and older patients: guidelines for the clinician. J Am Geriatr Soc 48:318–324, 2000

Cummings JH, Bingham SA: Diet and the prevention of cancer. BMJ 317:1636–1640, 1998

Daviglus ML, Stamler J, Orencia AJ, et al: Fish consumption and the 30-year risk of fatal myocardial infarction. N Engl J Med 336:1046–1053, 1997

Dawson-Hughes B, Harris SS, Krall EA, et al. Effect of calcium and vitamin D supplementation on bone density in men and women 65 years of age or older. N Engl J Med 337:670–676, 1997

de Lorgeril M, Salen P, Martin J-L, et al: Mediterranean diet, traditional risk factors, and the rate of cardiovascular complications after myocardial infarction. Final report of the Lyon Diet Heart Study. Circulation 99:779–785, 1999

Deyle GD, Henderson NE, Matekel RL, et al: Effectiveness of manual physical therapy and exercise in osteoarthritis of the knee. Ann Intern Med 132:173–181, 2000

Dunn AL, Marcus BH, Kampert JB, et al: Comparison of lifestyle and structured interventions to increase physical activity and cardiorespiratory fitness: a randomized trial. JAMA 281:327–334, 1999

Elliott P, Stamler J, Nichols R, et al: INTERSALT revisited: further analyses of 24 hour sodium excretion and blood pressure within and across populations. BMJ 312:1249–1253, 1996

Esselstyn CB Jr: Updating a 12-year experience with arrest and reversal therapy for coronary heart disease (an overdue requiem for palliative cardiology). Am J Cardiol 84:339–341, A8, 1999

Feskanich D, Singh V, Willett WC, et al: Vitamin A intake and hip fractures among postmenopausal women. JAMA 287:47–54, 2002

Fontijn-Tekamp GA, van't Hof MA, Slagter AP, et al: The state of dentition in relation to nutrition in elderly Europeans in the SENECA study of 1993. Eur J Clin Nutr 50 (suppl 2):S1172–S1122, 1996

Frost G, Leeds AA, Madeiros DS, et al: Glycaemic index as a determinant of serum HDL-cholesterol concentration. Lancet 353:1045–1048, 1999

Fuster V, Badimon L, Badimon JJ, et al: The pathogenesis of coronary artery disease and the acute coronary syndromes. N Engl J Med 326:242–250, 1992

Gardner AW, Katzel LI, Sorkin JD, et al: Improved functional outcomes following exercise rehabilitation in patients with intermittent claudication. J Gerontol A Biol Sci Med Sci 55:M570–M577, 2000

Gill TM, DiPietro L, Krumholz HM: Role of exercise stress testing and safety monitoring for older persons starting an exercise program. JAMA 284:342–349, 2000

Giovannucci E, Stampfer MJ, Colditz GA, et al: Multivitamin use, folate, and colon cancer in women in the Nurses' Health Study. Ann Intern Med 129:517–524, 1998

Godin G, Shephard RJ, Colantonio A: The cognitive profile of those who intend to exercise but do not. Public Health Rep 100:521–526, 1985

Hakim AA, Petrovitch H, Burchfiel CM, et al: Effects of walking on mortality among nonsmoking retired men. N Engl J Med 338:94–99, 1998

Harper CR, Jacobson TA: The fats of life: the role of omega-3 fatty acids in the prevention of coronary heart disease. Arch Intern Med 161:2185–2192, 2001

Hartman CA, Manos TM, Winter C, et al: Effects of t'ai chi training on function and quality of life indicators in older adults with osteoarthritis. J Am Geriatr Soc 48:1553–1559, 2000

Heart Outcomes Prevention Evaluation Study Investigators: Vitamin E supplementation and cardiovascular events in high-risk patients. N Engl J Med 342:154–160, 2000

Heiat A, Vaccarino V, Krumholz HM: An evidence-based assessment of Federal guidelines for overweight and obesity as they apply to elderly persons. Arch Intern Med 161:1194–1203, 2001

Hollenberg M, Ngo LH, Turner D, et al: Treadmill exercise testing in an epidemiologic study of elderly subjects. J Gerontol A Biol Sci Med Sci 53:B259–B267, 1998

Hu FB, Sigal RJ, Rich-Edwards JW, et al: Walking compared with vigorous physical activity and risk of type 2 diabetes in women: a prospective study. JAMA 282:1433–1439, 1999a

Hu FB, Stampfer MJ, Rimm EB, et al: A prospective study of egg consumption and risk of cardiovascular disease in men and women. JAMA 281:1387–1394, 1999b

Hu FB, Stampfer MJ, Colditz GA, et al: Physical activity and risk of stroke in women. JAMA 283:2961–2967, 2000

Hu FB, Manson JE, Stampfer MJ, et al: Diet, lifestyle, and the risk of type 2 diabetes mellitus in women. N Engl J Med 345:790–797, 2001

Joshipura KJ, Ascherio A, Manson JE, et al: Fruit and vegetable intake in relation to risk of ischemic stroke. JAMA 282:1233–1239, 1999

Kant AK, Schatzkin A, Graubard BI, et al: A prospective study of diet quality and mortality in women. JAMA 283:2109–2115, 2000

Kenney WL, Chiu P: Influence of age on thirst and fluid intake. Med Sci Sports Exerc 33:1524–1532, 2001

Kleiner SM: Water: an essential but overlooked nutrient. J Am Diet Assoc 99:200–206, 1999

Kolonel LN, Nomura AMY, Cooney RV: Dietary fat and prostate cancer: current status. J Natl Cancer Inst 91:414–428, 1999

Lemaitre RN, Siscovic DS, Raghunathan TE, et al: Leisure-time physical activity and the risk of primary cardiac arrest. Arch Intern Med 159:686–690, 1999

Manson JE, Hu FB, Rich-Edwards JW, et al: A prospective study of walking as compared with vigorous exercise in the prevention of coronary heart disease in women. N Engl J Med 341:650–658, 1999

Mazzeo RS, Cavanagh P, Evans WJ, et al: Exercise and physical activity for older adults. Med Sci Sports Exerc 30:992–1008, 1998

McCay L, Maynard L, Sperling G, et al: Retarded growth, life span, ultimate body size and age changes in the albino rat after feeding diets restricted in calories. J Nutr 18:1–13, 1939

McGinnis JM, Foege WH: Actual causes of death in the United States. JAMA 270:2207–2212, 1993

Michaud DS, Giovannucci E, Willett WC, et al: Physical activity, obesity, height, and the risk of pancreatic cancer. JAMA 286:921–929, 2001

Mokdad AH, Bowman BA, Ford ES, et al: The continuing epidemics of obesity and diabetes in the United States. JAMA 286:1195–1200, 2001

Nordin BE, Need AG, Steurer T, et al: Nutrition, osteoporosis and aging. Ann N Y Acad Sci 854:336–351, 1998

O'Keefe SJ: Food and the gut. S Afr Med J 85:261–268, 1995

Ornish D, Scherwitz LW, Billings JH, et al: Intensive lifestyle changes for reversal of coronary heart disease. JAMA 280:2001–2007, 1998

Pate RR, Pratt M, Blair SN, et al: Physical activity and public health: a recommendation from the Centers for Disease Control and Prevention and the American College of Sports Medicine. JAMA 273:402–407, 1995

Pedrini MT, Levey AS, Lau J, et al: The effect of dietary protein restriction on the progression of diabetic and nondiabetic renal diseases: a meta-analysis. Ann Intern Med 124:627–632, 1996

Pereira MA, Kriska AM, Day RD, et al: A randomized walking trial in postmenopausal women: effects of physical activity and health 10 years later. Arch Intern Med 158:1695–1701, 1998

Pollock ML, Gaessar GA, Butcher JD, et al: The recommended quantity and quality of exercise for developing and maintaining cardiorespiratory and muscular fitness, and flexibility in healthy adults. Med Sci Sports Exerc 30:975–991, 1998

Pollock ML, Franklin BA, Balady GJ, et al: AHA Science Advisory. Resistance exercise in individuals with and without cardiovascular disease: benefits, rationale, safety, and prescription: an advisory from the Committee on Exercise, Rehabilitation, and Prevention, Council on Clinical Cardiology, American Heart Association. Circulation 101:828–833, 2000

President's Council on Physical Fitness and Sports: Physical Fitness Research Digest, Series 1, No 1. Washington, DC, U.S. Government Printing Office, 1971

Riggs BL, Hodgson SF, O'Fallon WM, et al: Effect of fluoride treatment on the fracture rate in postmenopausal women with osteoporosis. N Engl J Med 322:802–809, 1990

Rissanen T, Voutilainen S, Nyyssonen K, et al: Fish oil-derived fatty acids, docasahexaenoic acid and docosaentaenoic acid, and the risk of acute coronary events. The Kuopio Ischaemic Heart Disease Risk Factor Study. Circulation 102:2677–2679, 2000

Roberts CW: High salt intake, its origins, its economic impact, and its effect on blood pressure. Am J Cardiol 88:1338–1346, 2001

Robinson K, Arheart K, Refsum H, et al: Low circulating folate and vitamin B6 concentrations: risk factors for stroke, peripheral vascular disease, and coronary artery disease. Circulation 97:437–443, 1998

Rock CL, Lampe JW, Patterson RE: Nutrition, genetics, and risks of cancer. Annu Rev Public Health 21:47–64, 2000

Russell RG, Croucher PI, Rogers MJ: Bisphosphonates: pharmacology, mechanisms of action and clinical uses. Osteoporos Int 2 (suppl):S66–S80, 1999

Sacks FM, Svetkey LP, Vollmer WM, et al: Effects on blood pressure of reduced dietary sodium and the dietary approaches to stop hypertension (DASH) diet. N Engl J Med 344:3–10, 2001

Schiffman SS: Taste and smell losses in normal aging and disease. JAMA 278:1357–1362, 1997

Sergi G, Perini P, Bussolotto M, et al: Body composition study in the elderly: comparison between tritium dilution method and dual photon absorptiometry. J Gerontol 48:M244–M248, 1993

Seshadri S, Beiser A, Selhum J, et al: Plasma homocysteine as a risk factor for dementia and Alzheimer's disease. N Engl J Med 346:476–483, 2002

Shephard RJ: Does insistence on medical clearance inhibit adoption of physical activity in the elderly? Journal of Aging and Physical Activity 8:301–311, 2000

Singh NA, Clements KM, Singh MAF: The efficacy of exercise as a long-term antidepressant in elderly subjects: a randomized controlled trial. J Gerontol A Biol Sci Med Sci 56:M497–M504, 2001

Stampfer MJ, Hu FB, Manson JE, et al: Primary prevention of coronary heart disease in women through diet and lifestyle. N Engl J Med 343:16–22, 2000

Tice JA, Ross E, Coxson PG, et al: Cost-effectiveness of vitamin therapy to lower plasma homocysteine levels for the prevention of coronary heart disease: effect of grain fortification and beyond. JAMA 286:936–943, 2001

Tuomilehto J, Lindstrom J, Ericsson JG, et al: Prevention of type 2 diabetes mellitus by changes in lifestyle among subjects with impaired glucose tolerance. N Engl J Med 344:1343–1350, 2001

Ulijaszek SJ, Kerr DA: Anthropometric measurement error and the assessment of nutritional status. Br J Nutr 82:165–177, 1999

U.S. Public Health Service: Physical activity and health: a report of the Surgeon General. Atlanta, GA, Centers for Disease Control and Prevention, National Center for Chronic Disease Prevention and Health Promotion, 1996

van Baar ME, Assendelft WJ, Dekker J, et al: Effectiveness of exercise therapy in patients with osteoarthritis of the hip or knee. A systematic review of randomized clinical trials. Arthritis Rheum 42:1361–1369, 1999

van Dam RM, Rimm EB, Willett WC, et al: Dietary patterns and risk for type 2 diabetes mellitus in U.S. men. Ann Intern Med 136:201–209, 2002

Velie E, Kulldorff M, Schairer C, et al: Dietary fat, fat subtypes, and breast cancer in postmenopausal women: a prospective cohort study. J Natl Cancer Inst 92:833–839, 2000

Wannamethee SG, Shaper AG, Walker M: Changes in physical activity, mortality, and incidence of coronary heart disease in older men. Lancet 351:1603–1608, 1998

Whelton PK, He J, Cutler JA, et al: Effects of oral potassium on blood pressure: meta-analysis of randomized controlled clinical trials. JAMA 277:1624–1632, 1997

Willett WC, Stampfer MJ: What vitamins should I be taking, doctor? N Engl J Med, 345:1819–1824, 2001

Williams PT: Relationship of distance run per week to coronary heart disease risk factors in 8,283 male runners: the National Runners' Health Study. Arch Intern Med 157:191–198, 1997

Individual and Group Psychotherapy

Thomas R. Lynch, Ph.D.

Ann K. Aspnes

Psychotherapy has been shown to be an effective treatment for a number of mental disorders seen in older adults. As a treatment modality it can be particularly useful for older adult psychiatric patients who cannot or will not tolerate medication or who are dealing with stressful conditions, interpersonal difficulties, limited levels of social support, or recurrent episodes of the disorder. However, it has been estimated that only 10% of older adults in need of psychiatric services actually receive professional care, and there has been minimal utilization of mental health services in this age group (Abrahams and Patterson 1978; Friedhoff 1994; Weissman et al. 1981).

Many practitioners assume that older adults have negative attitudes toward psychotherapy. Although research on attitudes toward treatment in elderly samples is not conclusive, contrary to clinical lore, growing descriptive research suggests that older adults may prefer counseling over medication treatment. In a community sample of 462 nondepressed older adults, 68% agreed with a statement that professional counseling or therapy helps most depressed people feel better. Interestingly, 56% of the same sample reported that they believed antidepressant medications to be addictive, and only 4% disagreed (Vitt et al. 1999). Older adults have also been shown to report a greater number of positive attitudes toward mental health professionals and to be less concerned than younger adults with stigmas attached to seeking treatment for depression (Rokke and Scogin 1995). Regardless, attitudinal barriers to treatment occur in samples of both younger and older adults (Allen et al. 1998), and patient preferences or biases toward treatment should be considered before referral for psychotherapy.

In this chapter we review the theoretical and empirical evidence for psychotherapy in older adults. The material is organized by type of disorder and, for each disorder, type of therapy. We begin by reviewing what is known about common factors that influence outcome across modalities. When possible, we evaluate the evidence with respect to quality of data, generalizability, and long-term effects of treatment.

Common Factors

Simply stated, the goals of psychotherapy are to enhance human coping and to reduce human suffering. In fact, a recurring issue in psychotherapy research is the attempt to understand the unique and shared factors associated with empirically tested interventions. Beutler (2000) and colleagues have been attempting to create a therapy that is based on the common curative factors associated with all treatments. Of course, this therapy then becomes a new type of treatment, requiring the same empirical validation as other treatments (Rounsaville and Carroll 2002). Thus, there is no shortcut to determining the best psychotherapeutic approach.

Most therapies consist of some type of therapeutic feedback to enhance patient awareness or to change patient behavior (Goldfried et al. 1997, 1998). Therapist feedback may help patients by influencing cognitive and attentional biases for problematic stimuli (Beck et al. 1979; Hayes et al. 1996; Klerman et al. 1984; Strupp and Binder 1984). Thus, therapists can be seen to work toward helping patients refocus attention toward aspects of themselves that have previously been avoided or over-attended so that they can gain new perspectives about themselves or improve their ability to solve problems (Goldfried et al. 1997). Therapeutic feedback may function optimally when corrective information regarding ineffective behavior is balanced by validation of behavior that is effective (Linehan 1993).

Therapy also typically occurs within the context of some type of interpersonal relationship. Some have argued that relationship factors account for as much as 80% of the variance in treatment outcomes (Andrews 1998). However, research has not confirmed this assertion. Contrary to the belief that the therapeutic relationship is the salient curative feature, relationship variables have been shown to produce only 10% of the variance in outcomes, essentially equivalent to the variance attributed to specific therapeutic approaches (Horvath and Symonds 1991; Luborsky et al. 2002; Martin et al. 2000).

In an attempt to reconfirm their classic box-score analysis, Luborsky and colleagues (2002) conducted a meta-meta-analysis. They concluded that all psychotherapies are essentially equivalent in their ability to produce therapeutic gain. However, a number of methodological flaws were associated with their study, including the following: 1) the authors mixed together studies with both random and nonrandom assignment (D.F. Klein 2002); 2) many of the studies included in the analysis constituted poor comparison groups for the psychotherapy condition being examined; 3) the assumption that aggregated effect sizes would be independent was invalidated by the inclusion of 14 studies that were in more than one of the aggregated meta-analyses (Chambless 2002); and 4) the exclusion of studies comparing dynamic and experiential therapy from the meta-analysis by Svartberg and Stiles (1991) resulted in the omission of studies that showed poor effects for psychodynamic research (Chambless 2002).

In addition, to conclude that all psychotherapy works the same for all patients one must assume that average differences between all types of therapy can reasonably represent the differences between treatments on specific disorders (Chambless 2002). For example, depression research has generally shown minimal effect size differences between divergent treatments (Chambless and Ollendick 2001), which suggests that the type of therapy sought by a depressed patient may be relatively unimportant. However, the meta-meta-analysis by Luborsky et al. (2002) was heavily loaded with depression studies, which consequently diminished the differences (Beutler 2002). In addition, a comparison analysis has shown that even within the same therapeutic modality (e.g., cognitive-behavioral treatment), treatments with a common profile

can have significantly different elements, which calls into question the validity of broadly collapsing therapies—even those with similar theoretical origins or labels (Beutler 2002; Malik et al. 2000).

Psychotherapy outcome studies may also be influenced by therapy allegiance effects. In fact, some have argued that nearly 70% of the variance in outcome can be explained by allegiance to the therapy (Messer and Wampold 2002). However, conclusions in this realm are hampered by competence issues related to adherence, such as the concept that therapists who believe in a therapy are more likely to administer it competently.

Therefore, although some common factors have been identified across treatment modalities that likely influence outcome (e.g., strength of therapeutic relationship, therapeutic feedback, allegiance effects), to date the debate regarding unique and shared features associated with therapeutic progress remains unresolved. In addition, there has been a dearth of research addressing these issues among older adults. In general, older adults will respond to many of the therapeutic interventions used with younger populations. The pace of therapy should be slower, and fonts for written material should be larger. In addition, providing memory aids can be very helpful. For example, in our work we audiotape each session and ask the patient to review the session during the week before the next meeting. Additional areas to consider are listed below.

- Medical illness or problematic medicines can exacerbate symptoms of a mental disorder. During assessment it is important to obtain a medical history and a medication list.
- Social desirability factors should be considered when obtaining self reports. A nonjudgmental stance on the part of the clinician will likely help disclosure.
- The clinician should actively work against stereotypes of elderly persons as being withdrawn, rigid, lonely, dependent, or unable to learn.
- Older adults may have difficulty remembering troublesome events. The clinician should consider consulting family members or longtime friends.
- Some patients may avoid feedback about their problems as a way to reduce anxiety. Patients should be advised that change will likely involve some discomfort as they learn to cope differently (e.g., being assertive if normally avoidant).
- Cognitive deficits can impede learning speed and memory. Therapists may need to slow the pace when teaching skills and may need to ask patients to summarize issues covered.

Depression

Cognitive-Behavioral Therapy

Cognitive-behavioral therapy (CBT) techniques currently in use generally combine earlier work that used either solely cognitive or solely behavioral therapies and now encompass a wide variety of treatment protocols. There has been ongoing debate in the literature as to whether strictly behavioral or strictly cognitive strategies have greater treatment utility. However, regardless of mechanistic explanations of change, cognitive-behavioral interventions have been the most frequently studied therapies and have repeatedly been found useful in treating depression in older adults (Koder et al. 1996; Scogin and McElreath 1994; Thompson and Gallagher 1984; Thompson et al. 1987).

Cognitive therapies focus on problematic thoughts that may perpetuate depression. The goal is to change and adapt cognitive patterns away from negative thoughts that have become automatic. By changing the thoughts, therapists hope to change underlying dysfunctional attitudes that are hypothesized to result in relapse (Floyd and Scogin 1998). However, research supporting the process by which cognitive therapy reduces depressive relapse has not been well articulated (Barber and DeRubeis 1989; Teasdale et al. 2002). Recent component analysis research suggests that behavioral activation and automatic thought modification have equal effectiveness and that both components together are no more effective in preventing relapse than when used alone (Gortner et al. 1998; Jacobson et al. 1996). In addition, an increasing amount of data suggests that the salient mechanism of change in cognitive therapy is the development of metacognition (i.e., responding to negative thoughts as transitory events rather than as an inherent aspect of self or as necessarily true) rather than change in the dysfunctional attitude per se (Teasdale et al. 2002).

More purely behavioral interventions are derived from classic learning theory in which problem behaviors are viewed as the result of specific antecedent stimuli and consequential events that reinforce, punish, or maintain behavioral responses (e.g., Dougher and Hackbert 1994). Genetics and biology are considered to play important roles in the development of psychopathology; however, theorists believe that biological predispositions can be mediated by skill acquisition and learning that occurs throughout the lifespan. This therapeutic approach views depression as a state in which there is a relative shift toward an increase in dysphoric or hopeless affective reactions and a concomitant reduction in the frequency of reinforcing overt activities. Problem behaviors are analyzed functionally. For example, dysphoric responses (e.g., sad facial expressions, self-denigration) may function to reduce hostility or increase sympathy by caregivers, yet over time the lack of recovery or recurrent depression may be seen as aversive to caregivers (Biglan 1991; Coyne 1976; Dougher and Hackbert 1994). Behavioral techniques include monitoring behavior and affect patterns, assigning pleasant events, stimulus control, limiting worry and depressive ruminations with time limits, behavioral exposure, and skills training (relaxation, problem-solving, interpersonal skills).

Using a form of behavioral activation, Blumenthal et al. (1999) studied the effects of exercise on depression in older adults. In a sample of 156 adults ages 55 and older, participants were randomly assigned to supervised exercise therapy, medication (sertraline) alone, or combined exercise and medication therapy. All three groups reported significant improvements in depressive symptoms. There were no significant differences between treatment groups, which suggests that exercise training might be comparable to the use of medication in older adults. Interestingly, follow-up assessment at 10 months showed lower rates of depression in the exercise-training group than in the medication or combined treatment groups (Babyak et al. 2000). However, the sample as a whole was slightly younger than what is normally considered the minimum age for an older adult (mean age was 57, with range 50–77), which may limit generalization to older-older adults.

In a study comparing cognitive, behavioral, and brief psychodynamic therapy to waiting-list control subjects, Thompson and colleagues (1987) found that all of the treatment modalities led to comparable and clinically significant reductions of depression. All three treatment regimens included individual treatment twice weekly for 4 weeks and weekly thereafter, totaling 16–20 sessions. Overall, 52% of the sample attained complete remission after treatment, and 18% showed significant improvement with some enduring depressive symptoms. These rates are comparable to treatment outcomes in younger adult populations and response to pharmacotherapy (O'Rourke and Hadjistavropoulos 1997; Thompson et al. 1987). Follow-up research indicated that at 12 months after treatment, 58% of the sample was depression free and that at 24 months, 70% of the sample was not depressed. Like in acute treatment, no differences were found between treatment modalities at follow-up (Gallagher-Thompson et al. 1990), although in previous research with a smaller sample size depressed geriatric patients in cognitive and behavioral therapies maintained the gains longer than those treated with brief psychodynamic therapy (Gallagher and Thompson 1982).

In the first known randomized trial examining CBT as a medication augmentation strategy, Thompson et al. (2001) assessed 102 depressed older adults. Patients were assigned to one of three treatment conditions: 1) CBT alone, 2) medication alone, or 3) combined CBT and medication. Although all three groups showed improvements in depressive symptoms over 16–20 weeks of treatment, the combined-therapy group had the greatest improvements. A significant difference was found between the combined-therapy and the medication-only groups. The CBT-alone group showed similar improvements as the combined-therapy group, but the superiority of CBT alone over medication alone did not reach a significant level. This study supports conclusions by Reynolds et al. (1999) that a combined medication plus psychotherapy approach may be optimal for the treatment of depression in older adults.

A related therapy for elderly depression that utilizes elements associated with both cognitive and behavioral interventions described above examines problems associated with social problem solving. Social problem-solving therapy (PST) is based on a model in which ineffective coping under stress is hypothesized to lead to a breakdown of problem-solving abilities and subsequent depression (Nezu 1987; Thompson and Gallagher 1984). Patients are taught a structured format for solving problems that considers problem details, present goals, multiple solutions, specific solution advantages, and assessing the final solution in context. PST ideally refines and augments patients' present strategies to improve their ability to handle day-to-day problems. Like interpersonal psychotherapy, PST bolsters an area of weakness in individuals with depression. PST attempts to increase coping and buffer factors that maintain and aggravate depression (Hegel et al. 2002a). One of the attractions of PST is that it can be delivered in a limited space of time. A positive trend in the research examines adaptations of PST to be used in primary care facilities. Because many older adults do not seek treatment for depression beyond their primary care health providers, this is an ideal place to deliver psychotherapies for depression in older adults.

Arean et al. (1993) examined the efficacy of PST in a randomized, controlled trial of 74 clinically depressed older adults (age 55 or older). Patients were assigned to one of three treatment conditions: PST, reminiscence therapy, or a waiting-list control condition. After 12 weekly sessions, both therapies showed significant reductions in depressive symptoms at posttreatment and at a 3-month follow-up relative to control subjects. However, a significantly greater number of patients in the PST group than in the reminiscence therapy group were classified as improved or in remission after treatment.

Several studies have evaluated the adaptation of problem-solving treatment in primary care (PST-PC) (Hegel et al. 2002a; Mynors-Wallis 2001; Unutzer et al. 2001; Williams et al. 2000). In one study, primary care treatment options were compared in a population of older adults with depression or dysthymia (Williams et al. 2000). Subjects were randomly assigned to treatment with an antidepressant, treatment with a placebo, or PST-PC. Subjects who received PST-PC did not show significant improvements over subjects who received placebos. The antidepressant treatment group did show significant improvements over placebo. These findings suggest that the ideal use of PST-PC for older adults might include augmentation with medication.

PST-PC has advantages because it requires only brief training and has been shown to be almost equally effective whether delivered by a nurse practitioner or a medical doctor (Mynors-Wallis 2001). However, in a recent study, previous training of therapists in cognitive-behavioral interventions proved to be a significant predictor of treatment improvement (Hegel et al. 2002b). This difficulty may be mitigated in primary care multidisciplinary teams by placing a point person trained in cognitive-behavioral interventions within each team.

Interpersonal Psychotherapy

Interpersonal psychotherapy (IPT) is a manualized treatment that focuses on four components that are hypothesized to lead to or maintain depression. Whatever its etiology, depression is seen to persist in a social context. The four components of treatment focus are 1) grief (e.g., death of spouse); 2) interpersonal disputes (e.g., conflict with adult children); 3 role transitions (e.g., retirement); and 4) interpersonal deficits (e.g., lack of assertiveness skills). Techniques utilized in treatment include role-playing, communication analysis, clarification of the patient's wants and needs, and links between affect and environmental events (Hinrichsen 1997). Frank and colleagues (1993) developed separate treatment manuals for interpersonal therapy in late life and interpersonal maintenance therapy for older patients. These manuals include adaptations specific for use in elderly patients, including flexibility in length of sessions, long-standing role disputes, and the need to help the patient with practical problems.

Controlled trials in populations of depressed adults have demonstrated the efficacy of IPT for the treatment of acute depression (Frank and Spanier 1995; Hinrichsen 1997). Interpersonal therapy has also been found to be as effective in the acute treatment of major depressive disorder in elderly patients as nortriptyline (Sloane et al.

1985). Of additional importance are findings that elderly patients in IPT treatment were less likely to drop out of treatment than were those taking nortriptyline because of the medication's side effects.

IPT in combination with nortriptyline has been shown to be an effective treatment for depression in geriatric samples (Reynolds et al. 1992, 1994). In an attempt to understand more about the treatment of elderly patients with recurrent depression, Reynolds et al. (1992) selected patients only if they reported at least one prior episode of depression. Seventy-eight percent (116 of 148) remitted during the acute phase of treatment (8–14 weeks). During the continuation phase, 15% (18 of 116) experienced relapse of major depression; therefore, a total of 66% of patients recovered fully (Reynolds et al. 1992, 1994). The authors concluded that older patients with recurrent major depression can be successfully treated with a combination of antidepressant medication and IPT and that older patients respond as well, albeit more slowly, as middle-aged patients (Reynolds et al. 1997).

Psychodynamic Psychotherapy

Psychodynamic psychotherapy is based on psychoanalytical theory, which views current interpersonal and emotional experience as having been influenced by early childhood experience (Bibring 1952). Revised conceptualizations have emphasized how relationships are internalized and transformed into a sense of self (e.g., Kernberg 1976; M. Klein 1952; Kohut and Wolf 1978; Mahler 1952). Psychopathology is theorized as being related to arrestments in the development of the self, and depression is viewed as a symptom state resulting from unresolved intrapsychic conflict that may be activated by life events such as loss. During therapy patients are encouraged to develop insight into their past experience and how this experience influences their current relationships.

Although short-term psychodynamic therapy has been less studied than other treatments for older adults (e.g., CBT, IPT), there have been several indications that short-term psychodynamic therapy, particularly as conducted by Thompson, Gallagher-Thompson, and colleagues, is an effective means to treat depression in samples of older adults. In studies with random assignment to a waiting-list control condition, short-term psychodynamic therapy, or cognitive-behavioral therapy, no significant differences were found between the types of psychotherapy at the end of treatment nor at 12- and 24-month follow-ups (Gallagher-Thompson et al. 1990; Thompson et al. 1987). Additional research on depressed caregivers demonstrated an interaction between the mode of therapy and length of caregiving, such that those who had been providing care for less than 44 months appeared to achieve greater improvement with dynamic therapy, whereas longer-term caregivers seemed to obtain greater benefit from CBT (Gallagher-Thompson and Steffen 1994). The authors suggested that the long-term caregivers needed the skills learned in CBT to care for family members with more pronounced deficits and requiring more complicated care. These interesting results call for additional controlled trials comparing different treatment modalities, continued component analysis research, and continued research that examines which type of treatment works best with which type of patient.

Life Review and Reminiscence Psychotherapy

Life review and reminiscence psychotherapy are both based on the patient reexperiencing personal memories and significant life experiences. In life review, individuals are encouraged to acknowledge past conflicts and to consider their meaning in their life as a whole. Reminiscence psychotherapy focuses more on positive memories in group settings to improve self-esteem and social cohesiveness.

However, empirical support for life review and reminiscence psychotherapy as a treatment for depression is sparse. Much of the research in this area focuses on case studies, qualitative reports, and general functioning. Early work by Fry (1983) specifically assessed the use of reminiscence therapy in older adults with depression and addressed the degree of structure required to define clinically helpful reminiscence therapy. Study participants in structured or unstructured reminiscence therapy reported improvement in depression symptoms over a no-treatment control group. Those who participated in the structured reminiscence therapy also showed significantly greater improvement in depression symptoms than those who participated in the unstructured reminiscence therapy.

As reported above (see "Cognitive-Behavioral Therapy"), Arean et al. (1993) conducted a randomized trial comparing reminiscence psychotherapy, social PST, and a waiting-list control condition in older adults with major depression. The reminiscence psychotherapy protocol in this study emphasized acceptance of past events and development of personal goals. Social PST was associated with significantly greater improvements in depressive symptoms compared with reminiscence therapy. Therefore, although reminiscence psychotherapy at first blush appeared to have theoretical and practical treatment utility for older adults, to date empirical results fail to support its use.

Group Psychotherapy

Our review of the literature found seven published reports on controlled studies of group treatments for noncognitively impaired elderly persons with depression. Perrotta and Meacham (1982) reported that group reminiscence therapy was no more effective than a waiting-list control condition. In contrast, self-management therapy and education groups were both equally effective and were superior to a waiting-list control condition (Rokke et al. 1999). In comparisons with medications, one nonrandomized controlled study found that cognitive-behavioral and psychodynamic group therapies were both more effective than placebo pill but less effective than tricyclics (Jarvik et al. 1982) and that although the cognitive-behavioral and psychodynamic groups were equivalent on most measures of depression and anxiety, the CBT group had lower posttreatment scores on one depression measure (Steuer 1984). A randomized, controlled study found that cognitive therapy with or without alprazolam (an anxiolytic) was more effective than alprazolam alone (Beutler et al. 1987). Also, the addition of behavioral group therapy to standard hospital care (which presumably included medication) led to higher remission rates among inpatients than standard care alone (Brand and Clingempeel 1992). In a recent study, antidepressant medication plus clinical management alone was compared with the same therapy with the addition of dialectical behavior therapy (DBT) skills training and scheduled telephone coaching sessions (Lynch et al. 2003). At 6-month follow-up, 73% of medication plus DBT patients were in remission, compared with only 38% of medication-only patients, a significant difference. Only patients receiving DBT showed significant improvements from pretreatment to posttreatment on scores of dependency and adaptive coping, which are theorized to create vulnerability to depression (Lynch et al. 2003).

In summary, certain group therapy interventions, particularly cognitive-behavioral groups, appear promising for use with depressed older adults. Group therapy may also offer advantages for many elders; it is generally less expensive than individual treatment, and the social network provided by group therapy may provide significant therapeutic benefits to elders experiencing a loss of interpersonal relationships through the death of friends and spouses.

Bibliotherapy

Bibliotherapy, or book therapy, emphasizes a skills acquisition approach via selected readings from books. For example, Scogin and his associates (Jamison and Scogin 1995; Scogin et al. 1987, 1989, 1990) have done a series of controlled, randomized studies to test the efficacy of bibliotherapy for mild to moderate depression in older adults. Individuals with depression read books to enhance behavioral skills that combat depression or to modify dysfunctional thoughts.

In one of the early studies, the use of bibliotherapy was assessed in a population of 29 mildly to moderately depressed adults ages 60 or older (Scogin et al. 1989). Subjects were assigned to one of three groups: the cognitive bibliotherapy group read a self-help book called *Feeling Good* (Burns 1980), which explains cognitive strategies used to decrease depression, the control bibliotherapy group read a psychoeducational book that did not describe specific therapeutic strategies, and the waiting-list control group received cognitive bibliotherapy after a no-treatment period. Subjects in the cognitive bibliotherapy group reported a significant decrease in depression symptoms between a pretreatment assessment and a posttreatment assessment. At 2-year follow-up, those who had completed the cognitive bibliotherapy showed no significant changes in depressive symptoms from the initial posttreatment gains (Scogin et al. 1990). Cognitive bibliotherapy participants appeared to retain their original treatment gains for 2 years. However, the lack of differences between bibliotherapy conditions and the use of weekly supportive telephone calls within the bibliotherapy condition weaken conclusions regarding the efficacy of the bibliotherapy component.

However, in a subsequent study, Jamison and Scogin (1995) compared cognitive bibliotherapy to a waiting-list control condition. The cognitive bibliotherapy group showed significant improvement in both self-reported and clinician-rated depression symptoms compared with the waiting-list control group. At 3-month follow-up assessment, cognitive bibliotherapy participants had maintained their treatment gains. In terms of clinical efficacy, after treatment 70% of the original cognitive bibliotherapy group no longer met criteria for a major depressive episode, in comparison to only 3% of the waiting-list control group. After they received treatment, 73% of the control group no longer met criteria for depression.

Bibliotherapy has advantages for older adults. Because the intervention is delivered in a book format, adults with late-life depression are able to read and process material at their own pace. In addition, bibliotherapy can be privately self-administered, and consequently fears about stigmatization can be avoided. Also, for older adults who have limited mobility, these interventions do not require as many visits to a clinical site, and clinicians can monitor their progress intermittently through telephone calls. The optimal use of bibliotherapy appears to be as an adjunct to pharmacotherapy or individual therapy, and even bibliotherapy alone should be conducted under the care of a trained clinician. In addition, bibliotherapy obviously would not be appropriate for older adults who cannot read or who have poor eyesight or cognitive deficits that prevented them from attending to the book.

Anxiety Disorders

Anxiety Symptoms

According to epidemiological sampling, anxiety disorders are the most prevalent mental disorders diagnosed among community-dwelling older adults (Regier et al. 1988). The prevalence of anxiety disorders among younger adults was estimated at 7.3% of the population; a slightly lower rate of 5.5% was reported among older adults (Regier et al. 1988). Review of these reports, however, suggests that the rate of anxiety disorders in older adults may be underestimated due to older adults' reluctance to report symptoms, confusion of anxiety symptoms with symptoms of physical illness, and a lack of measurement instruments validated for geriatric populations. A review of eight community surveys revealed that prevalence rates for anxiety disorders in older adults ranged from 0.7% to 18.6% (Flint 1994). Another possible explanation for the range in reported prevalence rates is that the symptomatic makeup of anxiety disorders in older adults differs from that seen in younger adults. Indeed, older adults tend to report anxiety symptoms that do not necessarily fit a specific disorder. A naturalistic survey of primary care patients found that in older adults diagnosed with anxiety disorders, the most prevalent diagnosis was anxiety disorder not otherwise specified (Stanley et al. 2001). A portion of the empirical work on the psychotherapeutic treatment of anxiety in older adults focuses on symptoms rather than specific diagnostic categories.

The most frequently used and the most well-substantiated treatments for anxiety in older adults are based on behavioral therapies. Specifically, a variety of relaxation training techniques have been pilot tested as a treatment strategy for older adults. Preliminary work by DeBerry (1982a, 1982b) showed that progressive muscle relaxation and meditation relaxation techniques reduced anxiety symptoms more effectively than treatment control conditions in older adults. Scogin and associates (1992) assessed the use of progressive muscle relaxation and imaginal relaxation, with mixed results. Both relaxation training groups showed improvements in state anxiety and anxiety symptoms after training, but there was no

significant improvement in state anxiety. In a 1-year follow-up assessment (Rickard et al. 1984) of older adults who had responded to relaxation training with a significant decrease in anxiety symptoms, the improvements from the pretraining assessment to the 1-year follow-up in state anxiety, trait anxiety, psychological symptoms, and relaxation level were all significant. Study participants also showed a nonsignificant trend of continuing treatment gains from posttreatment to 1-year follow-up. Given the small sample size of 26 study participants, these results indicate the possibility of promise in using relaxation strategies to treat distinct anxiety symptoms.

Relaxation training does have some advantages for treating mild anxiety in older adults. The strategies can be taught in brief individual or group sessions. Theoretically, the strategies can be delivered during a regular visit to a primary care physician. Like many behavioral strategies, relaxation training has the advantage of masquerading as skills training for patients who might avoid traditional psychotherapy. Also, patients with cognitive deficits, who may have difficulty with more cognitive strategies, may benefit from purely behavioral strategies.

CBT is a potentially useful treatment for anxiety symptoms. Unfortunately, the bulk of literature assessing CBT for anxiety in older adults describes case reports or suffers from problematic methodology. An exception is a randomized trial conducted by Barrowclough and colleagues (2001) comparing CBT and supportive counseling delivered in patients' homes for the treatment of anxiety symptoms in older adults (over age 55) who met criteria for a range of anxiety disorders. Despite a strong effort in the recruitment phase of this study, which originally identified 179 potentially eligible older adults, only 55 individuals qualified. Further attrition due to dropouts or changes in health status among study participants reduced the final sample to 33. Participants who received CBT showed significantly greater decreases in self-reported anxiety symptoms after treatment than did participants who received supportive counseling. Although the CBT participants also showed a stronger decreasing trend from posttreatment to 12-month follow-up in clinician-rated anxiety symptoms, the differences between the two treatment groups on this measure did not reach statistical significance ($P < 0.08$). At the 12-month follow-up, the number of participants in the CBT group who attained criteria for treatment response was significantly higher than in the supportive counseling group. Despite some of the weaknesses of this study, the results did support the efficacy of CBT for anxiety in older adults and did so in comparison to supportive counseling rather than a weaker treatment comparison, such as standard care.

Certainly, more empirical support is needed to establish the efficacy of CBT as a treatment for anxiety symptoms in older adults. Barrowclough and colleagues have shown at the very least that the use of CBT in an older population deserves further investigation.

Generalized Anxiety Disorder

Among older adults, generalized anxiety disorder (GAD) is the most commonly diagnosed anxiety disorder. Based on Epidemiological Catchment Area surveys, it is estimated that up to 1.9% of older adults currently experience GAD (Blazer et al. 1991). Although researchers tend to agree that rates of GAD are lower in older adults than in younger populations, several researchers have suggested that GAD is still underdiagnosed in this population (Fuentes and Cox 1997; Palmer et al. 1997; Stanley and Novy 2000). Diagnostic criteria for GAD in younger adults may fail to take into account different ways that older adults experience anxiety. Older adults may focus on different targets of worry and on somatic symptoms that can be confused with medical illness. Evidence also suggests that GAD often appears in conjunction with depressive symptoms, which confuse both diagnostic criteria and the focal point for treatment strategies. One study reported that 91% of individuals with GAD diagnoses also met criteria for depression (Lindesay et al. 1989). In a sample of older adults, 60% of those who met criteria for GAD also endorsed comorbid depressive episodes. The problems of variant symptom presentations, overemphasis on somatic symptoms, and depressive comorbidity create confusion in both diagnoses and treatment choices.

Given the issue of comorbidity with depression, the previously reported success of CBT in the treatment of depression in older adults makes it a logical area of treatment research for GAD in older adults. Because of the nature of CBT, this treatment will also theoretically expose a variety of cognitive patterns of worry regardless of content and the cognitive and behavioral antecedents that link anxiety to somatic symptoms. CBT appears to be the best-equipped form of psychotherapy to manage the diagnostic and treatment issues that exist in older populations with GAD. Treatment research on GAD in late life is limited. Not surprisingly, though, the bulk of this literature focuses on the efficacy of CBT in this population (Stanley and Novy 2000; Stanley et al. 1996; Stanley et al., in press; Wetherell et al. 2003).

In a randomized trial, Stanley et al. (2003) compared the efficacy of CBT to that of a minimal contact condition. The researchers' treatment protocol included education training, relaxation training, cognitive restructuring, and exposure to anxiety-provoking stimuli. Compared with the minimal contact condition, participation in CBT was associated with significantly greater improvements over time in GAD severity, anxiety, and depression. These marked improvements in depression and anxiety symptoms were demonstrated in both self-report measures and clinician ratings. CBT participants reported a significant within-group improvement in the severity of GAD symptoms from the point of their assessment immediately after the completion of the treatment protocol to an assessment 12 months after treatment completion. These findings suggest that CBT may not only provide effective immediate therapy but may also promote long-term gains in the management of GAD.

Because of the tendency for older adults to seek treatment for mental disorders in primary care facilities, current research is exploring an adaptation of CBT protocols that can be delivered in primary care. A pilot study by Stanley and associates (in press) presents a shortened CBT protocol for use in a primary care setting. This therapy was administered in eight sessions, either within the medical clinic or in the patients' homes. The treatment focused on six issues: education, relaxation training, cognitive therapy, problem-solving strategies, gradual exposure treatment, and sleep management. Further details may be found in the treatment manual (Stanley et al., in press). Compared with a usual-care control condition, CBT was associated with significant decreases in GAD severity, anxiety symptoms, and depression symptoms. Although the sample size was very small (N = 12), the positive results provide preliminary utility for the use of CBT in primary care settings.

Although CBT has strong promise for treating GAD in older adults, further empirical research must be conducted to verify its efficacy in this population. Adapting CBT to use in primary care facilities is a logical step that, it is hoped, will prove efficacious. Primary care treatment will provide treatment where older adults are most likely to look for it, and it facilitates collaboration between CBT therapists and prescription providers. This integration may also be a cost-effective treatment option, as has been the case in primary care psychotherapy for depression.

Substance Use Disorders

Limited research is available on the prevalence of substance use disorders in older people, much less on the treatment of substance use disorders. With the exception of alcohol use, most substance use in late life is thought to be an extension of substance use from earlier periods of life into late life (Oslin et al. 2000). Although medical comorbidity becomes an increasing factor in older adults, most substance use in late life is presumed to differ from younger populations' use more because of cohort differences than developmental differences. Treatment research on substance use in this population is nearly absent but is greatly needed.

The only substance whose use has been studied comprehensively in older adults is alcohol. Alcohol dependence is estimated to be lower in older adults than in younger cohorts. According to Epidemiological Catchment Area surveys, current alcohol dependence and abuse prevalence rates ranged from 1.4% in North Carolina to 3.7% in Maryland in adults over age 65 in comparison to a prevalence rate of 8.6% in all adult Americans (Adams et al. 1993). Regular alcohol use that falls below diagnostic criteria can still be problematic in older adults. Given the possibility of interactions with prescription medications and increased risk of physical illness, lower levels of alcohol can be potentially dangerous for older adults (Fingerhood 2000; Moore et al. 1999).

Research on effective therapy for alcohol-related disorders in older adults is sparse. In the review literature, standard treatment for older adults is to "mainstream" them into therapeutic groups for adults of any age, such as Alcoholics Anonymous. This treatment choice has not been empirically validated for older adults, and in fact some researchers suggest that older adults will demonstrate better treatment gains in peer support groups and age-specific treatment protocols (Dupree et al. 1984; Schonfeld et al. 2000).

Schonfeld and colleagues (2000) compared the success of veterans age 60 and above who completed a cognitive-behavioral treatment for substance abuse with veterans who dropped out of the treatment program. Although the dropouts do not constitute an unbiased treatment control comparison group, the dropouts do allow some level of comparison between those who received full treatment and those who did not. Of the 110 veterans who enrolled in the program, 61 dropped out. The treatment program consisted of 22 weekly group sessions, including components of health education, cognitive-behavioral treatment, and self-management strategies. The cognitive-behavioral and self-management strategies focused especially on identifying and managing situations that were risky for substance abuse, coping with depression and anxiety without substance abuse, and reestablishing goals after a relapse. Analysis found that the veterans who completed treatment were significantly more likely to have remained abstinent even after a brief relapse than were those who had dropped out of treatment.

Veterans who dropped out of treatment were more likely to have died, to have evaded location, or to have returned to substance abuse. This study has several limitations, including a lack of division between alcohol abuse and other substance abuse and a biased control comparison group. However, given the positive preliminary findings, especially in a difficult-to-treat population in which 34.2% were homeless, this study shows a clear incentive to investigate the use of age-specific cognitive-behavioral treatments for substance abuse in older adults.

As in other Axis I disorders such as depression and generalized anxiety disorder, brief interventions in primary care have received increasing attention for the treatment of alcohol use in older adults. Because primary care physicians are most likely to identify overuse of alcohol in their patients, this is a natural area in which to develop treatment protocols. In a recent study, adults age 65 and older either received a brief cognitive-behavioral intervention from their physician or just a general health booklet (Fleming et al. 1999). The intervention consisted of two 10- to 15-minute counseling sessions in which the physician discussed consequences of alcohol consumption and personal cues for alcohol consumption. The physician also instructed the patient to keep a diary card of his or her drinking behavior and made a drinking agreement with each patient to control his or her alcohol consumption. The researchers found that at 3-month and 12-month follow-ups, the patients who had received the intervention drank significantly less than those who received only a health booklet. Patients who participated in the intervention also had significantly less binge drinking and excessive drinking than those who did not receive the intervention.

The empirical studies described above provide groundwork for further research in this area. Age-specific cognitive-behavioral treatment techniques show promise for the treatment of alcohol abuse in older adults. One avenue of research might examine group interventions to take advantage of peer support, whereas a second avenue of research might investigate primary care interventions to take advantage of older adults' relationships with their physicians.

Axis II Disorders

According to the DSM-IV and DSM-IV-TR (American Psychiatric Association 1994, 2000), a personality disorder is an enduring pattern of inner experience (e.g., cognition, affect, impulse control) and behavior (e.g., interpersonal difficulties) that has an onset in adolescence or early adulthood, is stable over time, deviates considerably from normal cultural expectations, and causes distress or impairment in functioning. Although a recent meta-analysis concludes that rates of personality disorders among older adults are essentially equivalent to rates observed in younger age groups (Abrams and Horowitz 1999), others contend that rates of personality disorders decline over age (Solomon 1981; Tyrer 1988).

Growing empirical evidence suggests that elderly depressed patients with comorbid personality disorder are generally less responsive to treatment, including antidepressant medications and psychotherapy (Abrams 1996; Abrams et al. 1994; Pilkonis and Frank 1988; Thompson et al. 1988; Vine and Steingart 1994; also see Gradman et al. 1999 for a review). However, with the exception of case studies, no published outcome study has specifically focused on treating late-life personality disorders.

Gradman et al. (1999) reviewed seven treatment studies of older adults in which personality disorder was examined. However, only one of these studies included a randomized control. In their randomized, controlled trial, Thompson et al. (1988) examined 75 elderly outpatients who met diagnostic criteria for major depression. The researchers then compared the outcomes of short-term cognitive (Beck et al. 1979), behavioral (Lewinsohn et al. 1973), and psychodynamic therapy (Horowitz et al. 1980). Therapy sessions were held twice a week for the first 4 weeks and once a week for the remaining 16–20 sessions. Although it was not the specific focus of the study, the authors examined the effect of personality disorder on outcome using the Structured Interview for DSM-III Personality Disorders (Stangl et al. 1985). Results indicated that the likelihood of treatment failure was approximately four times greater for patients diagnosed with personality disorders (37%) than for those without (9.5%). In addition, the authors reported that individuals with passive-aggressive or compulsive personality disorders were more likely to experience treatment failure, whereas those with dependent or avoidant personality disorders were more likely to have their treatment succeed. A 2-year follow-up of this study concluded that patients with avoidant and mixed personality disorders were at a higher risk of relapse (Rose et al. 1991).

Methodological differences across studies also limit the ability to make strong conclusions. Treatments were often not clearly defined, standardized instruments varied across studies or were not used at all, and measures of treatment adherence were not obtained. Gradman et al. (1999) concluded that disorders such as dependent and avoidant personality disorder may respond better to treatment because patients with these disorders are more likely to comply with suggestions by the therapist and to

work in a collaborative way. However, as Morse and Lynch (2000) point out, rates of Cluster A disorders may be higher than previously thought among older adults, and consequently treatments that specifically target noncompliance may prove more relevant (e.g., DBT).

As mentioned above (see "Group Psychotherapy"), DBT has been successfully modified to treat depression in older adults using a group skills training format (Lynch et al. 2003). Extending this work, Lynch and colleagues at Duke University are examining DBT as a medication augmentation for depressed older adults with personality disorders. Patients are selected for depression and the presence of personality disorder pathology, are tested prospectively for lack of response to a selective serotonin reuptake inhibitor antidepressant, and are then randomized to treatments. Interestingly, to date 50% of participants randomized were assessed to have obsessive-compulsive personality disorder. At this time results are too premature for any definitive conclusions regarding treatments.

Treatments for Dementia

The development of psychosocial interventions for dementia is a complicated area of research. Unlike some of the other disorders discussed in this chapter, dementia is unlikely to remit as a result of psychotherapy. Researchers in this area have struggled to find distinct goals and outcomes to focus on. Because the dementia as a whole is not expected to abate, researchers have chosen specific variables to focus on in older adults with dementia, such as global quality of life, affective states, disruptive behavioral symptoms, functional impairment, and prevention of self-harm.

Another concern is whom to target in psychosocial interventions. Dementia is a disease with social consequences. The families of older adults with dementia gradually lose their loved ones to the disease and learn to cope with the demands of caring for an individual with dementia. In addition, individuals with dementia are also institutionalized. Consensus is lacking on what is the best program of care in an inpatient facility. For example, patients with dementia may cause social distress in patients without dementia but may also benefit from social contact with other patients (Lawton 1996). Because of the social impact of dementia, interventions for it may be delivered directly to treat the individual patient, to alter the individual's environment, or to help an individual's caregiver.

Because of the cognitive deterioration experienced, most empirical research on interventions for dementia is based on behavioral strategies. Numerous behavioral strategies have been tested for the management of dementia, but the goals have not been cohesive. Studies of psychosocial interventions can be categorized by the treatment outcome goals and by the intervention targets.

In one study of behavioral management, the patients' environment was altered but no therapeutic intervention was delivered to the individual patients (Dickinson et al. 1995). In this study, researchers targeted the behavior of leaving care wards because patients are at greater risk for injury outside their protected wards. When views of areas outside the wards were obscured using blinds and cloth coverings, patients were significantly less likely to try to exit their area than when these views were left uncovered. Inpatient care facilities as well as community caregivers could benefit from future research on environmental design strategies to manage patients' problem behaviors.

Cognitive symptoms such as disorientation and confusion can cause distress and injury in patients and increased stress in caregivers. One proposed psychotherapeutic technique to cope with the cognitive symptoms of dementia is reality orientation therapy. The purpose of this therapy is to continuously reorient patients' attention to the present situation and surroundings by repeating who they are and where they are. Reality orientation is often augmented by group classes that provide reorienting information. In a randomized treatment-control study, inpatients with Alzheimer's disease completed either a series of reality orientation therapy cycles or standard care (Zanetti et al. 1995). Patients who completed reality orientation therapy showed significantly better cognitive outcomes than those in the control condition at an 8-month checkpoint. However, participants in reality orientation therapy did not differ in terms of affect measures or decline in their ability to complete normal activities of daily living. One concern in the use of this therapy is that reality orientation may itself be distressing to confused patients. One patient in the treatment group did become emotionally distressed and was subsequently removed from the treatment protocol. In some patients, though, reality orientation may be a positive component to include in a wider behavioral treatment protocol to target cognitive decline in patients with dementia.

Individuals with dementia are often at risk for anxiety, depression, or other negative affective states. Successful treatments of noncognitive affective symptoms in dementia can be thought to have one of two goals: to increase positive affect or to decrease negative affect. Many of the treatments that have been proposed to promote positive experience in individuals with dementia, such as art therapy, music therapy, religious participation, or social participation, lack empirical validation (Lawton 1996). Treatment research on decreasing negative affective states, such as depression, has a stronger empirical base.

Certain behavioral therapies directly target depressive symptoms in patients. One such therapy was evaluated in a study by Teri and colleagues (1997). Two therapy protocols were assessed: behavior therapy with pleasant events and behavior therapy with problem solving. In both therapies, the therapists helped the caregiver develop behavioral strategies in response to the patient's behavior. Participants in the pleasant-events group were also encouraged to increase pleasant activities. Participants in the problem-solving group were taught systematic problem-solving strategies along with the behavior therapy. Immediately after treatment, there were no significant improvements. However, at 6 months, both therapy groups showed significant improvements over baseline measures in patients' depressive symptoms and patients' cognitive status scores. Both problem solving around problem behaviors and introducing more pleasant events into patients' experience may function as successful behavioral management strategies for depressive moods in patients with dementia.

Behavioral therapy in general has a strong history in controlling problem behaviors in patients, such as aggression or resistance. These therapies generally train those who care for the individuals with dementia—whether in the community or in inpatient facilities—to manage patient behavior using principles of operant conditioning. However, other treatments exist with a less clearly defined theoretical foundation and less empirical support.

One example of a popular, but not empirically well-validated therapy, is validation therapy. The premise of validation therapy is that patients who experience dementia use their remaining cognitive abilities to communicate with others. When communication efforts are validated through simple speech, empathetic voice tone, and attempts to reflect speech and behavior, the hypothesized result is a reduction in negative behavior and affect.

A nonrandomized example study that examined the use of validation therapy in a nursing home with a group of patients with dementia revealed only mildly positive effects (Toseland et al. 1997). After participation in a validation therapy group, nurses reported significant decreases in verbal and physical aggression. They also reported significantly greater confidence in their ability to manage problem behaviors. Similar results were obtained at 3- and 12-month follow-ups. According to ratings by trained observers, though, there was not a significant decrease in agitation or a significant increase in positive behavior. The researchers also compared validation therapy with a social contact control. Treatment gains from validation therapy were not significantly different from those found in the social contact condition. There is no strong support for validation therapy having greater efficacy than other interventions such as social support. However, validation therapy remains a popular therapeutic intervention in practical care.

Other behavioral strategies in which the caregivers receive training have produced more successful results. In a treatment efficacy study with Alzheimer's disease patients and their spouses (Bourgeois et al. 2002), 63 spousal caregivers were assigned to one of three test conditions: patient change, self-change, or control. Subjects in the patient-change group assessed individual problem behaviors in their spouses and then individually developed behavioral management strategies, such as distracting the patient or using physical prompts. The self-change intervention focused on teaching the caregivers specific strategies to manage personal stress, including increasing pleasant activities, enhancing problem-solving strategies, and practicing relaxation techniques. Patients whose spouses participated in the patient-change group showed a significant decrease in the frequency of problem behaviors from a pretreatment baseline to evaluations after treatment, at 3 months, and at 6 months. Both intervention groups showed significant decreases in aggressive behavior at 3 months and 6 months, as well as significant improvements in the caregivers' moods after treatment and at 6 months. These findings suggest that interventions for caregivers that combine self-care and behavioral management strategies might prove most effective.

Although different behavioral interventions have shown success in either promoting positive outcomes or decreasing negative outcomes, each intervention appears to target a limited number of symptoms experienced by patients with dementia. Further research should examine more comprehensive treatment interventions that take advantage of behavioral management through controlling the environment, delivering direct interventions to patients, and educating caregivers on how to use behavioral strategies to manage patient behavior. Comprehensive treatments may also contain different behavioral components that target different symptoms of dementia. For example, one intervention might include increasing pleasant events to reduce depression, reality orientation to increase cognitive function, and caregiver training to promote effective care for patients.

Conclusion

It is becoming increasingly evident that psychotherapy offers significant promise for the treatment of psychopathology in elderly persons and at times may be the treatment of choice in terms of both efficacy and patient preference. We encourage practitioners to select treatments

that have been tested using randomized clinical trials not based on theoretical preference or ease of application. Use of treatments without this type of empirical support can slow or reduce recovery. For example, reminiscence, life review, and bibliotherapy have readily apparent face validity. Yet, research to date has failed to support the use of these therapies in isolation.

Future research should continue to examine the beneficial effects of strategies combining medication and psychotherapy. In addition, research examining the mechanisms of change and issues associated with treatment response by disorder and type of therapy remain to be more fully developed. Finally, continued research needs to focus on populations with treatment-resistant illness (e.g., personality disorders and comorbid disorders).

References

Abrahams RB, Patterson RD: Psychological distress among the community elderly: prevalence, characteristics and implications for service. Int J Aging Hum Dev 9:1–18, 1978

Abrams RC: Personality disorders in the elderly. Int J Geriatr Psychiatry 11:759–763, 1996

Abrams RC, Horowitz SV: Personality disorders after age 50: a meta-analytic review of the literature, in Personality Disorders in Older Adults: Emerging Issues in Diagnosis and Treatment. Edited by Rosowsky E, Abrams RC. Mahwah, NJ, Erlbaum, 1999, pp 55–68

Abrams RC, Rosendahl E, Card C, et al: Personality disorder correlates of late and early onset depression. J Am Geriatr Soc 42:727–731, 1994

Adams WL, Yuan Z, Barboriak JJ, et al: Alcohol-related hospitalizations of elderly people: prevalence and geographic variation in the United States. JAMA 270:1222–1225, 1993

Allen R, Walker Z, Shergill P, et al: Attitudes to depression in hospital inpatients: a comparison between older and younger subjects. Aging Ment Health 2:36–39, 1998

American Psychiatric Association: Diagnostic and Statistical Manual of Mental Disorders, 4th Edition. Washington, DC, American Psychiatric Association, 1994

American Psychiatric Association: Diagnostic and Statistical Manual of Mental Disorders, 4th Edition, Text Revision. Washington, DC, American Psychiatric Association, 2000

Andrews HB: The myth of the scientist-practitioner: a reply. Aust Psychol 35:60–63, 1998

Arean PA, Perri MG, Nezu AM, et al: Comparative effectiveness of social problem-solving therapy and reminiscence therapy as treatments for depression in older adults. J Consult Clin Psychol 61:1003–1010, 1993

Babyak M, Blumenthal JA, Herman S, et al: Exercise treatment for major depression: maintenance of therapeutic benefit at 10 months. Psychosom Med 62:633–638, 2000

Barber JP, DeRubeis RJ: On second thought: where the action is in cognitive therapy for depression. Cognit Ther Res 13:441–457, 1989

Barrowclough C, King P, Colville J, et al: A randomized trial of the effectiveness of cognitive-behavioral therapy and supportive counseling for anxiety symptoms in older adults. J Consult Clin Psychol 69:756–762, 2001

Beck AT, Rush AJ, Shaw BF, et al: Cognitive Therapy of Depression. New York, Guilford, 1979

Beutler LE: David and Goliath: when empirical and clinical standards of practice meet. Am Psychol 55:997–1007, 2000

Beutler LE: The dodo bird is extinct. Clinical Psychology Science and Practice 9:30–34, 2002

Beutler LE, Scogin F, Kirkish P, et al: Group cognitive therapy and alprazolam in the treatment of depression in older adults. J Consult Clin Psychol 55:550–556, 1987

Bibring E: The problem of depression. Psyche 6:81–101, 1952

Biglan A: Distressed behavior and its context. Behav Anal 14:157–169, 1991

Blazer D, George LK, Hughes D: The epidemiology of anxiety disorders: an age comparison, in Anxiety in the Elderly: Treatment and Research. Edited by Salzman C, Lebowitz BD. New York, Springer, 1991, pp 17–30

Blumenthal JAP, Babyak MAP, Moore KAP, et al: Effects of exercise training on older patients with major depression. Arch Intern Med 159:2349–2356, 1999

Bourgeois MS, Schulz R, Burgio LD, et al: Skills training for spouses of patients with Alzheimer's disease: outcomes of an intervention study. Journal of Clinical Geropsychology 8:53–73, 2002

Brand E, Clingempeel WG: Group behavioral therapy with depressed geriatric inpatients: an assessment of incremental efficacy. Behav Ther 23:475–482, 1992

Burns D: Feeling Good. New York, New American Library, 1980

Chambless DL: Beware the dodo bird: the dangers of overgeneralization. Clinical Psychology Science and Practice 9:13–16, 2002

Chambless DL, Ollendick TH: Empirically supported psychological interventions: controversies and evidence. Annu Rev Psychol 52:685–716, 2001

Coyne JC: Depression and the response of others. J Abnorm Psychol 85:186–193, 1976

DeBerry S: The effects of meditation-relaxation on anxiety and depression in a geriatric population. Psychotherapy: Theory, Research and Practice 19:512–521, 1982a

DeBerry S: An evaluation of progressive muscle relaxation on stress related symptoms in a geriatric population. Int J Aging Hum Dev 14:255–269, 1982b

Dickinson JI, McLain-Kark J, Marshall-Baker A: The effects of visual barriers on exiting behavior in a dementia care unit. Gerontologist 35:127–130, 1995

Dougher MJ, Hackbert L: A behavior-analytic account of depression and a case report using acceptance-based procedures. Behav Anal 17:321–334, 1994

Dupree LW, Broskowski H, Schonfeld LI: The Gerontology Alcohol Project: a behavioral treatment program for elderly alcohol abusers. Gerontologist 24:510–516, 1984

Fingerhood M: Substance abuse in older people. J Am Geriatr Soc 48:985–995, 2000

Fleming MFM, Manwell LB, Barry KLP, et al: Brief physician advice for alcohol problems in older adults: a randomized community-based trial. J Fam Pract 48:378–384, 1999

Flint AJ: Epidemiology and comorbidity of anxiety disorders in the elderly. Am J Psychiatry 15:640–649, 1994

Floyd M, Scogin F: Cognitive-behavior therapy for older adults: how does it work? Psychotherapy 35:459–463, 1998

Frank E, Spanier C: Interpersonal psychotherapy for depression: overview, clinical efficacy, and future directions. Clinical Psychology Science and Practice 2:349–369, 1995

Frank E, Frank N, Cornes C, et al: Interpersonal psychotherapy in the treatment of late-life depression, in New Applications of Interpersonal Psychotherapy. Edited by Klerman GL, Weissman MM. Washington, DC, American Psychiatric Press, 1993, pp 167–198

Friedhoff AJ: Consensus Development Conference statement: diagnosis and treatment of depression in late life, in Diagnosis and Treatment of Depression in Late Life: Results of the NIH Consensus Development Conference. Edited by Schneider LSM, Reynolds CF III, Lebowitz BD, et al. Washington, DC, American Psychiatric Press, 1994, pp 491–511

Fry PS: Structured and unstructured reminiscence training and depression among the elderly. Clin Gerontol 1:15–37, 1983

Fuentes K, Cox BJ: Prevalence of anxiety disorders in elderly adults: a critical analysis. J Behav Ther Exp Psychiatry 28:269–279, 1997

Gallagher DE, Thompson LW: Treatment of major depressive disorder in older adult outpatients with brief psychotherapies. Psychotherapy: Theory, Research and Practice 19:482–490, 1982

Gallagher-Thompson D, Steffen AM: Comparative effects of cognitive-behavioral and brief psychodynamic psychotherapies for depressed family caregivers. J Consult Clin Psychol 62:543–549, 1994

Gallagher-Thompson D, Hanley-Peterson P, Thompson LW: Maintenance of gains versus relapse following brief psychotherapy for depression. J Consult Clin Psychol 58:371–374, 1990

Goldfried MR, Castonguay LG, Hayes AM, et al: A comparative analysis of the therapeutic focus in cognitive-behavioral and psychodynamic-interpersonal sessions. J Consult Clin Psychol 65:740–748, 1997

Goldfried MR, Raue PJ, Castonguay LG: The therapeutic focus in significant sessions of master therapists: a comparison of cognitive-behavioral and psychodynamic-interpersonal interventions. J Consult Clin Psychol 66:803–810, 1998

Gortner ET, Gollan JK, Dobson KS, et al: Cognitive-behavioral treatment for depression: relapse prevention. J Consult Clin Psychol 66:377–384, 1998

Gradman TJ, Thompson LW, Gallagher-Thompson D: Personality disorders and treatment outcome, in Personality Disorders in Older Adults: Emerging Issues in Diagnosis and Treatment. Edited by Rosowsky E, Abrams RC. Mahwah, NJ, Erlbaum, 1999, pp 69–94

Hayes AM, Castonguay LG, Goldfried MR: Effectiveness of targeting the vulnerability factors of depression in cognitive therapy. J Consult Clin Psychol 64:623–627, 1996

Hegel MTP, Barrett JE, Cornell JE, et al: Predictors of response to problem solving treatment of depression in primary care. Behav Ther 33:511–527, 2002a

Hegel MT, Imming J, Cyr-Provost M, et al: Role of allied behavioral health professionals in a collaborative stepped care treatment model for depression in primary care: Project IMPACT. Families, Systems and Health 20:265–277, 2002b

Hinrichsen GA: Interpersonal psychotherapy for depressed older adults. J Geriatr Psychiatry 30:239–257, 1997

Horowitz MJ, Wilner N, Kaltreider N, et al: Signs and symptoms of posttraumatic stress disorder. Arch Gen Psychiatry 37:85–92, 1980

Horvath AO, Symonds BD: Relation between working alliance and outcome in psychotherapy: a meta-analysis. J Couns Psychol 38:139–149, 1991

Jacobson NS, Dobson KS, Truax PA, et al: A component analysis of cognitive-behavioral treatment for depression. J Consult Clin Psychol 64:295–304, 1996

Jamison C, Scogin F: The outcome of cognitive bibliotherapy with depressed adults. J Consult Clin Psychol 63:644–650, 1995

Jarvik LF, Mintz J, Steuer JL, et al: Treating geriatric depression: a 26-week interim analysis. J Am Geriatr Soc 30:713–717, 1982

Kernberg OF: Technical considerations in the treatment of borderline personality organization. J Am Psychoanal Assoc 24:795–829, 1976

Klein DF: Dodo deliberations. Clinical Psychology Science and Practice 9:28–29, 2002

Klein M: The origins of transference. Int J Psychoanal 33:433–438, 1952

Klerman GL, Weissman MM, Rounsaville BJ, et al: Interpersonal Psychotherapy of Depression. New York, Basic Books, 1984

Koder DA, Brodaty H, Anstey KJ: Cognitive therapy for depression in the elderly. Int J Geriatr Psychiatry 11:97–107, 1996

Kohut H, Wolf ES: The disorders of the self and their treatment: an outline. Int J Psychoanal 59:413–425, 1978

Lawton MP: Behavioral problems and interventions in Alzheimer's disease: research needs. Int Psychogeriatr 8:95–98, 1996

Lewinsohn PM, Lobitz WC, Wilson S: "Sensitivity" of depressed individuals to aversive stimuli. J Abnorm Psychol 81:259–263, 1973

Lindesay J, Briggs K, Murphy E: The Guy's/Age Concern Survey: prevalence rates of cognitive impairment, depression and anxiety in an urban elderly community. Br J Psychiatry 155:317–329, 1989

Linehan MM: Cognitive-behavioral treatment of borderline personality disorder. New York, Guilford, 1993

Luborsky L, Rosenthal R, Diguer L, et al: The dodo bird verdict is alive and well—mostly. Clinical Psychology Science and Practice 9:2–12, 2002

Lynch TR, Morse JQ, Mendelson T, et al: Dialectical behavior therapy for depressed older adults: a randomized pilot study. Am J Geriatr Psychiatry 11:33–45, 2003

Mahler MS: On child psychosis and schizophrenia: autistic and symbiotic infantile psychoses. Psychoanal Study Child 7:286–305, 1952

Malik M, Alimohamed S, Holoway R, et al: Are all cognitive therapies alike? Validation of the TPRS. Paper presented at the 31st Annual Meeting of the Society for Psychotherapy Research, Chicago, IL, June 21–25, 2000

Martin DJ, Garske JP, Davis MK: Relation of the therapeutic alliance with outcome and other variables: a meta-analytic review. J Consult Clin Psychol 68:438–450, 2000

Messer SB, Wampold BE: Let's face facts: common factors are more potent than specific therapy ingredients. Clinical Psychology Science and Practice 9:21–25, 2002

Moore AA, Morton SC, Beck JC, et al: A new paradigm for alcohol use in older persons. Med Care 37:165–179, 1999

Morse JQ, Lynch TR: Personality disorders in late-life. Curr Psychiatry Rep 2:24–31, 2000

Mynors-Wallis LM: Pharmacotherapy is more effective than psychotherapy for elderly people with minor depression or dysthymia. Evidence-Based Healthcare 5:61, 2001

Nezu AM: A problem-solving formulation of depression: a literature review and proposal of a pluralistic model. Clin Psychol Rev 7:121–144, 1987

O'Rourke N, Hadjistavropoulos T: The relative efficacy of psychotherapy in the treatment of geriatric depression. Aging Ment Health 1:305–310, 1997

Oslin DW, Katz IR, Edell WS, et al: Effects of alcohol consumption on the treatment of depression among elderly patients. Am J Geriatr Psychiatry 8:215–220, 2000

Palmer BW, Jeste DV, Sheikh JI: Anxiety disorders in the elderly: DSM-IV and other barriers to diagnosis and treatment. J Affect Disord 46:183–190, 1997

Perrotta P, Meacham JA: Can a reminiscing intervention alter depression and self-esteem? Int J Aging Hum Dev 14:23–30, 1982

Pilkonis PA, Frank E: Personality pathology in recurrent depression: Nature, prevalence, and relationship to treatment response. Am J Psychiatry 145:435–441, 1988

Regier DA, Boyd JH, Burke JD, et al: One-month prevalence of mental disorders in the United States: based on five epidemiologic catchment area sites. Arch Gen Psychiatry 45:977–986, 1988

Reynolds CF 3rd, Frank E, Perel JM, et al: Combined pharmacotherapy and psychotherapy in the acute and continuation treatment of elderly patients with recurrent major depression: a preliminary report. Am J Psychiatry 149:1687–1692, 1992

Reynolds CF 3rd, Frank E, Perel JM, et al: Treatment of consecutive episodes of major depression in the elderly. Am J Psychiatry 151:1740–1743, 1994

Reynolds CF 3rd, Frank E, Houck PR, et al: Which elderly patients with remitted depression remain well with continued interpersonal psychotherapy after discontinuation of antidepressant medication? Am J Psychiatry 154:958–962, 1997

Reynolds CF 3rd, Frank E, Perel JM, et al: Nortriptyline and interpersonal psychotherapy as maintenance therapies for recurrent major depression: a randomized controlled trial in patients older than 59 years. JAMA 281:39–45, 1999

Rickard HC, Scogin F, Keith S: A one-year follow-up of relaxation training for elders with subjective anxiety. Gerontologist 34:121–122, 1984

Rokke PD, Scogin F: Depression treatment preferences in younger and older adults. Journal of Clinical Geropsychology 1:243–257, 1995

Rokke PD, Tomhave JA, Jocic Z: The role of client choice and target selection in self-management therapy for depression in older adults. Psychol Aging 14:155–169, 1999

Rose J, Schwarz M, Steffen AM, et al: Personality disorder and outcome in the treatment of depressed elders: two year follow-up. Poster presented at the 44th Annual Conference of the Gerontological Society of America, San Francisco, CA, November 22–26, 1991

Rounsaville BJ, Carroll KM: Commentary on dodo bird revisited: why aren't we dodos yet? Clinical Psychology Science and Practice 9:17–20, 2002

Schonfeld L, Dupree LW, Dickson-Fuhrmann E, et al: Cognitive-behavioral treatment of older veterans with substance abuse problems. J Geriatr Psychiatry Neurol 13:124–129, 2000

Scogin F, McElreath L: Efficacy of psychosocial treatments for geriatric depression: a quantitative review. J Consult Clin Psychol 62:69–73, 1994

Scogin F, Hamblin D, Beutler L: Bibliotherapy for depressed older adults: a self-help alternative. Gerontologist 27:383–387, 1987

Scogin F, Jamison C, Gochneaur K: Comparative efficacy of cognitive and behavioral bibliotherapy for mildly and moderately depressed older adults. J Consult Clin Psychol 57:403–407, 1989

Scogin F, Jamison C, Davis N: Two-year follow-up of bibliotherapy for depression in older adults. J Consult Clin Psychol 58:665–667, 1990

Scogin F, Rickard HC, Keith S, et al: Progressive and imaginal relaxation training for elderly persons with subjective anxiety. Psychol Aging 7:419–424, 1992

Sloane RB, Staples FR, Schneider LSM: Interpersonal therapy versus nortriptyline for depression in the elderly: case reports and discussion, in Clinical and Pharmacological Studies of Psychiatric Disorders. Edited by Burrows G, Norman TR, Dennerstein L. London, John Libbey, 1985, pp 344–346

Solomon K: Personality disorders and the elderly, in Personality Disorders: Diagnosis and Management. Edited by Lion JR. Baltimore, MD, Williams & Wilkins, 1981, pp 310–338

Stangl D, Pfohl B, Zimmerman M, et al: A structured interview for the DSM-III personality disorders—a preliminary report. Arch Gen Psychiatry 42:591–596, 1985

Stanley MA, Novy DM: Cognitive-behavior therapy for generalized anxiety in late life: an evaluative overview. J Anxiety Disord 14:191–207, 2000

Stanley MA, Beck JG, Glassco JD: Treatment of generalized anxiety in older adults: a preliminary comparison of cognitive-behavioral and supportive approaches. Behav Ther 27:565–581, 1996

Stanley MA, Roberts RE, Bourland SL, et al: Anxiety disorders among older primary care patients. Journal of Clinical Geropsychology 7:105–116, 2001

Stanley MA, Beck JG, Novy DM, et al: Cognitive behavioral treatment of late-life generalized anxiety disorder. J Consult Clin Psychol 71:309–319, 2003

Stanley MA, Diefenbach GJ, Hopko DR: Cognitive behavioral treatment for older adults with generalized anxiety disorder: a therapist manual for primary care settings. Behav Modif (in press)

Steuer JL: Cognitive-behavioral and psychodynamic group psychotherapy in treatment of geriatric depression. J Consult Clin Psychol 52:180–189, 1984

Strupp HH, Binder J: Psychotherapy in a New Key. New York, Basic Books, 1984

Svartberg M, Stiles TC: Comparative effects of short-term psychodynamic psychotherapy: a meta-analysis. J Consult Clin Psychol 59:704–714, 1991

Teasdale JD, Moore RG, Hayhurst H, et al: Metacognitive awareness and prevention of relapse in depression: empirical evidence. J Consult Clin Psychol 70:275–287, 2002

Teri L, Logsdon RG, Uomoto J, et al: Behavioral treatment of depression in dementia patients: a controlled clinical trial. J Gerontol B Psychol Sci Soc Sci 52:P159–P166, 1997

Thompson LW, Gallagher D: Efficacy of psychotherapy in the treatment of late-life depression. Advances in Behaviour Research and Therapy 6:127 139, 1984

Thompson LW, Gallagher D, Breckenridge JS: Comparative effectiveness of psychotherapies for depressed elders. J Consult Clin Psychol 55:385–390, 1987

Thompson LW, Gallagher D, Czirr R: Personality disorder and outcome in the treatment of late-life depression. J Geriatr Psychiatry 21:133–146, 1988

Thompson LW, Coon DW, Gallagher-Thompson D, et al: Comparison of desipramine and cognitive/behavioral therapy in the treatment of elderly outpatients with mild-to-moderate depression. Am J Geriatr Psychiatry 9:225–240, 2001

Toseland RW, Diehl M, Freeman K, et al: The impact of validation group therapy on nursing home residents with dementia. J Appl Gerontol 16:31–50, 1997

Tyrer P: Personality Disorders: Diagnosis, Management and Course. Kent, England, Wright/Butterworth Scientific, 1988

Unutzer JM, Katon WM, Williams JWJ, et al: Improving primary care for depression in late life: the design of a multicenter randomized trial. Med Care 39:785–799, 2001

Vine RG, Steingart AB: Personality disorder in the elderly depressed. Can J Psychiatry 39:392–398, 1994

Vitt CM, Idler EL, Leventhal H, et al: Attitudes toward treatment and help-seeking preferences in an elderly sample. Poster presented at the 52nd Annual Meeting of the Gerontological Society of America, San Francisco, CA, November 19–23, 1999

Weissman MM, Myers JK, Thompson WD: Depression and its treatment in a U.S. urban community—1975–1976. Arch Gen Psychiatry 38:417–421, 1981

Wetherell JL, Gatz M, Craske MG: Treatment of generalized anxiety disorder in older adults. J Consult Clin Psychol 71:31–40, 2003

Williams JW Jr, Barrett J, Oxman T, et al: Treatment of dysthymia and minor depression in primary care: a randomized controlled trial in older adults. JAMA 284:1519–1526, 2000

Zanetti O, Frisoni GB, De Leo D, et al: Reality orientation therapy in Alzheimer disease: useful or not? a controlled study. Alzheimer Dis Assoc Disord 9:132–138, 1995

Working With the Family of the Older Adult

Lisa P. Gwyther, M.S.W.

When you have worked with one family of an older adult, you have worked with one family of an older adult. It is axiomatic that individuals and families become more diverse as they age. Given this heterogeneity and the need for individualized family assessment and treatment, no single model exists for working with families of older adults. Despite the need for family-specific treatment, there are patterns of family issues based on consistent trajectories of psychiatric illness. Perhaps the most specific guidance in the literature comes from clinical research on families of older adults with progressive degenerative dementias (Haley 1997; Mittelman et al. 2002).

Over the course of an older adult's degenerative dementia, families will confront depression, delusions, agitation, behavioral changes, and other psychiatric symptoms in their cognitively impaired relatives (Lyketsos et al. 2000; Olin et al. 2002; Tractenberg et al. 2002). The burden on the family can be great, information can be insufficient, and doubt can be overwhelming (Gwyther 2000). Families caring for older members with dementia need reminders from psychiatrists to focus on maintaining family quality of life as well as quality of care within the constraints imposed by psychiatric, functional, and behavioral changes (Hughes et al. 1999).

This chapter takes a chronological approach to working with families over the course of the dementia of an older adult. Dementias are the focus because of ample evidence that dementia is more disruptive of family life, more likely to result in negative mental health outcomes

for family caregivers (especially females), and more likely to limit the patient's independent decision-making capacity compared with family care for other chronic conditions of late life (Ory et al. 1999). Compared with family caregivers of older adults with normal cognition, family caregivers of older adults with Alzheimer's disease spend more hours per week providing care, with measurable negative impacts on caregivers' mental health, personal and family time (Langa et al. 2001), and family relationships. Psychiatrists working with families of persons with dementia should expect to treat vulnerable primary family caregivers as well as families in conflict.

Family Care for Older Adults With Dementia

Older adults with dementia are cared for first by an available spouse (primarily in Caucasian families), next by a daughter or daughter-in-law, and (more commonly in African American families) by a network of extended kin. Families provide the bulk of care over the course of a dementia (Rabins 1998). The estimated value of that care soars above national spending for nursing home care and home health care combined (Arno et al. 1999). Half of family caregivers live with the older adult over a disease course of 3–20 years. Despite the high rates of shared

I gratefully acknowledge support for preparing this manuscript from grant 5P50 AG0 5128 from the National Institute on Aging to the Joseph and Kathleen Bryan Alzheimer's Disease Research Center at Duke University Medical Center and from grant 5R01 AG19605, "Stress, Serotonin Genes and Health Disparities," from the National Institute on Aging to the Duke University Behavioral Medicine Research Center.

residence, increasing evidence suggests that 20% of older adults with moderate to severe dementia live alone, often with extensive supervision and assistance from local and long-distance family caregivers.

Certain trends emerge from studies of family care in dementia. First, dementia family care is an increasingly common experience for families as older adults become more likely to survive to the age of greatest risk for dementia. A shift is occurring away from the direct provision of care by families toward more long-distance care or family care coordination. Dementia care may precipitate moves by retired adult children or a move by the older person to be closer to adult children. More female family caregivers are employed full- or part-time, and employment appears to have unanticipated benefits as well as commonly assumed burdens associated with role overload. Dementia care frequently precipitates the family's first experience seeking help from public or private agencies and even from other family members. Finally, increasing evidence shows that the lack of an affordable, available long-term-care system is pushing the limits of family capacity and solidarity.

Family care is universally preferred, based in strong family values that cross cultural and ethnic lines. Yet exclusive reliance on family care has well-documented social costs. Family caregivers may become overwhelmed, exhausted, depressed, or anxious. Many family caregivers report loss of pleasure, motivation, friends, activities, privacy, intimacy, or identity. Gradual and sometimes sudden loss of the person as he or she once was can precipitate significant anticipatory grief in older adults with dementia and their family members.

Research even documents that premature death is associated with spousal caregiver strain in the care of persons with Alzheimer's disease, suggesting an urgent public health preventive or protective focus for work with spouses of older adults with dementia (Schulz and Beach 1999).

Despite this apparent investment of families in care for older adults, family care is not necessarily synonymous with adequate, effective, or quality care. Inadequate family care may result in a family that has exceeded its knowledge or tolerance limits. For example, some families never comprehend minimal safety risks associated with dementia care. Elder mistreatment—whether abuse or passive or active neglect—may be associated with exceeding these family limits (American Medical Association 1999). Families may feel powerless and overwhelmed when they cannot predictably control the symptoms and course of dementia. The role of the psychiatrist with the family becomes one of assessment of tolerance limits, education, treatment of psychiatric

consequences of caregiver burden, and management of family expectations of the disease course and of themselves.

Despite a research focus on primary family caregivers, multiple family members are affected by dementia in one member. Often a change in primary caregiver occurs when a spouse dies or when siblings pass a cognitively impaired parent among themselves in a futile attempt to equalize responsibility. Children and teenagers living with an impaired parent or grandparent may react with school problems or behavioral changes.

Increasing dependency, loss, and grief are realities of family care in Alzheimer's disease, but not all family outcomes are negative or burdensome. Although depression is the most frequently reported psychiatric symptom among caregivers of Alzheimer's disease patients, some families express pride in their care as a legacy of commitment to family values. Despite some family caregivers' reports of feeling misunderstood or unappreciated, other families report deriving a sense of meaning in living up to obligations (Noonan and Tennstedt 1997).

The following clinical reminders about family care may prove useful in working with families of older adults:

1. Family care is an adaptive challenge: the family is not necessarily the problem, nor is the family necessarily the obstacle to effective care. Few incentives (financial, religious, or counseling) will make an unwilling family assume care. The reverse is equally true. Few disincentives will keep a determined spouse or child from honoring his or her commitment.
2. The family is rarely one voice. Different perceptions and expectations of close and distant family members frequently precipitate family conflict. There is no perfectly fair and equal division of family care responsibility. Families can expect a permanent imbalance in the normal give and take of family relationships while working toward a more equitable sharing of responsibility.
3. Few families have the luxury of one person needing care at a time. There is much less manipulation by dependent elders than there are real unmet dependency needs. There is more underreporting of burden and underutilization of services than the reverse.
4. There is no one right or ideal way or place to offer family care. Many families are forced to choose between equally unacceptable options. Successful family caregivers gather information, take direct action when possible, and often reframe things they cannot change in more positive terms. ("It could be worse—at least she is still with me.")

5. Successful family caregivers are flexible in adjusting expectations of themselves, of the older adult, and of other family members to fit the needs and capacities of all. Coping with family care is facilitated by a sense of humor; a strong faith, belief, or value system; creativity; practical problem-solving skills; and emotional support from other family members or friends.

6. Families caring for older adults with dementia must define and negotiate complex situations, perform physically intimate tasks, manage emotions and communication, modify expectations, and capitalize on the older adult's preserved capacities.

7. A family caregiver's knowledge of an available service, need for the service, and access to the service do not necessarily lead to appropriate and timely use of that service.

8. There is no perfect control in a family care situation. Families are better off if they work on their reactions to stress or lack of control.

9. Denial is a common defense of family caregivers. Some people need to deny the inevitable outcome (loss of a beloved spouse or eventual placement of a parent in a nursing home) to provide hopeful, consistent daily care.

10. A primary caregiver at home is efficient and preferred. Primary caregivers need breaks and backup people and services to supplement their personalized care. Even in ideal situations, contingency plans are necessary.

Goals in Working With Families of Older Adults

Clinical goals with families of older adults will vary with presenting problems and family resources. Common goals in working with families of older adults with dementia are to normalize variability, to address safety and security issues, to mobilize secondary family support, to facilitate appropriate decision making at care transitions, and to help family members accept help or let go of direct care as necessary. In essence, the family is forced to adapt to a new normal in family life, often with active resistance from the member with dementia. Well-timed psychiatric help in interpreting the family's and the elder's reluctance to accept new realities can promote appropriate decision making.

Other goals in working with family caregivers include treatment of affective, substance abuse, and anxiety disorders of the caregiver and individual or family treatment

around issues of grief, loss, or conflict in family relationships that limit the effectiveness of care. In general, family work should enhance the effectiveness of family care and coping, enhance the self-efficacy of caregivers (Fortinsky 2002a), and enhance the family's satisfaction with their preferred levels of involvement.

Psychiatrists working with family caregivers over time will monitor the quality of family care; the mental health, capacity, and vulnerability of caregivers; and the impact of the demands of care on family relationships (Yates et al. 1999). Psychiatrists should be especially alert to escalating anxiety, self-neglect, suicidal ideation, depression, or anger in caregivers and abuse or neglect of the patient. These indications should prompt immediate recommendations for treatment, respite, or relinquishment of primary care responsibility. Negative caregiver outcomes on which to focus therapeutic efforts include decrements in mental health, social participation, and personal or family time and loss of privacy.

Interdisciplinary Partnerships

Focused work with families of older adults holds great potential for positive outcomes, particularly in the context of an interdisciplinary partnership or team (Fortinsky 2002b). Research suggests that social workers' individual and family counseling with family caregivers can mobilize and sustain community and secondary family support, reduce primary caregiver depression, and even delay nursing home placement (Mittelman et al. 1996).

Psychiatrists may work collaboratively with social workers or nurses. These mental health professionals can provide sustained or timely assistance at care transitions. The psychiatrist's role is to assess and treat a family caregiver's psychiatric illness and to treat the cognitively impaired patient's psychiatric symptoms. The social worker or nurse may provide care coordination or case management, monitoring family capacity and tolerance while educating the family about common symptoms and care transitions over time.

Some families will resist referrals to social workers. These families may respond to descriptions of the social worker as an expert consumer guide or family consultant. A family consultant can offer assessment and intervention as well as information. Families can learn from family consultants how to be their own case managers with minimal professional support at key care transitions. The family consultant at any one time may be a teacher, coach, advocate, counselor, cheerleader, peer, or support person who can provide energy and a fresh perspective to promote family resilience.

Referrals to well-developed and validated psychoedu-cational group treatment programs have demonstrated equally positive results (Ostwald et al. 1999). Participation in peer counseling or support groups can have positive outcomes for active caregiver participants (Pillemer and Suitor 1996).

Another way to monitor goals in the psychiatric treatment of families of older adults is to base treatment on known precipitants of nursing home placement resulting from the breakdown of family care. Major precipitants of placement include both patient and caregiver factors (Yaffe et al. 2002). One of the patient factors that strongly predicts placement is disruptive psychiatric and behavioral symptoms. Changes in behavior and personality are also major causes of caregiver burden and depression. To the extent that psychiatric consultation is available to the older adult for treatment of psychiatric symptoms and to the extent the family can be taught nonpharmacological approaches (see Chapter 23, "Agitation and Suspiciousness"), the health of the family and caregivers and effective home care for the older adult can be preserved.

Other predictors of family care breakdown are affective, substance abuse, or anxiety disorders of the primary caregiver and unresolved family conflict, all of which are amenable to psychiatric treatment of families of older adults. Treating depression in a family caregiver generally has a positive impact on the mood, function, and behavior of the cognitively impaired older adult (Brodaty and Luscombe 1998), and the reverse is equally true.

The Family as Information Seeker

Families are more likely than older adults with dementia to initiate and seek psychiatric care throughout the course of the illness. The stigma of psychiatric illness often delays psychiatric diagnosis, and ethnic and cultural beliefs that equate cognitive decline with normal aging can produce the same result. Psychiatrists must remind families that a specific diagnosis suggests treatment options. Stigma is best addressed by correcting misconceptions or lack of information. An unconvinced family can be told that Alzheimer's disease is a brain disorder that can and does happen to anyone. The brain becomes the vulnerable organ in dementia, and psychiatric symptoms are brain symptoms just as angina is a symptom of a heart disorder. When damaged, both organs require special diagnosis and care.

Many family caregivers do not seek a diagnosis until the patient's psychiatric symptoms (such as suspiciousness) or the patient's personality changes (such as uncharacteristic irritability) disrupt family life. Unfortunately, the patient is most likely to resist an evaluation once psychiatric and behavioral symptoms are present, and psychiatrists are understandably reluctant to talk to family members without the consent of the patient. An evaluation can be facilitated if the psychiatrist agrees to see the older adult about a less threatening symptom such as headaches, loss of interest, or low energy.

Diagnostic Office Visits

Although the older adult is entitled to initial time alone with the psychiatrist, later time alone with family informants will be invaluable to the psychiatrist in assessing the impact of functional loss and other family stressors. Most family caregivers prefer to talk privately with the psychiatrist to avoid confronting the older adult with his or her symptoms or decline. It may be helpful to have two family members accompany the patient for an evaluation. One family member can distract or sit with the older adult while another family member has a private conversation with the psychiatrist.

Initial Communication With Older Adults and Their Families

Initial communication with older adults diagnosed with dementia and their families will be in response to common emotional reactions to a degenerative diagnosis. Elders and family members may express doubts about the diagnosis. Rather than confront the doubt and denial, it is often more helpful to suggest that the family behave as if the diagnosis of Alzheimer's disease had been confirmed while awaiting confirmation based on progression. Asking directly about common early changes such as difficulty handling money or increased irritability may highlight expectable changes and offer a preview of psychiatric expertise. Sometimes, explanations of apathy and loss of executive function help families understand why efforts to get the elder to try harder to function effectively may prove frustrating and futile.

Initial family sessions often elicit fear from both elders and family caregivers. Elders may express fears of embarrassment, loss of control, and abandonment. Family members may fear for their interdependent future or genetic risk. A psychiatrist's offer of active symptom treatment, regular monitoring, and willingness to see the family through the illness is always appreciated. Some families need to take action to address overwhelming fears and may respond best to proactive referrals of the older adult to an early-stage support group or a clinical trial.

Frustration is another common theme that emerges in early family treatment. The elder may be frustrated by perceptions of unrealistic demands. Family caregivers frequently express frustration with the elder's obsessive need for repetition and reassurance. Clearing up misconceptions about the presumed intentionality of the elder's resistance or the elder's confabulations to fill in gaps in memory helps families cope with these changes. Encouraging the family to get angry at the disease rather than at professionals, services, or each other can be extremely helpful. Families should be reminded that conflict among their members will only limit needed help. It is important for the family to understand that the elder's realistic dependency does not imply weakness of character or will.

Fatigue and exhaustion are common themes in work with families of older adults. Encouraging rest, exercise, and energy economies can be helpful for the elder and for family members. Guilt is another common theme in family work. Family members express guilt at losing patience, and elders express guilt about being a burden or not contributing to family life. Family members of older adults appreciate reminders from psychiatrists that everyone experiences regret based on unique but certain limits.

Key themes, tailored to the family's capacity to understand them, should be highlighted and repeated in writing to distant or absent family members after a psychiatric evaluation. The examples of specific messages listed in Table 28–1 are best delivered to the older adult and the family caregiver together, to reduce the older adult's suspiciousness about the physician and family talking behind his or her back. Older couples in first marriages are generally more comfortable facing threatening health information together. Spouses of older adults with Alzheimer's disease are often put off by attempts to separate them from their impaired spouse. Providing the same information at the same time helps older couples preserve their couple identity and accept the psychiatric recommendations as a mutual adaptive challenge. Even if the older adult patient forgets what was said, he or she is likely to remember being treated with respect in an adult manner and being included.

Family Expectations of Psychiatrists

Although families of older adults may never seek psychiatric services, it is useful to consider the expectations of health professionals that family members may have when they are faced with care for an older family member with dementia. Vulnerable family caregivers may notice office amenities first. These family members seek a private place and time, undivided professional attention, and the comfort of familiar initial polite small talk. Families want psychiatrists to listen without a rush to implied understanding or suggestions. Families of older adults expect to be asked what they have tried in coping with their relative's impairment. Even more, these families appreciate the psychiatrist asking about what else is going on within the family.

Families of older adults expect psychiatrists to be thoroughly knowledgeable about geriatric medicine, including symptoms and treatment of common chronic conditions of late life. Some families seek a psychiatrist as an authoritative specialist, but others may simply seek a psychiatrist as a support, coach, or advocate. If families are seeking a coach, they want tentative suggestions for short-term trials or reflective responses such as "I wonder if you have considered...."

Older spouse caregivers may expect advice from an authoritative expert and immediate cures for the dementia patient's most disruptive symptoms. These older spouse caregivers expect explanations about why antipsychotic medications do not "treat" wandering as well as environmental and activity strategies do. They need specific referrals to the Alzheimer's Association's Safe Return identification system as well as help in coping with the toll created by the prolonged hypervigilance needed to protect a wandering spouse.

Families of older adults want psychiatrists to tailor information and education relevant to their immediate, pressing concerns. Sometimes families need help breaking down an overwhelming problem to prioritized, pragmatic steps. For example, a family concerned about the increasingly combative behavior of an older adult male may be helped by a psychiatrist who responds, "First, let's get the guns out of the house" (Spangenberg et al. 1999). Other families need specific suggestions about how to communicate or visit with their impaired family member (Strauss 2001).

When depleted primary caregivers are confronting the range of behavioral symptoms of older adults with Alzheimer's disease, they may look to the psychiatrist to lend energy, a proactive attitude, and perspective. Later, families want acknowledgement of their contributions to the older adult's quality of life, or absolution or forgiveness for what they were unable to achieve despite their best intentions. The psychiatrist must be careful with well-intentioned efforts to commend families for doing "a great job." Some family caregivers are quick to point out, "I am not her caregiver—I am her husband and I promised to take care of her in sickness and in health."

TABLE 28–1. Key messages for older adults and their families

1. You have a brain disorder. It will be more difficult to do things that used to be easy for you. It is not your fault, and trying harder will not always work. It is best to ask for help or reminders.
2. Alzheimer's disease gets worse over time but progresses at different rates in different people. Not everyone has all the same changes in behavior, mood, or symptoms. We can treat your disease and your symptoms as they occur, but there is no going back to the way you were before, and there is no stopping the disease in its tracks forever.
3. You will have good days when things seem easier. You will retain some skills for quite some time, and you will always retain the capacity to enjoy life.
4. Simplify what you must remember. Ask for reminders, reassurance, labels, or cues. Assume that it will take longer to complete daily chores and that you will not do well if you are rushed.
5. You will feel better if you rely on trusted family members or friends. Now is the time to decide who should help with decisions about your health care and your money. Keeping track of money is a skill that is damaged early in your disease. Start talking to each other about whom you would choose to make your financial and health care decisions, and make those arrangements now while you are in charge.
6. Tell people that you have a memory problem. They will not be able to tell just by looking at you. It takes too much energy to hide your symptoms, and being honest saves embarrassment and frustration. People may offer too much or too little help. Accept help even though it is hard.
7. Thinking and remembering will tire you more easily. You may want to build in more breaks. You will feel less upset when you are rested.
8. Regular medical care, good nutrition, sleep, regular exercise, and treating your other illnesses will keep your symptoms from looking worse than they are. Be sure to get dental, vision, and hearing care. Your family members should be equally attentive to preventive health behaviors.
9. Develop and follow a predictable daily routine to limit the number of new situations that may confuse or upset you. Stay connected to groups that are important to you and your family. You and your family members need social time as well as rest.
10. The better you and your family understand what is happening to you and why, the better you will cope with it. Your family may want to read a firsthand account of what it is like to have Alzheimer's disease (Harris 2002). Call the Alzheimer's Association, join a support group, or go online to learn more.
11. Alzheimer's disease does not happen overnight, and it progresses slowly. You have time to adjust to living with it. Life will be different, but your care will not take much time each day. Find new or old activities you like to do, and make sure you do the things you enjoy often.

Families also appreciate preventive self-care reminders from psychiatrists, but vague suggestions that caregivers need to take care of themselves often frustrate overwhelmed families that have few resources (Burton et al. 1997). Family members need help translating principles of respite in ways that are congruent with their personal values and cultural expectations. Specific examples may help. For example, some husbands respond to statements such as "family care without respite is like expecting your car to run on empty. It doesn't." Respite options can be presented as opportunities to "recharge your battery."

Also, increasing evidence shows that encouraging physical activity (King and Brassington 1997) and actively assessing and treating sleep disorders in older adults and their family caregivers are associated with positive care and family outcomes (McCurry et al. 1998).

Families also look to psychiatrists for decisional support or help in mobilizing other family members. Psychiatric expertise in family systems and family communication is extremely relevant at these points. Family caregivers expect psychiatrists to let them express and learn how to manage unacceptable feelings, such as anger toward the older adult, toward other family members or service providers, or toward God. These families appreciate psychiatrists who create new choices by reframing the problem or situation. The primary family caregiver may seek permission from the psychiatrist to be less than perfect or a good-enough-for-now family caregiver. At such times, a psychiatrist's use of humor and compassion can produce dramatic results.

Assessing the Family of an Older Adult

Psychiatrists are comfortable making standard psychiatric assessments of affective, anxiety, substance abuse, and other psychiatric symptoms of primary family caregivers or older adults. Often, however, family assessment is overlooked. A targeted assessment of the family of an older adult may result in referrals to Alzheimer's Association services, private or public geriatric care management, family or peer counseling, home help, day programs, assisted living, or nursing home care. Cultural values, expectations, and health beliefs will influence how and when families decide to pursue referrals, as well as their receptivity to family treatment by psychiatrists.

One of the most useful ways to elicit a picture of family functioning is to ask the family to describe a typical day, highlighting family concerns about how the older adult spends his or her day. Clues about how much time the patient is left alone and about potential safety risks come from such open-ended questions. The psychiatrist should probe further if the caregiver hints about increased use of alcohol or psychoactive medications in response to stress. Older husband caregivers are particularly at risk of increased alcohol use in response to care demands.

The psychiatrist should be alert for positive activities such as regular exercise, social stimulation, and secondary family support. A husband caring for his wife may be frustrated by her loss of interest in cooking. A suggestion to try regular restaurant meals at a familiar diner may conserve his energy and better meet the couple's nutritional and social needs.

Questions about a typical day often elicit family anger at the patient's apathy and withdrawal or a family's lack of awareness of safety issues. The family may complain that the cognitively impaired older adult is becoming more irritable and jealous of grandchildren. Probing may reveal that the impaired grandparent is still providing child care despite significant declines in judgment or function.

It is wise to assess the home and neighborhood environment. People with dementia are easy targets for exploitation by telephone and mail fraud and people who come to the door. High-crime neighborhoods pose additional risks. An older adult who spends his time at the corner store buying alcohol and cigarettes may be especially vulnerable to excessive disability and malnutrition if living alone.

The psychiatrist should ask specifically about the primary caregiver's health. Although a spouse caregiver may be reluctant to focus on himself or herself, the psychiatrist should be alert to offhand comments such as "I'm fine as long as he can drive me to chemotherapy." The caregiver should be asked about his or her sleep and how it is affected by the older adult's sleep pattern. The mobility and stamina of the primary caregiver determines the viability of home care. Many family caregivers will report being frustrated, overwhelmed, edgy, or exhausted but will deny having depression, anxiety, or psychiatric symptoms. Although psychiatrists are well advised to respond promptly to poorly controlled rage or suicidal or violent threats, skillful probing may be required to elicit frank symptoms.

A brief review of family relationships may further elicit new or resurfacing family conflict that can complicate care. A distant, estranged sister may insist that her local sister is exaggerating their mother's dependency needs in an attempt to take control. The psychiatrist's written explanation of the mother's need for constant supervision may mobilize support from the distant daughter or at least may reassure the local daughter that her supervision is in fact what her mother needs. The psychiatrist must be alert to reports by family caregivers of exacerbated somatic symptoms or chronic illnesses that may not be attributed to caregiver burden.

Another key to effective family assessment is to ask about other family commitments. Poor or minority families may consider Alzheimer's disease care the least of their problems. A daughter backing up her mother's care of her father may be distracted by anxiety about her husband's failing business or a child's drug addiction. Her mother may know nothing about her daughter's family problems and may assume that her daughter is just putting her job ahead of her family. Again, cultural expectations must be carefully assessed along with each family member's subjective perceptions of financial resources. In some Asian American families, use of any formal services may be viewed as a moral failure of the family. When paid or formal services are needed, family decision making is often related to subjective perceptions of future financial adequacy rather than the objective cost or affordability of services. Some family members may be saving for a rainy day, whereas others may value preserving their inheritance above meeting the elder's current care needs.

It is wise to assess family styles, strengths, and goals. Some families cope well with end-of-life care for an immobile or incontinent older adult but are unable to tolerate the disruptive behaviors or sleep patterns of persons with moderate dementia. Older spouses in particular are often willing to sacrifice their own health care to preserve their goal of maintaining couplehood, even with a partner who no longer recognizes them. Families who have coped with chronic mental illness or substance abuse in other members may have well-developed coping strategies or support systems such as Alcoholics Anonymous that help them adapt to care for an impaired elder.

Finally, assessment should include some review of the family's experience with previous and current help, both family help and help from paid services. Previous family conflict over elder care will limit the family's willingness to ask for help. If the last home care worker stole from them or never showed up, the family is unlikely to accept another home health referral. If Uncle John thought the adult day center patronized or belittled him, the family will be unlikely to try it again. Key questions about previous and current help are about adequacy, quality, and dependability. If a family believes the help they give each other is adequate, dependable, or sufficient, they are often unwilling to consider formal services.

Selecting Interventions for Families of Older Adults

Families of persons with dementia need a continuing source of reliable information. Referrals to the Alzheimer's Association (800-272-3900; http://www.alz.org) and the Alzheimer's Disease Education and Referral Center of the National Institute on Aging (800-438-4380; http://www.alzheimers.org) meet this need.

Combined interventions have been shown to enhance positive caregiver outcomes. Combining individual and family counseling, family education, support group participation, and sustained availability of a care manager are associated with decreased caregiver burden and depression; decreases in the elder's disruptive symptoms; and increased caregiver satisfaction, subjective well-being, and self-efficacy (Sorensen et al. 2002). Psychoeducational and psychotherapeutic interventions produce the most consistent short-term effects on all outcome measures. Although interventions with dementia caregivers appear effective in meta-analyses, effects are small and domain-specific rather than global. For example, a reasonable multimodal approach to treating an elder's disruptive agitation could include treatment of depression in the elder or in the family caregiver with pharmacological and nonpharmacological strategies, participation by the family caregiver in psychoeducational, skills training, or caregiver support groups, and participation by the elder and the family caregiver in structured exercise programs.

Nonpharmacological approaches to the treatment of depression in elder-care family dyads could be based on increasing the frequency of individually selected pleasant events (Teri et al. 1997). The categories of pleasant events for Alzheimer's disease patients defined by Teri and colleagues include activities related to nature, socialization, pleasant thoughts and feelings, recognition from others, giving to others, and leisure pursuits. Rituals or religious activities may also be pleasant events for patients. Once the elder and caregiver have identified which activities are the most enjoyable, the goal becomes one of increasing the frequency and duration of these activities relative to less enjoyable daily activities.

Referrals to support groups should be balanced and not oversold. Research on participation in support groups documents specific benefits from experiential similarity, consumer information, coping and survivor models, expressive or advocacy outlets, and (for some participants) the creation of substitute family or social outlets. Indeed, early studies of support group participation showed that participants knew more about Alzheimer's disease and services (although participants did not necessarily use that information) and that participants felt less isolated and misunderstood than nonparticipants. There are, however, realistic limits to the benefits of support group participation.

One support group does not fit all. African Americans frequently do not understand the need to talk about family business among strangers. In an open mutual help group with revolving membership, not all participants will be dealing with the same care issues. The exclusive focus on Alzheimer's disease as just one aspect of family life may not meet family needs. Some families cannot get to meetings regularly, and some groups are not consistently available. These factors limit the benefits of such a minimalist intervention. The benefits of participation can be enhanced by encouraging families to shop around for a group that best meets their needs and by reminding them that they may be able to obtain comparable social support from groups to which they already belong, such as a church or retiree organization, or even from online sources such as discussion boards and online discussion groups dedicated to Alzheimer's disease.

Educational Strategies With Families of Older Adults

Family members and families differ in literacy levels, ethnicity, culture, and capacity to apply information, and these differences matter when selecting approaches to family education. Many families are too overwhelmed at a first psychiatric consultation to absorb information or instructions. It is best to tailor information to the family's tolerance and capacity to understand and to their current need to know. Teachable moments with families come at crisis points with specific psychiatric symptoms such as accusations of family theft or spousal infidelity or when the older adult asks his or her spouse to find his "real" wife or husband.

A medicine metaphor is appropriate. The timing and "dosing" of information may enhance effective use of that information in adapting care over time. Some families have read or heard inaccurate or partially correct information about symptoms that can be easily corrected, such as myths about all older men with dementia becoming sexual predators. Just like medication management in geriatrics, the maxim "start low and go slow" applies equally well to family education about dementia. Overwhelming families with too many treatment suggestions or referrals is just as likely to lead to poor compliance as is changing multiple medication regimens all at once. Finally, information should be presented in hopeful terms, such as "treating your depression should have positive effects on your husband's mood as well" or "many families surprise themselves with their resilience."

The presentation of information in a timed and dosed manner also offers opportunities for repetition of key themes. The key messages for family caregivers listed in Table 28–2 can be presented at intervals and in "doses" that are based on the frequency of contact with the family, the family's need to know, and the family's capacity to understand.

Responding to Families Over the Course of Progressive Impairment

Over the course of a dementia, family caregivers become not only information seekers but also care managers, consumer advocates, surrogate decision makers, and health care providers. It is difficult enough to negotiate these complex roles, and it is even more difficult if the family caregiver is burdened by role overload. Assessing caregiver vulnerability can be facilitated by asking family members to self-assess their pressure points, or signs of increasing caregiver overload (Kaufer et al. 1998). Examples of caregiver pressure points and overload indicators include the following:

- You cannot turn your back for a minute
- You are taking your frustration out on the older adult or yourself
- You see nothing beyond care tasks
- You have no lifestyle
- You resent everything, and it is all too much
- Your best efforts are not making him or her behave
- You do everything, but it is never enough
- Your family is critical of you
- You have no time to think
- You are drinking, eating, sleeping, or taking more pills than before
- You have fantasies about disappearing, running away, or just letting the older adult go if he or she wants to
- You feel like a failure
- You see no end in sight
- You cannot remember loving, pleasant times

Other clinical red flags may signal imminent danger resulting from the caregiver's precarious health. Unsubtle hints may be comments such as "after my last stroke," "before he totaled the car," or "sometimes I feel like just letting him wander away." Pursuing these threads with standard clinical protocols is certainly warranted.

TABLE 28–2. Key messages for family caregivers

1. Be willing to listen to the older adult, but understand that you cannot fix or do everything he or she may want or need. Know that it will not necessarily get easier, but things will change, and the experience will change you forever.

2. You are living with a situation you did not create, and your choices are limited by circumstances beyond your control. Seek options that are good enough for now.

3. You can only do what seems best at the time. Identify what you can and will tolerate, then set limits and call in reinforcements. Doubts are inevitable.

4. Find someone with whom you can be brutally honest, express those feelings, and move on.

5. Solving problems is much easier than living with the solutions. It is tempting for distant relatives to second-guess or criticize. Hope for the best but plan for the worst.

6. It is not always possible to compare how one person handles things to how another relative would handle it if the positions were reversed.

7. The older adult is not unhappy or upset because of what you have done. He or she is living with unwanted dependency. Sick people often take out their frustration on close family members.

8. Considering what is best for your family involves compromise among competing needs, loyalties, and commitments. Everyone may get some of what he or she needs. Think twice before giving up that job, club, or church group. Make realistic commitments, and avoid making promises that include the words *always*, *never*, or *forever*.

9. Find ways to let your older relative give to or help you. He or she needs to feel purposeful, appreciated, and loved.

10. Take time to celebrate small victories when things go well.

Other issues surface when working with families of moderately impaired older adults. Isolation of the caregiver and elder is common as friends drop off in response to disruptive behavioral symptoms or the need for constant supervision of the older adult. Adults with dementia may feel lonely and misunderstood in a world that no longer makes sense, and their family members may feel equally misunderstood as the elder becomes less able to predict the effects of his or her behavior on others. When people with dementia feel threatened, they are most likely to take it out on those they depend on. Families need to be reminded that being vulnerable does not make older people grateful or lovable and that cabin fever among co-residing elders and family caregivers is a real threat to mental health and safety. Families are especially sensitive to elders who confuse or mistake family identities or suggest that family members are impostors. Making suggestions that family caregivers say something like "I'll try to do it like your mother would" may help them to understand.

Family members need to be warned not to give up cherished activities—social engagement has positive mental health effects at any age, and maintenance of a strong religious faith or community has been shown to have positive effects on elders and family caregivers. Expressive outlets such as sports, the arts, or advocacy can help families cope with frustration and anger. Prayer, meditation, exercise, massage, and yoga in combination with active treatment of depression or anxiety are all worthy treatment recommendations. Participation at an adult day center can be presented to the elder as an opportunity to help others and can be presented to the family as a source of social stimulation for the elder and a stress-reduction strategy for the family caregiver (Zarit et al. 1998).

Helping Families Assess Capacity of Older Adults

Many families turn to psychiatrists to assess the judgment and decision-making capacity of older adults, whether it is related to handling money, health decisions, living alone, or driving.

Handling money and health care decisions should be addressed soon after diagnosis to ensure time for patients to select a surrogate. Often families seek psychiatric consultation when family conflict surfaces over the patient's selection of a surrogate or the surrogate's handling of the older adult's funds. Questions about whether the patient had sufficient capacity at the time he or she wrote a will or assigned power of attorney can become adversarial and unrelated to family treatment.

Effective work with families regarding capacity is done early with a preventive focus. Families must be reminded that financial judgment is impaired early in dementia. It is wise for one family member to make sure bills are paid. This can be done with different levels of involvement of the patient, from decision making about which bills to pay to signing checks. If bills are forwarded to another family member, the patient should be ensured access to regular mail and to enough cash to meet adult dignity and identity needs.

Assessment and Limitations on Driving

Families can be encouraged to assess driving capacity based on observations of current driving, with reminders that dementia affects judgment, reaction time, and problem solving. Psychiatric assessment of the patient along with current observations from the family will provide direction on when driving should be limited. Unfortunately, by the time there is evidence of a decline in driving abilities, many patients cannot adequately report or judge their safety on the road. Anonymous reports to the department of motor vehicles may lead to required testing or removal of the patient's license, but the absence of a license rarely stops a determined older adult with dementia. Driving is one area in which the family must be encouraged and prepared to assess capacity over time. The signs listed in Table 28–3 may guide family observations and reports to the psychiatrist.

Psychiatrists may suggest a range of successful ways to limit driving, such as the following:

TABLE 28–3. Signs of decline in driving skills

Incorrect signaling

Trouble navigating turns

Moving into the wrong lane

Confusion on exits

Parking in inappropriate places

Driving at inappropriate speed

Delayed responses to unexpected situations

Failure to anticipate dangerous situations

Scrapes or dents on car, garage, or mailbox

Becoming lost in familiar places

Arriving unusually late for a short-distance drive

Receiving moving violations or warnings about near misses

Confusing the brake and accelerator

Stopping in traffic for no apparent reason

- A prescription reminder to stop driving can be tempered with a qualifier such as "until the end of your treatment." The patient's forgetfulness can be put to work for the psychiatrist. However, patients have been known to keep driving, making comments such as "That doctor doesn't know anything."
- Shaving the patient's keys, substituting another key, removing a distributor cap, or otherwise disabling a car can sometimes reduce the need to confront the patient with lost skills. However, patients have been known to fix the car, replace the keys, or even buy a new car while the old one was "in the shop."
- The car could be sold, moved to an undisclosed location, or put up on blocks. One family of a taxi driver put the taxi on blocks in the backyard to help the patient remember that it was broken.
- The family can also work on solutions that limit the need for driving—delivery services, senior vans, or offers of regular rides to church or for visits. Some families find that a taxi charge account works best.

Addressing Questions of Capacity to Live Alone

Families may go to extremes to keep an older adult with dementia in a familiar environment, allowing values of autonomy and choice to temporarily trump safety. In addition to psychiatric assessment of the patient's cognition, judgment, functional impairment, and decision-making capacity, the psychiatrist can suggest that the family consider the following questions:

- Can he or she use the telephone to call for help from a family member or to call 911? Will he or she respond inappropriately to telemarketers? Have mysterious packages or bills for unusual items begun appearing? Does he or she make repetitive calls every few minutes to the police or the same family member at work or at home?
- Can he or she get to the store or to regular activities? Does he or she overbuy or underbuy certain items?
- Can he or she handle money and pay bills, or is he or she willing to let others do this for him or her?
- Can he or she take medicine appropriately, on time, and in correct doses? Does he or she self-medicate or risk overdoses of unnecessary medications?
- Is he or she bathing, changing clothes, and dressing appropriately for the weather?
- Is he or she leaving the house after dark or traveling in dangerous areas alone? Does he or she let strangers in or buy from or contribute to questionable causes based on visits to his or her home?

- Is he having problems positioning his body to use a toilet, or is he urinating in wastebaskets or outdoors?
- Is he or she falling or getting lost by wandering outside a safe area?
- Are there significant changes in his or her appetite, weight, sleep, appearance, or eating habits?
- Is discreet surveillance by neighbors, friends, or family readily available?

The question of discreet surveillance is paramount. Persons with moderate dementia may live alone successfully if they have regular contact with, surveillance by, or checking from neighbors or family members. Environmental demand varies considerably and must be assessed along with patient variables.

Families and Institutionalization of the Older Adult

Not only does family stress not stop at the door of the nursing home, but ample evidence shows that families experience the greatest burden, disruption, and conflict in the time immediately before and after nursing home placement. Family members may seek psychiatric services to deal with guilt, anticipatory grief, and often anger toward the nursing facility, reimbursement system, and each other. Many families are disappointed by the lack of medical or psychiatric treatment available to residents of nursing homes. Families should be encouraged to work with the facility and the nursing home ombudsman while dealing with their affective, anxiety, and grief symptoms. Families should be reminded that their choices are often limited to equally unacceptable options. The advice given in Table 28–4 from family caregivers may reassure families facing placement of an older adult.

TABLE 28–4. Family caregiver affirmations

My choices may be limited and beyond my control.

There are no perfect elder care solutions and no perfect families.

If I had selected another course of action, I might now be having doubts about that as well.

Things probably would have been worse if I had done nothing.

Many others in similar situations have come to similar conclusions.

New problems are not necessarily related to what I did or did not do.

Conclusion

Work with families of older adults is about adaptation to change and loss. Much of psychiatric treatment of families helps them modify expectations for new dependency while learning to forgive themselves and others for inevitable doubts and mistakes. Interdisciplinary partnerships and teamwork with the Alzheimer's Association or with nurses or social workers offer the most effective and efficient models for psychiatric services to families of older adults. There is often as much need for "timed and dosed" patient and family education as there is need for treatment of specific psychiatric symptoms or syndromes of the elder or family members. Families will expect psychiatrists to provide active treatment and monitoring of psychiatric symptoms, reassurance, interpretation of information, and referrals. In addition, it is always helpful to acknowledge losses and contributions to care by individual family members, to encourage caregiver self-care, to offer authoritative absolution for inevitable mistakes, and to offer decisional support, especially with transitions in care or with end-of-life care.

References

American Medical Association: Diagnosis, Management and Treatment of Dementia: A Practical Guide for Primary Care Physicians. Chicago, IL, AMA Press, 1999

Arno PS, Levine C, Memmott MM: The economic value of informal caregiving. Health Aff (Millwood) 18:182–188, 1999

Brodaty H, Luscombe G: Psychological morbidity in caregivers is associated with depression in patients with dementia. Alzheimer Dis Assoc Disord 1:62–70, 1998

Burton LC, Newsom JT, Schulz R, et al: Preventive health behaviors among spousal caregivers. Prev Med 26:162–169, 1997

Fortinsky RH, Kercher K, Burant CJ: Measurement and correlates of family caregiver self-efficacy for managing dementia. Aging Ment Health 6:153–160, 2002a

Fortinsky RH, Unson CG, Garcia RI: Helping family caregivers by linking primary care physicians with community-based dementia care services. Dementia 1(2):227–240, 2002b

Gwyther LP: Family issues in dementia: finding a new normal. Neurol Clin 18:993–1010, 2000

Haley WE: The family caregiver's role in Alzheimer's disease. Neurology 48 (suppl 6):S25–S29, 1997

Harris PB (ed): The Person With Alzheimer's Disease: Pathways to Understanding the Experience. Baltimore, MD, Johns Hopkins University Press, 2002

Hughes SL, Giobie-Hurder A, Weaver FM, et al: Relationships between caregiver burden and health-related quality of life. Gerontologist 39:534–545, 1999

Kaufer DI, Cummings JL, Christine D, et al: Assessing the impact of neuropsychiatric symptoms in Alzheimer's disease: the Neuropsychiatric Inventory Caregiver Distress Scale. J Am Geriatr Soc 46:210–215, 1998

King AC, Brassington G: Enhancing physical and psychological functioning in older family caregivers: the role of regular physical activity. Ann Behav Med 19:91–100, 1997

Langa KM, Chernew ME, Kabeto MU, et al: National estimates of the quantity and cost of informal caregiving for the elderly with dementia. J Gen Intern Med 16:770–776, 2001

Lyketsos CG, Steinberg M, Tschanz JT: Mental and behavioral disturbances in dementia: findings from the Cache County Study on Memory in Aging. Am J Psychiatry 157:708–714, 2000

McCurry SM, Logsdon RG, Vitiello MV, et al: Successful behavioral treatment of reported sleep problems in elderly caregivers of dementia patients. J Gerontol B Psychol Sci Soc Sci 53:122–129, 1998

Mittelman MS, Ferris SH, Shulman E, et al: A family intervention to delay nursing home placement of patients with Alzheimer disease: a randomized controlled trial. JAMA 276:1725–1731, 1996

Mittelman MS, Epstein C, Pierzchala A: Counseling the Alzheimer's Caregiver: A Resource for Healthcare Professionals. Chicago, IL, American Medical Association, 2002

Noonan AE, Tennstedt SL: Meaning in caregiving and its contribution to caregiver well-being. Gerontologist 37:785–794, 1997

Olin JT, Schneider LS, Katz IR, et al: Provisional diagnostic criteria for depression of Alzheimer's disease. Am J Geriatr Psychiatry 10:125–128, 2002

Ory MG, Hoffman RR, Yee JL, et al: Prevalence and impact of caregiving: a detailed comparison between dementia and nondementia caregivers. Gerontologist 39:177–185, 1999

Ostwald SK, Hepburn KW, Caron W, et al: Reducing caregiver burden: a randomized psychoeducational intervention for caregivers of persons with dementia. Gerontologist 39:299–309, 1999

Pillemer K, Suitor JJ: "It takes one to help one": effects of similar others on the well-being of caregivers. J Gerontol B Psychol Sci Soc Sci 51:S250–S257, 1996

Rabins PV: The caregiver's role in Alzheimer's disease. Dement Geriatr Cogn Disord 9 (suppl 3):25–28, 1998

Schulz R, Beach SR: Caregiving as a risk factor for mortality: the Caregiver Health Effects Study. JAMA 282:2215–2219, 1999

Sorensen S, Pinquart M, Duberstein P, et al: How effective are interventions with caregivers? An updated meta-analysis. Gerontologist 42:356–372, 2002

Spangenberg KB, Wagner MT, Hendrix S, et al: Firearm presence in households of patients with Alzheimer's disease and other dementias. J Am Geriatr Soc 47:1183–1186, 1999

Strauss CJ: Talking to Alzheimer's. Oakland, CA, New Harbinger Publications, 2001

Teri L, Logsdon RG, Uomoto J, et al: Behavioral treatment of depression in dementia patients: a controlled clinical trial. J Gerontol B Psychol Sci Soc Sci 52:P159–P166, 1997

Tractenberg RE, Weiner MF, Thal LJ: Estimating the prevalence of agitation in community-dwelling persons with Alzheimer's disease. J Neuropsychiatry Clin Neurosci 14:11–18, 2002

Yaffe K, Fox P, Newcomer R, et al: Patient and caregiver characteristics and nursing home placement in patients with dementia. JAMA 287:2090–2097, 2002

Yates ME, Tennstedt S, Chang BH: Contributors to and mediators of psychological well-being for informal caregivers. J Gerontol B Psychol Sci Soc Sci 54:P12–P22, 1999

Zarit SH, Stephens MA, Townsend A, et al: Stress reduction for family caregivers: effects of adult day care use. J Gerontol B Psychol Sci Soc Sci 53:S267–S277, 1998

Clinical Psychiatry in the Nursing Home

Joel E. Streim, M.D.

Ira R. Katz, M.D., Ph.D.

Nursing homes provide long-term care for elderly patients with chronic illness and disability as well as rehabilitation and convalescent care for those recovering from acute illness. As documented in recent reviews (Katz et al. 2000; Streim et al. 1996), clinical studies have consistently provided evidence that the diagnosis, management, and treatment of mental disorders is an important component of nursing home care. At present, the delivery of mental health services is being shaped by several factors, including growing scientific knowledge, availability of new treatments, evolving federal regulations, public dissemination of survey data, and changes in the medical marketplace. In this chapter we review current information on the psychiatric problems that are common in the nursing home, discuss current trends affecting clinical care, and present a conceptual model for the organization of mental health services.

Nursing Home Populations

According to the 1995 National Nursing Home Survey (Gabrel and Jones 2000), 4.13% of Americans age 65 years or older—1.4 million people—resided in 16,700 long-term-care facilities. Compared with 1985 survey data (National Center for Health Statistics 1987), this percentage represents a 0.5% decline in the proportion of adults over age 65 residing in nursing homes and probably reflects the increased availability of long-term-care services at home and in assisted living facilities. However, during the same period, the mean age of nursing home residents increased by 0.9 year, and the proportion of residents age 85 years and older increased from 49% to 56%

for women and from 29% to 33% for men. Persons living in these institutions tend to be very disabled: 96% of residents required assistance with bathing, 86% with dressing, 57% with toileting, and 45% with feeding. Thirty percent had ambulatory dysfunction, and 24% required assistance getting in and out of bed. The proportion needing help with three or more activities of daily living (ADLs) was 83.3%, and only 8% were independent in all ADLs (Krauss and Altman 1998; Rhoades and Krauss 1999). Among residents age 65 years and older, 27% had visual impairment and 23% had hearing impairment. Approximately half of nursing home residents had some incontinence of both bladder and bowel. These statistics show that nursing home residents are characterized by extreme old age and high levels of disability. It is predicted that the future nursing home population will be composed of increasingly older, sicker, and more functionally dependent residents (J.M. Evans et al. 1995).

Prevalence of Psychiatric Disorders

Epidemiological studies conducted over the past 15 years have uniformly reported high prevalence rates for psychiatric disorders among nursing home residents. Rovner and colleagues (1990a) reported the prevalence of psychiatric disorders among persons newly admitted to a proprietary chain of nursing homes to be 80.2%. Parmelee and associates (1989) found psychiatric disorders diagnosed according to DSM-III-R (American Psychiatric Association 1987) criteria in 91% of the residents of a large urban geriatric center. On the basis of psychiatric interviews of subjects in randomly selected samples, other investigators found prevalence rates of DSM-III (American Psychiatric Association 1980) or DSM-III-R disorders to be as high as 94% (Chandler and Chandler 1988; Rovner et al. 1986; Tariot et al. 1993). Although some studies reported lower rates, those investigations used less rigorous methods for sampling or diagnosis (Burns et al. 1988; Custer et al. 1984; German et al. 1986; National Center for Health Statistics 1987; Teeter et al. 1976). In one study, Rovner and colleagues (1990a) found that 67.4% of residents had dementia, 10.4% had depressive disorders, and 2.4% had schizophrenia or other psychotic disorders. More recent data from the Medical Expenditures Panel Survey (MEPS) reveal that 70%–80% of residents have cognitive impairment and 20% have a diagnosis of a depressive disorder (Krauss and Altman 1998). Although the MEPS data were not derived from clinical interviews, they indicate prevalence rates of dementia and depression that are greater than the prevalence rates found in nursing home studies a decade ago.

These prevalence data also suggest that nursing homes are de facto neuropsychiatric institutions, although they were not originally intended for this purpose. The challenge of providing long-term-care services in nursing homes is therefore complicated by the extensive psychiatric comorbidity found in this setting.

Cognitive Disorders and Behavioral Disturbances

In all studies, the most common psychiatric disorder was dementia, with prevalence rates of 50%–75% (Chandler and Chandler 1988; Katz et al. 1989; Parmelee et al. 1989; Rovner et al. 1986, 1990a; Tariot et al. 1993; Teeter et al. 1976). Alzheimer's disease (DSM-III-R primary degenerative dementia) accounted for about 50%–60% of cases of dementia, and vascular dementia accounted for about 25%–30% (Barnes and Raskind 1980; Rovner et al. 1986, 1990a). Other causes of dementia were reported with lower prevalence and greater variability between sites. The prevalence of Lewy body dementia has not been ascertained in nursing home populations.

Delirium is common in nursing homes and occurs primarily in patients made more vulnerable by a dementing illness. Available studies indicated that approximately 6%–7% of residents were delirious at the time of evaluation (Barnes and Raskind 1980; Rovner et al. 1986, 1990a). However, this figure probably underestimates the number of patients who have reversible toxic or metabolic components in their cognitive impairment. In one study,

investigators found that nearly 25% of impaired residents had potentially reversible conditions (Sabin et al. 1982); in another study it was found that 6%–12% of residential care patients with dementia actually improved in cognitive performance over the course of 1 year (Katz et al. 1991). In the nursing home, as in other settings, the most common reversible cause of cognitive impairment may be cognitive toxicity from drugs used to treat medical or psychiatric disorders.

The clinical features of dementing disorders include treatable psychiatric symptoms—such as hallucinations, delusions, and depression—that can contribute to disability. Psychotic symptoms have been reported in approximately 25%–50% of residents with a primary dementing illness (Berrios and Brook 1985; Chandler and Chandler 1988; Rovner et al. 1986, 1990a; Teeter et al. 1976). Clinically significant depression is seen in approximately 25% of patients with dementia; one-third of such patients exhibit symptoms of secondary major depression (Parmelee et al. 1989; Rovner et al. 1986, 1990a).

MEPS data revealed that 30% of residents exhibit behavioral problems, including 11.8% with verbal abuse, 9.1% with physical abuse, 14.5% with socially inappropriate behavior, 12.5% with resistance to care, and 9.4% with wandering (Krauss and Altman 1998). In earlier studies, behavioral disturbances were found in up to 75% of residents, and multiple behavior problems were found in at least half (Chandler and Chandler 1988; Cohen-Mansfield 1986; National Center for Health Statistics 1979; Rovner et al. 1986, 1990a; Tariot et al. 1993; Zimmer et al. 1984). It is likely that the lower rates reported in MEPS reflect a different method of case ascertainment, rather than improvement in behavioral management leading to a recent decrease in prevalence. In addition to impaired ability to perform ADLs, disturbances of behavior have been identified as the most common reasons that patients with dementia are admitted to nursing homes (Steele et al. 1990), and disruptive behaviors frequently complicate care after admission (Cohen-Mansfield et al. 1989; Teeter et al. 1976; Zimmer et al. 1984). The majority of psychiatric consultations in long-term-care settings are for the evaluation and treatment of behavioral disturbances (Loebel et al. 1991) such as pacing and wandering, verbal abusiveness, disruptive shouting, physical aggression, and resistance to necessary care. Behavioral disturbances most frequently occur in patients with dementia, often in those with psychotic symptoms—an association that remains even after controlling for level of cognitive impairment (Rovner et al. 1990b). Agitation and hyperactivity can also be caused by agitated depression, delirium, sensory deprivation or overload, occult physical illness, pain, constipation, urinary retention, and adverse drug effects (including akathisia due to neuroleptics) (Cohen-Mansfield and Billig 1986).

In addition to agitation, symptoms such as apathy, inactivity, and withdrawal occur among nursing home residents. Although these symptoms are less disturbing to staff and less frequently lead to psychiatric consultation, they can be disabling and may be associated with decreases in socialization and self-care.

Depression

Depressive disorders represent the second most common psychiatric diagnosis in nursing home residents. Most studies in United States nursing homes show depression prevalence rates of 15%–50%, depending on the population studied and the instruments used, whether major depression or depressive symptoms are being reported, and whether primary depression and depression occurring secondary to dementia are considered together or separately (Baker and Miller 1991; Chandler and Chandler 1988; Hyer and Blazer 1982; Katz et al. 1989; Lesher 1986; Parmelee et al. 1989; Rovner et al. 1986, 1990a, 1991; Tariot et al. 1993; Teeter et al. 1976). Studies from other countries have shown similar rates (Ames 1990, 1991; Ames et al. 1988; Harrison et al. 1990; Horiguchi and Inami 1991; Mann et al. 1984; Snowdon 1986; Snowdon and Donnelly 1986; Spagnoli et al. 1986; Trichard et al. 1982). Thus, the high rates of depression in the United States cannot be attributed solely to problems in this country's approach to long-term care for elderly persons. Approximately 6%–10% of all nursing home residents, and 20%–25% of those who are cognitively intact, meet DSM-III or DSM-III-R criteria for major depression; the latter figure is an order of magnitude greater than rates among community-dwelling elderly persons (Blazer and Williams 1980; Kramer et al. 1985).

The prevalence of less severe but clinically significant (e.g., minor or subsyndromal) depression is even higher. In one study, Parmelee and associates (1992a) reported that the 1-year incidence of major depression was 9.4% and that patients with preexisting minor depression were at increased risk; the incidence of minor depression among those who were euthymic at baseline was 7.4%. Other smaller-scale studies have shown comparable rates (Foster et al. 1991; Katz et al. 1989). These data show that minor depression in nursing home residents appears to be a risk factor for major depression and might represent an opportunity for preventive treatment in this population.

Depression among nursing home residents tends to be persistent. Although there may be moderate decreases in self-rated depression in the initial 2 weeks after nursing home admission (Engle and Graney 1993), Ames et al.

(1988) found that only 17% of patients with diagnosable depressive disorders had recovered after an average 3.6 years of follow-up. Evidence for morbidity associated with depression comes from studies that showed an increase in pain complaints among residents with depression (Parmelee et al. 1991) and an association between depression and biochemical markers of subnutrition (Katz et al. 1993). In addition to its association with morbidity, depression has been found to be associated with an increase in mortality rate, with effect sizes ranging from 1.6 to 3 (Ashby et al. 1991; Katz et al. 1989; Parmelee et al. 1992b; Rovner et al. 1991). There is, however, controversy about the mechanism involved. Whereas Rovner and colleagues (1991) reported that the increased mortality rate remained apparent after controlling for the patients' medical diagnoses and level of disability, Parmelee and associates (1992a) found that the effect could be attributed to the interrelationships among depression, disability, and physical illness. Resolution of this issue will require further study.

The literature on depression as it presents in patients with significant medical illness is marked by recurring questions about the extent to which diagnostic criteria developed in younger and healthier adults remain valid among patients with significant psychiatric-medical comorbidity. It might seem logical to expect that the somatic and vegetative symptoms that characterize major depression in other populations lose their diagnostic value among long-term-care residents and that long-term-care patients who have symptoms consistent with a diagnosis of major depressive disorder may instead be experiencing a combination of medical symptoms and an existential reaction to disease, disability, and residential care placement. However, it has been demonstrated that DSM diagnostic criteria remain valid as predictors of treatment response and that the symptoms of major depression in frail elderly patients characterize a disease similar to that which occurs among younger adult psychiatric patients (Katz et al. 1990), even though most nursing home patients have concurrent medical illnesses and disabilities that complicate diagnosis and treatment.

In addition to the high level of complexity that characterizes major depression among nursing home residents, there is evidence for heterogeneity in these patients that may reflect the existence of clinically relevant subtypes of depression. The treatment study by Katz and colleagues (1990) demonstrated that measures of self-care deficits and serum levels of albumin were highly intercorrelated and that both predicted a lack of response to treatment with nortriptyline. Therefore, although this study demonstrated that major depression is a specific, treatable disorder—even in long-term-care patients with medical comorbidity—there is also evidence in this setting for a treatment-relevant subtype of depression characterized by high levels of disability and low levels of serum albumin. This latter condition may be related to failure to thrive in infants, as discussed by Braun and colleagues (1988) and by Katz et al. (1993).

Progress in Treatment of Psychiatric Disorders in the Nursing Home

As described above, the high levels of psychiatric morbidity in nursing home residents did not diminish over the last 15 years of the twentieth century. However, during the 1990s and beyond, there was significant progress in the development and evaluation of treatments for psychiatric disorders in nursing homes. An appreciation of the unique characteristics of nursing home populations—particularly the extremes of old age and the high prevalences of cognitive impairment, psychiatric-medical comorbidity, and disability, all in the context of residential long-term-care institutions—has led to increased recognition that results of efficacy studies conducted in general adult outpatient populations may not be readily generalizable to nursing home residents. This recognition points to the need for treatment studies conducted specifically with nursing home patients. Although the number of randomized controlled studies is limited, there is a growing body of literature on treatment outcomes in the nursing home.

Nonpharmacological Management of Behavioral Disturbances

Since 1990, more than 40 studies have been published describing nonpharmacological interventions for behavioral disturbances associated with dementia in the nursing home setting. Few are randomized controlled trials. The reader is referred to comprehensive reviews of these studies by Cohen-Mansfield (2001) and Snowden et al. (2003). Several nonpharmacological interventions have been shown to be effective. One promising approach combined enhanced activities, guidelines for the use of psychotropic medication, and educational rounds for nursing home staff (Rovner et al. 1996). In a randomized clinical trial, this approach was shown to reduce the prevalence of problem behaviors and the use of antipsychotic drugs and physical restraints. Individualized consultation for staff nurses about the management of patients with dementia was also shown to diminish the use of physical

restraints (L.K. Evans et al. 1997). Reductions in agitation were also observed in a study of a daytime physical activity intervention combined with a nighttime program to decrease noise and sleep-disruptive nursing care practices (Alessi 1999). Other programs decrease behavioral difficulties through modifications in the physical environment. Research on individualized behavioral interventions for patients with behavioral disturbances of dementia has been limited to case series and small-scale controlled trials that are often difficult to replicate, although some of the results are promising (Allen-Burge et al. 1999).

Psychotherapy

The growing evidence for the efficacy of psychotherapy in other settings suggests that it may be of value for treating mental disorders of aging in patients whose cognitive abilities allow them to participate. However, a search of the MEDLINE and PsycINFO databases for the terms *psychotherapy* and *nursing homes* from 1987 to the time of writing this chapter identified only a small number of controlled studies of the effectiveness of specific psychotherapeutic modalities, individual or group, for nursing home residents (Table 29–1). Controlled research on psychotherapeutic interventions has included studies of task-oriented versus insight-oriented therapy (Moran and Gatz 1987); reality orientation (Baines et al. 1987); reminiscence groups (Baines et al. 1987; Goldwasser et al. 1987; McMurdo and Rennie 1993; Orten et al. 1989; Rattenbury and Stones 1989; Youssef 1990); exercise, activity, and progressive relaxation groups (Bensink et al. 1992; McMurdo and Rennie 1993); supportive group psychotherapy (Goldwasser et al. 1987; Williams-Barnard and Lindell 1992); validation therapy (Toseland et al. 1997); cognitive or cognitive-behavioral group therapies (Abraham et al. 1992; Zerhusen et al. 1991); focused visual imagery therapy (Abraham et al. 1997); and a psychosocial activity intervention (Beck et al. 2002). With the exception of the investigations by Abraham and colleagues, patients in most of these studies were not selected on the basis of specific psychiatric symptoms or syndromes, but rather on the basis of age, cognitive status, or mobility.

Some of these studies reported improvements on measures of communication, behavior, cognitive performance, mood, social withdrawal, physical function, somatic preoccupation, self-esteem, perceived locus of control, and life satisfaction. Case reports and demonstration projects by experienced clinicians also documented the value of psychotherapy for treating depressed nursing home residents (Leszcz et al. 1985; Sadavoy 1991).

TABLE 29–1. Randomized controlled studies of the outcomes of psychotherapeutic interventions in elderly nursing home residents

Study	Type of intervention	Sample	Outcome measures	Results and comments
Moran and Gatz (1987)	Task-oriented group vs. insight-oriented group vs. waiting room control group	$N=59$; mean age, 76.3 years; mobile conversant,	Self-reported psychosocial competence in (a) sense of control, (b) trust, (c) active coping, (d) striving for social approval; life satisfaction	Task group improved on all measures except trust. Task group had significant increase in life satisfaction compared with insight and control groups. Insight group improved on sense of control and trust.
Baines et al. (1987)	Reality orientation vs. reminiscence therapy vs. no-therapy control group (crossover design)	$N=15$; mean age, 81.5 years; moderately to severely cognitively impaired	Cognitive function; life satisfaction; communication; behavior; staff knowledge of residents	Only the group that received reality orientation first, followed by reminiscence therapy, showed sustained improvement in communication and behavior and nonsustained improvement in function (information/orientation). No improvement was found in other groups. Intervention was associated with improved staff knowledge of residents.
Goldwasser et al. (1987)	Reminiscence group therapy vs. supportive group therapy vs. no-treatment control group	$N=27$; demented (MMSE range, 1–22; mean, 10.4)	Depression; cognitive function; behavioral/ADL function	Reminiscence group showed nonsustained improvement in self-reported depression on BDI. Neither intervention showed significant effects on cognitive or behavioral function.
Orten et al. (1989)	Reminiscence group vs. control group	$N=56$; mean age, 82.6 years; moderately confused	Social behavior; ADL function; agitation; somatic complaining; attitude	Significant improvement for 1 of 3 experimental groups; no improvement when all groups were analyzed together. Investigators suggest that therapist skills are an important variable.
Rattenbury and Stones (1989)	Reminiscence group vs. current topics discussion group vs. no group	$N=24$; mean ages of groups, 83–87 years; judged by nursing home staff not to be cognitively impaired	Psychological well-being (happiness-depression scale); activity level; functional level; mood	Both intervention groups improved on happiness-depression scale. No improvement on other measures, including mood scale. Positive correlation between happiness scores and increased verbal activity level between first and fourth weeks.

TABLE 29–1. Randomized controlled studies of the outcomes of psychotherapeutic interventions in elderly nursing home residents (*continued*)

Study	Type of intervention	Sample	Outcome measures	Results and comments
Youssef (1990)	Group reminiscence counseling for young-old subjects vs. group reminiscence counseling for old-old subjects vs. control group	N = 60, all women; young-old, 65–74 years; old-old, ≥75 years	Depression	Young-old group had significant improvement in depression scores on BDI. Old-old group showed improvement only on social withdrawal and somatic preoccupation items but not on total BDI scores. Control condition was not described.
Ames (1990)	Psychogeriatric team recommendations vs. routine clinical care	N = 93; mean age, 82.3 years	Depression; ADL performance	No difference between intervention and control groups. Only 27 of 81 recommended interventions were actually implemented (e.g., medication changes, referral for mental health services). Role of psychogeriatric services in management of the facilities and medical care of the residents was not clearly defined.
Zerhusen et al. (1991)	Group cognitive therapy vs. music group (control) vs. routine clinical care (control)	N = 60; mean age, 77 years	Depression; performance ratings of group leaders	Cognitive therapy group had 30% improvement in self-rated depression scores on BDI; no significant improvement in control subjects. Group gains did not vary with group leader ratings.
Williams-Barnard and Lindell (1992)	Group therapy with high nurse prizing vs. group therapy with low nurse prizing vs. control group (control had 3 meetings vs. 16 meetings for experimental groups)	N = 73; age ≥65 years	Self-concept	Self-concept improved in 68.4% of residents in high-prizing group, 29.4% of residents in low-prizing groups, and 10.8% of residents in control group. Self-concept declined in 40% of low-prizing group and 5.3% of high-prizing group.
Bensink et al. (1992)	PR group vs. activity group (control)	N = 28; age ≥65 years; mean age, 77 years; MMSE score ≥20	Locus of control; self-esteem	Only PR group showed increase in perceived internal locus of control. Both PR and activity groups showed improvement in self-esteem, with greater effect in PR group.
Abraham et al. (1992)	CB group therapy vs. FVI group therapy vs. control groups (control had 3 meetings vs. 16 meetings for experimental groups)	N = 76; mean age, 84 years; depressed and mildly to moderately cognitively impaired	Cognitive function; depression; hopelessness; life satisfaction	No effects of group therapy on geriatric depression, hopelessness, or life satisfaction. Both CB and FVI groups showed improved cognitive function on modified MMSE, with greater gains in FVI participants. No significant cognitive change in ED control groups.

TABLE 29–1. Randomized controlled studies of the outcomes of psychotherapeutic interventions in elderly nursing home residents (*continued*)

Study	Type of intervention	Sample	Outcome measures	Results and comments
McMurdo and Rennie (1993)	Exercise sessions vs. reminiscence groups	N = 49; mean age, 81 years	Physical function; ADL performance; depression; life satisfaction; cognitive function	Physical function improved in exercise group, declined in reminiscence group. Self-reported depression (BDI scores) declined in both groups; exercise group showed significantly greater improvement than reminiscence group.
Abraham et al. (1997)	CB group therapy vs. FVI group therapy vs. control groups	N = 76; mean age, 84 years; depressed with mild to moderate cognitive impairment	Depression factors; cognitive factors	Secondary analyses. Both CB and FVI reduced depressive symptoms over 24 weeks.
Toseland et al. (1997)	VT group vs. social contact group (control) vs. usual care group (control)	N = 88; mean age, 87 years; dementia	Behavioral disturbances; depression; use of physical restraints; use of psychotropic medication	VT group had less physical and verbal aggression and less depression than social contact or usual care group. VT not effective in reducing physical restraints or psychotropic drug use. Social contact and usual care groups had great reductions in nonaggressive behavioral problems.
Beck et al. (2002)	ADL group vs. psychosocial activity intervention, vs. both, vs. placebo, vs. no intervention	N = 127; mean age, 83 years; mean MMSE = 10; with disruptive behaviors	Positive and negative affect; frequency of disruptive behaviors	Significantly more positive affect in treatment groups; no decrease in negative affect and no change in disruptive behaviors.

Note. ADL = activities of daily living; BDI = Beck Depression Inventory (Beck et al. 1961); CB = cognitive-behavioral; ED = education-discussion; FVI = focused visual imagery; MMSE = Mini-Mental State Exam (Folstein et al. 1975); PR = progressive relaxation; VT = validation therapy.

Overall, there is a paucity of research on the outcomes of well-described psychotherapies among nursing home residents who have well-characterized psychiatric disorders. Nevertheless, the available evidence from nursing home research, considered together with outcomes of psychotherapy for older adults in other clinical settings, suggests that psychotherapy should be regarded as an important component of mental health treatment for the more cognitively intact nursing home residents with depression.

Pharmacotherapy

Pharmacological treatments are commonly used in nursing homes for dementia and its psychiatric and behavioral complications and for depression. Before 1985 there were few randomized, placebo-controlled clinical trials of psychotropic drugs that were conducted specifically in nursing home populations; those that have been published since that time are summarized in Table 29–2. Some of the earlier studies provided evidence for the efficacy of antipsychotic drugs in managing agitation and related symptoms in nursing home residents with dementia, but the effect sizes were often modest, and high placebo response rates were common (Barnes et al. 1982; Schneider et al. 1990). More recently, two multicenter, randomized, double-blind, placebo-controlled clinical trials have demonstrated the efficacy of risperidone, an atypical antipsychotic agent, for the treatment of psychotic symptoms and agitated behavior in nursing home residents with dementia (Brodaty et al. 2003); DeDeyn et al. 1999; Katz et al. 1999). The results showed that risperidone had antipsychotic effects and also had independent effects on aggression or agitation. The study by DeDeyn and colleagues included a comparison group treated with haloperidol. Follow-up studies suggested that risperidone may cause less tardive dyskinesia than do typical antipsychotic agents (Jeste et al. 2000). A randomized clinical trial of olanzapine versus placebo in nursing home residents showed efficacy similar to risperidone (Street et al. 2000). Randomized controlled trials of aripiprazole and quetiapine in nursing home patients with dementia complicated by psychosis or agitation were completed but not yet published at the time this chapter was written.

These controlled clinical trials have examined only the acute effects of treatment, typically for 6–12 weeks of treatment, and little is known about the effectiveness of treatment for longer periods. However, there is evidence to suggest that the need for and benefit from antipsychotic drug treatment changes over the course of months in nursing home patients with dementia. Two recent double-blind, placebo-controlled studies of antipsychotic drug discontinuation demonstrated that the

majority of patients who had been receiving longer-term treatment could be withdrawn from these agents without reemergence of psychosis or agitated behaviors (Bridges-Parlet et al. 1997; Cohen-Mansfield et al. 1999). This finding is consistent with findings from previous discontinuation studies (Barton and Hurst 1966; Risse et al. 1987). Therefore, it is important to reevaluate on a regular basis the need for continuing antipsychotic drug treatment.

Two randomized clinical trials evaluated the efficacy of mood-stabilizing anticonvulsant drugs for the treatment of agitation and aggression in nursing home residents. The first was a study of carbamazepine that showed it to be effective for agitation and aggression but not for psychotic symptoms such as delusions and hallucinations (Tariot et al. 1998). In this study, nursing reports indicated that less staff time was required for patient care in the group treated with carbamazepine. Another placebo-controlled study evaluated divalproex and found evidence for its efficacy in reducing agitated behavior (Porsteinsson et al. 2001), although sedation and diminished oral intake may be problems in elderly nursing home residents with dementia.

Acetylcholinesterase inhibitors have been shown to delay the decline in cognitive function in patients with mild to moderate Alzheimer's disease. However, little is known about the effects of these agents in more advanced dementia, which is commonly found in nursing home populations. One randomized clinical trial of donepezil in nursing home residents showed effects on cognitive performance that were comparable to those observed in less impaired outpatients (Tariot et al. 2001). A few studies have examined the effects of acetylcholinesterase inhibitors on behavioral disturbances, usually as a secondary outcome measure in outpatients, and some findings suggested that these agents may be useful for treating such disturbances (Kaufer et al. 1998; J.C. Morris et al. 1998). Prospective trials are needed to evaluate effects on behavioral disturbances in nursing home populations. There have been only four randomized clinical trials evaluating the effects of antidepressants in nursing home residents. The first study, which was placebo controlled, showed a positive response to nortriptyline for treatment of major depression in a long-term-care population with high levels of medical comorbidity (Katz et al. 1990). In the second study, patients were randomized to receive regular or low-dosage nortriptyline, and significant plasma level–response relationships were demonstrated in cognitively intact patients (Streim et al. 2000). These findings again confirmed the validity of the diagnosis of depression in nursing home residents in the context of significant medical comorbidity and disability. However, in patients with dementia, the plasma level–response relationship was significantly different, suggesting that the

TABLE 29–2. Randomized, placebo-controlled studies of the efficacy of psychotropic medications in elderly nursing home residents

Study	Medication and dosage (mg/day)	Sample	Efficacy measures	Results and comments
Beber (1965)	Oxazepam (10–80) vs. placebo	$N=100$; mean age, 79 years; nonpsychotic with chronic brain syndrome ($n=28$), mixed anxiety/depression ($n=26$), anxiety ($n=43$), or depression ($n=3$)	Anxiety and tension; depression, lethargy, and autonomic reactions; irritability, insomnia, agitation, phobic reactions	Improvement in all parameters was significantly greater in oxazepam-treated group than in placebo-treated group; 44 subjects received concomitant treatment with other drugs, including neuroleptics, antidepressants, hypnotics, antiparkinsonian agents, and analgesics.
Barnes et al. (1982)	Thioridazine (mean, 62.5) vs. loxapine (mean, 10.5) vs. placebo	$N=53$; mean age, 83 years; dementia and three or more behavioral symptoms	BPRS; SCAG; NOSIE; CGI	Total scores and global ratings showed modest efficacy with thioridazine and loxapine, not statistically better than placebo; high placebo response rate; significant improvement in anxiety, excitement, emotional lability, and uncooperativeness in active treatment groups, but no significant differences in overall efficacy between thioridazine and loxapine; significant improvement on BPRS and SCAG only in subjects with high-severity baseline scores.
Stotsky (1984)	Thioridazine (10–200) vs. diazepam (20–40) vs. placebo	$N=237$ nursing home patients; mean age, 80 years; all nonpsychotic with cognitive impairment, emotional lability, and ADL dysfunction and agitation, anxiety, depressed mood, or sleep disturbance (also studied were 273 patients on geriatric wards of state hospitals)	Modified Ham-A; modified NOSIE; global evaluations	Thioridazine was well tolerated with few side effects. Thioridazine-treated group improved significantly more than placebo group on all Ham-A items (74% vs. 42%) and global evaluations. Thioridazine-treated group improved significantly more than diazepam group on NOSIE and global ratings. Insomnia responded better to diazepam, but there was more overall improvement on Ham-A rating with thioridazine.
Dehlin et al. (1985)	Alaproclate (400) (serotonin reuptake inhibitor) vs. placebo	$N=40$; mean age, 82 years; primary degenerative, multi-infarct, or mixed dementia; not selected on the basis of affective or behavioral symptoms	Intellectual function; motor function (ADL); emotional function (including depressive symptoms); clinical global evaluation	No difference in efficacy between alaproclate and placebo. Severity of dementia ranged from mild to severe. Behavioral problems not described.

TABLE 29–2. Randomized, placebo-controlled studies of the efficacy of psychotropic medications in elderly nursing home residents *(continued)*

Study	Medication and dosage (mg/day)	Sample	Efficacy measures	Results and comments
Katz et al. (1990)	Nortriptyline (mean, 65.25) vs. placebo	$N = 30$ residents of nursing home or congregate housing; mean age = 84 years; major depression (Ham-D scores ≥18)	Ham-D; Geriatric Depression Scale; CGI	Significant improvement in patients treated with nortriptyline compared with placebo on Ham-D and CGI but not on Geriatric Depression Scale. Location (in nursing home vs. congregate housing) not significantly related to response. Trend toward decreased nortriptyline response in nursing home related to higher levels of disability and lower serum albumin in nursing home patients.
Nyth et al. (1990)	Citalopram (10–30; mean, 25) vs. placebo	$N = 98$; mean age, 77.6 years; primary degenerative (Alzheimer's disease) or multi-infarct dementia (vascular dementia)	GBS; CGI; MADRS	Compared to controls, Alzheimer's disease patients in citalopram group had significant reduction in irritability and depressed mood on GBS. From baseline to week 4, Alzheimer's disease patients in citalopram group improved significantly on MADRS and on GBS emotional blunting, confusion, irritability, anxiety, fear-panic, depressed mood, and restlessness. No treatment benefits found in vascular dementia patients. Placebo group worsened on CGI. Few adverse effects, with no drug–placebo differences.
Finkel et al. (1995)	Thiothixene (0.25–18; mean, 4.6) vs. placebo	$N = 33$; mean age, 85 years; dementia with agitated or aggressive behavior	CMAI; MMSE; GDS; ADLs	Thiothixene-treated group had significantly greater reduction in agitation than placebo group after 11 weeks of treatment and 6 weeks after crossover from placebo; no between-group differences on MMSE, GDS, ADLs.
Tariot et al. (1998)	Carbamazepine (modal dose, 300; mean serum level, 5.3 µg/mL) vs. placebo	$N = 51$; dementia with agitation	BPRS; CGI; agitation; aggression; cognition; functional status; staff time	Carbamazepine-treated group had significantly greater improvement on BPRS compared with placebo group at 6 weeks. Global improvement in 77% of patients taking carbamazepine and in 22% of those taking placebo. Secondary analyses showed that improvement was attributable to decreased agitation and aggression. Nurses reported perception of decreased time required to manage agitation in carbamazepine group.

TABLE 29–2. Randomized, placebo-controlled studies of the efficacy of psychotropic medications in elderly nursing home residents *(continued)*

Study	Medication and dosage (mg/day)	Sample	Efficacy measures	Results and comments
DeDeyn et al. (1999)	Risperidone (0.5–4; mean, 1.1) vs. haloperidol (0.5–4; mean, 1.2) vs. placebo	N = 344; dementia	CMAI; BEHAVE-AD; MMSE	Reduction in BEHAVE-AD and CMAI aggression scores was significantly greater with risperidone than with placebo. Extrapyramidal symptoms were significantly greater with haloperidol (22%) than with risperidone (15%) or placebo (11%). Slight but significant decline in MMSE scores in haloperidol group.
Katz et al. (1999)	Risperidone (0.5–2) vs. placebo	N = 625; mean age, 82.7 years; psychotic and behavioral symptoms and Alzheimer's disease, vascular dementia, or mixed Alzheimer's disease and vascular dementia	BEHAVE-AD; CMAI; CGI; MMSE; FAST; PSMS	Significantly greater reductions in BEHAVE-AD total scores and in Aggressiveness and Psychosis subscale scores with risperidone 1 mg and 2 mg compared with placebo. More extrapyramidal symptoms and somnolence with 2 mg than 1 mg of risperidone; 1 mg appears to be optimal dose for nursing home patients with severe dementia.
Street et al. (2000)	Olanzapine (5, 10, 15) vs. placebo	N = 206; mean age, 83.8 years; Alzheimer's disease with psychotic and/or behavioral symptoms	NPI-NH (including Occupational Disruptiveness scores); BPRS; MMSE	Olanzapine 5 mg and 10 mg produced significant improvement in summary measures of agitation, aggression, and psychosis. Olanzapine 5 mg significantly reduced disruptive effects on caregivers compared with placebo. Olanzapine was associated with somnolence and gait disturbance but not with increased extrapyramidal symptoms, central anticholinergic effects, or cognitive impairment compared with placebo.
Magai et al. (2000)	Sertraline vs. placebo	N = 31; all women with late-stage Alzheimer's disease and depression	Depression; facial affect	Both groups were improved at 8 weeks; sertraline had no significant benefits over placebo. "Knit-brow" facial response approached significance for treatment × time effect.
Porsteinsson et al. (2001)	Divalproex (mean, 826; mean serum level, 45.4 µg/mL) vs. placebo	N = 56; mean age, 85.0 years; probable or possible Alzheimer's disease, vascular dementia, or mixed dementia with agitation	BPRS; CGI	Divalproex group showed significant improvement on BPRS at 6 weeks compared with placebo; 68% of divalproex group and 52% of placebo group had reduced agitation on CGI (NS). Significantly more side effects in divalproex vs. placebo group (68% vs. 33%), generally mild.

TABLE 29–2. Randomized, placebo-controlled studies of the efficacy of psychotropic medications in elderly nursing home residents *(continued)*

Study	Medication and dosage (mg/day)	Sample	Efficacy measures	Results and comments
Tariot et al. (2001)	Donepezil (5–10) vs. placebo	*N* = 208; mean age, 85.7 years; probable or possible Alzheimer's disease or Alzheimer's disease with cerebrovascular disease (mean MMSE, 14.4)	NPI-NH; CDR-SB; MMSE; PSMS	Both groups improved on NPI-NH, with no significant difference between donepezil and placebo. Significantly greater improvement with donepezil than with placebo on CDR-SB at week 24 and on MMSE at weeks 8, 16, 20, but not on PSMS. Improvement not influenced by advanced age. No difference in adverse events between drug and placebo.
Brodaty et al. (2003)	Risperidone (0.5–2; mean, 0.95) vs. placebo	*N* = 345; mean age, 83 years; Alzheimer's, vascular, or mixed dementia, with aggressive behavior	CMAI; BEHAVE-AD; CGI-S (severity); CGI-C (change)	Compared to placebo group, risperidone group had significant improvement on CMAI total aggression and non-aggressive agitation scores, on BEHAVE-AD total scores and psychosis subscale, and on CGI severity and change scores. More somnolence, urinary tract infections, and cerebrovascular adverse events in risperidone group but no drug–placebo difference in extrapyramidal side effects.

Note. ADL = activities of daily living; BEHAVE-AD = Behavioral Pathology in Alzheimer's Disease (Reisberg et al. 1996); BPRS = Brief Psychiatric Rating Scale (Overall and Gorham 1962); CDR-SB = Clinical Dementia Rating (Nursing Home Version)–Sum of the Boxes (Hughes et al. 1982); CGI = Clinical Global Impression Scale (Guy 1976); CMAI = Cohen-Mansfield Agitation Inventory (Cohen-Mansfield et al. 1989); FAST = Functional Assessment Staging (Reisberg 1988); GBS = Gottfries-Brane-Steen Geriatric Rating Scale (Gottfries et al. 1982); GDS = Global Deterioration Scale (Reisberg et al. 1988); Ham-A = Hamilton Anxiety Scale (Hamilton 1959); Ham-D = Hamilton Rating Scale for Depression (Hamilton 1960); MADRS = Montgomery-Åsberg Depression Rating Scale (Montgomery and Åsberg 1979); MMSE = Mini-Mental State Exam (Folstein et al. 1975); NPI-NH = Neuropsychiatric Inventory–Nursing Home Version (Woods et al. 2000); NOSIE = Nurses' Observation Scale for Inpatient Evaluation (Honigfeld et al. 1966); PSMS = Physical Self-Maintenance Scale (Lawton and Brody 1966); SCAG = Sandoz Clinical Assessment–Geriatric (Shader et al. 1974).

depression occurring in dementia might be a treatment-relevant subtype of depression or a distinct disorder. A controlled antidepressant trial in nursing home residents with late-stage Alzheimer's disease showed no significant benefits of sertraline over placebo (Magai et al. 2000). Available open-label studies of the efficacy of serotonin reuptake inhibitors (SRIs) in nursing home residents with depression have had mixed results, some consistent with the findings of Magai and coworkers, suggesting that SRIs may be less effective for depression in patients with dementia than in those who are cognitively intact (Oslin et al. 2000; Rosen et al. 2000; Trappler and Cohen 1996, 1998).

Although the SRIs might be expected to be well tolerated by frail elderly nursing home patients because of their side-effect profile, there is evidence that these drugs can cause serious adverse events in this population. Thapa et al. (1998) demonstrated that the use of SRIs was associated with a nearly twofold increase in the risk of falls in nursing home residents, comparable to the risk found with tricyclic antidepressant drugs. Investigators in the United Kingdom reported that antidepressant use was associated with better physical functioning but also with greater frequency of falls in residential care patients (Arthur et al. 2002). A recently completed randomized trial found that venlafaxine was less well tolerated compared with sertraline in frail nursing home patients without conferring more treatment benefits, as might be expected from an agent with mixed serotoninergic and noradrenergic effects (Oslin et al. 2003).

Deficient Mental Health Care as an Impetus for Nursing Home Reform

Although psychiatric disorders are extraordinarily common among nursing home residents, and efficacious treatments exist, psychiatric services are often not adequate. Historically, nursing home design, staffing, programs, services, and funding have not evolved to meet the needs of patients with mental disorders (Streim and Katz 1994). In the 1980s, it was estimated that as many as two-thirds of nursing home residents with psychiatric disorders were misdiagnosed (German et al. 1986; Sabin et al. 1982) and that as little as 5% of nursing home residents' needs for mental health services were being met (Burns and Taube 1990). This mismatch of psychiatric needs and available treatment led not only to neglect but also to inappropriate treatment, in which psychiatric problems were often mismanaged by using physical or chemical restraints.

Physical Restraints

A 1977 survey of American nursing home residents showed that 25% of 1.3 million people were restrained by geriatric chairs, cuffs, belts, or similar devices, primarily in an attempt to control behavioral symptoms (National Center for Health Statistics 1979). Other early surveys demonstrated rates of restraint as high as 85%. Patient factors predicting the use of restraints, in addition to agitation and behavior problems, include age, cognitive impairment, risk of injuries to self (e.g., from falls) or others (e.g., from combative behavior), physical frailty, the presence of monitoring or treatment devices, and the need to promote body alignment. Institutional and systemic factors associated with restraint use include pressure to avoid litigation, staff attitudes, insufficient staffing, and the availability of restraint devices. Potential adverse effects include an increased risk of falls and other injuries (Capezuti et al. 1996), as well as functional decline, skin breakdown, physiological effects of immobilization stress, disorganized behavior, and demoralization. Although mechanical restraints have frequently been used in attempts to control agitation, they do not, in fact, decrease behavioral disturbances (Werner et al. 1989), and cross-national studies indicated that it is possible to manage nursing home residents without such measures (Cape 1983; Evans and Strumpf 1989; Innes and Turman 1983).

Misuse of Psychotropic Drugs

Concerns about inadequate and inappropriate care have also focused on the overuse of psychotropic drugs in nursing home residents, especially the misuse of these drugs as "chemical restraints" to control patient behaviors. Studies in the 1970s and 1980s reported that approximately 50% of residents had orders for psychotropic medications, with 20%–40% taking antipsychotic drugs, 10%–40% taking anxiolytics or hypnotics, and 5%–10% taking antidepressants (Avorn et al. 1989; Beers et al. 1988; Buck 1988; Burns et al. 1988; Cohen-Mansfield 1986; Custer et al. 1984; DeLeo et al. 1989; Ray et al. 1980; Teeter et al. 1976; Zimmer et al. 1984). Psychotropic drugs were frequently prescribed without adequate regard for the residents' psychiatric diagnosis or medical status. In one study, Zimmer and coworkers (1984) reported that only 15% of residents being given psychotropic drugs had received a psychiatric consultation. Other studies reported that 21% of patients without a psychiatric diagnosis were receiving psychotropic medication (Burns et al. 1988), that physicians'—as opposed to patients'—characteristics predicted drug dosages (Ray et al. 1980), and that psychotropic drugs were often prescribed in the absence of any documentation of the patients' mental status in the clinical record (Avorn et al. 1989).

The greatest concerns about inappropriate overprescribing of medications have related to the misuse of neuroleptics as chemical restraints to control resident behaviors. Despite evidence for the efficacy of antipsychotic drugs in managing psychosis and agitation in nursing home residents with dementia, patients with nonpsychotic behavioral problems may be appropriately managed with other medications, behavioral treatments, interpersonal approaches, or environmental interventions. Moreover, it is important to note that whereas all the evidence for the efficacy of antipsychotic medications comes from short-term studies, these medications are frequently prescribed for long-term treatment. In this context, concerns about overuse of antipsychotic drugs were supported by findings from drug discontinuation studies (cited above). One classic double-blind study of neuroleptic withdrawal showed that only 16% of patients who had been receiving medications on a chronic basis exhibited significant deterioration when the drugs were withdrawn (Barton and Hurst 1966). A subsequent, small-scale withdrawal study in patients who had been receiving neuroleptics for several months showed that 22% experienced increased agitation on withdrawal, indicating a need for continued treatment, but that 22% were unchanged and 55% actually showed improvement (Risse et al. 1987).

Inadequate Treatment of Depression

Although the focus of public concern and regulatory scrutiny in the 1970s and 1980s was on overprescription of antipsychotic medications in patients with dementia, undertreatment of other psychiatric conditions in the nursing home has also been a serious problem. The Institute of Medicine (1986) report "Improving the Quality of Care in Nursing Homes," which did much to stimulate nursing home reform, highlighted problems both in the overuse of antipsychotic drugs and in the underuse of antidepressants for treatment of affective disorders. Similarly, in reviewing epidemiological studies on the use of psychotropics in nursing homes, Murphy (1989) noted that antidepressants were the one class of drugs that appeared to be underused and that as a result, major depression in this setting often remained untreated.

Federal Regulations and Psychiatric Care in the Nursing Home

The misuse of physical and chemical restraints was a rallying point for advocacy groups that urged the federal government to institute a process of nursing home reform. In addition, the U.S. General Accounting Office was concerned that states were admitting patients with chronic and severe psychiatric problems to Medicaid-certified nursing homes not because patients needed this type of care but because admission would shift a substantial portion of the costs of patients' care from the state to the federal government. Apparently in response to both sets of concerns, Congress enacted the Nursing Home Reform Act as part of the Omnibus Budget Reconciliation Act of 1987 (OBRA-87), Public Law 100-203. This legislation provided for government regulation of the operation of nursing facilities and of the care that they provide (Elon and Pawlson 1992). This legislation directed the Health Care Financing Administration (HCFA) to issue regulations (Health Care Financing Administration 1991) that operationalize the laws and to develop guidelines that assist federal and state surveyors in interpreting the regulations (Health Care Financing Administration 1992a). Mental health screening, assessment, care planning, and treatment are addressed under sections of the regulations that pertain to resident assessment, resident rights and facility practices, and quality of care.

The regulations include provisions for preadmission screening and annual resident review that require assessment of each resident before admission to any nursing facility that receives federal funds (Health Care Financing Administration 1992b). When an initial first-stage screening reveals that a serious mental disorder (other than dementia) might be present, a second-stage assessment that includes a psychiatric evaluation must be made in order to ascertain whether the patient has a mental disorder, to make a specific psychiatric diagnosis, and to determine whether there is a need for acute psychiatric care that precludes adequate or appropriate treatment in a nursing home. Patients found to have dementia on the initial screen are exempt from the preadmission psychiatric evaluation. Thus, preadmission screening is intended 1) to prevent inappropriate admission to nursing homes of patients who do not have dementia but who have severe psychiatric disorders and 2) to help ensure that patients with disabilities due in large part to treatable psychiatric disorders (such as depression) are not placed in long-term-care facilities before they receive the benefits of adequate psychiatric treatment. For eligible patients who are admitted to a nursing home, an annual reassessment must be made in order to determine whether nursing home care remains appropriate. Regulations requiring comprehensive assessment for all residents (Health Care Financing Administration 1991) have led to development of a uniform Resident Assessment Instrument, which includes the Minimum Data Set (MDS) (J.N. Morris et al. 1990). This instrument must be administered on a regular basis by members of an interdisciplinary health care team; usually a nurse—and ultimately the nursing home administrator—is responsible for its completion (Health Care Financing Administration 1992c). Areas of assessment relevant to mental illness and behavior include mood, cognition, communication, functional status, medications, and other treatments.

Responses on the MDS suggesting that there may be a need to reevaluate a patient's clinical status and treatment plan serve as triggers for completing Resident Assessment Protocols (RAPs). These protocols 1) define medical conditions, psychiatric disorders, adverse treatment effects, functional impairments, and disabilities that are common among nursing home residents, 2) note differential diagnoses and potential causal and aggravating factors, 3) outline procedures for evaluation, and 4) list key elements of management or treatment (Health Care Financing Administration 1992c). The MDS and RAPs together are designed as a two-stage assessment system, with a screening survey followed by a focused clinical evaluation. RAP problem areas related to mental disorders and behavior include delirium, cognitive loss and dementia, psychosocial well-being, mood state, behavior problems, psychotropic drug use, and physical restraints. The individual RAPs are designed to 1) help nursing home staff recognize common signs and symptom clusters that are indicators of clinically significant problems, 2) conduct evaluations that use standardized algorithms, and 3) determine whether it is necessary to alter the treatment plan. The regulations hold facilities responsible for ensuring that RAPs are followed appropriately. Although physicians have no mandated role in this process, physician involvement is clearly necessary for proper diagnosis and treatment of conditions covered by the RAPs (Elon and Pawlson 1992). Psychiatric consultation may be needed when RAPs indicate a need for the evaluation of problems related to mental health.

Regulations related to resident rights and facility practices restrict the use of physical restraints and antipsychotic drugs when they are "administered for purposes of discipline or convenience and not required to treat the resident's medical symptoms" (Health Care Financing Administration 1991, p. 48,875 [tag F204]). Regulations related to quality of care further require that residents not receive "unnecessary drugs" and specify that antipsychotic drugs may not be given "unless these are necessary to treat a specific condition as diagnosed and documented in the clinical record" (p. 48,910 [tag F307]). An unnecessary drug is defined as any drug used 1) in excessive dose (including duplicate therapy), 2) for excessive duration, 3) without adequate monitoring, 4) without adequate indications for its use, 5) in the presence of adverse consequences that indicate that it should be reduced or discontinued, or 6) for any combination of the first five reasons (Health Care Financing Administration 1991). The guidelines based on these regulations further limit the use of antipsychotic drugs, antianxiety agents, sedative-hypnotics, and related drugs (Health Care Financing Administration 1992a). For each of these classes, the guidelines specify a list of acceptable indications, upper limits for daily doses, requirements for monitoring treatment and adverse effects, and time frames for attempting dose reductions and discontinuation. These guidelines were updated in 2000 to reflect new clinical knowledge and the availability of new drugs approved by the U.S. Food and Drug Administration (Health Care Financing Administration 2000).

To minimize concerns about federal interference with medical practice, the current guidelines include qualifying statements that recognize cases in which strict adherence to prescribing limits is "clinically contraindicated." Although the focus is on limiting the use of psychotropic drugs, the guidelines acknowledge that appropriate medical treatment can entail psychotropic drug regimens that depart from these limits. The guidelines instruct surveyors monitoring nursing facilities to allow the facilities the opportunity to present a rationale for the use of drugs prescribed outside the guidelines, and to explain why such use is in the best interest of the resident, before finding that the facility is not in compliance with regulations. Thus, the physician's options for treating nursing home residents need not be restricted by the regulations if the clinical rationale—explaining that the benefits of treatment (in terms of symptom relief, improved health status, or improved functioning) outweigh the risks—is clearly documented in the medical record. Although the facility, not the physician, is accountable for compliance with the regulations, the physician's clinical reasoning and judgment play a critical role in the process of ensuring quality care.

In addition to addressing the use of psychotropic drugs, the interpretive guidelines also outline conditions for the use of physical restraints. According to the guidelines, restraints may not be used unless there is documentation that 1) efforts were made to identify and correct preventable or treatable factors that cause or contribute to the problem, 2) prior attempts to use less restrictive measures failed, and 3) use of restraints enables the resident to achieve or maintain the highest practicable level of function. Physical or occupational therapists must be consulted if restraints are deemed necessary to enhance body positioning or improve mobility.

Although much of the emphasis of the federal regulations is on eliminating inappropriate treatment, there are also requirements for the provision of necessary and appropriate care for residents with mental health problems. Under the provisions designed to ensure quality of care, federal regulations define a need for geriatric psychiatry services in nursing homes, requiring that "the facility must ensure that a resident who displays mental or psychosocial adjustment difficulties receives appropriate services to correct the assessed problem" (Health Care Financing Administration 1991, p. 48,896 [tag F272]). More recently, within the scope of its responsibility as a payer, HCFA developed a system for assessing the quality of care provided in United States nursing homes. To enable surveyors to compare individual facilities within the same state, HCFA introduced quality indicators (QIs) derived from MDS data (Clark 1999). There are 24 QIs in 11 different domains, including behavior and emotional problems, cognitive patterns, and psychotropic drug use.

The domain of behavioral and emotional patterns covers the prevalence of behavioral symptoms affecting others (e.g., verbally or physically abusive, socially inappropriate, or disruptive behavior), prevalence of symptoms of depression, and prevalence of depression without antidepressant therapy. The cognitive pattern domain examines the incidence of cognitive impairment when consecutive MDS assessments reveal new onset of impairments in short-term memory or decision-making capacity. The psychotropic drug use domain includes the prevalence of antipsychotic use for patients without psychotic conditions, the prevalence of anxiolytic and hypnotic use, and the prevalence of hypnotic use more than twice in a 7-day period. QIs that are indirectly related to mental disorders and their treatment include the use of nine or more different medications and the prevalence of falls, weight loss, daily application of physical restraints, and little or no activity.

Whenever a review in any of these areas results in a citation of deficiency, a plan of correction must be developed and submitted for approval. This system is a first step in monitoring quality of care, although the face validity of some of the QIs has been questioned and the results of quality surveys may be difficult to interpret. Nevertheless, the results from every nursing home surveyed

are available for public inspection, and consumers of nursing home services (and their families) are beginning to pay attention to the QI reports.

Changing Patterns of Psychiatric Care

Since the implementation of the Nursing Home Reform Act in 1990, there have been significant changes in nursing home care, including mental health care. Some of these changes may be attributed to the process of conducting surveys and enforcing federal regulations; however, several other factors appear to have contributed, including the dissemination of information about regulatory requirements, availability and marketing of new medications, advances in scientific knowledge from nursing home research, and cumulative effects of professional education regarding good clinical practice. Increasing consumer awareness is also likely to have played a role.

Shifts in Antipsychotic Drug Use

Studies of the effect of federal regulations in the early years after implementation showed a substantial decline in the use of antipsychotic drugs (Shorr et al. 1994) and physical restraints (Hawes et al. 1997) and increases in antidepressant use (Lantz et al. 1996). One study reported that greater reductions in antipsychotic use during this period were found in nursing facilities with an emphasis on psychosocial care, a less severe case mix, and a higher nurse-to-resident ratio (Svarstad et al. 2001). Soon after the regulations were introduced, several investigators developed educational programs for physicians, nurses, and aides, teaching practice principles consistent with federal guidelines. Studies evaluating these educational interventions demonstrated reductions of 23%–72% in the use of antipsychotic drugs (Avorn et al. 1992; Meador et al. 1997; Ray et al. 1993; Rovner et al. 1992; Schnelle et al. 1992). Siegler and colleagues (1997) examined the effect of OBRA regulations on appropriateness of antipsychotic use and found that the percentage of residents who were taking antipsychotics and who lacked an OBRA-approved indication declined from 21.3% to 14.6%. Another study of pharmacy records in eight nursing homes found that, of the 17.7% of residents receiving antipsychotic medications, 70.9% had an OBRA-approved diagnostic indication, 90.4% had documentation of appropriate target symptoms, and 90.1% were taking doses within the recommended limits in the HCFA guidelines, suggesting relatively high rates of compliance with the OBRA regulations (Llorente et al. 1998).

Although the changes found by the studies were generally interpreted as an indication of improvement in care, the studies did not examine health care outcomes or the effect on residents' quality of life (Snowden and Roy-Byrne 1998) and did not address concerns that reductions in medication use might have an adverse effect on patients who required antipsychotic treatment. A retrospective study in a single nursing facility, which described attempts to discontinue or lower the dose of antipsychotic drugs in 75% of subjects studied, found that residents with appropriate indications for antipsychotic use according to the federal regulations were significantly less likely to have their antipsychotic agents stopped (Semla et al. 1994). Nevertheless, for 20% of residents whose antipsychotic was discontinued or reduced in dose, the agent was subsequently resumed or its dose was increased. This result, which is consistent with reports from earlier discontinuation studies, suggests that the finding of a reduction in overall rates of antipsychotic use may reflect a beneficial trend for a majority of patients, but this result cannot be interpreted as an indication of across-the-board improvement in the quality of residents' care (Lantz et al. 1996).

In contrast to the declining rates of antipsychotic use in the early 1990s, Online Survey Certification and Reporting (OSCAR) data showed a reversal in this trend from 1995 to 1999, with the national rate for antipsychotic drug use in nursing homes increasing from 16% to 19.4% during that period (American Society of Consultant Pharmacists 2000). Despite this increase, a survey conducted by the Office of the Inspector General of the Department of Health and Human Services, based on data from the year 2000, found that psychotropic drugs were appropriately prescribed in 85% of 485 cases reviewed (Office of Inspector General 2001c). However, it should be noted that, since Borson and Doane's (1997) review of publications on psychotropic drug use after the implementation of OBRA-87, there are still no pharmacoepidemiological studies that have examined the effect of compliance with the federal guidelines or of the changing rates of psychotropic drug use on resident outcomes such as symptom control, functional status, and quality of life.

Increase in Antidepressant Drug Use

Despite the decline in use of antipsychotic drugs in the early 1990s, it has been estimated that the overall use of psychotherapeutic medications in United States nursing homes actually increased, from 21.7% in 1991 to 46.1%

in 1997 (Health Care Financing Administration 1998). This increase was in part the net result of a decrease in the use of antipsychotic medications from 33.7% to 16.1% (a 52.2% decrease) and an increase in the use of antidepressants from 12.6% to 24.9% (a 97.6% increase) during that period. Since the mid-1990s, there has been emerging evidence of further increases in the prevalence of antidepressant use. A retrospective chart review of psychiatric referrals in seven Massachusetts nursing homes during 1995–1996 found that 61% of patients were taking antidepressants and 53% were taking serotonin reuptake inhibitors (Lasser and Sunderland 1998). Rates of antidepressant use also increased in the United Kingdom, from 11% in 1990 to 18.9% in 1997 (Arthur et al. 2002). According to OSCAR data (American Society of Consultant Pharmacists 2000), 35.5% of United States nursing home patients had prescriptions for antidepressant medication in 2001, ranging from 27.9% in Hawaii to 62.7% in Utah. A study of five Pennsylvania nursing homes similarly found that 47.6% of residents were taking antidepressants (Datto et al. 2002). Before 1990, fewer than 15% of residents with a known diagnosis of depression were receiving antidepressant medication (Heston et al. 1992).

Considered together, these data represent an extraordinary change in the pattern of drug use in a population that has traditionally received inadequate pharmacotherapy for depression. The dramatic increase in antidepressant prescriptions is probably due in part to the wide availability of newer antidepressants that are thought to be well tolerated by elderly nursing home residents with medical-psychiatric comorbidity. Aggressive marketing to primary care physicians may also play a role. With current antidepressant drug use rates that appear comparable to or greater than the estimated prevalence of depression in nursing homes, it is possible that a significant proportion of antidepressant prescriptions are intended for indications other than depression, such as sleep, pain, or agitation. Research is needed to determine whether the reported changes in prescribing have had a positive effect on the mental health of nursing home residents with depression.

Decline in Physical Restraint Use

Although questions remain about the interpretation of trends in psychotropic drug use (Lantz et al. 1996), the effect of the federal regulations on restraints appears to be positive, with several studies showing significant reductions in the use of physical restraints (Castle et al. 1997). One study found restraint use rates of 37.4% in 1990 (before OBRA-87 implementation in October 1990) and 28.1% in 1993 (after introduction of the standardized Resident Assessment Instrument required by OBRA-87) (Hawes et al. 1997). Siegler et al. (1997) enrolled three nursing homes in a clinical trial of educational and consultation interventions that would support OBRA mandates to reduce physical restraint use. The study found that restraint use declined significantly in the home that received the combined educational and consultation program, and none of these interventions was associated with an increase in antipsychotic or benzodiazepine use. There are no published studies showing an increase in fall-related injuries associated with lower rates of physical restraint use.

Special Care Units

Encouraged by consumer demand to better meet the needs of nursing home residents with dementia, 10% of United States nursing homes had established special care units (SCUs) by 1991. A decade later, it was estimated that 22% of nursing homes had designated SCUs for patients with dementia. Research on the effectiveness of SCUs is difficult to interpret and generalize because of the heterogeneity of these facilities (Office of Technology Assessment 1992; Ohta and Ohta 1988). In an effort to characterize the population served by these units, Holmes et al. (1990) reported that SCU patients had more severe cognitive, behavioral, and functional deficits than non-SCU patients with dementia who lived in the same nursing home. More than 90% of residents in SCUs have behavior problems (Wagner et al. 1995).

Some studies indicate that the facilities, services, and programs offered by SCUs may not be significantly better than those available on conventional nursing home units. A study of Minnesota nursing homes described unit and facility characteristics, noting that the designation of SCU was not associated with more services or more individualized dementia care than were units without the designation; however, the study found that some dementia-specific features were less likely to be found in regular units of nursing homes that had designated SCUs (Grant et al. 1995). This sample of SCUs had a higher proportion of residents with dementia and fewer residents with acute problems.

A case-control study of 625 patients in 31 SCUs and 32 traditional units found that residence in an SCU was associated with reduced use of physical restraints but not with less use of "pharmacological restraints" (Sloane et al. 1991). A recent study that included data on more than 1,100 residents in 48 SCUs reported that the use of

physical restraints was not different, and the likelihood of psychotropic medication use was actually greater, for patients on SCUs than for their counterparts on traditional units (Phillips et al. 2000). These authors suggested that residents of SCUs might even receive a poorer quality of care than that provided to similar residents in traditional units. Although evidence suggests that mobility may be maintained for longer among residents of SCUs (Saxton et al. 1998), others have found that the rate of decline in ADL function is not significantly slower for SCU residents (Phillips et al. 1997). Studies showing benefits of SCUs for behavioral disturbances are limited, and randomized clinical trials reporting positive outcomes of SCU residency have been limited to reduced frequency of catastrophic reactions (Swanson et al. 1993)—sudden agitated behavior in response to overwhelming external stimuli. Some studies have demonstrated psychological benefits not only for patients (Lawton et al. 1998) but also for caregivers (Kutner et al. 1999; Wells and Jorm 1987), with evidence of increased family involvement (Hansen et al. 1988; Sloane et al. 1998).

Studies have also examined the extent to which agitation is associated with aspects of the treatment environment in SCUs. Independent correlates of low agitation levels in these units included low rates of physical restraint use, a high proportion of residents in bed during the day, small unit size, fewer comorbid conditions, low levels of functional dependency, and favorable scores on measures of physical environment and unit activities. Despite the efforts of these investigators, there is still insufficient knowledge about the essential elements of treatment in SCUs, and evidence for the effectiveness of these units has not been adequately demonstrated.

Subacute Care in Nursing Homes

Since 1983, when the Medicare Prospective Payment System established reimbursement for acute-care hospitals on the basis of diagnosis-related groups rather than number of inpatient days, hospitals have had a strong incentive to limit lengths of stay by discharging patients earlier. Over the past 20 years, therefore, many patients have been discharged to nursing homes that serve as step-down facilities, providing subacute medical treatment, convalescent care, and rehabilitation services. Subsequently, the trend toward decreasing lengths of stay in hospitals and the transfer of subacute-care patients to nursing homes has been reinforced by additional efforts on the part of insurers and health maintenance organizations to contain hospital costs. In response both to heavy demand and to nursing home reimbursement rates that were substantially higher for short-stay patients with rehabilitation needs (compared with the per diem rates for long-term-care patients), the availability of nursing home beds designated for subacute care increased dramatically in the mid-1990s. It was estimated that subacute-care patients constituted about one-third of nursing home admissions during that period. Medicare reimbursement rates for the first 100 days of nursing home care, computed according to the Resource Utilization Groups (RUGs) system, combined with increased use of the facilities, resulted in significant increases in Medicare spending on subacute care patients in the nursing home setting. Alarm about the increase in spending occurring in the late 1990s prompted changes in Medicare reimbursement that resulted in dramatic reductions in payments to nursing homes from the late 1990s up to the time of writing this chapter.

Depending on the extent to which these trends affect the policies of specific institutions, the clinical characteristics of patients who are admitted to nursing homes and their needs for mental health care will change. In general, short-stay residents—patients who, after relatively brief stays in nursing homes, are discharged to the community or die—differ from long-term-care patients in that they are younger; more likely to be admitted directly from an acute-care hospital; less likely to have irreversible cognitive impairment, incontinence, or ambulatory dysfunction; and more likely to have a primary diagnosis of hip fracture, stroke, or cancer. The objectives of mental health care for short-stay patients are related not so much to managing behavior problems associated with dementia as to helping patients cope with disease and disability, to searching for reversible causes of cognitive impairment, and to treating disorders such as depression and anxiety that can be impediments to rehabilitation and recovery. In short, the objectives of mental health care for these patients are similar to the goals of traditional consultation-liaison psychiatry in the general hospital. As the opportunities for psychiatric intervention follow these patients from the acute-care hospital into the nursing homes, the services required may need to be more frequent or intensive than those usually available to long-term-care residents. Enhanced mental health services will increase opportunities for tradeoffs in which an investment in psychiatric care can lead to more independent functioning and more rapid discharge to the community. It is hoped that the benefits of mental health care, in terms of both cost offsets and improved quality of life, will provide a strong incentive for insurers, public and private, to establish reimbursement policies that facilitate such treatment.

Adequacy of Care

The high prevalence of psychiatric problems and the federal mandate to ensure quality of care define a need for geriatric mental health services in nursing homes (Smith et al. 1990). Although the OBRA regulations are having the intended impact (Snowden and Roy-Byrne 1998) and have resulted in measurable improvements in patient care, it has not been shown that the federal requirements for assessment and treatment of mental disorders have led to improved case identification, access to mental health care, receipt of appropriate care, or improved health care outcomes. Medicare claims data in 1992, 2 years after implementation of the Nursing Home Reform Act of 1987, indicated that only 26% of all nursing home residents and 36% of residents with a mental illness received psychiatric services (Smyer et al. 1994), and evidence shows continued low levels of mental health treatment in nursing homes (Shea et al. 2000). Although Medicare payments for psychiatric services in nursing facilities increased in the mid-1990s, expenditures declined from $221 million in 1996 to $194 million in 1999 (Office of Inspector General 2001a).

Borson and coworkers (1997) found that the required preadmission assessment is inadequate for identifying nursing home applicants who require mental health services. This inadequate assessment occurs, in part, because patients with dementia are exempt from initial psychiatric evaluation; therefore, a large number of patients with psychiatric disturbances secondary to dementia are not identified. Although 88% of patients in the sample in this study were appropriately placed on the basis of their personal and nursing care needs, 55% had unmet mental health needs. There are also concerns that required assessments using the MDS *after* admission do not provide adequate detection of depression (Brown et al. 2002; Office of Inspector General 2001b; Schnelle et al. 2001). In examining the data from 1,492 nursing homes across five states, Brown and coworkers (2002) found that 11% of residents were identified on the MDS as depressed, half the rate that was expected on the basis of epidemiological studies that used direct clinical assessments. Of the 11% detected, only 55% received antidepressant therapy. Thus, even when mental disorders are identified, detection does not routinely result in treatment.

Limited access to care appears to be at least part of the problem. In a survey of nursing homes across six states, conducted by Reichman et al. (1998), 47.6% of 899 respondents indicated that the frequency of on-site psychiatric consultation was inadequate. Directors of nursing judged 38% of nursing home residents as needing a psychiatric evaluation, but more than one-fourth of rural facilities and more than one-fifth of small facilities reported that no psychiatric consultant was available to them. Meeting the demand for mental health treatment may also be more difficult for nursing facilities that are part of a chain or contain Medicaid beds (Castle and Shea 1997). Thus, there is evidence that the federal requirement that patients receive services to "attain or maintain the highest practicable physical, mental, and psychosocial well-being" has not remedied the problem of access to mental health services in United States nursing homes (Colenda et al. 1999). Despite this evidence for the continuing lack of available services, the Office of the Inspector General reported in 2001 that 27% of mental health services provided in nursing homes and paid for by Medicare were "medically unnecessary" (Office of Inspector General 2001a). However, it is important to recognize that many of the services identified as resulting in "inappropriate" payments were specifically for excessive psychological testing and group psychotherapy for patients with severe cognitive impairment who were determined by reviewers to be incapable of benefiting from these specific procedures. This survey by the Office of the Inspector General did not examine the adequacy of appropriate, medically necessary psychiatric care.

Even among patients whose mental disorders are recognized and for whom treatment is initiated, there is evidence that treatment is often inadequate. A report by Brown et al. (2002) indicated that, of nursing home residents known to be depressed and receiving antidepressants, 32% were taking doses less than the manufacturers' recommended minimum effective dose for treating depression. In a survey of five nursing homes, Datto and colleagues (2002) found 47% of patients were taking antidepressants, but nearly half of these patients were still depressed. Although a small proportion of these residents may have been in the early stages of treatment, before a treatment response could reasonably be expected, it appears likely that many residents did not receive proper follow-up care with required dose adjustments or changes in therapy for those who were not responsive to initial treatment. This finding points to a need for nursing home providers to improve adherence to practice guidelines for the follow-up care of depression.

These findings also raise questions about the face validity of the federal QI based on rates of depression treated with antidepressants. This QI implies that the prescription of an antidepressant for a depressed resident is an indicator of good-quality care. Indeed, initiation of treatment suggests that depression has been recognized and diagnosed and that the first step has been taken to manage it. However, persistence of depression in a patient who is receiving an antidepressant drug suggests that the treatment may not be adequate. Thus, if the proportion of depressed patients receiving antidepressants is high, it may indicate that the facility is doing a good job of recognizing depression and initiating treatment, but it may also suggest it is not doing an adequate job of monitoring patients' response to treatment and modifying treatments as needed to produce optimal outcomes. Clearly, there is a need to refine the federal QIs for depression care in the nursing home.

Mental Health Care in Nursing Homes: A Model for Service Delivery

The high prevalence of psychiatric disorders in nursing homes argues for the importance of establishing systems that incorporate mental health into the basic services provided (Borson et al. 1987). In addition, several factors argue for the importance of the professional components of care: 1) the complex nature of the psychiatric disorders exhibited by nursing home residents, 2) the need to evaluate medical as well as social and environmental factors as causes of mental health problems, 3) the potential benefits of specific treatments, and 4) the need for careful monitoring to assess treatment responses and prevent serious adverse effects of medications. Thus, clinical needs demand that mental health services in nursing homes have two distinct but interacting systems: one that is intrinsic to the facility and contextual, another that is professional and concerned primarily with the delivery of specific treatments.

It has been suggested that mental health training should be provided to facility staff to develop basic skills in assessment and clinical management that can help staff handle problems that occur when specific professional services are lacking. However, it is important to recognize that the intrinsic and the professional systems cannot readily replace each other and that adequate care requires both. Although there is a real need for staff training, a realistic goal is to develop staff skills that complement rather than replace the activities of mental health professionals. This two-system model has obvious implications with respect to the financing of mental health services in nursing homes: it demonstrates the need to fund mental health care both as a necessary part of the per diem costs of nursing home care and as a reimbursable professional service.

Although the intrinsic and the professional systems for mental health services are distinct, they must interact: Geriatric psychiatrists and psychologists and gero-psychiatric nurse-practitioners can play important intrinsic roles as administrative and staff consultants, in-service educators, moderators of case conferences, participants in interdisciplinary team meetings, and contributors in other activities familiar to the consultation-liaison psychiatrist. Facility staff must be effective in recognizing problems, facilitating referral, supporting treatment, and monitoring outcome to enable the professional system to function optimally.

Intrinsic System

The intrinsic system of mental health care in nursing homes can be conceptualized as including a wide range of components: design of the environment; implementation of psychosocial programs; formulation of institutional policies and procedures for assessment, care delivery, monitoring, and quality improvement; and optimization of the ways in which staff and residents interact. The importance of the intrinsic system is recognized in nursing home regulations that require training of nursing aides; in the nursing staff assessments required for completion of the MDS and RAPs; and in OBRA requirements that nursing homes provide assessments, treatment planning, and services to attain or maintain the highest practicable level of mental and physical well-being for each resident. Because psychiatric disorders are common in nursing homes, nurses and aides should be knowledgeable about the nature of the cognitive and functional deficits associated with dementia and the manifestations of delirium and depression. Staff members should understand how to modify their approach to working with residents when cognitive impairment or communication deficits interfere with care. Staff should also know how to apply basic principles of behavioral psychology to identify the causes of agitation and related behavioral symptoms in patients with dementia, as well as how to plan environmental and behavioral interventions.

A number of approaches to providing such staff training have been developed. Evaluation studies have demonstrated that improved mental health care through staff training is an attainable goal and have identified barriers that must be overcome (Smyer et al. 1992). As mental health care is incorporated into the basic fabric of the nursing home, it must include provisions for patients with variable degrees of cognitive impairment and depression in both the extent of residents' autonomy and the design of activities.

The concept that several key components of mental health services are intrinsic to the nursing home is per-haps best developed in the design of SCUs for patients with dementing illnesses. Nonetheless, the need for these services applies to all patients, not only to those with dementia. Moreover, the potential benefits of such services are not limited to their effects on residents with diagnosed disorders; there is also the potential for prevention. For example, evidence indicates that contextual interventions designed to encourage a sense of empowerment in residents can have positive effects on both mental and physical health.

Knowledge of the benefits of encouraging autonomy is derived from the classic study by Langer and Rodin (1976), who evaluated a controlled intervention designed to increase nursing home residents' sense of control over day-to-day events. Residents were randomized to either 1) a treatment group in which staff gave the message that residents were expected to be responsible for making decisions for themselves or 2) a control condition in which the message conveyed was that staff were responsible for residents' care. Both immediately after the intervention and at 18-month follow-up, the treatment groups exhibited benefits in mood, alertness, and active participation. The effects of control-enhancing interventions have been confirmed in a number of other studies (for example, Banziger and Roush 1983; Schulz 1976; Thomasma et al. 1990) and have been discussed in terms of "learned helplessness" models (Avorn and Langer 1982).

Benefits of interventions designed to enhance the predictability of the environment have also been confirmed (Krantz and Schulz 1980). In summary, these studies demonstrate that the social environment within which care is provided can have a significant effect on nursing home residents; environmental design should be viewed as a component of mental health care.

Professional System

The intrinsic system for mental health services as described above is necessary but not sufficient to meet the needs of nursing home residents. In addition, the services of mental health professionals are important in evaluating the interactions between medical and mental health problems, in establishing psychiatric diagnoses, and in planning and administering specific treatments for mental disorders. This component of the professional system must encompass medically oriented psychiatric care, including psychopharmacological treatment. A position statement by the major provider groups in this field (American Association for Geriatric Psychiatry et al. 1992) acknowledged the history of misuse of psychotropic drugs in nursing homes, but the statement emphasized that psychopharmacological treatment of diagnosed mental disorders is an important part of the medical and mental health care of nursing home residents. The evidence base for the appropriate use of psychotropic medications in the nursing home setting is described earlier in the chapter, in the section titled "Pharmacotherapy." The complexity of psychopharmacological treatment in frail nursing home residents with medical comorbidity requires that the skills of psychiatrists knowledgeable in geriatrics be an integral part of the professional system.

The professional system should include care with a psychosocial as well as a biomedical focus. For example, psychiatrists, psychologists, and psychiatric nurse-practitioners with specific expertise in behavioral treatment may be successful in evaluating the antecedents and causes of agitation and related symptoms among patients with dementia and in developing environmental and behavioral interventions, even when efforts by the facility's nursing staff have proven ineffective. As described earlier in this chapter, psychotherapy may be of value for residents whose cognitive abilities allow them to participate. Further research is needed in order to determine how existing treatments should be modified and how they can be administered to optimize their effectiveness in the nursing home. However, despite the need for more research, psychotherapy for the more cognitively intact nursing home residents with depression should be considered an important treatment among the professional mental health services made available to nursing home residents.

Integration of the professional and intrinsic components of mental health care in the nursing home is required because of the inherent interdependence of these systems. To conduct valid assessments and make diagnoses, mental health professionals must rely on nursing home staff to report their shift-by-shift observations of residents' behavior and other clinical signs. Mental health professionals must also depend on nursing home staff to implement and monitor the treatments they prescribe. Conversely, to succeed in providing appropriate mental health care to nursing home residents, staff members in the intrinsic system must have access to ongoing consultation from, and must receive direct support from, mental health professionals who are knowledgeable in geriatrics.

References

Abraham IL, Neundorfer MM, Currie LJ: Effects of group interventions on cognition and depression in nursing home residents. Nurs Res 41:196–202, 1992

Abraham IL, Onega LL, Reel SJ, et al: Effects of cognitive group interventions on depressed frail nursing home residents, in Depression in Long Term and Residential Care: Advances in Research and Treatment. Edited by Rubinstein RL, Lawton MP. New York, Springer, 1997, pp 154–168

Alessi CA: A randomized trial of a combined physical activity and environmental intervention in nursing home residents: do sleep and agitation improve? J Am Geriatr Soc 47:784–791, 1999

Allen-Burge R, Stevens AB, Burgio LD: Effective behavioral interventions for decreasing dementia-related challenging behavior in nursing homes. Int J Geriatr Psychiatry 14:213–228, 1999

American Association for Geriatric Psychiatry, American Geriatrics Society, American Psychiatric Association: Psychotherapeutic medications in the nursing home. J Am Geriatr Soc 40:946–949, 1992

American Psychiatric Association: Diagnostic and Statistical Manual of Mental Disorders, 3rd Edition. Washington, DC, American Psychiatric Association, 1980

American Psychiatric Association: Diagnostic and Statistical Manual of Mental Disorders, 3rd Edition, Revised. Washington, DC, American Psychiatric Association, 1987

American Society of Consultant Pharmacists: Fact Sheet. Alexandria, VA, American Society of Consultant Pharmacists, September, 2000

Ames D: Depression among elderly residents of local-authority residential homes: its nature and the efficacy of intervention. Br J Psychiatry 156:667–675, 1990

Ames D: Epidemiological studies of depression among the elderly in residential and nursing homes. Int J Geriatr Psychiatry 6:347–354, 1991

Ames D, Ashby D, Mann AH, et al: Psychiatric illness in elderly residents of part III homes in one London borough: prognosis and review. Age Ageing 17:249–256, 1988

Arthur A, Matthews R, Jagger C, et al: Factors associated with antidepressant treatment in residential care: changes between 1990 and 1997. Int J Geriatr Psychiatry 17:54–60, 2002

Ashby D, Ames D, West CR, et al: Psychiatric morbidity as prediction of mortality for residents of local authority homes for the elderly. Int J Geriatr Psychiatry 6:567–575, 1991

Avorn J, Langer E: Induced disability in nursing home patients: a controlled trial. J Am Geriatr Soc 30:397–400, 1982

Avorn J, Dreyer P, Connelly K, et al: Use of psychoactive medication and the quality of care in rest homes: findings and policy implications of a statewide study. N Engl J Med 320:227–232, 1989

Avorn J, Soumerai SD, Everitt DE, et al: A randomized trial of a program to reduce the use of psychoactive drugs in nursing homes. N Engl J Med 327:168–173, 1992

Baines S, Saxby P, Ehlert K: Reality orientation and reminiscence therapy. Br J Psychiatry 151:222–231, 1987

Baker FM, Miller CL: Screening a skilled nursing home population for depression. J Geriatr Psychiatry Neurol 4:218–221, 1991

Banziger G, Roush S: Nursing homes for the birds: a control-relevant intervention with bird feeders. Gerontologist 23: 527–531, 1983

Barnes RD, Raskind MA: DSM-III criteria and the clinical diagnosis of dementia: a nursing home study. J Gerontol 36: 20–27, 1980

Barnes R, Veith R, Okimoto J, et al: Efficacy of antipsychotic medications in behaviorally disturbed dementia patients. Am J Psychiatry 139:1170–1174, 1982

Barton R, Hurst L: Unnecessary use of tranquilizers in elderly patients. Br J Psychiatry 112:989–990, 1966

Beber CR: Management of behavior in the institutionalized aged. Dis Nerv Syst 26:591–596, 1965

Beck AT, Ward CH, Mendelson M, et al: An inventory for measuring depression. Arch Gen Psychiatry 4:561–571, 1961

Beck CK, Vogelpohl TS, Rasin JH, et al: Effects of behavioral interventions on disruptive behavior and affect in demented nursing home residents. Nurs Res 51:219–228, 2002

Beers M, Avon J, Soumerai SB, et al: Psychoactive medication use in intermediate-care facility residents. JAMA 260:3016–3020, 1988

Bensink GW, Godbey KL, Marshall MJ, et al: Institutionalized elderly: relaxation, locus of control, self-esteem. J Gerontol Nurs 18:30–36, 1992

Berrios GE, Brook P: Delusions and psychopathology of the elderly with dementia. Acta Psychiatr Scand 75:296–301, 1985

Blazer DG, Williams CD: Epidemiology of dysphoria and depression in an elderly population. Am J Psychiatry 137: 439–444, 1980

Borson S, Doane K: The impact of OBRA-87 on psychotropic drug prescribing in skilled nursing facilities. Psychiatr Serv 48:1289–1296, 1997

Borson S, Liptzin B, Nininger J, et al: Psychiatry and the nursing home. Am J Psychiatry 144:1412–1418, 1987

Borson S, Loebel JP, Kitchell M, et al: Psychiatric assessments of nursing home residents under OBRA-87: should PASARR be reformed? Pre-Admission Screening and Annual Review. J Am Geriatr Soc 45:1173–1181, 1997

Braun JV, Wykle MH, Cowling WR: Failure to thrive in older persons: a concept derived. Gerontologist 28:809–812, 1988

Bridges-Parlet S, Knopman D, Steffes S: Withdrawal of neuroleptic medications from institutionalized dementia patients: results of a double-blind, baseline-treatment-controlled pilot study. J Geriatr Psychiatry Neurol 10:119–126, 1997

Brodaty H, Ames D, Snowdon J, et al: A randomized placebo-controlled trial of risperidone for the treatment of aggression, agitation, and psychosis of dementia. J Clin Psychiatry 64:134–143, 2003

Brown MN, Lapane KL, Luisi AF: The management of depression in older nursing home residents. J Am Geriatr Soc 50: 69–76, 2002

Buck JA: Psychotropic drug practice in nursing homes. J Am Geriatr Soc 36:409–418, 1988

Burns BJ, Taube CA: Mental health services in general medical care and in nursing homes, in Mental Health Policy for Older Americans: Protecting Minds at Risk. Edited by Fogel BS, Furino A, Gottlieb GL. Washington, DC, American Psychiatric Press, 1990, pp 63–84

Burns BJ, Larson DB, Goldstrom ID, et al: Mental disorder among nursing home patients: preliminary findings from the National Nursing Home Survey Pretest. Int J Geriatr Psychiatry 3:27–35, 1988

Cape RD: Freedom from restraint. Gerontologist 23:217, 1983

Capezuti E, Evans L, Strumpf N, et al: Physical restraint use and falls in nursing home residents. J Am Geriatrics Soc 44:627–633, 1996

Castle NG, Shea D: Institutional factors of nursing homes that predict the provision of mental health services. J Ment Health Adm 24:44–54, 1997

Castle NG, Fogel B, Mor V: Risk factors for physical restraint use in nursing homes: pre- and post-implementation of the Nursing Home Reform Act. Gerontologist 37:737–747, 1997

Chandler JD, Chandler JE: The prevalence of neuropsychiatric disorders in a nursing home population. J Geriatr Psychiatry Neurol 1:71–76, 1988

Clark TR (ed): Nursing Home Survey Procedures and Interpretive Guidelines. A Resource for the Consultant Pharmacist. Alexandria, VA, American Society of Consultant Pharmacists, 1999, pp 1–8

Cohen-Mansfield J: Agitated behaviors in the elderly: preliminary results in the cognitively deteriorated. J Am Geriatr Soc 34:722–727, 1986

Cohen-Mansfield J: Nonpharmacologic interventions for inappropriate behaviors in dementia: a review, summary, and critique. Am J Geriatr Psychiatry 9:361–381, 2001

Cohen-Mansfield J, Billig N: Agitated behaviors in the elderly: a conceptual review. J Am Geriatr Soc 34:711–721, 1986

Cohen-Mansfield J, Marx MS, Rosenthal AS: A description of agitation in a nursing home. J Gerontol 44:M77–M84, 1989

Cohen-Mansfield J, Lipson S, Werner P, et al: Withdrawal of haloperidol, thioridazine, and lorazepam in the nursing home: a controlled, double-blind study. Arch Intern Med 159:1733–1740, 1999

Colenda CC, Streim JE, Greene JA, et al: The impact of the Omnibus Budget Reconciliation Act of 1987 (OBRA '87) on psychiatric services in nursing homes. Am J Geriatr Psychiatry 7:12–17, 1999

Custer RL, Davis JE, Gee SC: Psychiatric drug usage in VA nursing home care units. Psychiatr Ann 14:285–292, 1984

Datto C, Oslin D, Streim J, et al: Pharmacological treatment of depression in nursing home residents: a mental health services perspective. J Geriatr Psychiatry Neurol 15:141–146, 2002

DeDeyn PP, Rabheru K, Rasmussen A, et al: A randomized trial of risperidone, placebo, and haloperidol for behavioral symptoms of dementia. Neurology 53:946–955, 1999

Dehlin O, Hedenrud B, Jansson P, et al: A double-blind comparison of alaproclate and placebo in the treatment of patients with senile dementia. Acta Psychiatr Scand 71:190–196, 1985

DeLeo D, Stella AG, Spagnoli A: Prescription of psychotropic drugs in geriatric institutions. Int J Geriatr Psychiatry 4:11–16, 1989

Elon R, Pawlson LG: The impact of OBRA on medical practice within nursing facilities. J Am Geriatr Soc 40:958–963, 1992

Engle VF, Graney MJ: Stability and improvement of health after nursing home admission. J Gerontol 48:S17–S23, 1993

Evans LK, Strumpf NE: Tying down the elderly: a review of the literature on physical restraint. J Am Geriatr Soc 37:65–74, 1989

Evans JM, Chutka DS, Fleming KC, et al: Medical care of nursing home residents. Mayo Clin Proc 70:694–702, 1995

Evans LK, Strumpf NE, Allen-Taylor SL, et al: A clinical trial to reduce restraints in nursing homes. J Am Geriatr Soc 45:675–681, 1997

Finkel SI, Lyons JS, Anderson RL, et al: A randomized, placebo-controlled trial of thiothixene in agitated, demented nursing home patients. Int J Geriatr Psychiatry 10:129–136, 1995

Folstein MF, Folstein SE, McHugh PR: Mini-Mental State: a practical method for grading the cognitive state of patients for the clinician. J Psychiatr Res 12:189–198, 1975

Foster JR, Cataldo JK, Boksay IJE: Incidence of depression in a medical long-term care facility: findings from a restricted sample of new admissions. Int J Geriatr Psychiatry 6:13–20, 1991

Gabrel C, Jones A: The National Nursing Home Survey: 1995 Summary. Vital Health Stat 13(146):1–83, 2000

German PS, Shapiro S, Kramer M: Nursing home study of eastern Baltimore epidemiologic catchment area, in Mental Illness in Nursing Homes: Agenda for Research. Edited by Harper MS, Lebowitz BD. Rockville, MD, National Institute of Mental Health, 1986, pp 21–40

Goldwasser AN, Auerbach SM, Harkins SW: Cognitive, affective, and behavioral effects of reminiscence group therapy of demented elderly. Int J Aging Hum Dev 25:209–222, 1987

Gottfries CG, Brane G, Gullberg B, et al: A new rating scale for dementia syndromes. Arch Gerontol Geriatr 1:311–330, 1982

Grant LA, Kane RA, Stark AJ: Beyond labels: nursing home care for Alzheimer's disease in and out of special care units. J Am Geriatr Soc 43:569–576, 1995

Guy W (ed): ECDEU Assessment Manual for Psychopharmacology, Revised (DHEW Publ No ADM-76-388). Rockville, MD, U.S. Department of Health, Education and Welfare, 1976

Hamilton M: The assessment of anxiety states by rating. Br J Med Psychol 32:50–55, 1959

Hamilton M: A rating scale for depression. J Neurol Neurosurg Psychiatry 23:56–62, 1960

Hansen SS, Patterson MA, Wilson RW: Family involvement on a dementia unit: the Resident Enrichment and Activity Program. Gerontologist 28:508–510, 1988

Harrison R, Savla N, Kafetz K: Dementia, depression, and physical disability in a London borough: a survey of elderly people in and out of residential care and implications for future developments. Age Ageing 19:97–103, 1990

Hawes C, Mor V, Phillips CD, et al: The OBRA-87 nursing home regulations and implementation of the Resident Assessment Instrument: effects on process quality. J Am Geriatr Soc 45:977–985, 1997

Health Care Financing Administration: Medicare and Medicaid: Requirements for Long Term Care Facilities, Final Regulations. Fed Regist 56:48865–48921, 1991

Health Care Financing Administration: Medicare and Medicaid Programs: Preadmission Screening and Annual Resident Review. Fed Regist 57:56450–56504, 1992a

Health Care Financing Administration: Medicare and Medicaid: Resident Assessment in Long Term Care Facilities. Fed Regist 57:61614–61733, 1992b

Health Care Financing Administration: State Operations Manual: Provider Certification (Transmittal No 250). Washington, DC, Health Care Financing Administration, 1992c

Health Care Financing Administration: Report to Congress: Study of Private Accreditation (Deeming) of Nursing Homes, Regulatory Incentives and Non-Regulatory Incentives, and Effectiveness of the Survey and Certification System. Washington, DC, Health Care Financing Administration, 1998. Available at http://cms.hhs.gov/medicaid/reports/default.asp. Accessed July 17, 2003.

Health Care Financing Administration: Appendix PP: Guidance to Survivors—Long Term Care Facilities, in Medicare State Operations Manual: Provider Certification (Transmittal No 15). Washington, DC, Health Care Financing Administration, April 2000, pp 121–164. Available at http://cms.hhs.gov/manuals/pm_trans/R15SOM.pdf. Accessed October 19, 2003.

Heston LL, Garrard J, Makris L, et al: Inadequate treatment of depressed nursing home elderly. J Am Geriatr Soc 40:1117–1122, 1992

Holmes D, Teresi J, Weiner A, et al: Impact associated with special care units in long-term care facilities. Gerontologist 30:178–181, 1990

Honigfeld G, Roderic D, Klett JC: NOSIE-30: a treatment-sensitive ward behavior scale. Psychol Rep 19:180–182, 1966

Horiguchi J, Inami Y: A survey of the living conditions and psychological states of elderly people admitted to nursing homes in Japan. Acta Psychiatr Scand 83:338–341, 1991

Hughes CD, Berg L, Danziger L, et al: A new clinical scale for the staging of dementia. Br J Psychiatry 140:566–572, 1982

Hyer L, Blazer DG: Depressive symptoms: impact and problems in long term care facilities. International Journal of Behavioral Gerontology 1:33–44, 1982

Innes EM, Turman WG: Evolution of patient falls. Q Rev Biol 9:30–35, 1983

Institute of Medicine, Committee on Nursing Home Regulation: Improving the Quality of Care in Nursing Homes. Washington, DC, National Academy Press, 1986

Jeste DV, Okamoto A, Napolitano, et al: Low incidence of persistent tardive dyskinesia in elderly patients with dementia treated with risperidone. Am J Psychiatry 157:1150–1155, 2000

Katz IR, Lesher E, Kleban M, et al: Clinical features of depression in the nursing home. Int Psychogeriatr 1:5–15, 1989

Katz IR, Simpson GM, Curlik SM, et al: Pharmacological treatment of major depression for elderly patients in residential care settings. J Clin Psychiatry 51 (suppl):41–48, 1990

Katz IR, Parmelee P, Brubaker K: Toxic and metabolic encephalopathies in long-term care patients. Int Psychogeriatr 3: 337–347, 1991

Katz IR, Beaston-Wimmer P, Parmelee PA, et al: Failure to thrive in the elderly: exploration of the concept and delineation of psychiatric components. J Geriatr Psychiatry Neurol 6:161–169, 1993

Katz IR, Jeste DV, Mintzer JE, et al: Comparison of risperidone and placebo for psychosis and behavioral disturbances associated with dementia: a randomized, double-blind trial. J Clin Psychiatry 60:107–115, 1999

Katz IR, Streim JE, Smith BD: Psychiatric aspects of long-term care, in Kaplan and Sadock's Comprehensive Textbook of Psychiatry, 7th Edition, Vol 2. Edited by Sadock BJ, Sadock VA. Philadelphia, PA, Lippincott Williams & Wilkins, 2000, pp 3145–3150

Kaufer D, Cummings JL, Christine D: Differential neuropsychiatric symptom responses to tacrine in Alzheimer's disease: relationship to dementia severity. J Neuropsychiatry Clin Neurosci 10:55–63, 1998

Kramer M, German PS, Anthony JC, et al: Patterns of mental disorders among the elderly residents of eastern Baltimore. J Am Geriatr Soc 33:236–245, 1985

Krantz DS, Schulz PR: Personal control and health: some applications to crises of middle and old age. Advances in Environmental Psychology 2:23–57, 1980

Krauss NA, Altman BM: Characteristics of Nursing Home Residents—1996. MEPS Research Findings No 5 (AHCPR Publ No 99-0006). Rockville, MD, Agency for Health Care Policy and Research, 1998

Kutner N, Mistretta E, Barnhart H, et al: Family members' perceptions of quality of life change in dementia SCU residents. J Appl Gerontol 18:423–439, 1999

Langer E, Rodin J: The effects of choice and enhanced personal responsibility for the aged: a field experiment in an institutional setting. J Pers Soc Psychol 34:191–198, 1976

Lantz MS, Giambanco V, Buchalter EN: A ten-year review of the effect of OBRA-87 on psychotropic prescribing practices in an academic nursing home. Psychiatr Serv 47:951–955, 1996

Lasser RA, Sunderland T: Newer psychotropic medication use in nursing home residents. J Am Geriatr Soc 46:202–207, 1998

Lawton MP, Brody EM: Assessment of older people: self-maintaining and instrumental activities of daily living. Gerontologist 9:179–186, 1969

Lawton MP, Van Haitsma K, Klapper J, et al: A stimulation-retreat special care unit for elders with dementing illness. Int Psychogeriatr 10:379–395, 1998

Lesher E: Validation of the Geriatric Depression Scale among nursing home residents. Clinics in Gerontology 4:21–28, 1986

Leszcz M, Sadavoy J, Feigenbaum E, et al: A men's group psychotherapy of elderly men. Int J Group Psychother 33:177–196, 1985

Llorente MD, Olsen EJ, Leyva O, et al: Use of antipsychotic drugs in nursing homes: current compliance with OBRA regulations. J Am Geriatr Soc 46:198–201, 1998

Loebel JP, Borson S, Hyde T, et al: Relationships between requests for psychiatric consultations and psychiatric diagnoses in long-term care facilities. Am J Psychiatry 148:898–903, 1991

Magai C, Kennedy G, Cohen CI, et al: A controlled clinical trial of sertraline in the treatment of depression in nursing home patients with late-stage Alzheimer's disease. Am J Geriatr Psychiatry 8:66–74, 2000

Mann AH, Graham N, Ashby D: Psychiatric illness in residential homes for the elderly: a survey in one London borough. Age Ageing 13:257–265, 1984

McMurdo MET, Rennie L: A controlled trial of exercise by residents of old people's homes. Age Ageing 22:11–15, 1993

Meador KG, Taylor JA, Thapa PB, et al: Predictors of antipsychotic withdrawal or dose reduction in a randomized controlled trial of provider education. J Am Geriatr Soc 45:207–210, 1997

Montgomery SA, Åsberg M: A new depression scale designed to be sensitive to change. Br J Psychiatry 134:381–382, 1979

Moran JA, Gatz M: Group therapies for nursing home adults: an evaluation of two treatment approaches. Gerontologist 27:588–591, 1987

Morris JC, Cyrus PS, Orazem J, et al: Metrifonate benefits cognitive, behavioral, and global function in patients with Alzheimer's disease. Neurology 50:1222–1230, 1998

Morris JN, Hawes C, Fries BE, et al: Designing the national resident assessment instrument for nursing homes. Gerontologist 30:293–307, 1990

Murphy E: The use of psychotropic drugs in long-term care (editorial). Int J Geriatr Psychiatry 4:1–2, 1989

National Center for Health Statistics: The National Nursing Home Survey (DHEW Publ No PHS-79-1794). Hyattsville, MD, National Center for Health Statistics, 1979

National Center for Health Statistics: Use of nursing homes by the elderly: preliminary data from the 1985 National Nursing Home Survey (DHHS Publ No PHS-87-1250). Hyattsville, MD, National Center for Health Statistics, 1987

Nyth AL, Gottfries CG: The clinical efficacy of citalopram in treatment of emotional disturbances in dementia disorders. A Nordic multicentre study. Br J Psychiatry 157:894–901, 1990

Office of Inspector General: Medicare Payments for Psychiatric Services in Nursing Homes: A Follow-Up (Publ No OEI-02-99-00140). Washington, DC, U.S. Department of Health and Human Services, 2001a. Available at http://oig.hhs.gov/oei/reports/oei-02-99-00140.pdf. Accessed July 17, 2003.

Office of Inspector General: Nursing Home Resident Assessment, Quality of Care (Publ No OEI-02-99-00040). Washington, DC, U.S. Department of Health and Human Services, 2001b. Available at http://oig.hhs.gov/oei/reports/oei-02-99-00040.pdf. Accessed July 17, 2003.

Office of Inspector General: Psychotropic Drug Use in Nursing Homes (Publ No OEI-02-00-00490). Washington, DC, U.S. Department of Health and Human Services, 2001c. Available at http://oig.hhs.gov/oei/reports/oei-02-00-00490.pdf. Accessed July 17, 2003.

Office of Technology Assessment: Special Care Units for People With Alzheimer's and Other Dementias: Consumer Education, Research, Regulatory, and Reimbursement Issues (OTA-H-543). Washington, DC, U.S. Government Printing Office, August 1992

Ohta RJ, Ohta BM: Special units for Alzheimer's disease patients: a critical look. Gerontologist 28:803–808, 1988

Omnibus Budget Reconciliation Act of 1987, Pub. L. No. 100-203. Subtitle C: Nursing home reform. Washington, DC

Orten JD, Allen M, Cook J: Reminiscence groups with confused nursing center residents: an experimental study. Soc Work Health Care 14:73–86, 1989

Oslin DW, Streim JE, Katz IR, et al: Heuristic comparison of sertraline with nortriptyline for the treatment of depression in frail elderly patients. Am J Geriatr Psychiatry 8:141–149, 2000

Oslin DW, Ten Have TR, Streim JE, et al: Probing the safety of medications in the frail elderly: evidence from a randomized clinical trial of sertraline and venlafaxine in depressed nursing home residents. J Clin Psychiatry 64:875–882, 2003

Overall JE, Gorham DR: The Brief Psychiatric Rating Scale. Psychol Rep 10:799–812, 1962

Parmelee PA, Katz IR, Lawton MP: Depression among institutionalized aged: assessment and prevalence estimation. J Gerontol 44:M22–M29, 1989

Parmelee PA, Katz IR, Lawton MP: The relation of pain to depression among institutionalized aged. J Gerontol 46:P15–P21, 1991

Parmelee PA, Katz IR, Lawton MP: Depression and mortality among institutionalized aged. J Gerontol 47:P3–P10, 1992a

Parmelee PA, Katz IR, Lawton MP: Incidence of depression in long-term care settings. J Gerontol 47:M189–M196, 1992b

Phillips CD, Sloane PD, Hawes C, et al: Effects of residence in Alzheimer's disease special care units on functional outcomes. JAMA 278:1340–1344, 1997

Phillips CD, Spry KM, Sloane PD, et al: Use of physical restraints and psychotropic medications in Alzheimer special care units in nursing homes. Am J Public Health 90:92–96, 2000

Porsteinsson AP, Tariot PN, Erb R, et al: Placebo-controlled study of divalproex sodium for agitation in dementia. Am J Geriatr Psychiatry 9:58–66, 2001

Rattenbury C, Stones MJ: A controlled evaluation of reminiscence and current topics discussion groups in a nursing home context. Gerontologist 29:768–771, 1989

Ray WA, Federspiel CF, Schaffner W: A study of antipsychotic drug use in nursing homes: epidemiologic evidence suggesting misuse. Am J Public Health 70:485–491, 1980

Ray WA, Taylor JA, Meador KG, et al: Reducing antipsychotic drug use in nursing homes. A controlled trial of provider education. Arch Intern Med 153:713–721, 1993

Reichman WE, Coyne AC, Borson S, et al: Psychiatric consultation in the nursing home. A survey of six states. Am J Geriatr Psychiatry 6:320–327, 1998

Reisberg B: Functional Assessment Staging (FAST). Psychopharmacol Bull 24:653–659, 1988

Reisberg B, Ferris SH, deLeon MJ, et al: Global Deterioration Scale (GDS). Psychopharmacol Bull 24:661–663, 1988

Reisberg B, Auer SR, Monteiro IM: Behavioral Pathology in Alzheimer's Disease (BEHAVE-AD) rating scale. Int Psychogeriatr 8 (suppl 3):301–308, 1996

Rhoades J, Krauss N: Nursing Home Trends, 1987 and 1996. MEPS Chartbook No 3 (AHCPR Publ No 99-0032). Rockville, MD, Agency for Health Care Policy and Research, 1999

Risse SC, Cubberley L, Lampe TH, et al: Acute effects of neuroleptic withdrawal in elderly dementia patients. Journal of Geriatric Drug Therapy 2:65–77, 1987

Rosen J, Mulsant BH, Pollock BG: Sertraline in the treatment of minor depression in nursing home residents: a pilot study. Int J Geriatr Psychiatry 15:177–180, 2000

Rovner BW, Kafonek S, Filipp L, et al: Prevalence of mental illness in a community nursing home. Am J Psychiatry 143:1446–1449, 1986

Rovner BW, German PS, Broadhead J, et al: The prevalence and management of dementia and other psychiatric disorders in nursing homes. Int Psychogeriatr 2:13–24, 1990a

Rovner BW, Lucas-Blaustein J, Folstein MF, et al: Stability over one year in patients admitted to a nursing home dementia unit. Int J Geriatr Psychiatry 5:77–82, 1990b

Rovner BW, German PS, Brant LJ, et al: Depression and mortality in nursing homes. JAMA 265:993–996, 1991

Rovner BW, Edelman BA, Cox MP, et al: The impact of antipsychotic drug regulations (OBRA 1987) on psychotropic prescribing practices in nursing homes. Am J Psychiatry 149:1390–1392, 1992

Rovner BW, Steele CD, Shmuely Y, et al: A randomized trial of dementia care in nursing homes. J Am Geriatr Soc 44:7–13, 1996

Sabin TD, Vitug AJ, Mark VH: Are nursing home diagnosis and treatment inadequate? JAMA 248:321–322, 1982

Sadavoy J: Psychotherapy for the institutionalized elderly, in Practical Psychiatry in the Nursing Home: A Handbook for Staff. Edited by Conn DK, Herrman N, Kaye A, et al. Toronto, ON, Canada, Hogrefe & Huber, 1991, pp 217–236

Saxton J, Silverman M, Ricci E, et al: Maintenance of mobility in residents of an Alzheimer's special care facility. Int Psychogeriatr 10:213–224, 1998

Schneider LS, Pollack VE, Lyness SA: A meta-analysis of controlled trials of neuroleptic treatment in dementia. J Am Geriatr Soc 38:553–563, 1990

Schnelle JF, Newman DR, White M, et al: Reducing and managing restraints in long-term-care facilities. J Am Geriatr Soc 40:381–385, 1992

Schnelle JF, Wood S, Schnelle ER, et al: Measurement sensitivity and the Minimum Data Set depression quality indicator. Gerontologist 41:401–405, 2001

Schulz PR: Effect of control and predictability on the psychological well-being of the institutionalized aged. J Pers Soc Psychol 33:563–573, 1976

Semla TP, Palla K, Poddig B, et al: Effect of the Omnibus Reconciliation Act 1987 on antipsychotic prescribing in nursing home residents. J Am Geriatr Soc 42:648–652, 1994

Shader RI, Harmatz JS, Salzman C: A new scale for clinical assessment in geriatric populations: Sandoz Clinical Assessment—Geriatric (SCAG). J Am Geriatr Soc 22:107–113, 1974

Shea DG, Russo PA, Smyer MA: Use of mental health services by persons with a mental illness in nursing facilities: initial impacts of OBRA 87. J Aging Health 12:560–578, 2000

Shorr RI, Fought RL, Ray WA: Changes in antipsychotic drug use in nursing homes during implementation of the OBRA-87 regulations. JAMA 271:358–362, 1994

Siegler EL, Capezuti E, Maislin G, et al: Effects of a restraint reduction intervention and OBRA '87 regulations on psychoactive drug use in nursing homes. J Am Geriatr Soc 45:791–796, 1997

Sloane PD, Mathew LS, Scarborough M, et al: Physical and pharmacologic restraint of nursing home patients with dementia: impact of specialized units. JAMA 265:1278–1282, 1991

Sloane PD, Mitchell CM, Preisser JS, et al: Environmental correlates of resident agitation in Alzheimer's disease special care units. J Am Geriatr Soc 46:862–869, 1998

Smith M, Buckwalter KC, Albanese M: Geropsychiatric education programs. Providing skills and understanding. J Psychosoc Nurs Ment Health Serv 28:8–12, 1990

Smyer M, Brannon D, Cohn M: Improving nursing home care through training and job redesign. Gerontologist 32:327–333, 1992

Smyer MA, Shea DG, Streit A: The provision and use of mental health services in nursing homes: results from the National Medical Expenditure Survey. Am J Public Health 84:284–287, 1994

Snowden M, Roy-Byrne P: Mental illness and nursing home reform: OBRA-87 ten years later. Omnibus Budget Reconciliation Act. Psychiatr Serv 49:229–233, 1998

Snowden M, Sato K, Roy-Byrne P: Assessment and treatment of nursing home residents with depression or behavioral symptoms associated with dementia: a review of the literature. J Am Geriatr Soc 51:1305–1317, 2003

Snowdon J: Dementia, depression, and life satisfaction in nursing homes. Int J Geriatr Psychiatry 1:85–91, 1986

Snowdon J, Donnelly N: A study of depression in nursing homes. J Psychiatr Res 20:327–333, 1986

Spagnoli A, Forester G, MacDonald A, et al: Dementia and depression in Italian geriatric institutions. Int J Geriatr Psychiatry 1:15–23, 1986

Steele C, Rovner BW, Chase GA, et al: Psychiatric symptoms and nursing home placement in Alzheimer's disease. Am J Psychiatry 147:1049–1051, 1990

Stotsky B: Multicenter study comparing thioridazine with diazepam and placebo in elderly, nonpsychotic patients with emotional behavioral disorders. Clin Ther 6:546–559, 1984

Street JS, Clark WS, Gannon KS, et al: Olanzapine treatment of psychotic and behavioral symptoms in patients with Alzheimer disease in nursing care facilities, a double-blind, randomized, placebo-controlled trial. Arch Gen Psychiatry 57:968–976, 2000

Streim JE, Katz IR: Federal regulations and the care of patients with dementia in the nursing home. Med Clin North Am 78:895–909, 1994

Streim JE, Rovner BW, Katz IR: Psychiatric aspects of nursing home care, in Comprehensive Review of Geriatric Psychiatry—II, 2nd Edition. Edited by Sadavoy J, Lazarus LW, Jarvik LF, et al. Washington, DC, American Psychiatric Press, 1996, pp 907–936

Streim JE, Oslin DW, Katz IR, et al: Drug treatment of depression in frail elderly nursing home residents. Am J Geriatr Psychiatry 8:150–159, 2000

Svarstad BL, Mount JK, Bigelow W: Variations in the treatment culture of nursing homes and responses to regulations to reduce drug use. Psychiatr Serv 52:666–672, 2001

Swanson E, Maas M, Buckwalter K: Catastrophic reactions and other behaviors of Alzheimer's residents: special unit compared with traditional units. Arch Psychiatr Nurs 7:292–299, 1993

Tariot PN, Podgorski CA, Blazina L, et al: Mental disorders in the nursing home: another perspective. Am J Psychiatry 150:1063–1069, 1993

Tariot PN, Erb R, Podgorski CA, et al: Efficacy and tolerability of carbamazepine for agitation and aggression in dementia. Am J Psychiatry 155:54–61, 1998

Tariot PN, Cummings JL, Katz IR, et al: A randomized, double-blind, placebo-controlled study of the efficacy and safety of donepezil in patients with Alzheimer's disease in the nursing home setting. J Am Geriatr Soc 49:1590–1599, 2001

Teeter RB, Garetz FK, Miller WR, et al: Psychiatric disturbances of aged patients in skilled nursing homes. Am J Psychiatry 133:1430–1434, 1976

Thapa PB, Gideon P, Cost CW, et al: Antidepressants and the risk of falls among nursing home residents. N Engl J Med 339:875–882, 1998

Thomasma M, Yeaworth R, McCabe B: Moving day: relocation and anxiety in institutionalized elderly. J Gerontol Nurs 16:18–24, 1990

Toseland RW, Diehl M, Freeman K, et al: The impact of validation group therapy on nursing home residents with dementia. J Appl Gerontol 61:31–50, 1997

Trappler B, Cohen CI: Using fluoxetine in "very old" depressed nursing home residents. Am J Geriatr Psychiatry 4:258–262, 1996

Trappler B, Cohen CI: Use of SSRIs in "very old" depressed nursing home residents. Am J Geriatr Psychiatry 6:83–89, 1998

Trichard L, Zabow A, Gillis LS: Elderly persons in old age homes: a medical, psychiatric and social investigation. S Afr Med J 61:624–627, 1982

Wagner AW, Teri L, Orr-Rainey N: Behavior problems of residents with dementia in special care units. Alzheimer Dis Assoc Disord 9:121–127, 1995

Wells Y, Jorm FA: Evaluation of a special nursing home unit for dementia suffers: a randomized controlled comparison with community care. Aust N Z J Psychiatry 21:524–531, 1987

Werner P, Cohen-Mansfield J, Braun J, et al: Physical restraint and agitation in nursing home residents. J Am Geriatr Soc 37:1122–1126, 1989

Williams-Barnard CL, Lindell AR: Therapeutic use of "prizing" and its effect on self-concept of elderly clients in nursing homes and group homes. Issues Ment Health Nurs 13:1–17, 1992

Woods S, Cummings JL, Hsu MA, et al: The use of the neuropsychiatric inventory in nursing home residents: characterization and measurement. Am J Geriatr Psychiatry 8:75–83, 2000

Youssef FA: The impact of group reminiscence counseling on a depressed elderly population. Nurse Pract 15:32–38, 1990

Zerhusen JD, Boyle K, Wilson W: Out of the darkness: group cognitive therapy for depressed elderly. J Psychosoc Nurs Ment Health Serv 29:16–21, 1991

Zimmer JG, Watson N, Treat A: Behavioral problems among patients in skilled nursing facilities. Am J Public Health 74:1118–1121, 1984

The Continuum of Care

Movement Toward the Community

George L. Maddox, Ph.D.

Elise J. Bolda, M.S.P.H., Ph.D.

From 1980 to the present time, the conversation among health care policy analysts, care providers, and consumers about the role of communities in chronic care over the long term has changed significantly. A primary stimulus for this change has been increased awareness of how badly the currently dominant medical model of hospital care is mismatched with increasingly obvious needs for more effective care of chronic conditions in nonhospital settings. This mismatch in the United States has been stated dramatically in a recent report issued by the Institute of Medicine of the National Academy of Sciences, *Crossing the Quality Chasm: A New Health System for the 21st Century* (Institute of Medicine 2001).

More than two decades ago James Fries (1980) argued persuasively that the demographics of the aging population in the United States were being misunderstood. Although the population was demonstrably aging, the onset of chronic illness and of disabling chronic illness was apparently being delayed, in part by a variety of successful social, psychological, and biomedical interventions. Fries correctly anticipated that the implications of these epidemiological changes would include delayed use of institutional forms of care for chronic conditions and greater use of care in the community. Whereas in 1980 these conclusions were only informed guesses, evidence has increasingly tended to confirm them (Fries 2001). (For an illustration online of the practical implications of Fries's argument, see http://healthproject.stanford.edu/mission/index.html.) Recent confirming evidence also indicates that disability in the United States population has apparently been declining at a rate of about 1% a year over the past several decades (Cutler 2001). Further-

more, since 1983, the occupancy rate of available nursing home beds has also declined. The disparity between the care needed in the long term (as demonstrated by evidence) and the care currently provided by the dominant medical-hospital care system has continued to grow—hence the reference by the Institute of Medicine to a "quality chasm."

The demonstrable and anticipated long-term-care needs of aging populations have been a prominent driver of the observed change in the conversation among policy analysts and care providers. But another factor has more recently contributed to this change: the voices of younger adults and their advocates, whose chronic conditions typically appear to be well served—if not better served—by community-based services and care than by typical institutional alternatives. The voices of younger consumers of long-term care for chronic conditions, encouraged by the Americans With Disabilities Act of 1990 (P.L. 101-336; Vachon 2001), have over time encouraged older adults with chronic conditions and their advocates to join in a demand for community alternatives for care in the long term. In a logical extension of the right to more care in the community, chronically disabled adults and their advocates have demonstrated increased interest in and demand for consumer-directed care in the provision of personal assistance services, which is discussed in more detail later in this chapter (see the subsection "Consumer-Directed Care").

In the United States, health care policy is often influenced, if not mandated, by legal decisions. In their decision in *Olmstead v. L.C.* (1999), the U.S. Supreme Court interpreted the Americans With Disabilities Act of

1990 to cover an institutionalized person who claimed the right to obtain alternative appropriate, cost-effective community-based care. Because research suggests that at least a significant minority of persons with chronic conditions living in institutions could be appropriately placed in the community, and vice versa, the legal challenge could not be easily dismissed. How the full implications of the *Olmstead* decision will play out remains to be seen. But states are taking great care to certify that they intend to be in compliance. The gauntlet has been thrown down; the routine, convenient assignment of persons with chronic conditions to existing institutional care services rather than to community-based care services is now subject to legal challenge. Communities as well as state and federal policymakers have both incentives and opportunities to consider again the case for community-based services for persons with chronic conditions.

Long-Term-Care Policy in the United States: Muddling Through

To the despair of policy analysts who believe that health care policy making should be and can be a rational, evidence-based enterprise, health care policy in the United Kingdom since the creation of the National Health Service in 1948 has rather consistently appeared to be adequately described as "muddling through" (Maddox 1971). Muddlers respond to their critics by noting that muddling—or pragmatism—just may be the policy strategy of choice in the rapidly changing circumstances of democratic societies with complex and sometimes conflicting values. This strategy is further reinforced by the observation of organizational theorists that no single correct way to implement desired policy outcomes exists.

Successful policy implementations, however, depend substantially on societal context and leadership. One example of the importance of context and leadership in policy implementation is the origin and recent history of long-term-care policy in the United States since 1965.

As Theodore Marmor (2000) argued in his account of the creation of Medicare and Medicaid in 1965, the enabling legislation was a marvelously complex political creation. Proponents of broad health care services underwritten by public dollars faced not only opposing medical and hospital interests but also—which was perhaps more daunting—deeply held public values favoring keeping health care in the private sector and favoring personal responsibility for long-term care (Maddox 1992). The muddling outcome of this complex political contest was the decision to make public dollars available to private-sector entrepreneurs to create what is now observed as a

hospital-like system of nursing homes whose facilities are frequently described in terms of numbers of "beds" to be occupied by "patients" and serviced by medical directors, nurses, and their various aides.

Medicare was initially intended to provide services predominantly to older adults, as indicated by the nearly universal association of age 65 with eligibility for the program. Yet there has never been any provision for Medicare to underwrite long-term care beyond limited post-hospitalization care, most often provided initially in nursing homes. More recently, limited care at home has been permitted. The welfare component of Medicare was made a separate program, Medicaid, for persons with incomes at or below the federal poverty level. Over time, Medicaid has come to serve a large number of nonelderly mothers and children, whereas the support of services for poor older adults has been substantially directed toward underwriting the cost of institutional long-term care.

This characterization of long-term care in the United States has remained largely accurate since the 1960s. Interestingly, in the mid-1990s, when the Clinton administration was promising large-scale health care reform, no significant change in the structure and function of long-term-care policy was proposed. Recently, there has been increasing pressure to provide some coverage of prescribed drugs under Medicare, as has already occurred under Medicaid. The future of such a proposal remains in doubt, not only because of concern about the cost of its implementation but also because political uneasiness appears to increase whenever a broad promise is made to underwrite personal health care costs with public dollars in the absence of demonstrated financial need. The issue of the cost of alternative forms of caring in the long term warrants a brief commentary.

For decades, the United States has ranked at the top of international comparisons of investment in formal health care. In recent years such investment has reached 14% of gross domestic product. Although doctors, hospitals, and drug companies have not typically been singled out for pointed and sustained public criticism in discussions of health care policy, discussions of the public financing of Medicare and Medicaid have included criticism of all three. For Medicare, federal legislation has continually ratcheted down the fees that physicians and hospitals can charge for older patients; Medicaid legislation has permitted states to limit the eligibility of indigent persons for access to publicly supported health care services provided in institutions or in the community.

With the United States' history of interest in cost control, the cost of alternative types of long-term-care services tends to appear early and often in discussion of long-term-care policy and programs. Proponents of long-term-care services in the community expect to be asked, and in fact typically are asked, "But is it cheaper than institutional care in the medical-hospital tradition?" One might argue that although this question is legitimate, it may be the wrong question. A better question might be "What if consumers of community-based long-term care prefer such care and the evidence indicates that care is not cheaper but is not more costly?" Would consumer preference outweigh evidence that community care might be more costly or equally costly?

All evidence indicates that most adults with chronic conditions requiring sustained care prefer to be served in noninstitutional settings and in the community. But evidence that response to community-based care preferences is cheaper is equivocal at best—not merely because of inadequate research, although that is part of the problem. Longitudinal evidence on the cost of serving chronically impaired adults when their needs are appropriately specified is rare because of the complexity of measuring service use and the difficulty of establishing true cost across care settings. Compared with nursing home care, serving high-need chronically impaired persons in the community costs more—and paradoxically, the cost of community care can seem deceptively low because it is substantially funded not by public dollars but by private family resources. In fact, research indicates that about 80% of community-based care is provided informally by family and friends.

In sum, health care policy in the United States has historically focused on the development and financing of medicine and hospitals. Continuing this focus has not apparently displeased most consumers, who appear to accept the idea that good medicine is typically high-technology medicine. Long-term-care policy has remained muddled nationally. Personal responsibility for care in the long term remains the dominant preference. And when alternative forms of care compete with medical and hospital care, the issue of cost arises early and often.

Such an environment is not congenial for bridging the quality chasm between the existing care system designed to manage needs for acute care and a care system capable of managing the increasing prevalence of needs for chronic care. The dominant national policy response to managing long-term chronic conditions retains its institutional and medical focus. For older adults, this policy reaffirms the use of nursing homes as the dominant long-term response to chronic conditions and serious illness—a response financed substantially out of pocket for individuals with assets or by Medicaid for low-income individuals.

However, concentrating solely, and pessimistically, on inertia at the federal level misses a new dynamic—one

that is generating innovations in existing long-term-care regulation and within communities that are exploring alternative ways to provide care in the long term. The new dynamic does not flow primarily from federal policy initiatives but reflects pragmatic (muddling, if you prefer) private initiatives of professional organizations such as the Institute of Medicine, population change, and state and community initiatives for housing and caring for frail and disabled persons.

Care in the Community: A New Dynamic

These changing dynamics, reflected in conversations about new structures and strategies for long-term care of persons with chronic conditions and illness, have become increasingly obvious. These new conversations focus less on issues, such as the relative cost of alternatives to institutional care, and more on the potential beneficial effects on health if those who need assistance are empowered to participate in choices regarding their care. Evidence now makes it unmistakably clear that frail and chronically disabled individuals exhibit an extraordinary variety of capabilities for participating in selecting and implementing the care they receive, that some chronically disabling conditions are modifiable, and that how a care system is organized and implemented is itself an important variable in achieving and sustaining maximum functioning of chronically disabled individuals (Maddox 2000).

One indication of the importance of consumer empowerment as a variable in health care effectiveness is the emergence of *self-efficacy* as a key concept in health care research. The concept is studied particularly in intervention research intended to enhance individual capacity for psychological and social functioning. Self-efficacy refers to specific judgments by individuals that they can perform competently and capably in given situations. Recognition of the specific nature of self-efficacy is important; it is not a global concept but a situationally grounded judgment that varies across activity domains, task demands, and situational characteristics (Bandura 1997).

In intervention research, self-efficacy has become one of the most powerful predictors of beneficial changes in health behavior, in health, and in functioning (Schulz et al. 1998). An important extrapolation of self-efficacy is provided by the concept of *collective efficacy*, which has been usefully applied in social survey research to identify collectivities such as neighborhood and community characterized by a shared sense of trust and the reliable availability of help (Kawachi and Berkman 2000; Maddox 2001). One outcome of enhanced self- and collective efficacy that might be expected is a sense of both individual and community empowerment that in turn would enhance a population's level of functional capacity and sense of well-being.

The importance of efficacy will be apparent in interpreting each of the six initiatives, discussed below, that illustrate notable innovations in community-based long-term care: hospice, chronic care management, consumer-directed care, assisted living housing, empowerment and community in mental health initiatives, and collaborative partnerships of community care for elders. None of these innovations was the product of a federal policy initiative. One is an initiative of the Institute of Medicine, National Academy of Sciences; one was an import from abroad; one is an outcome of decisions in the housing industry; and four are initiatives supported in part by a private foundation. All have helped fill a void in federal policy on long-term care in the United States. In the brief discussion of each of these notable innovations, illustrative recent literature references will be cited, with the expectation that relevant background and historical material will be found within the recent references. In addition, useful information sources on the Web are provided for each innovation.

Six Illustrative Innovations in Community-Based Long-Term Care

Hospice

Hospice is an ancient provision of community care for dying persons and their families that reemerged in the modern era with the establishment of St. Christopher's Hospice outside London in 1967. The idea migrated to the United States in the 1970s, but with a difference (Mor and Allen 2001). Whereas the English hospice was a community of caring for the dying within institutional walls, the American version has emphasized home care, or "hospice without walls." The inadequacy of care at the end of life, particularly in hospital and nursing home settings, has been widely documented (Institute of Medicine 1997; Meier and Morrison 1999). The Institute of Medicine review (1997) reported by Field and Cassel documents widespread neglect of dying patients and their families on hospital wards, in nursing homes, and in medical education. The perceived inadequacy of care at the end of life in hospital settings, disenchantment with the unfulfilled promise of curative medicine, and a new sensitivity to the possibility of better care at the end of life

have combined to promote the implementation in hospice of a new philosophy about care at the end of life. The philosophy emphasizes the importance of a homelike environment for terminal care, effective pain control, the absence of high-technology medical and surgical interventions characteristic of hospitals, and emotional support for dying patients and their families.

Hospice care is designed to maximize a sense of self-efficacy in managing as much as possible one's final transition in a minimally medical environment, with the promise of a collective assurance that social support will remain reliably available. The life-prolonging high-technology interventions characteristic of hospitals are simply not present; and this, economists have conjectured, is one likely explanation of the low cost of hospice in comparison with hospitalization.

Hospice is one of the innovations in long-term care that has been extensively evaluated. This strategy of terminal care, which since the mid-1980s has been covered by Medicare, does tend to reduce cost of care at the end of life. And, overall, the quality of medical care provided within this low-technology environment compares favorably with the care that hospitals provide for comparable patients. Terminal care provided by hospice has become increasingly popular as a service. By the late 1990s, more than 1,000 hospices were serving more than 350,000 patients in the United States. Hospice, in sum, has become a major community alternative for terminal care—particularly for patients with cancer, and more recently for those with AIDS. Current information on hospice is available online at http://www.hospicefoundation.org.

Chronic Care Management

Curative medicine has produced the paradox of facilitating the survival of individuals who in an earlier day would have died young yet who in modern times are unable to manage their chronic conditions and illnesses effectively. A growing chorus of critics is pointing out that the dominant medical-hospital complex is proving inadequate in providing effective care for a population with increasing rates of chronic conditions and illness. The current health system, they conclude, cannot do the job.

The Institute of Medicine, National Academy of Sciences, has become a principal advocate of designing a new, more adequate health care system (Institute of Medicine 2001). An executive summary and the full text of the group's conclusions and proposal for corrective action are available online. Go to the National Academies Press Web site, http://www.nap.edu; then specify *Crossing the*

Quality Chasm. (All publications of the National Academies Press are available free online.)

An initiative of the Robert Wood Johnson Foundation, Chronic Care Management (CCM), provides a convincing demonstration of how a new way of thinking about caring for patients with chronic conditions can be implemented in health care organizations of various sizes (Wagner et al. 2001). An overview of the idea of CCM and its current implementation is available online at http://www.improvingchroniccare.org. CCM applies the principles of chronic care management identified as essential by the Institute of Medicine—for example, the importance of continuous relationships among members of a care team, the primacy of anticipating as well as recognizing patient needs, and having information about care options available to patients. The intention is not to make decisions for an uninformed patient but to provide decision support for an informed patient.

The principles of CCM are not new. Evidence of their effective implementation and of positive results in managing chronic conditions is new.

Consumer-Directed Care

Self-care is a typical first response when symptoms of acute illness appear. Self-care when chronic conditions occur is likely to involve consideration of health-promoting activities such as diet, exercise, rest, and stress control (DeFriese 2001). With either type of condition, the individual's emphasis is on self-management. In contrast, recent interest in consumer-directed care, particularly since the enactment of the Americans With Disabilities Act of 1990, focuses rather on the management of personal assistance services by the consumer of such services.

Disabled Americans of all ages require the assistance of some other person to function adequately in their daily lives. And about 80% of persons needing personal supportive care, a majority of whom are elderly, reside in the community, mostly at home.

Since about 1983, most personal care services have been provided and supervised by designated agencies and social service organizations. The 1990s, however, produced new programs in more than half the states that offer chronically disabled persons services they can employ and direct. Recent survey evidence reports that more than 12 million Americans of all ages need some kind of personal care over the long term and that about a third of these require personal assistance services.

Current consumer-directed services for frail and disabled persons have been modeled on earlier experience in providing personal services for younger adults with physical disabilities. Older consumers with disabilities and their advocates have increasingly expressed interest in consumer-directed personal care services.

Programs of consumer-directed personal care vary widely, both among countries and, in this country, among states. An overview article that displays with clarity the observed variety and issues is offered online by the Urban Institute (Cuellar et al. 2000). Prominent issues for older consumers include the competence of consumers to make decisions and manage finances, whether family members can be hired, whether cash and cash payments are under consumers' control, the availability of consumer training for care direction, the availability of appropriate care providers, and the provision of quality assurance. Although definitive answers are not yet available on these issues, consumer-directed personal assistance services continue to flourish internationally.

Consumer-directed care, like chronic care management, is consistent with current interest in the empowerment of health care consumers and with the enhancement of both self-efficacy and collective efficacy. The relatively passive and grateful patients of an earlier day are now encouraged to be involved and informed consumers, and sometimes directors, of their own health care.

In addition to the potential benefit of expanding the workforce, public officials might be expected to be interested in good-quality consumer-directed care if it is cost effective, which early evidence indicates it probably is. Early evidence also indicates that the risk of poor care is no higher for consumers who direct their own personal service care than for those using established service organizations. Evaluation research accompanying the Robert Wood Johnson Foundation's Cash and Counseling initiative promises to provide policymakers with more definite answers for key questions (see also Mahoney et al. 2001; Polivka 2000).

Consumer-directed personal service care does appear to enhance the competence of chronically disabled individuals to care for themselves, to increase their sense of self-efficacy in achieving a satisfactory quality of life, and to encourage communities to develop a sense of collective efficacy in providing reliably available compensatory services for chronically disabled persons.

Assisted Living Housing

A home locates families socially in a community and is the locale for reliably available social support when needed. For a minority, there is neither home nor family. Many elderly chronically disabled persons, even if other housing is available, live alone or in home settings they cannot negotiate safely. In earlier decades, frail chronically disabled adults were housed in homes for the poor and elderly. In more recent decades, such vulnerable individuals became patients in nursing homes or residents in adult care homes or similar nonmedical residential care settings. None of the typically available housing arrangements for frail chronically disabled elderly persons was designed to maintain or enhance their sense of self-efficacy, nor have the usually available housing arrangements promised reliably available compensatory care for frail disabled residents.

Fortunately, studies of housing and living arrangements in the United States indicate that, overall, older persons are among the best-housed adults in a well-housed nation. Only a minority of older adults (though a significant minority) live alone. Periodic reviews of housing in the United States have documented the quality of housing available, but only recently have these reviews questioned the appropriateness of that housing and of various housing alternatives for frail disabled adults. The medicalized environment of nursing homes provides reliably available nursing care for patients, but for a minority too much care is provided, increasing the risk of creating dependency. Nonmedical residential care homes for older adults have not typically provided reliably available care designed to meet the measured needs of residents.

For more information in this area, Maddox (2001) provides an overview of current Census of Housing information about housing and living arrangements in the United States, behavioral and social science theory, research about the significance of housing over the life course, and the recent availability of new forms of housing of importance for frail disabled adults.

In the midst of a clear mismatch between housing needs and availability for chronically disabled older adults, a distinctive new type of housing has appeared: assisted living housing. The four concepts of the philosophy of assisted living housing in its ideal form are: 1) offering a private, self-contained space of one's own, 2) matching reliably available services with measured individual need, 3) sharing responsibility for care among residents, family and staff, and 4) making information available to residents to promote informed choices and control of their lives. These concepts clearly resonate with the philosophy of the community care innovations discussed above: enhancement of self-efficacy and collective efficacy in responsive communities such as hospice, chronic care management, and consumer-directed services.

Currently, more than 28,000 assisted living housing facilities in the United States serve more than 600,000 residents. The number of these facilities and their residents continues to increase rapidly. Clearly, assisted living housing has appealed to economically secure elderly per-

sons who value the philosophy of this new form of housing. Affordability, however, is clearly a problem of the new housing option: the average annual income of current residents is $31,000. Despite a few innovative state efforts, a national commitment to subsidize such housing routinely for frail disabled adults is not in prospect. More information on affordable assisted living housing is available online at http://www.ncbdc.org.

Nevertheless, assisted living housing has attracted attention because its philosophy is so consistent with current values emphasizing self-efficacy, autonomy, and the reliable availability of needed compensatory services. Of particular interest in current theories of adult development is Paul and Margret Baltes' theory of selective optimization with compensation (Baltes and Baltes 1990). In brief, they argue that as energy and personal resources wane in late adulthood, autonomous individuals select how they will concentrate their resources, and they search for environments in which compensatory services are reliably available when needed. These are precisely the conditions that the philosophy of assisted living housing offers (Again, see Maddox 2001 for a review of the history of assisted living housing and a review of relevant research assessing its philosophy and its outcomes in practice.) The initial evidence suggests that this new form of housing does deliver the promised outcomes when its philosophy is implemented: autonomy, self-direction, social involvement, and enhanced well-being.

Mental Health Care: From Deinstitutionalization to Empowerment and Community

Mental health care has remained at the margins of the dominant medical and hospital care system in the United States. In the twentieth century, when chronic mood disorders ranked as the second most common disability among adults, mental health problems tended to be considered the problems of individuals and families until they became severe; then the response tended to be hospitalization.

Movement toward reform of mental health services was evident in the 1950s and 1960s, beginning with federal policy to deinstitutionalize persons in mental hospitals. In the 1950s, for example, the risk of placement in a mental institution fell from 339 to 29 per 100,000 adults. The most obvious outcome of returning behaviorally challenged individuals "to the community" turned out to be, for many, placement in nursing homes and adult care homes and, for some, homelessness on the street (e.g., Kahana 2001).

Mental health services in the community were enhanced in the mid-1970s by a federal mandate to create community health centers. And mental health services were broadened to include special populations such as mentally retarded and developmentally delayed persons and those with substance abuse problems. Mental health services for older adults were rarely featured in community programs.

In health services research on mental health in the United States, the issue of cost tends to be raised early and often. Discussion of mental health care in one of the most prestigious journals has focused on economic issues, such as 1) the concern of employers underwriting health care for employees that demand for mental health services might be limitless; 2) the concern of consumers and consumer advocates that insurance for mental health care might be arbitrarily limited; and 3) the concern of ethicists that mental health services, already marginalized and undercapitalized in today's dominant medicalized care system, may, in the interest of cost control, be even more inequitably treated. One symptom of the current interest in cost control of mental health services is the practice of the "carve-out" of such services from managed care insurance. This practice refers to contracting with behavioral health companies specifically to provide mental health services. This practice has demonstrably reduced cost by limiting the number of services provided and the number of hospital days allowed. Assessment of the quality of care provided remains to be demonstrated ("New Mental Health Care Market" 1999).

There is a relative dearth of current literature summarizing systematically the experience of moving mental health services from institutions toward the community and relating this movement to theory and research. A recent monograph, however, provides an adequately comprehensive review of research and theory underlying the movement of mental health toward the community: *Shifting the Paradigm in Community Mental Health* (Nelson et al. 2001) provides a particularly readable account of how mental health services in a midsize Canadian city were transformed to implement three primary values:

1. Enhancing the personal empowerment of individual consumers of mental health care
2. Effective integration of mental health organizations and programs through collaboration and partnering
3. More equitable distribution of community resources and social capital to mental health services

The monograph provides a clear statement of the history of movement of mental health services toward the community. In addition, theories of personal empowerment, of organizational collaboration, and of equitable distribution of social capital are discussed and are related to the research on interventions to enhance such values in Waterloo, a midsize Canadian city. Qualitative research strategies were used to demonstrate how the mental health services paradigm was shifted toward the community and how personal empowerment, organizational partnering, and interest in more equitable distribution of community resources and social capital were implemented. Movement toward the valued outcomes did appear to occur.

Although similar progress in the United States is emerging only slowly, it is heartening to find growing awareness of the gaps between community mental health services and supportive services for older adults. Examples of such awareness are the discussions of community mental health services for the elderly in *Mental Health: A Report of the Surgeon General* (U.S. Public Health Service 1999) and in the Administration on Aging (2001) report *Older Adults and Mental Health: Issues and Opportunities*. The surgeon general's report and other documents on mental health and aging services are available through the Mental Health and Aging link on the Administration on Aging Web site, http://www.aoa.gov/prof/notes/Docs/Mental_Health.pdf.

Although the Older Americans Act of 1965 (P.L. 89-73) specifically discusses mental health needs, federal funding in support of this legislation through the Administration on Aging has not included specific mandates for mental health funding. And, as noted earlier in the chapter, community mental health service agencies have had few incentives to serve older adults. Thus two distinct systems of service exist, with few mechanisms for coordinating or integrating services for older adults with physical and mental health needs. However, at the state and local levels, efforts are emerging to bridge this gap for persons with severe and persistent mental illness who are growing older and for adults who develop a need for mental health services in later life. Specifically, collaborative partnerships among professionals in the fields of aging and of mental health are being fostered through the American Society on Aging, the Mental Health and Aging Network, and the National Coalition on Mental Health and Aging. These organizations work to build state and community mental health and aging coalitions described online at the Administration on Aging's Web site, http://www.aoa.gov/prof/notes/Docs/Mental_Health.pdf.

In addition to community empowerment efforts, efforts to empower the individual are also beginning to surface. One example is the formation of an advocacy network seeking to provide a voice for older mental health consumers and for people with Alzheimer's disease with regard to public policies on home- and community-based services. A description of this network, Our Own Voice, is included at its link from the Web site http://www.bazelon.org/agingiss.html.

Collaborative Partnerships of Community Care for Elders

Another initiative emerged, beginning in the mid-1970s to the early 1980s and peaking in the 1990s, from a perceived crisis in lack of essential cohesion in communities. This initiative is a growing array of home and community care options, subsidized by federal and state funds, that developed in response to changes in family structure and a growing demand for community-based services. A pervasive crisis in confidence occurred when it was perceived that community cohesiveness and civic consciousness had waned (e.g., Putnam 2000). However, a countervailing interest in community building and civic leadership development has become increasingly apparent. For examples, see Partners for Livable Communities, at http://www.livable.com, and Pew Partnerships for Collaborative Community Leadership, at http://www.pew-partnership.org/collableadership/collableadership.html.

In the absence of a cohesive federal policy, responsibility for community care has largely devolved on the state, with mixed results. In light of the impending shift in the age structure of the population and already burdensome Medicaid and state program budgets, states are reluctant to expand public subsidies, and few states have successfully developed cohesive long-term-care policies and systems with community-based care services as an integral component. But most of such emerging policies and systems have mechanisms to encourage collaborative community partnerships designed to produce integrated long-term-care services. One of the most promising state-designed programs relying on communities is the managed long-term-care program in Arizona, described online at http://www.ahcccs.state.az.us/Services/altcs/altcspgm.htm. Several other states have created incentives for community innovation in health and supportive services for care in the long term; they include California, Minnesota, Texas, Wisconsin, and Vermont.

Elsewhere, municipal, county, and other substate groups have coalesced—responding to the unmet needs of their older neighbors and/or recognizing the economic impact of the aging of the baby-boom generation. These community partnerships between consumers, providers, and local civic and business leaders, as they seek to create a more elder-friendly community, are showing increasing concern about the need for care in the long term for residents of all income groups.

In response to the myriad challenges faced by collaborative community partnerships that are seeking solutions for their communities, the Robert Wood Johnson Foundation established the Community Partnership for Older Adults program in 2001. This national program is based on the powerful melding of the collective efficacy of collaborative community partnerships and the self-efficacy of knowledgeable consumers. The program's goals are 1) to mobilize the community to create greater awareness of the unique contributions and increasing needs of older community members, 2) to educate community members to be more knowledgeable consumers and more effective decision makers, 3) to promote a better quality of life and care by enhancing choices and decision making by older adults and their caregivers within both existing and new programs, and 4) to leverage public and private resources in response to identified community needs so that access to care will improve. Among the community care system improvements expected are a) the availability of more responsive and timely information for older adults and their caregivers; and b) increased communication and coordination among communities' disparate providers of health, long-term-care, and supportive services. For more information visit http://www.partnershipsforolderadults.org.

The notion of collective efficacy is further embraced by the program's promise to foster intercommunity information sharing, which can include lessons learned and barriers surmounted. As this program proceeds, information sharing among communities will be available through the "virtual community" established for this purpose. Combined with a technical assistance consortium—designed in response to communities' common needs for assistance with particularly complex or vexing challenges—the virtual community will include information to help communities communicate with their older residents and the general public to raise civic awareness and interest in issues of long-term caregiving. Through this means, communities can share their experiences with leadership development, consumer inclusion, employee assistance programs in the private sector, local tax levies devoted to aging services, and other financial and human resource development. In this way the program will provide information for community groups on partnership building and problem solving as they seek to improve systems that provide support services to vulnerable older adults. More information on these partnerships is available at http://partnershipsforolderadults.org.

The long-term objectives of this national initiative are to facilitate, monitor, evaluate, and share the experience of effective community partnering in the provision of community-based services. They are, at their best, learning laboratories illustrating how partnering enhances effective serving of older adults. Community partnerships become teachers of other communities as they develop as integrated *learning organizations* (Senge 1990).

Finally, because communities have widely varying resources and needs, there is almost no limit to the solutions that may be crafted through this and other community-guided innovations working to meet the challenges of providing care in the long term.

References

Administration on Aging: Older Adults and Mental Health: Issues and Opportunities. Washington, DC, U.S. Department of Health and Human Services, 2001

Americans With Disabilities Act of 1990, Pub. L. No. 101-336, 101st Congress (enacted 26 July 1990)

Baltes P, Baltes M: Psychological perspectives on successful aging: the model of selective optimization with compensation, in Successful Aging. Edited by Baltes PB, Baltes MM. New York, Cambridge University Press, 1990, pp 1–34

Bandura A: Self-Efficacy: The Exercise of Control. New York, WH Freeman, 1997

Chronic Care in America. Health Aff (Millwood) 20(6):1–286, 2001

Cuellar AE, Tilly J, Wiener JM: Consumer-directed home and community services programs in five countries: policy issues for older people and government. Washington, DC, Urban Institute, 2000. Available at http://www.urban.org/url.cfm?ID=410330. Accessed December 1, 2003.

Cutler DM: Declining disability among the elderly. Health Aff 20(6):1–27, 2001

DeFriese G: Self-care activities, in Encyclopedia of Aging, 3rd Edition. Edited by Maddox G. New York, Springer, 2001, pp 900–902

Fries J: Aging, natural death, and the compression of morbidity. N Engl J Med 303:130–135, 1980

Fries J: Compression of morbidity, in Encyclopedia of Aging, 3rd Edition. Edited by Maddox G. New York, Springer, 2001, pp 234–236

Institute of Medicine, Committee on Care at the End of Life: Approaching Death: Improving Care at the End of Life. Edited by Field MJ, Cassel CK. Washington, DC, National Academy Press, 1997

Institute of Medicine, Committee on Quality Health Care in America: Crossing the Quality Chasm: A New Health System for the 21st Century. Washington, DC, National Academy Press, 2001

Kahana E: De-institutionalization, in Encyclopedia of Aging, 3rd Edition. Edited by Maddox G. New York, Springer, 2001, pp 273–276

Kawachi I, Berkman L: Social cohesion, social capital, and health, in Social Epidemiology. Edited by Berkman L, Kawachi I. New York, Oxford University Press, 2000, pp 174–190

Maddox G: Muddling through: planning health services in England. Med Care 9:439–448, 1971

Maddox G: Long-term care in comparative perspective. Ageing Soc 12:335–368, 1992

Maddox G: Behavioral and social dynamics of aging well, in Promoting Health: Intervention Strategies From Social and Behavioral Research. Edited by Smedby B, Syme L. Washington, DC, National Academy Press, 2000, pp 322–336

Maddox G: Housing and living arrangements, in Handbook of Aging and the Social Sciences, 5th Edition. Edited by Binstock R, George L. San Diego, CA, Academic Press, 2001, pp 426–443

Mahoney K, Simon-Rasinowitz L, Mares L: Cash payments for care, in Encyclopedia of Aging, 3rd Edition. Edited by Maddox G. New York, Springer, 2001, pp 167–170

Marmor TR: The Politics of Medicare, 2nd Edition. New York, A de Gruyter, 2000

Meier D, Morrison R (eds): Care at the end of life: restoring a balance. Generations: Journal of the American Society on Aging 23(1), 1999

Mor V, Allen S: Hospice, in Encyclopedia of Aging, 3rd Edition. Edited by Maddox G. New York, Springer, 2001, pp 507–509

Nelson G, Lord J, Ochoocka J: Shifting the Paradigm in Community Mental Health: Towards Empowerment and the Community. Toronto, ON, Canada, University of Toronto Press, 2001

New Mental Health Care Market. Health Aff (Millwood) 18(5):1–255, 1999

Older Americans Act of 1965, Pub. L. No. 89-73, 89th Congress (enacted July 14, 1965)

Olmstead v L C (98-536) 527 US 581 (1999) 138 F3d 893, affirmed in part, vacated in part, and remanded.

Polivka L: The ethical and empirical basis for consumer-directed care for frail elderly. Contemporary Gerontology 7(2):50–52, 2000

Putnam R: Bowling Alone: The Collapse and Revival of American Community. New York, Simon & Schuster, 2000

Schulz R, Maddox G, Lawton P (eds): Interventions Research With Older Adults. Annu Rev Gerontol Geriatr 18, 1998

Senge P: The Fifth Discipline: The Art and Practice of Learning Organization. New York, Doubleday/Currency, 1990

U.S. Public Health Service: Mental Health: A Report of the Surgeon General. Rockville, MD, U.S. Department of Health and Human Services, 1999

Vachon A: Americans With Disabilities Act, in Encyclopedia of Aging, 3rd Edition. Edited by Maddox G. New York, Springer, 2001, pp 91–183

Wagner EH, Austin BT, Davis C, et al: Improving chronic illness care: translating evidence into action. Health Aff (Millwood) 20(6):64–78, 2001

Web Resources

Innovations in Community-Based Long-Term Care

Hospice

Current information on hospice is available online at http://www.hospicefoundation.org.

Chronic Care Management

To view a proposal for changes in the health care system from the Institute of Medicine, National Academy of Sciences, visit the National Academies Press Web site at http://www.nap.edu. Search for *Crossing the Quality Chasm* to view book excerpts.

An overview of the idea of chronic care management and its current implementation is available at http://www.improvingchroniccare.org.

Consumer-Directed Services

An overview of consumer-directed home and community services programs in five countries is available in an article from the Urban Institute's Web site at http://www.urban.org/url.cfm?ID=410330.

Assisted Living Housing

An introduction to assisted living housing from an industry perspective is available from The Assisted Living Federation of America at http://www.alfa.org.

For more information on affordable assisted living housing, see http://www.ncbdc.org. Select "Affordable Assisted Living" from the site's menu.

Mental Health Care Reform

Documents on mental health and aging services and on collaborative partnerships to build state and community mental health and aging coalitions are described at the Administration on Aging Web site, http://www.aoa.gov/prof/notes/Docs/Mental_Health.pdf.

For a description of an advocacy network, Our Own Voice, which seeks to provide a voice for older mental health consumers and people with Alzheimer's disease, visit http://www.bazelon.org/agingiss.html.

Collaborative Partnerships of Community Care

The following sites provide information on community building and civic leadership development: Partners for Livable Communities: http://www.livable.com; and Pew Partnerships for Collaborative Community Leadership: http://www.pew-partnership.org/collableadership/collableadership.html.

One of the most promising state-designed programs relying on communities is the managed long-term-care program in Arizona. The state's program description can be found online at http://www.ahcccs.state.az.us/Services/altcs/altcspgm.htm.

Brief descriptions of several elder-friendly community initiatives appear in the Grantmakers in Aging Annual Conference 2000 Report, *Elder-Friendly Communities: Opportunities for Creative Grantmaking*, at http://www.giaging.org/conference%20brochure.pdf.

To find information about partnerships and community care system improvements, visit the Web site for Community Partnerships for Older Adults at http://www.partnershipsforolderadults.org.

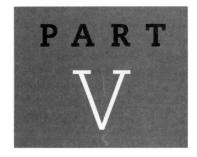

PART

V

Special Topics

Legal, Ethical, and Policy Issues

William E. Reichman, M.D.

Joel E. Streim, M.D.

J. Pierre Loebel, M.D.

With the explosive growth anticipated in the ranks of the elderly over the coming decades, clinicians, educators, researchers, patient advocates, and policy makers in the United States have become increasingly focused on society's ability to meet the anticipated health care needs of this population. That focus has involved ongoing reexamination of the financing structure and the workforce dedicated to supporting the health care of the nation's elderly. In addition, increasingly open dialogues on important related social themes have included the array of ethical issues that must be confronted and managed in caring for patients at the end of life (Institute for Health and Aging 1996). Reform and redesign of health care services to be directed to the care of an aging and increasingly infirm population is a dynamic and highly politicized process. The same holds true for discussions related to the social and ethical dimensions of geriatric health care. In the midst of this evolving and complex process, one particular conclusion has been widely embraced by all, especially interested stakeholders: the current United States mental health care system serves older patients with mental disorders poorly and is largely unprepared to meet what has been described as an upcoming crisis (Jeste et al. 1999).

This concern has been raised to such a high level of attention that a recent United States Surgeon General's Report on Mental Health highlighted in depth the challenges confronting those committed to ensuring the optimal provision of health care to elderly persons with psychiatric illness (U.S. Department of Health and Human Services 1999b). That seminal report concluded that there are barriers to access in the organization and financing of health care services for the aged. Specific problems exist with Medicare, Medicaid, nursing home funding, and managed care. In this chapter we review the dominant themes that have emerged in the present debate on how best to meet the growing mental health care needs of an aging population; we touch on legal, ethical, and policy concerns. We focus particular attention on the financing of mental health care for older patients, the clear imperative to train a larger workforce to meet the needs of this population, and the cardinal ethical issues that must be confronted when caring for older patients toward the end of life.

Geriatric Mental Health Policy

Financing of Mental Health Care for Older Adults

Policies on paying for mental health care for older adults in the United States have been shaped by the federal government since the inception of Medicare and Medicaid in the mid-1960s. These policies, which have been mirrored by private health insurance carriers, have consistently restricted coverage for mental health services more stringently than coverage for general medical care (Frank 2000).

Medicare

Between 1966 and 1988, Medicare Part B covered outpatient psychiatric services up to a maximum of $500, subject to a 50% copayment; thus, Medicare paid only $250 per year. The Omnibus Budget Reconciliation Act of 1987 (OBRA-87), raised the $500 cap for psychotherapy reimbursement to $2,200 per year but retained the 50% copayment; thus actual Medicare payments were limited to $1,100 per year. However, medical management of psychotropic medications was exempted from this limit, and the copayment for these services was reduced to 20% under OBRA-87. Although the Omnibus Budget Reconciliation Act of 1989 eliminated the cap on outpatient mental health services, the 50% copayment was retained for psychotherapy services, and that disparity with coverage for general medical care (which requires only a 20% copayment) remains as a matter of dispute in Congress at the time of this writing. Consumer and professional groups have lobbied to change this discriminatory policy. To date, several bills have been introduced in Congress that would provide mental health care coverage on a par with coverage for other medical and surgical care, but none have been enacted at the time of this writing.

In 1990, the Medicare Part B psychiatric benefit was expanded to allow licensed clinical psychologists and certified social workers to bill Medicare for mental health services. This led to a substantial increase in Medicare payments for mental health services, especially in nursing homes, during the early and mid-1990s, although it is not known whether the increased spending was associated with better access to appropriate care or with provision of mental health services for those most in need.

Despite increasing incentives to use outpatient rather than inpatient services in the private sector, Medicare payment policies for mental health care continue to encourage the use of acute inpatient services (Bartels and Colenda 1998). Traditional fee-for-service Medicare Part A coverage for inpatient psychiatric hospital care sets a 190-day lifetime limit for care rendered in freestanding psychiatric hospitals but no time limit on care rendered on psychiatric units in general hospitals. In 2000, Medicare paid for inpatient care up to 90 days during a benefit period, paying all but a 1-day deductible of $768 for the first 60 days and all but $192 for days 61–90 (Health Care Financing Administration 2000).

In the context of these reimbursement policies, outpatient service use remains low. Despite the 14%–17% prevalence of clinically significant mental disorders among older adults residing in community settings, it is estimated that only 6%–8% of older adults actually receive outpatient mental health services. Overall, Medicare expenditures for mental health care are similarly disproportionate to need. Although more than one-fourth of older adults residing in the community have mental health or substance abuse disorders, only 4.9% of total Medicare expenditures in 1996 were directed to this area (Witkin et al. 1998), and most of the expenditures were for hospital-based services.

The Balanced Budget Act of 1997 (P.L. 105-33) established Medicare Part C (Medicare Plus Choice), a managed care program offered through private insurance companies. Before 1997, Medicare's managed care products included Medicare risk contracting (MRC) plans, point-of-service (POS) options, social health maintenance organizations (S/HMOs) (Kane et al. 1997), and programs of all-inclusive care for the elderly (PACE) (Eng et al. 1997). The latter two were demonstration projects combining Medicare and Medicaid funding to provide a continuum of health services that included inpatient, outpatient, and long-term-care settings (Colenda et al. 1999). Medicare Plus Choice expanded managed care options to include medical savings accounts, point-of-service options that permit patients to select from a broader panel of practitioners outside the HMO network, religious fraternal benefit plans, and other coordinated care plans.

MRC plans typically "carve out" mental health benefits, which helps vendors manage costs and services. However, these programs might not contract with mental health providers who are geographically accessible to older adults, and communication between providers of general medical care and mental health care is more cumbersome, hampering the coordination of services. Some experts advocate a "carve-in" model for mental health services, which better integrates behavioral and medical care, reduces stigma, improves access, increases coordination of care, and produces cost offsets in general health expenditures in elderly patients with medical-psychiatric comorbidity (Bartels et al. 1999; Mechanic 1997).

Participation in Medicare Plus Choice plans declined in the late 1990s. In 2000, 16.4% of all Medicare beneficiaries were enrolled in these plans. Many managed care companies withdrew after 1999 because of low payment rates and heavy regulatory burdens ("Medicare Plus Choice" 1999). Despite predictions that a large proportion of Medicare beneficiaries would elect managed Medicare options because of enticements such as prescription drug coverage, preventive care, and optical benefits (Hogan et al. 2000; Langwell et al. 1999), the future of managed Medicare is uncertain.

Medicaid

Medicaid is the joint federal-state program that pays for long-term care in nursing homes and acute care services for poor patients. It is not possible to determine the proportion of Medicaid dollars that is spent on mental health care for patients older than age 65, and the effect of managed Medicaid enrollment on mental health service use by elders has not been evaluated (Colenda et al. 2002).

However, approximately 75% of Medicaid expenditures for the elderly are for long-term-care services. Approximately 40% of nursing home costs are paid for out of pocket by patients. Although some individuals have purchased long-term-care insurance policies in addition to their medical insurance, only a small proportion of nursing home costs are covered by private insurance. Many older adults spend down most of their life savings to pay for nursing home care, then become eligible for Medicaid benefits. Overall, the Medicaid program covers about 68% of nursing home residents and more than 59% of nursing home costs (Streim et al. 2002).

Reimbursement of Nursing Homes

Although Medicare pays for psychiatric services rendered in the nursing home by consulting physicians, psychologists, and nurse practitioners on a fee-for-service basis, the nursing facility is responsible for ensuring the psychosocial well-being of residents and the provision of other mental health care by nursing home staff as part of a bundled service package. Financial support for these nursing-home–based mental health services for long-term-care patients comes in large part from Medicaid payments made directly to nursing facilities on a per diem basis. This support decreased for many facilities after the federal Balanced Budget Act of 1997 repealed federal standards for reimbursing nursing homes under Medicaid, giving states the freedom to set payment rates. Nursing homes, therefore, must now rely on per diem reimbursement, with Medicaid rates that vary substantially across states, to cover nursing-home–based mental health care costs.

Department of Veterans Affairs

Another major provider of geriatric mental health care for older Americans is the Department of Veterans Affairs (VA) health care system. More than 9 million veterans are older than age 65, and 510,000 are age 85 or older. The VA currently supports an extensive system of care for older adults with mental disorders, including acute inpatient psychiatric hospitalization, outpatient mental health and substance abuse clinics, a network of more than 120 long-term-care facilities, and domiciliary care. Between 1990 and 2000, the number of veterans in the 45- to 54-year-old age group who received mental health services from the VA more than tripled. These were mostly Vietnam-era veterans, many of them the baby boomers who are now beginning to, and will continue to, swell the ranks of those needing geriatric care. However, the most rapid growth in demand during the same period was among the oldest of older veterans. During the years 1990–2000, the number of veterans ages 75–84 who received VA mental health services increased fourfold. To promote mental health care for veterans, Congress has authorized funding for eight Mental Illness Research, Education, and Clinical Centers (MIRECCs) to conduct research, disseminate findings, and translate new knowledge into practice.

Federal Regulation of Mental Health Care in Nursing Homes

The substantial role of the federal government in paying for health care has given Congress and the Centers for Medicare and Medicaid Services (CMS; formerly the Health Care Financing Administration, or HCFA, as of July 1, 2001) the license to impose stringent regulations on the delivery of mental health care to elderly patients residing in long-term-care facilities. Regulatory focus on nursing homes was prompted in the 1980s by a combination of factors: 1) concerns about the inappropriate use of physical and chemical restraints, 2) concerns about inadequate treatment of depression (Institute of Medicine 1986), and 3) cautions from the federal Office of Management and Budget that older adults with chronic mental illness were being discharged from state mental hospitals and admitted to nursing homes, thereby shifting the cost of their care from the states to the federal government. Congress responded by passing the Nursing Home Reform Act as part of OBRA-87. Mental health aspects of federally mandated nursing home reform are detailed earlier in this volume, in Chapter 29, "Clinical Psychiatry in the Nursing Home."

When it enacted OBRA-87, Congress directed HCFA to take steps to ensure that unmet mental health needs of nursing home residents were addressed. Those resultant HCFA regulations require preadmission assessment a) to identify nursing home applicants with mental illness who require acute psychiatric care; and b) to ensure that applicants are appropriately placed in residential or treatment settings (Health Care Financing Administration 1992b). For individuals admitted to a nursing home, the regulations require the facility to conduct periodic assessments of mental health and to "ensure that a resident who displays mental or psychosocial adjustment difficulties receives appropriate services to correct the assessed problem" (Health Care Financing Administration 1991, p. 48,896 [tag F272]), including treatment not otherwise provided for by the state (U.S. Department of Health and Human Services 2001). Together, these regulations provide a clear federal mandate for detection and treatment of mental illness in nursing home residents.

Quality of care is addressed in regulations intended to limit the inappropriate use of psychotropic medications.

Although after implementation of nursing home reforms the use of antipsychotic drugs and physical restraints declined (Rovner et al. 1992; Shorr et al. 1994) and the use of antidepressant drugs increased (Lantz et al. 1996; Lasser and Sunderland 1998), the effect of the federal regulations on symptom control, functional status, quality of life, and other important outcome measures has not been studied (Llorente et al. 1998; Semla et al. 1994; Streim et al. 2002).

Despite the federal mandate for assessment and treatment, 48% of nursing home administrators report that the frequency of on-site psychiatric consultation is inadequate (Reichman et al. 1998), leaving nursing home staff to provide mental health care without sufficient expert support. More than one-fourth of rural nursing homes and more than one-fifth of small nursing homes reported that no psychiatric consultant was available to them despite high rates of psychiatric problems among residents. Studies showed evidence that many nursing home patients still had undetected psychiatric symptoms (Snowden and Roy-Byrne 1998) and that 55% of residents still had unmet mental health service needs (Borson et al. 1997). Thus, the HCFA requirement that patients receive needed mental health care did not remedy the lack of access to mental health services in U.S. nursing homes (Colenda et al. 1999).

Federal Quality Improvement Initiatives

Nursing homes have also been the setting for new government efforts to use the regulatory and payment systems to encourage improvement in the quality of care for older adults. Assessment, survey, and payment data can be used to analyze the quality of care and, in turn, feedback can inform refinements in care (Nyman 1988). In 1999, HCFA introduced 24 quality indicators, derived from the standardized assessment data that all nursing homes are required to report, to enable facilities and surveyors to compare individual facility performance within the same state. Results are used to identify and address potential quality problems (Clark 1999) and also to inform consumers about the quality of individual nursing home performance. Quality indicators that pertain to geriatric mental health encompass behavior problems, emotional problems, cognitive patterns, and psychotropic drug use. Whenever a review in any of these areas results in a citation of a deficiency, a plan of correction must be developed and submitted to the state department of health for approval. This system is a first step in monitoring quality of care, although the face validity of some of the quality indicators has been questioned and the results of quality surveys may be difficult to interpret (Katz et al. 2002). Nevertheless, quality monitoring is a potent mecha-

nism by which the assessment data required by the payment system can drive quality improvement efforts (Institute of Medicine 2001).

Systems of Care for Older Adults With Serious Mental Illness

At least 1% of individuals over age 55 have serious mental illnesses, such as schizophrenia, schizoaffective disorder, and bipolar disorder; and this population of older adults is expected to double by the year 2030 (U.S. Department of Health and Human Services 1999b). In the 1970s and 1980s, with the widespread downsizing and closure of state mental hospitals and other facilities with long-term psychiatric inpatient units, many older patients were transferred to nursing home beds instead of being discharged to community-based care as were their younger counterparts. Despite the provisions of OBRA-87 that limit the use of nursing homes for people with severe mental illness who do not require skilled nursing facility care, inappropriate nursing home placement continues (U.S. Department of Health and Human Services 2001). To counter this trend, there has been increasing attention over the past decade to providing home- and community-based alternatives to long-term institutional care for older adults (Kane 1998; Meeks et al. 1990). These efforts have been bolstered by the 1999 *Olmstead v. L.C.* decision, which requires that states develop plans to end unnecessary institutionalization through creation of opportunities for community living (Williams 2000).

The challenge of caring for older adults with severe mental illness in community settings is substantial. Although patients with serious mental illness account for only 22% of older adults receiving services in community mental health centers, these patients account for 60% of mental health service costs. Among patients with schizophrenia, the greatest per capita expenditures for mental health care are for the youngest and the oldest patients (Cuffel et al. 1996).

Of particular concern is the high prevalence of medical comorbidity in this population of elderly patients (Dixon et al. 1999; Goldman 1999; Sheline 1990; Vieweg et al. 1995; Zubenko et al. 1997). However, there is disagreement about the ideal model for providing integrated medical and psychiatric care for these patients. Policies that encourage the provision of psychiatric services that are "carved into" general medical care may be more likely to result in coordinated care, but such policies have been criticized for failing to meet the specialized care needs of older adults with serious mental illness (Bartels and Colenda 1998; Mechanic 1997). On the other hand, policies that promote carved-out mental health services may result in higher quality specialized services but run the risk of fragmenting medical and psychiatric services. Regardless of the arrangement, Medicare and Medicaid pay for most health care for older adults with serious mental illness, and the cost of their health care is projected to grow exponentially over the next 10 years (Heffler et al. 2002). Alternatives to traditional financing of mental health care, such as PACE, S/HMOs, and Medicaid long-term-care waiver programs, are likely to increase the availability and use of home- and community-based services for the sickest elderly patients.

Workforce and Training Issues

There are currently about 2,500 board-certified geriatric psychiatrists in the United States, and fewer than 100 psychiatrists graduate from fellowship training programs in geriatrics each year. Thus, it is clear that the number of psychiatrists with subspecialty training and certification is insufficient to meet the growing need for geriatric psychiatric care in the United States. Most of the clinical training in geriatric psychiatry in the United States is funded by Medicare graduate medical education (GME) payments, plus support of some training positions from the VA and the Health Resources and Services Administration (HRSA) of the U.S. Department of Health and Human Services. Under current law, hospitals receive 100% GME reimbursement for initial residency training up to 5 years, depending on specialty board requirements. After that, programs receive only 50% of GME funding for subspecialty fellowship training. However, the law now includes a geriatric exception, under which programs training fellows in geriatric medicine or psychiatry are eligible to receive full funding for an additional 2 years beyond the initial residency. As of the time of writing of this chapter, legislation has been proposed but not passed that would also permit hospitals to add GME-funded geriatric fellowship positions beyond the 1996 cap on total positions for each facility. Even if such legislation were adopted, recruitment to the field of geriatric psychiatry is likely to lag behind the projected workforce needs at least until 2015.

Ethical Issues and End-of-Life Care

A good death does honor to a whole life.

Petrarch (1304–1374)

Concern about the quality of the end of life (i.e., "the good death," Webb 1997) is increasing rapidly and has

been subject to numerous reviews and position statements by professional organizations (Institute of Medicine 1997; Rabow et al. 2000; Sachs 2000). The American Geriatrics Society is one such organization that has thoughtfully addressed end-of-life issues. In the society's related position statement, emphasis is placed on the humanism that must be at the center of the care of terminally ill patients:

> Dying is the final portion of the life cycle for all of us. Providing excellent, humane care to patients near the end of life, when curative means are no longer possible or, on the whole, no longer desired by the patient, is an essential part of medicine.... Most people at the end of life desire to be treated as valued persons by health care professionals and to have skilled attention directed to maintaining dignity[,] foster[ing] independence[,] relieving symptoms[,] and maximizing comfort. Care of patients who are dying is more than just withholding burdensome treatments; it is the provision of a special form of medical care, one in which physicians can take pride and find fulfillment. Providing excellent care to dying patients and to their families is time-consuming and requires expertise as well as compassion. Making such care regularly available will require improvements in systems for service delivery and in professional education. (American Geriatrics Society 1998)

Uncertainty and disagreement exist, however, about the characteristics of "the good death." A recent study brought to light a wide variation in attitudes among patients, physicians, other professional care providers, and family members about the specific attributes of the concept (Steinhauser et al. 2000). Nevertheless, some common fundamentals have emerged (Table 31–1).

Despite a common awareness of needs, differing opinions remain on the extent to which care should appropriately continue to be mechanized and impersonal and what constitutes acceptable practices of intervention in assisting death to occur (Robert Wood Johnson Foundation 1998).

> The healthy and the mildly chronically ill want prevention and cure. Those with disabling, progressive, eventually fatal chronic illness have much broader priorities. For example, when patients are very sick, they want to be comfortable, retain control and dignity, leave a legacy, live longer, and bring closure to their lives. (Lynn 2001, p. 930)

Underlying all efforts must be the primary objective of enabling individuals "to live well on their own terms right up to the time of death" (Lynn 1997, p. 1635).

In addition to the American Geriatrics Society, other medical organizations have attempted to define the characteristics of good care at the end of life; these groups

TABLE 31–1. Fundamental aspects for consideration when providing end-of-life care

Advance planning and preparation for death
Quality of life
    Alleviation of suffering of physical and mental
       symptoms
    Autonomy
    Continuity of care, nonabandonment
    Education and training of caregivers
    Pain management
    Removal of regulatory barriers to access to care
    Respect and dignity
    Spirituality
    Support of family and caregivers before and after death of
       patient

include the American Medical Association (1986) and the American Psychiatric Association (1994; Steinberg and Youngner 1998). Working with representatives of several specialty societies, the Joint Commission on Accreditation of Healthcare Organizations developed a list of core principles for care at the end of life (Cassel and Foley 1999):

1. Respect the dignity of both patient and caregivers.
2. Be sensitive to and respectful of the patient's and family's wishes.
3. Use the most appropriate measures that are consistent with the patient's choices.
4. Encompass alleviation of pain and other physical symptoms.
5. Assess and manage psychological, social, and spiritual/religious problems.
6. Offer continuity (the patient should be able to continue to be cared for, if so desired, by his/her primary care and specialist providers).
7. Provide access to any therapy which may realistically be expected to improve the patient's quality of life, including alternative or nontraditional treatments.
8. Provide access to palliative care and hospice care.
9. Respect the right to refuse treatment.
10. Respect the physician's professional responsibility to discontinue some treatments when appropriate, with consideration for both patient and family preferences.
11. Promote clinical and evidence-based research on providing care at the end of life.

Collaborative Care

Quality end-of-life care relies on a well-coordinated collaboration between the patient, all treating professionals,

the patient's family, and involved clergy. A variety of programs have been developed by interested organizations that serve to alert and educate physicians and others about the numerous services that can assist them (home care, hospice programs, nursing homes, palliative care units) (e.g., The Robert Wood Johnson Foundation Last Acts™ [www.lastacts.org]; and the American Medical Association's Education for Physicians on End-of-life Care Project [www.ama-assn.org/ama/pub/category/2910.html]). It is important to ensure that in designing and offering these services, cultural and religious variants are taken into account (Kagawa-Singer and Blackhall 2001; Lo et al. 2002).

The Role of the Psychiatrist

Psychiatrists working with elderly patients are in a privileged position; their specialized training allows them to stand apart from the still prevailing attitude that the dying patient has in some way lost significance as a person. Psychiatric sensitivity to the interplay of multiple influences and the biopsychosocial paradigm, as well as to developmental stages and their dynamics, is valuable in enabling psychiatrists to make in-depth individualized assessment and give attention to the special requirements of the dying person. Table 31–2 lists some areas for consideration by the psychiatrist.

TABLE 31–2. Areas for consideration by the psychiatrist in end-of-life care

Quality of life
Pain and suffering
Diagnostic foci
    Decision-making capacity
    Axis I
    Axis II
Family conflict
Patient-physician relationship
Withholding or withdrawal of treatment
Assistance in dying
Treatment

Source. Data from American Psychiatric Association 1994; Larson and Tobin 2000; Quill 2000; Von Gunten 2000.

The American Association for Geriatric Psychiatry (2001) has developed its own position statement on care at the end of life. Two of these principles are of special interest to this discussion.

Principle 1 calls for respecting the dignity of both patient and caregiver. Give special attention to the changes in mental state and in psychodynamic and social functioning and behavior that are an integral part of the aging process; such changes are not to be considered psycho-pathological per se. The rationale for this principle is that "The mental state is affected not only by the terminal condition(s) but also by the aging process." The elderly patient's own perspective about this time of closure is an issue that must be assessed and knowledgeably managed. Other issues include support of psychodynamic defenses, life review, countering fears of helplessness and abandonment, and assistance with active conflicts (e.g., within the family).

Principle 4 involves giving high priority to the alleviation of pain and distress in psychological and social domains in addition to the physical arena. The rationale for this principle is that alleviating pain and distress includes sensitively working with elderly patients' "feelings of hopelessness (not necessarily arising in the context of depression), absence of self-worth when not productive, weariness with life, and a desire not to be a burden to others."

End-of-Life Care in Patients With Dementia

Evidence-based interventions. Volicer and colleagues (1994a, 1999) have been especially active in developing instruments to evaluate mood, level of engagement, activity level, and other behavioral characteristics of patients with late-stage dementia. The instruments rate the efficacy of interventions for improvement of these patients' psychological well-being, finding many interventions effective at earlier stages of dementia. These include engaging the person in the activities of daily living, maintenance of mobility, environmental modifications such as improving levels of illumination, and the provision of safe areas for ambulation. Importantly, for patients with advanced dementia, some specific types of stimulation have shown themselves to be of value. One such intervention is simulated presence therapy (Wood and Ashley 1995), in which an audiotape is keyed to an individual's long-term memories and is played repeatedly.

Hospice care and follow-up programs. There are still significant problems with access to hospice programs, despite a Medicare hospice benefit that is available (Hanrahan and Luchins 1995; Luchins 1995). One of the chief barriers to accessing these programs is the requirement that there be a prognosis of 6 months or less to live—which is problematic in view of the uncertain nature of the course and rate of decline of Alzheimer's disease. Another barrier is that some primary care physicians and other professionals have a limited appreciation of the contribution hospice programs can make to the care of

TABLE 31–3. Family needs during a member's terminal illness

Maintain timely communication
Maintain consistent communication
Gear communication to need
Refocus hope
Encourage planning
Be aware of family conflict
Remain available
Focus on the patient's wishes
Attend to the comfort of the patient
Accommodate the family's grief
Follow up with the family after death

persons in late stages of dementia and their families. The median length of stay in hospice programs in 1998 was only 19 days (National Hospice Organization 1999). In general, the rate of hospice use has been estimated as 15.5 per 100 deaths (Virnig et al. 2000), with considerable geographic variation.

However, a sense of the value of hospice care is growing for persons with late-stage dementia (Volicer and Hurley 1998) and of the value of the psychiatrist's special role in addressing the interplay of biological, social, and psychological elements. Hospice programs may be delivered both in institutional sites and at home. A wide array of interventions is offered, including medication, oxygen, companions and aides, spiritual counseling, advance planning, and support for the family (Health Care Financing Administration 2000; National Task Force on End-of-Life Care 1999). The efficacy of appropriately chosen and managed pharmacotherapy should not be underestimated, even in institutionalized patients with late-stage dementia (Volicer et al. 1994b).

During hospice care and in the aftermath of the patient's death, skilled, informed, compassionate support of the patient's family is essential (D.A. Gruenewald, personal communication, March 2000; Hanson et al. 1997; Prigerson and Jacobs 2001). For families, services can be continued for up to 1 year after the relative's death (Health Care Financing Administration 1992a). These services include bereavement counseling and assistance with an adjustment process that may be difficult after many years of social limitations imposed on the caregiver by the tasks of caregiving. Table 31–3 provides a concise summary of the core elements of such support of the family.

Treatment decisions for patients at the end of life. When determining what specific interventions should ultimately comprise the care of elderly patients at the end of life, a frequent suggestion is to do what is "best" for the patient. The patient's wishes and interests must take first place whenever possible. However, other persons concerned in providing treatment and care must have input in making decisions. For example, relatives, the attending physician, and other medical and nonmedical professionals involved in the patient's care are often significantly affected by such end-of-life decision making. How are the views and needs of the various stakeholders reconciled if they are at odds with one another or if the patient is unable to effectively express his or her desire? This situation may especially arise when the patient's own views are based on erroneous information, or the patient is unable by reasons of mental or physical incapacity to express preferences at all. Furthermore, the prognosis for the illness and outcomes of treatment may be far from certain.

Given these complicating factors, the search for answers in considering what is "best"—especially when the question is posed in the medical realm—must become a process of inquiry and decision making. In place of general questions, specific inquiries resolve dilemmas and conflicts; for example, what forms of help can be offered, for what conditions, affecting what individual, at what place and time in life, with what likely outcomes? In many instances the approach to these questions needs input from several informed and interested persons. As a result, ethics committees are increasingly found in both professional organizations and health care institutions (Winn and Cook 2000). Some broadly based basic guidelines have been suggested including beneficence, nonmaleficence, autonomy, justice, and fidelity (Kane 1999). For more detailed reviews, a number of other works may be consulted (Beauchamp and Childress 1989; Bloch and Chodoff 1991; Thornton and Winkler 1988).

Legal Decisions at the End of Life

Acceptance of the naturalness of dying, however, directly conflicts with the medicalization and legalization of death that characterizes modern society's treatment of dying elderly patients.

McCue 1995, p. 1039

Advance Directives for Health Care, Living Wills, and Powers of Attorney for Health Care

The Patient Self-Determination Act (PSDA 1991) requires hospitals, nursing homes, and organizations receiving Medicare and Medicaid funds from the federal government to notify patients of their right to express their wishes concerning life-sustaining care and of the laws of the relevant state with respect to advance directives. The law does not require patients to sign such a document.

Advance directives for health care should include the following:

1. *A living will.* In some states, witnesses to the signing are required.
2. *A power of attorney for health care.* In some states this document requires notarization. Power of attorney differs from guardianship in that the power of attorney is given by a competent individual, whereas guardianship is imposed on one deemed incompetent. The *durable* power of attorney is one that survives (or comes into existence upon) the disability of the principal.

In many states the living will relates only to 1) a terminal condition (incurable and irreversible); and 2) a permanently unconscious condition (persistent vegetative state). Hence, the living will is generally made in association with a durable power of attorney for health care, which confers wider scope on the decision-making right.

However, in spite of a long series of informational and legislative initiatives (Emanuel et al. 1991; Luptak and Boult 1994; Spears et al. 1993), only 10%–30% of all older adults, and a somewhat higher percentage of the nursing home population, have stated their preferences for life-sustaining treatment (Molloy et al. 2000; Sachs et al. 1992; "A controlled trial" 1995; Teno 2000; Teno et al. 1997). Factors contributing to such decision making include ethnicity, age, gender, socioeconomic status, level of education, and marital status (Vaughn et al. 2000).

Further complicating the implementation of this process is the observation that individuals' preferences change with time. These preferences may specifically change in concert with the patient's changing mood, experience of illness, and degree of hope (Menon et al. 2000). Another complicating factor is that the level of compliance by the health care profession with the preferences of patients, even when these have been explicitly stated, continues to be poor (Cantor 2000; Danis et al. 1991; Lee et al. 1998; McSkimming et al. 1999; Teno et al. 1998). When patients are unable to explicitly state their preferences, the process of *substituted judgment* may be operative. It occurs when a decision is being made by another person on the basis of what the patient's wishes would be if the patient were physically and mentally capable of choice and expression. One study assessed the congruence between patients' preferences for resuscitation and their spouses' and physicians' predictions of those preferences (Uhlmann et al. 1988). The proportion of correct predictions made by physicians did not exceed that due to chance. The same was true in about half of the spousal decisions. The direction of misjudgment between these two groups was significantly different, with physicians tending to underestimate the actual preferences of the patients for resuscitation, and spouses to overestimate this preference.

When no advance directive or legally appointed proxies exist, certain individuals, by virtue of their relationship with the patient, are authorized in terms of family consent laws to do surrogate decision making. Laws about this process are largely dictated by the state in which the patient resides. In Washington State, for example, family decision makers for health care are prioritized in order of spouse, adult children, parents, and adult siblings. Decisions by surrogates need to be informed by an understanding of the benefits, risks, and burdens of the course chosen, the criterion being the attainment of the "best interests" of the patient. This criterion is the broadest standard used in the United States as well as in the United Kingdom (Brahams 1989) but is not without difficulties (Wikler 1988). Assessment of best interests should include consideration of relief of suffering, preservation or restoration of function, and quality and extent of sustained life. Even with this broad standard, caveats are needed. For instance, judgments of quality of life need to take into consideration factors other than strictly medical ones (Pearlman and Uhlmann 1988, 1991).

One reason for the low level of compliance with individuals' preferences, even when explicit, may be that the advance directive must be transcribed into a doctor's orders format by a "do not resuscitate" (DNR) order so that it can be acted on (Teno and Lynn 1996). In most states, a DNR order is a physician's prerogative and cannot be simply incorporated into an advance directive by the patient, although the patient can express preferences. One Oregon project attempted to facilitate this process by developing a specialized form, the Physician Orders for Life-Sustaining Treatment (POLST) form (Lee et al. 2000). The form was designed to accompany the individual at all times and was accepted as dictating the care to be provided, even in an emergency. A study comparing care actually delivered with that mandated by the POLST documentation showed that in more technical interventions (e.g., cardiopulmonary resuscitation, antibiotics, intravenous fluids, feeding tubes) the care provided was generally in the direction requested. However, more loosely defined care ("medical interventions" at four different levels of invasiveness) was delivered as specified in less than half the cases. Overall, only 39% of patients had

all their POLST preferences followed. The reasons for these failures to conform more closely to patients' preferences remain uncertain.

The motivation for advance directives arises principally from considerations of the right of a mentally incapacitated patient to refuse or to withdraw from life-sustaining treatment (e.g., artificial hydration and nutrition). There have been historical changes in the public's concern with these questions, in clinical practice, and in the legal definitions of death (Sprung 1990). Although the right of mentally incapacitated persons and their properly appointed proxies to refuse or discontinue artificial hydration and nutrition has been affirmed by the U.S. Supreme Court (*Cruzan v. Director* 1990; *Washington v. Glucksberg* 1997), legal standards applied by states widely vary. It thus behooves the physician to be clear about the specifics of the standard applicable in each case. This variability in legal standards may have contributed to the considerable variation found by one review on the use of artificial hydration and nutrition, which ranged from an odds ratio of 1.00 for tube feeding in Maine to an odds ratio of 5.83 in Ohio (Ahronheim et al. 2001). Clearly, it is not unusual for conflicts of ethical judgment to arise between different physicians and between physicians and other professionals and family members. This situation is especially prone to arise for a patient with advanced dementia who is being cared for in the absence of an advance directive. In this event, the medical requirement for providing life-sustaining treatment conflicts with the reality that there can be no prospect of recovery. This type of dilemma may also arise in connection with an acute illness such as pneumonia during the course of late-stage dementia.

Catholic and Jewish religious groups have adopted the position that the right to refuse or discontinue life-sustaining treatment does apply to events in which such refusal could lead to death or in cases in which the patient is not terminally ill (National Conference of Catholic Bishops 1995; Rosin and Sonnenblick 1998). Courts have also legitimized the withdrawal of life-sustaining treatment, basing the decisions in part on rejection of the distinction between withholding and withdrawing treatment, with artificial feeding included in the category of treatment (*Barber v. Superior Court* 1983; *Brophy v. New England Sinai Hospital Inc.* 1986). It has been concluded that the right to refuse medical treatment, including artificial hydration and nutrition, outweighed states' interest in the preservation of life, the prevention of suicide, and the ethical integrity of the medical profession. The discontinuation of feeding has not been found to be suicide or active euthanasia; it has rather been viewed as allowing the underlying disease to take its natural course.

The American Medical Association (1999) has concurred with this interpretation.

Competency and Decision-Making Capacity

Much of the discussion in deciding that an individual is mentally incapacitated involves the concept of competency and the related one of informed consent. These concepts are especially invoked when a patient's cognitive abilities, by reason of dementia or other illnesses, are impaired and the need arises to make a will or to participate in treatment decisions. The concepts of competency and informed consent are legal doctrines that have undergone elaborate judicial evolution (Grisso and Appelbaum 1998). Competency requires a legal determination by a court. The standards applied in establishing competency vary with the purpose for which the evaluation is being performed. Making a will requires the lowest level of competency (Spar and Garb 1992), whereas higher levels are required for executing a power of attorney. Hence, the psychiatric evaluation should take into account the purpose for which a competency assessment is being sought (Feinberg and Whitlatch 2001; Overman and Stoudemire 1988). The basic requirement for the psychiatrist is to provide adequate information on the individual's mental status to enable the court to make a determination about the individual's decision-making capacity in the area of concern. The court may rely on the psychiatrist's written report or may require the psychiatrist to testify in person.

Considerations of competency and informed consent may also arise when an individual's participation is being sought for research purposes. A durable power of attorney may be of value when the potential research subject lacks the ability during the course of a research study to continue giving informed consent (Dukoff and Sunderland 1997). Further safeguards are being sought. One example consists of enhancement of the procedure for obtaining consent when the individual shows demonstrable improvements in comprehension (Dunn et al. 2001).

Conclusion

The number of older patients with mental disorders is expected to grow dramatically in coming decades. In response, a number of professional and consumer advocates, government agencies, policy analysts, policy planners, and university-based academics have opened a vigorous dialogue focused on how best to meet the mental health needs of the elderly. Preliminary but important discussions have begun on how best to structure and finance mental health care for older persons, how to strengthen an inadequate and undertrained workforce to deal with these issues, and how to resolve the ethical and legal questions that arise toward the end of life. What will probably emerge is a mandate to implement a research and policy agenda for aging and mental health that focuses on prevention, early detection, evidence-based intervention, and training. Without such forethought and planning, those stakeholders who predict a crisis in geriatric mental health in coming decades may prove correct.

References

A controlled trial to improve care for seriously ill hospitalized patients: the Study to Understand Prognoses and Preferences for Outcomes and Risks of Treatment (SUPPORT). Report by SUPPORT principal investigators. JAMA 274: 1591–1598, 1995

Ahronheim JC, Mulvihill M, Sieger C, et al: State practice variations in the use of tube feeding for nursing home residents with severe cognitive impairment. J Am Geriatr Soc 49: 148–152, 2001

American Association for Geriatric Psychiatry: End-of-life care: position statement of the American Association for Geriatric Psychiatry. Adopted by the AAGP Board of Directors, February 2001. Available at http://www.aagponline.org/prof/position_end.asp. Accessed December 2, 2003.

American Geriatrics Society: The Care of Dying Patients. Position Statement of the Ethics Committee. New York, The American Geriatrics Society, 1998. Available at http://www.americangeriatrics.org/products/positionpapers/careofd/shtml. Accessed August 15, 2003.

American Medical Association: Current opinions of the Council of Ethical and Judicial Affairs: withholding or withdrawing life-prolonging medical treatment. Chicago, IL, American Medical Association, 1986

American Medical Association: Medical futility in end-of-life care. Report of the Council on Ethical and Judicial Affairs. JAMA 281:937–941, 1999

American Psychiatric Association: The role of the psychiatrist in end-of-life decisions. Report of the subcommittee on psychiatric aspects of life-sustaining technology. Washington, DC, American Psychiatric Association, May 1994

Barber v Superior Court, 195 Cal Rptr 484, 147 Cal App 3d 1006 (1983)

Bartels SJ, Colenda CC: Mental health services for Alzheimer's disease: current trends in reimbursement and public policy, and the future under managed care. Am J Geriatr Psychiatry 6 (2 suppl):S85–S100, 1998

Bartels SJ, Levine KJ, Shea D: Community-based long-term care for older persons with severe and persistent mental illness in an era of managed care. Psychiatr Serv 50:1189–1197, 1999

Beauchamp T, Childress JF: Principles of Biomedical Ethics, 3rd Edition. New York, Oxford University Press, 1989

Bloch S, Chodoff P: Psychiatric Ethics, 2nd Edition. New York, Oxford University Press, 1991

Borson S, Loebel JP, Kitchell M, et al: Psychiatric assessments of nursing home residents under OBRA-87: should PASARR be reformed? Pre-Admission Screening and Annual Review. J Am Geriatr Soc 45:1173–1181, 1997

Brahams D. Sterilization of a mentally incapable woman. Lancet i:1275–1276, 1989

Brophy v New England Sinai Hospital Inc, 497 NE 2d 626 (Mass 1986)

Cantor MD: Improving advance care planning: lessons from POLST. J Am Geriatr Soc 48:1343–1344, 2000

Cassel CK, Foley KM: Principles for the care of patients at the end of life: an emerging consensus among the specialties of medicine. New York, Milbank Memorial Fund, 1999. Available at http://www.milbank.org/endoflife. Accessed July 1, 2003.

Clark TR (ed): Nursing Home Survey Procedures and Interpretive Guidelines. A Resource for the Consultant Pharmacist. Alexandria, VA, American Society of Consultant Pharmacists, 1999, pp 1–8

Colenda CC, Streim JE, Greene JA, et al: The impact of the Omnibus Budget Reconciliation Act of 1987 (OBRA '87) on psychiatric services in nursing homes. Am J Geriatr Psychiatry 7:12–17, 1999

Colenda CC, Bartels SC, Gottlieb GL: The North American System of Care in Principles and Practice of Geriatric Psychiatry, 2nd Edition. Edited by Copeland J, Abou-Saleh M, Blazer D. London, Wiley and Son, 2002, pp 689–696

Cuffel BJ, Jeste DV, Halpain M, et al: Treatment costs and use of community mental health services for schizophrenia by age cohorts. Am J Psychiatry 153:870–876, 1996

Cruzan v Director, Missouri Department of Health, 497 US 261, 279 (1990)

Danis M, Southerland LI, Garrett JM, et al: A prospective study of advance directives of life-sustaining care. N Engl J Med 324:882–888, 1991

Dixon L, Postrado L, Delahanty J, et al: The association of medical comorbidity in schizophrenia with poor physical and mental health. J Nerv Ment Dis 187:496–502, 1999

Dukoff R, Sunderland T: Durable power of attorney and informed consent with Alzheimer's disease patients: a clinical study. Am J Psychiatry 154:1070–1075, 1997

Dunn LB, Lindamer LA, Palmer BW, et al: Enhancing comprehension of consent for research in older patients with psychosis: a randomized study of a novel consent procedure. Am J Psychiatry 158:1911–1913, 2001

Emanuel LL, Barry MJ, Stoeckle JD, et al: Advance directives for medical care: a case for greater use. N Engl J Med 324: 889–895, 1991

Eng C, Pedulla J, Eleazer GP, et al: Program of all-inclusive care for the elderly (PACE): an innovative model of integrated geriatric care and financing. J Am Geriatr Soc 452:223–232, 1997

Feinberg LF, Whitlatch CJ: Are persons with cognitive impairment able to state consistent choices? Gerontologist 41:374–382, 2001

Frank RG: The creation of Medicare and Medicaid: the emergence of insurance and markets for mental health services. Psychiatr Serv 51:465–468, 2000

Goldman LS: Medical illness in patients with schizophrenia. J Clin Psychiatry 60 (suppl 21):10–15, 1999

Grisso T, Appelbaum PS: Assessing Competence to Consent to Treatment: A Guide for Physicians and other Health Professionals. New York, Oxford University Press, 1998

Hanrahan P, Luchins DJ: Access to hospice programs in end-stage dementia: a national survey of hospice programs. J Am Geriatr Soc 43:56–59, 1995

Hanson LC, Danis M, Garrett J: What is wrong with end-of-life care? opinions of bereaved family members. J Am Geriatr Soc 45:1339–1344, 1997

Health Care Financing Administration: Medicare and Medicaid: Requirements for Long-Term Care Facilities, Final Regulations. Federal Register 56:48865–48921, September 26, 1991

Health Care Financing Administration: Code of Federal Regulations, Part 418, Hospice Care. Washington, DC, National Archives and Records Administration, 1992a, pp 567–579

Health Care Financing Administration: Medicare and Medicaid Programs: Preadmission Screening and Annual Resident Review. Federal Register 57:56450–56504, November 30, 1992b

Health Care Financing Administration: Medicare and Your Mental Heath Benefits. Washington, DC, U.S. Government Printing Office, 2000

Heffler S, Smith S, Won G, et al: Health spending projections for 2001–2011: the latest outlook. Health Aff (Millwood) 21:207–218, 2002

Hogan C, Lynn J, Gabel J, et al: Medicare Beneficiaries' Costs and Use of Care in the Last Year of Life. Washington, DC, Medicare Payment Advisory Commission, 2000

Institute for Health and Aging: Chronic Care in America: A 21st Century Challenge. Princeton, NJ, Robert Wood Johnson Foundation, 1996

Institute of Medicine, Committee on Nursing Home Regulation: Improving the Quality of Care in Nursing Homes. Washington, DC, National Academy Press, 1986

Institute of Medicine, Committee on Care at the End of Life: Approaching Death: Improving Care at the End of Life. Edited by Field MJ, Cassel CK. Washington, DC, National Academy Press, 1997

Institute of Medicine, Committee on Improving Quality in Long-Term Care: Improving the Quality of Long-Term Care. Edited by Wunderlich GS, Kohler P. Washington, DC, National Academy Press, 2001, pp 235–247

Jeste DV, Alexopoulos GS, Bartels SJ, et al: Consensus statement on the upcoming crisis in geriatric mental health: research agenda for the next 2 decades. Arch Gen Psychiatry 56:848–853, 1999

Kagawa-Singer M, Blackhall L: Negotiating cross-cultural issues at the end of life: "You got to go where he lives." JAMA 286:2993–3001, 2001

Kane RL: Managed care as a vehicle for delivering more effective chronic care for older persons. J Am Geriatr Soc 46:1034–1039, 1998

Kane RL, Kane RA, Finch M, et al: S/HMOs, the second generation: building on the experience of the first social health maintenance organization demonstrations. J Am Geriatr Soc 45:101–107, 1997

Kane RL, Ouslander JG, Abrass IB: Essentials of Clinical Geriatrics, 4th Edition. New York, McGraw-Hill, 1999

Katz IR, Van Haitsma KS, Streim JE: Psychiatric services in long-term care, in Principles and Practice of Geriatric Psychiatry, 2nd Edition. Edited by Copeland JRM, Abou-Saleh MT, Blazer DG. Baltimore, MD, John Wiley & Sons, 2002

Langwell K, Topoleski C, Sherman D: Analysis of Benefits Offered by Medicare HMOs, 1999: Complexities and Implications. Menlo Park, CA, Henry J Kaiser Foundation, 1999

Lantz MS, Giambanco V, Buchalter EN: A ten-year review of the effect of OBRA-87 on psychotropic prescribing practices in an academic nursing home. Psychiatr Serv 47:951–955, 1996

Larson DG, Tobin DR: End-of-life conversations. JAMA 284:1573–1578, 2000

Lasser RA, Sunderland T: Newer psychotropic medication use in nursing home residents. J Am Geriatric Soc 46:202–207, 1998

Lee MA, Smith DM, Fenn DS, et al: Do patients' treatment decisions match advance statements of their preferences? J Clin Ethics 9:258–262, 1998

Lee MA, Brummel-Smith K, Meyer J, et al: Physician Orders for Life-Sustaining Treatment (POLST): Outcomes in a PACE Program. J Am Geriatr Soc 48:1219–1225, 2000

Llorente MD, Olsen EJ, Leyva O, et al: Use of antipsychotic drugs in nursing homes: current compliance with OBRA regulations. J Am Geriatr Soc 46:198–201, 1998

Lo B, Ruston D, Kates LW, et al: Discussing religious and spiritual issues at the end of life: a practical guide for physicians. JAMA 287:749–754, 2002

Luchins DJ: Access to hospice programs in end-stage dementia: a national survey of hospice programs. J Am Geriatr Soc 43:56–59, 1995

Luptak MK, Boult C: A method for increasing elders' use of advance directives. Gerontologist 34:409–412, 1994

Lynn J: Clinical crossroads: an 88-year-old woman facing the end of life. JAMA 277:1633–1640, 1997

Lynn J: Perspectives on care at the close of life: serving patients who may die soon and their families: the role of hospice and other services. JAMA 285:925–932, 2001

McCue J: The naturalness of dying. JAMA 276:1039–1043, 1995

McSkimming S, Hodges M, Super A, et al: The experience of life-threatening illness: patients' and their loved ones' perspectives. J Palliat Med 2:173–184, 1999

Mechanic D: Approaches for coordinating primary and specialty care for persons with mental illness. Gen Hosp Psychiatry 19:395–402, 1997

Medicare Plus Choice: a program in transition, in Medicare Payment Advisory Commission Report to Congress: Medicare Payment Policy. Washington, DC, Medicare Payment Advisory Commission (MedPAC), 1999, pp 27–46. Available at http://www.medpac.gov/publications. Click on "Reports," then select the report title (at the bottom of the page). Accessed October 16, 2003.

Meeks S, Carstensen LL, Stafford PB, et al: Mental health needs of the chronically mentally ill elderly. Psychol Aging 5:163–171, 1990

Menon AS, Campbell D, Ruskin P, et al: Depression, hopelessness, and the desire for life-saving treatments among elderly medically ill veterans. Am J Geriatr Psychiatry 8:333–342, 2000

Molloy DW, Guyatt GH, Russo R, et al: systematic implementation of an advance directive program in nursing homes: a randomized controlled trial. JAMA 283:1437–1443, 2000

National Conference of Catholic Bishops: Ethical and Religious Directives for Catholic Health Care Services. Washington, DC, U.S. Catholic Conference, 1995

National Hospice Organization: 1998 Length-of-Stay Fax-Back Survey, final report. NHO Newsline, May 1, 1999, p 6

National Task Force on End-of-Life Care in Managed Care: Meeting the Challenge: Twelve Recommendations for Improving End-of-Life Care in Managed Care. Newton, MA, Education Development Center, Inc., 1999

Nyman JA: Improving the quality of nursing home outcomes: are adequacy- or incentive-oriented policies more effective? Med Care 26:1158–1171, 1988

Omnibus Budget Reconciliation Act of 1987, Pub. L. No. 100–203. Available at http://thomas.loc.gov/cgi-bin/bdquery/z?d100:HR03545:|TOM:/bss/d100query.html. Accessed October 16, 2003.

Overman W Jr, Stoudemire A: Guidelines for legal and financial counseling of Alzheimer's disease patients and their families. Am J Psychiatry 145:1495–1500, 1988

Patient Self-Determination Act, Pub. L. No. 101-508, 1991

Pearlman RA, Uhlmann RF: Quality of life in elderly, chronically ill outpatients. Journal of Gerontology: Medical Sciences 46:M31–M38, 1991

Pearlman RA, Uhlmann RF: Quality of life in the elderly: comparisons between nursing home and community residents. J Appl Gerontol 3:316–330, 1988

Prigerson HG, Jacobs SC: Perspectives on care at the close of life: caring for bereaved patients: "All the doctors just suddenly go." JAMA 286:1369–1376, 2001

Quill TE: Initiating end-of-life discussions with seriously ill patients. JAMA 284:2502–2507, 2000

Rabow MW, Hardie GE, Fair JM, et al: End-of-life care content in 50 textbooks from multiple specialties. JAMA 283:771–778, 2000

Reichman W, Coyne A, Borson S, et al: Psychiatric consultation in the nursing home: a survey of six states. Am J Geriatr Psychiatry 6:320–327, 1998

Robert Wood Johnson Foundation: Death and Dying in America: Too Much Technology, Too Little Care. Princeton, NJ, Robert Wood Johnson Foundation, May 1998

Rosin AJ, Sonnenblick M: Autonomy and paternalism in geriatric medicine: the Jewish ethical approach to issues of feeding terminally ill patients, and to cardiopulmonary resuscitation. J Med Ethics 24:44–48, 1998

Rovner BW, Edelman BA, Cox MP, et al: The impact of antipsychotic drug regulations (OBRA 1987) on psychotropic prescribing practices in nursing homes. Am J Psychiatry 149:1390–1392, 1992

Sachs GA: A piece of my mind: sometimes dying still stings (editorial). JAMA 284:2423, 2000

Sachs GA, Stocking CB, Miles SH: Empowerment of the older patient? a randomized, controlled trial to increase discussion and use of advance directives. J Am Geriatr Soc 40:269–273, 1992

Semla TP, Palla K, Poddig B, et al: Effect of the Omnibus Reconciliation Act 1987 on antipsychotic prescribing in nursing home residents. J Am Geriatr Soc 42:648–652, 1994

Sheline YI: High prevalence of physical illness in a geriatric psychiatric inpatient population. Gen Hosp Psychiatry 12:396–400, 1990

Shorr RI, Fought RL, Ray WA: Changes in antipsychotic drug use in nursing homes during implementation of the OBRA-87 regulations. JAMA 271:358–362, 1994

Snowden M, Roy-Byrne P: Mental illness and nursing home reform: OBRA-87 ten years later: Omnibus Budget Reconciliation Act. Psychiatr Serv 49:229–233, 1998

Spar JE, Garb AS: Assessing competency to make a will. Am J Psychiatry 149:169–174, 1992

Spears R, Drinka PJ, Voeks SK: Obtaining a durable power of attorney for health care from nursing home residents. J Fam Pract 36:409–413, 1993

Sprung CL: Concepts in emergency and critical care: changing attitudes and practices in forgoing life-sustaining treatments. JAMA 263:2211–2216, 1990

Steinberg MD, Youngner SJ (eds): End-of-Life Decisions: A Psychosocial Perspective. Washington, DC, American Psychiatric Press, 1998

Steinhauser KE, Christakis NA, Clipp EC, et al: Factors considered important at the end of life by patients, family, physicians and other care providers. JAMA 284:2476–2482, 2000

Streim JE, Beckwith EW, Arapakos D, et al: Regulatory oversight, payment policy, and quality improvement in mental health care in nursing homes. Psychiatr Serv 53:1414–1418, 2002

Teno JM: Advance directives for nursing home residents: achieving compassionate, competent, cost-effective care. JAMA 283:1481–1482, 2000

Teno JM, Lynn J: Putting advance-care planning into action. J Clin Ethics 7:205–213, 1996

Teno JM, Lynn J, Wenger NS, et al: Advance directives for seriously ill hospitalized patients: effectiveness with the Patient Self-Determination Act and the SUPPORT intervention. J Am Geriatr Soc 45:500–507, 1997

Teno JM, Stevens M, Spernak S, et al: Role of written advance directives in decision making: insights from qualitative and quantitative data. J Gen Intern Med 13:439–446, 1998

Thornton JE, Winkler ER (eds): Ethics and Aging: The Right to Live, the Right to Die. Vancouver, BC, Canada, University of British Columbia Press, 1988

U.S. Department of Health and Human Services: Organizing and financing mental health services, in Mental Health: A Report of the Surgeon General. Bethesda, MD, National Institute of Mental Health, 1999a, pp 405–433. The report is available with a link for the chapter at http://www.surgeongeneral.gov/library/mentalhealth/home.html. Accessed October 16, 2003.

U.S. Department of Health and Human Services: Older adults and mental health, in Mental Health: A Report of the Surgeon General. Bethesda, MD, National Institute of Mental Health, 1999b, pp 335–401. The report is available with a link for the chapter at http://www.surgeongeneral.gov/library/mentalhealth/home.html. Accessed October 16, 2003.

U.S. Department of Health and Human Services, Office of the Inspector General: Medicare Payments for Psychiatric Services in Nursing Homes: A Follow-Up (DHHS Publ No OEI-02-99-00140). New York, Office of Evaluation and Inspections, 2001. Available at http://oig.hhs.gov/oei/reports/oci-02-99-00140.pdf. Accessed October 16, 2003.

Uhlmann RF, Pearlman RA, Cain KC: Physicians' and spouses' predictions of elderly patients' resuscitation preferences. Journal of Gerontology: Medical Sciences 43:M115–M121, 1988

Vaughn G, Kiyasu E, McCormick WC: Advance directive preferences among subpopulations of Asian nursing home residents in the Pacific Northwest. J Am Geriatr Soc 48:554–557, 2000

Vieweg V, Levenson J, Pandurangi A, et al: Medical disorders in the schizophrenic patient. Int J Psychiatry Med 25:137–172, 1995

Virnig BA, Kind S, McBean M, et al: Geographic variation in hospice use prior to death. J Am Geriatr Soc 48:1117–1125, 2000

Volicer L, Hurley A: Hospice Care for Patients With Advanced Progressive Dementia. New York, Springer, 1998

Volicer L, Hurley AC, Lathi DC, et al: Measurement of severity in advanced Alzheimer's disease. Journal of Gerontology: Medical Sciences 49:M223–M226, 1994a

Volicer L, Rheaume Y, Cyr D: Treatment of depression in advanced Alzheimer's disease using sertraline. J Geriatr Psychiatry Neurol 7: 227–229, 1994b

Volicer L, Hurley AC, Camberg L: A model of psychological well-being in advanced dementia. J Ment Health Aging 5:83–94, 1999

Von Gunten CF, Ferris FD, Emanuel LL: Ensuring competency in end-of-life care. JAMA 284:3051–3057, 2000

Washington v Glucksberg, 117 SC 2258, 2270 (1997)

Webb M: The Good Death. New York, Bantam, 1997

Wikler D: Patient interests: clinical implications of philosophical distinctions. J Am Geriatr Soc 36:951–958, 1988

Williams L: Long-term care after Olmstead v L.C.: will the potential of the ADA's integration mandate be achieved? J Contemp Health Law Policy 17:205–239, 2000

Winn P, Cook J: Ethics committees in long-term care: a user's guide to getting started. Annals of Long-Term Care 8:35–42, 2000

Witkin MJ, Atay JE, Manderscheid RW, et al: Highlights of organized mental health services in 1994 and major national and state trends, in Mental Health, United States 1998 (HHS Pub No 99-3285). Rockville, MD, Substance Abuse and Mental Health Services Administration, 1998

Woods P, Ashley J: Simulated presence therapy: using selected memories to manage problem behaviors in Alzheimer's disease patients. Geriatr Nurs 16:9–14, 1995

Young SN, Gauthier S: Is placebo control in geriatric psychopharmacology clinical trials ethical? International Journal of Geriatric Psychopharmacology 2:113–118, 2000

Zubenko GS, Marino LJ, Sweet RA, et al: Medical comorbidity in elderly psychiatric inpatients. Biol Psychiatry 41:724–736, 1997

The Past and Future of Geriatric Psychiatry

Dan G. Blazer, M.D., Ph.D.

David C. Steffens, M.D., M.H.S.

Ewald W. Busse, M.D.

The Path of Geriatric Psychiatry in the United States

The relatively recent emergence of geriatric psychiatry in North America is based on two centuries of interest and work by both Americans and non-Americans. For example, Benjamin Franklin (1706–1790) maintained a strong belief that science would eventually discover the aging process, control it, and be able to rejuvenate people. He apparently was convinced that if the patriarchs of the antediluvian era, described in the Hebrew Scriptures (Old Testament), could achieve extended life spans, so could the human of the future. Two of his inventions have contributed to the well-being of elderly persons: the Franklin stove and bifocal eyeglasses (Gruman 1966).

Benjamin Rush (1745–1830), a famous American physician, patron of the American Psychiatric Association, and signer of the Declaration of Independence, wrote extensively and lucidly on a variety of subjects, including old age. In 1805, he published "An Account of the State of the Body and Mind in Old Age: With Observations on Its Diseases and Remedies" (Butterfield 1976).

In the 1930s, increased interest was focused on age research. Walter R. Miles and his associates developed the Stanford Greater Maturity Project with the objective of investigating systematically the psychological aspects of aging. Medical research was enhanced by the publication of *Problems of Aging* by Edmund V. Cowdry (1938), which brought together discussions of physical and health-related problems in one volume. Cowdry played a major role in organizing the American Geriatrics Society, the Gerontological Society of America, and the International Association of Gerontology. Also in the late 1930s, two important sociologists, Leo Simmons and Ernest W. Burgess, independently published studies on social aspects of aging. In 1945, Simmons published a pioneer study of aging in 70 preliterate societies (Simmons 1945). Burgess and his associates at the University of Chicago developed instruments to measure personality adjustment in old age.

Nascher, who is frequently considered the father of geriatrics and who is thought to have coined the word *geriatric* with the publication of his text *Geriatrics: The Diseases of Old Age and Their Treatment* (Nascher 1914), published an article on the aging mind the month before his death in 1944 (Nascher 1944). In this article, Nascher tabulated the characteristics of chronic brain syndrome and suggested that the condition was a primary change of senescence. He suggested that it must have a familial determinant.

In 1946, the American Psychological Association created the division of later maturity in old age. In the same year, the first issue of the *Journal of Gerontology* was published by the Gerontological Society of America. The first national conference of that society was held in 1950 and was followed by several White House Conferences on Aging, the last occurring in 1995. Also in 1950, the International Association of Gerontology was organized in Liege, Belgium.

In 1969, one of the first American books on aging and psychiatry was published, *Behavior and Adaptation in Late Life,* edited by Ewald W. Busse and Eric Pfeiffer (Busse and Pfeiffer 1969). The book derived in large part from ongoing Duke University studies of the longitudinal aspects of normal aging. Another longitudinal study of normal aging, the Baltimore Longitudinal Study on Aging, was sponsored by the National Institutes of Health. Before the appearance of the Busse and Pfeiffer book, among the best-known texts in the English language about geriatric psychiatry were Felix Post's *The Clinical Psychiatry of Late Life* (Post 1965) and *Normal Psychology of the Aging Process* by Zinberg and Kaufman (1963).

The Emergence of Geriatric Psychiatry in Professional Organizations

Authorized by the constitution of the American Psychiatric Association (APA), the APA Council on Aging was established in 1979 to address six areas of activity: 1) evaluation and diagnosis, 2) training, 3) interface problems between psychiatry and other geriatric care disciplines, 4) design of services and third-party payment for psychiatric disorders in the elderly, 5) decisions made by government that influence the mental health of the aged, and 6) identifying and implementing research in the problems of geriatric psychiatry. The Council on Aging is responsible for developing and maintaining liaison with groups involved in the mental health care of aging Americans: other APA components, appropriate non-APA organizations, and federal agencies.

Psychiatrists have played leading roles in the activities of two major U.S. societies concerned with aging: the Gerontological Society of America and the American Geriatrics Society. The Gerontological Society of America, founded in 1945, is a multidisciplinary organization with four distinct sections: biological sciences, medical sciences, social sciences, and psychological sciences. Four psychiatrists have served as presidents of this organization during the past generation. The American Geriatrics Society, established in 1942, is composed largely of physicians and members of the health care professions. Psychiatrists have led this medical society.

The American Association for Geriatric Psychiatry was founded in 1978. Its membership now exceeds 1,700, including about 100 affiliates. Of the active members, about 800 have reported that they have Certification in the Subspecialty of Geriatric Psychiatry (formerly Added Qualifications in Geriatric Psychiatry) from the American Board of Psychiatry and Neurology. About 1,200 persons attend the annual meeting.

The American Association for Geriatric Psychiatry played a significant role in the effort to obtain recognition for geriatric psychiatry as a subspecialty and in establishing the certifying examination for this subspecialty by the American Board of Psychiatry and Neurology (ABPN). The first examination was given in 1991; more than 800 persons sat for the examination, and more than 500 passed it. Between 1991 and the end of calendar year 2000, ABPN issued 2,508 certificates in geriatric psychiatry. (However, only 83 certificates were issued in 2000— primarily because of the newer requirement that all psychiatrists who sit for the examination must have completed a 1-year fellowship in geriatric psychiatry, in contrast to the "grandfather clause" used for the earlier examinations and certifications). The original certification was for 10 years, and the first recertifying examination was given in 2001—an open-book examination, in contrast to the original closed-book examination. Recertifying examinations will continue to be given.

The Center for the Study of Mental Health of the Aging was established at the National Institute of Mental Health (NIMH) in 1975, but it later disbanded during reorganizational efforts by NIMH. In 1977, the center received funds to support and coordinate research, research training, and clinical training projects. Its original efforts focused primarily on research and clinical training, with long-term support of fellowship stipends for approved geriatric psychiatry training programs, which greatly increased the number of psychiatrists with specialty training. Recently, efforts have been renewed at NIMH to reinvigorate the research agenda of the institute. These efforts resulted in the release of a report, "Mental Health for a Lifetime: Research for Mental Health Needs of Older Americans" (National Institute of Mental Health 2003).

The National Institute on Aging (NIA) was established in May 1974 as part of the National Institutes of Health. The first director of NIA was a psychiatrist, Robert N. Butler, M.D. Enabling legislation was passed designating NIA as the chief federal agency responsible for promoting, coordinating, and supporting basic research and training relevant to the aging process and to the diseases and problems of the elderly. A unique aspect of NIA's mandate was that it was the first component of the National Institutes of Health to be formally charged by Congress with conducting research in the biological, biomedical, behavioral, and social sciences. This broad mandate has resulted in activities differing from those of other national research institutes. NIA has led the effort in Alzheimer's disease research, whereas research in other geriatric psychiatric disorders, especially major depression, has been led by NIMH.

For many years, medical and health care education related to geriatrics received little attention. The first training program in geriatric psychiatry supported by NIMH was established at Duke University Medical Center in 1965, and it was the only such program for almost a decade. However, a rapidly increasing number of geriatric psychiatry fellowship programs now exist, although few currently receive NIMH support. These programs have been funded primarily through the Department of Veterans Affairs (VA), state support, and support from individual medical centers. The establishment of these training programs and lobbying by groups (including the American Association for Geriatric Psychiatry) convinced the American Board of Psychiatry and Neurology to establish an examination for Added Qualifications in Geriatric Psychiatry (now called Certification in the Subspecialty of Geriatric Psychiatry), previously mentioned.

Geriatric Psychiatry: Present and Future

The geriatric psychiatrist, in relation to the general psychiatrist, the generalist physician, and the geriatrician, has made a significant and unique contribution to clarifying the role of psychiatry in relation to other specialties in caring for the elderly mentally ill. The current emphasis on primary care has challenged the viability of all medical specialties during the past few years. Nevertheless, geriatric psychiatry has established itself solidly on a foundation of knowledge and skill in caring for older persons with psychiatric disorders, using the most advanced technologies and clinically proven therapies. In most settings, the geriatric psychiatrist has established a unique and meaningful role on interdisciplinary teams caring for older adults.

Geriatric psychiatrists assume in many ways the role of primary care physicians. Not only must they maintain proficiency in general medicine, they must also apply special knowledge of epidemiology, as well as of behavioral and social factors, to patient care. For example, geriatric psychiatrists have no alternative but to recognize that many of the disorders they treat cannot currently be cured or prevented—such as Alzheimer's disease—but these clinicians know that the resultant suffering can be relieved and the disability reduced. Focusing on improving function encourages clinicians to make observations that can contribute to a better understanding of the course of chronic illness. These observations can also motivate investigations that may in the future lead to improved convalescence from, or even eradication of, such disorders when they are recognized earlier in the course of illness.

To achieve the goal of effective care of chronically ill older adults with psychiatric problems, geriatric psychiatrists must broaden their skills to include proficiency in geriatric medicine, neurology, and the neurosciences as well as focus their skills on advances in geriatric psychiatry. Proficient geriatricians and geriatric psychiatrists must be aware of aging changes that affect the human organism's capacity to respond to stress, disease, and trauma and that may eventually result in death (Busse and Blazer 1980). Specific procedures, such as the treatment of urinary tract infection, moderate hypertension, and peripheral edema, should not require that geriatric psychiatrists consult internists or geriatricians for appropriate management. The role of geriatric psychiatrists may indeed be such that specialty consultation is frequent and that combined management of the patient is conducted by a geriatrician and a geriatric psychiatrist (for example, in a tertiary-care center). However, the skill of geriatric psychiatrists should be such that in the absence of a geriatrician they can administer adequate medical care. As care moves increasingly from inpatient to ambulatory settings, the independent skills of geriatric psychiatrists will be required more and more.

At the same time, significant advances will emerge in the epidemiology, pathophysiology, diagnosis, and treatment of the most frequently encountered late-life psychiatric disorders. These disorders span at least the range described in this volume, and even a short list must include dementias, mood disorders, anxiety disorders, schizophrenic disorders, light disorders, sleep disorders, and psychological and social factors affecting medical conditions. Advances in the neuroscience and clinical management of dementia of the Alzheimer's type alone illustrate the substantial knowledge base on which geriatric psychiatry is practiced. Previous trends have been such that when a biological etiology has been identified for a behavioral disorder, that disorder is passed from psychiatry to another specialty, usually neurology. Surely this cannot be tolerated in the future by geriatric psychiatrists. For example, geriatric psychiatrists must maintain a central role in the clinical management of patients with dementia, especially because patients' primary problems are usually behavioral. To maintain this role, psychiatrists must have skills at a level that are not overshadowed by those of neurologists and geriatricians.

Geriatric psychiatry currently faces special problems in the future regarding referrals. Managed care systems discourage referrals (although managed care penetration of Medicare is still limited), and geriatric psychiatry must help identify for the primary care physician the cases in which the unique skills of the geriatric psychiatrist can contribute to cost-effective care of the older adult. Although geriatric psychiatry is a broad-based specialty, in practice it rarely receives primary referrals. Patients do not usually consider the psychiatrist as the coordinator or the provider of general medical care. The geriatric psychiatrist has special skills in the management of acute schizophrenia-like disorders, the more severe mood disorders, severe anxiety and panic disorders, behavioral disorders resulting from dementing illness, complex personality and behavioral disturbances that interfere with appropriate medical management, and severe problems with sleep. Appropriate referral by the primary care physician to the geriatric psychiatrist, especially if initial therapy by the primary care physician proves ineffective, can both prove cost-effective and provide relief of considerable suffering in the psychiatrically impaired older adult.

Therefore, geriatric psychiatrists in the twenty-first century find themselves in a paradoxical situation. On the one hand, they are better trained, and their training rests on a firmer knowledge base, than at any time in the past. Of more importance, advances in understanding of the diagnosis and treatment of psychiatric disorders in late life have led to significantly improved and cost-effective therapies for psychiatrically disturbed older adults. On the other hand, specialty care, in particular psychiatric care, could lose badly in the struggle for scarce health care resources. Administrators of fellowship programs in geriatric medicine as well as psychiatry are finding that recruitment to these programs has been more difficult in recent years. Training has never been better, and the original hesitation of many young physicians to treat older persons because of prejudices about aging has been largely overcome. Yet the uncertain future of medical specialties and the difficulty of receiving reimbursement for the care of older persons render geriatric medicine and geriatric psychiatry less desirable financially than procedure-driven medical specialties and primary care.

Financing Psychiatric Care for Older Adults

The future of health care financing, much less the financing of psychiatric care, is uncertain at the writing of this chapter. The federal government has shaped the financing of psychiatric care for older adults since the mid-1960s with the transfer of financial responsibility from state and private insurance to Medicare and Medicaid. Since that time, Medicare has tended to lead rather than

follow health care financing reform in this country. For example, the capitation of payments for certain illnesses via diagnosis-related groups (DRGs) was instituted in 1983, although DRGs have yet to be applied to inpatient psychiatric disorders.

The Omnibus Budget Reconciliation Act of 1987 (P.L. 100-203) increased coverage for outpatient psychiatric services from a total annual reimbursement of $500, with a 62.5% reimbursement of charges, to $2,200 annually for 1989. Services for the medical management of psychiatric disorders were exempted from this $2,200 limit. A 50% copayment for Part B services remains, however. The higher copayment required for mental health services has been and continues to be the subject of considerable debate regarding parity for mental health services with other health services paid for by Medicare. However, the Omnibus Budget Reconciliation Act of 1989 (P.L. 101-239) further improved outpatient psychiatric benefits: effective July 1, 1990, annual dollar limits for outpatient mental health services were eliminated.

Inpatient services have not been capitated in terms of reimbursement for individual hospitalizations, yet a 190-day lifetime psychiatric hospitalization limit remains in effect. This limit applies to freestanding psychiatric hospitals, not to psychiatric units in general hospitals. Medicare requires a one-time deductible of $768 for a hospital stay of up to 60 days and daily deductibles after 60 days until the 150th day of a hospitalization, and Medicare does not pay after day 150 of a single hospitalization. Recent legislation reduces average payments to all physicians by 5.4% below the 2001 level, which will undoubtedly jeopardize future care of older adults.

Two additional providers of care directly affect the delivery of health services to psychiatrically impaired older adults. First, the VA provides care for many older adults, primarily, although not exclusively, for men. The VA currently supports the most comprehensive system of care for mentally impaired older adults, including acute inpatient hospitalization, outpatient clinics, long-term-care facilities, and domiciliary care. Blurring of the boundaries between the VA and Medicare reimbursement for mental health services may occur, however, as length of stay decreases and outpatient care replaces inpatient care. In the future, the VA's extensive network of hospitals could be used for a broader constituency, with reimbursements from other health plans.

A second important sector of the health care delivery system for psychiatrically impaired elders is long-term care. Support for long-term care in existing health plans is limited. Therefore, many older adults must use their life savings to support long-term care until only a small sum remains, at which time the older person becomes eligible for Medicaid support. Medicare supports long-term care only for rehabilitation and only for 120 days.

The Medicaid system reimburses about 42% of all nursing home care for older adults. The development of humane and effective treatment facilities for persons with chronic psychiatric disorders, especially persons with Alzheimer's disease and chronic schizophrenia, will depend in large part on the availability of funds to support long-term care. Although some older persons are purchasing long-term-care insurance, the inability to actuate the needs of long-term care over the lifetimes of a cohort of older adults, coupled with the relatively short life of these insurance programs to date, does not ensure that long-term care will be adequately financed in the future.

Geriatric Psychiatrists and Public Health

The number of older persons in North America is ever increasing, and resources for the psychiatric care of these individuals are limited. Therefore, geriatric psychiatrists of the future must understand the prevalence and distribution of psychiatric disorders in the population and the delivery of psychiatric services to these older adults in order to advocate for humane and cost-effective mental health care for older adults. Most older adults with psychiatric disorders do not receive any care for their conditions. For those who do receive care, most of it is provided by primary care physicians (German et al. 1985).

In planning for more effective and efficient delivery of psychiatric services to older adults, the geriatric psychiatrist must consider interventions at one of three points in the natural course of a disorder. These points correspond to the three classic types of prevention described by public health specialists—primary, secondary, and tertiary (Last 1980). Primary prevention is prevention of the occurrence of disease or injury. Secondary prevention is early detection and intervention. Tertiary prevention minimizes the effects of disease and disability.

The geriatric psychiatrist can effect primary prevention by identifying potential stressful events and elements in the environment, both social and physical, of the older adult that contribute to the onset of a psychiatric disorder. For example, forced isolation and the absence of effective communication with other persons contribute to the onset of major depression and paranoid psychoses. Intervention would encourage social interaction. The appropriate use of psychotropic medications may

prevent the occurrence of acute organic brain syndromes in an older adult who is bereaved. This intervention would focus on education. Early supportive intervention has also been demonstrated to prevent the onset of major depression in the bereaved.

Secondary prevention requires the geriatric psychiatrist to intervene early enough in the course of an illness to facilitate the prescription of effective treatment to prevent a complicated convalescence. It is at this level that the geriatric psychiatrist may achieve the greatest success, given the limited resources available. For example, early diagnosis of major depression permits the psychiatrist to attempt a rational course of outpatient antidepressant therapy before the complications of excess medication or neglect of physical health ensue during the course of a depressive illness.

Tertiary prevention is directed toward preventing the disability that may result from mental illness. Rehabilitation techniques are important in long-term-care facilities, especially in the management of the patient with dementia. These techniques include reality orientation, adequate hygiene efforts, and maintenance of mobility. Although the activities themselves may not be the direct responsibility of geriatric psychiatrists, development of a comprehensive treatment and rehabilitation plan must involve these clinicians.

Geriatric Psychiatry and Successful Aging

Physicians have traditionally focused on illness, and the success of the practice of medicine, including psychiatry, has been determined by the removal of illness or disability. However, an interest in successful aging—an idea that has implicitly undergirded gerontological research since its inception—has assumed prime importance in gerontological circles since the 1980s. The construct arose primarily as a response to a perceived need to view aging as something other than loss, decline of functioning, and approaching death. In addition, physicians working with older adults have been faulted for not looking beyond the absence of disease as a marker for health (Baltes and Baltes 1990). Criteria that have been suggested as markers of successful aging include length of life, biological health, life satisfaction and morale, cognitive efficacy, social competence and productivity, personal control, and resiliency and adaptivity (Baltes and Baltes 1990; Nowlin 1977, 1985; Palmore 1979; Rowe and Kahn 1987). Rowe and Kahn (1987) emphasized the need to explore how greatly extrinsic factors can play positive as well as negative roles in the aging process. For example, they noted studies of social support demonstrating that the availability of perceived connectedness and membership in a network of family and friends decreases the likelihood of illness and mortality (Berkman and Syme 1979; Blazer 1982). Rodin (1986) emphasized the greater positive effects on health and well-being of older adults who were involved in and asserted more control over their environments compared with older adults who assumed a passive role.

Another theme that has traversed studies of successful aging is that of resiliency and adaptation. For example, Busse (1985) equated successful aging in part with the capacity to respond with resilience to challenges arising from changes within one's body, mind, and environment. A central task for older adults is to adopt effective strategies for dealing with losses and to be able to change goals and aspirations as either physical or psychosocial changes occur.

Baltes (1993) emphasized the importance of wisdom in successful aging, something that cannot be measured quantitatively. For example, he suggested that wisdom includes 1) factual knowledge (the data necessary to respond to a situation); 2) procedural knowledge (strategies of acquiring data, making decisions, and providing advice); 3) life-span contextualization (recognizing the inner relationships, tensions, and priorities of different life domains within the context of the life span); 4) value relativism (ability to separate one's own values from those of others); and 5) acceptance of uncertainty (recognizing that no perfect solution exists and optimizing the resolution of a situation as well as possible). Baltes notes that wisdom falls generally within the domain of cognitive pragmatics, or cognitive functioning that is primarily culture based and therefore potentially stable over time in persons who reach old age without specific brain pathology. In contrast, cognitive mechanics is roughly comparable to fluid intelligence and is primarily determined by the neurophysiological functioning of the brain.

Not all commentators have accepted the construct of successful aging. Cole (1991) noted that this change in perspective regarding late life may be secondary to the dramatic increase in the proportion of the adult population over age 65. Specifically, as more people have aged, it is less acceptable to view aging as a time of frailty, poor health, and death. Cole pointed out that questions about the quality of life of the oldest old (persons age 85 and older) remain at the center of the health care debate regarding ordinary versus extraordinary life-extending therapies and even health care monitoring. He suggested that our society does not apply the construct of success

to other stages of the life cycle and that the natural consequence of the construct of successful aging is the assumption that growing old presents a problem that must be solved "successfully." Aging continues to present many problems, not the least of which are the finitude of life, preservation of personal integrity, and quality of life. Yet Cole believes our culture has distanced itself from these troubling issues, in part through its emphasis on successful aging.

Baltes and Baltes (1990) proposed the third and fourth ages of the life cycle—the third age corresponding to our conceptions of the young old (for whom the construct of successful aging is quite pertinent) and the fourth age (after the age span of 80–85) being a period when a different construct may be needed. These authors suggested that this new construct be selection, optimization, and compensation. This model is based on a recognition of the realities of aging, including the recognition that 1) late-life development is a specialized and age-graded adaptation, 2) elderly persons experience a reduction in general reserve capacity, and 3) losses occur in specific functions. Such recognition leads to selection, optimization, and compensation, which in turn leads to a reduced and transformed life. In other words, self-efficacy results when the elderly person realistically accepts the limits of aging and at the same time compensates for these limits through a recognition of other potentials for happiness and productivity. Selection, optimization, and compensation ensure the efficacious life.

It is far from clear, however, that conflict is inevitable between the idea of successful aging and the care of frail elderly persons. For example, emphasis on successful aging has decreased fatalism about health and health habits in late life. Through diet, exercise, and strengthening (especially of the lower extremities), older persons can improve their balance, decrease their risk of falling, and improve their quality of life. On the other hand, when illness does occur that is chronic and about which outcomes are better known, there is no reason that health care professionals cannot realistically and seriously address the proper and realistic, not to mention the humane, care of these persons.

References

Baltes PB: The aging mind: potential and limits. Gerontologist 33:580–594, 1993
Baltes PB, Baltes MM: Successful Aging: Perspectives From the Behavioral Sciences. New York, Cambridge University Press, 1990

Berkman LF, Syme LS: Social network, host resistance, and mortality: a 9-year follow-up study of Alameda County residents. Am J Epidemiol 109:186–204, 1979

Blazer DG: Social support and mortality in an elderly community population. Am J Epidemiol 115:684–694, 1982

Busse EW: Mental health and mental illness, in Normal Aging, III. Edited by Palmore E, Busse EW, Maddox G, et al. Durham, NC, Duke University Press, 1985, p 81–91

Busse EW, Blazer DG (eds): Handbook of Geriatric Psychiatry. New York, Van Nostrand Reinhold, 1980

Busse EW, Pfeiffer E (eds): Behavior and Adaptation in Late Life. Boston, MA, Little, Brown, 1969

Butterfield LH: Benjamin Rush, the American Revolution and the American millennium. Harvard Medical Alumni Bulletin 50:16–22, 1976

Cole TR: The Journey of Life: A Cultural History of Aging in America. New York, Cambridge University Press, 1991

Cowdry EV: Problems of Aging: Biological and Medical Aspects. Baltimore, MD, Williams & Wilkins, 1938

German PS, Shapiro S, Skinner EA: Mental health of the elderly: use of health and mental health services. J Am Geriatr Soc 33:246–252, 1985

Gruman GJ: A history of ideas about the prolongation of life: the evolution of prolongevity hypotheses to 1800 (Transactions of the American Philosophical Society, Vol 56, Part 9). Philadelphia, PA, American Philosophical Society, 1966

Last JM (ed): Public Health and Preventive Medicine, 11th Edition. New York, Appleton-Century-Crofts, 1980

Nascher IL: Geriatrics: the diseases of old age and their treatment. Philadelphia, PA, P Blakiston's Sons, 1914

Nascher IL: The aging mind. Medical Record 157:669, 1944

National Institute of Mental Health: Mental Health for a Lifetime: Research for Mental Health Needs of Older Americans. Rockville, MD, National Institute of Mental Health, October 22, 2003

Nowlin JB: Successful aging. Black Aging 2:4–6, 1977

Nowlin JB: Successful aging, in Normal Aging, III. Edited by Palmore E, Busse EW, Maddox G, et al. Durham, NC, Duke University Press, 1985, pp 34–46

Omnibus Budget Reconciliation Act of 1987, Pub. L. No. 100–203

Omnibus Budget Reconciliation Act of 1989, Pub. L. No. 101–239

Palmore E: Predictors of successful aging. Gerontologist 19:427–431, 1979

Post F: The Clinical Psychiatry of Late Life. Oxford, UK, Pergamon, 1965

Rodin J: Aging and health: effects of the sense of control. Science 233:1271–1276, 1986

Rowe JW, Kahn RL: Human aging: usual and successful. Science 237:143–149, 1987

Simmons LW: The Role of the Aged in Primitive Societies. New Haven, CT, Yale University Press, 1945

Zinberg NE, Kaufman I: Normal Psychology of the Aging Process. New York, International Universities Press, 1963

Index

Page numbers printed in *boldface* type refer to tables or figures.

Agitation *(continued)*
  nonpharmacological approaches to
    (continued)
      common strategies, 379
      communication strategies,
        379–380
      family education, 378–379
      questions to guide problem
        solving, 379
      summary of, 380
    in nursing home residents, 474–475
    pharmacotherapy for, 382
      acetylcholinesterase inhibitors,
        382
      anticonvulsants, 382
      antipsychotics, 46, 218, 382
      β-blockers, 291, 382
      selective serotonin reuptake
        inhibitors, 288, 382, 389
      trazodone, 289, 382
Agnosia, acoustic, 62
Agoraphobia
  panic disorder with, 284
  without history of panic disorder,
    284
Agranulocytosis, drug-induced
  carbamazepine, 399
  clozapine, 180, 274
  mirtazapine, 391
Agraphesthesia, 236
Agraphia, 30
AIDS (acquired immune deficiency
    syndrome). *See* Human
    immunodeficiency virus infection
AIDS-related dementia vs. Alzheimer's
    disease, 180, **181**
AIMS (Abnormal Involuntary
    Movement Scale), 174, 277
Akathisia, 237
Akinetopsia, 63
Al-Anon, 360
Alaproclate, use in nursing homes, **481**
Alcohol abuse/dependence, 351–361
  addiction, 355–356
  amnestic disorder induced by,
    223–224
  cognitive functioning and,
    31, 354–355, 357
  dementia and, 223
  depression and, 256
  development of tolerance, 356
  diagnostic workup for, 356–358
  drug interactions with alcohol,
    355
  genetic predisposition to, 357
  interpersonal problems and, 357

longitudinal studies of risk factors
    for, 352–353
mortality related to, 355
motivational approaches to, 358
outcome of, 353
pharmacological properties of
    alcohol, 353–354
physical consequences of, 354–355
prevalence of, 21, **24**, 25, **26**,
    351–352, 451
sexual dysfunction and, 354
sleep problems and, 355
social factors affecting recovery
    from, 153
tardive dyskinesia and, 276
treatment of, 359–361
  case management, 360
  detoxification, 359
  disulfiram, 359–360
  family therapy, 360
  fluid management, 359
  integrated approach to, 361
  placement options for, 359
  psychotherapy, 451
  self-help groups, 360–361
Wernicke-Korsakoff syndrome and,
    223, 354
withdrawal from, 356, 359
Alcohol Use Disorders Identification
    Test (AUDIT), 357
Alcoholics Anonymous (AA),
    360–361, 451
Aldosterone, 41
Alexithymia, 299
Alien hand syndrome, 235
Allocortex, 60
Alprazolam, 400
Alprostadil, penile intracavernosal
    self-injection for erectile
    dysfunction, 311
ALS (amyotrophic lateral sclerosis), 196
Alzheimer's Association, 211, 466, 470
Alzheimer's disease (AD), 210–218.
    See also Dementia
  agitation in, 46, 218, 381–382
  vs. AIDS-related dementia, 180, **181**
  antemortem diagnosis of, 211–212
  caregiving for persons with, 130–131
  corticotropin-releasing factor in,
    98–100, **99**
  course and symptoms of,
    45, 208, 212
  depression and, 46, 254
  diagnostic criteria for, 210–211, **211**
  Down syndrome and, 30
  early symptomatic phase of, 189

electroencephalography in, 66, 185
epidemiology of, 212
genetic testing for, 115, 186
genetics of, 30, 109–113, 212–214
  β-amyloid precursor protein gene
    (APP), 110, 213
  apolipoprotein E ε4, 30, 73, 111,
    213–214
  autosomal dominant genes,
    110–111
  family and twin studies, 109–110
  low-density lipoprotein receptor-
    related protein gene *(LRP)*,
    111, 113
  α2-macroglobulin gene *(A2M)*,
    111, 113
  presenilin-1 gene *(PS1)*,
    110, 213, 214
  presenilin-2 gene *(PS2)*,
    110, 213, 214
  putative genes, 111–113
glutamate in, 96
incidence of, 27
magnetoencephalography in, 68
neuropathology of, 69–73, **70, 71,
    72**, 210–212
neuropsychological assessment of,
    189–199
neuropsychology of, 192–193,
    193, 194
NIA-Reagan diagnostic criteria
    for, 73
nitric oxide in, 102
vs. normal aging, 192–193, **193**
pathogenesis and pathophysiology of,
    212–215
  β-amyloid and tau proteins,
    110, 213
  apolipoprotein E ε4, 30, 73, 111,
    213–214
  hypothalamic-pituitary-adrenal
    axis, 213
  norepinephrine, 214
  presynaptic cholinergic deficit,
    86, 215
  serotonin, 214
personality changes in, 128
prevalence of, 21, **23**, 189, 212
psychosis of, 272–274
  compared with schizophrenia,
    273, **273**
  diagnostic criteria for, 274
  prevalence of, 272–273
  treatment of, 274–275
risk factors for, 30
seizures and, 67